Drug Eruption Reference Manual 2001

DERM

Drug Eruption Reference Manual 2001

DERM

Jerome Z. Litt, MD

Assistant Clinical Professor of Dermatology
Case Western Reserve University School of Medicine
Cleveland, Ohio, USA

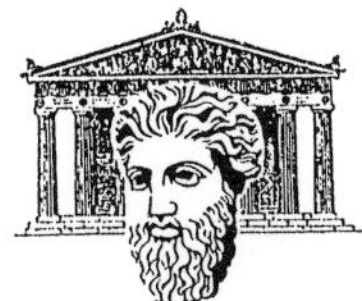

The Parthenon Publishing Group

International Publishers in Medicine, Science & Technology

NEW YORK LONDON

Library of Congress Cataloging-in-Publication Data

British Library Cataloguing in Publication Data

Data available on request

ISBN 1-84214-070-1

Published in the USA by
The Parthenon Publishing Group Inc.
One Blue Hill Plaza
PO Box 1564, Pearl River
New York 10965, USA

Published in the UK and Europe by
The Parthenon Publishing Group Limited
Casterton Hall, Carnforth
Lancs., LA6 2LA, UK

Typeset by Martin Lister Publishing Services, Carnforth, UK

Printed and bound by Bookcraft (Bath) Ltd., Midsomer Norton, UK

CONTENTS

INTRODUCTION

More and more people – primarily the older population – are taking more and more prescription and over-the-counter medications. New drugs are appearing in the medical marketplace on an almost daily basis. More and more drug reactions – in the form of cutaneous eruptions – are developing from all drugs. It has been reported that more than 100 000 hospitalized people in the United States died in 1999 as a result of medications.

Dermatologists and general physicians are often perplexed by the nature of some of these problems. The few sources that are available to identify the causes of many of these side-effects cannot be accessed by proprietary (trade, brand) names.

This Manual is a drug eruption reference guide that describes and catalogues the adverse cutaneous side-effects of more than 740 commonly prescribed and over-the-counter American generic drugs. The drugs have been listed and indexed by both their generic and trade (brand) names for easy accessibility.

Some of the fifty newer generic drugs in the past year that have been catalogued for this new edition include (the **trade/brand** name drugs are in bold):

Alosetron (**Lotronex**), bexarotene (**Targretin**), capecitabine (**Xeloda**), cilostazol (**Pletal**), denileukin (**Ontak**), dofetilide (**Tikosyn**), eflornithine (**Vaniqa**), entacapone (**Comtan**), eprosartan (**Teveten**), etanercept (**Enbrel**), gemtuzumab (**Mylotarg**), irinotecan (**Camptosar**), ketotifen (**Zaditor**), levetiracetam (**Keppra**), linezolid (**Zyvox**), meloxicam (**Mobic**), mifepristone (**Mifeprex**), moxifloxacin (**Avelox**), orlistat (**Xenical**), pantoprazole (**Protonix**), perindopril (**Aceon**), pioglitazone (**Actos**), rabeprazole (**Aciphex**), risendronate (**Actonel**), sirolimus (**Rapamune**), stavudine (**Zerit**), zonisamide (**Zonegran**), and others.

For each drug, I have listed all the known adverse side-effects – in the form of drug reactions – that can develop from the use of the corresponding drug. These side-effects include those that primarily involve the skin, the hair, the nails and the mucous membranes.

Appropriate references (author, journal or book, volume, date and page) for each side-effect for every drug have been cited. Where there is more than one reference to a particular side-effect, I have employed the most illustrative and most recent citation(s) in the literature. Citations in the English language predominate.

In this new, 2001 state-of-the-art seventh edition, I have cited more than 18 000 references and sources from journal articles, books and observations from dermatologists all over the world via the Internet.

The first part of the Manual lists, in alphabetical order, all the 740+ generic drugs that have been accessed. Next comes a listing of the various classes of drugs, and those generic drugs that belong to each class.

The major portion of the Manual – the body of the work – lists the 740+ generic drugs in alphabetical order and the adverse reactions that can arise from their use along with the appropriate references.

Following this is a section on the adverse reactions to various herbals and supplements that have been popular in the past few years.

The last parts of the Manual include a description of the 29 most common **reaction patterns**, as well as a listing of those drugs that can occasion more than 100 different reaction patterns, including, among others, **acne, acute exanthematous pustulosis, alopecia, aphthous stomatitis, bullous eruptions, bullous pemphigoid, erythema multiforme, erythema nodosum, exanthems, exfoliative dermatitis, fixed eruptions, lichenoid eruptions, lupus erythematosus, onycholysis, pemphigus, photosensitivity, pityriasis rosea, pruritus, psoriasis, purpura, pustular eruptions, Stevens–Johnson syndrome, toxic epidermal necrolysis, urticaria, and vasculitis**.

The new **Index** lists, alphabetically, the generic and trade names for easy access to the A–Z section – the main body of the Manual.

USAGE, STYLE & CONVENTIONS EMPLOYED IN THIS MANUAL

The generic drug name is given first in the tinted box. The **trade (brand) name(s)** are then listed alphabetically. When there are many **trade names**, the ten (or so) most commonly recognized ones are listed. This compilation lists and cross-references both the **trade** *and* **generic names** of all the catalogued drugs. Following the more **common trade name** drugs are recorded – in parentheses – the latest name of the pharmaceutical company that is marketing the drug. As a result of acquisitions, mergers, and other factors in the pharmaceutical industry, many of the names of the companies have changed from earlier editions of this Manual.

Beneath the **trade name** listing is a list of **other common trade names**, those drugs from other countries. Then appear the **indication(s)**, the **category** in which the drug belongs, and the **half-life** of each drug, when known. On occasion, an important or pertinent **note** will follow.

Reactions: These are the adverse reactions to the particular generic drug. They are classified in four **categories**: **skin**, **hair**, **nails**, and **other**. (**Other** refers to **mucous membrane**, **teeth**, **muscle** and various other forms of **reactions**.) **Reactions** are listed alphabetically in each **category**.

Under each **reaction pattern** are listed the **references** (the sources of the information). These are arranged in reverse chronological order – the most recent reference appearing first on the list.

References in the English language predominate. For the few foreign references, we have resorted to the summary or abstract. The majority of the citations come from *J Am Acad Dermatol, Arch Dermatol, Cutis, Int J Dermatol, Contact Dermatitis, Br J Dermatol, JAMA, Lancet, BMJ, Aust J Dermatol, N Engl J Med, Ann Intern Med*, and other prominent and easily accessible journals.

Many of the sources have been gathered from the following reference works:

(1998): Kauppinen K, et al, *Skin Reactions to Drugs*, CRC Press, Boca Raton etc.

(1996): Bruinsma W, *A Guide to Drug Eruptions*, The File of Medicines, PO Box 21, 1474 HJ Oosthuizen, The Netherlands.

(1994): Goldstein S & Wintroub BU, *Adverse Cutaneous Reactions to Medication*, CoMedica, New York.

(1992): Zürcher K & Krebs A, *Cutaneous Drug Reactions*, Karger, Basel.

(1992): Breathnach SM & Hintner H, *Adverse Drug Reactions and the Skin*, Blackwell, Oxford.

(1988): Bork K, *Cutaneous Side Effects of Drugs*, WB Saunders, Philadelphia.

Other references have been obtained from:

(2000): *Lexi-Comp's Clinical Reference Library*, Hudson, Ohio.

(1999): *Drug Facts & Comparisons*, St. Louis, Missouri.

(1999): *USP Dispensing Information*, Rockville, Maryland.

(1999): *PDR Generics*, Montvale, New Jersey.

Note: Most of the references from the above four sources are essentially the package inserts.

There are occasions when there are very few adverse reactions to a specific drug. These drugs are still included in the Manual since there is often a **positive significance in negative findings**.

As a departure from the official, conventional and established style guide, and as a function of space constraints, the order of each **reference** will appear as follows:

- The year in parentheses. The most recent citation appearing first.
- Last name and initial(s) of the principal author.
- A plus sign (+) after the author's name denotes one or more co-authors.
- Journal name (standard abbreviation where possible), *in italics*.
- Volume number (often followed by a parenthetical part or supplemental number).
- First page of the article
- Books when cited are in capitalized *italics* followed by the publisher and page number.

Other notes:

- (sic) means **just so**. This is how the authors designated the **reaction**.
  For example, **rash** (sic); **dermatitis** (sic); **skin rash** (sic)*
- I have used the term **passim** to mean "in passing." Forgive me.

There are occasional allusions to the incidence of many of the listed **reactions**. Percentages – which for the most part are essentially vague and meaningless – are obtained from articles, from Zürcher & Krebs, and from Bork.

I have simplified the references to the many **reaction patterns** by eliminating, for the most part, tags such as '-like' as in psoriasis-like, '-reactivation,' '-syndrome,' '-dissemination,' '-iform,' etc.

'Observation' means just that. Observations (read: Anecdotes) are derived from information obtained from reliable dermatologists from the Internet and from personal correspondence. And if you send me your observations, they will be catalogued and you will be given appropriate attribution and recognition in the next edition.

Enjoy!

Jerome Z. Litt, MD
December, 2000

*The term **skin rash** is a deplorable and reprehensible idiotism adored by non-dermatologists and the writers of the PDR (read package inserts). Can you have a **rash** on any other organ?

Classes of Drugs

ACE-inhibitors

benazepril
candesartan*
captopril
cilazapril
enalapril
eprosartan*
fosinopril
irbesartan
lisinopril
losartan*
moexipril
perindopril
quinapril
ramipril
spirapril
telmisartan*
trandolapril
valsartan*

*Angiotenin II receptor antagonist

Alpha adrenergic receptor inhibitors

doxazosin
phenoxybenzamine
phentolamine
prazosin
tamsulosin
terazosin

Alpha adrenoreceptor agonists

clonidine
guanabenz
guanethidine
guanfacine
tizanidine

Aminoglycosides

amikacin
ceftazidime
gentamicin
kanamycin
neomycin
netilmicin
streptomycin
tobramycin

Amphetamines

amphetamine sulfate
dexfenfluramine
dextroamphetamine
diethylpropion
fenfluramine
mazindol
methamphetamine
methylphenidate
phendimetrazine
phentermine

Antiarrhythmic agents and class

adenosine
amiodarone III
atropine
belladonna
beta-blockers II
bretylium III
chlorothiazide
digoxin
diltiazem IV
disopyramide IA
dofetilide III
edrophonium
esmolol II
flecainide IC
ibutilide III
indecainide IC
isoproterenol
lidocaine IB
magnesium sulfate
metoprolol
mexiletine IB
minoxidil
moricizine I
phenytoin IB
procainamide IA
propafenone IC
propranolol II
quinidine IA
sotalol III
tocainide IB
verapamil IV

Anticholinergic agents

albuterol
amantadine
atropine
belladonna
benztropine
biperiden
bromocriptine
carbidopa
clidinium
dicyclomine
diphenhydramine
glycopyrrolate
homatropine
hyoscyamine
ipratropium
levodopa
methantheline
orphenadrine
pergolide
physostigmine
procyclidine
propantheline
scopolamine
selegiline
tacrine
tolterodine
trihexiphenidyl

Anticoagulants [1]
Antiplatelets [2]
Thrombolytics [3]

abciximab [2]
alteplase [3]
anagrelide [2]
anistreplase [3]
ardeparin [1]
aspirin [2]
clopidogrel [2]
dalteparin [1]
danaparoid [1]
dipyridamole [2]
enoxaparin [1]
heparin [1]
reteplase [3]
streptokinase [3]
ticlopidine [2]
urokinase [3]
warfarin [1]

Anticonvulsants

acetazolamide
amobarbital
carbamazepine
chlorpromazine
clonazepam
clorazepate
diazepam
divalproex
ethosuximide
ethotoin
felbamate
fosphenytoin
gabapentin
hydroxyzine
lamotrigine
levetiracetam
lorazepam
mephenytoin
mephobarbital
methsuximide
oxazepam
oxcarbazepine
paraldehyde

paramethadione
pentobarbital
phenobarbital
phensuximide
phenytoin
primidone
thiopental
tiagabine
topiramate
trimethadione
valproic acid
vigabatrin
zonisamide

Antidepressants
Tricyclics I = 1st generation
Tricyclics II = 2nd generation
Tricyclics III = 3rd generation
amitriptyline I
amoxapine II
benactyzine
bupropion II
citalopram III
clomipramine I
desipramine I
divalproex
doxepin I
fluoxetine III
fluvoxamine III
imipramine I
isocarboxazid
lithium
loxapine
maprotiline II
methylphenidate
mirtazapine III
nefazodone III
nortriptyline I
paroxetine III
perphenazine
phenelzine
protriptyline I
sertraline III
thioridazine
tranylcypromine
trazodone II
trimipramine I
venlafaxine III

Antidiabetic agents
acarbose
acetohexamide
chlorpropamide
glimepiride
glipizide
glucagon
glyburide
insulin
metformin
miglitol
pioglitazone
repaglinide
rosiglitazone
tolazamide
tolbutamide
troglitazone

Antifungals
amphotericin B
clotrimazole
fluconazole
flucytosine
griseofulvin
itraconazole
ketoconazole
metronidazole
miconazole
nystatin
terbinafine

Antihypertensives
acebutolol
amiloride
amlodipine
atenolol
benazepril
bendroflumethiazide
benzthiazide
betaxolol
bisoprolol
captopril
carteolol
chlorothiazide
chlorthalidone
clonidine
cyclothiazide
diazoxide
diltiazem
doxazosin
enalapril
ethacrynic acid
felodipine
fosinopril
guanabenz
guanethidine
guanfacine
hydralazine
hydrochlorothiazide
hydroflumethiazide
indapamide
isradipine
labetalol
lisinopril
losartan
meclofenamate
methclothiazide
methyldopa
methylphenidate
metolazone
metoprolol
minoxidil
moexipril
nadolol
nicardipine
nifedipine
nimodipine
nisoldipine
nitroglycerin
penbutolol
phentolamine
pindolol
polythiazide
prazosin
propantheline
propranolol
quinapril
ramipril
reserpine
spironolactone
terazosin
timolol
torsemide
triamterene
trichlormethiazide
verapamil
yohimbine

Antimalarial agents
chloroquine
hydroxychloroquine
mefloquine
primaquine
pyrimethamine
quinacrine
quinine

Antimigraine drugs
5-HT, receptor agonists
naritriptan
rizatriptan
sumatritan
zolmitriptan

Antimycobacterial agents
aminosalicylic acid
capreomycin
clofazimine
cycloserine
dapsone
ethambutol
ethionamide
isoniazid
kanamycin
pyrazinamide
rifampin
streptomycin

Antineoplastics
aldesleukin
altretamine

azathioprine
asparaginase
bleomycin
busulfan
carboplatin
carmustine
chlorambucil
chlorotrianisene
cisplatin
clomiphene
cyclophosphamide
cyclosporine
cytarabine
dacarbazine
dactinomycin
danazol
daunorubicin
diethylstilbestrol
docetaxel
doxorubicin
estradiol
estramustine
etoposide
fluorouracil
fluoxymesterone
flutamide
gemcitabine
hydroxyprogesterone
hydroxyurea
ifosfamide
idarubicin
interferon
leucovorin
leuprolide
levamisole
lomustine
masoprocol
mechlorethamine
medroxyprogesterone
megestrol
melphalan
mercaptopurine
mesna
methotrexate
methyltestosterone
mitomycin
mitotane
nafarelin
octreotide
paclitaxel
pentostatin
plicamycin
procarbazine
progesterone
somastatin
streptozocin
tamoxifen
taxol
testosterone
thioguanine
thiotepa
topotecan
trimetrexate
vinblastine
vincristine
vinorelbine

Antiparkinsonian agents

amantadine
benztropine
bromocriptine
cabergoline
carbidopa
entacapone
levodopa/carbidopa
pergolide
pramipexole
procyclidine
ropinirole
selegiline
tolcapone
trihexyphenidyl

Antipsychotic agents

acetophenazine
chlorpromazine
chlorprothixene
clozapine
droperidol
fluphenazine
haloperidol
loxapine
mesoridazine
molindone
olanzapine
perphenazine
prochlorperazine
pimozide
promazine
quetiapine
riluzole
risperidone
sertindole
thioridazine
thiothixene
trifluoperazine

Antiretroviral agents

Nucleoside analog reverse transcriptase inhibitors (NRTIS)

abacavir
didanosine
lamivudine
stavudine
zalcitabine
zidovudine

Non-nucleoside reverse transcriptase inhibitors (NNRTIS)

delavirdine
efavirenz
nevirapine

Protease inhibitors

amprenavir
indinavir
lopinavir
nelfinavir
ritonavir
saquinavir

Anxiolytics, sedatives and hypnotics

alprazolam
amobarbital
aprobarbital
buspirone
butabarbital
chloral hydrate
chlordiazepoxide
chlormezanone
chlorzoxazone
clonazepam
clorazepate
diazepam
droperidol
estazolam
ethchlorvynol
fentanyl
flurazepam
glutethimide
hydroxzine
ketamine
lorazepam
mephobarbital
meprobamate
methohexital
midazolam
opium alkaloids
oxazepam
paraldehyde

Paroxetine

pentobarbital
phenobarbital
prazepam
prochlorperazine
promethazine
propofol
quazepam
secobarbital
sertraline
temazepam
thiopental
triazolam
trifluoperazine
zaleplon
zolpidem

Benzodiazepines

alprazolam
amitriptyline
chlordiazepoxide
clonazepam
clorazepate
diazepam
estazolam
flurazepam
halazepam

lorazepam
midazolam
olanzapine
oxazepam
prazepam
quazepam
temazepam
triazolam

Beta-blockers

acebutolol
atenolol
betaxolol
bisoprolol
carteolol
carvedilol
esmolol
labetalol
levobunolol
metipranolol
metoprolol
nadolol
penbutolol
pindolol
propranolol
sotalol
timolol

Beta-lactam antibiotics

aztreonam
cefixime
cefoxitin
imipenen/cilastin
loracarbef
meropenem
moxalactam
tazobactam

Bronchodilators

albuterol
aminophylline
atropine
bitolterol
ephedrine
epinephrine
ipratropium
isoetharine
isoproterenol
levalbuterol
metaproterenol
montelukast
pirbuterol
salmeterol
terbutaline
theophylline salts
zafirlukast
zileuton

Calcium channel blockers

amlodipine
bepridil
diltiazem
felodipine
isradipine
mibefradil
nicardipine
nifedipine
nimodipine
nisoldipine
verapamil

Cephalosporins

By generation

First generation

cefadroxil
cefazolin
cephalexin
cephalothin
cephapirin
cephradine

Second generation

cefaclor
cefamandole
cefmetazole
cefonicid
ceforanide
cefotetan
cefoxitin
cefprozil
cefuroxime
loracarbef

Third generation

cefdinir
cefixime
cefoperazone
cefotaxime
cefpodoxime
ceftazidime
ceftibuten
ceftizoxime
ceftriaxone

Fourth generation

cefepime

Diuretics

acetazolamide
amiloride
bendroflumethiazide
benzthiazide
bumetanide
chlorthalidone
chorothiazide
cyclothiazide
ethacrynic acid
furosemide
hydrochlorothiazide
hydroflumethiazide
indapamide
isosorbide
mannitol
methyclothiazide
metolazone
polythiazide
potassium chloride
quinethazone
spironolactone
torsemide
triamterene
trichlormethiazide
urea

Diuretics, loop

bumetanide
ethacrynic acid
furosemide
torsemide

Fluoroquinolones

alatrofloxacin
cinoxacin
ciprofloxacin
enoxacin
gatifloxacin
grepafloxacin
levofloxacin
lomefloxacin
moxifloxacin
norfloxacin
ofloxacin
sparfloxacin
trovafloxacin

H_2 antagonists

cimetidine
famotidne
nizatidine
ranitidine
roxatidine

HMG-CoA reductase inhibitors (statins)

atorvastatin
cerivastatin
fluvastatin
lovastatin
pravastatin
simvastatin

Hypnotics

aprobarbital
ethchlorvynol
flurazepam
glutethimide
L-tryptophan
methohexital
opium alkaloids
pentobarbital
phenobarbital
propofol
quazepam
secobarbital
temazepam

thiopental
triazolam
zolpidem

Hypolipidemic agents HMG-CoA reductase inhibitors
atorvastatin
cerivastatin
cholestyramine
clofibrate
colestipol
dextrothyroxine
fenofibrate
fluvastatin
gemfibrozil
lovastatin
niacin
pravastatin
probucol
simvastatin

Macrolides
azithromycin
clarithromycin
dirithromycin
erythromycin
troleandomycin

Monamine oxidase inhibitors
isocarboxazid
pargyline
phenelzine
tranylcypromine
narcotic agonists
alfentanil
buprenorphine
butorphanol
codeine
fentanyl
hydrocodone
hydromorphone
levorphanol
meperidine
methadone
morphine
nalbuphine
oxycodone
pentazocine
propoxyphene
remifentanil
sufentanil

Neuroleptics
amitriptyline
chlorpromazine
fluphenazine
haloperidol
lithium
loxapine
molindone
prochlorperazine
thioridazine
thiothixene
tranylcypromine
trifluoperazine

Neuromuscular blocking agents
tracurium
cisatracurium
doxacurium
gallimine
metocurine
mivacurium
pancuronium
pipecuronium
rocuronium
succinylcholine
tubocurarine
vecuronium

NSAIDs
aspirin
bromfenac
celecoxib
choline salicylate
diclofenac
diflunisal
etodolac
fenoprofen
flurbiprofen
ibuprofen
indomethacin
ketoprofen
ketorolac
magnesium salicylate
mefenamic acid
mesalamine
methotrexate
nabumetone
naproxen
olsalazine
oxaprozin
oxyphenbutazone
phenylbutazone
piroxicam
rofecoxib
salsalate
sodium salicylate
sulindac
tolmetin

Penicillin antibiotics
amoxicillin
ampicillin
carbenicillin
cloxacillin
dicloxacillin
methicillin
mezlocillin
nafcillin
oxacillin
penicillin
piperacillin
ticarcillin

Selective serotonin reuptake inhibitors (SSRIs)
citalopram
fluoxetine
fluvoxamine
nefazodone
paroxetine
sertraline
trazodone
venlafaxine

Sulfonamide derivatives
Antimicrobial agents
mafenide acetate
silver sulfadiazine
sodium sulfacetamide
sulfadiazine
sulfamethiazole
sulfamethoxazole
sulfisoxazole
Diuretic, carbonic anhydrase inhibitor
acetazolamide
dichlorphenamide
methazolamide
Diuretics, loop
bumetanide
furosemide
torsemide
Diuretics, thiazide
bendroflumethiazide
benzthiazide
chlorothiazide
chlorthalidone
cyclothiazide
hydrochlorothiazide
hydroflumethiazide
indapamide
methyclothiazide
metolazone
polythiazide
quinethazone
trichlormethiazide
Hypoglycemic agents, oral
acetohexamide
chlorpropamide
glipizide
glyburide
tolazamide
tolbutamide
Other agents
cyclamate
dorzolamide
saccharin
sulfasalazine

Tranquilizers
- amitriptyline
- buspirone
- chlordiazepoxide
- chlormezanone
- chlorpromazine
- clorazepate
- diazepam
- doxepin
- droperidol
- fluphenazine
- haloperidol
- hydroxyzine
- lorazepam
- loxapine
- meprobamate
- mesoridazine
- molindone
- oxazepam
- perphenazine
- pimozide
- prochlorperazine
- promazine
- promethazine
- reserpine
- risperidone
- thioridazine
- thiothixene
- trifluoperazine

Tetracycline antibiotics
- demeclocycline
- doxycycline
- minocycline
- oxytetracycline
- tetracycline

Vasodilators
- hydralazine
- isoxusprine
- minoxidil
- nitroglycerin
- nitroprusside
- Papaverine

ABACAVIR

Trade name: Ziagen (GlaxoWellcome)
Indications: HIV infections in combination with other antiretrovirals
Category: Antiretroviral; nucleoside reverse transcriptase inhibitor
Half-life: 1.5 hours
Clinically important, potentially serious interactions with: no data

Reactions

Skin

Edema
(1999): Spruance SL, *Skin and Allergy News* October, 37
Exanthems
(1999): Nathanson N, (from Internet) (observation) (generalized)
(1999): Spruance SL, *Skin and Allergy News* October, 37
Rash (sic) (10%)
(1999): Spruance SL, *Skin and Allergy News* October, 37 (69%)
(1999): Hughes W+, *Antimicrob Agents Chemother* 43, 609 (9%)
(1998): Foster RH+, *Drugs* 55, 729

Other

Anaphylactoid reaction
(1999): Walensky RP+, *AIDS* 13, 999
(1999): Spruance SL, *Skin and Allergy News* October, 37 (3–4%)
Hypersensitivity (5%)
(2000): GlaxoWellcome *Important Drug Warning*, July (severe or fatal)
(1998): Foster RH+, *Drugs* 55, 729 (2–3%)
Myalgia
(1999): Spruance SL, *Skin and Allergy News* October, 37
Oral ulceration
(1999): Spruance SL, *Skin and Allergy News* October, 37

ABCIXIMAB

Synonym: C7E3
Trade name: Reopro (Lilly)
Indications: Thrombotic arterial disease
Category: Non-nucleoside reverse transcriptase inhibitor, platelet aggregation inhibitor
Half-life: 10–30 minutes – given intravenously
Clinically important, potentially serious interactions with: anticoagulants, heparin, NSAIDs

Reactions

Skin

Cellulitis (0.3%)
Peripheral edema (1.6%)
Petechiae (0.3%)
Pruritus (0.3%)

Other

Anaphylactoid reaction
(1999): Guzzo JA+, *Catheter Cardiovasc Interv* 48, 71
Hypesthesia (1%)
Injection-site reaction (3.6%)
Myalgia (0.3%)
Myopathy (0.3%)

ACARBOSE

Trade name: Precose (Bayer)
Other trade names: *Glucobay; Glumida; Prandase*
Indications: Non-insulin dependent diabetes type II
Category: Oral antidiabetic (alpha-glucosidase inhibitor)
Half-life: 2.7–9 hours
Clinically important, potentially serious interactions with: beta-blockers, calcium channel blockers, corticosteroids, diuretics, estrogens, isoniazid, niacin, phenothiazines, phenytoin, sulfonylureas, thyroid

Reactions

Skin

Erythema (<1%)
Erythema multiforme
(1999): Kono T+, *Lancet* 354, 396 (generalized)
Urticaria (<1%)
Rash (sic)

Other

Ageusia
(1996): Martin Bun N+, *Med Clin (Barc)* (Spanish) 28, 399

ACEBUTOLOL

Trade name: Sectral (Wyeth)
Other common trade names: *Acecor; Acetanol; Alol; Apo-Acebutolol; Monitan; Neptal; Novo-Acebutolol; Nu-Acebutolol; Prent; Rhodiasectral; Rhotral*
Indications: Hypertension, angina, ventricular arrhythmias
Category: Cardioselective beta-adrenergic blocker; antiarrhythmic; antihypertensive
Half-life: 3–7 hours
Clinically important, potentially serious interactions with: calcium channel blockers, cimetidine, clonidine, diltiazem, insulin, NSAIDs, prazosin, reserpine, verapamil

Note: Cutaneous side-effects of beta-receptor blockaders are clinically polymorphous. They apparently appear after several months of continuous therapy. Atypical psoriasiform, lichen planus-like, and eczematous chronic rashes are mainly observed. (1983): Hödl St, *Z Hautkr* (German) 1:58, 17.

Reactions

Skin

Dermatitis (sic)
Diaphoresis
(1995): Schmutz JL+, *Dermatology* 190, 86
Edema (1–10%)
Erythema multiforme (<1%)
Exanthems (4%)
(1985): Singh BN+, *Drugs* 29, 531
Exfoliative dermatitis
Facial edema (<1%)
Hyperkeratosis (palms and soles)
Hyperpigmentation
Lichenoid eruption
(1982): Taylor AEM+, *Clin Exp Dermatol* 7, 219
(1978): Savage RL+, *BMJ* 1, 987
Lupus erythematosus (<1%)
(1997): Burlingame RW, *Clin Lab Med* 17, 367
(1992): Stevens MB, *Hosp Pract* 27, 27
(1992): Rubin RL+, *J Clin Invest* 90, 165
(1987): Doktor D, *Rev Fr Allergol Immunol* (French) 27, 77
(1985): Hourdebaight-Larrusse P+, *Ann Cardiol Angeiol* (Paris) (French) 34, 421
(1985): Singh BN+, *Drugs* 29, 531
(1984): Bigot MC+, *Therapie* (French) 39, 571
(1984): Meyer O+, *Rev Rhum Mal Osteoartic* (French) *51, 303*
(1983): Homberg JC+, *J Pharmacol* (French) 14, 61

(1982): Taylor AE+, *Clin Exp Dermatol* 7, 219
(1981): Simon P+, *Nouv Presse Med* (French) 10, 105
(1981): Record NB, *Ann Intern Med* 95, 326
Pityriasis rubra pilaris
(1978): Finlay AY+, *BMJ* 1, 987
Pruritus (<2%)
Psoriasis
(1986): Czernielewski J+, *Lancet* 1, 808
(1984): Arntzen N+, *Acta Derm Venereol* (Stockh) 64, 346
Rash (sic) (1–10%)
Raynaud's phenomenon
(1984): Eliasson K+, *Acta Med Scand* 215, 333
(1976): Marshall AJ+, *BMJ* 1, 1498
Toxic epidermal necrolysis
Urticaria
(1977): Ashford R+, *Lancet* 2, 462
Vasculitis
(1988): Bonnefoy M+, *Ann Dermatol Venereol* (French) 115, 27
(1977): Ashford R+, *Lancet* 2, 462
Xerosis

Hair

Hair – alopecia

Nails

Nails – bluish
Nails – dystrophy
Nails – onycholysis
Nails – pincer (reverse transverse curvature of the nails)
(1998): Greiner D+, *J Am Acad Dermatol* 39, 486

Other

Dysgeusia
Hyperesthesia (<2%)
Hypesthesia (<2%)
Myalgia (1–10%)
Oculo-mucocutaneous syndrome
(1982): Cocco G+, *Curr Ther Res* 31, 362
Oral lichenoid eruption
Peyronie's disease
(1979): Pryor JP+, *Lancet* 1, 331
Xerostomia (<1%)

ACETAMINOPHEN

Synonyms: APAP, paracetamol
Trade names: Anacin-3; Bromo-Seltzer; Darvocet-N; Datril; Dristan; Excedrin; Liquiprin; Lorcet; Mapap; Neopap; Panadol; Percogesic; Percoset; Phenaphen; Sinutab; Tylenol; Valadol; Vicodin; etc. (Various pharmaceutical companies.)
Other common trade names: *Abenol; Anaflon; Ben-U-Ron; Doliprane; Geluprane; Panadol*
Indications: Pain, fever
Category: Non-narcotic antipyretic analgesic
Half-life: 1–3 hours
Clinically important, potentially serious interactions with: alcohol, antacids, barbiturates, carbamazepine, cimetidine, hydantoins, phenothiazines, sulfinpyrazone

Note: Acetaminophen is the active metabolite of phenacetin.

Reactions

Skin

Acute generalized exanthematous pustulosis (AGEP)
(1998): Leger F+, *Acta Derm Venereol* 78, 222
(1996): DeConinck AL+, *Dermatology* 193, 338
(1995): Moreau A+, *Int J Dermatol* 34, 263 (passim)
(1991): Roujeau J-C+, *Arch Dermatol* 127, 1333
Angioedema (<1%)
(1997): de Almeida MA+, *Allergy Asthma Proc* 18, 313
(1990): Van Diem L+, *Eur J Clin Pharmacol* 38, 389
(1986): Idoko JA+, *Trans R Soc Trop Med Hyg* 80, 175
(1985): Stricker BH+, *BMJ* 291, 938
(1970): Henriques CC, *JAMA* 214, 2336
Contact dermatitis
(1997): Mathelier-Fusada P+, *Contact Dermatitis* 36, 267
(1996): Szczurko C+, *Contact Dermatitis* 35, 299
Dermatitis (sic)
(1995): Barbaud A+, *Lancet* 346, 902
Diaphoresis
Erythema (sic)
(1985): Stricker BH+, *BMJ* 291, 938
Erythema multiforme
(1995): Dubey NK+, *Indian Pediatr* 32, 1117
(1984): Hurvitz H+, *Isr J Med Sci* 20, 145
Erythema nodosum (<1%)
Exanthems
(1997): Foong H, Malaysia (from Internet) (observation)
(1985): Stricker BH+, *BMJ* 291, 938
(1985): Matheson I+, *Pediatrics* 76, 651
(1975): Michelson PA, *Ann Intern Med* 83, 374
(1970): Henriques CC, *JAMA* 214, 2336
Exfoliative dermatitis
(1984): Guerin C+, *Therapie* (French) 39, 47
Fixed eruption (<1%)
(2000): Galindo PA+, *J Investig Allergol Clin Immunol* 9, 399
(2000): Ozkaya-Bayazit E+, *Eur J Dermatol* 10, 288
(2000): Ko R+, *Clin Exp Dermatol* 25, 96
(1999): Sehgal VN, *Pediatr Dermatology* 16, 165 (multiple)
(1998): Litt JZ, Beachwood, OH, personal case (observation)
(1998): Hern S+, *Br J Dermatol* 139, 1129,
(1996): Laude TA, *Cosmetic Dermatology* 9, 7
(1996): Gomez-Martinez M+, *J Investig Allergol Clin Immunol* 6, 131
(1996): Kawada A+, *Int J Dermatol* 35, 148
(1995): Harris A+, *Br J Dermatol* 133, 790
(1994): Rademaker M+, *N Z Med J* 107, 295
(1992): Zemtsov A+, *Cutis* 50, 281
(1992): Cohen HA+, *Ann Pharmacother* 26, 1596
(1991): Thankappen TP+, *Int J Dermatol* 30, 867
(1990): Duhra P+, *Clin Exp Dermatol* 15, 293
(1990): Gaffoor PMA+, *Cutis* 45, 242 (passim)
(1989): Valsecchi R, *Dermatologica* 179, 51
(1988): Guin J+, *Cutis* 41, 107
(1987): Guin J+, *J Am Acad Dermatol* 17, 399
(1987): Bharija SC+, *Australas J Dermatol* 28, 85
(1986): Meyrick-Thomas RH+, *Br J Dermatol* 115, 357
(1985): Verbov J, *Dermatologica* 171, 60 (along with chlormezanone)
(1975): Wilson HTH, *Br J Dermatol* 92, 213
(1970): Henriques CC, *JAMA* 214, 2336
Flushing
(1985): Stricker BH+, *BMJ* 291, 938
Neutrophilic eccrine hidradenitis
(1988): Kuttner BJ+, *Cutis* 41, 403
Pemphigus
(1990): Brenner S+, *Acta Derm Venereol* 70, 357
Penile edema
(1997): Cabanes Higuero N+, *Med Clin (Barc)* (Spanish) 109, 685
Photosensitivity
(1999): Popescu C, Bucharest, Romania (from Internet) (observation)
Pityriasis rosea
(1993): Yosipovitch G+, *Harefuah* (Israel) 124, 198; 247
Progressive pigmentary purpura (Schamberg's disease)
(1992): Abeck D+, *J Am Acad Dermatol* 27, 123
Pruritus
(1985): Stricker BH+, *BMJ* 291, 938
Purpura
(1998): Kwon SJ+, *J Dermatol* 25, 756
(1993): Guccione JL+, *Arch Dermatol* 129, 1267
(1992): Abeck D+, *J Am Acad Dermatol* 27, 123
(1980): Miescher PA+, *Clin Haematol* 9, 505
(1977): Ameer B+, *Ann Intern Med* 87, 202
(1973): Skokan JD+, *Cleve Clin Quart* 40, 89
Purpura fulminans
(1993): Guccione JL+, *Arch Dermatol* 129, 1267
Rash (sic) (<1%)
Sensitivity (sic)
(1998): Mendizabal SL+, *Allergy* 53, 457
Stevens–Johnson syndrome
(1995): Kuper K+, *Ophthalmologue* (German) 92, 823

(1985): Ting HC+, *Int J Dermatol* 24, 587
Toxic epidermal necrolysis
(2000): Halevi A+, *Ann Pharmacother* 34, 32
(1991): Sakellariou G+, *Int J Artif Organs* 14, 634
(1986): Roupe G+, *Int Arch Allergy Appl Immunol* 80, 145
Urticaria
(2000): Samanta BB, *J Assoc Physicians India* 47, 464
(1997): de Almeida MA+, *Allergy Asthma Proc* 18, 313
(1997): Ownby DR, *J Allergy Clin Immunol* 99, 151
(1985): Cole TO, *Clin Exp Dermatol* 10, 404
(1985): Stricker BH+, *BMJ* 291, 938
(1975): Michelson PA, *Ann Intern Med* 83, 374
(1970): Henriques CC, *JAMA* 214, 2336
Vasculitis
(1995): Harris A+, *Br J Dermatol* 133, 790
(1988): Dussarat GV+, *Presse Med* (French) 17, 1587

Hair
Hair – alopecia
(1998): Litt JZ, Beachwood, OH, personal case (observation)

Nails
Nails – disorder (sic)
(1975): Michelson PA, *Ann Intern Med* 83, 374

Other
Anaphylactoid reaction
(1999): Spitz E, *Ann Allergy Asthma Immunol* 82, 591
(1999): Kumar RK+, *Hosp Med* 60, 66
(1998): Galindo PA+, *Allergol Immunopathol (Madr)* (Spanish) 26, 199
(1998): Huitema AD+, *Hum Exp Toxicol* 17, 406
(1990): Van Diem L+, *Eur J Clin Pharmacol* 38, 389
(1988): *Allergy Observer* (Janssen Pharmaceutica) 5(7), 1
(1985): Stricker BH+, *BMJ* 291, 938
Dysgeusia
(1976): Rollin H, *Laryngol Rhinol Otol* (Stuttgart) (German) 55, 873
Hypersensitivity (<1%)
(1999): Kivity S+, *Allergy* 54, 187
(1997): Vidal C+, *Ann Allergy Asthma Immunol* 79, 320
(1996): Ibanez MD+, *Allergy* 51, 121
(1993): Martin JA+, *Med Clin (Barc)* (Spanish) 100, 158

ACETAZOLAMIDE

Trade name: Diamox (Storz)
Other common trade names: *Acetazolam; Ak-Zol; Dazamide; Defiltran; Diuramid; Novo-Zolamide*
Indications: Epilepsy, glaucoma
Category: Anticonvulsant; carbonic anhydrase inhibitor; sulfonamide* diuretic
Half-life: 2–6 hours
Clinically important, potentially serious interactions with: amphetamines, cyclosporine, diflunisal, digoxin, methenamine, primidone, quinidine, salicylates

Reactions

Skin
Acute generalized exanthematous pustulosis (AGEP)
(1995): Moreau A+, *Int J Dermatol* 34, 263 (passim)
(1992): Ogoshi M+, *Dermatology* 184, 142
Bullous eruption (<1%)
(1957): Ellis FA, *Arch Dermatol* 75, 836
Erythema multiforme
(1961): Baer RL+, *Year Book of Dermatology*, Year Book Medical Publishers, 9
(1956): Spring M, *Ann Allergy* Jan/Feb, 41
Exanthems
(1967): Lockey SD, *Med Sci* 18, 43
(1956): Spring M, *Ann Allergy* Jan/Feb, 41
Lupus erythematosus
(1966): Cohen P+, *JAMA* 197, 817
Photosensitivity
Pruritus
Purpura
(1976): Underwood LC, *JAMA* 161, 1477
Pustular eruption
(1992): Ogoshi M+, *Dermatology* 184, 142
Pustular psoriasis
(1995): Kuroda K+, *J Dermatol* 22, 784
Rash (sic) (<1%)
Rosacea
(1993): Shah P+, *Br J Dermatol* 129, 647
Stevens–Johnson syndrome
Toxic epidermal necrolysis (<1%)
(1957): Ellis FA, *Arch Dermatol* 75, 836
Urticaria

Hair
Hair – hirsutism
(1974): Weiss IS, *Am J Ophthalmol* 78, 327

Other
Ageusia
Anaphylactoid reaction
(2000): Gerhards LJ+, *Ned Tijdschr Geneeskd* (Dutch) 144, 1228
(1998): Tzanakis N+, *Br J Ophthalmol* 82, 588
Anosmia
Dysgeusia (>10%) (metallic taste)
(1997): Martinez-Mir I+, *Ann Pharmacother* 31, 373
(1990): Miller LG+, *J Fam Pract* 31, 199
(1981): Lichter PR, *Ophthalmol* 88, 266
Extravasation
(1994): Callear A+, *Br J Ophthalmol* 78, 731
Paresthesias (<1%)
(1981): Lichter PR, *Ophthalmol* 88, 266
Xerostomia (<1%)

***Note:** Acetazolamide is a sulfonamide and can be absorbed systemically. Sulfonamides can produce severe, possibly fatal, reactions such as toxic epidermal necrolysis and Stevens–Johnson syndrome.

ACETOHEXAMIDE

Trade name: Dymelor (Lilly)
Other common trade names: *Dimelin; Dimelor*
Indications: non-insulin dependent diabetes type II
Category: Sulfonylurea* antidiabetic; oral hypoglycemic
Half-life: 1–6 hours
Clinically important, potentially serious interactions with: androgens, beta-blockers, chloramphenicol, clofibrate, fluconazole, hydantoin, MAO inhibitors, NSAIDs, phenylbutazones, probenecid, salicylates, sulfonamides, thiazides

Reactions

Skin
Eczema (sic)
Erythema (<1%)
Exanthems (<1%)
Diaphoresis
Lichenoid eruption
Photosensitivity (1–10%)
Pruritus (<1%)
Rash (sic) (1–10%)
Urticaria (1–10%)

Hair
Hair – alopecia
(1962): Boshell BR+, *Clin Pharmacol Ther* 3, 750

Other
Paresthesias
Porphyria cutanea tarda

***Note:** Acetohexamide is a sulfonamide and can be absorbed systemically. Sulfonamides can produce severe, possibly fatal, reactions such as toxic epidermal necrolysis and Stevens–Johnson syndrome.

ACITRETIN

Trade name: Soriatane (Roche)
Other common trade name: *Neotigason*
Indications: Psoriasis
Category: Antipsoriatic retinoid
Half-life: 49 hours
Clinically important, potentially serious interactions with: antidiabetics, estrogens, ethanol, methotrexate, phenytoin, tetracycline, vitamin A

Reactions

Skin

Atrophy (10–25%)
Bullous eruption (1–10%)
Cheilitis (>75%)
(1999): Katz HI+, *J Am Acad Dermatol* 41, S7 (>75%)
(1997): Buccheri L+, *Arch Dermatol* 133, 711 (100%)
(1996): Lacour M+, *Br J Dermatol* 134, 1023
(1991): Murray HE+, *J Am Acad Dermatol* 24, 598 (49%)
(1990): Ruzicka T+, *Arch Dermatol* 126, 482 (80%)
(1989): Gupta AK+, *J Am Acad Dermatol* 21, 1088 (100%)
(1988): Geiger J-M+, *Dermatologica* 176, 182 (82%)
Cold/clammy skin (1–10%)
Dermatitis (sic) (1–10%)
Diaphoresis (1–10%)
(1997): Buccheri L+, *Arch Dermatol* 133, 711 (18.2%)
(1988): Geiger J-M+, *Dermatologica* 176, 182 (9%)
Erythema (sic)
(1997): Buccheri L+, *Arch Dermatol* 133, 711 (18.2%)
Exanthems (10–25%)
(1999): Katz HI+, *J Am Acad Dermatol* 41, S7
(1990): Ruzicka T+, *Arch Dermatol* 126, 482 (2%)
Fissures (1–10%)
Milia
(1993): Chang A+, *Acta Derm Venereol* 73, 235
Palmoplantar desquamation
(1991): Murray HE+, *J Am Acad Dermatol* 24, 598 (29%)
(1990): Ruzicka T+, *Arch Dermatol* 126, 482 (20–25%)
(1989): Gupta AK+, *J Am Acad Dermatol* 21, 1088 (50–80%)
(1988): Geiger J-M+, *Dermatologica* 176, 182 (26%)
Peeling
(1999): Katz HI+, *J Am Acad Dermatol* 41, S7 (25–50%)
(1997): Buccheri L+, *Arch Dermatol* 133, 711 (36.4%)
Phototoxic reaction
(1999): Katz HI+, *J Am Acad Dermatol* 41, S7
Pruritus (25–50%)
(1999): Katz HI+, *J Am Acad Dermatol* 41, S7
(1997): Buccheri L+, *Arch Dermatol* 133, 711 (54.5%)
(1996): Lacour M+, *Br J Dermatol* 134, 1023
(1991): Murray HE+, *J Am Acad Dermatol* 24, 598 (32%)
(1990): Ruzicka T+, *Arch Dermatol* 126, 482 (37%)
(1989): Gupta AK+, *J Am Acad Dermatol* 21, 1088 (10–20%)
(1988): Geiger J-M+, *Dermatologica* 176, 182 (16%)
Psoriasis (1–10%)
Purpura (1–10%)
Pyogenic granuloma (1–10%)
Rash (sic) (>10%)
Seborrhea (1–10%)
Shaking (sic)
Stickiness (10–25%%)
(1999): Katz HI+, *J Am Acad Dermatol* 41, S7
(1997): Buccheri L+, *Arch Dermatol* 133, 711 (18.2)
(1991): Murray HE+, *J Am Acad Dermatol* 24, 598 (8%)
(1989): Schröder K+, *Acta Derm Venereol* (Stockh) 69, 111 (3%)
(1988): Geiger J-M+, *Dermatologica* 176, 182 (2.5%)
Sunburn (1–10%)
Ulceration (1–10%)
Urticaria
Xerosis (25–50%)
(1999): Katz HI+, *J Am Acad Dermatol* 41, S7 (15–25%)
(1997): Buccheri L+, *Arch Dermatol* 133, 711 (45.5%)
(1991): Murray HE+, *J Am Acad Dermatol* 24, 598 (24%)
(1990): Ruzicka T+, *Arch Dermatol* 126, 482 (48%)
(1989): Schröder K+, *Acta Derm Venereol* (Stockh) 69, 111 (65%)
(1989): Gupta AK+, *J Am Acad Dermatol* 21, 1088 (10–20%)
(1988): Geiger J-M+, *Dermatologica* 176, 182 (30%)

Hair

Hair – alopecia (50–75%)
(1999): Katz HI+, *J Am Acad Dermatol* 41, S7 (10–25%)
(1997): Buccheri L+, *Arch Dermatol* 133, 711 (45.5%)
(1991): Murray HE+, *J Am Acad Dermatol* 24, 598 (33%)
(1990): Ruzicka T+, *Arch Dermatol* 126, 482 (12%)
(1989): Schröder K+, *Acta Derm Venereol* (Stockh) 69, 111 (13%)
(1989): Gupta AK+, *J Am Acad Dermatol* 21, 1088 (30–70%)
(1988): Geiger J-M+, *Dermatologica* 176, 182 (20%)
Hair – alopecia universalis
(1998): Nadel RS, Springfield, MA (from Internet) (observation)
(1998): Haycox CL, Seattle, WA (from Internet) (observation)

Nails

Nails – disorder (sic) (25–50%)
Nails – fragility (sic)
(1991): Murray HE+, *J Am Acad Dermatol* 24, 598 (27%)
(1990): Ruzicka T+, *Arch Dermatol* 126, 482
(1988): Geiger J-M+, *Dermatologica* 176, 182 (10%)
Nails – paronychia (10–25%)
(1999): Katz HI+, *J Am Acad Dermatol* 41, S7
(1997): Buccheri L+, *Arch Dermatol* 133, 711 (18.2%)
(1991): Murray HE+, *J Am Acad Dermatol* 24, 598 (7%)
Nails – periungual granuloma
(1997): Buccheri L+, *Arch Dermatol* 133, 711 (9.1%)

Other

Bromhidrosis (1–10%)
(2000): Liss WA, Pleasanton, CA, (from Internet) (observation)
Gingival bleeding (1–10%)
Gingivitis (1–10%)
Gouty tophi
(1998): Vanhooteghem O+, *Clin Exp Dermatol* 23, 274
Hyperesthesia (10–25%)
(1999): Katz HI+, *J Am Acad Dermatol* 41, S7
Myopathy
(1996): Lister RK+, *Br J Dermatol* 134, 989
Oral mucosal lesions
(1988): Geiger J-M+, *Dermatologica* 176, 182 (6%)
Paresthesias (10–25%)
(1999): Katz HI+, *J Am Acad Dermatol* 41, S7
Pseudotumor cerebri
(1999): Katz HI+, *J Am Acad Dermatol* 41, S7
Sialorrhea (1–10%)
Stomatitis (1–10%)
Ulcerative stomatitis (1–10%)
Vulvovaginal candidiasis
(1995): Sturkenboom MC+, *J Clin Epidemiol* 48, 991
Xerostomia (10–25%)
(1999): Katz HI+, *J Am Acad Dermatol* 41, S7
(1997): Buccheri L+, *Arch Dermatol* 133, 711 (63.6%)
(1989): Schröder K+, *Acta Derm Venereol* (Stockh) 69, 111 (60%)
(1988): Geiger J-M+, *Dermatologica* 176, 182 (30%)

ACTINOMYCIN-D

(See DACTINOMYCIN)

ACYCLOVIR

Synonyms: aciclovir, ACV, acycloguanosine
Trade name: Zovirax (GlaxoWellcome)
Other common trade names: *Acifur; Acyclo-V; Acyvir; Avirax; Herpefug; Zyclir*
Indications: Herpes simplex; herpes zoster
Category: Antiviral, antiherpes drug (oral, parenteral and topical)
Half-life: 3 hours (adults)
Clinically important, potentially serious interactions with: meperidine, phenytoin, probenecid, valproic acid, zidovudine

Reactions

Skin

Acne (<3%)
Contact dermatitis
(2000): Serpentier-Daude A+, *Ann Dermatol Venereol* 127, 191
(1996): Bourezane Y+, *Allergy* 51, 755
(1995): Koch P, *Contact Dermatitis* 33, 255
(1991): Goday J+, *Contact Dermatitis* 24, 381
(1990): Baes H+, *Contact Dermatitis* 23, 200
(1990): Valsecchi R+, *Contact Dermatitis* 23, 372
(1989): Gola M+, *Contact Dermatitis* 20, 394
(1988): Camarasa JG+, *Contact Dermatitis* 19, 235
Dermatitis (sic)
(1989): O'Brien JJ+, *Drugs* 37, 233 (vesicular)
(1985): Robinson GE+, *Genitourin Med* 61, 62 (palms and soles)
Diaphoresis
Edema
(1991): Medina S+, *Int J Dermatol* 30, 305
Erythema nodosum
(1983): Richards DM+, *Drugs* 26, 378
Exanthems (1–5%)
(1991): Whitley R+, *N Engl J Med* 324, 444
(1985): Robinson GE+, *Genitourin Med* 61, 62
(1984): Strauss SE+, *N Engl J Med* 301, 1545
(1983): Richards DM+, *Drugs* 26, 378
(1983): Balfour HH+, *N Engl J Med* 308, 1448
Fixed eruption
(1997): Montoro J+, *Contact Dermatitis* 36, 225
Herpes zoster (recurrent)
(1993): Murphy F, *The Schoch Letter* 43, 28, #104 (observation)
Lichenoid eruption
(1985): Robinson GE+, *Genitourin Med* 61, 62
Peripheral edema
(1991): Medina S+, *Int J Dermatol* 30, 305
(1988): Hisler BM+, *J Am Acad Dermatol* 18, 1142
Pruritus (1–10%)
(1993): Goldberg LH+, *Arch Dermatol* 129, 582 (passim)
Rash (sic) (<3%)
(1985): Lundgren G+, *Scand J Infect Dis* Suppl 47, 137
(1983): Balfour HH+, *N Engl J Med* 308, 1448
(1983): Masaoka T+, *Gan To Kagaku Ryoho* (Japanese) 10, 944
Stevens–Johnson syndrome
(1995): Fazal BA+, *Clin Infect Dis* 21, 1038
Urticaria (1–5%)
(1985): Robinson GE+, *Genitourin Med* 61, 62
(1983): Richards DM+, *Drugs* 26, 378
(1982): Smith CI+, *Am J Med* 73, 267
(1981): Balfour HH+, *Minn Med* 64, 739
Vasculitis
(1983): Richards DM+, *Drugs* 26, 378
Vesicular eruption
(1993): Buck ML+, *Ann Pharmacother* 27, 1458

Hair

Hair – alopecia (<3%)

Other

Anaphylactoid reaction (<1%)
Dysgeusia (0.3%)
Injection-site inflammation (>10%)
(1989): O'Brien JJ+, *Drugs* 37, 233
Injection-site necrosis
(1987): Fayol J+, *Therapie* (French) 42(2), 249
Injection-site thrombophlebitis (9%)
(1988): Arndt KA, *J Am Acad Dermatol* 18, 188
Injection-site vesicular eruption
(1986): Sylvester RK+, *JAMA* 255, 385
Paresthesias (<1%)
(1993): Goldberg LH+, *Arch Dermatol* 129, 582 (passim)
Tremor
Vaginitis (candidal)
(1993): Goldberg LH+, *Arch Dermatol* 129, 582 (passim)

ALBENDAZOLE

Trade name: Albenza (SmithKline Beecham)
Other common trade names: *ABZ; Albezole; Alzol; Bendex; Eskazole; Vermin; Zentel*
Indications: Nematode infections; hydatid cyst disease
Category: Anthelmintic
Half-life: 8–12 hours
Clinically important, potentially serious interactions with: carbamazepine, cimetidine, dexamethasone, praziquantel. Also **food**

Reactions

Skin

Allergic reactions (sic) (<1%)
Contact dermatitis
(1991): Macedo NA+, *Contact Dermatitis* 25, 73
Fixed eruption
(1998): Mahboob A+, *JPMA J Pak Med Assoc* 48, 316
Pruritus (<1%)
Rash (sic) (<1%)
Stevens–Johnson syndrome
(1997): Dewardt S+, *Acta Derm Venereol* 77, 411
Urticaria (<1%)
(1991): Macedo NA+, *Contact Dermatitis* 25, 73

Hair

Hair – alopecia (<1%)
(1993): Tomas S+, *Enferm Infecc Microbiol Clin* (Spanish) 11, 113
(1990): Pilar-Garcia-Muret M+, *Int J Dermatol* 29, 669

Other

Xerostomia (<1%)

ALBUTEROL

Synonym: salbutamol
Trade names: Airet (Medeva); Combivent (Boehringer Ingelheim); Proventil (Schering); Ventolin (GlaxoWellcome); Volmax (Muro)
Other common trade names: *Asmaven; Broncho-Spray; Cobutolin; Salbulin; Ventoline*
Indications: Bronchospasm associated with asthma
Category: Beta$_2$ adrenergic agonist; bronchodilator (sympathomimetic)
Half-life: 3–6 hours
Clinically important, potentially serious interactions with: beta-blockers, digoxin, MAO inhibitors, sympathomimetic agents, tricyclic antidepressants

Combivent is albuterol and ipratropium

Reactions

Skin

Angioedema
Chills
Contact dermatitis
(1994): Smeenk G+, *Contact Dermatitis* 31, 123

Diaphoresis (1–10%)
(1989): Price AH+, *Drugs* 38, 77
Erythema (palmar) (with infusion)
(1992): Lebre C+, *Ann Dermatol Venereol* (French) 119, 293
(1990): Morin Leport LRM+, *Br J Dermatol* 122, 116
Exanthems
Flushing (1–10%)
Lupus erythematosus (pseudo-lupus)
(1987): Lacour JP+, *Presse Med* (French) 16, 1599
Pallor
Pruritus
(1991): Hatton MQ+, *Lancet* 337, 1169
Shakiness (sic)
Urticaria
(1991): Hatton MQ+, *Lancet* 337, 1169

Other

Dysgeusia (1–10%)
Tremor
Xerostomia (1–10%)

ALDESLEUKIN

Synonyms: IL-2, interleukin-2
Trade name: Proleukin (Chiron)
Other common trade names: *Aerovent; Atem; Atronase; Narilet; Tropium*
Indications: Metastatic renal cell carcinoma
Category: Antineoplastic; biological response modulator (parenteral)
Half-life: 6–85 minutes
Clinically important, potentially serious interactions with: analgesics, beta-blockers, narcotics, psychotropics, sedatives, tranquilizers

Reactions

Skin

Allergic granulomatous angiitis (Churg–Strauss syndrome)
(1997): Shiota Y+, *Inren Med* 36, 709
Allergic reactions (sic) (<1%)
Angioedema
(1992): Baars JW+, *Ann Oncol* 3, 243
Bullous eruption
(1991): Staunton MR, *J Natl Cancer Inst* 83, 56
Bullous pemphigoid
(1993): Fellner MJ, *Clin Dermatol* 11, 515
Dermatitis (sic)
(1989): Kerker BJ+, *Semin Dermatol* 8, 173
(1987): Gaspari AA+, *JAMA* 258, 1624 (1–5%)
Eczema reactivation
(1997): Cork MJ+, *Br J Dermatol* 136, 644
Edema (47%)
(1994): Rosenberg SA+, *JAMA* 271, 907
(1990): Chien CH+, *Pediatrics* 86, 937
Erythema (sic) (41%)
(1993): Wolkenstein P+, *J Am Acad Dermatol* 28, 66
(1992): Blessing K+, *J Pathol* 167, 313
(1988): Lee RE+, *Arch Dermatol* 124, 1811
(1987): Gaspari AA+, *JAMA* 258, 1624
Erythema nodosum
(1989): Kerker BJ+, *Semin Dermatol* 8, 173
(1987): Weinstein A+, *JAMA* 258, 3120
Erythroderma
(1992): Blessing K+, *J Pathol* 167, 313
(1991): Siegel JP+, *J Clin Oncol* 9, 694 (>5%)
(1989): Kerker BJ+, *Semin Dermatol* 8, 173
(1987): Gaspari AA+, *JAMA* 258, 1624
Exanthems
(1991): Siegel JP+, *J Clin Oncol* 9, 694 (>5%)
(1991): Dummer R+, *Dermatologica* 183, 95
(1989): Jost LM+, *Schweiz Med Wochenschr* (German) 119, 137
(1987): Gaspari AA+, *JAMA* 258, 1624
Exfoliative dermatitis (14%)
(1993): Larbre B+, *Ann Dermatol Venereol* (French) 120, 528
Graft-versus-host reaction
(1995): Costello R+, *Bone Marrow Transplant* 16, 199
Intertriginous cutaneous eruption (sic)
(1996): Prussick R+, *J Am Acad Dermatol* 35, 705
Kaposi's sarcoma
(1989): Krigel RL+, *J Biol Response Mod* 8, 359
Linear IgA bullous dermatosis
(1996): Tranvan A+, *J Am Acad Dermatol* 35, 865
(1993): Oeda E+, *Am J Hematol* 44, 213
(1990): Guillaume JC+, *Ann Dermatol Venereol* (French) 117, 899
Pemphigus
(1995): Wolkenstein P+, *Arch Dermatol* 130, 890
(1994): Prussick R+, *Arch Dermatol* 130, 890
(1989): Ramseur WL+, *Cancer* 63, 2005 (fatal)
Peripheral edema (1–10%)
Petechiae (4%)
Photosensitivity
(1992): Blessing K+, *J Pathol* 167, 313
Pruritus (48%)
(1995): Wahlgren CF+, *Arch Dermatol Res* 287, 572
(1994): Rosenberg SA+, *JAMA* 271, 907
(1993): Wolkenstein P+, *J Am Acad Dermatol* 28, 66
(1988): Lee RE+, *Arch Dermatol* 124, 1811
(1987): Gaspari AA+, *JAMA* 258, 1624
Psoriasis
(1991): Siegel JP+, *J Clin Oncol* 9, 694 (>5%)
(1989): Kerker BJ+, *Semin Dermatol* 8, 173
(1988): Lee RE+, *Arch Dermatol* 124, 1811 (exacerbation)
(1987): Gaspari AA+, *JAMA* 258, 1624
Purpura (4%)
(1989): Kerker BJ+, *Semin Dermatol* 8, 173
Rash (sic) (26%)
Scleroderma
(1994): Boni R, *Dermatology* 189, 330
(1994): Puett DW+, *J Rheumatol* 21, 752
Toxic epidermal necrolysis
(1992): Wiener JS+, *South Med J* 85, 656
Urticaria (2%)
(1993): Wolkenstein P+, *J Am Acad Dermatol* 28, 66
(1992): Baars JW+, *Ann Oncol* 3, 243
Vitiligo
(1996): Rosenberg SA+, *J Immunother Emphasis Tumor Immunol* 19, 81
(1995): Wolkenstein P+, *Arch Dermatol* 130, 890
(1994): Scheibenbogen C+, *Eur J Cancer* (30A) 8, 1209
Xerosis (15%)

Hair

Hair – alopecia (<1%)
(1989): Jost LM+, *Schweiz Med Wochenschr* (German) 119, 137
(1987): Gaspari AA+, *JAMA* 258, 1624 (10%)

Other

Aphthous stomatitis
(1987): Gaspari AA+, *JAMA* 258, 1624 (5%)
Dysgeusia (7%)
Glossitis
(1987): Gaspari AA+, *JAMA* 258, 1624 (30%)
Injection-site inflammation
(1999): Asadullah K+, *Arch Dermatol* 135, 187
Injection-site nodules
(1993): Klapholtz L+, *Bone Marrow Transplant* 11, 443
Injection-site panniculitis
(1992): Baars JW+, *Br J Cancer* 66, 698
Injection-site reactions (sic) (3%)
Myalgia (6%)
Necrosis
(1993): Wolkenstein P+, *J Am Acad Dermatol* 28, 66
(1988): Rosenberg SA+, *Ann Intern Med* 108, 853 (3%)
Oral mucosal eruption
(1989): Kerker BJ+, *Semin Dermatol* 8, 173
(1987): Gaspari AA+, *JAMA* 258, 1624
Oral ulceration
(1990): Chien CH+, *Pediatrics* 86, 937
Stomatitis (32%)

ALENDRONATE

Trade name: Fosamax (Merck)
Other common trade name: *Fosalan*
Indications: Osteoporosis in postmenopausal women, Paget's disease
Category: Inhibitor of bone resorption; biphosphonate
Half-life: >10 years
Clinically important, potentially serious interactions with: aspirin, calcium supplements, ranitidine

Reactions

Skin

Erythema (<1%)
(1996): Keen RW+, *Br J Clin Pract* 50, 211
Erythema multiforme
(2000): Madnani N, Bombay, India (from Internet) (observation)
Exanthem
(2000): Madnani N, Bombay, India (from Internet) (observation)
Fixed eruption
(1998): McCarthy J, Ft. Worth, TX (from Internet) (observation)
Peripheral edema
Petechiae
(1997): Berger R, St. George, UT (from Internet) (observation)
Pruritus (0.6%)
(2000): Madnani N, Bombay, India (from Internet) (observation)
(1997): Kyriakidou-Himonas M+, *Advances in Therapy* 14, 281
Rash (sic) (<1%)
(1997): Berger R, St. George, UT (from Internet) (observation)
(1996): Selby PL, *Osteoporosis Int* 6, S21
(1996): Keen RW+, *Br J Clin Pract* 50, 211
(1996): Freedholm D+, *Osteoporosis Int* 6, 261
(1995): Chestnut CH+, *Am J Med* 99, 144

Other

Dysgeusia (0.6%)
(1997): Kyriakidou-Himonas M+, *Advances in Therapy* 14, 281
Hypersensitivity
(1996): Kirk JK+, *Am Fam Physician* 54, 2053
Ocular inflammation
(1999): Mbekeani JN+, *Arch Ophthalmol* 117, 837
Oral ulceration
(1999): Demerjian N+, *Clin Rheumatol* 18, 349

ALFENTANIL

Trade name: Alfenta (Taylor)
Other trade name: *Rapifen*
Indications: General anesthesia; post-operative pain
Category: Narcotic agonist analgesic
Half-life: 83–97 minutes (adults)
Clinically important, potentially serious interactions with: beta-blockers, CNS depressants, diazepam, erythromycin, reserpine

Reactions

Skin

Clammy skin (<1%)
Pruritus (<1%)
(1999): Kyriakides K+, *Br J Anaesth* 82, 439
Rash (sic) (<1%)
Shivering (sic) (3–9%)
Urticaria (<1%)

Other

Dysesthesia

ALITRETINOIN

Trade name: Panretin (Ligand)
Indications: Kaposi's sarcoma cutaneous lesions
Category: Antineoplastic retinoic acid derivative (topical)
Half-life: no data
Clinically important, potentially serious interactions with: deet, methoxsalen

Reactions

Skin

Abrasions
Bullous eruption
Edema (3–8%)
Exfoliative dermatitis (3–9%)
Flushing
Pain (0–34%)
Photosensitivity
Pruritus (8–11%)
Rash (sic) (25–77%)
Skin disorder (sic) (0–8%)

Hair

Hair – alopecia

Other

Application-site reactions
(1999): Walmsley S+, *J Acquir Immune Defic Syndr* 22, 325
Myalgia
Paresthesias (3–22%)

ALLOPURINOL

Trade name: Zyloprim (Faro)
Other common trade names: *Allo 300; Alloprin; Allo-Puren; Atisuril; Bleminol; Caplenal; Hamarin; Novo-Purol; Purinol; Unizuric; Zyloric*
Indications: Gouty arthritis
Category: Uricosuric; anti-gout
Half-life: 1–3 hours
Clinically important, potentially serious interactions with: amoxicillin, ampicillin, azathioprine, chlorpropamide, cyclophosphamide, dicumarol, mercaptopurine, theophylline, thiazides, warfarin

Reactions

Skin

Acute generalized exanthematous pustulosis (AGEP)
(1995): Moreau A+, *Int J Dermatol* 34, 263 (passim)
Angiitis (<1%)
Angioedema
(1996): Yale SH+, *Hosp Pract Off Ed* 31, 92
Cutaneous reaction (severe) (sic)
(1999): Tanna SB+, *Ann Pharmacother* 33 1180
Chills (1–10%)
Diaphoresis (<1%)
Ecchymoses (<1%)
Edema (periorbital)
(1981): McInnes GT+, *Ann Rheum Dis* 40, 245
Erythema multiforme (<1%)
(1999): Fonseka MM+, *Ceylon Med J* 44, 190
(1996): Kumar A+, *BMJ* 312, 173
(1984): Pennell DJ+, *Lancet* 1, 463
(1979): Lupton GP+, *J Am Acad Dermatol* 1, 365
Exanthems (1–5%)
(1998): Dintiman B, Fairfax, VA (from Internet) (observation)
(1992): Fam AG+, *Am J Med* 93, 299
(1989): Chan SH+, *Dermatologica* 179, 32
(1987): Hoigné R+, *N Engl J Med* 316, 1217
(1984): Hande KR+, *Am J Med* 76, 47
(1981): McInnes GT+, *Ann Rheum Dis* 40, 245

(1981): Jick H+, *J Clin Pharmacol* 21, 456 (with ampicillin 14%)
(1979): Lang GP+, *South Med J* 72, 1361
(1979): Lupton GP+, *J Am Acad Dermatol* 1, 365
(1976): Utsinger PD+, *Am J Med* 61, 287
(1976): Lockard O+, *Ann Intern Med* 85, 333
(1971): Mills RM, *JAMA* 216, 799

Exfoliative dermatitis (>10%)
(1996): Sigurdsson V+, *J Am Acad Dermatol* 35, 53
(1996): Emmerson BT, *N Engl J Med* 334, 445
(1989): Chan SH+, *Dermatologica* 179, 32
(1984): Vinciullo C, *Aust J Dermatol* 25, 59
(1979): Lupton GP+, *J Am Acad Dermatol* 1, 365
(1979): Lang GP+, *South Med J* 72, 1361
(1977): Boyer TD+, *West J Med* 126, 143
(1976): McMenamin RA+, *Aust N Z J Med* 6, 583
(1975): Sisca TS, *J Clin Pharmacol* 15, 566
(1973): Feuerman EJ+, *Br J Dermatol* 89, 83
(1966): Rundles RW+, *Ann Intern Med* 64, 229

Fixed eruption (<1%)
(1999): Sehgal VN+, *J Dermatol* 26, 198 (transitory giant)
(1998): Umpierrez A+, *J Allergy Clin Immunol* 101, 286
(1996): Kelso JM+, *J Allergy Clin Immunol* 97, 1171
(1996): Gimbel Moral LF+, *Med Clin (Barc)* (Spanish) 106, 119
(1990): Audicana M+, *Clin Exp Allergy* 20, Supp 1, 121

Graft-versus-host reaction
(1998): Jappe U+, *Hautarzt* (German) 49, 126

Granuloma annulare (disseminated)
(1995): Becker D+, *Hautarzt* (German) 46, 343

Ichthyosis
(1968): Auerbach R+, *Arch Dermatol* 98, 104

Lichen planus (<1%)

Lupus erythematosus
(1978): Pereyo-Torrellas N, *Arch Dermatol* 114, 1097
(1975): Lee SL+, *Semin Arthritis Rheum* 5, 83

Lymphocytoma cutis
(1988): Raymond JZ+, *Cutis* 41, 323

Necrotizing angiitis

Perforating foot ulceration
(1997): Bouloc A+, *Clin Exp Dermatol* 21, 351

Petechiae
(1977): Chan HL+, *Aust N Z J Med* 7, 518

Photosensitivity
(1986): Lerman S, *Ophthalmology* 93, 304

Pruritus (<1%)
(1998): Dintiman B, Fairfax, VA (from Internet) (observation)
(1979): Lupton GP+, *J Am Acad Dermatol* 1, 365
(1979): Lang GP+, *South Med J* 72, 1361
(1965): Klinenberg JR+, *Ann Intern Med* 62, 639

Purpura (>10%)
(1979): Lang GP+, *South Med J* 72, 1361
(1977): Boyer TD+, *West J Med* 126, 143

Pustuloderma
(1994): Fitzgerald DA+, *Clin Exp Dermatol* 19, 243

Rash (sic) (>10%)
(1996): Yale SH+, *Hosp Pract Off Ed* 31, 92

Sensitivity (sic)
(1979): Haughey DB+, *Am J Hosp Pharm* 36, 1377

Stevens–Johnson syndrome (>10%)
(1995): Roujeau JC+, *N Engl J Med* 333, 1600
(1993): Leenutaphong V+, *Int J Dermatol* 32, 428
(1992): Goodglick TA+, *Ophthalmic Surg* 23, 557
(1989): Chan SH+, *Dermatologica* 179, 32
(1985): Renwick IG, *BMJ* 291, 485
(1985): Ting HC+, *Int J Dermatol* 24, 587
(1985): Edwards R+, *Dimens Crit Care Nurs* 4, 335
(1984): Pennell DJ+, *Lancet* 1, 463 (fatal)
(1979): Lupton GP+, *J Am Acad Dermatol* 1, 365
(1978): Assaad D+, *Can Med Assoc* 118, 154
(1977): Chan HL+, *Aust N Z J Med* 7, 518

Toxic epidermal necrolysis
(1999): Sorkin MJ, Denver, CO (from Internet) (observation)
(1995): Roujeau JC+, *N Engl J Med* 333, 1600
(1995): Wolkenstein P+, *Arch Dermatol* 131, 544
(1994): Alfandari S+, *Infection* 22, 365
(1993): Leenutaphong V+, *Int J Dermatol* 32, 428
(1993): Correia O+, *Dermatology* 186, 32
(1991): Sakellariou G+, *Int J Artif Organs* 14, 634
(1987): Guillaume JC+, *Arch Dermatol* 123, 1166
(1986): Kumar L, *Indian J Dermatol* 31, 53
(1985): Auboeck J+, *BMJ* 290, 1969
(1985): Renwick IG, *BMJ* 291, 485
(1985): Zakraoui L+, *Tunis Med* (French) 63, 167
(1984): Dan M+, *Int J Dermatol* 23, 142
(1984): Chan HL, *J Am Acad Dermatol* 10, 973
(1979): Lupton GP+, *J Am Acad Dermatol* 1, 365
(1979): Lang GP+, *South Med J* 72, 1361
(1978): Assaad D+, *Can Med Assoc* 118, 154
(1977): Chan HL+, *Aust N Z J Med* 7, 518
(1977): Bennett TO+, *Arch Ophthalmol* 95, 1362 (ocular)
(1976): Fellner MJ, *Arch Dermatol* 112, 1327
(1975): Trentham DE+, *N Engl J Med* 292, 870
(1975): Sisca TS, *J Clin Pharmacol* 15, 566
(1975): Ellman MH+, *Arch Dermatol* 111, 986
(1972): Stratigos JD+, *Br J Dermatol* 86, 564
(1970): Kantor GL, *JAMA* 212, 478 (fatal)

Toxic erythema
(1995): Rademaker M, *N Z Med J* 108, 165

Toxic pustuloderma
(1994): Boffa MJ+, *Br J Dermatol* 131, 447
(1994): Fitzgerald DA+, *Clin Exp Dermatol* 19, 243
(1993): Yu RC+, *Br J Dermatol* 128, 95

Urticaria (>10%)
(1999): Litt JZ, Beachwood, OH, personal case (observation)
(1992): Breathnach SM+, *Adverse Drug Reactions and the Skin*, Blackwell, Oxford, 193 (passim)
(1991): Anderson MH+, *Ann Allergy* 66, 207

Vasculitis (<1%)
(1998): Choi HK+, *Clin Exp Rheumatol* 16, 743
(1996): Emmerson BT, *N Engl J Med* 334, 445
(1977): Boyer TD+, *West J Med* 126, 143
(1976): Bailey RR+, *Lancet* 2, 907
(1971): Mills RM, *JAMA* 216, 799

Hair

Hair – alopecia (1–10%)
(1974): Lovatt GE, *Br J Dermatol* 91, 115
(1968): Auerbach R+, *Arch Dermatol* 98, 104

Nails

Nails – onycholysis (<1%)

Other

Dysgeusia

Hypersensitivity*
(1999): Morel D+, *Nephrol Dial Transplant* 14, 780
(1999): Melsom RD, *Rheumatology* 38, 1301 (familial)
(1999): Gillott TJ+, *Rheumatology* (Oxford) 38, 85
(1998): Schlienger RG+, *Epilepsia* 39, S3 (passim)
(1998): Pluim HJ+, *Neth J Med* 52, 107
(1998): Kluger E, *Ugeskr Laeger* (Danish) 160, 1179
(1997): Carpenter C, *Tenn Med* 90, 151
(1996): Kumar A+, *BMJ* 312, 173
(1995): Elasy T+, *West J Med* 162, 360
(1994): Lee SS+, *Chung Hua Min Kuo Wei Sheng Wu Chi Mien I Hsueh Tsa Chih* 27, 140
(1994): Salinas Martin A+, *Aten Primaria* (Spanish) 14, 694
(1989): Puig JG+, *J Rheumatol* 16, 842
(1988): McDonald J+, *J Rheumatol* 15, 865
(1985): Stein CM, *S Afr Med J* 67, 935
(1984): Vinciullo C, *Aust J Dermatol* 25, 59
(1984): Vinciullo C, *Med J Aust 141, 449*
(1979): Lupton GP+, *J Am Acad Dermatol* 1, 365
(1976): Utsinger PD+, *Am J Med* 61, 287

Mucocutaneous eruption

Myalgia
(1996): Ghanem BM+, *J Egypt Soc Parasitol* 26, 619

Myopathy (<1%)

Oral ulceration
(1984): Chau NY+, *Oral Surg Oral Med Oral Pathol* 58, 397 (lichenoid)
(1979): Lang GP+, *South Med J* 72, 1361

Paresthesias (<1%)

Polyarteritis nodosa
(1976): Bailey RR+, *Lancet* 2, 907
(1974): Young JL+, *Arch Intern Med* 134, 553
(1970): Jarzobski J+, *Am Heart J* 79, 116

Stomatitis
(1981): McInnes GT+, *Ann Rheum Dis* 40, 245
(1977): Chan HL+, *Aust N Z J Med* 7, 518 (ulcerative)
Thrombophlebitis (<1%)
Tongue edema (<1%)

***Note:** The antiepileptic drug hypersensitivity syndrome is a severe, occasionally fatal, disorder characterized by any or all of the following: pruritic exanthem, toxic epidermal necrolysis, Stevens–Johnson syndrome, exfoliative dermatitis, fever, hepatic abnormalities, eosinophilia, and renal failure.

ALOSETRON

Trade name: Lotronex (GlaxoWellcome)
Indications: Irritable bowel syndrome
Category: 5-HT_3 receptor antagonist
Half-life: 1.5 hours
Clinically important, potentially serious interactions with: hydralazine, isoniazid, procainamide

Reactions

Skin

Acne (<1%)
Allergic reactions (<1%)
Bacterial infections
Folliculitis (<1%)
Hematomas (<1%)

Other

Dysgeusia (<1%)
Parosmia (<1%)

ALPRAZOLAM

Trade name: Xanax (Pharmacia & Upjohn)
Other common trade names: *Alprox; APO-Alpraz; Cassadan; Kalma; Nu-Alprax; Ralozam; Tafil*
Indications: Anxiety, depression, panic attacks
Category: Benzodiazepine anxiolytic tranquilizer
Half-life: 11–16 hours
Clinically important, potentially serious interactions with: alcohol, cimetidine, clarithromycin, CNS depressants, digoxin, disulfiram, fluconazole, fluoxetine, itraconazole, ketoconazole, lithium, omeprazole, oral contraceptives, propoxyphene, ritonavir, theophyllines, grapefruit juice

Reactions

Skin

Acne
(1985): Levy MH+, *Semin Oncol* 12, 411
Allergic reactions (sic)
(1996): Bhatia MS, *Indian J Med Sci* 50, 285 (to the tartrazine dye)
Dermatitis (sic) (3.8%)
(1984): Elie R+, *J Clin Psychopharmacol* 4, 125
(1982): Fawcett JA+, *Pharmacotherapy* 2, 243
(1981): Kolin IS+, *J Clin Psychiatry* 42, 169
(1981): Evans RL, *Drug Intell Clin Pharm* 15, 633
(1976): Fabre LF, *Curr Ther Res* 19, 661
Diaphoresis (15.8%)
Edema (4.9%)
Exanthems
(1988): Warnock JK+, *Am J Psychiatry* 145, 425
Photosensitivity
(1999): Watanabe Y+, *J Am Acad Dermatol* 40, 832
(1998): Pazzagli L+, *Pharm World Sci* 20, 136 (along with fluoxetine)
(1994): Shelley WB+, *Cutis* 54, 70 (observation)
(1990): Kanwar AJ+, *Dermatologica* 181, 75
Phototoxic reaction
(1993): Litt JZ, Beachwood, OH, personal case (observation)
(1991): Shelley WB+, *Cutis* 48, 187 (observation)
Pruritus
(1988): Islas JA+, *Curr Ther Res* 43, 384
(1982): Chouinard G+, *Psychopharmacol* 77, 229
Purpura
Rash (sic) (10.8%)
(1987): Fyer AJ+, *Am J Psychiatry* 144, 303
(1985): Rush AJ+, *Arch Gen Psychiatry* 42, 1154
(1985): Jerram TC, *Side Eff Drugs Annu* 9, 39
(1983): Davison K+, *Psychopharmacol* 80, 308
Urticaria
Xerosis
(1982): Chouinard G+, *Psychopharmacol* 77, 229

Other

Dysgeusia (<1%)
(1982): Chouinard G+, *Psychopharmacol* 77, 229
Galactorrhea
Gynecomastia
Oral ulceration
Paresthesias (2.4%)
Pseudolymphoma
(1995): Magro CM+, *J Am Acad Dermatol* 32, 419
Sialopenia (32.8%)
Sialorrhea (4.2%)
Xerostomia (14.7%)
(1988): Islas JA+, *Curr Ther Res* 43, 384
(1984): Elie R+, *J Clin Psychopharmacol* 4, 125
(1982): Chouinard G+, *Psychopharmacol* 77, 229
(1982): Fawcett JA+, *Pharmacotherapy* 2, 243
(1981): Evans RL, *Drug Intell Clin Pharm* 15, 633

ALPROSTADIL

Synonyms: PGE; prostaglandin E_1
Trade names: Caverject (Pharmacia & Upjohn); Edex (Schwarz); Muse (Vivus); Prostin VR (Pharmacia & Upjohn)
Other common trade names: *Lyple; Minprog; Palux; Prostine VR; Prostivas*
Indications: Impotence; to maintain patent ductus arteriosus
Category: Prostaglandin; erectile dysfunction agent
Half-life: 5–10 minutes
Clinically important, potentially serious interactions with: anticoagulants, heparin

Reactions

Skin

Balanitis (<1%)
Diaphoresis (<1%)
Ecchymoses
(1996): Linet OI+, *N Engl J Med* 334, 873 (8%)
Edema (1%)
Flushing (>10%)
Lichen sclerosus (penile shaft hypopigmentation)
(1998): English JC+, *J Am Acad Dermatol* 39, 801
Penile edema (1%)
Penile pain (37%)
(1997): Padma-Nathan H+, *N Engl J Med* 336, 1 (32.7%)
(1996): Linet OI+, *N Engl J Med* 334, 873 (50%)
Penile pruritus (<1%)
Penile rash (1–10%)
Rash (sic) (<1%)
Toxic epidermal necrolysis
(1996): Lecorvaisier-Pieto C+, *J Am Acad Dermatol* 35, 112
Urticaria
(2000): Carter EL+, *Pediatr Dermatol* 17, 58

Other

Hypesthesia (<1%)

Injection-site ecchymoses (1–10%)
(1996): Linet OI+, *N Engl J Med* 334, 873 (8%)
Injection-site hematoma (3%)
Injection-site inflammation (<1%)
Injection-site pain (2%)
(1996): Hellstrom WJG, *Urology* 48, 851
Injection-site pruritus (<1%)
Priapism (4%)
(1999): Lue TF, *J Urol* 161, 725
(1998): Bettocchi C+, *Br J Urol* 81, 926
(1997): *Med Lett Drugs Ther* 39, 32
(1996): Linet OI+, *N Engl J Med* 334, 873 (1%)
(1996): Hellstrom WJG, *Urology* 48, 851
Xerostomia (<1%)

ALTEPLASE

Trade name: Activase (Genentech)
Other common trade names: *Actilyse; Activacin; Lysatec-rt-PA*
Indications: Acute myocardial infarction, acute pulmonary embolism
Category: Thrombolytic (tissue plasminogen activator)
Half-life: 30–45 minutes
Clinically important, potentially serious interactions with: anticoagulants, aspirin, dipyridamole, heparin, nitroglycerin, NSAIDs, ticlopidine

Reactions

Skin

Angioedema
(2000): Hill MD+, *CMAJ* 162, 1281
(2000): Rudolf J+, *Neurology* 55, 599
Ecchymoses (1–10%)
Rash (sic) (<0.02%)
Purpura (<1%)
(1990): De Trana+, *Arch Dermatol* 126, 690 (painful) (<1%)
Urticaria (<1%)
(1989): Collen D+, *Drugs* 38, 346

Other

Anaphylactoid reaction (<0.02%)
(2000): Hill MD+, *CMAJ* 162, 1281 (fatal)
(1999): Rudolf J+, *Stroke* 30, 1142
Gingival bleeding (<1%)

ALTRETAMINE

Synonym: hexamethylmelamine
Trade name: Hexalen (US Bioscience)
Other common trade names: *Hexamethylmelamin; Hexastat; Hexinawas*
Indications: Palliative treatment of recurrent ovarian cancer
Category: Antineoplastic
Half-life: 13 hours
Clinically important, potentially serious interactions with: antidepressants, cimetidine, MAO inhibitors, pyridoxine

Reactions

Skin

Dermatitis (sic)
Exanthems
Pruritus (<1%)
Rash (sic) (<1%)

Hair

Hair – alopecia (<1%)

Other

Mucocutaneous side effects (sic)
(1978): Levine LR, *Cancer Treat Rev* 5, 67
Tremor (<1%)

AMANTADINE

Trade names: Symadine; Symmetrel (Endo Lab)
Other common trade names: *Amixx; Endantadine; Grippin-Merz; Mantadix; PK-Merz; Protexin; Tregor*
Indications: Parkinsonism, influenza A viral infection
Category: Antiviral, antidyskinetic and antifatigue, antiparkinsonian
Half-life: 10–28 hours
Clinically important, potentially serious interactions with: amiloride, hydrochlorothiazide, triamterene, tricyclic antidepressants, trimethoprim

Note: Fifty to 90% of patients receiving amantadine for Parkinsonism develop "a more or less livedo reticularis."

Reactions

Skin

Ankle edema
(1972): Schwab RS+, *JAMA* 222, 792
(1972): Calne DB+, *Drugs* 4, 49
(1971): Vollum DI+, *BMJ* 2, 628
(1971): Parkes JD+, *Lancet* 1, 1085
Contact dermatitis
(1997): Jauregui I+, *J Invest Allergol Clin Immunol* 7, 260
(1990): Patruno C+, *Contact Dermatitis* 22, 187
(1988): van Ketel WG, *Derm Beruf Umwelt* (German) 36, 23
(1987): Miranda A+, *Contact Dermatitis* 17, 55
(1987): Angelini G+, *Contact Dermatitis* 15, 114
(1987): van Joost T+, *Ned Tijdschr Geneeskd* (Dutch) 131, 21
(1987): van Ketel WG, *Ned Tijdschr Geneeskd* (Dutch) 131, 461
(1985): Valsecchi R+, *Contact Dermatitis* 13, 341
(1985): Tosti A+, *Contact Dermatitis* 13, 339
(1984): Santucci B+, *Contact Dermatitis* 10, 317
(1984): Agathos M+, *Derm Beruf Umwelt* (German) 32, 157
(1984): Lembo G+, *Contact Dermatitis* 10, 317
(1983): Przybilla B, *J Am Acad Dermatol* 9, 165
(1982): Brandao FM+, *Contact Dermatitis* 8, 140
(1982): van Ketel WG, *Contact Dermatitis* 8, 71
(1982): van der Walle HB+, *Ned Tijdschr Geneeskd* (Dutch) 126, 1033
(1980): Przybilla B+, *MMW Munch Med Wochenschr* (German) 122, 1195
(1978): Miescher P+, *Hautarzt* (German) 29, 337
(1976): Fanta D+, *Contact Dermatitis* 2, 282
Dermatitis (sic) (0.1%)
(1972): Schwab RS+, *JAMA* 222, 792
Discoloration (sic)
(1971): Parkes JD+, *Lancet* 1, 1083
Eczematous eruption (sic)
(1983): Hellgren L+, *Dermatologica* 167, 267
Edema
(1975): Butzer JF+, *Neurology* 25, 603
Erythema multiforme
(2000): Mitchell D, Thomasville, GA, (from Internet) (observation)
Exanthems
(1971): Vollum DI+, *BMJ* 2, 627
Eyelid edema
Livedo reticularis (50–90%)
(2000): Litt JZ, Beachwood, OH, personal case (observation)
(1998): Loffler H+, *Hautarzt* (German) 49, 224
(1996): Eisner J, Mount Vernon, WA, (from Internet) (observation)
(1995): Paulson GW+, *Clin Neuropharmacol* 18, 466
(1975): Butzer JF+, *Neurology* 25, 603 (25%)
(1974): Kalsbeek GL+, *Ned Tijdschr Geneeskd* (Dutch) 118, 66
(1972): Silver DE+, *Neurology* 22, 665
(1972): Schwab RS+, *JAMA* 222, 792
(1971): Marchoul JC+, *Bull Soc Fr Dermatol Syphiligr* (French) 78, 236
(1971): Vollum DI+, *BMJ* 2, 627
(1971): Parkes JD+, *Lancet* 1, 1083 (90%)
(1970): Shealy CN+, *JAMA* 212, 1522 (55%)
Peripheral edema (1–10%)
Photosensitivity
(1983): van den Berg WH+, *Contact Dermatitis* 9, 165
(1974): van Ketel WG+, *Dermatologica* 148, 124
Pruritus (<1%)
(1972): Schwab RS+, *JAMA* 222, 792

Rash (sic) (<1%)
Urticaria

Hair

Hair – alopecia
(1975): Butzer JF+, *Neurology* 25, 603 (8%)
Hair – hypertrichosis
(1975): Butzer JF+, *Neurology* 25, 603

Nails

Nails – increased growth
(1975): Butzer JF+, *Neurology* 25, 603

Other

Xerostomia (1–10%)
(1972): Schwab RS+, *JAMA* 222, 792
(1971): Parkes JD+, *Lancet* 1, 1085

AMIFOSTINE

Synonyms: ethiofos; gammaphos
Trade name: Ethyol (Alza)
Other trade name: *Ethyol 500*
Indications: Nephrotoxicity prophylaxis
Category: Antidote (cisplatin); cytoprotective
Half-life: 9 minutes
Clinically important, potentially serious interactions with: antihypertensives, levamisole

Reactions

Skin

Allergic reactions (sic)
Chills (sic) (>10%)
(2000): Sriswasdi C+, *J Med Assoc Thai* 83, 374
Flushing (>10%)
(2000): Sriswasdi C+, *J Med Assoc Thai* 83, 374
Rash (sic) (<1%)
(1998): Buresh CM+, *J Pediatr Hematol Oncol* 20, 361

Other

Dysgeusia
(2000): Sriswasdi C+, *J Med Assoc Thai* 83, 374

AMIKACIN

Trade name: Amikacin Sulfate (Elkins-Sinn)
Other common trade names: *Amicacina; Amicasil; Amikan; Biclin; Biklin; Gamikal; Kanbine; Lukadin; Miacin; Yectamid*
Indications: Short-term treatment of serious infections due to gram-negative bacteria
Category: Aminoglycoside antibiotic (parenteral)
Half-life: 1.5–2.5 hours (adults)
Clinically important, potentially serious interactions with: aminoglycosides, amphotericin, bumetanide, carbenicillin, ethacrynic acid, furosemide, indomethacin, loop diuretics, succinylcholine, ticarcillin, torsemide, vancomycin

Reactions

Skin

Dermatitis (sic)
(1989): Rudzki E+, *Contact Dermatitis* 20, 391
(1985): Holdiness MR, *Int J Dermatol* 24, 280
Exanthems
(1977): Yu VL+, *JAMA* 238, 943 (3.7%)
(1977): Pollack AA+, *JAMA* 237, 562 (3.7%)
Pruritus
(1985): Holdiness MR, *Int J Dermatol* 24, 280
Rash (sic) (<1%)
(1995): Rodriguez-Noriega E+, *J Chemother* 7, 155
Urticaria

Other

Injection-site induration
Injection-site necrosis
(1993): Plantin P+, *Presse Med* (French) 22, 1366
Injection-site pain
Paresthesias (<1%)
Tremor (<1%)

AMILORIDE

Trade names: Midamor (Merck); Moduretic (Merck)
Other common trade names: *Amikal; Kaluril; Medamor; Midoride; Modamide; Nirulid; Ride*
Indications: Prevention of hypokalemia associated with kaliuretic diuretics and management of edema in hypertension
Category: Potassium-sparing antihypertensive diuretic
Half-life: 6–9 hours
Clinically important, potentially serious interactions with: ACE-inhibitors, amantadine, anticoagulants, indomethacin, lithium, NSAIDs, potassium salts, spironolactone, triamterene

Moduretic is amiloride and hydrochlorothiazide.

Reactions

Skin

Diaphoresis
Exanthems
(1972): *Drug Ther Bull* 10, 30
Flushing (>1%)
Photosensitivity
(1981): *Aust Prescriber* 5, 23
Pruritus (<1%)
Purpura
Rash (sic) (<1%)
Urticaria
Vasculitis
Xerosis (<1%)

Hair

Hair – alopecia (<1%)

Other

Anaphylactoid reaction
Dysgeusia (<1%)
Gynecomastia (1–10%)
Paresthesias (<1%)
Tremor
Xerostomia (<1%)

AMINOCAPROIC ACID

Trade name: Amicar (Immunex)
Other common trade names: *Capramol; Caproamin; Caprolisin; Ipron; Ipsilon; Resplamin*
Indications: To provide hemostasis in the treatment of fibrinolysis
Category: Antifibrinolytic; hemostatic
Half-life: 1–2 hours
Clinically important, potentially serious interactions with: estrogens, oral contraceptives, thrombolytic agents

Reactions

Skin

Bullous eruption
(1992): Brooke CP+, *J Am Acad Dermatol* 27, 880
Contact dermatitis
(2000): Miyamoto H+, *Contact Dermatitis* 42, 50
(1989): Shono M, *Contact Dermatitis* 21, 106

Dermatitis (systemic)
(1999): Villarreal O, *Contact Dermatitis* 40, 114
Eczematous eruption (sic)
(1989): Shono M, *Contact Dermatitis* 21, 106
Edema
Exanthems
(1995): Gonzalez-Gutierrez ML+, *Allergy* 50, 745
Kaposi's sarcoma
Pruritus
Purpura
(1985): Verstraete M, *Drugs* 29, 236
(1980): Chakrabarti A+, *BMJ* 281, 197
Rash (sic) (1–10%)
Systemic dermatitis (sic)
(1999): Villarreal O, *Contact Dermatitis* 40, 114
Urticaria

Other

Anaphylactoid reaction
Injection-site erythema
Injection-site phlebitis
Injection-site reaction (sic)
Muscle necrosis
Myalgia
Myopathy (1–10%)
(1988): Kane MJ+, *Am J Med* 85, 861
Thrombophlebitis

AMINOGLUTETHIMIDE

Trade name: Cytadren (Novartis)
Other common trade names: *Orimeten; Orimetene; Rodazol*
Indications: Suppression of adrenal function, metastatic carcinoma
Category: Antiadrenal and antineoplastic
Half-life: 7–15 hours
Clinically important, potentially serious interactions with: dexamethasone, oral anticoagulants, propranolol, theophylline, warfarin

Reactions

Skin

Angioedema
(1967): Horky K+, *Schweiz Med Wochenschr* (German) 98, 1843
Erythema
(1987): Williams DS+, *Br J Radiology* 60, 1226
Exanthems
(1990): Vanek N+, *Med Pediatr Oncol* 18, 162
(1987): Williams DS+, *Br J Radiology* 60, 1226
(1986): Leloire O+, *Presse Med* (French) 15, 34
(1984): Coltart RS, *Br J Radiol* 57, 531
(1982): Naysmith A+, *N Engl J Med* 306, 45 (26%)
(1982): Santen RJ+, *Ann Intern Med* 96, 94 (29%)
(1980): Savaraj N+, *Med Pediatr Oncol* 8, 251
(1967): Horky K+, *Schweiz Med Wochenschr* (German) 98, 1843 (4–30%)
Exfoliative dermatitis
(1967): Horky K+, *Schweiz Med Wochenschr* (German) 98, 1843
Lupus erythematosus (>10%)
(1980): McCraken M+, *BMJ* 281, 1254
Pruritus (5%)
Purpura
(1994): Stratakis CA+, *Am J Hosp Pharm* 51, 2589
Pustular psoriasis
(1984): Coltart RS, *Br J Radiol* 57, 531
Rash (>10%)
Urticaria

Hair

Hair – hirsutism (1–10%)

Other

Anaphylactoid reaction
(1986): Leloire O+, *Presse Med* (French) 15, 34
Myalgia (3%)
Oral mucosal eruption
(1984): Coltart RS, *Br J Radiol* 57, 531
(1967): Horky K+, *Schweiz Med Wochenschr* (German) 98, 1843
Oral ulceration
(1984): Coltart RS, *Br J Radiol* 57, 531

AMINOPHYLLINE

Synonym: theophylline ethylenediamine
Trade names: Aerolate; Aminophyllin; Bronkodyl; Choledyl; Elixophyllin; Norphyl; Phyllocontin; Quibron; Slo-Bid; Somophyllin; Theo-Dur; Truphylline (Various pharmaceutical companies.)
Other common trade names: *Corophyllin; Euphyllin; Palaron; Phyllotemp; Planphylline; Tefamin*
Indications: Prevention or treatment of reversible bronchospasm
Category: Xanthine bronchodilator
Half-life: 3–15 hours (in adult nonsmokers)
Clinically important, potentially serious interactions with: allopurinol, beta-blockers, calcium channel blockers, cimetidine, ciprofloxacin, corticosteroids, difulfiram, ephedrine, erythromycin, halothane, interferon, lithium, macrolide antibiotics, mexiletine, oral contraceptives, phenytoin, propranolol, quinolone antibiotics, rifampin, thyroid, etc., **St John's wort, cigarette smoking**

Reactions

Skin

Allergic reactions (sic) (<1%)
(1986): Cusano F+, *G Ital Dermatol Venereol* (Italian) 121, 443
(1985): Editorial, *Lancet* 1, 289
(1983): Hardy C+, *Br Med J (Clin Res Ed)* 286, 2051
(1983): Gibb W+, *Br Med J (Clin Res Ed)* 13, 501
Baboon syndrome
(1999): Guin JD+, *Contact Dermatitis* 40, 170
Contact dermatitis
(1994): Corazza M+, *Contact Dermatitis* 31, 328
(1984): *Lancet* 2, 1192
(1983): van den Berg WH+, *Ned Tijdschr Geneeskd* (Dutch) 127, 1801
(1983): Berman BA+, *Cutis* 31, 594
(1980): Vazquez Botet M, *Bol Asoc Med P R* (Spanish) 72, 14
(1959): Baer RL+, *Arch Dermatol* 79, 647
Cutaneous side effects (sic)
(1995): Simon PA+, *JAMA* 273, 1737
Dermatitis (sic)
(1985): Editorial, *Lancet* 2, 1192
(1978): Tsyrkunova LP+, *Gig Tr Prof Zabol* (Russian) October, 52
Diaphoresis
Exanthems
(1985): Editorial, *Lancet* 2, 1192
(1984): Thompson PJ+, *Thorax* 39, 600
(1983): Hardy C+, *BMJ* 286, 2051
(1981): de Shazo RD+, *Ann Allergy* 46, 152
(1980): Lawyer CH+, *J Allergy Clin Immunol* 65, 353
Exfoliative dermatitis
(1984): Thompson PJ+, *Thorax* 39, 600
(1982): Nierenberg DW+, *West J Med* 137, 328
(1981): Elias JA+, *Am Rev Respir Dis* 123, 550
(1979): Bernstein JE+, *Arch Dermatol* 115, 360
(1976): Petrozzi JW+, *Arch Dermatol* 112, 525
(1958): Tas J+, *Acta Allergologica* 12, 39
Flushing
Pruritus
(1980): Lawyer CH+, *J Allergy Clin Immunol* 65, 353
(1971): Davidson MB, *N Engl J Med* 285, 689
(1971): Wong D+, *J Allergy* 48, 165
Rash (sic) (<1%)
(1983): Hardy C+, *BMJ* 286, 2051
Shakiness (sic)
Stevens–Johnson syndrome
(1989): Hidalgo HA, *Pediatr Pulmonol* 6, 209 (theophylline)
Urticaria
(1994): Urbani CE, *Contact Dermatitis* 31, 198
(1985): Editorial, *Lancet* 2, 1192

(1984): Thompson PJ+, *Thorax* 39, 600
(1982): Neumann H, *Dtsch Med Wochenschr* (German) 107, 116
(1979): Booth BH+, *Ann Allergy* 43, 289
(1971): Wong D+, *J Allergy* 48, 165

Hair

Hair – alopecia

Other

Hypersensitivity
(1999): Yoshizawa A+, *Arerugi* (Japanese) 48, 1206 (from ethylenediamine)
(1985): Gibb WR, *Lancet* 1, 49
(1981): Elias JA+, *Am Rev Respir Dis* 123, 550
(1970): Foussereau J+, *Bull Soc Fr Dermatol Syphiligr* (French) 77, 415
(1967): Sonnischen N, *Allerg Asthma Leipz* (German) 13, 259
(1967): Sonnischen N, *Allerg Asthma Leipz* (German) 13, 215
Parosmia

AMINOSALICYLATE SODIUM

Synonyms: para-aminosalicylate sodium; PAS
Trade names: Paser Granules (Jacobus); Sodium P.A.S. (Lannett; Palisades); Tubasal
Other common trade names: *Aminox; Eupasal; Nemasol*
Indications: Tuberculosis
Category: Antimycobacterial; anti-inflammatory
Half-life: 45–60 minutes
Clinically important, potentially serious interactions with: cyanocobalamin, digoxin, rifampin

Reactions

Skin

Allergic reactions (sic)
(1988): Fardy JM+, *J Clin Gastroenterol* 10, 635
Angioedema
(1964): Lajouanine P+, *Ann Pédiatr Paris* (French) 40, 620
(1959): Bereston ES, *J Invest Dermatol* 33, 427
Bullous eruption
(1964): Lajouanine P+, *Ann Pédiatr Paris* (French) 40, 620
(1959): Bereston ES, *J Invest Dermatol* 33, 427
Eczematous eruption (sic) (<1%)
Erythema multiforme
(1963): Van Ketel WG, *Ned Tijdschr Geneeskd* (Dutch) 107, 952
Exanthems
(1988): Gron I+, *Ugeskr Laeger* (Danish) 150, 32
(1982): Nagaratnam N, *Postgrad Med J* 58, 729
(1968): Sarkany I, *Proc R Soc Med* 61, 891
(1964): Lajouanine P+, *Ann Pédiatr Paris* (French) 40, 620
(1964): Duncan JT, *Am Rev Respir Dis* 89, 103
(1963): Filoz-Diaz JA+, *Archos Méd Panama* (Spanish) 12, 68
(1960): Simpson DG+, *Am J Med* 29, 297 (1–5%)
(1959): Bereston ES, *J Invest Dermatol* 33, 427 (1–5%)
(1950): Cuthbert J, *Lancet* 2, 209
Exfoliative dermatitis
(1972): Kauppinen K, *Acta Derm Venereol* (Stockh) 52 (suppl), 68
(1967): Coleman WP, *Med Clin North Am* 51, 1073
(1965): Griffiths HED+, *J Bone Joint Surg* (Edinburgh) 47, 86
(1964): Bower G, *Am Rev Respir Dis* 89, 440
(1964): Lajouanine P+, *Ann Pédiatr Paris* (French) 40, 620
(1961): Gupta SK, *Indian J Dermatol* 6, 115
Fixed eruption
(1972): Levantine A+, *Br J Dermatol* 86, 604
(1965): Snelling MRJ+, *Tubercle* 46, 284
(1965): Laszczka C, *Gruzlica* (Polish) 33, 935
(1961): Welch AL+, *Arch Dermatol* 84, 1004
(1952): Warring FC+, *Am Rev Tuberc Pulm Dis* 65, 235
(1949): Kierland RR+, *Proc Staff Meet Mayo Clin* 24, 539
Lichenoid eruption
(1971): Almeyda J+, *Br J Dermatol* 95, 604
(1964): Baker H+, *Br J Dermatol* 76, 186
(1953): Shatin H+, *J Invest Dermatol* 21, 135
Lupus erythematosus
(1985): Holdiness MR, *Int J Dermatol* 24, 280
(1961): Bickers JN+, *N Engl J Med* 265, 131
Lymphoma (benign)
(1982): Nagaratnam N, *Postgrad Med J* 58, 729
Photosensitivity
(1972): Kuokkanen K, *Acta Allergol* 27, 407
(1971): Girard JP, *Helv Med Acta* 36, 3
(1964): Lajouanine P+, *Ann Pédiatr Paris* (French) 40, 620
Pruritus
(1968): No Author, *BMJ* 3, 664
(1964): Berté SJ+, *Am Rev Respir Dis* 90, 598
(1960): Simpson DG+, *Am J Med* 29, 297
Purpura
(1980): Miescher PA+, *Clin Haematol* 9, 505
(1963): Filoz-Diaz JA+, *Archos Méd Panama* (Spanish) 12, 68
(1959): Bereston ES, *J Invest Dermatol* 33, 427
(1952): Warring FC+, *Am Rev Tuberc Pulm Dis* 65, 235
Toxic epidermal necrolysis
(1963): Filoz-Diaz JA+, *Archos Méd Panama* (Spanish) 12, 68
Urticaria
(1964): Lajouanine P+, *Ann Pédiatr Paris* (French) 40, 620
(1961): Gupta SK, *Indian J Dermatol* 6, 115
(1960): Simpson DG+, *Am J Med* 29, 297
(1959): Bereston ES, *J Invest Dermatol* 33, 427
(1952): Warring FC+, *Am Rev Tuberc Pulm Dis* 65, 235
Vasculitis (<1%)
(1972): Levantine A+, *Br J Dermatol* 87, 646

Hair

Hair – alopecia
(1982): Kutty PK+, *Ann Intern Med* 97, 785
(1965): Griffiths HED+, *J Bone Joint Surg* (Edinburgh) 47, 86
(1960): Simpson DG+, *Am J Med* 29, 297
(1951): Grandjean LC, *Acta Derm Venereol* (Stockh) 31, 615

Other

Hypersensitivity
Oral lichenoid eruption
Oral mucosal eruption
(1964): Lajouanine P+, *Ann Pédiatr Paris* (French) 40, 620
(1960): Simpson DG+, *Am J Med* 29, 297

AMIODARONE

Trade names: Cordarone (Wyeth); Pacerone (Upsher-Smith)
Other common trade names: *Aratac; Corbionax; Cordarex; Cordarone X; Tachydaron*
Indications: Ventricular fibrillation; ventricular tachycardia
Category: Class III antiarrhythmic
Half-life: 26–107 days
Clinically important, potentially serious interactions with: anticoagulants, astemizole, beta-blockers, calcium channel blockers, cyclosporine, digoxin, diltiazem, fentanyl, flecainide, methotrexate, phenytoin, procainamide, quinidine, ritonavir, sparfloxacin, theophylline, tricyclic antidepressants, verapamil, warfarin

Reactions

Skin

Allergic reactions (sic)
(1989): Reingardene DI, *Klin Med Mosk* (Russian) 67, 128
Basal cell carcinoma
(1995): Monk BE, *Br J Dermatol* 133, 148
Cutaneous side effects (sic)
(1994): Shukla R+, *Postgrad Med J* 70, 492
Diaphoresis
(1985): Raeder EA+, *Am Heart J* 109, 979 (0.5%)
(1983): McGovern B+, *BMJ* 287, 175 (2.5%)
Ecchymoses (<1%)
Edema (1–10%)
Erythema nodosum (<1%)
(1983): Fogoros RN+, *Circulation* 68, 88 (1%)

(1976): Rosenbaum MB+, *Am J Cardiol* 38, 934
Exanthems
(1985): Raeder EA+, *Am Heart J* 109, 975 (0.9%)
(1984): Rotmensch HH+, *Ann Intern Med* 101, 462 (0.7%)
(1983): Harris L+, *Circulation* 67, 45
(1983): Fogoros RN+, *Circulation* 68, 88 (2%)
(1969): Kappart A, *Z Ther* (German) #8, 474
Exfoliative dermatitis
(1988): Moots RJ+, *BMJ* 296, 1332
Facial erythema (3.1%)
(1984): Rotmensch HH+, *Ann Intern Med* 101, 462
(1983): Harris L+, *Circulation* 67, 45
Flushing (1–10%)
Iododerma
(1997): Ricci C+, *Ann Dermatol Venereol* (French) 124, 260
(1975): Zantkuyl CF+, *Dermatologica* 151, 311
(1975): Porters JE+, *Arch Dermatol* 111, 1656
Keratosis pilaris
(1999): Capper N, Mobile, AL (from Internet) (observation)
Linear IgA bullous dermatosis
(1996): Tranvan A+, *J Am Acad Dermatol* 35, 865
(1996): Primka EJ+, *J Cutan Pathol* 23, 58
(1994): Primka EJ+, *J Am Acad Dermatol* 31, 809
(1990): Espagne E+, *Ann Dermatol Venereol* (French) 117, 898
Lupus erythematosus
(1999): Susano R+, *Ann Rheum Dis* 58, 655
(1985): Raeder EA+, *Am Heart J* 109, 979 (4.6%)
Photosensitivity (10–30%)
(2000): Burns KE+, *Can Respir* 7, 193 (passim)
(1997): O'Reilly FM+, American Academy of Dermatology Meeting, Poster #14
(1995): Zehender M, *Circulation* 92, 1665
(1995): Tisdale JE+, *J Clin Pharmacol* 35, 351
(1995): Collins P+, *Br J Dermatol* 132, 956
(1993): Ettler K+, *Sb Ved Pr Lek Fak Karlovy Univerzity Hradci Kralove Suppl (Czech) 36, 305 (9.4%)*
(1993): Allen JE, *Clin Pharm* 12, 580
(1992): Gosselink AT+, *JAMA* 267, 3289
(1992): Editorial, *JAMA* 267, 3322
(1990): Monk B, *Clin Exp Dermatol* 15, 319
(1989): Rappersberger K+, *J Invest Dermatol* 93, 201
(1988): Hyatt RH+, *Age Aging* 17, 116 (10%)
(1988): Parodi A, *Photodermatology* 5, 146
(1987): Roupe G+, *Acta Derm Venereol* (Stockh) 67, 76
(1987): Waitzer S+, *J Am Acad Dermatol* 16, 779
(1986): Ferguson J, *Br J Clin Pract Symp* Suppl 44, 63
(1986): Ljunggren B+, *Photodermatol* 3, 26
(1986): Toback AC+, *Dermatol Clin* 4, 223
(1986): Török L+, *Hautarzt* (German) 37, 507 (24%)
(1986): Boyle J, *Br J Dermatol* 115, 253
(1985): Vila Serra MD+, *Med Clin (Barc)* (Spanish) 84, 379
(1985): Ferguson J+, *Br J Dermatol* 113, 537
(1985): Raeder EA+, *Am Heart J* 109, 979 (4.6%)
(1985): Stäubli M, *Postgrad Med J* 61, 245
(1985): Mulrow JP+, *Ann Int Med* 103, 68
(1984): Zachary CB+, *Br J Dermatol* 110, 451
(1984): Walter JF+, *Arch Dermatol* 120, 1591
(1984): Ferguson J+, *Lancet* 2, 414
(1984): Guerciolini R+, *Lancet* 1, 962
(1984): Kaufmann G, *Lancet* 1, 51
(1984): Diffey BL+, *Clin Exp Dermatol* 9, 248
(1983): Fogoros RN+, *Circulation* 68, 88 (11%)
(1983): McGovern B+, *BMJ* 287, 175 (8.75%)
(1983): Nadamanee K+, *Ann Intern Med* 98, 577 (5.3%)
(1983): Harris L+, *Circulation* 67, 45 (57%)
(1982): Chalmers RJ+, *Br Med J Clin Res Ed* 285, 341
Pigmentation
(2000): Burns KE+, *Can Respir* 7, 193 (passim)
(1999): Karrer S+, *Arch Dermatol* 135, 251
(1997): Sivaram CA+, *N Engl J Med* 337, 1813
(1996): Kounis NG+, *Clin Cardiol* 19, 592
(1996): Ammann R+, *Hautarzt* (German) 47, 930
(1995): Tisdale JE+, *J Clin Pharmacol* 35, 351 (blue-gray)
(1993): Colquhoun JP, *Aust Fam Physician* 22, 2168
(1993): Ettler K+, *Sb Ved Pr Lek Fak Karlovy Univerzity Hradci Kralove Suppl (Czech) 36, 305 (9.4%)*
(1993): Balslev E+, *Ugeskr Laeger* (Danish) 155, 4014 (blue-gray)
(1992): Son En Ai+, *Klin Med Mosk* (Russian) 70, 46
(1992): Fitzpatrick JE, *Derm Clinics* 10, 19
(1992): Editorial, *JAMA* 267, 3322
(1991): Blackshear JL+, *Mayo Clin Proc* 66, 721
(1991): Fazekas T+, *Szent Gyorgyi Albert Orvostudomanyi Egyetem* (Hungarian) 132, 2157
(1990): Brazzelli V+, *G Ital Dermatol Venereol* (Italian) 125, 521
(1989): Reingardene DI, *Kardiologiia* (Russian) 29, 112
(1989): Klein AD+, *Arch Dermatol* 125, 417
(1989): Rappersberger K+, *J Invest Dermatol* 93, 201
(1988): Beukema WP+, *Am J Cardiol* 62, 1146
(1988): Zadionchenko VS+, *Klin Med Mosk* (Russian) 66, 126
(1987): Goldstein GD+, *Chest* 91, 772
(1987): Waitzer S+, *J Am Acad Dermatol* 16, 779
(1986): Török L+, *Hautarzt* (German) 37, 507
(1986): Dowson JH+, *Arch Dermatol* 122, 244
(1986): Rappersberger K+, *Br J Dermatol* 114, 189
(1985): Lakatos A, *Orv Hetil* (Hungarian) 126, 1343
(1985): Varotti C+, *G Ital Dermatol Venereol* (Italian) 120, 183
(1985): Alinovi A+, *J Am Acad Dermatol* 12, 563
(1984): Rotmensch HH+, *Ann Intern Med* 101, 462 (4.6%)
(1984): Miller RAW+, *Arch Dermatol* 120, 646
(1984): Weiss SR+, *J Am Acad Dermatol* 11, 898
(1984): Onofrey BE+, *J Am Optom Assoc* 55, 337
(1984): Zachary CB+, *Br J Dermatol* 110, 451
(1983): Trimble JW+, *Arch Dermatol* 119, 914
(1983): McGovern B+, *BMJ* 287, 175
(1983): Harris L+, *Circulation* 67, 45 (1.4%)
(1982): Quintanilla E+, *Med Cutan Ibero Lat Am* (Spanish) 10, 177
(1982): Ferrer I+, *Med Clin (Barc)* (Spanish) 79, 355
(1981): Korting HC+, *Hautarzt* (German) *32, 301*
(1981): Granstein RD+, *J Am Acad Dermatol* 5, 1 (blue-gray)
(1979): Nageli U+, *Schweiz Med Wochenschr* (German) 109, 1708
(1978): Cassilas-Ruiz JA+, *Rev Esp Cardiol* (Spanish) 31, 617
(1975): Lambert D+, *Ann Dermatol Syphiligr Paris* (French) 102, 277
(1975): Delage C+, *Can*
(1974): Olmos L+, *Med Cutan Ibero Lat Am* (Spanish) 2, 447
(1972): Balouet G+, *Arch Anat Pathol* (Paris) (French) 20, 265
(1971): Thiers H+, *Bull Soc Fr Dermatol Syphiligr* (French) 78, 548
(1971): Labouche F+, *Bull Soc Fr Dermatol Syphiligr* (French) 78, 27
Pruritus (1–5%)
(1969): Kappart A, *Z Ther* (German) #8, 474 (4.1%)
(1968): Leutenegger A+, *Schweiz Med Wochenschr* (German) 98, 2020 (4.1%)
Psoriasis
(1986): Abel EA+, *J Am Acad Dermatol* 15, 1007
(1982): Muir AD, *N Z Med J* 95, 711
Purpura (2%)
(1983): Fogoros RN+, *Circulation* 68, 88
Pustular psoriasis
(1982): Muir AD, *N Z Med J* 95, 711
Rash (sic) (<1%)
Rosacea
(1987): Reifler DM+, *Am J Ophthalmol* 103, 594
Stevens–Johnson syndrome (<1%)
Toxic epidermal necrolysis
(2000): Danby WF, Manchester, NH (from Internet) (observation)
(1985): Bencini PL+, *Arch Dermatol* 121, 838
Urticaria
(1983): McGovern B+, *BMJ* 287, 175 (1.25%)
Vasculitis (<1%)
(1994): Dootson G+, *Clin Exp Dermatol* 19, 422
(1994): Gutierrez R+, *Ann Pharmacother* 28, 537
(1985): Stäubli M, *Postgrad Med J* 61, 245
(1985): Starke ID+, *BMJ* 291, 940

Hair

Hair – alopecia (<1%)
(2000): Litt JZ, Beachwood, OH, personal case (observation) (after 2 weeks of therapy)
(1995): Ahmad S, *Arch Intern Med* 155, 1106
(1992): Samuel LM+, *Postgrad Med J* 68, 771
(1985): Raeder EA+, *Am Heart J* 109, 979 (4.1%)
(1984): Rotmensch HH+, *Ann Intern Med* 101, 462 (0.7%)
(1983): McGovern B+, *BMJ* 287, 175 (2.5%)
Hair – hypertrichosis
(1985): Ferguson J+, *Br J Dermatol* 113, 537

Other

Dysgeusia (1–10%)
(1983): McGovern B+, *BMJ* 287, 175
Paresthesias (4–9%)
Parosmia (1–10%)
Pseudoporphyria
(1988): Parodi A, *Photodermatology* 5, 146
Pseudotumor cerebri (<1%)
Sialorrhea (1–3%)
Tremor

AMITRIPTYLINE

Trade names: Elavil (AstraZeneca); Limbitrol (ICN)
Other common trade names: *Amineurin; Domical; Laroxyl; Lentizol; Levate; Novotriptyn; Saroten; Tryptanol; Tryptizol*
Indications: Depression
Category: Tricyclic antidepressant; antimigraine
Half-life: 10–25 hours
Clinically important, potentially serious interactions with: anticonvulsants, barbiturates, cimetidine, clonidine, CNS depressants, disulfiram, epinephrine, fluoxetine, guanethidine, MAO inhibitors, phenobarbital, SSRIs, valproic acid

Limbitrol is amitriptyline and chlordiazepoxide

Reactions

Skin

Acne
Allergic reactions (sic) (<1%)
Angioedema
(1999): Garcia-Doval I+, *Cutis* 63, 35 (passim)
Bullous eruption (<1%)
(1979): Herschthal D+, *Arch Dermatol* 115, 499
Dermatitis (sic)
(1966): Hollister LE+, *J Nerv Ment Dis* 142, 460
Dermatitis herpetiformis
(1969): Rhyner K, *Diss Zürich* (German)
Diaphoresis (1–10%)
(1995): Feder R, *J Clin Psychiatry* 56, 35
Erythema
Erythema annulare centrifugum
(1999): Garcia-Doval I+, *Cutis* 63, 35
Erythroderma
(1999): Garcia-Doval I+, *Cutis* 63, 35 (passim)
Exanthems
Exfoliative dermatitis
Facial edema
Fixed eruption
(1998): McCarthy J, Ft. Worth, TX (from Internet) (observation)
Flushing
Lichen planus
(1999): Garcia-Doval I+, *Cutis* 63, 35 (passim)
Lupus erythematosus
(1993): Dove FB, *Hosp Pract Off Ed* 28, 14
Necrosis
(1999): Fogarty BJ+, *Burns* 25, 768
Parkinsonism
Petechiae
Photosensitivity (<1%)
(1999): Garcia-Doval I+, *Cutis* 63, 35 (passim)
(1996): Taniguchi S+, *Am J Hematol* 53, 49
(1966): Hollister LE+, *J Nerv Ment Dis* 142, 460
Pigmentation
(1999): Garcia-Doval I+, *Cutis* 63, 35 (passim)
(1985): Basler RS+, *J Am Acad Dermatol* 12, 577
(1988): Warnock JK+, *Am J Psychiatry* 145, 425
Pruritus
(1999): Garcia-Doval I+, *Cutis* 63, 35 (passim)
(1988): Larrey D+, *Gastroenterology* 94, 200
(1966): Hollister LE+, *J Nerv Ment Dis* 142, 460
Purpura
(1999): Garcia-Doval I+, *Cutis* 63, 35 (passim)
(1971): Kozakova M, *Cesk Dermatol* (Czech) 46, 158
Rash (sic)
Urticaria
Vasculitis
(1969): Gisslén H+, *Dermatol Monatsschr* (German) 155, 783

Hair

Hair – alopecia (<1%)
(1992): Breathnach SM+, *Adverse Drug Reactions and the Skin*, Blackwell, Oxford, 196 (passim)

Other

Ageusia
Anaphylactoid reaction
Black tongue
Bromhidrosis
Dysgeusia (>10%)
Galactorrhea (<1%)
Glossitis
Gynecomastia (<1%)
Hypersensitivity
(2000): Milionis HJ, *Postgrad Med J* 76, 361
Lymphoid hyperplasia
(1995): Crowson AN+, *Arch Dermatol* 131, 925
Oral mucosal eruption
(1964): Pollack B+, *Am J Psychiatry* 121, 384
Paresthesias
Pseudolymphoma
(1995): Magro CM+, *J Am Acad Dermatol* 32, 419
(1995): Crowson AN+, *Arch Dermatol* 131, 925
Sialopenia
(1995): Loesche WJ+, *J Am Geriatr Soc* 43, 401
Sialorrhea
Stomatitis
(1988): Larrey D+, *Gastroenterology* 94, 200
Stomatopyrosis
Tongue edema
Tremor
Vaginitis
Xerostomia (>10%)
(1995): Loesche WJ+, *J Am Geriatr Soc* 43, 401
(1996): Rani PU+, *Anesth Analg* 83, 371
(1966): Hollister LE+, *J Nerv Ment Dis* 142, 467

AMLODIPINE

Trade names: Lotrel (Novartis); Norvasc (Pfizer)
Other common trade names: *Amdepin; Amlodin, Amlogard; Amlopin; Amlor; Istin; Norvas*
Indications: Hypertension, angina
Category: Calcium channel blocker; antianginal; antihypertensive
Half-life: 30–50 hours
Clinically important, potentially serious interactions with: beta-blockers, cyclosporine, fentanyl, **grapefruit juice**

Lotrel is amlodipine and benazepril

Reactions

Skin

Dermatitis (sic) (1–10%)
Diaphoresis (<1%)
Discoloration (sic) (<1%)
Edema (5–14%)
(1996): Corea L+, *Clin Pharmacol Ther* 60, 341
(1992): DiBianco R+, *Clin Cardiol* 15, 519
(1992): Johnson BF+, *Am J Hypertens* 5, 727
(1991): Elliott HL+, *Postgrad Med J* 67, S20
(1991): Murdoch D+, *Drugs* 41, 478
(1989): Estrada JN+, *Am Heart J* 118, 1130
(1989): Chahine RA+, *Am Heart J* 118, 1128

(1989): Osterloh I, *Am Heart J* 118, 1114
(1989): Doyle GD+, *Eur J Clin Pharmacol* 36, 205 (ankle)
(1988): Glasser SP+, *Am J Cardiol 62*, 518

Erythema multiforme
(1993): Bewley AP+, *BMJ* 307, 241

Exanthems (2–4%)
(1989): Doyle GD+, *Eur J Clin Pharmacol* 36, 205

Flushing (1–10%)
(1992): *Med Lett Drugs Ther* 34, 99
(1992): Johnson BF+, *Am J Hypertens* 5, 727
(1991): Murdoch D+, *Drugs* 41, 478
(1989): Osterloh I, *Am Heart J* 118, 1114

Lichenoid eruption
(1998): Silver B, Deerfield, Il (from Internet) (observation)

Peripheral edema (>10%)
(1994): Clavijo GA+, *Am J Hosp Pharm* 51, 59
(1993): Ellis JS+, *Lancet* 341, 1102

Petechiae (<1%)

Pruritus (2–4%)
(1998): Litt JZ, Beachwood, OH, personal case (observation)
(1997): Orme S+, *BMJ* 315, 463
(1994): Baker BA+, *Ann Pharmacother* 28, 118
(1993): Ellis JS+, *Lancet 341*, 1102

Purpura (<1%)
(1994): Dacosta A+, *Therapie* (French) 49, 515

Rash (sic) (1–10%)

Telangiectases (facial)
(1999): van der Vleuten CJ+, *Acta Derm Venereol* 79, 323
(1997): Basarab T+, *Br J Dermatol* 136, 974 (photo-induced)

Urticaria (<1%)

Vasculitis
(1995): del Rio Fermandez MC+, *Rev Clin Esp* (Spanish) 195, 738

Xerosis (<0.1%)

Hair

Hair – alopecia (<1%)

Other

Acute intermittent porphyria
(1997): Kepple A+, *Ann Pharmacother* 31, 253

Dysgeusia (<1%)

Gingival hyperplasia
(2000): James JA+, *J Clin Periodontol* 27, 109 (with cyclosporine)
(1999): Ellis JS+, *J Periodontol* 70, 63 (3.3%)
(1999): van der Vleuten CJ+, *Acta Derm Venereol* 79, 323
(1997): Infante-Cossio P+, *An Med Interna* (Spanish) 14, 83
(1997): Jorgensen MG, *J Periodontol* 68, 676
(1995): Salerno L+, *Clin Ter* (Italian) 146, 275
(1995): Wynn RL, *Gen Dent* 43, 218
(1994): Seymour RA+, *J Clin Periodontol* 21, 281
(1994): Juncadella Garcia E+, *Med Clin (Barc)* (Spanish) 103, 358
(1993): Smith RG, *Br Dent J* 175, 279
(1993): Ellis JS+, *Lancet* 341, 1102
(1991): Wynn RL, *Gen Dent* 39, 240

Gynecomastia
(1994): Zochling J+, *Med J Aust* 160, 807

Hypesthesia (<1%)

Paresthesias (<1%)

Parosmia (<0.1%)

Tendinitis
(1999): Zambanini A+, *J Hum Hypertens* 13, 565 (Achilles)

Tremor

Xerostomia (<1%)

AMOBARBITAL

Trade name: Amytal (Lilly)
Other common trade names: *Amytal Sodium; Isoamitil Sedante; Neur-Amyl; Novambarb; Sodium Amytal*
Indications: Insomnia, sedation
Category: Intermediate-acting barbiturate; anticonvulsant; hypnotic; sedative
Half-life: initial: 40 minutes; terminal: 20 hours
Clinically important, potentially serious interactions with: acetaminophen, anticoagulants, anticonvulsants, bepridil, calcium channel blockers, CNS depressants, diltiazem, estrogens, felbamate, felodipine, isradipine, MAO inhibitors, verapamil

Reactions

Skin

Acne

Angioedema

Bullous eruption

Erythema
(1979): Rudzki E, *Przegl Dermatol* (Polish) 66, 415

Exanthems

Exfoliative dermatitis (<1%)

Photosensitivity

Purpura

Rash (sic) (<1%)

Stevens–Johnson syndrome (<1%)

Toxic epidermal necrolysis
(1969): Strom J, *Scand J Infect Dis* 1, 209

Urticaria (<1%)

Other

Hypersensitivity

Injection-site pain (>10%)

Serum sickness

Thrombophlebitis (<1%)

AMOXAPINE

Trade name: Amoxapine (Watson)
Other common trade names: *Amoxan; Asendis; Defanyl; Demolox*
Indications: Depression
Category: Tricyclic antidepressant
Half-life: 11–30 hours
Clinically important, potentially serious interactions with: barbiturates, cimetidine, clonidine, epinephrine, fluoxetine, guanethidine, MAO inhibitors, tricyclic antidepressants

Reactions

Skin

Acne

Acute generalized exanthematous pustulosis (AGEP)
(1998): Loche F+, *Acta Derm Venereol* 78, 224
(1994): Larbre B+, *Ann Dermatol Venereol* (French) 121, 40

Allergic reactions (sic) (<1%)

Cutaneous side effects (sic) (5.1%)
(1982): Jue SG+, *Drugs* 24, 1

Dermatitis (sic)

Diaphoresis (1–10%)

Edema (>1%)

Erythema multiforme (observation)
(1982): Bishop L, *ADRRS* oral communication

Exanthems
(1996): Nagayama H+, *J Dermatol* 23, 899
(1982): Jue SG+, *Drugs* 24, 1

Flushing

Petechiae

Photosensitivity (<1%)

Pruritus (<1%)
(1988): Warnock JK+, *Am J Psychiatry* 145, 425
Pseudoparkinsonism (sic)
Purpura
Rash (sic) (>1%)
Toxic epidermal necrolysis
(1988): Warnock JK+, *Am J Psychiatry* 145, 425
(1983): Camisa C+, *Arch Dermatol* 119, 709
Urticaria (<1%)
Vasculitis (<1%)
(1988): Warnock JK+, *Am J Psychiatry* 145, 425
Xerosis

Hair

Hair – alopecia (<1%)

Other

Black tongue
Bromhidrosis
Dysgeusia (>10%)
Galactorrhea (<1%)
(1979): Gelenberg AJ+, *JAMA* 242, 1900
(1978): Jaffe K, *J Clin Psychiatry* 39, 821
Glossitis
Gynecomastia (<1%)
Paresthesias (<1%)
Sialorrhea
Stomatitis
Tremor
Vaginitis
Xerostomia (14%)
(1982): Jue SG+, *Drugs* 24, 1

AMOXICILLIN

Synonym: amoxycillin
Trade names: Amoxil (SmithKline Beecham); Augmentin (SmithKline Beecham); Prevpac (TAP)
Other common trade names: *A-Gram; Acimox; Almodan; Amodex; Apo-Amoxi; Clamoxyl; Eupen; Fisamox; Lin-Amnox; Novamoxin; Nu-Amoxi; Pro-Amox*
Indications: Infections of the respiratory tract, skin and urinary tract
Category: Aminopenicillin antibiotic
Half-life: 0.7–1.4 hours
Clinically important, potentially serious interactions with: allopurinol, aminoglycosides, anticoagulants, cyclosporine, disulfiram, methotrexate, oral contraceptives, tetracyclines

Augmentin is amoxicillin and clavulanate

Reactions

Skin

Acute generalized exanthematous pustulosis (AGEP)
(1997): Zabawski, E, Dallas, TX (from Internet) (observation)
(1997): Gibert-Agullo A+, *An Esp Pediatr* (Spanish) 46, 285
(1996): Wolkenstein P+, *Contact Dermatitis* 35, 234
(1995): Moreau A+, *Int J Dermatol* 34, 263 (passim)
(1991): Roujeau J-C+, *Arch Dermatol* 127, 1333
(1989): Epelbaum S+, *Pediatrie* (French) 44, 387
Angioedema (1–10%)
(1998): Minguez MA+, *Allergol Immunopathol (Madr)* (Spanish) 26, 43
(1994): Galindo-Bonilla PA+, *Contact Dermatitis* 31, 319
(1994): Vega JM+, *Allergy* 49, 317
(1989): Chopra R+, *Can Med Assoc J* 140, 921 (in children)
Baboon syndrome
(1996): Kohler LD+, *Int J Dermatol* 35, 502
(1994): Duve S+, *Acta Derm Venereol* 74, 480
(1993): Herfs H+, *Hautarzt* (German) 44, 466
Bullous pemphigoid
(1997): Miralles J+, *Int J Dermatol* 36, 42
(1988): Alcalay J+, *J Am Acad Dermatol* 18, 345
Contact dermatitis
(1996): Garcia R+, *Contact Dermatitis* 35, 116
(1995): Gamboa P+, *Contact Dermatitis* 32, 48 (occupational)
Cutaneous side effects (sic)
(1994): Paparello SF+, *AIDS* 8, 276
Diaper rash
(1988): Honig PJ+, *J Am Acad Dermatol* 19, 275
Ecchymoses
Edema
(1993): Echeverria-Arellano A+, *An Esp Pediatr* (Spanish) 39, 448
Erythema multiforme
(1999): Wakelin SH+, *Clin Exp Dermatol* 24, 71
(1999): Benjamin S+, *Ann Pharmacother* 33, 109
(1996): Webster GF, Philadelphia, PA (from Internet) (observation)
(1995): Wolkenstein P+, *Arch Dermatol* 131, 544
(1992): Gross AS+, *J Am Acad Dermatol* 27, 781
(1990): Chan HL+, *Arch Dermatol* 126, 43
(1990): Escallier F+, *Rev Med Interne* (French) 11, 73
(1989): Chopra R+, *Can Med Assoc J* 140, 921 (in children)
(1988): Platt R, *J Infect Dis* 158, 474
(1988): Massullo RE+, *J Am Acad Dermatol* 19, 358
(1986): Davidson NJ+, *BMJ* 292, 380
(1986): Dikland WJ+, *Pediatr Dermatol* 3, 135
(1982): Freeman T, *Can Med Assoc J* 127, 818
Exanthems (>5%)
(1999): Wakelin SH+, *Clin Exp Dermatol* 24, 71 (flexural)
(1997): Blumenthal HL, Beachwood, OH, personal case (observation)
(1997): Barbaud AM+, *Arch Dermatol* 133, 481
(1995): Wolkenstein P+, *Arch Dermatol* 131, 544
(1995): Romano A+, *Allergy* 50, 113
(1994): Litt JZ, Beachwood, OH, personal case (observation)
(1993): Romano A+, *J Invest Allergol Clin Immunol* 3, 53
(1993): Fellner MJ, *Int J Dermatol* 32, 308
(1990): Pauszek ME, *Indiana Med* 83, 330
(1989): Kennedy C+, *Contact Dermatitis* 20, 313
(1989): Battegay M+, *Lancet* 2, 1100
(1989): Chopra R+, *Can Med Assoc J* 140, 921 (in children)
(1986): Bigby M+, *JAMA* 256, 3358 (5.14%)
(1986): Sonntag MR+, *Schweiz Med Wochenschr* (German) 116, 142 (7%)
(1986): de Haan P+, *Allergy* 41, 75
(1985): Levine LR, *Pediatr Infect Dis* 4, 358
(1981): Odegaard OR, *Tidsskr Nor Laegeforen* (Norwegian) 101, 1973
(1977): Taylor B+, *BMJ* 2, 552 (3.7%)
(1975): Brogden RN+, *Drugs* 9, 88 (1–22%)
(1974): Wise PJ+, *J Infect Dis* 129 (Suppl), s266
(1973): Dubb S, *S A Med J* 47, 1218
Exfoliative dermatitis
Fixed eruption
(1997): Zabawski E, Dallas, TX (from Internet) (observation)
(1997): Jimenez I+, *Allergol Immunopathol (Madr)* 25, 247 (glans penis)
(1995): Arias J+, *Clin Exp Dermatol* 20, 339
(1995): Dhar S+, *Pediatr Dermatol* 12, 51 (tongue)
(1994): Gil-Garcia JF+, *Med Clin (Barc)* (Spanish) 102, 438
(1989): Shuttleworth D, *Clin Exp Dermatol* 14, 367 (pustular)
(1982): Chowdhury FH, *Practitioner* 226, 1450 (penile)
Hematomas
Intertrigo
(1992): Wolf B+, *Acta Derm Venereol* (Stockh) 72, 441
Jarisch–Herxheimer reaction
(1998): Maloy AL+, *J Emerg Med* 16, 437
Keratosis pilaris
(1997): Kay M, North Hollywood, CA (from Internet) (observation)
Pemphigus
(1997): Brenner S+, *J Am Acad Dermatol* 36, 919
(1997): Landau M+, *Am J Dermatopathol* 19, 411
(1991): Escallier F+, *Ann Dermatol Venereol* (French) 118, 381
(1983): Toan ND+, *Ann Dermatol Venereol* (French) 110, 917
Perleche
(1982): Arata J+, *Jpn J Antibiot* (Japanese) 35, 394
Petechiae (Rumpel–Leede sign)
(1992): Gross AS+, *J Am Acad Dermatol* 27, 781
Pruritus
(2000): Blumenthal HL, Beachwood, OH, personal case (observation)
(1996): Drouet M+, *Allerg Immunol Paris* (French) 28, 311
(1995): Shelley WB+, *Cutis* 55, 202 (observation)
(1993): Fellner MJ, *Int J Dermatol* 32, 308
(1989): Battegay M+, *Lancet* 2, 1100

Psoriasis
(1993): Litt JZ, Beachwood, OH, personal case (observation)
Purpura
Pustular eruption
(2000): Whittam LR+, *Clin Exp Dermatol* 25, 122
(1995): Wolkenstein P+, *Arch Dermatol* 131, 544
(1992): Trueb R+, *Hautarzt* (German) 43, 595
(1991): Roujeau J-C+, *Arch Dermatol* 127, 1333
(1991): Armster H+, *Hautarzt* (German) 42, 713
(1990): Guy C+, *Nouv Dermatol* (French) 9, 540
(1989): Epelbaum S+, *Pédiatrie* (French) 44, 387
(1989): Shuttleworth D, *Clin Exp Dermatol* 14, 367
Pustular psoriasis
(1987): Katz M, *J Am Acad Dermatol* 17, 918
Rash (sic) (1–10%)
(1997): Van Buchem FL+, *Lancet* 349, 683
(1989): Battegay M+, *Lancet* 2, 1100
(1982): Arata J+, *Jpn J Antibiot* (Japanese) 35, 394
(1982): Millard G, *Scott Med J* 27, S35
(1980): Porter J+, *Lancet* 1, 1037
Stevens–Johnson syndrome
(1999): Limauro DL+, *Ann Pharmacother* 33, 560
(1996): Cullimore KC, Westminster, CO (from Internet) (observation)
(1992): Martin Mateos MA+, *J Investig Allergol Clin Immunol* 2, 278
(1988): Platt R, *J Infect Dis* 158, 474
Toxic epidermal necrolysis
(1996): Blum L+, *J Am Acad Dermatol* 34, 1088
(1996): Surbled M+, *Ann Fr Anesth Reanim* (French) 15, 1095
(1993): Correia O+, *Dermatology* 186, 32
(1993): Romano A+, *J Invest Allergol Clin Immunol* 3, 53
(1988): Massullo RE+, *J Am Acad Dermatol* 19, 358
(1984): Herman TE+, *Pediatr Radiol* 14, 439
Toxic pustuloderma
(1992): Trueb R+, *Hautarzt* (German) 43, 595
(1991): Armster H+, *Hautarzt* (German) 42, 713
Urticaria (1–5%)
(2000): Blumenthal HL, Beachwood, OH, personal case (observation)
(1998): Minguez MA+, *Allergol Immunopathol (Madr)* (Spanish) 26, 43
(1997): Thaler, D, Monona WI (from Internet) (observation)
(1997): Delpre G+, *Dig Dis Sci* 42, 728
(1995): Litt JZ, Beachwood, OH, personal case (observation)
(1994): Vega JM+, *Allergy* 49, 317
(1990): Fraj J+, *Clin Exp Allergy* 20, 121
(1989): Chopra R+, *Can Med Assoc J* 140, 921 (in children)
(1989): Battegay M+, *Lancet* 2, 1100
(1985): Goolamali SK, *Postgrad Med J* 61, 925
Vasculitis
(1999): Garcia-Porrua C+, *J Rheumatol* 26, 1942
Vesicular eruption

Other

Anaphylactoid reaction
(1999): Salgado Fernandez J+, *Rev Esp Cardiol* (Spanish) 52, 622
(1998): Rich MW, *Tex Heart Inst J* 25, 194
(1994): Vega JM+, *Allergy* 49, 317
(1993): van der Klauw MM+, *Br J Clin Pharmacol* 35, 400
(1990): Fraj J+, *Clin Exp Allergy* 20, 121
(1988): Blanca M+, *Allergy* 43, 508
Black tongue
Dysgeusia
Glossitis
Glossodynia
Hypersensitivity
(1995): Mokry C, *N Engl J Med* 333, 1151
(1993): Romano A+, *Contact Dermatitis* 28, 190
(1989): Kennedy C+, *Contact Dermatitis* 20, 313
Injection-site pain
Oral candidiasis
Serum sickness (1–10%)
(1995): Martin J+, *N Z Med J* 108, 123
(1992): Stricker BH+, *J Clin Epidemiol* 45, 1177
(1990): Heckbert SR+, *Am J Epidemiol* 132, 336
(1989): Chopra R+, *Can Med Assoc J* 140, 921 (in children)
(1988): Platt R+, *J Infect Dis* 158, 474
Stomatitis
(1996): Drouet M+, *Allerg Immunol Paris* (French) 28, 311
Stomatodynia
Vaginitis (1%)
(1996): Drouet M+, *Allerg Immunol Paris* (French) 28, 311
(1978): Fang LST+, *N Engl J Med* 298, 413
Xerostomia

AMPHOTERICIN B

Trade names: Abelcet; AmBisome (Fujisawa); Amphocin (Pharmacia & Upjohn); Fungizone (Apothecon)
Other common trade names: *Ampho-Moronal; Fungilin; Fungizone*
Indications: Potentially life-threatening fungal infections
Category: Antifungal; antiprotozoal (parenteral)
Half-life: initial: 15–48 hours; terminal: 15 days
Clinically important, potentially serious interactions with: aminoglycosides, corticosteroids, cyclosporine, digoxin, vancomycin

Reactions

Skin

Angioedema
Burning (sic) (from topical)
Chills
Contact dermatitis
Diaphoresis
Erythema
Erythema multiforme
Exanthems (<1%)
(1999): Cesaro S+, *Support Care Cancer* 7, 284
(1976): Lorber B+, *Ann Intern Med* 84, 54
(1966): Beaty HN+, *Ann Intern Med* 65, 641
Exfoliative dermatitis
(1961): Sternberg TH+, *Med Clin North Am* 45, 781
Fixed eruption
(1969): Kandil E, *Dermatologica* 139, 37
Flushing (1–10%)
(1964): Martin WJ, *Med Clin North Am* 48, 255
(1961): Sternberg TH+, *Med Clin North Am* 45, 781
Pigmentation
Pruritus
(1999): Cesaro S+, *Support Care Cancer* 7, 284
(1966): Beaty HN+, *Ann Intern Med* 65, 641
Purpura
(1971): Costello MJ, *Arch Dermatol* 79, 184
(1966): Beaty HN+, *Ann Intern Med* 65, 641
(1961): Sternberg TH+, *Med Clin North Am* 45, 781
Rash (sic)
(1995): Oppenheim BA+, *Clin Infect Dis* 21, 1145
Raynaud's phenomenon (cyanotic)
(1997): Zernikow B+, *Mycoses* 40, 359
Red man syndrome
(1990): Ellis ME+, *BMJ 300*, 1468
Ulceration
Urticaria
Vesicular eruption
Xerosis

Hair

Hair – alopecia

Other

Anaphylactoid reaction
(1999): Cronin JE+, *Clin Infect Dis* 28, 1342
(1998): Schneider P+, *Br J Haematol* 102, 1108
Infusion-site pain
Infusion-site thrombophlebitis
(1995): Goodwin SD+, *Clin Infect Dis* 20, 755
Infusion-site toxicity
(2000): Karthaus M+. *Chemotherapy* 46, 293
Myalgia
Paresthesias (1–10%)
Stomatitis
Thrombophlebitis (1–10%)
(1993): Dietze R+, *Clin Infect Dis* 17, 981
Xerostomia

AMPICILLIN

Trade names: D-Amp; Marcillin; Omnipen (Wyeth); Polycillin (Mead Johnson); Principen (Bristol-Myers Squibb); Totacillin (Beecham)
Other common trade names: *Amfipen; Ampicin; Binotal; Penbritin; Penstabil; Pro-Ampi; Sinaplin; Taro-Ampicillin Trihydrate; Totapen; Vidopen*
Indications: Susceptible strains of gram-negative and gram-positive bacterial infections
Category: Aminopenicillin antibiotic
Half-life: 1–1.5 hours
Clinically important, potentially serious interactions with: allopurinol, anticoagulants, atenolol, cyclosporine, disulfiram, oral contraceptives, probenecid, tetracyclines

Note: Five to 10% of people taking ampicillin develop eruptions between the 5th and 14th day following initiation of therapy. Also, there is a 95% incidence of exanthematous eruptions in patients who are treated for infectious mononucleosis with ampicillin. The allergenicity of ampicillin appears to be enhanced by allopurinol or by hyperuricemia. Ampicillin is clearly the more allergenic of the two drugs when given alone.

Reactions

Skin

Acute generalized exanthematous pustulosis (AGEP)
(1995): Moreau A+, *Int J Dermatol* 34, 263 (passim)
(1994): Manders SM+, *Cutis* 54, 194
(1991): Roujeau J-C+, *Arch Dermatol* 127, 1333

Allergic reactions (sic) (1–10%)
(1993): Grover JK+, *Indian J Physiol Pharmacol* 37, 247 (2.9%)
(1974): Revuz J+, *Nouv Presse Med* (French) *3, 1169*

Angioedema (<1%)
(1982): Valsecchi R+, *Contact Dermatitis* 8, 278
(1980): Kraemer MJ+, *Pediatrics in Review* 1, 197

Baboon syndrome
(1993): Herfs H+, *Hautarzt* (German) 44, 466
(1985): Rasmussen LP+, *Ugeskr Laeger* (Danish) 147, 1341
(1984): Andersen KE+, *Contact Dermatitis* 10, 97

Bullous eruption (<1%)
(1982): Stepien B+, *Przegl Dermatol* (Polish) 69, 65

Bullous pemphigoid
(1990): Hodak E+, *Clin Exp Dermatol* 15, 50

Candidiasis
(1973): Bass JW+, *J Pediatrics* 83, 106

Contact dermatitis
(1997): Romano A+, *Clin Exp Allergy* 27, 1425
(1995): Gamboa P+, *Contact Dermatitis* 32, 48
(1988): Andersen KE, *Acta Derm Venereol* Suppl (Stockh) 135, 62 (systemic)
(1986): Pigatto PD+, *Contact Dermatitis* 14, 196
(1978): Bruevich TS+, *Vest Dermatol Venerol* (Russian) March, 74
(1970): Schulz KH+, *Berufsdermatosen* (German) 18, 132
(1969): Braun W+, *Ther Ggw* (German) 108, 250

Diaper rash
(1973): Bass JW+, *J Pediatrics* 83, 106 (4.5–13%)

Erythema annulare centrifugum
(1975): Gupta HL+, *J Indian Med Assoc* 65, 307

Erythema multiforme (<1%)
(1995): Dhar S+, *Dermatology* 191, 76
(1994): Garty BZ+, *Ann Pharmacother* 28, 730
(1990): Chan HL+, *Arch Dermatol* 126, 43
(1985): Konstantinidis AB+, *J Oral Med* 40, 168
(1984): Gebel K+, *Dermatologica* 168, 35
(1979): Gupta HL+, *J Indian Med Assoc* 72, 188
(1975): Böttiger LE+, *Acta Med Scand* 198, 229
(1972): Kauppinen K, *Acta Derm Venereol* (Stockh) 52, 68
(1970): Crow KD, *Trans A Rep St John's Hosp Dermatol Soc* 56, 35

Exanthems (>10%)
(1997): Romano A+, *Clin Exp Allergy* 27, 1425
(1996): Adcock BB+, *Arch Fam Med* 5, 301
(1996): Marra CA+, *Ann Pharacother* 30, 401
(1995): Romano A+, *Allergy* 50, 113
(1994): Shelley WB+, *Cutis* 53, 40 (observation)
(1994): Grayson ML+, *Clin Infect Dis* 18, 683
(1993): Warrington RJ+, *J Allergy Clin Immunol* 92, 626
(1993): Romano A+, *J Invest Allergol Clin Immunol* 3, 53
(1988): Hou SR, *Chung Hua Nei Ko Tsa Chih* (Chinese) 27, 36
(1987): Pavithran K, *Indian J Lepr* 59, 309
(1986): Cabo HA+, *Med Cutan Ibero Lat Am* (Spanish) 14, 177
(1986): de Haan P+, *Allergy* 41, 75
(1986): Sonntag MR+, *Schweiz Med Wochenschr* (German) 116, 142 (8%)
(1985): Bruynzeel DP+, *Dermatologica* 171, 429
(1985): Hefelfinger DC, *Ala Med* 55, 16
(1983): Scioli C+, *Boll Ist Sieroter Milan* (Italian) 62, 287
(1983): Bianchi C+, *Med Cutan Ibero Lat Am* (Spanish) 11, 113
(1982): Dourmischev AL+, *Dermatol Monatsschr* (German) 168, 469
(1982): Gatter KC+, *Clin Allergy* 12, 279
(1981): Lin CS+, *Arch Dermatol* 117, 282
(1981): Jick H+, *J Clin Pharmacol* 21, 456 (5.9%)
(1980): Scherzer W+, *Derm Beruf Umwelt* (German) 28, 175
(1980): Porter D+, *Lancet* 1, 1037
(1980): Kraemer MJ+, *Pediatrics in Review* 1, 197
(1979): Murphy TF, *Ann Intern Med* 91, 324
(1978): Geyman JP+, *J Fam Pract* 7, 493
(1978): Kouba K+, *Cesk Pediatr* (Czech) 33, 487
(1978): Pollowitz JA, *Am J Dis Child* 132, 819
(1977): Gupta HL+, *J Indian Med Assoc* 68, 33
(1977): Campbell AB+, *Pediatrics* 59, 638
(1977): Sokoloff B, *Pediatrics* 59, 637
(1976): Wuthrich B, *Dtsch Med Wochenschr* (German) 101, 470
(1976): Fellner MJ+, *N Y State J Med* 76, 101
(1976): Arndt KA+, *JAMA* 235, 918 (5.2%)
(1976): Morris J, *Lancet* 1, 423
(1975): Gleckman RA, *JAMA* 233, 427 (2.5%)
(1975): Lehnhoff B, *Monatsschr Kinderheilkd* (German) 123, 548
(1975): Editorial, *BMJ* 2, 708
(1975): Esten H+, *Med Welt* (German) 26, 296
(1975): Krsic B+, *Lijec Vjesn* (Serbo-Croatian-Roman) 97, 339
(1974): Webster AW+, *Clin Exp Immunol* 18, 553
(1974): Spitzy KH, *Acta Med Austriaca* (German) 2, 46
(1973): Gregg I, *BMJ* 1, 295
(1973): *BMJ*, 1, 7
(1973): *N Z Med J* 77, 105
(1973): Wemmer U, *Fortschr Med* (German) 91, 1232
(1973): Bass JW+, *J Pediatrics* 83, 106 (4.75%)
(1973): Kerns DL+, *Am J Dis Child* 125, 187
(1973): Boston Collaborative Drug Surveillance Program, *Arch Dermatol* 107, 74 (9.7%)
(1973): Zürcher K+, *Dermatologica* (German) 147, 1
(1972): Potter JPL, *BMJ* 1, 749
(1972): Harris JR+, *BMJ* 1, 687
(1972): Bierman CW+, *JAMA* 220, 1098
(1972): *N Engl J Med* 286, 1217
(1972): *BMJ* 1, 195
(1972): *BMJ* 1, 505
(1972): Weuta H, *Arzneimittelforschung* (German) 22, 1300
(1972): Steiniger U, *Dtsch Gesundheitsw* (German) 27, 1164
(1972): Balfour HH+, *Clin Pediatr Phila* 11, 417
(1972): Almeyda J+, *Br J Dermatol* 87, 293
(1972): Kuokkanen K, *Acta Allergol* 27, 407
(1972): Schulz KH, *Arch Dermatol Forsch* (German) 244, 309
(1971): Kroidon EaP, *Antibiotiki* (Russian) 16, 549
(1971): Pullen H, *BMJ* 2, 653
(1971): Beckmann H, *Munch Med Wochenschr* (German) 113, 1423
(1971): Speck WT, *Clin Pediatr Phila* 10, 59
(1971): Bronsert U, *Med Klin* (German) 66, 352
(1970): Kerrebijn KF, *Lancet* 1, 245
(1970): Jaffe IA, *Lancet* 1, 245
(1970): Crow KD, *Trans St Johns Hosp Dermatol Soc* 56, 35
(1970): Corless JD+, *South Med J* 63, 1341
(1970): Kronig B+, *Arzneimittelforschung* (German) 20, 1930
(1970): Fournier A+, *J Sci Med Lille* (French) 88, 529
(1970): Knudsen ET+, *BMJ* 1, 469
(1970): Shapiro S+, *Lancet* 1, 194 (9.5%)
(1970): Weary PE+, *Arch Dermatol* 101, 86
(1969): No Author, *Lancet* 2, 993
(1969): Sanders DY, *Clin Pediatr Phila* 8, 47
(1969): Hurwitz N+, *BMJ* 1, 531 (7.8%)
(1969): Shapiro S+, *Lancet* 2, 969 (7.7%)
(1968): Gabbert WR+, *J Ky Med Assoc* 66, 967
(1968): Loffler H+, *Med Welt* (German) 32, 1736
(1968): Levene G+, *Br J Dermatol* 80, 417
(1966): Stevenson J+, *BMJ* 1, 1359

Exfoliative dermatitis
(1985): Fong PH+, *Ann Acad Med Singapore* 14, 693
(1974): Tay C, *Asian J Med* 10, 223
Fixed eruption
(1990): Bharija SC+, *Dermatologica* 181, 237
(1990): Gaffoor PMA+, *Cutis* 45, 242
(1987): Sharma SN, *J Assoc Physicians India* 35, 608
(1986): Panagariya A, *J Ass Physicians India* 34, 458
(1986): Kanwar AJ+, *Dermatologica* 172, 315
(1984): Chan H-L, *Arch Dermatol* 120, 542
(1983): Chan H-L, *Int J Dermatol* 23, 607
(1970): Savin JA, *Br J Dermatol* 83, 546
Linear IgA bullous dermatosis
(1996): Tranvan A+, *J Am Acad Dermatol* 35, 865
(1981): Boffety B+, *Journées Dermatologiques de Paris* (French), 53–53a
Pemphigus
(1997): Brenner S+, *J Am Acad Dermatol* 36, 919
(1996): Takizawa H+, *Am J Gastroenterol* 91, 1654
(1993): Brenner S+, *Isr J Med Sci* 29, 44
(1986): Wilson JP+, *Drug Intell Clin Pharm* 20, 219
(1986): Brenner S+, *J Am Acad Dermatol* 14, 453
(1980): Fellner MJ+, *Int J Dermatol* 19, 392
Pityriasis rosea
(1987): Olumide Y, *Int J Dermatol* 26, 234
Pruritus (1–5%)
(1996): Adcock BB+, *Arch Fam Med* 5, 301
(1982): Bernhard JD+, *Cutis* 29, 158
(1973): Bass JW+, *J Pediatrics* 83, 106 (0.75%)
(1980): Kraemer MJ+, *Pediatrics in Review* 1, 197
Psoriasis
(1993): Litt JZ, Beachwood, OH, personal case (observation)
(1992): Breathnach SM+, *Adverse Drug Reactions and the Skin*, Blackwell, Oxford, 141 (passim)
(1990): Saito S+, *J Dermatol* 17, 677
(1988): Tsankov N+, *J Am Acad Dermatol* 19, 629
Purpura
(1993): Pang BK+, *Ann Acad Med Singapore* 22, 870
(1990): Hannedouche T+, *J Antimicrob Chemother* 20, 3
(1982): Beeching NL+, *J Antimicrob Chemother* 10, 479
(1981): Valman HB, *Br Med J Clin Res Ed* 283, 970
(1973): Croydon EAP+, *BMJ* 1, 7
(1971): Parker JC+, *Arch Intern Med* 127, 474
Pustular eruption
(1995): Lim JT+, *Cutis* 56, 163
(1994): Jay S+, *Arch Dermatol* 130, 787 (localized)
(1991): Roujeau J-C+, *Arch Dermatol* 127, 1333
(1990): Guy C+, *Nouv Dermatol* (French) 9, 540
Pustular psoriasis
(1987): Katz M+, *J Am Acad Dermatol* 17, 918
(1986): Verner E+, *Harefuah* (Hebrew) 110, 132
Rash (sic) (1–10%)
Stevens–Johnson syndrome
(1990): Cavanzo FJ+, *Gastroenterology* 99, 854
(1990): Chan HL+, *Arch Dermatol* 126, 43
(1987): Howell CG+, *J Pediatr Surg* 22, 994
(1985): Turck M, *Hosp Pract Off Ed* 20, 49
(1985): Ting HC+, *Int J Dermatol* 24, 587
(1979): Gupta HL+, *J Indian Med Assoc* 72, 188
(1978): Assaad D+, *Can Med Assoc* 118, 154
(1975): McArthur JE+, *N Z Med J* 81, 390
(1972): Kauppinen K, *Acta Derm Venereol* (Stockh) 52, 68
Toxic epidermal necrolysis (<1%)
(1997): Rodrigues-Ares MT+, *Int Ophthalmol* 21, 39
(1993): Romano A+, *J Invest Allergol Clin Immunol* 3, 53
(1991): Heng MC+, *J Am Acad Dermatol* 25, 778
(1985): Robbens EJ+, *Acta Clin Belg* 40, 115
(1983): Tagami H+, *Arch Dermatol* 119, 910
(1981): Berkel AI+, *Turk J Pediatr* 23, 37
(1980): Giuffre L+, *Minerva Pediatr* (Italian) 32, 633
(1979): Rosenthal AL+, *Cutis* 24, 437
(1978): Assaad D+, *Can Med Assoc* 118, 154
(1975): Schopf E+, *Z Haut* (German) 50, 865
(1975): McArthur JE+, *N Z Med J* 81, 390
(1975): Böttiger LE+, *Acta Med Scand* 198, 229
(1972): Carli-Basset C+, *Sem Hop* (French) 48, 497
Urticaria
(1997): Romano A+, *Clin Exp Allergy* 27, 1425
(1996): Adcock BB+, *Arch Fam Med* 5, 301
(1985): Goolamali SK, *Postgrad Med J* 61, 925
(1982): Valsecchi R+, *Contact Dermatitis* 8, 278
(1980): Kraemer MJ+, *Pediatrics in Review* 1, 197
(1977): Gupta HL+, *J Indian Med Assoc* 68, 33
(1975): Gleckman RA, *JAMA* 233, 427 (0.8%)
(1973): Croydon EAP+, *BMJ* 1, 7
(1972): Bierman CW+, *JAMA* 220, 1098
(1969): Coskey RJ+, *Arch Dermatol* 100, 717
(1969): Knudsen ET, *BMJ* 1, 846
(1969): Pullen H, *BMJ* 2, 247
(1963): Kennedy WPU+, *BMJ* 2, 962 (10%)
Vasculitis
(1991): Estrada-Rodriguez JL+, *J Investig Allergol Clin Immunol* 1, 69
(1990): Hannedouche T+, *J Antimicrob Chemother* 20, 3
(1975): Pevny I+, *MMW Munch Med Wochenschr* (German) 117, 9
(1974): Tay C, *Asian J Med* 10, 223

Other

Anaphylactoid reaction
(1998): Rich MW, *Tex Heart Inst J* 25, 194
(1997): Romano A+, *Clin Exp Allergy* 27, 1425
(1996): Adcock BB+, *Arch Fam Med* 5, 301
(1976): Fellner MJ, *Int J Dermatol* 15, 497
(1975): Pietzcker F+, *Z Hautkr* (German) 50, 437
(1973): Weck AL de, *Munch Med Wochenschr* (German) 115, 1650
(1972): Ohela K+, *Duodecim* (Finnish) 88, 1177
Black tongue
(1966): Meyler L (ed), *Side Effects of Drugs* 5th ed. Amsterdam, Excerpta Medica
Glossitis
Hypersensitivity
(1996): Torricelli R+, *Hautarzt* (German) 47, 392
(1993): Romano A+, *Contact Dermatitis* 28, 190
(1987): Ackerman Z+, *Postgrad Med J* 63, 55
(1970): Klemola E, *Scand J Infect Dis* 2, 29
Injection-site pain (>10%)
Oral candidiasis
Oral mucosal eruption
(1984): Gebel K+, *Dermatologica* 168, 35
Phlebitis
Serum sickness
(1974): Caldwell JR+, *JAMA* 230, 77
Stomatitis
Thrombophlebitis
Vaginal candidiasis

AMPRENAVIR

Trade name: Agenerase (GlaxoWellcome)
Indications: HIV infection
Category: Protease inhibitor*; sulfonamide**
Half-life: no data
Clinically important, potentially serious interactions with: amiodarone, astemizole, bepridil, cisapride, ketoconazole, lidocaine, midazolam, quinidine, rifabutin, sildenafil, triazolam, tricyclic antidepressants, warfarin

Reactions

Skin

Exanthems
Pruritus
Rash (sic) (25%)
Stevens–Johnson syndrome (4%)

Other

Buffalo hump
Dysgeusia (10%)
Gynecomastia
Hypesthesia
(1999): Sadler BM+, *Antimicrob Agents Chemother* 14, 1686
Paresthesias (perioral) (26%)

***Note:** Protease inhibitors cause dyslipidemia which includes elevated triglycerides and cholesterol and redistribution of body fat centrally to produce the so-called "protease paunch," breast enlargement, facial atrophy, and "buffalo hump."

****Note**: Amprenavir is a sulfonamide and can be absorbed systemically. Sulfonamides can produce severe, possibly fatal, reactions such as toxic epidermal necrolysis and Stevens–Johnson syndrome

AMYL NITRITE

Synonym: isoamyl nitrite
Trade name: Amyl Nitrite (Lilly)
Other trade name: *Nitrit*
Indications: Angina pectoris
Category: Antianginal; coronary vasodilator
Half-life: no data
Clinically important, potentially serious interactions with: alcohol, aspirin, calcium channel blockers, heparin

Reactions

Skin

Allergic reactions (sic)
(1989): Dax EM+, *Am J Med* 86, 732
Contact dermatitis
(1985): Bos JD+, *Contact Dermatitis* 12, 109
(1982): Romaguera C+, *Contact Dermatitis* 8, 266
Dermatitis (sic)
(1984): Fisher AA, *Cutis* 34, 118
Diaphoresis
Edema
Flushing (1–10%)
Pallor
Rash (sic) (<1%)

ANISTREPLASE

Synonym: APSAC
Trade name: Eminase (Roberts)
Other trade name: *Iminase*
Indications: Acute myocardial infarction
Category: Thrombolytic enzyme
Half-life: 70–120 minutes
Clinically important, potentially serious interactions with: anticoagulants, aspirin, dipyridamole, NSAIDs, plicamycin, valproic acid

Reactions

Skin

Allergic reactions (sic)
Angioedema
Chills (<1%)
Diaphoresis (<1%)
Ecchymoses
Exanthems
(1995): Dykewicz MS+, *J Allergy Clin Immunol* 95, 1020
Flushing
Livedo reticularis
(1994): Gianni R+, *Ann Ital Med Int* (Italian) 9, 105
Purpura
Rash (sic)
Ulcer
(1994): Gianni R+, *Ann Ital Med Int* (Italian) 9, 105
Urticaria
(1995): Dykewicz MS+, *J Allergy Clin Immunol* 95, 1020

Other

Anaphylactoid reaction (1–10%)
(1997): Cannas S+, *G Ital Cardiol* (Italian) 27, 278
Gingival hemorrhage
Hypersensitivity
(1993): Lee HS+, *Eur Heart J* 14, 1640
Myalgia
(1994): Gianni R+, *Ann Ital Med Int* (Italian) 9, 105
Serum sickness
(1993): Lee HS+, *Eur Heart J* 14, 1640
Vasculitis
(1994): Gianni R+, *Ann Ital Med Int* (Italian) 9, 105
(1992): Burrows N+, *J Am Acad Dermatol* 26, 508
(1990): Burrows N+, *Br Heart J* 64, 289
(1988): Bucknall C+, *Br Heart J* 59, 9
(1988): Gemmill JD+, *Br Heart J* 60, 361

ANTIRETROVIRAL AGENTS

(Please refer to individual generic drugs for reaction patterns)

PROTEASE INHIBITORS*
Generic names:
Amprenavir
Trade name: Agenerase (GlaxoWellcome)
Indinavir
Trade name: Crixivan (Merck)
lopinavir (ABT-378/r)
Trade name: Kaletra
Nelfinavir
Trade name: Viracept (Agouron)
Ritonavir
Trade name: Norvir (Abbott)
Saquinavir
Trade names: Invirase; Fortovase (Roche)

***Note:** Protease inhibitors cause dyslipidemia which includes elevated triglycerides and cholesterol and redistribution of body fat centrally to produce the so-called "protease paunch," breast enlargement, facial atrophy, and "buffalo hump."

NUCLEOSIDE ANALOG REVERSE TRANSCRIPTASE INHIBITORS (NRTIs)
Generic names:
Abacavir (ABC)
Trade name: Ziagen (GlaxoWellcome)
Didanosine (ddI)
Trade name: Videx (Bristol-Myers Squibb)
Lamivudine (3TC)
Trade names: Epivir, Combivir (GlaxoWellcome)
Stavudine (d4T)
Trade name: Zerit (Bristol-Myers Squibb)
Zalcitabine (ddc)
Trade name: ddC; Hivid (Roche)
Zidovudine (AZT)
Trade name: AZT; Retrovir (GlaxoWellcome)

Combivir is a combination of lamivudine and zidovudine

NON-NUCLEOSIDE REVERSE TRANSCRIPTASE INHIBITORS (NNRTIs)
Generic names:
Delavirdine
Trade name: Rescriptor (Pharmacia & Upjohn)
Efavirenz
Trade name: Sustiva (Dupont)
Nevirapine
Trade name: Viramune (Roxane)

NUCLEOSIDE REVERSE TRANSCRIPTASE INHIBITORS (NRTIs)
Tenofovir*

***Note:** Not FDA approved as yet

APRACLONIDINE

Trade name: Iopidine (Alcon)
Indications: Postsurgical intraocular pressure elevation
Category: $Alpha_2$ adrenergic agonist; sympathomimetic ophthalmic solution; vasoconstrictor
Half-life: 8 hours
Clinically important, potentially serious interactions with: topical beta-blockers; MAO inhibitors

Reactions

Skin

Allergic reactions (<1%)
(2000): Geyer O+, *Graefes Arch Clin Exp Ophthalmol* 238, 149
(1999): Britt MT+, *Br J Ophthalmol* 83, 992 (progressing to ectropion)
(1995): Butler P+, *Arch Ophthalmol* 113, 293
(1995): Feibel RM, *Arch Ophthalmol* 113, 1579
Burning
(1996): Stewart WC, *Klin Monatsbl Augenheilkd* (German) 209, A7
Contact dermatitis (<1%)
(1998): Armisen M+, *Contact Dermatitis* 39, 193
Dermatitis (sic) (<1%)
Edema (eyelids) (<3%)
Facial edema (<1%)
Pruritus (10%)
(1996): Stewart WC, *Klin Monatsbl Augenheilkd* (German) 209, A7
Xerosis

Other

Dysgeusia (3%)
Myalgia (0.2%)
Paresthesias (<1%)
Parosmia (0.2%)
Xerostomia (1–10%)
(1987): Abrams DA+, *Arch Ophthalmol* 105, 1205 (52%)

APROBARBITAL

Trade name: Alurate (Roche)
Indications: Short-term sedation, sleep induction
Category: Intermediate-acting barbiturate
Half-life: 14–34 hours
Clinically important, potentially serious interactions with: no data

Reactions

Skin

Angioedema
Exanthems
Exfoliative dermatitis
Purpura
Rash (sic)
Stevens–Johnson syndrome
Urticaria

Other

Serum sickness

APROTININ

Trade name: Trasylol (Bayer)
Indications: For prophylactic use to reduce blood loss in patients undergoing coronary artery bypass surgery
Category: Hemostatic agent (a natural protease inhibitor)
Half-life: 150 minutes
Clinically important, potentially serious interactions with: ACE inhibitors, alteplase, anistreplase, heparin, streptokinse, succinylcholine, urokinase

Reactions

Skin

Allergic reactions (sic) (0.5%)
(1994): Bayo M+, *Rev Esp Anestesiol Reanim* (Spanish) 41, 123
(1983): Freeman JG+, *Curr Med Res Opin* 8, 559 (2 cases)
Angioedema
Erythema
Exanthems
(2000): Beierlein W+, *Transfusion* 40, 302 (generalized)
Pruritus
Rash (sic)
Urticaria

Other

Anaphylactoid reaction (0.5%)
(2000): Laxenaire MC+, *Ann Fr Anesth Reanim* (French) 19, 96
(2000): Beierlein W, *Ann Thorac Surg* 69, 1298
(1999): Laxenaire MC, *Ann Fr Anesth Reanim* (French) 18, 796 (4 cases)
(1999): Cohen DM+, *Ann Thorac Surg* 67, 837
(1999): Ryckwaert Y+, *Ann Fr Anesth Reanim* (French) 18, 904
(1999): Ong BC+, *Anaesth Intensive Care* 27, 538
(1998): Scheule AM+, *Gastrointest Endosc* 48, 83
(1997): Orsel I+, *Ann Fr Anesth Reanim* (French) 16, 292
(1997): Dietrich W+, *J Thorac Cardiovasc Surg* 113, 194
(1997): Scheule AM+, *Ann Thorac Surg* 63, 242
(1996): Martinelli L+, *Ann Thorac Surg* 61, 1288
(1995): Ceriana P+, *J Cardiothorac Vasc Anesth* 9, 477
(1995): Diefenbach C+, *Anesth Analg* 80, 830
(1994): Kon NF+, *Masui* (Japanese) 43, 1606
(1993): Schulze K+, *Eur J Cardiothorac Surg* 7, 495 (2 patients)
(1993): Cottineau C+, *Ann Fr Anesth Reanim* (French) 12, 590
(1984): *BMJ* 289, 1696
(1984): LaFerla GA+, *BMJ* 289, 1176
(1976): Proud G+, *Lancet* 2, 48
(1971): Bauer J+, *Am J Gastroenterol* 56, 542
Hypersensitivity
(2000): Beierlein W+, *Transfusion* 40, 302
(1998): Dietrich W, *Ann Thoracic Surg* 65, S60 (1.8%)
(1975): Ariani G+, *Minerva Anestesiol* (Italian) 41, 138
Lipohypertrophy
(1985): Dandona P+, *Diabetes Res* 2, 213 (in a diabetic)
(1985): Boag F+, *N Engl J Med* 312, 245 (in a diabetic)
Phlebitis (1–10%)
Shock (sic)
(1971): Vashchuk VV, *Klin Med (Mosk)* (Russian) 49, 128

ARSENIC

Trade names: Trisonex (manufacturer: Cell Therapeutics); Fowler's Solution (rarely employed); found in pesticides and herbal medicines
Indications: Acute promyelocytic leukemia; psoriasis (in the early 1900s), devitalization of pulp in dental procedures
Category: Trace metal
Half-life: no data
Clinically important, potentially serious interactions with: no data

Reactions

Skin

Basal cell carcinoma
(1996): Maloney ME, *Dermatol Surg* 22, 301 (passim)
(1996): Matsumura Y+, *Int J Cancer* 65, 778
(1994): McNutt NS+, *Arch Dermatol* 130, 225
(1993): Ziegler A+, *Proc Natl Acad*
(1993): Alain G+, *Int J Dermatol* 32, 899 (passim)
(1992): Breathnach SM+, *Adverse Drug Reactions and the Skin*, Blackwell, Oxford, 236 (passim)
(1986): Munzberger H+, *Z Arztl Fortbild Jena* (German) 80, 985
(1985): Kastl J+, *Dermatol Monatsschr* (German) 171, 158
(1984): Schroeder P+, *Fortschr Med* (German) 102, 1128
(1980): Weiss J+, *Hautarzt* (German) 31, 654
(1974): Tay CH, *Aust J Dermatol* 15, 121 (6%)
(1973): Yeh S, *Human Path* 4, 469
(1967): Schulz EJ *S Afr Med J* 41, 819
(1965): Fierz U, *Dermatologica* 131, 41

Bowen's disease
(1998): Tsuruta D+, *Br J Dermatol* 139, 291
(1997): Ohnishi Y+, *J Dermatol* 24, 310
(1996): Maloney ME, *Dermatol Surg* 22, 301 (passim)
(1996): Person JR, *Cutis* 58, 65
(1994): Hsieh LL+, *Cancer Lett* 86, 59
(1993): Alain G+, *Int J Dermatol* 32, 899 (passim)
(1992): Breathnach SM+, *Adverse Drug Reactions and the Skin*, Blackwell, Oxford, 236 (passim)
(1989): Shannon RL+, *Hum Toxicol* 8, 99
(1989): Koh E+, *Eur Urol* 16, 398
(1988): Ismail R+, *J Dermatol* 15, 65
(1983): Heddle R+, *Chest* 84, 776
(1982): Rosen T+, *J Am Acad Dermatol* 7, 364
(1982): Ohyama K, *Dermatologica* 164, 161
(1979): Allen RB+, *Cutis* 23, 805
(1974): Tay CH, *Aust J Dermatol* 15, 121
(1973): Yeh S, *Human Path* 4, 469

Bullous eruption
(1993): Alain G+, *Int J Dermatol* 32, 899 (passim)
(1992): Breathnach SM+, *Adverse Drug Reactions and the Skin*, Blackwell, Oxford, 236 (passim)
(1988): Bork K, *Cutaneous Side Effects of Drugs*, WB Saunders, 114
(1968): Privat Y+, *Bull Soc Med Afr Noire Lang Fr* (French) 13, 195
(1955): Alexander HL, *Reactions with Drug Therapy*, WB Saunders

Cancer
(1997): Schwartz RA, *Int J Dermatol* 36, 241
(1995): Hsueh YM+, *Br J Cancer* 71, 109
(1995): Fawell J, *Hum Exp Toxicol* 14, 464
(1993): Urbach F, *Recent Results Cancer Res* 128, 243
(1992): Wong O+, *Int Arch Occup Environ Health* 64, 235
(1989): Bickley LK+, *N J Med* 86, 377
(1988): Durocher LP+, *Union Med Can* (French) 117, 345
(1988): Chen CJ+, *Lancet* 1, 414
(1976): Spoor HJ, *Cutis* 18, 631
(1970): Thivolet J+, *Lyon Med* (French) 223, 457
(1969): Thivolet J+, *Bull Soc Fr Dermatol Syphiligr* (French) 76, 892

Contact dermatitis
(1995): Barbaud A+, *Contact Dermatitis* 33, 272
(1986): Wahlberg JE+, *Derm Beruf Umwelt* (German) 34, 10
(1964): Gaffi A, *Gazz Int Med Chir* (Italian) 69, 3363

Dermatitis (sic)
(1955): Alexander HL, *Reactions with Drug Therapy*, WB Saunders

Dermatofibrosarcoma protuberans
(1986): Shneidman D+, *Cancer* 58, 1585

Erythema multiforme
(1990): Vassileva S+, *Int J Dermatol* 29, 381
(1988): Bork K, *Cutaneous Side Effects of Drugs*, WB Saunders, 145
(1967): Coleman WP, *Med Clin North Am* 51, 1073
(1955): Alexander HL, *Reactions with Drug Therapy*, WB Saunders
(1945): Fletcher MWC+, *J Pediatr* 27, 465

Erythema nodosum
(1988): Bork K, *Cutaneous Side Effects of Drugs*, WB Saunders, 148

Exanthems
(1993): Alain G+, *Int J Dermatol* 32, 899 (passim)
(1974): Tay CH, *Aust J Dermatol* 15, 121 (16%)
(1974): *Med Lett* 16, 11
(1955): Alexander HL, *Reactions with Drug Therapy*, WB Saunders
(1952): Sulzberger MB+, *Postgrad Med* 11, 549

Exfoliative dermatitis
(1993): Alain G+, *Int J Dermatol* 32, 899 (passim)
(1992): Breathnach SM+, *Adverse Drug Reactions and the Skin*, Blackwell, Oxford, 236 (passim)
(1973): Nicolis GD+, *Arch Dermatol* 108, 788
(1967): Coleman WP, *Med Clin North Am* 51, 1073
(1967): Lockey SD, *Med Sci* 18, 43
(1965): Fellner MJ+, *Med Clin North Am* 49, 709
(1963): Abrahams I+, *Arch Dermatol* 87, 96
(1955): Alexander HL, *Reactions with Drug Therapy*, WB Saunders

Fixed eruption
(1988): Bork K, *Cutaneous Side Effects of Drugs*, WB Saunders, 108
(1964): Browne SG, *BMJ* 2, 1041
(1961): Welsh AL, *The Fixed Drug Eruption*, Thomas, Springfield
(1955): Alexander HL, *Reactions with Drug Therapy*, WB Saunders

Follicular keratosis (sic)
(1952): Sulzberger MB+, *Postgrad Med* 11, 549

Freckles
(1995): Gritiyarangsan P+, *Photodermatol Photoimmunol Photomed* 11, 174

Hyperkeratosis (palms and soles) (40%)
(1996): Maloney ME, *Dermatol Surg* 22, 301 (passim)
(1965): Fierz U, *Dermatologica* 131, 41

Keratoses
(1999): Tondel M+, *Environmental Health Perspectives* 107, 727
(1998): Guha Mazumder DN+, *Int J Epidemiol* 27, 871
(1993): Alain G+, *Int J Dermatol* 32, 899 (passim)
(1992): Breathnach SM+, *Adverse Drug Reactions and the Skin*, Blackwell, Oxford, 236 (passim)
(1988): Bork K, *Cutaneous Side Effects of Drugs*, WB Saunders, 232
(1978): Reymann F+, *Arch Dermatol* 114, 378
(1969): Bartruff JK, *Arch Dermatol* 100, 382
(1965): Dobson RL+, *Arch Dermatol* 92, 553

Leukomelanoderma (sic)
(1999): Tondel M+, *Environmental Health Perspectives* 107, 727
(1993): Sass U+, *Dermatology* 186, 303
(1974): Tay CH, *Aust J Dermatol* 15, 121 (31%)
(1952): Sulzberger MB+, *Postgrad Med* 11, 549

Lichen planus (bullous)
(1970): Aguilera-Diaz LF, *Ann Dermatol Syphiligr Paris* (French) 97, 39

Livedo reticularis
(1974): Nagy G+, *Z Hautkr* (German) 25, 534

Melanoderma
(1992): Breathnach SM+, *Adverse Drug Reactions and the Skin*, Blackwell, Oxford, 236 (passim)

Melanoma
(1984): Philipp R+, *Br Med J Clin Res Ed* 288, 237
(1980): Evans S, *BMJ* 280, 403
(1980): Clough P, *BMJ* 280, 112
(1976): Grobe JW, *Berufsdermatosen* (German) 24, 167

Merkel cell carcinoma
(1999): Huang-Chun L+, *J Am Acad Dermatol* 41, 641
(1998): Tsuruta D+, *Br J Dermatol* 139, 291
(1997): Ohnishi Y+, *J Dermatol* 24, 310
(1991): Huang HP+, *J Formos Med Assoc* 90, 900

Morphea
(1952): Sulzberger MB+, *Postgrad Med* 11, 549

Palmar-plantar erythema
(1952): Sulzberger MB+, *Postgrad Med* 11, 549

Palmar-plantar hyperhidrosis
(1974): Tay CH, *Aust J Dermatol* 15, 121 (31%)

Palmar-plantar keratoderma
(1993): Sass U+, *Dermatology* 186, 303

(1987): Chakraborty AK+, *Indian J Med Res* 85, 326
(1974): Tay CH, *Aust J Dermatol* 15, 121 (65%)
(1972): Hadida E+, *Bull Soc Fr Dermatol Syphiligr* (French) 79, 287

Palmar-plantar punctate keratoses
(1996): Maloney ME, *Dermatol Surg* 22, 301 (passim)
(1992): Breathnach SM+, *Adverse Drug Reactions and the Skin*, Blackwell, Oxford, 236 (passim)

Parapsoriasis
(1952): Sulzberger MB+, *Postgrad Med* 11, 549

Photosensitivity
(1992): Breathnach SM+, *Adverse Drug Reactions and the Skin*, Blackwell, Oxford, 236 (passim)

Pigmentation
(1999): Tondel M+, *Environmental Health Perspectives* 107, 727
(1998): Guha Mazumder DN+, *Int J Epidemiol* 27, 871
(1996): Maloney ME, *Dermatol Surg* 22, 301 (passim)
(1993): Alain G+, *Int J Dermatol* 32, 899 (passim)
(1992): Breathnach SM+, *Adverse Drug Reactions and the Skin*, Blackwell, Oxford, 236 (passim)
(1989): Shannon RL+, *Hum Toxicol* 8, 99
(1981): Granstein RD+, *J Am Acad Dermatol* 5, 1 (bronze)
(1974): Tay CH, *Aust J Dermatol* 15, 121 (85%)
(1973): Levantine A+, *Br J Dermatol* 89, 105

Pityriasis rosea (from organic arsenic)
(1988): Bork K, *Cutaneous Side Effects of Drugs*, WB Saunders, 169
(1952): Sulzberger MB+, *Postgrad Med* 11, 549

Pruritus
(1967): Young AW, *J Am Geriatr Soc* 15, 750

Psoriasis
(1952): Sulzberger MB+, *Postgrad Med* 11, 549

Purpura
(1988): Bork K, *Cutaneous Side Effects of Drugs*, WB Saunders, 191
(1955): Alexander HL, *Reactions with Drug Therapy*, WB Saunders

Squamous cell carcinoma
(1996): Maloney ME, *Dermatol Surg* 22, 301 (passim)
(1993): Alain G+, *Int J Dermatol* 32, 899 (passim)
(1992): Breathnach SM+, *Adverse Drug Reactions and the Skin*, Blackwell, Oxford, 236 (passim)
(1989): Shannon RL+, *Hum Toxicol* 8, 99
(1988): Ismail R+, *J Dermatol* 15, 65
(1988): Scholz S+, *Z Arztl Fortbild Jena* (German) 82, 1201
(1979): Brownstein MH+, *Int J Dermatol* 18, 1
(1979): Southwick GJ+, *J Surg Oncol* 12, 115
(1974): Tay CH, *Aust J Dermatol* 15, 121
(1973): Yeh S, *Human Path* 4, 469

Stevens–Johnson syndrome
(1990): Vassileva S+, *Int J Dermatol* 29, 381
(1967): Coleman WP, *Med Clin North Am* 51, 1073
(1945): Fletcher MWC+, *J Pediatr* 27, 465

Urticaria
(1955): Alexander HL, *Reactions with Drug Therapy*, WB Saunders

Vitiligo
(1989): Bickley LK+, *N J Med* 86, 377

Hair

Hair – alopecia
(1993): Alain G+, *Int J Dermatol* 32, 899 (passim)
(1992): Breathnach SM+, *Adverse Drug Reactions and the Skin*, Blackwell, Oxford, 236 (passim)
(1988): Bork K, *Cutaneous Side Effects of Drugs*, WB Saunders, 249
(1974): Tay CH, *Aust J Dermatol* 15, 121 (5%)

Nails

Nails – leukonychia
(1988): Bork K, *Cutaneous Side Effects of Drugs*, WB Saunders, 262

Nails – pigmentation
(1988): Bork K, *Cutaneous Side Effects of Drugs*, WB Saunders, 261
(1978): Shah PC+, *Br J Dermatol* 98, 675 (passim)

Nails – transverse white bands
(1993): Alain G+, *Int J Dermatol* 32, 899 (passim)
(1993): Sass U+, *Dermatology* 186, 303

Other

Foetor ex ore (halitosis)
(1988): Bork K, *Cutaneous Side Effects of Drugs*, WB Saunders, 310

Gangrene
(1952): Sulzberger MB+, *Postgrad Med* 11, 549

Gynecomastia
(1992): Breathnach SM+, *Adverse Drug Reactions and the Skin*, Blackwell, Oxford, 237 (passim)

Hyperhidrosis
(1993): Alain G+, *Int J Dermatol* 32, 899 (passim)

Oral mucosal eruption (8%)
(1974): Tay CH, *Aust J Dermatol* 15, 121
(1966): Dummett CO, *J Oral Ther Pharmacol* 1, 106
(1952): Sulzberger MB+, *Postgrad Med* 11, 549

Oral mucosal pigmentation
(1988): Bork K, *Cutaneous Side Effects of Drugs*, WB Saunders, 288

Stomatitis
(1966): Dummett CO, *J Oral Ther Pharmacol* 1, 106

ASCORBIC ACID

Synonym: vitamin C
Trade names: Ascorbicap; Cebid; Cecon; Cemill; Cetane; Cevalin (Lilly); Cevi-Bid; Dull-C; Sunkist; Vita-C
Other common trade names: *Apo-C; Ce-Vi-Sol; Cebion; Cetebe; Laroscorbine; Potent C; Pro-C; Redoxon*
Indications: Prevention of scurvy
Category: Water-soluble nutritional supplement
Half-life: no data
Clinically important, potentially serious interactions with: aspirin, iron, oral contraceptives, propranolol

Reactions

Skin

Angioedema
(1980): Bilyk MA+, *Vrach Delo* (Russian) May, 81

Cutaneous side effects (sic)
(1992): Breathnach SM+, *Adverse Drug Reactions and the Skin*, Blackwell, Oxford, 265 (passim)
(1980): Bilyk MA+, *Vrach Delo* (Russian) May, 81

Eczema (sic)
(1980): Metz J+, *Contact Dermatitis* 6, 172

Erythema

Flushing (<1%)

Other

Injection-site irritation

ASPARAGINASE

Synonym: L-asparaginase
Trade name: Elspar (Merck)
Other common trade names: *Crasnitin; Erwinase; Kidrolase; Laspar; Leunase*
Indications: Acute lymphocytic leukemia, lymphoma
Category: Antineoplastic; protein synthesis inhibitor (parenteral)
Half-life: 8–30 hours (IV); 39–49 hours (IM)
Clinically important, potentially serious interactions with: cyclophosphamide, mercaptopurine, methotrexate, prednisone, vincristine

Reactions

Skin

Angioedema
(1983): Bronner AK+, *J Am Acad Dermatol* 9, 645 (15%)
(1981): Weiss RB+, *Ann Intern Med* 94, 66
(1971): Jacquillat C+, *Med Welt* (German) 22, 503 (<1.0%)

Chills

Diaphoresis

Edema

Exanthems

Flushing
(1983): Bronner AK+, *J Am Acad Dermatol* 9, 645 (15%)
Pruritus (<1%)
(1981): Weiss RB+, *Ann Intern Med* 94, 66
Rash (sic) (<1%)
Toxic epidermal necrolysis
(1989): Stern RS+, *J Am Acad Dermatol* 21, 317
(1980): Rodriguez AR, *J Med Assoc Ga* 69, 355
Urticaria (<1%)
(1983): Bronner AK+, *J Am Acad Dermatol* 9, 645 (15%)
(1981): Weiss RB+, *Ann Intern Med* 94, 66
(1979): Ertel IJ+, *Cancer Res* 39, 3893
(1971): Jacquillat C+, *Med Welt* (German) 22, 503 (<0.5%)

Hair

Hair – alopecia

Other

Anaphylactoid reaction (10–40%)
(1983): Bronner AK+, *J Am Acad Dermatol* 9, 645 (15%)
(1982): Dunagin WG, *Semin Oncol* 9, 14 (3%)
(1979): Ertel IJ+, *Cancer Res* 39, 3893
Aphthous stomatitis (1–10%)
Hypersensitivity (10–40%)
(1998): Larson RA+, *Leukemia* 12, 660
(1998): Bonno M+, *J Allergy Clin Immunol* 101, 571
(1992): Weiss RB, *Semin Oncol* 19, 458
(1982): Dunagin WG, *Semin Oncol* 9, 14 (33%)
(1981): Weiss RB+, *Ann Intern Med* 94, 66 (6–43%)
(1978): Levine N+, *Cancer Treat Res* 5, 67 (5–20%)
(1974): Levantine A+, *Br J Dermatol* 90, 239
Injection-site erythema
Oral mucosal lesions (26%)
Serum sickness
(1983): Bronner AK+, *J Am Acad Dermatol* 9, 645 (15%)

ASPARTAME

Trade names: Equal; Nutrasweet*
Indications: No data
Category: Low-calorie artificial sweetener
Half-life: no data
Clinically important, potentially serious interactions with: no data

Reactions

Skin

Allergic reactions (sic)
(1996): Roberts HJ, *Arch Intern Med* 156, 1027
(1998): Garriga MM+, *Ann Allergy* 61, 63
Angioedema
(1992): Downham TF, *Clin Cases in Dermatol* 4, 12 (observation)
(1988): Metcalfe DD, *Skin and Allergy News* 19, 52 (observation)
Dermatitis (sic)
(1992): Downham TF, *Clin Cases in Dermatol* 4, 12 (observation)
Exanthems
(1986): *Arzneimittelinformation ATI Berlin GmbH* (German) 12, 121
Pruritus
(1994): Shelley WB+, *Cutis* 53, 77 (observation)
(1988): Metcalfe DD, *Skin and Allergy News* 19, 52 (observation)
Pruritus ani
(1994): Shelley WB+, *Cutis* 53, 237 (observation)
Purpura
(1992): Downham TF, *Clin Cases in Dermatol* 4, 12 (observation)
(1999): Leal G, Fortaleza, Brazil (from Internet) (observation)
Rash (sic)
(1988): Metcalfe DD, *Skin and Allergy News* 19, 52 (observation)
Urticaria
(1995): Kulczycki A, *J Allergy Clin Immunol* 95, 639
(1992): Downham TF, *Clin Cases in Dermatol* 4, 12 (observation)
(1988): Metcalfe DD, *Skin and Allergy News* 19, 52 (observation)
(1986): Kulczycki A, *Ann Intern Med* 104, 207
Vasculitis
(1992): Downham TF, *Clin Cases in Dermatol* 4, 12 (observation)

Other

Anaphylactoid reaction
(1996): Roberts HJ, *Arch Intern Med* 156, 1027
Panniculitis
(1992): Geha RS, *J Am Acad Dermatol* 26, 277 (lobular)
(1991): McCauliffe DP+, *J Am Acad Dermatol* 24, 298 (lobular)
(1985): Novick NL, *Ann Intern Med* 102, 206 (granulomatous)

***Note:** Aspartame can be found in instant breakfasts, breath mints, cereals, sugar-free chewing gum, cocoa mixes, coffee beverages, frozen desserts, gelatin desserts, juice beverages, laxatives, multivitamins, milk drinks, pharmaceuticals and supplements, shake mixes, soft drinks, tabletop sweeteners, tea beverages, instant teas and coffees, topping mixes, wine coolers, yogurt.

ASPIRIN

Synonyms: acetylsalicylic acid; ASA
Trade names: Aggrenox (Boehringer Ingelheim); Alka-Seltzer; Anacin; Ascriptin; Aspergum; Bufferin; Coricidin D; Darvon Compound; Ecotrin; Empirin; Equagesic; Excedrin; Fiorinal; Gelprin; Halfprin; Measurin; Norgesic; Percodan; Robaxisal; Soma Compound; Talwin Compound; Vanquish; etc. (Various pharmaceutical companies.)
Other common trade names: *ASA; ASS; Aspro; Bex; Caprin; Claragine; Disprin; Ecotrin; Novasen; Rhonal; etc.*
Indications: Pain, fever, inflammation
Category: Nonsteroidal anti-inflammatory (NSAID) analgesic; salicylate
Half-life: 15–20 minutes
Clinically important, potentially serious interactions with: acetohexamide, acetazolamide, alcohol, anticoagulants, heparin, hypoglycemics, insulin, methotrexate, NSAIDs, phenytoin, valproic acid, warfarin

Aggrenox is aspirin and dipyridamole

Reactions

Skin

Acute generalized exanthematous pustulosis (AGEP)
(1993): Ballmer-Weber BK+, *Schweiz Med Wochenschr (German)* 123, 542
Allergic reactions (sic) (<1%) (with dipyridamole)
Angioedema (1–5%)
(2000): Wong JT+, *J Allergy Clin Immunol* 105, 997
(2000): Pradalier A+, *Rev Med Interne* (French) 21, 75
(1998): Quiralte J, *Ann Allergy Asthma Immunol* 81, 459 (periorbital)
(1998): Grzelewska-Rzymowska I, *Pol Merkuriusz Lek* (Polish) 4, 233
(1997): Tomaz EM+, *Allergy Asthma Proc* 18, 319
(1996): Chan TY, *Br J Clin Pract* 50, 412
(1993): Grzelewska-Rzymowska I+, *Pneumonol Alergol Pol* (Polish) 61, 29
(1988): Botey J+, *Allergol Immunopathol Madr* (Spanish) 16, 43
(1984): Botey J+, *Ann Allergy* 53, 265
(1981): Juhlin L, *Br J Dermatol* 104, 369
(1977): Abrishami MA+, *Ann Allergy* 39, 28
(1977): Szczeklik A+, *J Allergy Clin Immunol* 60, 276
(1974): Schlumberger HD+, *Acta Med Scand* 196, 451
(1972): Kauppinen K, *Acta Derm Venereol* (Stockh) 52 (Suppl) 68
(1970): Baker H+, *Br J Dermatol* 82, 319
(1969): Girard JP+, *Helv Med Acta* 35, 86
(1967): Moore-Robinson M+, *BMJ* 4, 263
Bullous eruption (<1%)
(1972): Kauppinen K, *Acta Derm Venereol* (Stockh) 52 (Suppl) 68
(1960): Hejier A+, *Acta Derm Venereol* (Stockh) 40, 35
Dermatitis herpetiformis
(1966): Brannen M+, *Tex State J Med* 62, 58
Dermatomyositis
(1964): Shelley WB, *JAMA* 189, 986
Diaphoresis
Erythema multiforme (<1%)
(1998): Lee SG+, *Eur J Dermatol* 8, 280
(1985): Ting HC+, *Int J Dermatol* 24, 587
(1982): Bailin PL+, *Clin Rheum Dis* 8, 493 (passim)
(1977): Davis JD+, *Clin Pharm Ther* 21, 52

(1975): Bottiger LE+, *Acta Med Scand* 198, 229
(1968): Bianchine JR+, *Am Med J* 44, 390
(1966): Brannen M+, *Tex State J Med* 62, 58
(1960): Hejier A+, *Acta Derm Venereol* (Stockh) 40, 35

Erythema nodosum (<1%)
(1994): Fernandes NC+, *Rev Inst Med Trop Sao Paulo* (Portuguese) 36, 507
(1982): Bailin PL+, *Clin Rheum Dis* 8, 493 (passim)
(1970): Baker H+, *Br J Dermatol* 82, 319
(1966): Brannen M+, *Tex State J Med* 62, 58
(1964): Shelley WB, *JAMA* 189, 985

Erythroderma
(1974): Tay C, *Asian J Med* 10, 223

Exanthems
(1989): Hass WK+, *N Engl J Med* 321, 501 (5.2%)
(1982): Morley PA+, *Drugs* 23, 250 (5%)
(1987): Castles JJ+, *Arch Intern Med* 138, 362 (2.8%)
(1977): Chalem F+, *Curr Ther Res* 22, 769
(1977): Davis JD+, *Clin Pharm Ther* 21, 52 (1–5%)
(1975): Bowers DE+, *Ann Intern Med* 83, 470 (18%)
(1975): Blechman WJ+, *JAMA* 233, 336 (2.5%)
(1972): Kauppinen K, *Acta Derm Venereol* (Stockh) 52 (Suppl) 68
(1960): Hejier A+, *Acta Derm Venereol* (Stockh) 40, 35

Exfoliative dermatitis
(1969): Girard JP+, *Helv Med Acta* 35, 86

Fixed eruption (<1%)
(1997): Bhargava P+, *Int J Dermatol* 36, 236
(1992): Hatzis J+, *Cutis* 50, 50
(1991): Thankappen TP+, *Int J Dermatol* 30, 867 (1.7%)
(1990): Gaffoor PMA+, *Cutis* 45, 242
(1990): Bharija SC+, *Dermatologica* 181, 237
(1989): Shiohara T+, *Arch Dermatol* 125, 1371
(1986): Kanwar AJ, *Dermatologica* 172, 315
(1985): Kauppinen K+, *Br J Dermatol* 112, 575
(1985): Gomez B+, *Allergol Immunopathol Madr* (Spanish) 13, 87
(1984): Boyle J+, *Br Med J Clin Res Ed* 289, 802
(1984): Chan HL, *Int J Dermatol* 23, 607
(1982): Bailin PL+, *Clin Rheum Dis* 8, 493 (passim)
(1981): Shukla SR, *Dermatologica* 163, 160
(1975): Gimenez-Camarasa JM+, *N Engl J Med* 292, 819
(1974): Kuokkanen K, *Int J Dermatol* 13, 4
(1972): Kauppinen K, *Acta Derm Venereol* (Stockh) 52 (Suppl) 68
(1970): Savin JA, *Br J Dermatol* 83, 546

Flushing
(1964): Shelley WB, *JAMA* 189, 986

Genital herpes
(1964): Shelley WB, *JAMA* 189, 986

Graft-versus-host reaction
(1998): Jappe U+, *Hautarzt* (German) 49, 126 (passim)

Jitters (sic)

Lichenoid eruption
(1988): Bharija SC+, *Dermatologica* 177, 19
(1966): Brannen M+, *Tex State J Med* 62, 58

Parapsoriasis
(1966): Brannen M+, *Tex State J Med* 62, 58

Pemphigus
(1986): Pisani M+, *G Ital Dermatol Venereol* (Italian) 121, 39

Periorbital edema
(1993): Katz Y+, *Allergy* 48, 366
(1997): Price KS+, *Ann Allergy Asthma Immunol* 79, 420

Petechiae
(1997): Blumenthal HL, Beachwood, OH, personal case (observation)

Photo-recall
(1998): Lee SG+, *Eur J Dermatol* 8, 280

Pigmented purpuric eruption
(1999): Lipsker D+, *Ann Dermatol Venereol* (French) 126, 321

Pityriasis rosea
(1993): Yosipovitch G+, *Harefuah* (Hebrew) 124, 198; 247
(1966): Brannen M+, *Tex State J Med* 62, 58

Pruritus
(1981): Settipane GA, *Arch Intern Med* 141, 328
(1977): Chalem F+, *Curr Ther Res* 22, 769 (1–5%)
(1977): Davis JD+, *Clin Pharm Ther* 21, 52 (>5%)
(1975): Blechman WJ+, *JAMA* 233, 336 (2%)
(1969): Girard JP+, *Helv Med Acta* 35, 86
(1967): Moore-Robinson M+, *BMJ* 4, 263

Psoriasis
(1966): Brannen M+, *Tex State J Med* 62, 58
(1964): Shelley WB, *JAMA* 189, 986

Purpura
(1997): Sola-Alberich R+, *Ann Intern Med* 126, 665
(1989): Hass WK+, *N Engl J Med* 321, 501 (2%)
(1980): Miescher PA+, *Clin Haematol* 9, 505
(1976): Karchmer AW+, *N Engl J Med* 295, 451
(1972): Kauppinen K, *Acta Derm Venereol* (Stockh) 52 (Suppl) 68
(1971): Davis SL+, *Nebraska St Med J* 56, 432

Pustular psoriasis
(1976): Lindgren S+, *Acta Derm Venereol* (Stockh) 56, 139
(1964): Shelley WB, *JAMA* 189, 985

Rash (sic) (1–10%)

Stevens–Johnson syndrome
(1993): Leenutaphong V+, *Int J Dermatol* 32, 428
(1968): Bianchine JR+, *Am Med J* 44, 390
(1966): Brannen M+, *Tex State J Med* 62, 58

Toxic epidermal necrolysis (<1%)
(1993): Leenutaphong V+, *Int J Dermatol* 32, 428
(1988): Dahle MG, *Tidsskr Nor Laegeforen* (Norwegian) 108, 1917
(1987): Guillaume JC+, *Arch Dermatol* 123, 1166
(1970): Ocheret'ko MP, *Pediatriia* (Russian) 49, 86
(1967): Lyell A, *Br J Dermatol* 79, 662
(1967): Lowney ED+, *Arch Dermatol* 95, 359

Ulceration (<1%) (with dipyridamole)

Urticaria (1–10%)
(2000): Wong JT+, *J Allergy Clin Immunol* 105, 997
(2000): Pradalier A+, *Rev Med Interne* (French) 21, 75
(1998): Ohnishi-Inoue Y+, *Br J Dermatol* 138, 483
(1998): Grzelewska-Rzymowska I, *Pol Merkuriusz Lek* (Polish) 4, 233
(1997): Tomaz EM+, *Allergy Asthma Proc* 18, 319
(1995): Grzelewska-Rzymowska I+, *J Invest Allergol Clin Immunol* 5, 272
(1995): Gebhardt M+, *Z Rheumatol* (German) 54, 405
(1994): Paul E+, *Hautarzt* (German) 45, 12
(1994): Smith RJ+, *Br J Dermatol* 131, 583
(1993): Grzelewska-Rzymowska I+, *Pneumonol Alergol Pol* (Polish) 61, 29
(1992): Grzelewska-Rzymowska I+, *J Invest Alergol Clin Immunol* 2, 39
(1989): Alanko K+, *Acta Derm Venereol* (Stockh) 69, 223 (1–5%)
(1989): Grzelewska-Rzymowska I, *Allergol Immunopathol Madr* (Spanish) 16, 231
(1989): Hass WK+, *N Engl J Med* 321, 501 (0.3%)
(1988): Botey J+, *Allergol Immunopathol Madr* (Spanish) 16, 43
(1987): Asad SI+, *Ann Allergy* 59, 219
(1986): Finzi AF+, *Minerva Med* (Italian) 77, 1401
(1986): Wojnerowicz-*Grajewska M+*, *Przegl Dermatol* (Polish) 73, 115
(1986): Dupont C, *Int J Dermatol* 25, 334
(1984): Kauppinen K+, *Allergy* 39, 469
(1984): Botey J+, *Ann Allergy* 53, 265
(1983): Kaplan AP, *Postgrad Med* 74, 209
(1982): Kirchhof B+, *Dermatol Monatsschr* (German) 168, 513
(1981): Juhlin L, *Br J Dermatol* 104, 369
(1981): Settipane GA, *Arch Intern Med* 141, 328
(1980): Wuthrich B+, *Z Hautkr* (German) 55, 102
(1980): Settipane RA+, *Allergy* 35, 149
(1978): Hofmann C+, *Munch Med Wochenschr* (German) 120, 65
(1977): Doeglas HM, *Dermatologica* 154, 308
(1977): Rudzki E, *Przegl Dermatol* (Polish) 64, 163
(1977): Szczeklik A+, *J Allergy Clin Immunol* 60, 276
(1977): Abrishami MA+, *Ann Allergy* 39, 28
(1977): Chalem F+, *Curr Ther Res* 22, 769
(1976): Stubb S, *Acta Derm Venereol* (Stockh) 56 (Suppl 76), 16
(1976): Ros AM+, *Br J Dermatol* 95, 19
(1975): Doeglas HM, *Br J Dermatol* 93, 135
(1975): Blechman WJ+, *JAMA* 233, 336 (0.5%)
(1974): Schlumberger HD+, *Acta Med Scand* 196, 451
(1973): Samter M, *Hosp Pract* 8, 85
(1972): Kauppinen K, *Acta Derm Venereol* (Stockh) 52 (Suppl) 68
(1971): Davis SL+, *Nebraska St Med J* 56, 432
(1970): Baker H+, *Br J Dermatol* 82, 319
(1970): James J+, *Br J Dermatol* 82, 204
(1970): Naess K, *Tidsskr Nor Laegeforen* (Norwegian) 90, 112
(1969): Champion RH+, *Br J Dermatol* 81, 588
(1969): Girard JP+, *Helv Med Acta* 35, 86
(1967): Moore-Robinson M+, *BMJ* 4, 262
(1966): Brannen M+, *Tex State J Med* 62, 58
(1960): Warin RP, *Br J Dermatol* 72, 350
(1960): Hejier A+, *Acta Derm Venereol* (Stockh) 40, 35

Vasculitis
(1999): Crutchfield CE+, *Skin and Aging* May, 84 (leukocytoclastic)
(1984): Ekenstam E+, *Arch Dermatol* 120, 484
(1971): Meszaros C, *Börgyogy Vener Sz* (Hungarian) 47, 20

Hair

Hair – alopecia
(1968): Rawnsley HM+, *Lancet* 1, 561

Other

Ageusia (< 1%) (with dipyridamole)
Anaphylactoid reaction (1–10%)
(1984): Stevenson DD, *J Allergy Clin Immunol* 74, 617
Aphthous stomatitis
(1982): Bailin PL+, *Clin Rheum Dis* 8, 493 (passim)
(1966): Brannen M+, *Tex State J Med* 62, 58
Dysgeusia
Gingival bleeding (< 1%) (with dipyridamole)
Granulomata
(1982): Cozzutto C+, *Virchows Arch A Pathol Anat Histol* 397, 61
Myalgia (1.2%) (with dipyridamole)
Oral lichen planus
(1989): Espana-Alonso A+, *An Med Interna* (Spanish) 6, 219
Oral burn (sic)
(1998): Dellinger TM+, *Ann Pharmacother* 32, 1107
Oral mucosal eruption
(1988): Bork K, *Cutaneous Side Effects of Drugs*, WB Saunders, 283
(1966): Brannen M+, *Tex State J Med* 62, 58
(1964): Shelley WB, *JAMA* 189, 986
Oral ulceration
(1975): Kawashima Z+, *JADA* 91, 130
(1974): Glick GL+, *N Y St Dent J* 40, 475
(1970): Baker H+, *Br J Dermatol* 82, 319
(1967): Claman HN, *JAMA* 202, 651
Paresthesias (< 1%) (with dipyridamole)

ASTEMIZOLE*

Trade name: Hismanal (Janssen)
Other common trade names: *Adistan; Alestol; Astemina; Astimal; Astizol; Histamen; Pollon-Eze; Simprox; Stemiz*
Indications: Urticaria, allergic rhinitis
Category: Histamine H_1-receptor antagonist; non-sedating antihistamine
Half-life: 0.9–2.3 days
Clinically important, potentially serious interactions with: amiodarone, azithromycin, bepridil, bretylium, clarithromycin, disopyramide, diuretics, erythromycin, fluconazole, fluoxetine, fluvoxamine, indinavir, itraconazole, ketoconazole, metronidazole, miconazole, nefazodone, probucol, procainamide, protease inhibitors, quinidine, quinine, ritonavir, saquinavir, sotalol, SSRIs, terfenadine, troleandomycin, zileuton, **grapefruit juice**

Reactions

Skin

Angioedema (< 1%)
Dermatitis (sic)
(1984): Richards DM+, *Drugs* 28, 38
Eczema (sic)
(1983): Janssen Pharmaceutica, unpublished study
Edema (< 1%)
(1996): Berkowitz RB+, *Ann Allergy Asthma Immunol* 76, 363 (eyelid)
(1985): Wilson W+, Clinical, unpublished study
Exanthems (1.2%)
(1984): Richards DM+, *Drugs* 28, 38
Photosensitivity (< 1%)
(1996): Berkowitz RB+, *Ann Allergy Asthma Immunol* 76, 363
Pityriasis lichenoides et varioliformis acuta (PLEVA)
(1993): Stosiek N+, *Hautarzt* (German) 44, 235
Pruritus
(1985): Wilson W+, Clinical, unpublished study
(1984): *The Medicine Publishing Foundation*, Oxford, 63
(1983): Pattyn J+, Clinical, unpublished study
(1983): Bateman DN+, *European J Clin Pharmacol* 25, 547
Rash (sic) (< 1%)
(1989): Juniper EF+, *J Allergy Clin Immunol* 83, 627
(1983): D'Souza M+, Clinical, unpublished study
(1983): Pattyn J, Clinical, unpublished study
(1983): Janssen Pharmaceutica, unpublished study
Stevens–Johnson syndrome
(1995): Cunliffe NA+, *Postgrad Med J* 71, 383
Urticaria
(1983): Bateman DN+, *European J Clin Pharmacol* 25, 547

Hair

Hair – alopecia
(1987): Kailasam V+, *J Am Acad Dermatol* 16, 797
Hair – color change (sic)
(1989): Huerter CJ+, *Cleve Clin J Med* 56, 263

Other

Anaphylactoid reaction
Dysgeusia
(1987): Kailasam V+, *J Am Acad Dermatol* 16, 797
Myalgia (< 1%)
Oral mucosal eruption (5–15%)
(1984): Richards DM+, *Drugs* 28, 38
Paresthesias (< 1%)
(1990): Kaufman HS+, *N Engl J Med* 323, 684
(1988): Oei HD, *Ann Allergy* 61, 436
Sore nipples (sic)
(1989): Huerter CJ+, *Cleve Clin J Med* 56, 263
Xerostomia (5.2%)
(1995): Breneman D+, *J Am Acad Dermatol* 33, 192
(1991): Humphreys F+, *Br J Dermatol* 125, 364
(1989): Juniper EF+, *J Allergy Clin Immunol* 83, 627
(1984): Richards DM+, *Drugs* 28, 38
(1983): D'Souza M+, Clinical, unpublished study
(1983): Pattyn J+, Clinical, unpublished study

***Note:** Astemizole has been withdrawn in the USA as of 1999

ATENOLOL

Trade names: Tenormin (AstraZeneca); Tenoretic (AstraZeneca)
Other common trade names: *Antipressan; Apo-Atenol; AteHexal; Atendol; Evitocor; Noten; Novo-Atenol; Nu-Atenol; Taro-Atenol; Tenolin; Tenormine*
Indications: Angina, hypertension, acute myocardial infarction
Category: Beta-adrenergic blocker; antianginal; antihypertensive
Half-life: 6–7 hours (adults)
Clinically important, potentially serious interactions with: ampicillin, calcium channel blockers, ciprofloxacin, clonidine, diltiazem, flecainide, hydralazine, nifedipine, NSAIDs, oral contraceptives, prazosin, quinidine, reserpine, verapamil

Tenoretic is atenolol and chlorthalidone

Reactions

Skin

Acrocyanosis
(1987): Naeyaert JM+, *Br J Dermatol* 117, 371
Dermatitis (sic)
(1979): Harrison PV+, *Clin Exp Dermatol* 4, 547
Diaphoresis
Edema
Erythema multiforme
Exanthems
Facial edema
Fixed eruption
(1999): Palungwachira P+, *J Med Assoc Thai* 82, 1158
Grinspan's syndrome*
(1990): Lamey PJ+, *Oral Surg Oral Med Oral Pathol* 70, 184
Hyperkeratosis (palms and soles)
Lichenoid eruption
(1978): Savage RL+, *BMJ* 1, 987

Lupus erythematosus
(1997): McGuiness M+, *J Am Acad Dermatol* 37, 298
(1986): Gouet D+, *J Rheumatol* 13, 446
Necrosis
(1979): Rees PJ, *BMJ* 1, 955
(1979): Gokal R+, *BMJ* 1, 721
(1977): Simpson WT, *Postgrad Med J* 53, 162
Papular and nodular eruption
(1992): Shelley WB+, *Cutis* 50, 87 (observation)
Photosensitivity
Pityriasis rubra pilaris
(1978): Finlay AY+, *BMJ* 1, 987
Pruritus (1–5%)
Psoriasis
(1990): Wolf R, *Dermatologica* 181, 51
(1990): Wakefield PL+, *Arch Dermatol* 126, 968 (exacerbation)
(1988): Gold MH+, *J Am Acad Dermatol* 19, 837
(1988): Heng MCY+, *Int J Dermatol* 27, 619
(1986): Abel EA+, *J Am Acad Dermatol* 15, 1007
(1984): Gawkrodger DJ+, *Clin Exp Dermatol* 9, 92
Purpura
Pustular psoriasis
(1990): Wakefield PE+, *Arch Dermatol* 126, 968
Rash (sic)
(1987): Bolzano K+, *J Cardiovasc Pharmacol* 9 (Suppl 3), S43
Raynaud's phenomenon
(1976): Marshall AJ+, *BMJ* 1, 1498 (35%)
Toxic epidermal necrolysis
Urticaria
(1989): Wolf R+, *Cutis* 43, 231
(1988): Howard PJ+, *Scott Med J* 33, 344
Vasculitis
(1989): Wolf R+, *Cutis* 43, 231
Vitiligo
Xerosis

Hair

Hair – alopecia
(1991): Shelley WB+, *Cutis* 48, 368 (observation)

Nails

Nails – bluish
Nails – dystrophy
Nails – onycholysis
Nails – splinter hemorrhages
(1987): Naeyaert JM+, *Br J Dermatol* 117, 371

Other

Anaphylactoid reaction
(1988): Howard PJ+, *Scott Med J* 33, 344
Oculo-mucocutaneous syndrome
(1982): Cocco G+, *Curr Ther Res* 31, 362
Oral lichenoid eruption
(1990): Lamey PJ+, *Oral Surg Oral Med Oral Pathol* 70, 184
Peyronie's disease
Pseudolymphoma
(1990): Henderson CA+, *Clin Exp Dermatol* 15, 119

***Note:** Grinspan's syndrome: the triad of oral lichen planus, diabetes mellitus, and hypertension.

ATORVASTATIN

Trade name: Lipitor (Parke-Davis; Pfizer)
Indications: Hypercholesterolemia
Category: HMG-CoA reductase inhibitor; antihyperlipidemic
Half-life: 14 hours
Clinically important, potentially serious interactions with: anticoagulants, azole antifungals, clofibrate, cyclosporine, digoxin, erythromycin, gemfibrozil, itraconazole, niacin, oral contraceptives, warfarin

Reactions

Skin

Acne (<2%)
Allergic reactions (<2%)
Cheilitis (<2%)
Contact dermatitis (<2%)
Diaphoresis (<2%)
Ecchymoses (<2%)
Eczema (sic) (<2%)
Edema (<2%)
Exanthems
Facial edema (<2%)
Flu-like syndrome (sic)
Lichenoid eruption
(1998): Silver B, Deerfield, Il (from Internet) (observation)
Petechiae (<2%)
Photosensitivity (<2%)
Pruritus (<2%)
Rash (sic) (>3%)
Seborrhea (<2%)
Toxic epidermal necrolysis
(1998): Pfeiffer CM+, *JAMA* 279, 1613
Ulceration (<2%)
Urticaria (<2%)
Xerosis (<2%)

Hair

Hair – alopecia (<2%)
(1999): Oakley A, Hamilton, New Zealand (from Internet) (observation)
(1997): Litt JZ, Beachwood, OH, personal case (observation)

Other

Ageusia (<2%)
Dysgeusia (<2%)
Glossitis (<2%)
Gynecomastia (<2%)
Myalgia (>3%)
(1998): Malinowski JM, *Am J Health Syst Pharm* 55, 2253
Oral ulceration (<2%)
Paresthesias (<2%)
Parosmia (<2%)
Stomatitis (<2%)

ATOVAQUONE

Trade name: Mepron (GlaxoWellcome)
Other common trade name: *Wellvone*
Indications: *Pneumocystis carinii* infection
Category: Antiprotozoal
Half-life: 2.2–2.9 days
Clinically important, potentially serious interactions with: rifampin, zidovudine. Also **high fat content food**

Reactions

Skin

Diaphoresis (10%)
Erythema multiforme

Exanthems
(1993): Haile LG+, *Ann Pharmacother* 27, 1488
Pruritus (11%)
(1996): Radloff PD+, *Lancet* 347, 1511
Rash (sic) (23%)
(1993): Artymowicz RJ+, *Clin Pharm* 12, 563

Other

Dysgeusia (3%)
Oral candidiasis (1–10%)

ATRACURIUM

Trade name: Tracrium (GlaxoWellcome)
Indications: Neuromuscular blockade, endotracheal intubation
Category: Neuromuscular blocking agent; skeletal muscle relaxant
Half-life: initial: 2 minutes; terminal: 20 minutes
Clinically important, potentially serious interactions with: aminoglycosides, antibiotics, calcium channel blockers, cisplatin, corticosteroids, cyclosporine, diuretics, procainamide, quinidine, succinylcholine

Reactions

Skin

Allergic reactions (sic)
(1985): Aldrete JA, *Br J Anaesth* 57, 929
(1983): Mirakhur RK+, *Anaesthesia* 38, 818
Edema
Erythema (<1%)
Flushing (1–10%)
Pruritus (<1%)
Urticaria (<1%)

Other

Injection-site reaction

ATROPINE SULFATE

Trade names*: Belladenal; Bellergal-S; Butibel; Donnagel; Donnatal; Donnazyme; Hycodan; Isopto Atropine; Lofene; Logen; Lomanate; Lomotil; Urised; etc. (Various pharmaceutical companies.)
Other common trade names: *Atropine Martinet; Atropt; Chibro-Atropine; Isopto; Tropyn Z; Vitatropine*
Indications: Salivation, sinus bradycardia, uveitis, peptic ulcer
Category: Anticholinergic and antispasmodic
Half-life: 2–3 hours
Clinically important, potentially serious interactions with: amantadine, anticholinergics, atenolol, digoxin, haloperidol, phenothiazines, thiazides

Reactions

Skin

Allergic reactions (sic)
(1997): Moyano P+, *Rev Esp Anestesiol Reanim* (Spanish) 44, 290
Bullous eruption
(1967): Coleman WP, *Med Clin North Am* 51, 1073
Contact dermatitis
(1988): Gutierrez-Ortega MC+, *Med Cutan Ibero Lat Am* (Spanish) 16, 430
(1987): van der Willigen AH+, *Contact Dermatitis* 17, 56 (periocular)
(1985): Yoshikama K+, *Contact Dermatitis* 12, 56
(1982): Gallasch G+, *Klin Monatsbl Augenheilkd* (German) 181, 96 (periocular)
Eccrine hidrocystomas
(1992): Masri-Fridling GD+, *J Am Acad Dermatol* 26, 780
Erythema multiforme (<1%)
(1979): Guill MA, *Arch Dermatol* 115, 742
(1967): Coleman WP, *Med Clin North Am* 51, 1073
Exanthems
Exfoliative dermatitis
(1955): Alexander HL, *Reactions with Drug Therapy*, Saunders, Philadelphia
Eyelid edema
Fixed eruption
(1961): Welsh AL, *The Fixed Eruption*, Thomas, Springfield
Flushing
(1992): Amitai Y+, *JAMA* 268, 630
Hypohidrosis (>10%)
Photosensitivity (1–10%)
Pruritus
Rash (sic) (<1%)
Sheet-like erythema
Stevens–Johnson syndrome
(1967): Coleman WP, *Med Clin North Am* 51, 1073
Urticaria
(1986): Bigby M+, *JAMA* 256, 3358
Xerosis

Other

Dry mucous membranes (sic)
(1992): Amitai Y+, *JAMA* 268, 630
Dysgeusia
Injection-site irritation (>10%)
Tremor
Xerostomia (>10%)

***Note:** Many of the above trade name drugs contain phenobarbital, scopolamine, hyoscyamine, hydrocodone, methenamine, etc.

AURANOFIN

(See GOLD)

AUROTHIOGLUCOSE

(See GOLD)

AZATADINE

Trade names: Rynatan (Wallace); Trinalin (Key)
Other common trade names: *Idulamine; Idulian; Lergocil; Nalomet; Verben; Zadine*
Indications: Allergic rhinitis, urticaria
Category: H_1-receptor antihistamine
Half-life: 9 hours
Clinically important, potentially serious interactions with: alcohol, MAO inhibitors, procarbazine, tricyclic antidepressants

Reactions

Skin

Angioedema (<1%)
Diaphoresis
Edema (<1%)
Exanthems
Flushing
Photosensitivity (<1%)
Purpura
Rash (sic) (<1%)
Urticaria

Other

Myalgia (<1%)
Paresthesias (<1%)
Xerostomia (1–10%)
(1990): Small P+, *Ann Allergy* 64, 129

AZATHIOPRINE

Trade name: Imuran (Faro)
Other common trade names: *Azamedac; Azamune; Azatrilem; Imuprin, Imurek; Imurel; Thioprine*
Indications: Lupus nephritis, psoriatic arthritis, rheumatoid arthritis, autoimmune diseases, kidney transplant patients
Category: Immunosuppressant and antineoplastic
Half-life: 12 minutes
Clinically important, potentially serious interactions with: ACE-inhibitors, allopurinol, carbamazepine, chlorambucil, clozapine, co-trimoxazole, cyclophosphamide, methotrexate, phenothiazines, zidovudine

Reactions

Skin

Acanthosis nigricans
(1980): L'Eplattenier JL+, *Schweiz Med Wochenschr* (German) 110, 1307 (0.5%)
(1974): Koranda FC+, *JAMA* 229, 419 (10%)
Acne
(1983): Schmoeckel C+, *Hautarzt* (German) 34, 413
Allergic reactions (sic)
(1996): Parnham AP+, *Lancet* 348, 542
Angioedema
(1988): Saway PA+, *Am J Med* 84, 960 (passim)
Cancer (sic)
(1992): Taylor AE+, *Acta Derm Venereol* 72, 115
Chills (>10%)
Contact dermatitis
(1996): Soni BP+, *Am J Contact Dermat* 7, 116
(1992): Burden AD+, *Contact Dermatitis* 27, 329
Cutaneous infections (sic)
(1978): Bergfeld WF+, *Cutis* 22, 169 (62%)
(1974): Koranda FC+, *JAMA* 229, 419 (>5%)
(1973): Haim S+, *Br J Dermatol* 89, 169 (100%)
Erythema multiforme
(1995): Knowles SR+, *Clin Exp Dermatol* 20, 353 (passim)
(1988): Saway PA+, *Am J Med* 84, 960 (passim)
Erythema nodosum
(1995): Knowles SR+, *Clin Exp Dermatol* 20, 353 (passim)
(1988): Saway PA+, *Am J Med* 84, 960 (passim)
Exanthems (<1%)
(1995): Knowles SR+, *Clin Exp Dermatol* 20, 353 (passim)
(1990): Jeurissen ME+, *Ann Rheum Dis* 49, 25 (4%)
(1988): Bergman SM+, *Ann Intern Med* 109, 83
(1988): Saway PA+, *Am J Med* 84, 960
(1978): Franchmont P+, *J Rheumatol* 5 (Suppl 4), 85 (5.4%)
(1972): King JO+, *Med J Aust* 2, 939
(1972): Decker JL, *Ann Intern Med* 76, 619
(1971): Harris J+, *BMJ* 4, 463 (1–5%)
(1969): Mason M+, *BMJ* 1, 420 (1–5%)
(1967): Adams DA+, *JAMA* 199, 459
Fixed eruption
(1990): Black AK+, *Br J Dermatol* 123, 277 (observation)
Fungal infection
(1980): L'Eplattenier JL+, *Schweiz Med Wochenschr* (German) 110, 1307 (42%)
Herpes simplex
(1980): L'Eplattenier JL+, *Schweiz Med Wochenschr* (German) 110, 1307 (27%)
(1979): Spencer ES+, *BMJ* 2, 829
(1974): Koranda FC+, *JAMA* 229, 419 (35%)
Herpes zoster
(1991): Callen JP+, *Arch Dermatol* 127, 515
(1982): Speerstra F+, *Ann Rheum Dis* 41, Suppl 37
(1980): L'Eplattenier JL+, *Schweiz Med Wochenschr* (German) 110, 1307 (27%)
(1974): Koranda FC+, *JAMA* 229, 419 (13%)
(1966): Rifkind D, *J Lab Clin Med* 68, 463 (8%)
Kaposi's sarcoma
(1997): Aebischer MC+, *Dermatology* 195, 91
(1997): Vandercam B+, *Dermatology* 194, 180
(1997): Halpern SM+, *Br J Dermatol* 137, 140
(1997): Lesnoni-La-Parola I+, *Dermatology* 194, 229
(1996): Ozen S+, *Nephrol Dial Transplant* 11, 1162
(1991): Almog Y+, *Clin Exp Dermatol* 9, 285
(1984): Luderschmidt C+, *Klin Wochenschr* (German) 62, 803
(1982): Weiss VC+, *Arch Dermatol* 118, 183
(1980): Iversen OH+, *Scand J Urol Nephrol* 14, 125
(1974): Faye I+, *Bull Soc Fr Dermatol Syphiligr* (French) 81, 379
(1973): Haim S+, *Br J Dermatol* 89, 169
Keratoacanthoma
(1971): Walder BK+, *Lancet* 2, 1282
Lichenoid eruption
(1979): Beaaff D+, *Arch Dermatol* 115, 498
Pellagra
(1996): Oakley A, Hamilton, New Zealand (from Internet) (observation)
Photosensitivity
Pigmentation (sun-exposed skin)
(1974): Koranda FC+, *JAMA* 229, 419 (37%)
Porokeratosis
(1997): Matsushita S+, *J Dermatol* 24, 110 (disseminated superficial actinic)
(1988): Neumann RA+, *Br J Dermatol* 119, 375 (disseminated superficial actinic)
(1987): Tatnall FM+, *J R Soc Med* 80, 180 (Mibelli)
(1974): Macmillan AL+, *Br J Dermatol* 90, 45
Purpura
Pyoderma gangrenosum
(1976): Haim S+, *Dermatologica* 153, 44
Rash (sic) (1–10%)
(1997): Lavaud F+, *Dig Dis Sci* 42, 823
(1990): Jeurissen ME+, *Ann Rheum Dis* 49, 25
(1975): Goldenberg DL+, *J Rheumatol* 2, 346
(1972): King JO+, *Med J Aust* 2, 939
Raynaud's phenomenon
Sarcoma
(1996): Csuka ME+, *Arch Intern Med* 156, 1573
Scabies
(1980): L'Eplattenier JL+, *Schweiz Med Wochenschr* (German) 110, 1307 (1%)
(1978): Bricklin AS+, *Cutis* 22, 81
(1976): Anolik MA+, *Arch Dermatol* 112, 73
(1973): Paterson WD+, *BMJ* 4, 211
Scleroderma
(1993): Choy E+, *Br J Rheumatol* 32, 160
Skin peeling syndrome (sic)
(1997): Hermanns-Le T+, *Dermatology* 194, 175
Squamous cell carcinoma
(1995): Bottomley WW+, *Br J Dermatol* 133, 460
(1993): Nachbar F+, *Acta Derm Venereol* 73, 217
(1992): McCain J, *Nurs Pract* 17, 13
(1988): Krickeberg H, *Z Hautkr* (German) 63, 773
(1973): Westburg SP+, *Arch Dermatol* 107, 893
(1971): Walder BK+, *Lancet* 2, 1282
Tinea corporis
(1980): L'Eplattenier JL+, *Schweiz Med Wochenschr* (German) 110, 1307 (3%)
(1974): Koranda FC+, *JAMA* 229, 419 (2%)
Tinea versicolor
(1981): Burkhart CG+, *Cutis* 27, 56
(1974): Koranda FC+, *JAMA* 229, 419 (18%)
Toxic epidermal necrolysis
(1990): Black AK+, *Br J Dermatol* 123, 277 (observation)
Tumors (sic)
(1986): Gupta AK+, *Arch Dermatol* 122, 1288 (5.3%) (malignant)
(1982): Bailin PL+, *Clin Rheum Dis* 8, 493 (passim)
(1980): L'Eplattenier JL+, *Schweiz Med Wochenschr* (German) 110, 1307 (2.9%) (benign); (4.3%) (malignant)
(1978): Bergfeld WF+, *Cutis* 22, 169 (4.6%) (malignant)
(1974): Koranda FC+, *JAMA* 229, 419 (3.5%) (malignant)
(1973): Westburg SP+, *Arch Dermatol* 107, 893
(1973): Wishart J, *Arch Dermatol* 108, 563 (reticulosarcoma)
(1971): Walder BK+, *Lancet* 2, 1282 (>5%) (malignant)
Urticaria
(1995): Knowles SR+, *Clin Exp Dermatol* 20, 353 (passim)
(1990): Wijnands MJ+, *Scand J Rheumatol* 19, 167
(1988): Saway PA+, *Am J Med* 84, 960 (passim)
(1972): Decker JL, *Ann Intern Med* 76, 619

(1970): Drinkard JP+, *Medicine* (Baltimore) 49, 411

Vasculitis
  (1995): Knowles SR+, *Clin Exp Dermatol* 20, 353 (passim)
  (1995): Blanco R+, *Arthritis Rheum* 39, 1016
  (1988): Bergman SM+, *Ann Intern Med* 109, 83

Viral infections
  (1980): L'Eplattenier JL+, *Schweiz Med Wochenschr* (German) 110, 1307 (45%)
  (1974): Koranda FC+, *JAMA* 229, 419 (43%)

Warts
  (1991): Callen JP+, *Arch Dermatol* 127, 515
  (1980): L'Eplattenier JL+, *Schweiz Med Wochenschr* (German) 110, 1307 (21%)

Hair

Hair – alopecia (<1%)
  (1982): Bailin PL+, *Clin Rheum Dis* 8, 493 (passim)
  (1980): L'Eplattenier JL+, *Schweiz Med Wochenschr* (German) 110, 1307 (27%)
  (1974): Koranda FC+, *JAMA* 229, 419 (54%)

Hair – curly
  (1996): van der Pijl JW+, *Lancet* 348, 622 (with isotretinoin)

Nails

Nails – discoloration (red lunulae)
  (1974): Koranda FC+, *JAMA* 229, 419 (2%)

Nails – onychomycosis
  (1980): L'Eplattenier JL+, *Schweiz Med Wochenschr* (German) 110, 1307 (1%)
  (1974): Koranda FC+, *JAMA* 229, 419 (5%)

Other

Anaphylactoid reaction
  (1993): Jones JJ+, *J Am Acad Dermatol* 29, 795

Aphthous stomatitis (<1%)

Formication
  (1992): Shelley WB+, *Advanced Dermatologic Diagnosis*, WB Saunders, 1042 (passim)

Hypersensitivity (<1%)*
  (1999): Korelitz BI+, *J Clin Gastroenterol* 28, 341
  (1998): Schlienger RG+, *Epilepsia* 39, S3 (passim)
  (1998): Fields CL+, *South Med J* 91, 471
  (1998): Garey KW+, *Ann Pharmacother* 32, 425
  (1997): Knowles S+, *Muscle Nerve* 20, 1467
  (1997): Caramaschi P+, *Lupus* 6, 616
  (1996): Compton MR+, *Arch Dermatol* 132, 1254 (with rhabdomyolysis)
  (1995): Knowles SR+, *Clin Exp Dermatol* 20, 353
  (1982): Mosbech H+, *Ugeskr Laeger* (Danish) 144, 2424
  (1975): Goldenberg DL+, *J Rheumatol* 2, 346
  (1972): King JO+, *Med J Aust* 2, 939

Lymphoproliferative disease
  (1987): Pitt PI+, *J R Soc Med* 80, 428
  (1987): Phillips T+, *Clin Exp Dermatol* 12, 444
  (1982): Ulreich A+, *Z Rheumatol* (German) 41, 73

Myalgia (<1%)

Non-Hodgkin's lymphoma
  (2000): Lewis JD+, *Gastroenterology* 118, 1018

Oral ulceration

Rheumatoid nodules
  (1991): Langevitz P+, *Arthritis Rheum* 34, 123

Serum sickness

Stomatitis
  (1982): Bailin PL+, *Clin Rheum Dis* 8, 493 (passim)

Xerostomia

***Note:** The antiepileptic drug hypersensitivity syndrome is a severe, occasionally fatal, disorder characterized by any or all of the following: pruritic exanthem, toxic epidermal necrolysis, Stevens–Johnson syndrome, exfoliative dermatitis, fever, hepatic abnormalities, eosinophilia, and renal failure.

AZELASTINE

Trade name: Astelin (Wallace)
Other common trade names: *Allergodil; Azeptin*
Indications: Allergic rhinitis
Category: Antihistamine; intranasal H_1-blocker
Half-life: 22 hours
Clinically important, potentially serious interactions with: alcohol, cimetidine, CNS depressants

Reactions

Skin

Allergic reactions (sic) (<2%)

Contact dermatitis (<2%)

Eczema (sic) (<2%)

Exanthems
  (1989): McTavish D+, *Drugs* 38, 19

Flushing (<2%)

Folliculitis (<2%)

Furunculosis (<2%)

Herpes simplex (<2%)

Other

Ageusia (<2%)

Aphthous stomatitis (<2%)

Dysgeusia (bitter taste) (19.7%)
  (1993): Davies RJ+, *Rhinology* 31, 159
  (1990): Tinkelman DG+, *Am Rev Respir Dis* 141, 569 (30–52%)
  (1988): Weiler JM+, *J Allergy Clin Immunology* 82, 801 (19.7%)

Glossitis (<2%)

Hypesthesia (<2%)

Mastodynia (<2%)

Myalgia (1.5%)

Oral dryness
  (1989): McTavish D+, *Drugs* 38, 19

Oral mucosal eruption
  (1989): McTavish D+, *Drugs* 38, 19

Stomatitis (ulcerative) (<2%)

Xerostomia (2.8%)
  (1990): Tinkelman DG+, *Am Rev Respir Dis* 141, 569 (4–6%)

AZITHROMYCIN

Trade name: Zithromax (Pfizer)
Other common trade names: *Azenil; Azitrocin; Azitromax; Zeto; Zitromax*
Indications: Infections of the upper and lower respiratory tract, skin infections, sexually-transmitted diseases
Category: Macrolide antibiotic
Half-life: 68 hours
Clinically important, potentially serious interactions with: astemizole, bromocriptine, carbamazepine, cyclosporine, digoxin, disopyramide, loratadine, phenytoin, pimozide, tacrolimus, terfenadine, theophylline, triazolam, warfarin

Reactions

Skin

Allergic granulomatous angiitis (Churg–Strauss syndrome)
  (1998): Dietz A+, *Laryngorhinootologie* (German) 77, 111
  (1997): Kranke B+, *Lancet* 350, 1551

Allergic reactions (sic) (<1%)
  (1998): Salit IE+, *Infect Med* 15, 773 (0.4%)

Angioedema (<1%)

Cutaneous side effects (sic)
  (1993): Hopkins S, *J Antimicrob Chemother* 31 (Suppl E) 111

Diaper rash
  (1997): Arguedas A+, *Infections in Medicine* October, 807

Edema

Erythema
(1991): Felstead SJ+, *J Int Med Res* 19, 363
Exanthems
(2000): Schissel DJ+, *Cutis* 65, 123 (in a patient with infectious mononucleosis)
Facial edema
Fixed eruption
(1999): Smith KC, Niagara Falls, Ontario (from Internet) (observation)
Photosensitivity (1%)
Pruritus
(2000): Schissel DJ+, *Cutis* 65, 123 (in a patient with infectious mononucleosis)
Pustular eruption
(1994): Trevis P+, *Clin Exp Dermatol* 19, 280
Rash (sic) (<1%)
(1991): Hopkins S, *Am J Med* 91, 36s
(1991): Felstead SJ+, *J Int Med Res* 19, 363
Stevens–Johnson syndrome
(1998): Smith KC, Niagara Falls, Ontario (from Internet) (observation)
Toxic pustuloderma
(1994): Trevisi P+, *Clin Exp Dermatol* 19, 280
Urticaria
(1991): Hopkins S, *Am J Med* 91, 36s

Other

Anaphylactoid reaction
Hypersensitivity (0.6%)
(1998): Salit IE+, *Infect Med* 15, 773
Infusion-site erythema
(1997): Luke DR+, *Ann Pharmacother* 31, 965
Infusion-site tenderness
(1997): Luke DR+, *Ann Pharmacother* 31, 965
Vaginitis (2%)
(1991): Hopkins S, *Am J Med* 91, 36s

AZTREONAM

Synonym: azthreonam
Trade name: Azactam (Dura)
Other common trade names: *Primbactam; Urobactam*
Indications: Aerobic gram-negative bacillary infections
Category: Synthetic narrow spectrum antibiotic (monobactam) (parenteral)
Half-life: 1.4–2.2 hours
Clinically important, potentially serious interactions with: cefoxitin, furosemide, imipenem/cilastin, probenecid

Reactions

Skin

Angioedema
(1990): Soto Alvarez J+, *Lancet* 335, 1094
Diaphoresis
Erythema multiforme
(1997): Epstein ME+, *J Am Acad Dermatol* 37, 149 (passim)
Exanthems
(1990): Fekete T+, *Drug Intell Clin Pharm* 24, 438 (1–5%)
(1990): Adkinson NF, *Am J Med* 88 (Suppl 3C), 12S (1.6%)
(1988): Pazmiño P, *Am J Nephrol* 8, 68
(1986): Brogden RN+, *Drugs* 18, 241 (1.8%)
Exfoliative dermatitis
(1997): Epstein ME+, *J Am Acad Dermatol* 37, 149 (passim)
Petechiae
(1997): Epstein ME+, *J Am Acad Dermatol* 37, 149 (passim)
Pruritus
(1997): Epstein ME+, *J Am Acad Dermatol* 37, 149 (passim)
(1990): Adkinson NF, *Am J Med* 88 (Suppl 3C), 12S
(1986): Brogden RN+, *Drugs* 18, 241 (1.8%)
Purpura
(1997): Epstein ME+, *J Am Acad Dermatol* 37, 149 (passim)
(1990): Adkinson NF, *Am J Med 88* (Suppl 3C), 12S (0.1%)
Rash (sic) (1–10%)
(1985): Newman TJ+, *Rev Infect Dis* 7, S648
Toxic epidermal necrolysis
(1997): Epstein ME+, *J Am Acad Dermatol* 37, 149 (passim)
(1992): McDonald BJ+, *Ann Pharmacother* 26, 34
Urticaria
(1997): Epstein ME+, *J Am Acad Dermatol* 37, 149 (passim)
(1993): de la Fuente-Prieto R+, *Allergy* 48, 634
(1991): Hantson P+, *BMJ* 302, 294
(1990): Adkinson NF, *Am J Med* 88 (Suppl 3C), 12S (0.2%)
(1990): Soto Alvarez J+, *Lancet* 335, 1094

Other

Anaphylactoid reaction (<1%)
Aphthous stomatitis (<1%)
Dysgeusia (<1%)
Foetor ex ore (halitosis) (<1%)
Hypersensitivity
Injection-site pain (1–10%)
Injection-site phlebitis (1–10%)
Injection-site reactions
(1985): Newman TJ+, *Rev Infect Dis* 7, S648
Mastodynia (<1%)
Myalgia (<1%)
Oral ulceration (<1%)
Paresthesias
Thrombophlebitis (1–10%)
Tongue numb (sic) (<1%)
Vaginal candidiasis
Vaginitis (<1%)

BACAMPICILLIN

Synonym: carampicillin
Trade name: Spectrobid (Pfizer)
Other common trade names: *Albaxin; Ambacamp; Ambaxin; Bacacil; Bacampicine; Penglobe*
Indications: Respiratory tract infections, urinary tract infections, gonorrhea
Category: Beta-lactamase-sensitive aminopenicillin
Half-life: 65 minutes
Clinically important, potentially serious interactions with: allopurinol, anticoagulants, cyclosporine, disulfiram, oral contraceptives

Reactions

Skin

Acute generalized exanthematous pustulosis (AGEP)
(1990): Guy C+, *Nouv Dermatol* (French) 9, 540
Angioedema
Contact dermatitis
(1986): Stejskal VD+, *J Allergy Clin Immunol* 77, 411
Ecchymoses
Erythema multiforme
Exanthems
(1989): Alanko K+, *Acta Derm Venereol* (Stockh) 69, 223
(1988): Kohl PK+, *Aktuel Dermatol* 14, 104
(1986): Pauwels R+, *J Int Med Res* 14, 110
Exfoliative dermatitis
Fixed eruption
(1984): Chan HL, *Arch Dermatol* 120, 542
Hematomas
Jarisch–Herxheimer reaction
Pruritus
Pustular eruption
(1998): Isogai Z+, *J Dermatol* 25, 612
Rash (sic) (<1%)
Stevens–Johnson syndrome
Urticaria

Other

Anaphylactoid reaction
Black tongue
Dysgeusia
Glossitis
Glossodynia
Hypersensitivity (<1%)
Injection-site pain
Oral candidiasis
Serum sickness
Stomatitis
Stomatodynia
Vaginitis
Xerostomia

BACLOFEN

Trade name: Baclofen (Watson)
Other common trade names: *Alpha-Baclofen; Baclon; Baclosal; Baklofen; Clofen; Dom-Baclofen; Gen-Baclofen; Lebic; Nu-Baclo; Pacifen; PMS-Baclofen; Spinax*
Indications: Spasticity resulting from multiple sclerosis
Category: Antispastic and analgesic; skeletal muscle relaxant
Half-life: 2.5–4 hours
Clinically important, potentially serious interactions with: alcohol, antidiabetic agents, CNS depressants, clindamycin, lithium, morphine, tricyclic antidepressants

Reactions

Skin

Ankle edema
(1993): Albright AL+, *JAMA*, 270, 2475
Cutaneous side effects (sic) (1–2%)
(1972): Birkmayer W, *Aspeckte der Muskelspastik Int Symp Wien.* (German) Bern, Huber
Dermatitis (sic)
Diaphoresis
Exanthems
(1983): Lynde CW+, *Ann Neurol* 13, 216
Facial edema
Flushing
Pruritus
Rash (1–10%)
Urticaria
(1972): Birkmayer W, *Aspeckte der Muskelspastik Int Symp Wien.* (German) Bern, Huber (2%)

Other

Dysgeusia (<1%)
(1976): Rollin H, *Laryngol Rhinol Otol* (Stuttgart) (German) 55, 873
Paresthesias (<1%)
Xerostomia (<1%)

BENACTYZINE

Trade name: Deprol (Wallace)
Indications: Depression, anxiety
Category: Antidepressant
Half-life: no data
Clinically important, potentially serious interactions with: no data

Deprol is benactyzine and meprobamate

Note: Most of the adverse reactions are due to meprobamate (which see)

Reactions

Skin

Angioedema
Bullous eruption
Ecchymoses
Edema
Erythema multiforme
Exanthems
(1964): Welsh AL, *Med Clin North Am* 48, 459
Exfoliative dermatitis
Fixed eruption
Petechiae
Pruritus
Urticaria

Other

Anaphylactoid reaction
Paresthesias
Stomatitis
Xerostomia

BENAZEPRIL

Trade names: Lotensin (Novartis); Lotensin-HCT (Novartis); Lotrel (Novartis)
Other common trade names: *Cibace; Cibacen; Cibacene*
Indications: Hypertension
Category: Angiotensin-converting enzyme (ACE) inhibitor; antihypertensive and vasodilator
Half-life: 11–12 hours
Clinically important, potentially serious interactions with: alcohol, allopurinol, captopril, digoxin, lithium, NSAIDs, phenothiazines, thiazide diuretics

Lotrel is benazepril and amlodipine; Lotensin-HCT is benazepril and hydrochlorothiazide

Reactions

Skin

Angioedema (<1%)
(1996): O'Mara NB+, *Pharmacotherapy* 16, 675
(1992): Kuhn M, *Clin Issues Crit Care Nurs* 3, 461
(1991): Balfour JA+, *Drugs* 42, 511
(1991): MacNab M+, *Clin Cardiol* 14, IV33
(1991): Anon, *Med Lett Drugs Ther* 33, 83
Ankle edema
(1990): Mirvis DM+, *Am J Med Sci* 300, 354
Dermatitis (sic)
Diaphoresis (<1%)
(1991): Morant J+ (eds), *Arzneimittel-Kompendium der Schweiz*, Basel (German), Documed, 1990
Exanthems
(1991): Morant J+ (eds), *Arzneimittel-Kompendium der Schweiz*, Basel (German), Documed, 1990
Flushing
(1991): Morant J+ (eds), *Arzneimittel-Kompendium der Schweiz*, Basel (German), Documed, 1990
Peripheral edema
Photosensitivity (<1%)
Pruritus
(1991): Morant J+ (eds), *Arzneimittel-Kompendium der Schweiz*, Basel (German), Documed, 1990
Rash (sic) (<1%)
(1991): MacNab M+, *Clin Cardiol* 14, IV33
Urticaria
(1991): Moser M+, *Clin Pharmacol Ther* 49, 322

Other

Ageusia
Dysgeusia
(1991): MacNab M+, *Clin Cardiol* 14, IV33
Hypersensitivity
Myalgia (<1%)
Paresthesias (<1%)

BENDROFLUMETHIAZIDE

Trade name: Corzide (Bristol-Myers Squibb)
Other common trade names: *Aprinox; Berkozide; Centyl; Naturine; Neo-Naclex; Pluryle*
Indications: Edema, diabetes insipidus, hypertension
Category: Thiazide* diuretic; antihypertensive
Half-life: 8.5 hours
Clinically important, potentially serious interactions with: digoxin, lithium, MAO inhibitors

Corzide is bendroflumethiazide and nadolol

Reactions

Skin

Allergic reactions (sic)
Contact dermatitis
(1997): Pereira F+, *Contact Dermatitis* 35, 303
Diaphoresis
Exanthems
(1991): Morant J+ (eds), *Arzneimittel-Kompendium der Schweiz*, Basel (German), Documed, 1990
Exfoliative dermatitis
Facial edema
Grinspan's syndrome**
(1990): Lamey PG+, *Oral Surg Oral Med Oral Pathol* 70, 184
Pemphigoid (sic)
Photosensitivity
(1989): Diffey BL+, *Arch Dermatol* 125, 1355
Phototoxicity
(1997): Selvaag E+, *In Vivo* 11, 103
(1997): Selvaag E, *Arzneimittelforschung* (German) 47, 97
Pruritus
(1991): Morant J+ (eds), *Arzneimittel-Kompendium der Schweiz*, Basel (German), Documed, 1990
Purpura
Rash (sic)
Urticaria
Vasculitis

Hair

Hair – alopecia

Other

Anaphylactoid reaction
Gynecomastia
Paresthesias
Xanthopsia
Xerostomia

***Note:** Bendroflumethiazide is a sulfonamide and can be absorbed systemically. Sulfonamides can produce severe, possibly fatal, reactions such as toxic epidermal necrolysis and Stevens–Johnson syndrome.

****Note:** Grinspan's syndrome: the triad of oral lichen planus, diabetes mellitus, and hypertension.

BENZTHIAZIDE

Trade names: Aquatag; Exna (Robins); Hydrex; Marazide; Proaqua
Other common trade names: *Diurin; Fovane; Regulon*
Indications: Hypertension
Category: Thiazide* diuretic; antihypertensive
Half-life: no data
Clinically important, potentially serious interactions with: digoxin, furosemide, lithium

Reactions

Skin
Allergic reactions (sic) (<1%)
Photosensitivity
Purpura
Rash (sic)
Urticaria
Vasculitis

Other
Dysgeusia
Paresthesias (<1%)
Xanthopsia

***Note:** Benzthiazide is a sulfonamide and can be absorbed systemically. Sulfonamides can produce severe, possibly fatal, reactions such as toxic epidermal necrolysis and Stevens–Johnson syndrome.

BENZTROPINE

Trade name: Cogentin (Merck)
Other common trade names: *Akitan; Apo-Benzthioprine; Cogentine; Cogentinol; Phatropine; PMS-Benztropine*
Indications: Parkinsonism
Category: Antidyskinetic and anticholinergic; antiparkinsonian
Duration of action: 6–48 hours
Clinically important, potentially serious interactions with: amantadine, anticholinergics, antipsychotics, benztropine, haloperidol, MAO inhibitors, narcotic analgesics, quinidine, tricyclic antidepressants

Reactions

Skin
Exanthems
Hypohidrosis (>10%)
Photosensitivity (1–10%)
Pruritus
Rash (sic) (<1%)
Urticaria
Xerosis (>10%)

Other
Black tongue
(2000): Heymann WR, *Cutis* 66, 25
Dysgeusia
(2000): Heymann WR, *Cutis* 66, 25
Glossodynia
Paresthesias
Stomatodynia
Xerostomia (>10%)
(2000): Heymann WR, *Cutis* 66, 25
(1989): Gelenberg AJ+, *J Clin Psychopharmacol* 9, 180

BEPRIDIL

Trade name: Vascor (McNeil)
Other common trade names: *Bapadin; Bepricol; Cordium; Cruor*
Indications: Angina pectoris
Category: Calcium channel blocker; antianginal
Half-life: 24 hours
Clinically important, potentially serious interactions with: beta-blockers, carbamazepine, cyclosporine, digoxin, procainamide, quinidine, ritonavir

Reactions:

Skin
Diaphoresis (<2%)
Dysgeusia (<1%)
Edema (1–10%)
Irritation (sic)
Peripheral edema (<1%)
Rash (sic) (<2%)
(1988): Sharma MK+, *Am J Cardiol* 61, 1210

Other
Dysgeusia (<1%)
Myalgia (<1%)
Paresthesias (2.5%)
Tremor (<9%)
Xerostomia (1–10%)
(1988): Krusell LR+, *Eur J Clin Pharmacol* 34, 221
(1988): Hasegawa GR, *Clin Pharm* 7, 97

BETA-CAROTENE

Trade name: Solatene (Merck)
Other common trade names: *Betavin; B-Tene; Carotaben; Solvin*
Indications: Photosensitivity reactions
Category: Fat-soluble vitamin supplement; photosensitivity reaction suppressant
Half-life: no data
Clinically important, potentially serious interactions with: vitamin A

Reactions

Skin
Carotenemia (>10%)
(2000): Frieling UM+, *Arch Dermatol* 136, 179 (15.9%)
Dermatitis (sic)
(1992): Zürcher K and Krebs A, *Cutaneous Drug Reactions*, Karger, 280
Ecchymoses (<1%)
Purpura (<1%)

BETAXOLOL

Trade names: Betoptic [Ophthalmic] (Alcon); Kerlone (Searle)
Other common trade names: *Betoptic S; Betoptima; Kerlon; Optipres*
Indications: Open-angle glaucoma, hypertension
Category: Beta-adrenergic blocker; antihypertensive
Half-life: 14–22 hours
Clinically important, potentially serious interactions with: barbiturates, calcium channel blockers, ciprofloxacin, clonidine, diuretics, flecainide, hydralazine, insulin, nifedipine, NSAIDs, oral contraceptives, prazosin, quinidine, rifampin, salicylates, sulfinpyrazone, verapamil

Note: Cutaneous side-effects of beta-receptor blockaders are clinically polymorphous. They apparently appear after several months of continuous therapy. Atypical psoriasiform, lichen planus-like, and eczematous chronic rashes are mainly observed. (1983): Hödl St, *Z Hautkr* 1:58, 17.

Reactions

Skin
Acne
Allergy (sic) (<2%)
Angioedema
Cold extremities (sic)
Contact dermatitis
(1993): O'Donnell BF+, *Contact Dermatitis* 28, 121
Diaphoresis (<2%)
Edema (1.3%)
Erythema (1–10%)
Exanthems
Exfoliative dermatitis
Facial edema
Flushing (<2%)
Lupus erythematosus
(1997): Hardee JT+, *West J Med* 167, 106
Photosensitivity
Pigmentation (palms)
(1997): Adams DR+, *Am J Contact Dermat* 8, 183
Pruritus (1–10%)
Psoriasis
Purpura
Rash (sic) (1.2%)
(1989): Burris JF+, *Arch Intern Med* 149, 2437
Raynaud's phenomenon
Toxic epidermal necrolysis
Urticaria
Xerosis

Hair
Hair – alopecia (following topical use) (<2%)
(1990): Buckley MMT+, *Drugs* 40, 75
Hair – hypertrichosis (<2%)

Nails
Nails – pigmentation (bluish)

Other
Ageusia (<2%)
Anaphylactoid reaction
Dysgeusia (<2%)
Glossitis (following topical use)
Mastodynia (<2%)
Myalgia (3.2%)
Myasthenia gravis
(1997): Khella SL+, *Muscle Nerve* 20, 631
Oral ulceration (<2%)
Paresthesias (1.9%)
Peyronie's disease (<2%)
Sialorrhea (<2%)
Xerostomia (<2%)

BETHANECHOL

Trade name: Urecholine (Merck)
Other common trade names: *Muscaran; Myocholine-Glenwood; Myotonine Chloride; Urocarb*
Indications: Nonobstructive urinary retention
Category: Urinary tract cholinergic stimulant
Duration of action: up to 6 hours
Clinically important, potentially serious interactions with: cholinergic and anticholinesterase agents, ganglionic blockers, procainamide, quinidine

Reactions

Skin
Diaphoresis (1–10%)
Flushing (<1%)
Miliaria
(1967): Rochmis PG+, *Arch Dermatol* 95, 499

Other
Sialorrhea (<1%)

BEXAROTENE

Trade name: Targretin (Ligand)
Indications: Cutaneous T-cell lymphoma (CTCL), (mycosis fungoides)
Category: Retinoid (rexinoid)
Half-life: 7 hours
Clinically important, potentially serious interactions with: atorvastatin, erythromycin, fluvoxamine, gemfibrozil, itraconazole, ketoconazole, nefazodone, phenobarbital, phenytoin, quinine, rifampin, sulfonylureas, vitamin A, **grapefruit juice**

Reactions

Skin
Acne (<10%)
Bacterial infection (1.2–13.2%)
Cellulitis
Cheilitis (<10%)
Chills (9.5%)
Cold hand and feet
(2000): Bedikian AY+, *Oncol Rep* 7, 883
Exanthems (<10%)
Exfoliative dermatitis (10–28%)
Flu-like syndrome (sic) (3.6–13.2%)
Nodule (sic) (<10%)
Peripheral edema (13.1%)
Photosensitivity
Pruritus (20–30%)
(2000): Duvic M, *Dermatology Times*, August, 3 (25%)
Pustular eruption
Rash (sic) (16.7%)
Ulceration (<10%)
Vesiculobullous eruption (<10%)
Xerosis (10.7%)

Hair
Hair – alopecia (4–11%)

Other
Gingivitis (<10%)
Hyperesthesia (<10%)
Hypesthesia
Mastodynia (<10%)
Myalgia (<10%)
(2000): Bedikian AY+, *Oncol Rep* 7, 883
Xerostomia (<10%)

BICALUTAMIDE

Trade name: Casodex (AstraZeneca)
Indications: Metastatic prostatic carcinoma
Category: Antiandrogen antineoplastic
Half-life: up to 10 days
Clinically important, potentially serious interactions with: warfarin

Reactions

Skin

Diaphoresis (6%)
Edema (2–5%)
Exanthems (<1%)
Hot flashes (49%)
(1996): Bales GT+, *Urology* 47, 38
(1995): Lunglmayr G, *Anticancer Drugs* 6, 508
(1994): Eri LM+, *Eur Urol* 26, 219
(1990): Mahler C+, *J Steroid Biochem Mol Biol* 37, 921
Peripheral edema (8%)
Paresthesias (6%)
Pruritus (2–5%)
Rash (sic) (6%)
Xerosis (2–5%)

Hair

Hair – alopecia (2–5%)

Other

Gynecomastia (38%)
(1998): Goa KL+, *Drugs Aging* 12, 401
(1996): Kotake T+, *Hinyokika Kiyo* (Japanese) 42, 157
(1996): Bales GT+, *Urology* 47, 38
(1995): Lunglmayr G, *Anticancer Drugs* 6, 508
(1994): Eri LM+, *Eur Urol* 26, 219
(1990): Mahler C+, *J Steroid Biochem Mol Biol* 37, 921
Injection-site reaction (2–5%)
Mastodynia (39%)
(1998): Goa KL+, *Drugs Aging* 12, 401
(1996): Kotake T+, *Hinyokika Kiyo* (Japanese) 42, 157
(1996): Bales GT+, *Urology* 47, 38
(1995): Lunglmayr G, *Anticancer Drugs* 6, 508
(1994): Eri LM+, *Eur Urol* 26, 219
(1990): Mahler C+, *J Steroid Biochem Mol Biol* 37, 921
Myalgia (2–5%)
Paresthesias (6%)
Xerostomia (2–5%)

BIPERIDEN

Trade name: Akineton (Knoll)
Other common trade names: *Biperen; Bipiden; Dekinet; Desiperiden; Dyskinon*
Indications: Parkinsonism
Category: Anticholinergic; antiparkinsonian
Half-life: 18–24 hours
Clinically important, potentially serious interactions with: amantadine, anticholinergics, digoxin, haloperidol, meperidine, phenothiazines, quinidine, tricyclic antidepressants

Reactions

Skin

Contact dermatitis
(1995): Torinuki W, *Tohoku J Exp Med* 176, 249
Exanthems
Flushing
Rash (sic)
Urticaria

Other

Glossodynia
Paresthesias
Stomatodynia
Xerostomia

BISACODYL

Trade names: Carter's Little Pills; Biscolax; Dacody; Dulcagen; Dulcolax (Novartis); Fleet Laxative (Fleet)
Other trade names: *Apo-Bisacodyl; Dulcolan; Laxit*
Indications: Constipation
Category: Irritant/stimulant laxative
Onset of action: 6–10 hours
Clinically important, potentially serious interactions with: antacids, cimetidine, famotidine, **milk**, ranitidine

Reactions

Skin

Diaphoresis
Exanthems
Fixed eruption
(1997): Burrow WH, Jackson, MS (from Internet) (observation)
(1961): Welsh AL+, *Arch Dermatol* 84, 1004
Urticaria

BISOPROLOL

Trade names: Zebeta (Lederle); Ziac (Lederle)
Other common trade names: *Concor; Cordalin; Detensiel; Emcor; Fondril; Monocor; Soprol*
Indications: Hypertension
Category: Beta-adrenergic blocker
Half-life: 9–12 hours
Clinically important, potentially serious interactions with: cimetidine, clonidine, diuretics, flecainide, insulin, nifedipine, NSAIDs, prazosin, salicylates, sulfonylureas, verapamil

Ziac is bisoprolol and hydrochlorothiazide

Reactions

Skin

Acne
Angioedema
Ankle edema (1–10%)
Diaphoresis (1%)
Eczema (sic)
Edema (3%)
Exanthems
Exfoliative dermatitis
Facial edema
Flushing
Lupus erythematosus
Photosensitivity
Pigmentation
Pruritus
Psoriasis
Purpura
Rash (sic) (1–10%)
Raynaud's phenomenon (1–10%)
Urticaria
Xerosis

Hair

Hair – alopecia

Nails

Nails – bluish

Other

Anaphylactoid reaction
Dysgeusia
Hypesthesia (1.5%)
Myalgia (1–10%)
Paresthesias
Peyronie's disease
Xerostomia (1.3%)

BLEOMYCIN

Synonyms: bleo; BLM
Trade name: Blenoxane (Bristol-Myers Squibb)
Other common trade names: *Bleo; Bleocin; Bleomycine; Bleomycinum; BLM*
Indications: Melanomas, sarcomas, lymphomas, testicular carcinoma
Category: Antineoplastic antibiotic
Half-life: 1.3–9 hours
Clinically important, potentially serious interactions with: amphotericin B, CCNU, cisplatin, digoxin, NSAIDs, phenytoin

Reactions

Skin

Acral erythema
(1982): Burgdorf WHC+, *Ann Intern Med* 97, 61
Acral gangrene
(1998): Reiser M+, *Eur J Clin Microbiol Infect Dis* 17, 58
(1997): Hladunewich M+, *J Rheumatol* 24, 2371
Acral sclerosis
(1984): Snauwaert J+, *Dermatologica* 169, 172
Acrocyanosis
(1983): Bork K+, *Hautarzt* (German) 34, 10
Angioedema
(1984): Khansur T+, *Arch Intern Med* 144, 2267
Bullous eruption (1–5%)
Chills (>10%)
Cutaneous toxicity (sic)
(1998): Yeo W+, *J Clin Oncol* 16, 1626
(1998): Mullai N+, *J Clin Oncol* 16, 1625
Dermatitis (sic)
Digital necrosis
(1997): Sibilia J+, *Presse Med* (French) 26, 1564
(1997): Emmerich J, *Presse Med* (French) 26, 1580
Exanthems
(1993): Haerslev T+, *Cutis* 52, 45 (linear and symmetrical)
(1980): Lincke-Plewig H, *Hautarzt* (German) 31, 616
(1976): Werner Y+, *Acta Derm Venereol* (Stockh) 56, 155
Flagellate erythema
(1999): Rubeiz NG+, *Int J Dermatol* 38, 140 (urticarial)
(1998): Yamamoto T+, *Dermatology* 197, 399
(1997): Polsky D+, New York, American Academy of Dermatology Meeting (SF), (gross and microscopic)
(1995): Watanabe T+, *Dermatology* 190, 230
(1994): Mowad CM+, *Br J Dermatol* 131, 700
(1994): Zaki I+, *Clin Exp Dermatol* 19, 366
(1992): Jolin-Garijo L+, *An Med Interna* (Spanish) 9, 520
(1992): Barduagni O+, *Dermatol Clin* (Italian) 3, 169
(1991): Duhra P+, *Clin Exp Dermatol* 16, 216
(1990): Miori L+, *Am J Dermatopathol* 12, 598
(1990): Miori L+, *Dermatologica* 181, 238
(1990): Cortina P+, *Dermatologica* 180, 106
(1987): Lindae ML+, *Arch Dermatol* 123, 395
Flagellate pigmentation
(1993): Tsuji T+, *J Am Acad Dermatol* 28, 503
(1993): Lincke-Plewig H, *Hautarzt* (German) 44, 331
(1992): Albig J+, *Hautarzt* (German) 43, 376
(1990): Vicente MA+, *Med Cutan Ibero Lat Am* (Spanish) 18, 148
(1986): Polla BS+, *J Am Acad Dermatol* 14, 690
(1985): Fernandez-Obregon AC+, *J Am Acad Dermatol* 13, 464
Gangrene (digital)
(1998): Reiser M+, *Eur J Clin Microbiol Infect Dis* 17, 58
(1993): Vayssairat M+, *J Rheumatol* 20, 921
Hyperkeratosis (palms and soles)
(1976): Werner Y+, *Acta Derm Venereol* (Stockh) 56, 155
(1971): de Bast C+, *Arch Dermatol* 104, 509
Ichthyosis
(1971): de Bast C+, *Arch Dermatol* 104, 509
Intertrigo
(1971): de Bast C+, *Arch Dermatol* 104, 509
Linear streaking (sic)
(1989): Vignini M+, *Clin Exp Dermatol* 14, 261
(1988): Lazar A+, *Cutis* 42, 397
(1987): Rademaker M+, *Clin Exp Dermatol* 12, 457
(1975): Lowitz BB, *N Engl J Med* 292, 1300
Lymphangitis
(1998): Allen AL+, *J Am Acad Dermatol* 39, 295
Neutrophilic eccrine hidradenitis
(1988): Scallan PJ+, *Cancer* 62, 2532
Nodular eruption
(1997): Polsky D+, New York, American Academy of Dermatology Meeting (SF), (gross and microscopic)
Painful erythema (elbows, knees, palms)
(1980): Lincke-Plewig H, *Hautarzt* (German) 31, 616
(1976): Werner Y+, *Acta Derm Venereol* (Stockh) 56, 155
Palmar nodules
(1993): Haerslev T+, *Cutis* 52, 45
Palmoplantar erythema
(1990): Pagliuca A+, *Postgrad Med J* 66, 242
Pigmentation (~50%)
(1998): Behrens S+, *Hautarzt* (German) 49, 725
(1993): Tsuji T+, *J Am Acad Dermatol* 28, 503 (in striae distensae)
(1992): Gallais V+, *Ann Dermatol Venereol* (French) 119, 471
(1990): Wright AL+, *Dermatologica* 181, 255 (reticulate)
(1988): Massone L+, *G Ital Dermatol Venereol* (Italian) 123, 225 (striae)
(1986): Guillet G+, *Arch Dermatol* 122, 381 (in stripes)
(1985): Polla L+, *Ann Dermatol Venereol* (French) 112, 821
(1984): Schuler G+, *Hautarzt* (German) 35, 383 (linear)
(1983): Bork K+, *Hautarzt* (German) 34, 10
(1982): Kukla LJ+, *Cancer* 50, 2283
(1981): Nixon DW+, *Cutis* 27, 181
(1981): Granstein RD+, *J Am Acad Dermatol* 5, 1 (brown-black)
(1978): Perrot H+, *Arch Dermatol Res* 261, 245
(1973): Kiefer O, *Dermatologica* 146, 229
(1973): Cohen IS+, *Arch Dermatol* 107, 553
Pruritus (>5%)
(1990): Caumes E+, *Lancet* 336, 1593
Radiation recall
(1993): Stelzer KJ+, *Cancer* 71, 1322
Raynaud's phenomenon (>10%)
(1998): Reiser M+, *Eur J Clin Microbiol Infect Dis* 17, 58
(1997): Emmerich J, *Presse Med* (French) 26, 1580
(1997): Sibilia J+, *Presse Med* (French) 26, 1564 (12.6%)
(1997): Hladunewich M+, *J Rheumatol* 24, 2371
(1996): Munn SE+, *Br J Dermatol* 135, 969
(1996): Epstein Ernst, *The Schoch Letter* 46, 34 (observation)
(1993): von Gunten CF+, *Cancer* 72, 2004
(1992): Gregg LJ, *J Am Acad Dermatol* 26, 279
(1992): de Pablo P+, *Acta Derm Venereol* (Stockh) 72, 465
(1991): Epstein E, *J Am Acad Dermatol* 24, 785
(1985): Epstein E, *J Am Acad Dermatol* 13, 468
(1985): Bovenmyer DA, *J Am Acad Dermatol* 13, 470
(1985): Adoue D+, *Ann Dermatol Venereol* (French) 112, 151
(1984): Adoue D+, *Ann Intern Med* 100, 770
(1984): Snauwaert J+, *Dermatologica* 169, 172
(1981): Kukla LJ+, *Arch Dermatol* 117, 604
Scleroderma
(2000): D'Cruz D, *Toxicol Lett* 112 and 421
(1999): Passiu G+, *Clin Rheumatol* 18, 422
(1998): Behrens S+, *Hautarzt* (German) 49, 725 (pseudoscleroderma)
(1997): Komosinska K+, *Postepy Hig Med Dosw* (Polish) 51, 285
(1994): Marck Y+, *Ann Dermatol Venereol* (French) 121, 712,
(1992): Kerr LD+, *J Rheumatol* 19, 294
(1991): Guseva NG, *Revmatologiia Mosk* (Russian) 1, 33
(1991): Bourgeois P+, *Baillieres Clin Rheumatol* 5, 13
(1985): Haustein UF+, *Int J Dermatol* 24, 147
(1984): Rush PJ+, *J Rheumatol* 11, 262

(1983): Bork K+, *Hautarzt* (German) 34, 10
(1980): Finch WR+, *J Rheumatol* 7, 651
(1973): Cohen IS+, *Arch Dermatol* 107, 533
(1971): de Bast C+, *Arch Dermatol* 104, 509
Stevens–Johnson syndrome
(1989): Brodsky A+, *J Clin Pharmacol* 29, 821
(1986): Giaccone G+, *Tumori* 72, 331
Thickening (sic)
Urticaria
Xerosis
(1973): Cohen IS+, *Arch Dermatol* 107, 555, 556

Hair

Hair – alopecia (~50%)
(1992): Breathnach SM+, *Adverse Drug Reactions and the Skin*, Blackwell, Oxford, 292 (passim)
(1990): Siegel RD+, *Chest* 98, 507
(1982): Kukla LJ+, *Cancer* 50, 2283
(1973): Cohen IS+, *Arch Dermatol* 107, 553
(1973): Kiefer O, *Dermatologica* 146, 229
(1971): de Bast C+, *Arch Dermatol* 104, 509
Hair – gray

Nails

Nails – Beau's lines (transverse nail bands)
(1994): Ben-Dyan D+, *Acta Haematol* 91, 89
Nails – dystrophy
(1984): Miller RAW, *Arch Dermatol* 120, 963
Nails – growth reduced
(1971): de Bast C+, *Arch Dermatol* 104, 509
Nails – loss
(1986): Gonzalez FU+, *Arch Dermatol* 122, 974
Nails – onychodystrophy
(1985): Baran R, *Ann Dermatol Venereol* (French) 112, 463
Nails – onycholysis
(1998): Roussou P+, *Acta Derm Venereol* 78, 303
(1984): Snauwaert J+, *Dermatologica* 169, 172
Nails – pigmentation (banding)
(1977): Shetty MR, *Cancer Treatment Reports* 61, 501
Nails – shedding
(1973): Cohen IS+, *Arch Dermatol* 107, 553

Other

Anaphylactoid reaction (<1%)
Calcinosis
(1983): Bork K+, *Hautarzt* (German) 34, 10
(1975): Ihde DC+, *Cancer Chemother* 59, 1039 (penis)
Digital gangrene
(1998): Surville-Barland J+, *Eur J Dermatol* 8, 221
Glossitis
(1992): Breathnach SM+, *Adverse Drug Reactions and the Skin*, Blackwell, Oxford, 292 (passim)
Hyperesthesia
Hypersensitivity (1–10%)
(1992): Weiss RB, *Semin Oncol* 19, 458
Injection-site phlebitis (1–10%)
Oral papillomatosis
(1978): Hagedorn M+, *Hautarzt* (German) 29, 425
Oral ulceration
(1992): Breathnach SM+, *Adverse Drug Reactions and the Skin*, Blackwell, Oxford, 292 (passim)
(1971): de Bast C+, *Arch Dermatol* 104, 509
Paresthesias
Stomatitis (>10%)
(1993): Haerslev T+, *Cutis* 52, 45
(1990): Siegel RD+, *Chest* 98, 507
(1983): Bronner AK+, *J Am Acad Dermatol* 9, 645
(1976): Werner Y+, *Acta Derm Venereol* (Stockh) 56, 176
(1975): Khlebnov AV+, *Klin Med Mosk* (Russian) 52, 78
(1973): Kiefer O, *Dermatologica* 146, 229
(1973): Cohen IS+, *Arch Dermatol* 107, 553
Tongue erosions
(1973): Cohen IS+, *Arch Dermatol* 107, 553

BRETYLIUM

Trade name: Bretylol (Abbott)
Other trade names: *Bretylate, Critifib*
Indications: Ventricular tachycardia and fibrillation
Category: Antiarrhythmic class III
Half-life: 4–17 hours
Clinically important, potentially serious interactions with: antihypertensives, digoxin, sparfloxacin

Reactions

Skin

Diaphoresis (<1%)
Flushing (<1%)
Rash (sic) (<1%)

Other

Injection-site atrophy (<1%)
Injection-site necrosis (<1%)

BROMFENAC*

Trade name: Duract (Wyeth-Ayerst)
Indications: Pain
Category: Nonsteroidal anti-inflammatory agent (NSAID)
Half-life: 1.3 hours
Clinically important, potentially serious interactions with: anticoagulants, cimetidine, cyclosporine, lithium, phenytoin, warfarin

Reactions

Skin

Diaphoresis (<1%)
Ecchymoses (<1%)
Edema (<1%)
Exanthems (<1%)
Facial edema (<1%)
Generalized edema (<1%)
Pruritus (<1%)
Rash (sic) (<1%)
Seborrhea (<1%)
Ulceration (<1%)
Urticaria (<1%)

Hair

Hair – alopecia (<1%)

Other

Anaphylactoid reaction
Dysgeusia (<1%)
Mastodynia (<1%)
Myalgia (<1%)
Paresthesias (<1%)
Phlebitis (<1%)
Stomatitis (<1%)
Xerostomia (<1%)

***Note:** Bromfenac has been withdrawn in the USA

BROMOCRIPTINE

Trade name: Parlodel (Novartis)
Other common trade names: *Apo-Bromocriptine; Bromed; Cryocriptina; Kripton; Parilac; Pravidel; Serocryptin*
Indications: Amenorrhea, parkinsonism, infertility
Category: Dopamine agonist; antihyperprolactinemic; infertility therapy adjunct; lactation inhibitor; antidyskinetic; growth hormone suppressant; ergot alkaloid; antiparkinsonian
Half-life: initial: 6–8 hours; terminal: 50 hours
Clinically important, potentially serious interactions with: alcohol, amitriptyline, ergot alkaloids, erythromycin, imipramine, MAO inhibitors, methyldopa, metoclopramide, phenothiazines, reserpine, sympathomimetics

Reactions

Skin

Erythromelalgia
(1983): Dupont E+, *Neurology* 33, 670
(1981): Eisler T+, *Neurology* 31, 1368
(1979): Eisler T+, *Neurology* 29, 571
(1978): Calne DB+, *Lancet* 1, 735 (11%)
Exanthems
Flushing
(1992): Shelley WB+, *Advanced Dermatologic Diagnosis*, WB Saunders, 582 (passim)
Livedo reticularis
(1985): Hoehn MMM+, *Neurology* 35, 199
(1978): Calne DB+, *Lancet* 1, 735
(1978): Lees AJ+, *Arch Neurol* 35, 503 (2%)
Morphea
(1989): Leshin B+, *Int J Dermatol* 28, 177
Pedal edema
Purpura
Rash (sic)
Raynaud's phenomenon (1–10%)
(1987): Quagliarello J+, *Fertility and Sterility* 48, 877
(1978): Lees AJ+, *Arch Neurol* 35, 503 (5%)
(1978): Pearce I+, *BMJ* 1, 1402
(1976): Duvoisin RC, *Lancet* 2, 204
(1976): Wass JAH+, *Lancet* 1, 1135
Scleroderma
(1989): Leshin B+, *Int J Dermatol* 28, 177
(1983): Dupont E+, *Neurology* 33, 670
Urticaria
Vasculitis
(1978): Lees AJ+, *Arch Neurol* 35, 503

Hair

Hair – alopecia
(1993): Fabre N+, *Clin Neuropharmacol* 16, 266
(1980): Blum I+, *N Engl J Med* 303, 1418

Other

Anaphylactoid reaction
(1980): Parkes S, *N Engl J Med* 302, 750
Dysgeusia (metallic taste)
Paresthesias
(1985): Hoehn MMM+, *Neurology* 35, 199
Priapism (clitoral)
Stomatopyrosis
(1985): Hoehn MMM+, *Neurology* 35, 199
Xerostomia (4–10%)
(1985): Hoehn MMM+, *Neurology* 35, 199
(1982): Gauthier G+, *Eur Neurol* 21, 217

BROMPHENIRAMINE

Trade name: Dimetane (Robins)
Other common trade names: *Bromine; Brommine; Bromphen; Dimegan; Ilvin; Kinmedon; Nasahist; ND-Stat; Neo-Meton*
Indications: Allergic rhinitis, urticaria
Category: Antihistamine, H_1 blocker
Half-life: 12–48 hours
Clinically important, potentially serious interactions with: alcohol, CNS depressants, MAO inhibitors, tricyclic antidepressants

Reactions

Skin

Angioedema (<1%)
Exanthems (<1%)
Photosensitivity (<1%)
Rash (sic) (<1%)

Other

Myalgia (<1%)
Paresthesias (<1%)
Xerostomia (1–10%)

BUCLIZINE

Trade names: Bucladin-S (Stuart); Vibazine
Other common trade names: *Aphilan; Buclixin; Longifene; Odetin; Postafeno; Vibazina*
Indications: Motion sickness, nausea/vomiting
Category: Antihistamine; anticholinergic, antiemetic/antivertigo
Half-life: no data
Clinically important, potentially serious interactions with: CNS depressants, MAO inhibitors, tricyclic antidepressants

Reactions

Other

Tremor
Xerostomia

BUMETANIDE

Trade name: Bumetanide (Baxter)
Other common trade names: *Bumedyl; Burinex; Fondiuran; Fontego; Lunetoron; Miccil; Primex*
Indications: Edema associated with congestive heart failure
Category: Sulfonamide* loop diuretic; antihypertensive
Half-life: 1–1.5 hours
Clinically important, potentially serious interactions with: ACE-inhibitors, amiloride, aminoglycosides, amphotericin, cisplatin, digoxin, indomethacin, lithium, metolazone, NSAIDs, probenecid, salicylates, spironolactone, thiazide diuretics

Reactions

Skin

Allergic reactions (sic)
Bullous eruption
(1990): Leitao EA+, *J Am Acad Dermatol* 23, 129
Bullous pemphigoid
(1998): Boulinguez S+, *Br J Dermatol* 138, 549
Contact dermatitis
(1989): Moller NE+, *Contact Dermatitis* 20, 393
Cutaneous side effects (sic) (1.1%)
(1984): Ward A+, *Drugs* 28, 426 (1–5%)
Diaphoresis (0.1%)

Edema (periorbital)
(1981): Handler B+, *J Clin Pharmacol* 21, 691
Erythema multiforme (<1%)
(1975): Ring-Larsen H, *Acta Med Scand* 195, 411
Exanthems
Exfoliative dermatitis
(1981): Handler B+, *J Clin Pharmacol* 21, 691
Photosensitivity
(1990): Leitao EA+, *J Am Acad Dermatol* 23, 129
Pruritus (<1%)
(1992): Shelley WB+, *Cutis* 50, 17 (observation)
(1984): Ward A+, *Drugs* 28, 426 (1–5%)
Purpura
Rash (sic) (0.2%)
Urticaria (0.2%)
(1981): Handler B+, *J Clin Pharmacol* 21, 691
Vasculitis

Other

Nipple tenderness (0.1%)
Pseudoporphyria
(1990): Leitao EA+, *J Am Acad Dermatol* 23, 129
Xerostomia (0.1%)

***Note:** Bumetanide is a sulfonamide and can be absorbed systemically. Sulfonamides can produce severe, possibly fatal, reactions such as toxic epidermal necrolysis and Stevens–Johnson syndrome.

BUPROPION

Trade names: Wellbutrin (GlaxoWellcome); Zyban (GlaxoWellcome)
Indications: Depression, aid to smoking cessation
Category: Heterocyclic antidepressant; aid to smoking cessation
Half-life: 14 hours
Clinically important, potentially serious interactions with: alcohol, carbamazepine, cimetidine, lithium, MAO inhibitors, phenelzine, phenobarbital, phenytoin, rifampin, ritonavir, selegiline, trazodone, tricyclic antidepressants

Reactions

Skin

Acne (1–10%)
Angioedema
Diaphoresis
Ecchymoses (<0.1%)
Edema (>1%)
(1999): Peloso PM+, *JAMA* 282, 1817
Erythema multiforme
Exanthems (<0.1%)
(1983): Fabre LF+, *J Clin Psychiatry* 44, 88
(1981): Halaris AE+, *Psychopharmacol Bull* 17, 140
Exfoliative dermatitis
Diaphoresis (5%)
(1983): Feighner JP, *J Clin Psychiatry* 44, 49
(1981): Halaris AE+, *Psychopharmacol Bull* 17, 140
Flushing (4%)
Hot flashes
Lupus panniculitis
(1986): Ottuso P, *The Schoch Letter*, 46, 37 (observation)
Peripheral edema
(1999): Peloso PM+, *JAMA* 282, 1817
Photosensitivity (<0.1%)
Pruritus (4%)
(1983): Cato AE+, *J Clin Psychiatry* 44, 187
Rash (sic) (4%)
(2000): McCollom RA+*Ann Pharmacother* 34, 471
(1985): Golden RN+, *Am J Psychiatry* 142, 1459 (vascular)
Stevens–Johnson syndrome
Urticaria
(1999): Peloso PM+, *JAMA* 282, 1817
(1983): Mendels J+, *J Clin Psychiatry* 44, 118
(1983): Feighner JP, *J Clin Psychiatry* 44, 49
(1983): Cato AE+, *J Clin Psychiatry* 44, 187
(1983): Fabre LF+, *J Clin Psychiatry* 44, 88
(1978): Fann WE+, *Curr Ther Res* 23, 222
Xerosis (1–10%)

Hair

Hair – alopecia (<1%)
Hair – color change (sic) (<1%)
Hair – hirsutism (1–10%)

Other

Anaphylactoid reaction
Bromhidrosis
Bruxism (<0.1%)
Dysgeusia (4%)
(1999): Berigan TR, *JAMA* 281, 233 (letter)
Gingivitis
Glossitis
Gynecomastia (<1%)
Hypesthesia (<0.1%)
Myalgia (6%)
(1999): Peloso PM+, *JAMA* 282, 1817
Oral edema (<1%)
Painful erection
Paresthesias (2%)
Priapism
(1995): Levenson JL, *Am J Psychiatry* 152, 813
Serum sickness
(2000): McCollom RA+*Ann Pharmacother* 34, 471
(1999): Peloso PM+, *JAMA* 282, 1817
(1999): Tripathi A+, *Ann Allergy Asthma Immunol* 83, 165
(1999): Yolles JC+, *Ann Pharmacother* 33, 931
Sialorrhea
Stomatitis (>1%)
Tongue edema (0.1%)
(2000): McCollom RA+*Ann Pharmacother* 34, 471
Tremor (>10%)
Twitching (2%)
Vaginitis
Xerostomia (up to 64%)
(1999): Settle EC+, *Clin Ther* 21, 454
(1997): Hurd RD+, *N Engl J Med* 337, 1195
(1991): James WA+, *South Med J* 84, 222
(1986): Feighner JP+, *J Clin Psychopharmacol* 6, 27
(1983): Feighner JP, *J Clin Psychiatry* 44, 49
(1981): Halaris AE+, *Psychopharmacol Bull* 17, 140
(1983): Chouinard G, *J Clin Psychiatry* 44, 121

BUSPIRONE

Trade name: BuSpar (Bristol-Myers Squibb)
Other common trade names: *Ansail; Apo-Buspirone; Bespar; Biron; Busirone; Bustab; Kallmiren; Narol; Neurosine; Nu-Buspirone*
Indications: Anxiety
Category: Nonbenzodiazepine anxiolytic tranquilizer; serotonin antagonist
Half-life: 2–3 hours
Clinically important, potentially serious interactions with: aspirin, CNS depressants, digoxin, diltiazem, erythromycin, ethanol, fluoxetine, flurazepam, haloperidol, MAO inhibitors, SSRIs, trazodone, verapamil

Reactions

Skin

Acne (<0.1%)
Bullous eruption (<1%)
Diaphoresis
(1986): Newton RE+, *Am J Med* 3B:80, 17
Ecchymoses
Edema

Exanthems
Facial edema (1%)
Flushing
Pruritus (1%)
Purpura (1%)
Radiation recall
(1989): Vassal G+, *Cancer Chemother Pharmacol* 23, 117
Rash (sic) (<1%)
Seborrheic dermatitis
(1993): Litt JZ, Beachwood, OH, personal case (observation)
Sicca syndrome
(1977): Sidi Y+, *JAMA* 238, 1951
Urticaria (<1%)
Xerosis (1%)

Hair

Hair – alopecia (1%)
(2000): Mercke Y+, *Ann Clin Psychiatry* 12, 35
(1995): Ljungman P+, *Bone Marrow Transplant* 15, 869

Nails

Nails – thinning (<0.1%)

Other

Dysgeusia (<1%)
Galactorrhea (<0.1%)
Glossodynia
Glossopyrosis
Myalgia
Paresthesias (1%)
(1986): Newton RE+, *Am J Med* 3B:80, 17
Parosmia (1%)
Sialorrhea
Xerostomia (3%)

BUSULFAN

Trade name: Myleran (GlaxoWellcome)
Other common trade names: *Citosulfan; Leukosulfan; Mablin; Misulban*
Indications: Chronic myelogenous leukemia, bone marrow disorders
Category: Antineoplastic
Half-life: 3.4 hours (after first dose)
Clinically important, potentially serious interactions with: thioguanine

Reactions

Skin

Bullous eruption
(1970): Dosik H+, *Blood* 35, 543
Cheilitis
(1980): Wintroub B+, *Clinical Cancer Medicine*, GK Hall and Company, 206
(1961): Haut A+, *Blood* 17, 1
Eccrine squamous syringometaplasia
(1997): Valks R+, *Arch Dermatol* 133, 873
Erythema (macular) (sic) (>10%)
(1985): Hymes SR+, *J Cutan Pathol* 12, 125
Erythema multiforme (<1%)
(1981): Weiss RB+, *Ann Intern Med* 94, 66
(1980): Adrian RM+, *CA* 30, 143
(1978): Levine N+, *Cancer Treat Rev* 5, 67
(1974): Levantine A+, *Br J Dermatol* 90, 239
(1970): Dosik H+, *Blood* 35, 543
Erythema nodosum (<1%)
(1978): Levine N+, *Cancer Treat Rev* 5, 67
(1961): Kyle BA+, *Blood* 18, 497
(1956): Marinko HM+, *Arq Brasil Med* (Portuguese) 46, 161
Exanthems
(1992): Fitzpatrick JE, *Derm Clinics* 10, 19 (passim)
(1978): Leyden MJ+, *Lancet* 2, 797
Kaposi's sarcoma
(1998): Roszkiewicz A+, *Cutis* 61, 137
Pigmentation (1–10%) ("busulfan tan")
(1999): Simonart T+, *Ann Dermatol Venereol* (French) 126, 439
(1992): Fitzpatrick JE, *Derm Clinics* 10, 19 (passim)
(1985): Hymes SR+, *J Cutan Pathol* 12, 125
(1983): Bronner AK+, *J Am Acad Dermatol* 9, 645
(1981): Granstein RD+, *J Am Acad Dermatol* 5, 1 (brown-black)
(1980): Adam BA+, *J Dermatol* 7, 405
(1971): Burns WA+, *Med Ann DC* 40, 567
(1966): Harrold BP, *BMJ* 1, 463
(1966): Sprunt JG+, *BMJ* 5489, 736
(1965): Desai RG, *N Engl J Med* 272, 808
(1963): Marchal G+, *Sem Ther* (French) 39, 565
(1961): Kyle RA+, *Blood* 18, 497
(1961): Haut A+, *Blood* 17, 1
Purpura
Urticaria (>10%)
(1981): Weiss RB+, *Ann Intern Med* 94, 66
(1981): Spiegel RJ, *Cancer Treat Rev* 8, 197
(1978): Levine N+, *Cancer Treat Rev* 5, 67
(1961): Kyle BA+, *Blood* 18, 497
(1960): Ducach C+, *Rev Med Chile* (Spanish) 88, 36
Vasculitis
(1992): Breathnach SM+, *Adverse Drug Reactions and the Skin*, Blackwell, Oxford, 288 (passim)
(1982): Weiss RB, *Sem Oncology* 9, 5
(1967): Coleman WP, *Med Clin North Am* 51, 1073
Xerosis
(1961): Haut A+, *Blood* 17, 1

Hair

Hair – alopecia (>10%)
(2000): Tran D+, *Australas J Dermatology* 41, 106
(1995): Ljungman P+, *Bone Marrow Transplant* 15, 869
(1993): Vowels M+, *Bone Marrow Transplant* 12, 347
(1977): Moschella S, *Cutis* 19, 603
(1975): Dreizen S+, *Postgrad Med* 58, 150
(1961): Haut A+, *Blood* 17, 1

Nails

Nails – pigmentation

Other

Anhidrosis
(1961): Haut A+, *Blood* 17, 1
Dysgeusia
(1961): Haut A+, *Blood* 17, 1
Gynecomastia (<1%)
(1979): Harrington WJ, *Adv Intern Med* 24, 141
(1979): White DR+, *N C Med J* 40, 73
(1977): Moschella SL, *Cutis* 19, 603
Oral mucosal pigmentation
(1965): Desai RG, *N Engl J Med* 272, 808
Porphyria cutanea tarda
(1983): Bronner AK+, *J Am Acad Dermatol* 9, 645
(1964): Kyle BA+, *Blood* 23, 776
Stomatitis

BUTABARBITAL

Trade names: Butalan; Buticaps; Butisol (Wallace)
Other common trade names: *Butalan; Buticaps; Day-Barb*
Indications: Sedation
Category: Sedative-hypnotic barbiturate
Half-life: 40–140 hours
Clinically important, potentially serious interactions with: benzodiazepines, carbamazepine, chloramphenicol, CNS depressants, methylphenidate, phenytoin, propoxyphene, valproic acid, warfarin

Reactions

Skin

Acneform eruption
Angioedema (<1%)
Bullous eruption
(1970): Groeschel D+, *N Engl J Med* 283, 409

Erythema multiforme
(1975): Böttiger LE, *Acta Med Scand* 198, 229
Exanthems
(1943): Davison TC, *Curr Res Anesth Analg* 22, 52
Exfoliative dermatitis (<1%)
(1944): Potter JK+, *Ann Intern Med* 21, 1041
Fixed eruption
(1970): Savin JA, *Br J Dermatol* 83, 546
Herpes simplex
Lupus erythematosus
(1967): Williams DI, *Proc R Soc Med* 60, 299
(1951): Grant Peterkin GA, *Edinb Med J* 58, 41
Necrosis
(1972): Almeyda J+, *Br J Dermatol* 86, 313
Photosensitivity
(1939): Stryker GV, *J Mo Med Assn* 36, 484
Pruritus
Purpura
(1946): Grant Peterkin GA, *BMJ* 2, 52
Rash (sic) (<1%)
Stevens–Johnson syndrome (<1%)
Toxic epidermal necrolysis
(1973): Stüttgen G, *Br J Dermatol* 88, 291
Urticaria
Vasculitis

Other

Oral ulceration
Porphyria variegata
Thrombophlebitis (<1%)

BUTALBITAL

Trade name: Fiorinal (Novartis)
Other trade names: *Amaphen; Anoquan; Axotal; Butace; Fioricet; Marnal; Medigesic; Phrenilin; Tecnal*
Indications: Tension headaches
Category: Sedative and analgesic barbiturate
Half-life: 35 hours
Clinically important, potentially serious interactions with: benzodiazepines, chloramphenicol, CNS depressants, haloperidol, methylphenidate, phenothiazines, propoxyphene, valproic acid, warfarin

Reactions

Skin

Bullous eruption
(1970): Groeschel D+, *N Engl J Med* 283, 409
Erythema multiforme
(1984): Gebel K+, *Dermatologica* 168, 35
(1975): Böttiger LE, *Acta Med Scand* 198, 229
Exanthems
(1943): Davison TC, *Curr Res Anesth Analg* 22, 52
Exfoliative dermatitis (<1%)
(1944): Potter JK+, *Ann Intern Med* 21, 1041
Fixed eruption
(1970): Savin JA, *Br J Dermatol* 83, 546
Herpes simplex
Lupus erythematosus
(1967): Williams DI, *Proc R Soc Med* 60, 299
(1951): Grant Peterkin GA, *Edinb Med J* 58, 41
Necrosis
(1972): Almeyda J+, *Br J Dermatol* 86, 313
Photosensitivity
(1939): Stryker GV, *J Mo Med Assn* 36, 484
Pruritus
Purpura
(1946): Grant Peterkin GA, *BMJ* 2, 52
Rash (sic) (1–10%)
Stevens–Johnson syndrome (<1%)
Toxic epidermal necrolysis
(1973): Stüttgen G, *Br J Dermatol* 88, 291
Urticaria
(1993): Litt JZ, Beachwood, OH, personal case (observation)
Vasculitis

Other

Anaphylactoid reaction (1–10%)
Oral erythema multiforme
(1984): Gebel K+, *Dermatologica* 168, 35
Oral ulceration
Porphyria variegata

BUTORPHANOL

Trade name: Stadol (Bristol-Myers Squibb)
Other common trade names: *Biforal; Busphen; Stadol NS*
Indications: Pain, migraine
Category: Narcotic, analgesic
Half-life: 2.5–4 hours
Clinically important, potentially serious interactions with: alcohol, CNS depressants, cimetidine, MAO inhibitors, opiates, phenothiazines, ranitidine, ritonavir, tricyclic antidepressants

Reactions

Skin

Clammy skin (sic)
Diaphoresis (1–10%)
Edema (<1%)
Exanthems
Flushing (1–10%)
Gooseflesh (sic)
Pruritus (1–10%)
(1989): Ackerman WE+, *Can J Anaesth* 36, 388
(1981): Bernstein JE+, *J Am Acad Dermatol* 5, 227
Rash (sic) (<1%)
Urticaria (<1%)

Other

Dysgeusia (3–9%)
Injection-site reactions
Paresthesias
Xerostomia (3–9%)

CABERGOLINE

Trade name: Dostinex (Pharmacia & Upjohn)
Indications: Hyperprolactinemia; parkinsonism
Category: Dopamine receptor agonist, ergot alkaloid
Half-life: 63–69 hours
Clinically important, potentially serious interactions with: butyrophenones, metoclopramide, phenothiazines, thioxanthines

Reactions

Skin
Acne (1%)
(1997): Rademaker M, New Zealand (from Internet) (observation)
Ankle edema (1%)
Facial edema (1%)
Fixed eruption
(1997): Rademaker M, New Zealand (from Internet) (observation)
Flu-like syndrome (sic) (1%)
Hot flashes (3%)
Periorbital edema (1%)
Peripheral edema (1%)
Pruritus (1%)

Other
Mastodynia (2%)
Paresthesias (5%)
Toothache (1%)
Xerostomia (2%)

CALCITONIN
(HUMAN and SALMON)

Trade names: Calcimar (Aventis); Miacalcin (Novartis)
Other common trade names: *Caltine; Cibacalcine; Clasynar; Miacalcic*
Indications: Paget's disease of bone
Category: Calcium regulator; osteoporosis therapy adjunct; bone resorption inhibitor
Half-life: 70–90 minutes
Clinically important, potentially serious interactions with: calcium salts, vitamin D

Reactions

Skin
Edema of feet
Exanthems
Flushing (>10%)
(1995): Kobayashi T+, *J Endocrinol* 146, 431
(1975): Goldsmith RS, *JAMA* 232, 1156
(1975): Med Lett, 17, 97
Granuloma annulare
(1993): Goihman YM, *Int J Dermatol* 32, 150
Pruritus
Rash (sic) (<1%)
Tender palms and soles (sic)
Urticaria (<1%)
(1975): Med Lett, 17, 97

Other
Anaphylactoid reaction
Dysgeusia (metallic or salty)
Hypersensitivity
Injection-site edema (>10%)
Injection-site inflammation (>10%)
(1975): Goldsmith RS, *JAMA* 232, 1156
(1975): Med Lett, 17, 97
Injection-site pain
(1988): Warrell RP+, *Ann Intern Med* 108, 669 (62%)
Paresthesias (<1%)

CALFACTANT

Trade name: Infasurf (Forest)
Indications: Prevention of respiratory distress syndrome
Category: Lung surfactant (intratracheal)
Half-life: no data
Clinically important, potentially serious interactions with: aminoglycosides, amphotericin B, ceftazidime, pentamidine, vancomycin

Reactions

None

CANDESARTAN

Trade name: Atacand (AstraZeneca)
Other trade name: *Amias*
Indications: Hypertension
Category: Angiotensin II receptor antagonist, antihypertensive
Half-life: 9 hours
Clinically important, potentially serious interactions with: none

Reactions

Skin
Angioedema
Diaphoresis (>0.5%)
Edema
Exanthems (<1%)
Peripheral edema (>1%)
Rash (sic) (>0.5%)

Other
Myalgia (>0.5%)
Paresthesias (>0.5%)

CAPECITABINE

Trade name: Xeloda (Roche)
Indications: Metastatic breast cancer
Category: Antineoplastic, antimetabolite (a prodrug of 5-FU)
Half-life: 0.5–1 hour
Clinically important, potentially serious interactions with: antacids, anticoagulants, fluorouracil, immunosuppressives, leucovorin, NSAIDs, salicylates, warfarin

Reactions

Skin
Acral erythema
Blistering
Dermatitis (37%)
(1999): Dooley M+, *Drugs* 58, 69
Diaphoresis (0.2%)
Edema (9%)
(1996): Bajetta E+, *Tumori* 82, 450
Erythema
Exfoliative dermatitis (31–37%)
Infections (sic) (<1%)
Palmar-plantar erythrodysesthesia (hand-foot syndrome) (57%)
(1999): Dooley M+, *Drugs* 58, 69
(1999): Blum JL+, *J Clin Oncol* 17, 485 (10%)
(1999): Blum JL, *Oncology* 57, 16
(1999): Mrozek-Orlowski ME+, *Oncol Nurs Forum* 26, 753
(1998): Budman DR+, *J Clin Oncol* 16, 1795
Photosensitivity (<1%)
Pruritus
Purpura (0.2%)

Radiation recall (< 1%)
Xerosis

Hair

Hair – alopecia (< 1%)

Nails

Nail – disorder (sic) (7%)

Other

Hypersensitivity (< 1%)
Myalgia (9%)
Oral candidiasis (0.2%)
Oral ulceration
Paresthesias (21%)
Stomatitis (24%)
Thrombophlebitis (0.2%)

CAPTOPRIL

Synonym: ACE
Trade names: Capoten (Bristol-Myers Squibb); Capozide (Bristol-Myers Squibb)
Other common trade names: *Acenorm; Acepril; Adocor; APO-Capto; Captolane; Captoril; Lopirin; Lopril; Nu-Capto; Precaptil*
Indications: Hypertension
Category: Angiotensin-converting enzyme (ACE) inhibitor; antihypertensive and vasodilator
Half-life: <3 hours
Clinically important, potentially serious interactions with: alcohol, allopurinol, antacids, aspirin, digoxin, diuretics, heparin, indomethacin, insulin, lithium, mercaptopurine, NSAIDs, phenothiazines, probenecid, salicylates, **food**

Capozide is captopril and hydrochlorothiazide

Reactions

Skin

Angioedema (< 1%)
(1998): Smoger SH+, *South Med J* 91, 1060
(1997): Brown NJ+, *JAMA* 278, 232
(1997): Tisch M+, *Anaesthesiol Intensivmed Notfallmed Schmerzther* (German) 32, 122
(1996): Pillans PI+, *Eur J Clin Pharmacol* 51, 123
(1996): Ekborn A+, *Lakartidningen* (Swedish) 93, 468
(1995): Bauwens LJ+, *Ned Tijdschr Geneeskd* (Dutch) 139, 674
(1995): Kozel MM+, *Clin Exp Dermatol* 20, 60
(1993): Chu TJ+, *Ann Intern Med* 118, 314
(1993): Thompson T+, *Laryngoscope* 103, 10
(1992): Diehl KL+, *Dtsch Med Wochenschr* (German)117, 727
(1992): Dobroschke B+, *Anasthesiol Intensivmed Notfallmed Schmerzther* (German) 27, 510
(1992): Sanchez-Hernandez J+, *An Med Interna* (Spanish) 9, 572
(1992): Jason DR, *J Forensic Sci* 37, 1418 (fatal)
(1992): Hedner T+, *BMJ* 304, 941
(1991): Roberts JR+, *Ann Emerg Med* 20, 555
(1991): Pek F, HNO (German) 39, 410
(1990): Seidman MD+, *Otolaryngol Head Neck Surg* 102, 727
(1990): DiNardo LJ+, *Trans Pa Acad Ophthalmol Otolaryngol* 42, 998
(1990): Gannon TH+, *Laryngoscope* 100, 1156
(1990): Cameron DI, *Can J Cardiol* 6, 265
(1990): Zech J+, *HNO* (German) 38, 143
(1990): McAreavey D+, *Drugs* 40, 326
(1990): Motel PJ, *J Am Acad Dermatol* 23, 124
(1989): Werber JL+, *Otolaryngol Head Neck Surg* 101, 96
(1989): Barna JS+, *Va Med* 116, 147
(1988): Wernze H, *Z Kardiol* (German) 77, 61
(1988): Brogden RN+, *Drugs* 36, 540
(1988): Slater EE+, *JAMA* 260, 967 (0.1%)
(1987): Wood SM+, *BMJ* 294, 91
(1987): Ferner RE+, *BMJ* 294, 1119
(1987): Edwards IR+, *Br J Clin Pharmacol* 23, 529
(1987): No Author, *Am J Med 82*, 576
(1986): Suarez M+, *Am J Med* 81, 336
(1984): Smit AJ+, *Clin Allergy* 14, 413 (2%)
(1984): Materson BJ+, *Ann Intern Med* 144, 1947 (2.1%)
(1984): Jett GK, *Ann Emerg Med* 13, 489
(1982): Vidt DG+, *N Engl J Med* 306, 214 (passim)
(1980): Wilkin JK+, *Arch Dermatol* 116, 903 (15%)
Bullous eruption
(1989): Klein LE+, *Cutis* 44, 393
Bullous pemphigoid
(1993): Fitzgerald DA, *Clin Exp Dermatol* 18, 196
(1989): Mallet L+, *Drug Intell Clin Pharm* 23, 63
Contact dermatitis
(1990): Cnudde F+, *Contact Dermatitis* 23, 375
Cutaneous reaction (sic)
(1998): Lluch-Bernal M+, *Contact Dermatitis* 39, 316
Erythroderma
(1989): Allegue F+, *Rev Clin Esp* (Spanish) 184, 210
(1985): Goodfield MJ+, *BMJ* 290, 1111
Exanthems (4–7%)
(1993): Fitzgerald DA, *Clin Exp Dermatol* 18, 196 (passim)
(1990): McAreavey D+, *Drugs* 40, 326 (0.5–4%)
(1990): Cnudde F+, *Contact Dermatitis* 23, 375
(1990): Motel PJ, *J Am Acad Dermatol* 23, 124
(1989): Clemens G+, *Verh Dtsch Ges Inn Med* (German) 95, 721
(1989): Gomez-Martino-Arroyo JR+, *Rev Clin Esp* (Spanish) 184, 497
(1988): Brogden RN+, *Drugs* 36, 540 (0.5–4%)
(1988): Warner NJ+, *Drugs* 35 (Suppl 5) 89 (4–7%)
(1988): Bretin N+, *Dermatologica* 177, 11
(1985): Goodfield MJ+, *BMJ* 290, 1111
(1985): Todd PA+, *Drugs* 31, 198
(1984): Smit AJ+, *Clin Allergy* 14, 413 (7%)
(1983): Romankiewicz JA+, *Drugs* 25, 6 (4.6%)
(1983): Steinman TI+, *Am J Med* 75, 154
(1982): Vidt DG+, *N Engl J Med* 306, 214 (passim)
(1982): Luderer JR+, *J Clin Pharm* 22, 151
(1980): Heel RC+, *Drugs* 20, 409 (8–14%)
(1980): Wilkin JK+, *Arch Dermatol* 116, 903
(1978): Gavras H+, *N Engl J Med* 298, 991 (10%)
Exfoliative dermatitis (<2%)
(1990): Motel PJ, *J Am Acad Dermatol* 23, 124
(1989): O'Neill PG+, *Tex Med* 85, 40
(1988): Lai KN+, *Singapore Med J* 29, 526
(1982): Solinger AM, *Cutis* 29, 437
Flushing (< 1%)
(1989): Healy LA+, *N Engl J Med* 321, 763
(1987): Ferner RE+, *Br Med J Clin Res Ed* 294, 1119
Graft-versus-host reaction
(1998): Jappe U+, *Hautarzt* (German) 49, 126 (passim)
Kaposi's sarcoma
(1991): Larbre JP, *J Rheumatol* 18, 476
(1990): Puppin D+, *Lancet* 336, 1251
Lichenoid eruption
(1996): Revenga-Arranz F+, *Rev Clin Esp* (Spanish) 196, 412
(1994): Phillips WG+, *Clin Exp Dermatol* 19, 317
(1992): Wong SS+, *Acta Derm Venereol* (Stockh) 72, 358
(1992): Perez-Roldan E+, *Rev Clin Esp* (Spanish) 191, 501
(1990): Pascual J+, *Nephron* 56, 110
(1989): Rotstein E+, *Australas J Dermatol* 30, 9
(1989): Cox NH+, *Br J Dermatol* 120, 319
(1988): Bretin N+, *Dermatologica* 177, 11
(1984): Smit AJ+, *Clin Allergy* 14, 413 (1%)
(1983): Bravard P+, *Ann Dermatol Venereol* (French) 110, 433
(1983): Bravard P+, *Presse Med* (French) 12, 577
(1983): Reinhardt LA+, *Cutis* 31, 98
Lichen planus (pemphigoides)
(1986): Flageul B+, *Dermatologica* 173, 248
Linear IgA bullous dermatosis
(1998): Friedman IS+, *Int J Dermatol* 37, 608
(1994): Kuechle MK+, *J Am Acad Dermatol* 30, 187
(1989): Klein LE+, *Cutis* 44, 393
Lupus erythematosus
(1995): Fernandez-Diaz ML+, *Lancet* 345, 398
(1993): Pelayo M+, *Ann Pharmacother* 27, 1541
(1993): Bertin P+, *Clin Exp Rheumatol* 11, 695
(1990): Sieber C+, *BMJ* 301, 669
(1985): Patri P+, *Acta Derm Venereol* (Stockh) 65, 447
Mycosis fungoides

(1995): Carroll J+, *Cutis* 56, 276 (pustular)
(1986): Furness PN+, *J Clin Pathol* 39, 902

Palmar-plantar pustulosis
(1995): Eriksen JG+, *Ugeskr Laeger* (Danish) 157, 3335

Pemphigus (<2%)
(1995): Butt A+, *Br J Dermatol* 132, 315
(1994): Trinidad-Paz JM+, *Rev Clin Esp* (Spanish) 194, 999
(1994): Kuechle MK+, *Mayo Clin Proc* 69, 1166
(1992): Kaplan RP+, *J Am Acad Dermatol* 26, 364
(1992): Pinto GM+, *J Am Acad Dermatol* 27, 281 (vegetans)
(1992): Ruocco V+, *Int J Dermatol* 31, 33
(1991): Beaulieu P+, *Ann Dermatol Venereol* (French) 118, 547
(1991): Korman NJ+, *J Invest Dermatol* 96, 273
(1990): Motel PJ, *J Am Acad Dermatol* 23, 124
(1990): Black AK+, *Br J Dermatol* 123, 277
(1990): Ruocco V+, *Arch Dermatol* 126, 965
(1988): Blanken R+, *Acta Derm Venereol* (Stockh) 68, 456
(1988): Bretin N+, *Dermatologica* 177, 11
(1987): Katz RA+, *Arch Dermatol* 123, 20
(1987): Arnoux D+, *Ann Dermatol Venereol* (French) 114, 1241
(1986): Ricci G+, *Recenti Prog Med* (Italian) 77, 321
(1985): Bernard P+, *Ann Dermatol Venereol* (French) 112, 661
(1982): Ruocco V+, *Arch Dermatol Res* 274, 123
(1982): Christeler A+, *Schweiz Med Wochenschr* (German) 112, 1483
(1981): Clement MI, *Arch Dermatol* 117, 525
(1980): Parfrey PS+, *BMJ* 281, 194

Penile ulcers
(1983): Romankiewicz JA+, *Drugs* 25, 6 (4.6%)
(1981): Nicholls MG+, *Ann Intern Med* 94, 695

Photosensitivity
(1994): Shelley WB+, *Cutis* 54, 70 (observation)
(1990): Motel PJ, *J Am Acad Dermatol* 23, 124
(1988): Mauduit G+, *Ann Dermatol Venereol* (French) 115, 167

Phototoxic reaction (<2%)

Pigmentation
(1990): Black AK+, *Br J Dermatol* 123, 277
(1987): O'Neill MB+, *BMJ* 295, 33

Pityriasis rosea (<2%)
(1990): Motel PJ, *J Am Acad Dermatol* 23, 124
(1990): Ghersetich I+, *G Ital Dermatol Venereol* (Italian) 125, 457
(1990): Wolf R+, *Dermatologica* 181, 51
(1988): Bretin N+, *Dermatologica* 177, 11
(1983): Reinhardt LA+, *Cutis* 31, 98
(1982): Wilkin JK+, *Arch Dermatol* 118, 186

Pruritus (4–7%)
(1992): Shelley WB+, *Cutis* 49, 391 (observation)
(1990): Motel PJ, *J Am Acad Dermatol* 23, 124
(1984): Materson BJ+, *Ann Intern Med* 144, 1947 (0.2%)
(1983): Romankiewicz JA+, *Drugs* 25, 6 (4%)
(1983): Daniel F+, *Ann Dermatol Venereol* (French) 110, 441 (10%)
(1983): Steinman TI+, *Am J Med* 75, 154
(1982): Vidt DG+, *N Engl J Med* 306, 214 (passim)
(1982): Liebau G, *Klin Wochenschr* (German) 60, 107
(1980): Luderer JR+, *Clin Res* 28, 589A

Psoriasis
(1995): Ikai K, *J Am Acad Dermatol* 32, 819
(1993): Coulter DM+, *N Z Med J* 106, 392
(1992): Shelley WB+, *Cutis* 50, 87 (observation)
(1990): Sieber C+, *BMJ* 301, 669
(1990): Wolf R+, *Dermatologica* 181, 51
(1987): Wolf R+, *Cutis* 40, 162
(1987): Hamlet DW+, *BMJ* 295, 1352
(1986): Hauschild TT+, *Hautarzt* (German) 37, 274

Purpura
(1989): Grosbois B+, *BMJ* 298, 189

Rash (sic) (4–7%)
(1990): Kahan A+, *Clin Pharmacol Ther* 47, 483
(1985): Jenkins AC+, *J Cardiovasc Pharmacol* 7, S96
(1984): Martin MF+, *Lancet* 1, 1325
(1984): Kubo SH+, *Ann Intern Med* 100, 616
(1983): Steinman TI+, *Am J Med* 75, 154
(1983): Rotmensch HH+, *Pharmacotherapy* 3, 131
(1983): Romankiewicz JA+, *Drugs* 25, 6
(1982): Liebau G, *Klin Wochenschr* (German) 60, 107
(1982): Rosendorff C, *S Afr Med J* 62, 593
(1981): Luderer JR+, *Am J Med* 71, 493

Stevens–Johnson syndrome
(1984): Pennell DJ+, *Lancet* 1, 463 (fatal)

Toxic epidermal necrolysis
(1999): Winfred RI+, *South Med J* 92, 918
(1983): Sala F+, *G Ital Dermatol Venereol* (Italian) 118, 89

Urticaria
(1996): Pillans PI+, *Eur J Clin Pharmacol* 51, 123
(1993): Fitzgerald DA, *Clin Exp Dermatol* 18, 196 (passim)
(1988): Bretin N+, *Dermatologica* 177, 11
(1988): Slater EE+, *JAMA* 260, 967
(1987): Wood SM+, *BMJ* 294, 91
(1985): Goodfield MJD+, *BMJ* 290, 1111
(1984): Materson BJ+, *Ann Intern Med* 144, 1947 (1.4%)
(1984): Smit AJ+, *Clin Allergy* 14, 413 (7%)
(1980): Wilkin JK+, *Arch Dermatol* 116, 902

Vasculitis
(1994): Dorman RL+, *AJR Am J Roentgenol* 163, 840
(1990): Black AK+, *Br J Dermatol* 123, 277 (fatal)
(1988): Miralles R+, *Ann Intern Med* 109, 514
(1988): Lotti T+, *G Ital Dermatol Venereol* (Italian) 123, 657
(1987): Laaban J+, *European Heart J* 8, 319
(1984): Goodfield MJD+, *Lancet* 2, 517
(1984): Smit AJ+, *Clin Allergy* 14, 413

Xerosis
(1983): Smit AJ+, *Nephron* 34, 196

Hair

Hair – alopecia (<2%)
(1994): Shelley WB+, *Cutis* 52, 264 (observation)
(1990): Motel PJ, *J Am Acad Dermatol* 23, 124
(1984): Leaker B+, *Aust N Z J Med* 14, 866
(1984): Smit AJ+, *Clin Allergy* 14, 413 (3%)
(1983): Smit AJ+, *Nephron* 34, 196

Nails

Nails – dystrophy
(1984): Brueggemeyer CD+, *Lancet* 1, 1352
(1983): Smit AJ+, *Nephron* 34, 196

Nails – onycholysis
(1986): Borders JV, *Ann Intern Med* 105, 305
(1984): Brueggemeyer CD+, *Lancet* 1, 1352

Other

Ageusia (2–4%)
(1997): Acanfora D+, *Am J Ther* 4, 181
(1993): Fitzgerald DA, *Clin Exp Dermatol* 18, 196 (passim)
(1987): Edwards IR+, *Br J Clin Pharmacol* 23, 529
(1984): Martin MF+, *Lancet* 1, 1325
(1983): Smit AJ+, *Nephron* 34, 196
(1982): Liebau G, *Klin Wochenschr* (German) 60, 107
(1982): Vidt DG+, *N Engl J Med* 306, 214 (passim)
(1979): McNeil JJ+, *BMJ* 6204, 1555
(1979): Vlasses PH+, *Lancet* 2, 526

Anaphylactoid reaction (during hemodialysis)

Aphthous stomatitis (<2%)
(1983): Daniel F+, *Ann Dermatol Venereol* (French) 110, 441
(1982): Vidt DG+, *N Engl J Med* 306, 214 (passim)
(1980): Heel RC+, *Drugs* 20, 409
(1979): Seedat YK, *Lancet* 2, 1297

Dysgeusia (2–4%) (metallic or salty taste)
(2000): Zervakis J+, *Physiol Behav* 68, 405
(1993): Zazgornik J+, *Lancet* 341, 1542
(1993): Boyd I, *Lancet* 342, 304
(1990): Kahan A+, *Clin Pharmacol Ther* 47, 483
(1985): Jenkins AC+, *J Cardiovasc Pharmacol* 7, S96
(1985): Mauersberger H+, *Lancet* 1, 517
(1983): Kayanakis JG+, *Arch Mal Coeur Vaiss* (French) 76, 1065
(1983): Romankiewicz JA+, *Drugs* 25, 6
(1979): McNeil JJ+, *BMJ* 6204, 1555

Glossitis
(1989): Drucker CR+, *Arch Dermatol* 125, 1437 (atrophic)
(1983): Romankiewicz JA+, *Drugs* 25, 6
(1981): Nicholls MG+, *Ann Intern Med* 94, 659

Glossopyrosis
(1989): Drucker CR+, *Arch Dermatol* 125, 1437

Gynecomastia
(2000): Hugues FC+, *Ann Med Interne (Paris)* (French) 151, 10 (passim)
(1990): Nakamura Y+, *BMJ* 300, 541
(1988): Markusse HM+, *BMJ* 296, 1262

Lymphadenopathy
(1981): Aberg H+, *BMJ* 283, 1297
Myalgia
Oral mucosal eruption
(1989): Firth NA+, *Oral Surg Oral Med Oral Pathol* 67, 41 (lichenoid)
(1985): Todd PA+, *Drugs* 31, 198
(1980): Heel RC+, *Drugs* 20, 409
Oral ulceration
(1993): Fitzgerald DA, *Clin Exp Dermatol* 18, 196 (passim)
(1982): Viraben R+, *Arch Dermatol* 118, 959
Paresthesias (<2%)
Scalded mouth (sic)
(1982): Vlasses PH+, *BMJ* 284, 1672
Tongue ulceration
(1982): Viraben R+, *Arch Dermatol* 118, 959
(1982): Vlasses PH+, *BMJ* 284, 1672 (passim)
(1981): Nicholls MG+, *Ann Intern Med* 94, 659
Xerostomia (<2%)

CARBAMAZEPINE

Trade names: Carbatrol (Shire Richwood); Tegretol (Novartis)
Other common trade names: *Apo-Carbamazepine; Atreol; Foxsalepsin; Kodapan; Lexin; Mazepine; Sirtal; Tegretol XR; Teril; Timonil*
Indications: Epilepsy, pain or trigeminal neuralgia
Category: Anticonvulsant, antineuralgic, antimanic, antidiuretic and antipsychotic
Half-life: 18–55 hours
Clinically important, potentially serious interactions with: anticoagulants, barbiturates, cimetidine, danazol, diltiazem, erythromycin, felbamate, felodipine, haloperidol, hydantoins, isoniazid, lithium, primidone, propoxyphene, SSRIs, theophylline, tricyclic antidepressants, troleandomycin, valproic acid, verapamil, warfarin

Reactions

Skin

Acne keloid
(1990): Grunwald MH+, *Int J Dermatol* 29, 559
Acute generalized exanthematous pustulosis (AGEP)
(1999): Lachgar T, *Allerg Immunol* (Paris) (French) 31, 151
(1999): Poster Exhibit #163, AAD Meeting, March 1999 (Reported by ED and WB Shelley)
(1996): Wolkenstein P+, *Contact Dermatitis* 35, 234
(1995): Moreau A+, *Int J Dermatol* 34, 263 (passim)
(1991): Roujeau J-C+, *Arch Dermatol* 127, 1333
Allergic reactions (sic)
(1999): Pasmans SG+, *Allergy* 54, 649
(1995): Tijhuis GJ+, *Ned Tijdschr Geneeskd* (Dutch) 139, 2265 (42 cases)
(1993): Beran RG, *Epilepsia* 34, 163
(1992): Dzianott A+, *Wiad Lek* (Polish) 45, 465
(1985): Moore NC+, *Am J Psychiatry* 142, 974
Angioedema (<1%)
(1977): Houwerzijl J+, *Clin Exp Immunol* 29, 272
(1971): Virolainen M, *Clin Exp Immunol* 9, 429
(1967): Livingston S+, *JAMA* 200, 204
Ankle edema
Bullous eruption (<1%)
(1990): Gebauer K+, *Australas J Dermatol* 31, 89 (passim)
(1988): Warnock JK+, *Am J Psychiatry* 145, 425
(1983): Godden DJ+, *Postgrad Med J* 59, 336
Collagen disease (sic)
(1966): Simpson JR, *BMJ* 2, 1434
Contact dermatitis
(1992): Duhra P+, *Contact Dermatitis* 27, 325
(1991): Rodriguez-Mosquera M+, *Contact Dermatitis* 25, 137
(1991): Ljunggren B+, *Contact Dermatitis* 24, 259
Cutaneous side effects (sic)
(1994): Jones M+, *Dermatology* 188, 18 (4%)
(1967): Livingston S+, *JAMA* 200, 204 (4.5%)
Dermatitis (sic)
(1992): Duhra P+, *Contact Dermatitis* 27, 325
(1989): Malanin G+, *Duodecim* (Finnish) 105, 784
(1989): Terui T+, *Contact Dermatitis* 20, 260
(1981): Roberts DL+, *Arch Dermatol* 117, 273
(1967): Arieff AJ+, *Dis Nerv Syst* 28, 820
Diaphoresis (1–10%)
Eczematous eruption (sic)
(1999): Ozkaya-Bayazit E+, *J Eur Acad Dermatol Venereol* 12, 182
(1992): Duhra P+, *Contact Dermatitis* 27, 325
Edema
Eosinophilic pustular folliculitis (Ofuji's disease)
(1998): Mizoguchi S+, *J Am Acad Dermatol* 38, 641
Epidermolysis bullosa
(1992): Kong LN, *Chung Hua Hu Li Tsa Chih* (Chinese) 27, 495
Erythema multiforme
(1999): Frederickson K, (from Internet) (observation)
(1994): Friedmann PS+, *Arch Dermatol* 130, 598
(1993): Bruynzeel I+, *Br J Dermatol* 129, 45
(1993): Alanko K, *Contact Dermatitis* 29, 254
(1992): Chevenet C+, *Ann Dermatol Venereol* (French) 119, 929
(1989): Alanko K+, *Acta Derm Venereol* (Stockh) 69, 223
(1989): Busch RL, *N Engl J Med* 321, 692
(1988): Warnock JK+, *Am J Psychiatry* 145, 425
(1988): McDanal CE, *J Clin Psychiatr* 49, 369
(1987): Fawcett RG, *J Clin Psychiatry* 48, 416
(1986): Green ST, *Clin Neuropharmacol* 9, 561
(1985): Delafuente JC, *Drug Intell Clin Pharm* 19, 114
(1985): Patterson JF, *J Clin Psychopharmacol* 5, 185
(1984): Meisel S+, *Clin Pharm* 3, 15
(1975): Böttiger LE+, *Acta Med Scand* 198, 229
Erythema nodosum (<1%)
Erythroderma
(1998): Tayoro J+, *Therapie* 53, 513
(1996): Okuyama R+, *J Dermatol* 23, 489
(1995): Koga T+, *Contact Dermatitis* 33, 275
(1993): Blasco-Sarramian A+, *An Med Interna* (Spanish) 10, 341
(1990): Ruiz-Ezquerro JJ+, *An Med Interna* (Spanish) 31, 89
(1989): Romaguera C+, *Contact Dermatitis* 20, 304
(1987): Granier F+, *Rev Med Interne* (French) 8, 206
(1986): Silva R+, *Contact Dermatitis* 15, 254
(1982): Chennebault JM+, *Therapie* (French) 37, 106
(1980): Gaulier A+, *Nouv Presse Med* (French) 9, 1388
Exanthems (>5%)
(1999): Lombardi SM+, *Ann Pharmacother* 33, 571
(1998): Nathan D+, *J Am Acad Dermatol* 38, 806
(1997): Hyson C+, *Can J Neurol Sci* 24, 245
(1995): Wolkenstein P+, *Arch Dermatol* 131, 544
(1993): Konishi T+, *Eur J Pediatr* 152, 605
(1993): Hermle L+, *Nervenarzt* (German) 64, 208 (generalized)
(1993): Alanko K, *Contact Dermatitis* 29, 254
(1990): Garavelli PL+, *Minerva Med* (Italian) 81, 115
(1990): Gebauer K+, *Australas J Dermatol* 31, 89 (passim)
(1989): Eames P, *Lancet* 1, 509
(1988): Shear NH+, *J Clin Invest* 82, 1826
(1988): Warnock JK+, *Am J Psychiatry* 145, 425
(1984): Chadwick D+, *J Neurol Neurosurg Psychiatry* 47, 642 (17%)
(1982): Breathnach SM+, *Clin Exp Dermatol* 7, 585 (4%)
(1981): Sillanpää M, *Acta Neurol Scand* 64 (Suppl 88), 145
(1981): Taylor MW+, *Practitioner* 225, 219
(1977): Houwerzijl J+, *Clin Exp Immunol* 29, 272
(1974): Livingston S+, *Dis Nerv Syst* 35, 103 (2.7%)
(1972): Levantine A+, *Br J Dermatol* 87, 646 (3–4%)
(1971): Virolainen M, *Clin Exp Immunol* 9, 429
Exfoliative dermatitis
(1999): Lombardi SM+, *Ann Pharmacother* 33, 571
(1996): Sigurdsson V+, *J Am Acad Dermatol* 35, 53
(1996): Troost RJ+, *Pediatr Dermatol* 13, 316
(1995): Corazza M+, *Contact Dermatitis* 33, 447
(1995): Koga T+, *Contact Dermatitis* 32, 181
(1995): Bahamdan KA+, *Int J Dermatol* 34, 661
(1993): Alanko K, *Contact Dermatitis* 29, 254
(1991): Blin O+, *Therapie* (French) 46, 91
(1990): Gebauer K+, *Australas J Dermatol* 31, 89 (passim)
(1989): Alanko K+, *Acta Derm Venereol* (Stockh) 69, 223
(1989): Vaillant L+, *Arch Dermatol* 125, 299
(1989): Romaguera C+, *Contact Dermatitis* 20, 304
(1988): Cox NH+, *Postgrad Med J* 64, 249
(1987): Granier F+, *Rev Med Interne* 8, 206
(1987): Gimenez Garcia RM+, *Rev Clin Esp* (Spanish) 181, 542
(1985): Camarasa JG, *Contact Dermatitis* 12, 49

(1984): Shuttleworth D+, *Clin Exp Dermatol* 9, 421
(1982): Reed MD+, *Clin Pharm* 1, 78
(1981): Roberts DL+, *Arch Dermatol* 117, 273
(1977): Houwerzijl J+, *Clin Exp Immunol* 29, 272
(1968): Ford GR+, *N Z Med J* 68, 386

Facial edema

Fixed eruption (<1%)
(1997): Chan HL+, *J Am Acad Dermatol* 36, 259
(1997): de Argila D+, *Allergy* 52, 1039
(1993): Alanko K, *Contact Dermatitis* 29, 254
(1990): Gaffoor PMA+, *Cutis* 45, 242 (passim)
(1989): Stubb S+, *Br J Dermatol* 120, 583
(1988): Warnock JK+, *Am J Psychiatry* 145, 425
(1988): Bhariga JC+, *Sex Transm Dis* 15, 177
(1985): Kauppinen K+, *Br J Dermatol* 112, 575
(1984): Shuttleworth D+, *Clin Exp Dermatol* 9, 424

Lichenoid eruption
(1994): Thompson DF+, *Pharmacotherapy* 14, 561
(1990): Gebauer K+, *Australas J Dermatol* 31, 89 (passim)
(1990): Atkin SL+, *Clin Exp Dermatol* 15, 382
(1989): Ohtsuyama M+, *Nishinihon J Dermatol* (Japanese) 51, 958
(1988): Yasuda S+, *Photodermatology* 5, 206 (photosensitive)
(1981): Roberts DL+, *Arch Dermatol* 117, 273

Lupus erythematosus
(1998): Toepfer M+, *Eur J Clin Pharmacol* 54, 193 (late onset)
(1998): Bachmeyer C+, *Presse Med* (French) 27, 966
(1997): Reiffers-Mettelock J+, *Dermatology* 195, 306
(1997): Milesi-Lecat AM+, *Mayo Clin Proc* 72, 1145
(1996): Ghorayeb I+, *Rev Med Interne* (French) 17, 503
(1993): Ohashi T+, *Rinsho Shinkeigaku* (Japanese) 33, 1094
(1993): Drory VE+, *Clin Neuropharmacol* 16, 19 (passim)
(1992): Yust I+, *Intern Med* 31, 1303
(1992): Kanno T+, *Intern Med* 31, 1303
(1992): Boon DM+, *Ned Tijdschr Geneeskd* (Dutch) 136, 2085 (disseminated)
(1992): Schmidt S+, *Br J Psychiatry* 161, 560
(1991): Jain KK, *Drug Saf* 6, 350
(1991): De Giorgio CM+, *Epilepsia* 32, 128
(1990): Oner A+, *Clin Neurol Neurosurg* 92, 261
(1990): Gebauer K+, *Australas J Dermatol* 31, 89 (passim)
(1989): Drory VE+, *Clin Neuropharmacol* 12, 115
(1987): Alballa S+, *J Rheumatol* 14, 599
(1986): Leyh F+, *Z Haut* (German) 61, 611
(1985): *Br Med J Clin Res Ed* 291, 1125
(1985): Lovisetto P+, *Recenti Prog Med* (Italian) 76, 84
(1985): Bateman DE, *Br Med J Clin Res Ed* 291, 632
(1985): McNicholl B, *BMJ* 291, 1126
(1983): Kolstee HJ, *Ned Tijdschr Geneeskd* (Dutch) 127, 1588
(1976): Takigawa M+, *Arch Dermatol* 112, 845
(1974): Livingston S+, *Dis Nerv Syst* 35, 103 (2.7%)
(1969): Gayford JJ+, *Proc R Soc Med* 62, 615
(1967): Livingston S+, *JAMA* 200, 204
(1966): Simpson JR, *BMJ* 2, 1434

Mucocutaneous lymph node syndrome (Kawasaki syndrome)
(1990): Gebauer K+, *Australas J Dermatol* 31, 89 (passim)
(1987): Hicks RA+, *Pediatr Infect Dis J* 7, 525

Mycosis fungoides
(1991): Rijlaarsdam U+, *J Am Acad Dermatol* 24, 216
(1990): Welykyi S+, *J Cutan Pathol* 17, 111

Pellagra
(1998): Heyer G+, *Hautarzt* (German) 49, 123

Petechiae
(1993): Konishi T+, *Eur J Pediatr* 152, 605

Photosensitivity
(1991): Ljunggren B+, *Contact Dermatitis* 24, 259
(1990): Gebauer K+, *Australas J Dermatol* 31, 89 (passim)
(1989): Terui T+, *Contact Dermatitis* 20, 260
(1988): Warnock JK+, *Am J Psychiatry* 145, 425
(1988): Yasuda S+, *Photodermatology* 5, 206
(1986): Silva R+, *Contact Dermatitis* 15, 54
(1981): Sillanpää M, *Acta Neurol Scand* 64 (Suppl 88), 145
(1972): Levantine A+, *Br J Dermatol* 87, 646

Pigmentation

Pruritus (<1%)
(1969): Davis EH, *Headache* 9, 77
(1967): Livingston S+, *JAMA* 200, 204
(1964): Spillane D, *Practitioner* 192, 71

Psoriasis
(1994): Brenner S+, *Isr J Med Sci* 30, 283

Purpura
(1988): Warnock JK+, *Am J Psychiatry* 145, 425
(1984): Staughton RCD+, *J R Soc Med* 77 (Suppl 4), 6
(1972): Levantine A+, *Br J Dermatol* 87, 646
(1969): Peterkin GAG+, *Practitioner* 202, 117
(1967): Livingston S+, *JAMA* 200, 204
(1967): Harman RRM, *Br J Dermatol* 79, 500
(1964): Spillane D, *Practitioner* 192, 71

Pustular eruption
(1991): Kleier RS+, *Arch Dermatol* 127, 1361
(1990): Gebauer K+, *Australas J Dermatol* 31, 89 (passim)
(1988): Commens CA+, *Arch Dermatol* 124, 178
(1984): Staughton RCD+, *J R Soc Med* 77 (Suppl 4), 6

Rash (sic) (>10%)
(1999): van Ginneken EE+, *Neth Med J* 54, 158
(1998): Cates M+, *Ann Pharmacother* 32, 884
(1996): Puig L+, *Contact Dermatitis* 34, 435
(1996): Boyle N+, *Am J Psychiatry* 152, 1234
(1994): Kramlinger KG+, *J Clin Psychopharmacol* 14, 408 (12%)
(1993): Hosoda N+, *Jpn J Psychiatry Neurol* 47, 300
(1993): Konishi T+, *Eur J Pediatr* 152, 605
(1991): Frederick TE, *Neurology* 41, 1328
(1991): Murphy JM+, *Neurology* 41, 144
(1990): Garavelli PL+, *Minerva Med* (Italian) 81, 115
(1983): Vick NA, *N Engl J Med* 309, 1193
(1983): Ponte CD, *Drug Intell Clin Pharm* 17, 642

Schamberg's disease

Sheet-like erythema

Toxic-allergic shock (sic)
(1979): Rummel GL, *ZFA (Stuttgart)* 55, 627

Stevens–Johnson syndrome (1–10%)
(2000): Straussberg R+, *Pediatr Neurol* 22, 231
(2000): Suarez Moro R+, *An Med Interna* (Spanish) 17, 105
(1999): Petter G+, *Hautarzt* (German) 50, 884
(1999): Dhar S+, *Dermatology* 199, 194
(1999): Ruble R+, *CNS Drugs* 12, 215
(1999): Rzany B+, *Lancet* 353, 2190
(1995): Wolkenstein P+, *Arch Dermatol* 131, 544
(1995): Hughes-Davies L, *N Engl J Med* 332, 959
(1995): Keating A+, *Ann Pharmacother* 29, 538
(1995): Huang SC+, *Gen Hosp Psychiatry* 17, 458
(1993): Pagliaro LA+, *Hosp Community Psychiatry* 44, 999
(1993): Konishi T+, *Eur J Pediatr* 152, 605
(1993): Leenutaphong V+, *Int J Dermatol* 32, 428
(1993): Server Climent M, *Aten Primaria* (Spanish) 11, 377
(1992): Chevenet C+, *Ann Dermatol Venereol* (French) 119, 929 (with brain irradiation)
(1990): Hoang-Xuan K+, *Neurology* 40, 1144 (with cranial irradiation)
(1990): Wong KE, *Singapore Med J* 31, 432
(1990): Gebauer K+, *Australas J Dermatol* 31, 89 (passim)
(1990): Khe HX+, *Neurology* 40, 1144
(1989): Alanko K+, *Acta Derm Venereol* (Stockh) 69, 223
(1988): McDanal CE, *J Clin Psychiatr* 49, 369
(1988): Warnock JK+, *Am J Psychiatry* 145, 425
(1987): Fawcett RG, *J Clin Psychiatry* 48, 416
(1975): Böttiger LE+, *Acta Med Scand* 198, 229 (4 of 77 cases)
(1965): Inglis W, *Med J Aust* 2, 94
(1965): Coombs BW, *Med J Aust* 1, 895

Toxic epidermal necrolysis (1–10%)
(1999): Petter G+, *Hautarzt* (German) 50, 884
(1999): Dhar S+, *Dermatology* 199, 194
(1999): Rzany B+, *Lancet* 353, 2190
(1999): Ruble R+, *CNS Drugs* 12, 215
(1997): Belgodere X+, *Arch Pediatr* (French) 4, 1020
(1997): Jarrett P+, *Clin Exp Dermatol* 22, 146
(1996): Blum L+, *J Am Acad Dermatol* 34, 1088
(1995): Wolkenstein P+, *Arch Dermatol* 131, 544
(1995): Sterker M+, *Int J Clin Pharmacol Ther* 33, 595
(1995): Urbanowski S+, *Wiad Lek* (Polish) 48, 154
(1994): Friedmann PS+, *Arch Dermatol* 130, 598
(1993): Leenutaphong V+, *Int J Dermatol* 32, 428
(1993): Pagliaro LA+, *Hospital and Community Psychiatry* 44, 999
(1993): Correia O+, *Dermatology* 186, 32
(1992): Weller M+, *Am J Psychiatry* 149, 1114
(1992): Weller M+, *Nervenarzt* (German) 63, 308
(1992): Park BK+, *Br J Clin Pharmacol* 34. 377

(1991): Sakellariou G+, *Int J Artif Organs* 14, 634
(1990): Roujeau JC+, *Arch Dermatol* 126, 37
(1990): Gebauer K+, *Australas J Dermatol* 31, 89 (passim)
(1988): Shear NH+, *J Clin Invest* 82, 1826
(1987): Guillaume JC+, *Arch Dermatol* 123, 1166
(1986): Rusciani L+, *G Ital Dermatol Venereol* (Italian) 121, 149
(1984): Husegaard HC+, *Ugeskr Laeger* (Danish) 146, 2784
(1984): Staughton RCD+, *J R Soc Med* 77 (Suppl 4), 6
(1982): Breathnach SM+, *Clin Exp Dermatol* 7, 585
(1977): Houwerzijl J+, *Clin Exp Immunol* 29, 272
(1976): Mutina ES+, *Klin Med Mosk* (Russian) 54, 124
(1972): Carli-Basset C+, *Sem Hop* (French) 48, 497

Toxicoderma (sic)
(1983): Rozov VD+, *Vestn Dermatol Venerol* (Russian) September, 48

Toxic pustuloderma (sic) (probably AGEP [ed])
(1990): Gebauer K+, *Australas J Dermatol* 31, 89
(1988): Commens CA+, *Arch Dermatol* 124, 178
(1984): Staughton RCD+, *J R Soc Med* 77 (Suppl 4), 6

Urticaria
(1993): Konishi T+, *Eur J Pediatr* 152, 605
(1993): Alanko K, *Contact Dermatitis* 29, 254
(1990): Gebauer K+, *Australas J Dermatol* 31, 89 (passim)
(1988): Warnock JK+, *Am J Psychiatry* 145, 425
(1987): Johannessen AC+, *Ugeskr Laeger* (Danish) 149, 376
(1984): Staughton RCD+, *J R Soc Med* 77 (Suppl 4), 6
(1977): Houwerzijl J+, *Clin Exp Immunol* 29, 272
(1976): Al-Ubaidy SS+, *Br J Oral Surg* 13, 289 (4.2%)
(1969): Rull JA+, *Diabetologia* 5, 215 (6.6%)
(1967): Arieff AJ+, *Dis Nerv Syst* 28, 820
(1964): Spillane D, *Practitioner* 192, 71

Vasculitis
(1993): Drory VE+, *Clin Neuropharmacol* 16, 19 (passim)
(1990): Gebauer K+, *Australas J Dermatol* 31, 89 (passim)
(1987): Harats N+, *J Neurol Neurosurg Psychiatry* 50, 1241
(1978): Nieme KM+, *Acta Derm Venereol* (Stockh) 58, 337
(1967): Harman RRM, *Br J Dermatol* 79, 500

Hair

Hair – alopecia
(2000): Mercke Y+, *Ann Clin Psychiatry* 12, 35 (~6%)
(1997): Ikeda A+, *J Neurol Neurosurg Psychiatry* 63, 549
(1996): McKinney PA+, *Ann Clin Psychiatry* 8, 183
(1988): Warnock JK+, *Am J Psychiatry* 145, 425
(1985): Shuper A+, *Drug Intell Clin Pharm* 19, 924
(1982): Breathnach SM+, *Clin Exp Dermatol* 7, 585

Nails

Nails – discoloration (bluish-black)
(1989): Mishra D+, *Int J Dermatol* 28, 460

Nails – hypoplasia
(1985): Niesen M+, *Neuropediatrics* 16, 167

Nails – lichen planus
(1989): Ohtsuyama M+, *Nishinihon J Dermatol* (Japanese) 51, 958

Nails – loss (sic)
(1982): Breathnach SM+, *Clin Exp Dermatol* 7, 585

Nails – onychomadesis
(1989): Mishra D+, *Int J Dermatol* 28, 460

Other

Acute intermittent porphyria
(1984): Doss M+, *Lancet* 1, 1026
(1983): Shanley BC, *Lancet* 1, 1229
(1983): Yeung Laiwah AACY+, *Lancet* 1, 790
(1983): Rideout JM+, *Lancet* 2, 464
(1983): Liawah AC+, *Lancet* 1, 1442

Dyschromatopsia
(2000): Nousiainen I+, *Ophthalmology* 107, 884

Dysgeusia
(1976): Rollin H, *Laryngol Rhinol Otol* (Stuttgart) (German) 55, 873

Fetal anticonvulsant syndrome
(2000): Moore SJ+, *J Med Genet* 37, 489

Glossitis

Hypersensitivity*
(2000): Ivry S+, *Harefuah* (Hebrew) 138, 545
(2000): Straussberg R+, *Pediatr Neurol* 22, 231
(2000): Elstner S+, *Fortschr Neurol Psychiatr* (German) 68, 188
(1999): Mesec A+, *J Neurol Neurosurg Psychiatry* 66, 249
(1999): Balasubrananian S+, *Indian Pediatr* 36, 98
(1999): Hamer HM+, *Seizure* 8, 190
(1999): Moss DM+, *J Emerg Med* 17, 503
(1999): Brown KL+, *Dev Med Child Neurol* 41, 267
(1999): Lombardi SM+, *Ann Pharmacother* 33, 571
(1998): Dertinger S+, *J Hepatol* 28, 356
(1998): Schlienger RG+, *Epilepsia* 39, S3 (passim)
(1997): Morkunas AR+, *Crit Care Clin* 13, 727
(1997): Tennis P+, *Neurology* 49, 542
(1997): Stein J+, *Dtsch Med Wochenschr* (German) 122, 314
(1997): Pichler WJ+, *New Engl J Med* 336, 377
(1997): Waagner DC, *New Engl J Med* 336, 376
(1996): *New Engl J Med* 335, 577
(1996): Callot V+, *Arch Dermatol* 132, 1315
(1996): Oakley A, Hamilton, New Zealand (from Internet) (observation)
(1996): Koopman R, Enschede, The Netherlands (from Internet) (observation)
(1996): Knowles SR+, *J Clin Psychopharmacol* 16, 263
(1995): De Vriese AS+, *Medicine Baltimore* 74, 144
(1995): Bellman B+, *J Am Acad Child Adolesc Psychiatry* 34, 1405
(1995): Periole B+, *Ann Dermatol Venereol (French)* 122, 121
(1994): Gall H+, *Hautarzt* (German) 45, 494
(1994): Naranjo CA+, *Clin Pharmacol Ther* 56, 564
(1994): Alldredge BK+, *Pediatr Neurol* 10, 169
(1993): Handfield-Jones SE+, *Br J Dermatol* 129, 175
(1993): Scerri L+, *Clin Exp Dermatol* 18, 540
(1993): Parha S+, *Eur J Pediatr* 152, 1040
(1991): Hosoda N+, *Arch Dis Child* 66, 722
(1991): Baguena F+, *Med Clin (Barc)* (Spanish) 96, 237
(1989): Malanin G+, *Duodecim* (Finnish) 105, 784
(1983): Bernstein DI+, *Clin Pediatr* (Phila) *22, 524*
(1978): Stephan WC+, *Chest* 74, 463 (pneumonitis)

Lymphoproliferative disease
(1992): Sigal-Nahum M+, *Br J Dermatol* 127, 545
(1992): Schlaifer D+, *Eur J Dermatol* 48, 274
(1990): Katzin WE+, *Arch Pathol Lab Med* 114, 1244
(1987): Severson GS+, *Am J Med* 83, 597
(1984): Shuttleworth D+, *Clin Exp Dermatol* 9, 421

Mucocutaneous eruption
(1999): Edwards SG+, *Postgrad Med J* 75, 680
(1993): Konishi T+, *Eur J Pediatr* 152, 605
(1979): Pollack MA+, *Ann Neurol* 5, 262
(1975): Böttiger LE+, *Acta Med Scand* 198, 229

Oral lichenoid eruption
(1989): Ohtsuyama M+, *Nishinihon J Dermatol* (Japanese) 51, 958

Oral mucosal eruption
(1964): Spillane D, *Practitioner* 192, 71

Porphyria cutanea tarda
(1996): Leo RJ+, *Am J Psychiatry* 153, 443

Pseudolymphoma
(1999): Saeki H+, *J Dermatol* 26, 329
(1998): Nathan D+, *J Am Acad Dermatol* 38, 806
(1998): d'Incan M+, *Ann Dermatol Venereol* 125, 52
(1997): Paramesh H+, *Indian Pediatr* 34, 829
(1997): Kim ST+, Korea, American Academy of Dermatology Meeting (SF), Poster #82
(1996): Callot V+, *Arch Dermatol* 132, 1315
(1995): Magro CM+, *J Am Acad Dermatol* 32, 419
(1993): Sigal M+, *Ann Dermatol Venereol* (French) 120, 175
(1993): Rondas AA+, *Ned Tijdschr Geneeskd* (Dutch) 137, 1258
(1990): Sinnige HAM+, *J Intern Med* 227, 355
(1986): Yates P+, *J Clin Pathol* 39, 1224
(1984): Shuttleworth D+, *Clin Exp Dermatol* 9, 424

Serum sickness
(1993): Igarashi M+, *Int Arch Allergy Immunol* 100, 378

Stomatitis

Thrombophlebitis

Tongue ulceration
(1998): Melgarejo Moreno PJ+, *An Otorrinolaringol Ibero Am* (Spanish) 25, 167
(1964): Spillane D, *Practitioner* 192, 71

Xerostomia

***Note:** The antiepileptic drug hypersensitivity syndrome is a severe, occasionally fatal, disorder characterized by any or all of the following: pruritic exanthem, toxic epidermal necrolysis, Stevens–Johnson syndrome, exfoliative dermatitis, fever, hepatic abnormalities, eosinophilia, and renal failure.

CARBENICILLIN

Trade name: Geocillin (Pfizer)
Other common trade names: *Carbecin; Carbelin; Geopen; Pyopen*
Indications: Urinary tract infections
Category: Penicillinase-sensitive penicillin
Half-life: 1.0–1.5 hours
Clinically important, potentially serious interactions with: aminoglycosides, anticoagulants, oral contraceptives, probenecid, tetracyclines

Reactions

Skin

Allergic reactions (sic)
(1994): Pleasants RA+, *Chest* 106, 1124 (in patients with cystic fibrosis)
Angioedema
Bullous eruption
Ecchymoses
Edema
Erythema multiforme
Erythema nodosum
Exanthems
Exfoliative dermatitis
Hematomas
Jarisch–Herxheimer reaction
Pruritus
Purpura
(1976): Karchmer AW+, *N Engl J Med* 295, 451
(1970): McClure PD+, *Lancet* 2, 1307
Rash (sic) (<1%)
Stevens–Johnson syndrome
Toxic epidermal necrolysis
(1984): Westly ED+, *Arch Dermatol* 120, 721
Urticaria (<1%)
Vasculitis
Vesicular eruption

Other

Anaphylactoid reaction
Black tongue
Dysgeusia (1–10%)
Glossitis (1–10%)
Glossodynia
Hypersensitivity
Injection-site pain
Oral candidiasis
Serum sickness
Stomatitis
Stomatodynia
Thrombophlebitis (<1%)
Tongue, furry
Vaginitis (<1%)
Xerostomia

CARBIDOPA

(See LEVODOPA)

CARBOPLATIN

Trade name: Paraplatin (Bristol-Myers Squibb)
Other common trade names: *Carboplat; Carbosin; Ercar; Oncocarbin; Paraplatine*
Indications: Various carcinomas and sarcomas
Category: Antineoplastic
Half-life: terminal: 22–40 hours
Clinically important, potentially serious interactions with: aldesleukin, cisplatin, mesna, phenytoin

Reactions

Skin

Depigmentation
(1990): Costello SA+, *Clin Oncol R Coll Radiol* 2, 182
Erosion of body folds (sic)
(1996): Prussick R+, *J Am Acad Dermatol* 35, 705
Erythema (2%)
(1995): Inbar M+, *Anticancer Drugs* 6, 775
Exanthems
(1995): Inbar M+, *Anticancer Drugs* 6, 775
(1992): Beyer J+, *Bone Marrow Transplant* 10, 491
(1989): Wagstaff AJ+, *Drugs* 37, 162
Facial edema
(1992): Beyer J+, *Bone Marrow Transplant* 10, 491
Pigmentation
(1992): Beyer J+, *Bone Marrow Transplant* 10, 491
(1991): Singal R+, *Pediatr Dermatology* 8, 231
Pruritus (2%)
Rash (sic) (2%)
Urticaria (2%)
(1996): Broome CB+, *Med Pediatr Oncol* 26, 105
(1995): Sredni B+, *J Clin Oncol* 13, 2342

Hair

Hair – alopecia (3%)
(1989): Wagstaff AJ+, *Drugs* 37, 162

Other

Anaphylactoid reaction (<1%)
Hypersensitivity (2%)
(1999): Menczer J+, *Eur J Gynaecol Oncol* 20, 214 (4 patients)
(1999): Schiavetti A+, *Med Pediatr Oncol* 32, 183 (9.2%)
(1999): Shukunami K+, *Gynecol Oncol* 72, 431
(1998): Kook H+, *Bone Marrow Transplant* 21, 727
(1996): Broome CB+, *Med Pediatr Oncol* 26, 105
Injection-site pain (>10%)
Oral mucosal lesions
(1989): Wagstaff AJ+, *Drugs* 37, 162
Stomatitis (>10%)

CARISOPRODOL

Synonyms: carisoprodate; isobamate
Trade name: Soma (Wallace)
Other common trade names: *Artifar; Carisoma; Myolax; Sanoma; Sodol; Somadril; Soridol*
Indications: Painful musculoskeletal disorders
Category: Skeletal muscle relaxant
Half-life: 4–6 hours
Clinically important, potentially serious interactions with: alcohol, CNS depressants, clindamycin, MAO inhibitors, phenothiazines

Reactions

Skin

Angioedema (1–10%)
Diaphoresis
(1983): Rollings HE+, *Curr Ther Res* 34, 926

Edema
(1983): Rollings HE+, *Curr Ther Res* 34, 926
Erythema multiforme (<1%)
Exanthems
(1962): Honeycutt WM+, *JAMA* 180, 691 (passim)
Fixed eruption (<1%)
(1965): Gore HC, *Arch Dermatol* 91, 627
(1962): Honeycutt WM+, *JAMA* 180, 691
Flushing (1–10%)
Photosensitivity
(1994): Hazen PG, *J Am Acad Dermatol* 31, 498
Pruritus (<1%)
Rash (sic) (<1%)
Urticaria (<1%)
(1962): Honeycutt WM+, *JAMA* 180, 691 (passim)

Other

Anaphylactoid reaction
Paresthesias
(1983): Rollings HE+, *Curr Ther Res* 34, 926
Pseudoporphyria
(1994): Hazen PG, *J Am Acad Dermatol* 31, 498
Trembling (sic) (1–10%)
Xerostomia
(1983): Rollings HE+, *Curr Ther Res* 34, 926

CARMUSTINE

Synonym: BCNU
Trade names: BiCNU (Bristol-Myers Squibb); Gliadel Wafer (Aventis)
Other common trade names: *Bcnu; Becenun; BiCNU; Carmubris; Nitrumon*
Indications: Brain tumors, Hodgkin's disease, multiple myeloma
Category: Antineoplastic
Half-life: initial: 1.4 minutes; secondary: 20 minutes
Clinically important, potentially serious interactions with: amphotericin B, cimetidine, etoposide

Reactions

Skin

Contact dermatitis
(1994): Zackheim HS, *Semin Dermatol* 13, 202
(1990): Zackheim HS+, *J Am Acad Dermatol* 22, 802
Eccrine squamous syringometaplasia
(1997): Valks R+, *Arch Dermatol* 133, 873
Dermatitis (sic) (<1%)
Erythema
(1992): Breathnach SM+, *Adverse Drug Reactions and the Skin*, Blackwell, Oxford, 292
Exanthems
(1978): Levine N+, *Cancer Treat Rev* 5, 67
Flushing (1–10%)
(1978): Levine N+, *Cancer Treat Rev* 5, 67
(1971): Young RC+, *N Engl J Med* 285, 475
Pigmentation (on accidental contact)
(1982): Dunagin WG, *Semin Oncol* 9, 14
(1966): Frost P+, *Arch Dermatol* 94, 265
Skin tenderness (sic)
(1992): Breathnach SM+, *Adverse Drug Reactions and the Skin*, Blackwell, Oxford, 292
Telangiectases
(1994): Zackheim HS, *Semin Dermatol* 13, 202
(1992): Breathnach SM+, *Adverse Drug Reactions and the Skin*, Blackwell, Oxford, 292

Hair

Hair – alopecia (1–10%)

Other

Gynecomastia
Injection-site burning (>10%)
Injection-site necrosis
(1987): Dufresne RG, *Cutis* 39, 197
Injection-site pain
Stomatitis (1–10%)

CARTEOLOL

Trade names: Cartrol (Abbott); Ocupress (ophthalmic) (Otsuka)
Other common trade names: *Arteolol; Arteoptic; Calte; Carteol; Endak; Mikelan; Teoptic*
Indications: Glaucoma, hypertension
Category: Beta-adrenergic blocker
Half-life: 6 hours
Clinically important, potentially serious interactions with: albuterol, calcium channel blockers, clonidine, digoxin, diltiazem, diuretics, epinephrine, ergot alkaloids, flecainide, insulin, nifedipine, NSAIDs, oral contraceptives, prazosin, salicylates, sulfonylureas, theophylline, verapamil

Note: Cutaneous side-effects of beta-receptor blockaders are clinically polymorphous. They apparently appear after several months of continuous therapy. Atypical psoriasiform, lichen planus-like, and eczematous chronic rashes are mainly observed. (1983): Hödl St, *Z Hautkr* (German) 1:58, 17.

Reactions

Skin

Acne
Angioedema
Ankle edema (<1%)
Cold extremities (sic)
Contact dermatitis (eye-drops)
(2000): Quiralte J+, *Contact Dermatitis* 42, 245
Dermatitis (sic)
Diaphoresis (<1%)
(1997): Schmutz JL+, *Dermatology* 194, 197 (from topical)
Edema
Exanthems
Exfoliative dermatitis
Facial edema
Flushing
Lupus erythematosus
Peripheral edema (1.7%)
Photosensitivity
Pigmentation
Pruritus
Psoriasis
Purpura (<1%)
Rash (sic) (2.5%)
Raynaud's phenomenon (<1%)
Vesiculobullous eruption
Xerosis

Hair

Hair – alopecia

Nails

Nails – discoloration (bluish)

Other

Anaphylactoid reaction
Dysgeusia (from topical application)
Myalgia
Paresthesias (2%)
Peyronie's disease
Xerostomia

CARVEDILOL

Trade name: Coreg (SmithKline Beecham)
Other common trade names: *Dibloc; Dilatrend; Dimitone; Kredex; Querto*
Indications: Hypertension
Category: Beta-adrenergic blocker; antihypertensive
Half-life: 7–10 hours
Clinically important, potentially serious interactions with: antidiabetics, calcium channel blockers, cimetidine, clonidine, digoxin, diltiazem, diuretics, flecainide, fluoxetine, MAO inhibitors, nifedipine, oral contraceptives, quinidine, rifampin, tacrine, verapamil

Reactions

Skin

Allergy (sic) (<1%)
Angioedema
(1988): Ogihara G+, *Drugs* 36, 75 (<1%)
Cutaneous reaction (sic)
(1998): Simpson SH+, *Can J Cardiol* 14, 1277
Diaphoresis (2.9%)
Edema (generalized)(5.1%)
Exanthems (<1%)
(2000): Litt JZ, Beachwood, OH, personal case (observation)
(1988): Ogihara G+, *Drugs* 36, 75 (2%)
Exfoliative dermatitis (<1%)
Infection (sic) (2.2%)
Pain (8.6%)
Peripheral edema (1.4%)
Photosensitivity (<1%)
Pruritus (<1%)
(2000): Litt JZ, Beachwood, OH, personal case (observation)
Psoriasis (<1%)
Purpura (1–10%)
Rash (sic) (<1%)
Stevens–Johnson syndrome
(1997): Kowalski BJ+, *Am J Cardiol* 80, 669

Hair

Hair – alopecia (<0.1%)

Other

Anaphylactoid reaction (<1%)
Hypesthesia (<1%)
Myalgia (3.4%)
Paresthesias (2%)
Xerostomia (<1%)

CEFACLOR

Trade name: Ceclor (Lilly)
Other common trade names: *Alfatil; Apo-Cefaclor; CEC 500; Cefabiocin; Distaclor; Kefolor; Panoral; Sigacefal*
Indications: Various infections caused by susceptible organisms
Category: Second-generation cephalosporin
Half-life: 0.6–0.9 hours
Clinically important, potentially serious interactions with: aminoglycosides, anticoagulants, chloramphenicol, cimetidine, erythromycin, furosemide, heparin, probenecid, tetracycline, vancomycin

Note: Penicillin and cephalosporins share a common beta-lactam structure. People who are allergic to penicillin are approximately 4 times more likely to develop an allergic reaction to a cephalosporin than those people who have no penicillin allergy. (From 5 to 16% of patients allergic to penicillin develop reactions to cephalosporins.)

Reactions

Skin

Acute generalized exanthematous pustulosis (AGEP)
(1995): Moreau A+, *Int J Dermatol* 34, 263 (passim)
(1992): Ogoshi M+, *Dermatology* 184, 142
Angioedema (<1%)
(1998): Litt JZ, Beachwood, OH, personal case (observation)
Dermatitis (sic)
(1986): Hirata M+, *Kokyu To Junkan* (Japanese) 34, 791
Edema
(1995): Dark DS+, *Infections in Medicine* October, 551
Erythema multiforme
(2000): Ibia EO+, *Arch Dermatol* 136, 849
(1999): Joubert GI+, *Can J Clin Pharmacol* 6, 197 (17 cases)
(1988): Platt R+, *J Infect Dis* 158, 474 (0.6%)
(1985): Levine LR, *Ped Infect Dis* 4, 358 (0.6%)
(1982): Lovell SJ+, *Can Med Assoc J* 126, 1032
(1980): Murray DL+, *N Engl J Med* 303, 1003
Exanthems
(2000): Ibia EO+, *Arch Dermatol* 136, 849
(1996): Nagayama H+, *J Dermatol* 23, 899
(1994): Litt JZ, Beachwood, OH, personal case (observation)
(1994): Shelley WB+, *Cutis* 53, 40 (observation)
(1987): Norrby SR, *Drugs* 34 (Suppl 2), 105 (1–5%)
(1986): Ascher H, *Lakartidningen* (Swedish) 83, 411
(1985): Murray DL+, *Pediatr Infect Dis* 4, 706
(1983): Johnson T, *J Ark Med Soc* 80, 110
(1982): Lovell SJ+, *Can Med Assoc J* 126, 1032
(1981): Ackley AM+, *Southern Med J* 74, 1550
(1980): Murray DL+, *N Engl J Med* 303, 1003
Flushing
Pruritus (<1%)
(1998): Litt JZ, Beachwood, OH, personal case (observation)
(1988): Platt R+, *J Infect Dis* 158, 474
(1982): Lovell SJ+, *Can Med Assoc J* 126, 1032
(1981): Ackley AM+, *Southern Med J* 74, 1550
(1980): Murray DL+, *N Engl J Med* 303, 1003
Purpura
(1980): Murray DL+, *N Engl J Med* 303, 1003
Pustular eruption
(1992): Ogoshi M+, *Dermatology* 184, 142
Rash (sic) (1–1.5%)
Stevens–Johnson syndrome (<1%)
(1988): Platt R+, *J Infect Dis* 158, 474
Toxic epidermal necrolysis
(1987): Guillaume JC+, *Arch Dermatol* 123, 1166
Urticaria (<1%)
(2000): Ibia EO+, *Arch Dermatol* 136, 849
(1999): Joubert GI+, *Can J Clin Pharmacol* 6, 197 (26 cases)
(1998): Litt JZ, Beachwood, OH, personal case (observation)
(1995): Blumenthal HL, Beachwood, OH, personal case (observation)
(1994): Litt JZ, Beachwood, OH, personal case (observation)
(1993): Litt JZ, Beachwood, OH, 2 personal cases (observation)
(1991): Hebert AA+, *J Am Acad Dermatol* 25, 805
(1985): Levine LR, *Pediatr Infect Dis* 4, 358 (1–5%)
(1982): Lovell SJ+, *Can Med Assoc J* 126, 1032

Other

Anaphylactoid reaction (<1%)
(1999): Grouhi M+, *Pediatrics* 103, e50
(1986): Nishioka K+, *J Dermatol* 13, 226
Candidiasis (vaginal)
(1992): Stotka JL+, *Postgrad Med J* 68, S73
Dysgeusia
(1995): Dark DS+, *Infections in Medicine* October, 551
Glossitis
Hypersensitivity
Oral candidiasis
Paresthesias
Serum sickness (<1%)
(2000): Ibia EO+, *Arch Dermatol* 136, 849
(1999): Joubert GI+, *Can J Clin Pharmacol* 6, 197 (31 cases)
(1999): Phillips R, *Aust Fam Physician* 28, 539
(1999): Parshuram CS+, *J Paediatr Child Health* 35, 223
(1998): Kearns GL+, *Clin Pharmacol Ther* 63, 686 (10 patients)
(1998): Boyd IW, *Med J Aust* 169, 443
(1997): Szalai Z+, *Orv Hetil* (Hungarian) 138, 855
(1996): Grammer LC, *JAMA* 275, 1152
(1996): *Can Med Assoc J* 155, 913
(1996): Reynolds RD, *JAMA* 276, 950
(1995): Martin J+, *N Z Med J* 108, 123

(1995): Kearns GL+, *J Pediatr* 125, 805
(1992): Stricker BH+, *J Clin Epidemiol* 45, 1177
(1992): Parra FM+, *Allergy* 47, 439
(1992): Vial T+, *Ann Pharmacother* 26, 910
(1991): Hebert AA+, *J Am Acad Dermatol* 25, 805
(1990): Heckbert SB+, *Am J Epidemiol* 132, 336
(1988): Platt R+, *J Infect Dis* 158, 474
(1987): Norrby SR, *Drugs* 34 (Suppl 2), 105 (1–5%)
(1985): Levine LR, *Ped Infect Dis* 4, 358 (0.5%)
(1985): Callahan CW+, *J Am Osteopath* Assoc *85, 450*
(1985): Murray DL+, *Pediatr Inf Dis* 4, 706
(1983): Johnson T+, *J Ark Med Soc* 80, 110
(1982): Lovell SJ+, *Can Med Assoc J* 126, 1032

Vaginitis
(1992): Stotka JL+, *Postgrad Med J* 68, S73 (candidiasis)

CEFADROXIL

Trade name: Duricef (Bristol-Myers Squibb)
Other common trade names: *Baxan; Bidocef; Cedrox; Cefamox; Duracef; Moxacef; Oracefal; Sumacef*
Indications: Various infections caused by susceptible organisms
Category: First-generation cephalosporin antibiotic
Half-life: 1.2–1.5 hours
Clinically important, potentially serious interactions with: aminoglycosides, anticoagulants, chloramphenicol, cimetidine, erythromycin, furosemide, heparin, probenecid, tetracycline, vancomycin

Note: Penicillin and cephalosporins share a common beta-lactam structure. People who are allergic to penicillin are approximately 4 times more likely to develop an allergic reaction to a cephalosporin than those people who have no penicillin allergy. (From 5 to 16% of patients allergic to penicillin develop allergic reactions to cephalosporins.)

Reactions

Skin

Angioedema (<1%)
Candidiasis
Erythema
(1986): Tanrisever B+, *Drugs* 32 (Suppl 3), 1, 21, 43
Erythema multiforme (<1%)
Exanthems (<1%)
(1986): Tanrisever B+, *Drugs* 32 (Suppl 3), 1, 21, 43 (0.3%)
Pemphigus
(1986): Wilson JP+, *Drug Intell Clin Pharm* 20, 219
Pruritus (<1%)
(1986): Tanrisever B+, *Drugs* 32 (Suppl 3), 1, 21, 43 (0.3%)
Rash (sic) (<1%)
Stevens–Johnson syndrome (<1%)
Toxic epidermal necrolysis
Urticaria (<1%)
(1993): Shelley WB+, *Cutis* 52, 262 (observation)
(1986): Tanrisever B+, *Drugs* 32 (Suppl 3), 1, 21, 43 (0.1%)

Other

Anaphylactoid reaction (<1%)
Glossitis
(1986): Tanrisever B+, *Drugs* 32 (Suppl 3), 1, 21, 43
Hypersensitivity
Oral candidiasis
Oral mucosal eruption
(1986): Tanrisever B+, *Drugs* 32 (Suppl 3), 1, 21, 43 (0.1%)
Oral ulceration
(1986): Wilson JP+, *Drug Intell Clin Pharm* 20, 219
Serum sickness (<1%)
Vaginitis (<1%)
(1986): Tanrisever B+, *Drugs* 32 (Suppl 3), 1, 21, 43

CEFAMANDOLE

Trade name: Mandol (Lilly)
Other common trade names: *Cedol; Cefadol; Kefadol; Kefdole; Mancef; Mandokef*
Indications: Various infections caused by susceptible organisms
Category: Second-generation cephalosporin
Half-life: 0.5–1.0 hours
Clinically important, potentially serious interactions with: alcohol, aminoglycosides, anticoagulants, cimetidine, ethanol, furosemide, heparin, probenecid, warfarin

Note: Penicillin and cephalosporins share a common beta-lactam structure. People who are allergic to penicillin are approximately 4 times more likely to develop an allergic reaction to a cephalosporin than those people who have no penicillin allergy. (From 5 to 16% of patients allergic to penicillin develop allergic reactions to cephalosporins.)

Reactions

Skin

Acne
Diaper rash
Diaphoresis
Edema
Erythema multiforme
(1987): Argenyi ZB+, *Cleve Clin J Med* 54, 445
Exanthems
(1985): Richards DM+, *Drugs* 29, 281 (1.7%)
(1985): Sanders CV+, *Ann Intern Med* 103, 70 (2%)
Flushing
Linear IgA bullous dermatosis
(1987): Argenyi ZB+, *Cleve Clin J Med* 54, 445
Pruritus (<1%)
Purpura
Rash (sic) (<1%)
Stevens–Johnson syndrome (<1%)
Toxic epidermal necrolysis
(1985): Sanders CV+, *Ann Intern Med* 103, 70 (2%)
(1982): Seifter EJ+, *Johns Hopkins Med J* 151, 326
Toxic erythema
(1995): Rademaker M, *N Z Med J* 108, 165
Urticaria (<1%)

Other

Anaphylactoid reaction (<1%)
Dysgeusia
Glossitis
Hypersensitivity
Injection-site burning
Injection-site cellulitis
Injection-site edema
Injection-site inflammation
Injection-site pain (<1%)
(1985): Sanders CV+, *Ann Intern Med* 103, 70 (7%)
Injection-site thrombophlebitis (1–10%)
(1985): Sanders CV+, *Ann Intern Med* 103, 70 (15%)
Oral candidiasis (<1%)
Paresthesias
Serum sickness (<1%)
Vaginal candidiasis
Vaginitis

CEFAZOLIN

Trade names: Ancef (SmithKline Beecham); Kefzol (Lilly)
Other common trade names: *Basocef; Cefacidal; Cefamezin; Elzogram; Gramaxin; Kefarin; Totacef; Zolin*
Indications: Various infections caused by susceptible organisms
Category: First-generation cephalosporin antibiotic
Half-life: 1.4–1.8 hours
Clinically important, potentially serious interactions with: aminoglycosides, anticoagulants, cimetidine, heparin, probenecid, tetracycline, vancomycin

Note: Penicillin and cephalosporins share a common beta-lactam structure. People who are allergic to penicillin are approximately 4 times more likely to develop an allergic reaction to a cephalosporin than those people who have no penicillin allergy. (From 5 to 16% of patients allergic to penicillin develop allergic reactions to cephalosporins.)

Reactions

Skin

Acute generalized exanthematous pustulosis (AGEP)
(1995): Moreau A+, *Int J Dermatol* 34, 263 (passim)
(1994): Manders SM+, *Cutis* 54, 194 (with metronidazole)
Allergic reactions (sic)
(1994): Pleasants RA+, *Chest* 106, 1124 (in patients with cystic fibrosis)
(1993): Faulk D+, *Nurse Anesth* 4, 188 (3–5%)
Contact dermatitis
(2000): Straube MD+, *Contact Dermatitis* 42, 44
Erythema multiforme
Exanthems
(1990): Flax SH+, *Cutis* 46, 59
(1988): Fayol J+, *J Am Acad Dermatol* 19, 571
(1986): Szylit JA+, *Cutis* 37, 390
Fixed eruption (linear)
(1988): Sigal-Nahum M+, *Br J Dermatol* 118, 849
Pemphigus
(1997): Brenner S+, *J Am Acad Dermatol* 36, 919
Photo recall phenomenon (sic)
(1990): Flax SH+, *Cutis* 46, 59
Photosensitivity
(1990): Flax SH+, *Cutis* 46, 59
Pruritus (<1%)
(1987): Stough D+, *J Am Acad Dermatol* 16, 1051
Pruritus ani
Pustular eruption
(1990): Rustin MHA+, *Br J Dermatol* 123, 119
(1988): Fayol J+, *J Am Acad Dermatol* 19, 571
(1987): Stough D+, *J Am Acad Dermatol* 16, 1051
Rash (sic) (<1%)
Stevens–Johnson syndrome (<1%)
Toxic epidermal necrolysis
(1994): Julsrud ME, *J Foot Ankle Surg* 33, 255
Urticaria (<1%)

Other

Anaphylactoid reaction (<1%)
(1996): Warrington RJ+, *J Allergy Clin Immunol* 98, 460
Hypersensitivity
Injection-site induration
Injection-site pain (<1%)
Injection-site phlebitis (<1%)
Oral candidiasis (<1%)
Phlebitis
Serum sickness (<1%)
Vaginitis (<1%)

CEFDINIR

Synonym: CFDN
Trade name: Omnicef (Parke-Davis)
Indications: Community-acquired pneumonia and various infections caused by susceptible organisms
Category: Third-generation cephalosporin
Half-life: 1–2 hours
Clinically important, potentially serious interactions with: aminoglycosides, antacids, anticoagulants, cimetidine, cyclosporine, famotidine, heparin, iron supplements, nizatidine, omeprazole, probenecid, ranitidine

Note: Penicillin and cephalosporins share a common beta-lactam structure. People who are allergic to penicillin are approximately 4 times more likely to develop an allergic reaction to a cephalosporin than those people who have no penicillin allergy. (From 5 to 16% of patients allergic to penicillin develop allergic reactions to cephalosporins.)

Reactions

Skin

Candidiasis (1%)
Erythema multiforme
Erythema nodosum
Exanthems (0.2%)
Exfoliative dermatitis
Facial edema
Pruritus (0.2%)
Purpura
Rash (sic) (3%)
Stevens–Johnson syndrome (<1%)
Toxic epidermal necrolysis
Urticaria (<1%)
Vasculitis

Other

Anaphylactoid reaction
Serum sickness (<1%)
Stomatitis
Vaginal candidiasis (5%)
Vaginitis (1%)

CEFEPIME

Trade name: Maxipime (Dura)
Other common trade name: *Maxcef*
Indications: Various infections caused by susceptible organisms
Category: Fourth-generation cephalosporin
Half-life: 2–2.3 hours
Clinically important, potentially serious interactions with: aminoglycosides, probenecid

Note: Penicillin and cephalosporins share a common beta-lactam structure. People who are allergic to penicillin are approximately 4 times more likely to develop an allergic reaction to a cephalosporin than those people who have no penicillin allergy. (From 5 to 16% of patients allergic to penicillin develop allergic reactions to cephalosporins.)

Reactions

Skin

Angioedema
Candidiasis (<1%)
Erythema multiforme
Exanthems (1.8%)
Pruritus (1–10%)
Rash (sic) (51%)
(2000): Sheng WH+, *J Microbiol Immunol Infect* 33, 109
(1996): Holloway WJ+, *Am J Med* 100, 52S

(1994): Okamoto MP+, *Am J Hosp Pharm* 51, 463
Stevens–Johnson syndrome
Toxic epidermal necrolysis
Urticaria (1.8%)

Other

Anaphylactoid reaction
Hypersensitivity
Injection-site inflammation (0.6%)
Injection-site pain (0.6%)
Injection-site phlebitis (1.3%)
Injection-site rash (1.1%)
Oral candidiasis
Vaginitis (<1%)

CEFIXIME

Trade name: Suprax (Lederle)
Other common trade names: *Cefspan; Cephoral; Fixime; Oroken; Supran; Uro-cephoral*
Indications: Various infections caused by susceptible organisms
Category: Third-generation cephalosporin antibiotic
Half-life: 3–4 hours
Clinically important, potentially serious interactions with: aminoglycosides, anticoagulants, carbamazepine, cimetidine, furosemide, heparin, probenecid

Note: Penicillin and cephalosporins share a common beta-lactam structure. People who are allergic to penicillin are approximately 4 times more likely to develop an allergic reaction to a cephalosporin than those people who have no penicillin allergy. (From 5 to 16% of patients allergic to penicillin develop allergic reactions to cephalosporins.)

Reactions

Skin

Candidiasis
Erythema multiforme (<2%)
Pruritus (<2%)
(1987): Tally FP+, *Pediatr Infect Dis J* 6, 976
Pruritus ani
Rash (sic) (<2%)
(1987): Tally FP+, *Pediatr Infect Dis J* 6, 976
Stevens–Johnson syndrome (<2%)
Urticaria (<2%)
(1987): Tally FP+, *Pediatr Infect Dis J* 6, 976

Other

Anaphylactoid reaction
(1996): Vilas Martinez F+, *Med Clin (Barc)* (Spanish) 106, 439
Hypersensitivity
Pseudolymphoma
(1998): Jabbar A+, *Br J Haematol* 101, 209
Serum sickness (<2%)
(1987): Tally FP+, *Pediatr Infect Dis J* 6, 976
Xerostomia
(1987): Tally FP+, *Pediatr Infect Dis J* 6, 976
Vaginal candidiasis
Vaginitis (<2%)

CEFMETAZOLE

Trade name: Zefazone (Pharmacia & Upjohn)
Other common trade names: *Cefmetazon; Cefotazol; Cemetol; Cetazone; Gomcefa; Metalin*
Indications: Various infections caused by susceptible organisms
Category: Second-generation cephalosporin antibiotic
Half-life: 72 minutes
Clinically important, potentially serious interactions with: alcohol, aminoglycosides, anticoagulants, furosemide, probenecid

Note: Penicillin and cephalosporins share a common beta-lactam structure. People who are allergic to penicillin are approximately 4 times more likely to develop an allergic reaction to a cephalosporin than those people who have no penicillin allergy. (From 5 to 16% of patients allergic to penicillin develop allergic reactions to cephalosporins.)

Reactions

Skin

Candidiasis (<1%)
Cutaneous reactions (sic)
(1989): Saito A, *J Antimicrob Chemother* 23, 131
Disulfiram-like reaction*
(1989): Saito A, *J Antimicrob Chemother* 23, 131
Hot flashes (<1%)
Periorbital edema
Pruritus (<1%)
Purpura
Rash (sic) (1–10%)
Urticaria (<1%)
Stevens–Johnson syndrome (<1%)
Toxic epidermal necrolysis

Other

Anaphylactoid reaction
(1989): Saito A, *J Antimicrob Chemother* 23, 131
Dysgeusia
Hypersensitivity
Injection-site edema
Injection-site induration
Injection-site pain
Injection-site thrombophlebitis (<1%)
Phlebitis (<1%)
Serum sickness (<1%)
Vaginitis (<1%)

***Note:** The disulfiram-like reaction consists of facial flushing, diaphoresis, tachycardia, and pounding headache.

CEFONICID

Trade name: Monocid (SmithKline Beecham)
Other trade names: *Dinacid; Monocef; Monocidur*
Indications: Various infections caused by susceptible organisms
Category: Second-generation cephalosporin antibiotic
Half-life: 3–6 hours
Clinically important, potentially serious interactions with: alcohol, aminoglycosides, anticoagulants, furosemide, probenecid

Note: Penicillin and cephalosporins share a common beta-lactam structure. People who are allergic to penicillin are approximately 4 times more likely to develop an allergic reaction to a cephalosporin than those people who have no penicillin allergy. (From 5 to 16% of patients allergic to penicillin develop allergic reactions to cephalosporins.)

Reactions

Skin

Allergic reactions (sic)
(1994): Martin JA+, *Ann Allergy* 72, 341

Candidiasis (<1%)
Disulfiram-like reaction*
(1990): Marcon G+, *Recenti Prog Med* (Italian) 81, 47
Erythema (<1%)
Erythema multiforme
Pruritus (<1%)
Purpura
Rash (sic) (<1%)
Urticaria (<1%)
Stevens–Johnson syndrome (<1%)
Toxic epidermal necrolysis

Other

Anaphylactoid reaction (<1%)
Hypersensitivity
Injection-site edema (>1%)
Injection-site induration (>1%)
Injection-site pain (5.7%)
Injection-site phlebitis (>1%)
Myalgia
Serum sickness (<1%)
(1995): Ortega Calvo M+, *An Med Interna* (Spanish) 12, 289
Vaginitis

***Note:** The disulfiram-like reaction consists of facial flushing, diaphoresis, tachycardia, and pounding headache.

CEFOPERAZONE

Trade name: Cefobid (Pfizer)
Other trade names: *CPZ, Cefobis, Cefogram, Cefozone, Mediper, Tomabef, Zoncef*
Indications: Various infections caused by susceptible organisms
Category: Third-generation cephalosporin antibiotic
Half-life: 1.6–2.6 hours
Clinically important, potentially serious interactions with: alcohol, aminoglycosides, anticoagulants, furosemide

Note: Penicillin and cephalosporins share a common beta-lactam structure. People who are allergic to penicillin are approximately 4 times more likely to develop an allergic reaction to a cephalosporin than those people who have no penicillin allergy. (From 5 to 16% of patients allergic to penicillin develop allergic reactions to cephalosporins.)

Reactions

Skin

Candidiasis (<1%)
Disulfiram-like reaction*
(1981): Vonhogen LH+, *Ned Tijdschr Geneeskd* (Dutch) *125, 1610*
(1980): Foster TS+, *Am J Hosp Pharm* 37, 858
Erythema multiforme
Exanthems (<1%)
Pruritus (<1%)
Rash (sic) (2%)
(1983): Lyon JA, *Drug Intell Clin Pharm* 17, 7
Stevens–Johnson syndrome (<1%)
Toxic epidermal necrolysis
Urticaria (<1%)
(1983): Lyon JA, *Drug Intell Clin Pharm* 17, 7

Other

Hypersensitivity (>2%)
Injection-site induration (<1%)
Injection-site pain (<1%)
(1983): Lyon JA, *Drug Intell Clin Pharm* 17, 7
Phlebitis (<1%)
(1983): Lyon JA, *Drug Intell Clin Pharm* 17, 7
Serum sickness (<1%)
Thrombophlebitis

***Note:** The disulfiram-like reaction consists of facial flushing, diaphoresis, tachycardia, and pounding headache.

CEFOTAXIME

Trade name: Claforan (Aventis)
Other common trade names: *Alfotax; Benaxima; Biosint; Cefaxim; Cefotax; Molelant; Oritaxim; Primafen; Spirosine; Zariviz*
Indications: Various infections caused by susceptible organisms
Category: Third-generation, broad-spectrum, cephalosporin
Half-life: adults: 60 minutes
Clinically important, potentially serious interactions with: aminoglycosides, anticoagulants, cimetidine, furosemide, heparin, probenecid, tobramycin

Note: Penicillin and cephalosporins share a common beta-lactam structure. People who are allergic to penicillin are approximately 4 times more likely to develop an allergic reaction to a cephalosporin than those people who have no penicillin allergy. (From 5 to 16% of patients allergic to penicillin develop allergic reactions to cephalosporins.)

Reactions

Skin

Candidiasis
Erythema multiforme
(1990): Todd PA+, *Drugs* 40, 608
(1986): Green ST+, *Postgrad Med J* 62, 415
Exanthems
(1990): Todd PA+, *Drugs* 40, 608
(1984): Smith CR+, *Ann Intern Med* 101, 469 (3.4%)
(1983): Carmine AA+, *Drugs* 25, 223 (2%)
Pruritus (2.4%)
(1990): Todd PA+, *Drugs* 40, 608
(1983): Carmine AA+, *Drugs* 25, 223 (2%)
Rash: (sic) (2.4%)
(1982): LeFrock JL+, *Clin Ther* 5, 19
Stevens–Johnson syndrome
Toxic epidermal necrolysis
Urticaria (2.4%)

Other

Anaphylactoid reaction (2.4%)
Hypersensitivity
(1993): Papakonstantinou G+, *Clin Investig* 71, 165
Injection-site inflammation (4.3%)
(1983): Carmine AA+, *Drugs* 25, 223 (5%)
Injection-site pain (1–10%)
(1983): Carmine AA+, *Drugs* 25, 223 (32%)
Injection-site thrombophlebitis
Paresthesias
Phlebitis (<1%)
Serum sickness
Vaginitis (<1%)

CEFOTETAN

Trade name: Cefotan (AstraZeneca)
Other common trade names: *Apacef; Apatef; Ceftenon; Cepan; Yamatetan*
Indications: Various infections caused by susceptible organisms
Category: Second-generation cephalosporin antibiotic
Half-life: 3–5 hours
Clinically important, potentially serious interactions with: aminoglycosides, anticoagulants, furosemide, heparin, warfarin

Note: Penicillin and cephalosporins share a common beta-lactam structure. People who are allergic to penicillin are approximately 4 times more likely to develop an allergic reaction to a cephalosporin than those people who have no penicillin allergy. (From 5 to 16% of patients allergic to penicillin develop allergic reactions to cephalosporins.)

Reactions

Skin
Candidiasis (<1%)
Erythema multiforme
Exanthems
Pruritus (<1%)
Rash (sic) (<1%)
Stevens–Johnson syndrome (<1%)
Toxic epidermal necrolysis
Urticaria (<1%)

Other
Anaphylactoid reaction (<1%)
(1990): Faro S+, *Am J Obstet Gynecol* 162, 296
(1988): Bloomberg RJ, *Am J Obstet Gynecol* 159, 125
Hypersensitivity (1.2%)
Injection-site pain (<1%)
Phlebitis (<1%)
Serum sickness (<1%)
Thrombophlebitis

CEFOXITIN

Trade name: Mefoxin (Merck)
Other common trade names: *Cefmore; Cefoxin; Lephocin; Mefoxil; Mefoxitin*
Indications: Various infections caused by susceptible organisms
Category: Second-generation, broad-spectrum cephalosporin
Half-life: 40–60 minutes
Clinically important, potentially serious interactions with: aminoglycosides, anticoagulants, cimetidine, furosemide, heparin, probenecid, vancomycin

Note: Penicillin and cephalosporins share a common beta-lactam structure. People who are allergic to penicillin are approximately 4 times more likely to develop an allergic reaction to a cephalosporin than those people who have no penicillin allergy. (From 5 to 16% of patients allergic to penicillin develop allergic reactions to cephalosporins.)

Reactions

Skin
Angioedema (<1%)
Candidiasis (<1%)
Exanthems
(1979): Brogden RN+, *Drugs* 17, 1 (2.2%)
Exfoliative dermatitis (<1%)
(1987): Norrby SR, *Drugs* 34 (Suppl 2) 105
(1985): Sanders CV+, *Ann Intern Med* 103, 70 (2%)
(1983): Tietze KJ+, *Clin Pharmacy* 2, 582
(1982): Kannangara DW+, *Arch Intern Med* 142, 1031
Flushing
(1985): Sanders CV+, *Ann Intern Med* 103, 70
Pruritus (<1%)
(1983): Tietze KJ+, *Clin Pharmacy* 2, 582
(1979): Brogden RN+, *Drugs* 17, 1
Purpura
(1990): Burstein M+, *Drug Intell Clin Pharm* 24, 206
Pustular eruption
(1994): Spencer JM+, *Br J Dermatol* 130, 514
Rash (sic) (<1%)
Stevens–Johnson syndrome (<1%)
Toxic epidermal necrolysis (<1%)
Urticaria

Other
Anaphylactoid reaction (<1%)
Injection-site induration
Injection-site pain
(1985): Sanders CV+, *Ann Intern Med* 103, 70 (10%)
(1979): Brogden RN+, *Drugs* 17, 1 (>5%)
Injection-site tenderness
Serum sickness (<1%)
(1986): Panwalker AP+, *Drug Intell Clin Pharm* 20, 953
Thrombophlebitis

CEFPODOXIME

Trade name: Vantin (Pharmacia & Upjohn)
Other common trade names: *Cefodox; Celance; Orelox; Podomexef*
Indications: Various infections caused by susceptible organisms
Category: Third-generation cephalosporin
Half-life: 2.1–2.8 hours
Clinically important, potentially serious interactions with: aminoglycosides, antacids, anticoagulants, cimetidine, furosemide, heparin, probenecid

Note: Penicillin and cephalosporins share a common beta-lactam structure. People who are allergic to penicillin are approximately 4 times more likely to develop an allergic reaction to a cephalosporin than those people who have no penicillin allergy. (From 5 to 16% of patients allergic to penicillin develop allergic reactions to cephalosporins.)

Reactions

Skin
Acne
Candidiasis (<1%)
Diaper rash (12.1%)
Diaphoresis
Edema
Erythema multiforme
Flushing (<1%)
Pruritus (<1%)
Rash (sic) (1.4%)
Skin peeling (sic) (<1%)
Stevens–Johnson syndrome (<1%)
Toxic epidermal necrolysis
Urticaria (<1%)

Other
Anaphylactoid reaction (<1%)
Dysgeusia (<1%)
Glossitis
Hypersensitivity
Injection-site burning
Injection-site cellulitis
Injection-site edema
Injection-site inflammation
Injection-site thrombophlebitis
Oral candidiasis
Paresthesias
Serum sickness (<1%)
Sialopenia (<1%)
Vaginal candidiasis (<1%)
Vaginitis
(1991): Tack KJ+, *Drugs* 42, 51

CEFPROZIL

Trade name: Cefzil (Bristol-Myers Squibb)
Indications: Various infections caused by susceptible organisms
Category: Second-generation cephalosporin antibiotic
Half-life: 1.3 hours
Clinically important, potentially serious interactions with: aminoglycosides, furosemide, probenecid, vancomycin

Note: Penicillin and cephalosporins share a common beta-lactam structure. People who are allergic to penicillin are approximately 4 times more likely to develop an allergic reaction to a cephalosporin than those people who have no penicillin allergy. (From 5 to 16% of patients allergic to penicillin develop allergic reactions to cephalosporins.)

Reactions

Skin

Angioedema (<1%)
Diaper rash (1.5%)
Candidiasis
Erythema multiforme (<1%)
Exanthems
Pruritus
Rash (sic) (<1%)
Stevens–Johnson syndrome (<1%)
Toxic epidermal necrolysis
Urticaria (<1%)

Other

Anaphylaxis (<1%)
Genital pruritus (1.6%)
Glossitis
Hypersensitivity
Oral candidiasis
Paresthesias
Serum sickness (<1%)
(1994): Lowery N+, *J Pediatr* 125, 325
Vaginitis (1.6%)

CEFTAZIDIME

Trade names: Ceptaz (GlaxoWellcome); Fortaz (GlaxoWellcome); Tazicef (SmithKline Beecham); Tazidime (Lilly)
Other common trade names: *Ceftazim; Fortum; Tagal; Taloken; Waytrax*
Indications: Various infections caused by susceptible organisms
Category: Third-generation cephalosporin
Half-life: 1–2 hours
Clinically important, potentially serious interactions with: aminoglycosides, anticoagulants, cimetidine, furosemide, heparin, probenecid

Note: Penicillin and cephalosporins share a common beta-lactam structure. People who are allergic to penicillin are approximately 4 times more likely to develop an allergic reaction to a cephalosporin than those people who have no penicillin allergy. (From 5 to 16% of patients allergic to penicillin develop allergic reactions to cephalosporins.)

Reactions

Skin

Acne
Allergic reactions (sic)
(1994): Pleasants RA+, *Chest* 106, 1124 (in patients with cystic fibrosis)
Angioedema (2%)
Candidiasis (<1%)
Diaper rash
Diaphoresis
Edema
Erythema multiforme (2%)
(1983): Pierce TH+, *J Antimicrob Chemother* 12 (Suppl A), 21
Exanthems
(1985): Richards DM+, *Drugs* 29, 105 (1.6%)
Flushing
Pemphigus erythematosus (sic)
(1993): Pellicano R+, *Int J Dermatol* 32, 675
(1993): Iannantuono M+, *Int J Dermatol* 32, 675
Photosensitivity
(1993): Vinks SA+, *Lancet* 341, 1221
Pruritus (2%)
(1996): Holloway WJ+, *Am J Med* 100, 52S
(1985): Richards DM+, *Drugs* 29, 105
Rash (sic) (2%)
(1996): Holloway WJ+, *Am J Med* 100, 52S
Stevens–Johnson syndrome (2%)
Toxic epidermal necrolysis (2%)
Toxic erythema
(1995): Rademaker M, *N Z Med J* 108, 165
Toxic pustuloderma
(1990): Rustin MHA+, *Br J Dermatol* 123, 119
Urticaria (<1%)

Other

Anaphylactoid reaction (2%)
(1985): Richards DM+, *Drugs* 29, 105
Dysgeusia
Glossitis
Hypersensitivity (2%)
Injection-site burning
Injection-site cellulitis
Injection-site edema
Injection-site inflammation (2%)
Injection-site pain (1.4%)
(1989): Gaut PL+, *Am J Med* 87 (Suppl 5A), 169S
Injection-site thrombophlebitis (2%)
Oral candidiasis
Paresthesias (<1%)
Phlebitis (<1%)
Serum sickness
Vaginal candidiasis
Vaginitis (1%)

CEFTIBUTEN

Trade name: Cedax (Schering)
Other common trade names: *Ceten; Cilecef; Keimax; Seftem*
Indications: Various infections caused by susceptible organisms
Category: Third-generation cephalosporin
Half-life: 2 hours
Clinically important, potentially serious interactions with: aminoglycosides, anticoagulants, cimetidine, heparin, probenecid

Note: Penicillin and cephalosporins share a common beta-lactam structure. People who are allergic to penicillin are approximately 4 times more likely to develop an allergic reaction to a cephalosporin than those people who have no penicillin allergy. (From 5 to 16% of patients allergic to penicillin develop allergic reactions to cephalosporins.)

Reactions

Skin

Candidiasis (<1%)
Diaper rash (<1%)
Pruritus (0.3%)
Rash (sic) (0.3%)
Stevens–Johnson syndrome (<1%)
Toxic epidermal necrolysis
Urticaria (<1%)

Other

Dysgeusia (<1%)

Hypersensitivity
Oral candidiasis
Paresthesias (<1%)
Serum sickness (<1%)
Vaginitis (<1%)
Xerostomia (<1%)

CEFTIZOXIME

Trade name: Cefizox (Fujisawa)
Other trade names: *Ceftix; Ceftrax; Epocelin; Lyceft; Rocephin; Tefidox; Ultracef*
Indications: Various infections caused by susceptible organisms
Category: Third-generation cephalosporin antibiotic
Half-life: 1.6 hours
Clinically important, potentially serious interactions with: alcohol, aminoglycosides, anticoagulants, furosemide, probenecid

Note: Penicillin and cephalosporins share a common beta-lactam structure. People who are allergic to penicillin are approximately 4 times more likely to develop an allergic reaction to a cephalosporin than those people who have no penicillin allergy. (From 5 to 16% of patients allergic to penicillin develop allergic reactions to cephalosporins.)

Reactions

Skin

Candidiasis (<1%)
Pruritus (1–5%)
Rash (sic) (1–5%)
Urticaria (<1%)
Stevens–Johnson syndrome (<1%)
Toxic epidermal necrolysis

Other

Anaphylactoid reaction (<1%)
Injection-site edema
Injection-site induration
Injection-site pain (1–5%)
Injection-site phlebitis (1–5%)
Oral candidiasis
Paresthesias (1–5%)
Phlebitis (<1%)
Serum sickness (<1%)
Vaginitis (<1%)

CEFTRIAXONE

Trade name: Rocephin (Roche)
Other common trade names: *Benaxona; Cefaxona; Cefaxone; Rocefin; Rocephalin; Rocephine; Tacex; Triaken; Zefone*
Indications: Various infections caused by susceptible organisms
Category: Third-generation cephalosporin
Half-life: 5–9 hours
Clinically important, potentially serious interactions with: aminoglycosides, anticoagulants, cimetidine, cyclosporine, heparin, probenecid

Note: Penicillin and cephalosporins share a common beta-lactam structure. People who are allergic to penicillin are approximately 4 times more likely to develop an allergic reaction to a cephalosporin than those people who have no penicillin allergy. (From 5 to 16% of patients allergic to penicillin develop allergic reactions to cephalosporins.)

Reactions

Skin

Angioedema
(1984): Richards DM+, *Drugs* 27, 469
Candidiasis (sic) (5%)
(1983): Harrison CJ+, *Am J Dis Child* 137, 1048 (superficial) (sic) (5%)
(1983): Bittner MJ+, *Antimicrob Agents Chemother* 23, 261 (superficial) (sic)
Chills (<1%)
Cutaneous side effects (sic) (3%)
(1984): Richards DM+, *Drugs* 27, 469
Dermatitis (sic)
(1989): Baba S+, *Jap J Antibiotics* 42, 212 (4%)
(1984): Richards DM+, *Drugs* 27, 469 (0.4%)
Diaphoresis (0.2%)
(1984): Moskowitz BL, *Am J Med* 77 (Suppl 4C) 84
Erythema multiforme
(1984): Richards DM+, *Drugs* 27, 469
Exanthems
(1990): Schaad UB+, *N Engl J Med* 322, 141 (4%)
(1988): Richards DM+, *Drugs* 35, 604
(1985): Judson FN+, *JAMA* 253, 1417 (1.2%)
(1984): Richards DM+, *Drugs* 27, 469 (1.4%)
(1984): Moskowitz BL, *Am J Med* 77 (Suppl 4C), 84 (1.74%)
(1983): Eron LJ+, *J Antimicrob Chemother* 12, 65 (6%)
Flushing (<1%)
(1984): Moskowitz BL, *Am J Med* 77 (Suppl 4C), 84 (0.15%)
(1983): Harrison CJ+, *Am J Dis Child* 137, 1048
Jarisch–Herxheimer reaction
(1994): Strominger MB+, *J Neuroophthalmol* 14, 77
Pemphigus
(1992): Ruocco V+, *Acta Derm Venereol* (Stockh) 72, 48
Pruritus (<1%)
(1984): Richards DM+, *Drugs* 27, 469 (0.3%)
(1984): Moskowitz BL, *Am J Med* 77 (Suppl 4C) 84 (0.34%)
Purpura
Rash (sic) (1.7%)
(1992): Francioli P+, *JAMA* 267, 264
(1983): Eron LJ+, *J Antimicrob Chemother* 12, 65
Stevens–Johnson syndrome
Toxic epidermal necrolysis
Urticaria (0.1%)
(1984): Richards DM+, *Drugs* 27, 469

Other

Anaphylactoid reaction
(1984): Richards DM+, *Drugs* 27, 469
Dysgeusia (<1%)
(1992): Francioli P+, *JAMA* 267, 264
Glossitis
(1984): Moskowitz BL, *Am J Med* 77 (Suppl 4C), 84
(1984): Richards DM+, *Drugs* 27, 469
Hypersensitivity
(2000): Demoly P+, *Allergy* 55, 418 (immediate)
(2000): Romano A+, *Allergy* 55, 415 (immediate)
Injection-site induration
Injection-site pain (1–10%)
(1992): Francioli P+, *JAMA* 267, 264
(1984): Richards DM+, *Drugs* 27, 469 (1–15%)
(1984): Moskowitz BL, *Am J Med* 77 (Suppl 4C), 84 (1%)
Injection-site phlebitis (<1%)
(1984): Moskowitz BL, *Am J Med* 77 (Suppl 4C), 84 (0.95%)
(1984): Richards DM+, *Drugs* 27, 469
Oral mucosal eruption
(1984): Richards DM+, *Drugs* 27, 469
Serum sickness
(1984): Moskowitz BL, *Am J Med* 77 (Suppl 4C), 84 (0.04%)
Vaginitis (<1%)

CEFUROXIME

Trade names: Ceftin (GlaxoWellcome); Kefurox (Lilly); Zinacef (GlaxoWellcome)
Other common trade names: *Cefuril; Cepazine; Elobact; Froxal; Kefurox; Zinacet; Zinat; Zinnat; Zoref*
Indications: Various infections caused by susceptible organisms
Category: Second-generation cephalosporin
Half-life: 1–2 hours
Clinically important, potentially serious interactions with: aminoglycosides, anticoagulants, chloramphenicol, cimetidine, erythromycin, heparin, probenecid, tetracycline, vancomycin

Note: Penicillin and cephalosporins share a common beta-lactam structure. People who are allergic to penicillin are approximately 4 times more likely to develop an allergic reaction to a cephalosporin than those people who have no penicillin allergy. (From 5 to 16% of patients allergic to penicillin develop allergic reactions to cephalosporins.)

Reactions

Skin

Acute generalized exanthematous pustulosis (AGEP)
(1995): Moreau A+, *Int J Dermatol* 34, 263 (passim)
Angioedema (<1%)
Erythema multiforme (<1%)
Exanthems
(1997): Litt JZ, Beachwood, OH, personal case (observation)
(1990): Schaad UB+, *N Engl J Med* 332, 141 (6%)
(1979): Brogden RN+, *Drugs* 17, 233 (4.4–6.7% in penicillin-allergic patients)
Jarisch–Herxheimer reaction
(1992): Nadelman RB+, *Ann Intern Med* 117, 273
Pemphigus
(1997): Brenner S+, *J Am Acad Dermatol* 36, 919
Perianal thrush
(1987): Carson JWK+, *J Antimicrob Chemother* 19, 109
Pruritus (<1%)
Purpura
Pustular eruption
(1990): Rustin MHA+, *Br J Dermatol* 123, 119
Rash (sic) (<1%)
(1988): *Med Lett* 30, 57
Stevens–Johnson syndrome (<1%)
Toxic epidermal necrolysis (<1%)
(1997): Yossepowitch O+, *Eur J Med Res* 2, 182
(1993): Correia O+, *Dermatology* 186, 32
Urticaria (<1%)
(1995): Litt JZ, Beachwood, OH, personal case (observation)
(1987): Parish LC+, *Int J Dermatol* 26, 389

Other

Anaphylactoid reaction (<1%)
Hypersensitivity
(1998): Romano A+, *J Allergy Clin Immunol* 101, 564
(1992): Romano A+, *Contact Dermatitis* 27, 270
(1991): Powell DA+, *Drug Intell Clin Pharm* 25, 1236
Injection-site pain (<1%)
Oral candidiasis
(1985): Cooper TJ+, *J Antimicrobial Chemother* 16, 373
Serum sickness (<1%)
Thrombophlebitis (1–10%)
Vaginitis (<1%)
(1988): *Med Lett* 30, 57

CELECOXIB

Trade name: Celebrex (Pfizer; Searle)
Indications: Osteoarthritis; rheumatoid arthritis
Category: A benzene-sulfonamide NSAID (Cox-2 inhibitor)*
Half-life: 11 hours
Clinically important, potentially serious interactions with: ACE-inhibitors; fluconazole; furosemide; lithium, warfarin

Reactions

Skin

Allergic reactions (sic) (<2%)
Bacterial infection (sic) (<2%)
Candidiasis (<2%)
(1999): McClain SA, Bronx, NY (from Internet) (observation)
Dermatitis (sic) (<2%)
Diaphoresis (<2%)
Ecchymoses (<2%)
Erythema multiforme
(1999): Puritz E, Smithtown, NY (from Internet) (observation)
Exanthems (<2%)
(1999): Fisher BJ, Toronto, Ontario (from Internet) (observation)
(1999): Litt JZ, Beachwood, OH, personal case (observation)
(1999): Graedon J+, *People's Pharmacy* (anecdote from a reader)
(1999): Jaffe PG, Columbia, SC (from Internet) (observation) patient had "trouble" with sulfa years back
(1999): Rudolph RI, Wyomissing, PA (from Internet) (observation)
Facial edema (<2%)
Generalized edema (<2%)
Herpes simplex (<2%)
Herpes zoster (<2%)
Hot flashes (sic) (<2%)
Peripheral edema (2.1%)
(2000): Fetterman MR, Miami, FL (from Internet) (observation) (leg)
(2000): Panagotacos PJ, San Francisco, CA (from Internet) (observation) (pedal)
(1999): Simon LS+, *JAMA* 282, 1921
Photoreactions
(1999): Zabawski E, Dallas, TX (from Internet) (observation)
Photosensitivity (<2%)
Pruritus (<2%)
(1999): Rudolph RI, Wyomissing, PA (from Internet) (observation)
Psoriasis (palmoplantar)
(2000): Catalano PM, Bradenton, FL (from Internet) (observation)
Rash (sic) (2.2%)
Skin nodule (sic) (<2%)
Soft tissue infection (sic) (<2%)
Stevens–Johnson syndrome
(1999): Puritz E, Smithtown, NY (from Internet) (observation)
Toxic epidermal necrolysis
Urticaria (<2%)
Viral infection (sic) (<2%)
Xerosis (<2%)

Hair

Hair – alopecia (<2%)

Nails

Nails – disorder (sic) (<2%)

Other

Application site cellulitis (<2%)
Application site reaction (<2%)
Dysgeusia (<2%)
Hypesthesia (<2%)
Mastodynia (<2%)
Myalgia (<2%)
Paresthesias (<2%)
Stomatitis (<2%)
Tendinitis (<2%)
Thrombophlebitis (<0.1%)

Tooth disorder (sic) (<2%)
Vaginal candidiasis (<2%)
Vaginitis (<2%)
Xerostomia (<2%)

***Note:** Celecoxib is a sulfonamide and can be absorbed systemically. Sulfonamides can produce severe, possibly fatal, reactions such as toxic epidermal necrolysis and Stevens–Johnson syndrome.

CEPHALEXIN

Trade names: Keflex (Dista); Keftab (DJ Pharma)
Other common trade names: *Apo-Cephalex; Biocet; Ceforal; Ceporex; Ceporexine; Kefarol; Keftab; Novo-Lexin; Ospexin*
Indications: Various infections caused by susceptible organisms
Category: First-generation cephalosporin
Half-life: 0.9–1.2 hours
Clinically important, potentially serious interactions with: amikacin, aminoglycosides, anticoagulants, chloramphenicol, cimetidine, erythromycin, gentamicin, heparin, probenecid, tetracycline, vancomycin

Note: Penicillin and cephalosporins share a common beta-lactam structure. People who are allergic to penicillin are approximately 4 times more likely to develop an allergic reaction to a cephalosporin than those people who have no penicillin allergy. (From 5 to 16% of patients allergic to penicillin develop allergic reactions to cephalosporins.)

Reactions

Skin

Acute generalized exanthematous pustulosis (AGEP)
(1995): Moreau A+, *Int J Dermatol* 34, 263 (passim)
Angioedema (<1%)
(1971): Griffith RS+, *Lancet* 1, 452 (0.7%)
Contact dermatitis
(1986): Milligan A+, *Contact Dermatitis* 15, 91
Cutaneous side effects (sic) (2%)
(1972): Speight TM+, *Drugs* 3, 9
(1971): Griffith RS+, *Lancet* 1, 452 (0.9%)
Erythema multiforme (<1%)
(1998): Blumenthal HL, Beachwood, OH, personal case (observation)
(1992): Murray KM+, *Ann Pharmacotherapy* 26, 1230
(1988): Platt R+, *J Infect Dis* 158, 474
(1987): Norrby SR, *Drugs* 34 (Suppl 2), 105
Exanthems
(1999): Litt JZ, Beachwood, OH, personal case (observation)
(1997): McCloskey GL+, *Cutis* 59, 251
(1995): Litt JZ, Beachwood, OH, personal case (observation)
(1972): Speight TM+, *Drugs* 3, 9
(1970): *Drug Ther Bull* 8, 18 (1–5%)
Fixed eruption
(1991): Baran R+, *Br J Dermatol* 125, 592
Pemphigus
(1992): Vaillant L+, *Int J Dermatol* 31, 67
(1991): Wolf R+, *Int J Dermatol* 30, 213
Pruritus
(1999): Litt JZ, Beachwood, OH, personal case (observation)
(1988): Kumar A+, *Antimicrob Agents Chemother* 32, 882
(1977): Okita K+, *Jpn J Antibiot* (Japanese) 30, 911
(1971): Griffith RS+, *Lancet* 1, 452 (0.7%)
Pruritus ani et vulvae
Purpura
Pustular eruption
(1994): Spencer JM+, *Br J Dermatol* 130, 514
(1988): Jackson H+, *Dermatologica* 177, 292
Rash (sic) (<1%)
Stevens–Johnson syndrome (<1%)
(1992): Murray KM+, *Ann Pharmacother* 26, 1230
(1988): Platt R+, *J Infect Dis* 158, 474
(1975): McArthur JE+, *N Z Med J* 81, 390
Toxic epidermal necrolysis (<1%)
(1995): Jick H+, *Pharmacotherapy* 15, 428
(1991): Dave J+, *J Antimicrob Chemotherapy* 28, 477
(1987): Hogan DJ+, *J Am Acad Dermatol* 17, 852
(1987): Harnar TJ+, *J Burn Care Rehabil* 8, 554
Urticaria (<1%)
(1993): Litt JZ, Beachwood, OH, personal case (observation)
(1971): Griffith RS+, *Lancet* 1, 452 (0.7%)

Nails

Nails – paronychia
(1991): Baran R+, *Br J Dermatol* 125, 592

Other

Anaphylactoid reaction (<1%)
Hypersensitivity
Oral candidiasis
Serum sickness (<1%)
(1988): Platt R+, *J Infect Dis* 158, 474
Vaginitis

CEPHALOTHIN

Trade names: Keflin (Lilly); Kefzol (Lilly)
Other common trade names: *Ceftina; Ceporacin; Cepovenin; Keflin-N; Keflin Neutral; Keflin Neutro; Practogen*
Indications: Various infections caused by susceptible organisms
Category: First-generation, broad-spectrum cephalosporin
Half-life: 30–50 minutes
Clinically important, potentially serious interactions with: aminoglycosides, amphotericin B, anticoagulants, bleomycin, cimetidine, erythromycin, furosemide, gentamicin, heparin, penicillin, probenecid, ranitidine

Note: Penicillin and cephalosporins share a common beta-lactam structure. People who are allergic to penicillin are approximately 4 times more likely to develop an allergic reaction to a cephalosporin than those people who have no penicillin allergy. (From 5 to 16% of patients allergic to penicillin develop allergic reactions to cephalosporins.)

Reactions

Skin

Allergic reactions (sic)
(1975): Braun WP, *Contact Dermatitis* 1, 190
(1966): Thoburn R+, *JAMA* 198, 345 (8%)
Candidiasis (<1%)
Erythema multiforme
(1996): Munoz-D+, *Contact Dermatitis* 34, 227
Exanthems (<1%)
(1974): Sanders WE+, *N Engl J Med* 290, 424 (>5%)
(1966): Thoburn R+, *JAMA* 198, 345 (5.5%)
(1966): Merrill SL+, *Ann Intern Med* 64, 1 (1–5%)
(1964): Weinstein L+, *JAMA* 189, 829 (1–5%)
(1964): Griffith RS+, *JAMA* 189, 823 (5%)
Pruritus (<1%)
(1966): Beaty HN+, *Ann Intern Med* 65, 641
Purpura
(1980): Miescher PA+, *Clin Haematol* 9, 505
(1968): Sheiman L+, *JAMA* 203, 601
Rash (sic)
Stevens–Johnson syndrome (<1%)
Toxic epidermal necrolysis
(1988): Dreyfuss DA+, *Ann Plast Surg* 20, 146
Urticaria
(1979): Branch DR+, *JAMA* 241, 495
(1966): Thoburn R+, *JAMA* 198, 345 (4%)
(1966): Beaty HN+, *Ann Intern Med* 65, 641
(1966): Perkins RL+, *Ann Intern Med* 64, 13 (>5%)

Other

Anaphylactoid reaction
(1987): Norrby SR, *Drugs* 34 (Suppl 2) 105
(1974): Spruell FG+, *JAMA* 229, 440
Injection-site induration (<1%)
Injection-site pain (<1%)

Phlebitis
(1980): Meguro S+, *Jpn J Antibiot* 33, 1163
(1976): Sorrentino AP+, *Am J Hosp Pharm* 33, 642
(1973): Carrizosa J+, *Antimicrob Agents Chemother* 3, 306
(1973): Inagaki J+, *Curr Ther Res Clin Exp* 15, 37
(1973): Lane AZ+, *Antimicrob Agents Chemother* 2, 234
Serum sickness (<1%)
(1974): Sanders WE+, *N Engl J Med* 290, 424

CEPHAPIRIN

Trade name: Cefadyl (Bristol-Myers Squibb)
Other common trade names: *Brisfirina; Cefaloject; Cefatrex; Cefatrexyl; Lopitrex; Unipirin*
Indications: Various infections caused by susceptible organisms
Category: First-generation cephalosporin antibiotic
Half-life: 36–60 minutes
Clinically important, potentially serious interactions with: aminoglycosides, anticoagulants, furosemide, probenecid

Note: Penicillin and cephalosporins share a common beta-lactam structure. People who are allergic to penicillin are approximately 4 times more likely to develop an allergic reaction to a cephalosporin than those people who have no penicillin allergy. (From 5 to 16% of patients allergic to penicillin develop allergic reactions to cephalosporins.)

Reactions

Skin
Candidiasis (<1%)
Erythema multiforme
Pruritus (1–5%)
Rash (sic) (1–5%)
Urticaria (<1%)
Stevens–Johnson syndrome (<1%)
Toxic epidermal necrolysis

Other
Anaphylactoid reaction
(1979): Barnett AS+, *Anesth Analg* 58, 337
Hypersensitivity
Injection-site pain (1–5%)
Injection-site phlebitis (1–5%)
Paresthesias (1–5%)
Phlebitis
(1980): Meguro S+, *Jpn J Antibiot* 33, 1163
(1976): Sorrentino AP+, *Am J Hosp Pharm* 33, 642
(1973): Carrizosa J+, *Antimicrob Agents Chemother* 3, 306
(1973): Inagaki J+, *Curr Ther Res Clin Exp* 15, 37
(1973): Lane AZ+, *Antimicrob Agents Chemother* 2, 234
Serum sickness (<1%)
Vaginitis

CEPHRADINE

Trade name: Velosef (Bristol-Myers Squibb)
Other common trade names: *Anspor; Cefro; Celex; Doncef; Eskacef; Maxisporin; Opebrin; Sefril; Veracef*
Indications: Various infections caused by susceptible organisms
Category: First-generation cephalosporin
Half-life: 1–2 hours
Clinically important, potentially serious interactions with: aminoglycosides, anticoagulants, cimetidine, heparin, probenecid

Note: Penicillin and cephalosporins share a common beta-lactam structure. People who are allergic to penicillin are approximately 4 times more likely to develop an allergic reaction to a cephalosporin than those people who have no penicillin allergy. (From 5 to 16% of patients allergic to penicillin develop allergic reactions to cephalosporins.)

Reactions

Skin
Acute generalized exanthematous pustulosis (AGEP)
(1995): Moreau A+, *Int J Dermatol* 34, 263 (passim)
Erythema multiforme
Exanthems
(1976): Brillinberg Wurth GH+, *Curr Res Med Opin* 4, 139
Pruritus (<1%)
Purpura
Pustular eruption
(1986): Kalb RE+, *Cutis* 38, 58
Rash (sic) (<1%)
Stevens–Johnson syndrome (<1%)
Toxic epidermal necrolysis
(1990): Balcar-Boron A+, *Wiad Lek* (Polish) 43, 988
Toxic pustuloderma
(1990): Rustin MHA+, *Br J Dermatol* 123, 119
Urticaria (<1%)

Other
Anaphylactoid reaction
Hypersensitivity
Injection-site pain (<1%)
Injection-site phlebitis (<1%)
Serum sickness
Vaginitis

CERIVASTATIN

Synonyms: BAY W6228; rivastatin
Trade name: Baycol (Bayer)
Indications: Elevated cholesterol
Category: HMG-CoA reductase inhibitor; antihyperlipidemic
Half-life: 2–3 hours
Clinically important, potentially serious interactions with: amprenavir, clarithromycin, cyclosporine, danazol, diltiazem, erythromycin, fluconazole, fluvoxamine, gemfibrozil, indinavir, itraconazole, kaolin, ketoconazole, mibefradil, miconazole, nefazodone, nelfinavir, niacin, ritonavir, saquinavir, troleandomycin, verapamil

Reactions

Skin
Angioedema
Dermatomyositis
Edema
Erythema multiforme
Flushing
Lupus erythematosus
Nodules (sic)
Peripheral edema (2%)
Photosensitivity

Pigmentation
Pruritus
Purpura
Rash (sic) (3.4%)
Stevens–Johnson syndrome
Toxic epidermal necrolysis
Urticaria
Vasculitis
Xerosis

Hair
Hair – alopecia
Hair – changes (sic)

Nails
Nails – changes (sic)

Other
Anaphylactoid reaction
Dysgeusia
Gynecomastia
Hypersensitivity
Myalgia (2.7%)
Myopathy
Paresthesias
Xerostomia

CETIRIZINE

Synonyms: P-071; UCB-P071
Trade name: Zyrtec (Pfizer)
Other common trade names: *Alercet; Alerid; Cetrine; Cezin; Reactine; Triz; Virlix; Zirtin*
Indications: Allergic rhinitis, urticaria
Category: Antihistamine
Half-life: 8–11 hours
Clinically important, potentially serious interactions with: alcohol, anticholinergics, barbiturates, CNS depressants, opiate agonists

Reactions

Skin
Acne (<2%)
Angioedema (<2%)
Bullous eruption (<2%)
Dermatitis (sic)(<2%)
Diaphoresis (<2%)
Edema (periorbital, facial, ankle, generalized, peripheral)
Exanthems (<2%)
(1998): Rehbein H, Jacksonville, FL (generalized) (from Internet) (observation)
(1997): Stingeni L+, *Contact Dermatitis* 37, 249
Flushing (<2%)
Furunculosis (<2%)
Hyperkeratosis (<2%)
Photosensitivity (<2%)
Phototoxic reaction (<2%)
Pruritus (<2%)
Purpura (<2%)
Rash (sic) (<2%)
Seborrhea (<2%)
Urticaria (<2%)
(1999): Karamfilov T+, *Br J Dermatol* 140, 979
(1997): Stingeni L+, *Contact Dermatitis* 37, 249
Xerosis (<2%)

Hair
Hair – alopecia (<2%)
(1998): Reed BR, Denver, CO (from Internet) (observation)
Hair – hypertrichosis (<2%)

Other
Ageusia (<2%)
Anaphylactoid reaction (<2%)
Dysgeusia (<2%)
Hyperesthesia (<2%)
Hypesthesia (<2%)
Mastodynia (<2%)
Myalgia (<2%)
Paresthesias (<2%)
Parosmia (<2%)
Sialorrhea (<2%)
Stomatitis (<2%)
Tongue discoloration (<2%)
Tongue edema (<2%)
Vaginitis (<2%)
Xerostomia (5.7%)
(1995): Breneman D+, *J Am Acad Dermatol* 33, 192

CEVIMELINE

Trade name: Exovac (SnowBrand)
Indications: Sicca syndrome in patients with Sjøgren's syndrome
Category: Muscarinic agonist; cholinergic agent
Half-life: 3–4 hours
Clinically important, potentially serious interactions with: amiodarone, diltiazem, erythromycin, fluoxetine, itraconazole, ketoconazole, paroxetine, quinidine, ritonavir, verapamil

Reactions

Skin
Allergy (sic) (1–10%)
Bullous eruption (<1%)
Dermatitis (sic) (<1%)
Diaphoresis (20%)
Eczema (<1%)
Edema (1–10%)
Exanthems (1–10%)
Flu-like syndrome (sic) (1–10%)
Fungal infection (sic) (1–10%)
Genital pruritus (<1%)
Hot flashes (2%)
Peripheral edema (1–10%)
Photosensitivity (<1%)
Pruritus (1–10%)
Rash (sic) (4%)
Ulceration (<1%)
Xerosis (<1%)

Hair
Hair – alopecia (<1%)

Other
Dysgeusia (<1%)
Gingival hyperplasia (<1%)
Hypesthesia (1–10%)
Myalgia (1–10%)
Paresthesias (<1%)
Parosmia (<1%)
Sialorrhea (2%)
Stomatitis (<1%)
Tendinitis (<1%)
Thrombophlebitis (<1%)
Tongue discoloration (<1%)
Tongue ulceration (<1%)
Tooth disorder (sic) (1–10%)
Tremor (1–10%)
Ulcerative stomatitis (1–10%)
Vaginitis (1–10%)
Vasculitis (<1%)
Xerostomia (1–10%)

CHLORAL HYDRATE

Synonyms: chloral; hydrated chloral
Trade names: Aquachloral (Alcon); Noctec (Bristol-Myers Squibb)
Other common trade names: *Chloraldurat; Medianox; Novochlorhydrate; Somnox; Welldorm*
Indications: Insomnia, sedation
Category: Sedative hypnotic
Half-life: 8–11 hours
Clinically important, potentially serious interactions with: alcohol, CNS depressants, furosemide, oral anticoagulants, phenytoin, warfarin

Reactions

Skin

Acne
(1967): Hitch JM, *JAMA* 200, 879
(1956): Christianson HB+, *Arch Dermatol* 74, 232
Angioedema
(1973): Almeyda J+, *Br J Dermatol* 86, 313
(1956): Christianson HB+, *Arch Dermatol* 74, 232
Bullous eruption
(1967): Coleman WP, *Med Clin North Am* 51, 1073
Dermatitis (sic)
(1987): de Groot AC+, *Contact Dermatitis* 16, 229
(1956): Christianson HB+, *Arch Dermatol* 74, 232
Eczematous eruption (sic)
(1956): Christianson HB+, *Arch Dermatol* 74, 232
Erythema
(1956): Christianson HB+, *Arch Dermatol* 74, 232
Erythema multiforme
(1991): Porteous DM+, *Arch Dermatol* 127, 740 (in AIDS)
(1956): Christianson HB+, *Arch Dermatol* 74, 232
Exanthems
(1990): Lindner K+, *Dermatol Monatsschr* (German) 176, 483
(1976): Arndt KA+, *JAMA* 235, 918 (0.02%)
(1956): Christianson HB+, *Arch Dermatol* 74, 232
Fixed eruption
(1973): Almeyda J+, *Br J Dermatol* 86, 313
(1972): Verbov J, *Br J Dermatol* 86, 438
(1966): Miller LH+, *Arch Dermatol* 94, 60
(1961): Welsh AL+, *Arch Dermatol* 84, 1004
(1956): Christianson HB+, *Arch Dermatol* 74, 232
Flushing
(1956): Christianson HB+, *Arch Dermatol* 74, 232
Lichenoid eruption
(1956): Christianson HB+, *Arch Dermatol* 74, 232
Pruritus
(1990): Lindner K+, *Dermatol Monatsschr* (German) 176, 483
(1956): Christianson HB+, *Arch Dermatol* 74, 232
Purpura
(1973): Almeyda J+, *Br J Dermatol* 86, 313
(1956): Christianson HB+, *Arch Dermatol* 74, 232
Rash (sic) (1–10%)
Ulceration
(1956): Christianson HB+, *Arch Dermatol* 74, 232
Urticaria (1–10%)
(1973): Almeyda J+, *Br J Dermatol* 86, 313
(1956): Christianson HB+, *Arch Dermatol* 74, 232

Other

Acute intermittent porphyria
Dysgeusia
Hypersensitivity
Oral mucosal lesions
(1956): Christianson HB+, *Arch Dermatol* 74, 232
Oral ulceration
(1956): Christianson HB+, *Arch Dermatol* 74, 232
Stomatitis
(1956): Christianson HB+, *Arch Dermatol* 74, 232

CHLORAMBUCIL

Trade name: Leukeran (GlaxoWellcome)
Other common trade names: *Chloraminophene; Linfolysin*
Indications: Chronic lymphocytic leukemia, lymphomas, carcinomas
Category: Antineoplastic
Half-life: 1.5 hours
Clinically important, potentially serious interactions with: azathioprine, barbiturates

Reactions

Skin

Angioedema
(1977): Millard LG+, *Arch Dermatol* 113, 1298
Cutaneous necrosis
(1972): Decker JL, *Ann Intern Med* 76, 619
Cutaneous side effects (sic)
(1968): Moore GE+, *Cancer Chemother Abstr* 52, 661 (20%)
Edema
Erythema multiforme
(1987): Hitchens RN+, *Aust N Z J Med* 17, 600
Exanthems
(1992): Breathnach SM+, *Adverse Drug Reactions and the Skin*, Blackwell, Oxford, 289 (passim)
(1987): Hitchens RN+, *Aust N Z J Med* 17, 600
(1986): Peterman A+, *Arch Dermatol* 122, 1358
(1978): Franchimont P+, *J Rheumatol* 5, 85 (1.3%)
(1977): Millard LG+, *Arch Dermatol* 113, 1298
(1971): Knisely RE+, *Arch Dermatol* 104, 77
(1968): Vissian L+, *Bull Soc Fr Dermatol Syphiligr* (French) 75, 570
Exfoliative dermatitis
(1987): Hitchens RN+, *Aust N Z J Med* 17, 600
Facial erythema
(1986): Peterman A+, *Arch Dermatol* 122, 1358
Herpes simplex
(1984): Sahgal SM+, *J R Soc Med* 77, 144
(1971): Degos R+, *Bull Soc Fr Dermatol Syphiligr* (French) 78, 631
Herpes zoster
(1972): Decker JL, *Ann Intern Med* 76, 619 (>5%)
Kaposi's sarcoma
(1974): Faye I+, *Bull Soc Fr Dermatol Syphiligr* (French) 81, 379
Lupus erythematosus
(1986): Peterman A+, *Arch Dermatol* 122, 1358
Pellagra
(1987): Schmutz JL+, *Ann Dermatol Venereol* (French) 114, 569
Periorbital edema
(1992): Breathnach SM+, *Adverse Drug Reactions and the Skin*, Blackwell, Oxford, 289 (passim)
(1986): Peterman A+, *Arch Dermatol* 122, 1358
(1977): Millard LG+, *Arch Dermatol* 113, 1298
Photosensitivity
(1987): Schmutz JL+, *Ann Dermatol Venereol* (French) 114, 569
Pruritus
(1971): Knisely RE+, *Arch Dermatol* 104, 77
(1968): Vissian L+, *Bull Soc Fr Dermatol Syphiligr* (French) 75, 570
Psoriasis (exacerbation)
(1968): Vissian L+, *Bull Soc Fr Dermatol Syphiligr* (French) 75, 570
Purpura
(1990): Pietrantonio F+, *Cancer Lett* 54, 109
Rash (sic) (1–10%)
Sezary syndrome
(1981): Ferme F+, *Leuk Res* 5, 169
Stevens–Johnson syndrome
Toxic epidermal necrolysis
(1997): Aydogdu I+, *Anticancer Drugs* 8, 468
(1990): Pietrantonio F+, *Cancer Lett* 54, 109
(1990): Barone C+, *Eur J Cancer* 26, 1262
(1968): Vissian L+, *Bull Soc Fr Dermatol Syphiligr* (French) 75, 570
Urticaria
(1992): Breathnach SM+, *Adverse Drug Reactions and the Skin*, Blackwell, Oxford, 289 (passim)
(1977): Millard LG+, *Arch Dermatol* 113, 1298
(1971): Knisely RE+, *Arch Dermatol* 104, 77
(1968): Vissian L+, *Bull Soc Fr Dermatol Syphiligr* (French) 75, 570

Hair

Hair – alopecia
(1992): Breathnach SM+, *Adverse Drug Reactions and the Skin*, Blackwell, Oxford, 289 (passim)
(1978): Franchimont P+, *J Rheumatol* 5, 85 (1.3%)
(1978): Levine N+, *Cancer Treat Rev* 5, 67
(1973): Snaith ML+, *BMJ* 2, 197

Other

Acute intermittent porphyria
Hypersensitivity (<1%)
(1971): Knisley RE+, *Arch Dermatol* 104, 77
Oral mucosal lesions
(1968): Moore GE+, *Cancer Chemother Abstr* 52, 661 (2%)
Oral ulceration (<1%)
(1987): Hitchens RN+, *Aust N Z J Med* 17, 600
Stomatitis

CHLORAMPHENICOL

Trade names: AK-Chlor (Alcon); Chloromycetin (Parke-Davis); Chloroptic (Allergan); Ophthochlor (Parke-Davis)
Other common trade names: *Aquamycetin; Cebenicol; Diochloram; Kloramfenicol; Oleomycetin; Pentamycetin; Sopamycetin; Tifomycine*
Indications: Various infections caused by susceptible organisms
Category: Broad-spectrum antibiotic
Half-life: 1.5–3.5 hours
Clinically important, potentially serious interactions with: antidiabetics, anticoagulants, anticonvulsants, barbiturates, chlorpropamide, clindamycin, cyanocobalamin, erythromycin, penicillin, phenytoin, rifampin, sulfonylureas, tolbutamide, warfarin

Reactions

Skin

Acute generalized exanthematous pustulosis (AGEP)
(2000): Lee AY+, *Acta Derm Venereol* 79, 412
(1995): Moreau A+, *Int J Dermatol* 34, 263 (passim)
Angioedema (<1%)
(1985): Schewach-Millet M+, *Arch Dermatol* 121, 587
Bullous eruption
(1963): Ory EM+, *JAMA* 185, 273
Contact dermatitis
(1998): Le Coz CJ+, *Contact Dermatitis* 38, 108 (face)
(1996): Moyano JC+, *Allergy* 51, 67
(1992): Urrutia I+, *Contact Dermatitis* 26, 66
(1991): Vincenzi C+, *Contact Dermatitis* 25, 64
(1987): Kubo Y+, *Contact Dermatitis* 17, 245
(1987): Raulin C+, *Derm Beruf Umwelt* 35, 64
(1986): Rebandel P+, *Contact Dermatitis* 15, 92
(1986): van Joost T+, *Contact Dermatitis* 14, 176
(1985): Linss G+, *Dermatol Monatsschr* (German) 171, 250
(1978): Blondeel A+, *Contact Dermatitis* 4, 270
(1976): Rudzki E+, *Contact Dermatitis* 2, 181
(1975): Braun WP, *Contact Dermatitis* 1, 241
(1975): Wereide K, *Contact Dermatitis* 1, 271
(1973): Ebner H, *Wien Klin Wochenschr* (German) 85, 203
(1967): Schubert H, *Allerg Asthma Leipz* (German) 13, 25
(1966): Eberhartinger C+, *Arch Klin Exp Dermatol* (German) 224, 463
(1966): Korossy S+, *Z Haut Geschlechtskr* (German) *41, 375*
Dermatitis
Eczematous eruption (sic)
Erythema multiforme (<1%)
(1996): Lazarov A+, *Cutis* 58, 263 (from eyedrops)
(1986): Fisher AA, *Cutis* 37, 158 (topical application)
(1969): Ting HC+, *Int J Dermatol* 24, 587
(1967): Coleman WP, *Med Clin North Am* 51, 1073
(1965): Mathé P+, *J Med Bordeaux* (French) 42, 1367
(1965): Pieris EV, *Ceylon Med J* 10, 67
Exanthems (1–5%)
(1992): Breathnach SM+, *Adverse Drug Reactions and the Skin*, Blackwell, Oxford, 157 (passim)
(1972): Kauppinen K, *Acta Derm Venereol* (Stockh) 52, (Suppl) 68
(1969): Török H, *Dermatol Int* 8, 57
(1951): Usndek HE+, *Arch Dermatol* 64, 217
(1951): Altemeier WA+, *JAMA* 145, 489 (1.7%)
Fixed eruption
(1985): Pandhi RK+, *Australasian J Dermatol* 26, 88
Gray syndrome*
Leucoderma
(1980): Chalfin J+, *Ophthalmic Surg* 11, 194 (eyelid)
Pellagra
Pruritus (<1%)
(1992): Breathnach SM+, *Adverse Drug Reactions and the Skin*, Blackwell, Oxford, 157 (passim)
Purpura
(1967): Singh S+, *Indian J Pediatr* 4, 451
(1965): Horowitz HI+, *Semin Hematol* 2, 287
Pustular eruption
(1973): Macmillan AL, *Dermatologica* 146, 285
(1971): Stevanovic DN, *Br J Dermatol* 85, 134
Rash (sic) (<1%)
Sensitization (sic)
(1992): Urrutia I+, *Contact Dermatitis* 26, 66
(1986): van Joost T+, *Contact Dermatitis* 14, 176
Sheet-like erythema (sic)
Stevens–Johnson syndrome
(1965): Pieris EV, *Ceylon Med J* 10, 67
Systemic eczematous contact dermatitis
Toxic epidermal necrolysis (<1%)
(1975): Munstermann M+, *Dtsch Med Wochenschr* (German) 100, 2337
(1965): Mathé P+, *J Med Bord* (French) 142, 1367
Urticaria
(1992): Breathnach SM+, *Adverse Drug Reactions and the Skin*, Blackwell, Oxford, 157 (passim)
(1987): Perkins JB+, *Drug Intell Clin Pharm* 21, 343
(1985): Schewach-Millet M+, *Arch Dermatol* 121, 587
Vasculitis
(1965): McCombs RP, *JAMA* 194, 1059

Hair

Hair – alopecia
(1977): Kapp JP+, *Clinical Pediatrics* 16, 64

Nails

Nails – photo-onycholysis
(1985): Kechijian P, *J Am Acad Dermatol* 12, 552
(1984): Daniel CR+, *J Am Acad Dermatol* 10, 250

Other

Acute intermittent porphyria
Anaphylactoid reaction
(1976): Kozakova M, *Cesk Dermatol* (Slovak) 51, 82
Black tongue
(1954): Annotations, *Lancet* 2, 179
Glossitis
(1951): Altemeier WA+, *JAMA* 145, 489
Hypersensitivity
(1978): Simon N, *Z Hautkr* (German) 53, 341
(1974): Hegyi E+, *Cesk Dermatol* (Slovak) 49, 96
Oral mucosal eruption
(1951): Altemeier WA+, *JAMA* 145, 489
Oral ulceration
Paresthesias
(1988): Ramilo O+, *Pediatr Infect Dis* 7, 358
Porphyria
(1976): Panica D+, *Folia Med Plovdiv* 18, 161
Stomatitis (<1%)
Xerostomia

***Note:** Gray syndrome: toxic reactions in premature infants and newborns. Signs and symptoms include: abdominal distension, blue-gray skin color, low body temperature, and uneven breathing.

CHLORDIAZEPOXIDE

Trade names: Libritabs (ICN); Librium (ICN); Limbitrol (ICN)
Other common trade names: *Corax; Huberplex; Medilium; Mitran; Multum; Novopoxide; Psicofar; Reposans-10; Solium; Tropium*
Indications: Anxiety
Category: Benzodiazepine; antianxiety, sedative-hypnotic, antipanic and antitremor agent
Half-life: 6–25 hours
Clinically important, potentially serious interactions with: alcohol, barbiturates, cimetidine, ciprofloxacin, clarithromycin, clozapine, digoxin, diltiazem, disulfiram, erythromycin, fluconazole, fluoxetine, fluvoxamine, isoniazid itraconazole, ketoconazole, labetalol, levodopa, loxapine, MAO inhibitors, metoprolol, metronidazole, nefazodone, omeprazole, oral anticoagulants, phenytoin, probenecid, rifabutin, rifampin, tricyclic antidepressants, valproic acid, verapamil, **cigarette smoking**

Limbitrol is amitriptyline and chlordiazepoxide

Reactions

Skin
Angioedema (<1%)
(1971): Almeyda J, *Br J Dermatol* 84, 299
(1964): Welsh AL, *Med Clin North Am* 48, 459
Dermatitis (sic) (1–10%)
Diaphoresis (>10%)
Edema (1–10%)
Erythema multiforme (<1%)
(1992): Breathnach SM+, *Adverse Drug Reactions and the Skin*, Blackwell, Oxford, 200 (passim)
(1985): Kauppinen K+, *Br J Dermatol* 112, 575
(1981): Edwards JG, *Drugs* 22, 495 (passim)
(1974): Tay C, *Asian J Med* 10, 223
(1971): Almeyda J, *Br J Dermatol* 84, 299
Erythema nodosum (<1%)
(1981): Edwards JG, *Drugs* 22, 495 (passim)
(1971): Almeyda J, *Br J Dermatol* 84, 299
Exanthems
(1976): Arndt KA+, *JAMA* 235, 918 (0.42%)
(1971): Almeyda J, *Br J Dermatol* 84, 299
Fixed eruption (<1%)
(1990): Gaffoor PMA+, *Cutis* 45, 242 (passim)
(1981): Edwards JG, *Drugs* 22, 495 (passim)
(1974): Blair HM, *Arch Dermatol* 109, 914
(1970): Savin JA, *Br J Dermatol* 83, 546
(1964): Welsh AL, *Med Clin North Am* 48, 459
(1961): Gaul LE, *Arch Dermatol* 83, 1010
Lupus erythematosus
(1973): McCarthy J, *Arch Dermatol* 108, 733 (discussion)
(1973): Hicks JH, *Cutis* 11, 33
(1965): Grupper CH+, *Bull Soc Franc Derm Syphiligr* (French) 72, 714
Photosensitivity
(1986): Morliere P, *Biochemie* 68, 849
(1981): Edwards JG, *Drugs* 22, 495 (passim)
(1980): Bjellerup M+, *J Invest Dermatol* 75, 228
(1973): Torre D, *Arch Dermatol* 108, 733 (discussion)
(1971): Almeyda J, *Br J Dermatol* 84, 299
(1965): Luton EF+, *Arch Dermatol* 91, 362
Pigmented purpuric eruption
(1989): Nishioka K+, *J Dermatol* (Tokio) 16, 220
Pruritus
(1977): Ghosh JS, *BMJ* 1, 902
Purpura
(1981): Edwards JG, *Drugs* 22, 495 (passim)
(1977): Celada A+, *BMJ* 1, 268
(1971): Almeyda J, *Br J Dermatol* 84, 299
(1967): Copperman IJ, *BMJ* 4, 485
Rash (sic) (>10%)
(1960): Tobin JM, *JAMA* 174, 1242
Urticaria
(1981): Edwards JG, *Drugs* 22, 495 (passim)
(1974): Tay C, *Asian J Med* 10, 223
(1971): Almeyda J, *Br J Dermatol* 84, 299
(1964): Welsh AL, *Med Clin North Am* 48, 459
Vasculitis
(1989): Nishioka K+, *J Dermatol* 16, 220
(1971): Almeyda J, *Br J Dermatol* 84, 299

Hair

Hair – alopecia
(1977): Celada A+, *BMJ* 1, 268
(1973): Hicks JH, *Cutis* 11, 33
(1965): Luton EF+, *Arch Dermatol* 91, 362

Other

Acute intermittent porphyria
(1967): de Matteis F, *Pharmacol Rev* 19, 523
Galactorrhea
(1971): Almeyda J, *Br J Dermatol* 84, 299
(1961): Hooper JH+, *JAMA* 178, 506
(1956): Marshall WK+, *Lancet* 1, 152
Gynecomastia
(1965): Vavala V+, *Endocr Metabol* 36, 43
Injection-site phlebitis
Paresthesias
Porphyria
(1983): Eubanks SW+, *Int J Dermatol* 22, 337
Sialopenia (>10%)
Sialorrhea (1–10%)
Xerostomia (>10%)

CHLORHEXIDINE

Trade names: BactoShield; Betasept; Dyna-Hex; Exidine Scrub; Hibiclens; Hibistat; Peridex; PerioChip; Periogard (Various pharmaceutical companies.)
Other trade names: *Alcloxidine; Bactoscrub; Chlorhexamed; Corsodyl; Hibident; Hibiscrub; Hexol; Hibidil; Hibitane; Savlon; Spectro Gram*
Indications: Skin antisepsis, gingivitis
Category: Topical anti-infective; oral rinse
Half-life: no data
Clinically important, potentially serious interactions with: none

Reactions

Skin

Allergic reactions (sic)
(1995): Yong D+, *Med J Aust* 162, 257
(1992): Ramselaar CG+, *Br J Urol* 70, 451
(1985): Cheung J+, *Anaesth Intensive Care* 13, 429
(1982): Staab W+, *Stomatol DDR* (German) 32, 700
Contact dermatitis
(1998): Ebo DG+, *J Allergy Clin Immunol* 101, 128
(1995): Stingeni L+, *Contact Dermatitis* 33, 172
(1990): Reynolds NJ+, *Contact Dermatitis* 22, 103
(1988): Bergqvist-Karlsson A, *Contact Dermatitis* 18, 84
(1987): Osmundsen PE+, *Ugeskr Laeger* (Danish) *149, 3048*
(1985): Lasthein Andersen B+, *Contact Dermatitis* 13, 307 (5.4%)
(1983): Shoji A, *Contact Dermatitis* 9, 156
(1982): Osmundsen PE, *Contact Dermatitis* 8, 81
(1981): Roberts DL+, *Contact Dermatitis* 7, 326
(1972): Neering H+, *Ned Tijdschr Geneeskd* (Dutch) *116, 1742*
(1972): Ljunggren B+, *Acta Derm Venereol* (Stockh) 52, 308
Dermatitis (sic)
(1998): Thune P, *Tidsskr Nor Laegeforen* (Norwegian) 118, 3295
Facial edema (<1%)
Fixed eruption
(1991): Moghadam BK+, *Oral Surg Oral Med Oral Pathol* 71, 431
Photosensitivity
(1971): Wahlberg JE+, *Dermatologica* 143, 376
Urticaria
(1998): Stables GI+, *Br J Urol* 82, 756
(1990): Wong WK+, *Contact Dermatitis* 22, 52 (contact)
(1989): Fisher AA, *Cutis* 43, 17
(1988): Bergqvist-Karlsson A, *Contact Dermatitis* 18, 84

Other

Anaphylactoid reaction
(2000): Pham NH+, *Clin Exp Allergy* 30, 1001
(1999): Autegarden JE+, *Contact Dermatitis* 40, 215
(1999): Snellman E+, *J Am Acad Dermatol* 40, 771
(1998): Olivieri J+, *Schweiz Med Wochenschr* 128, 1508
(1998): Ebo DG+, *J Allergy Clin Immunol* 101, 128
(1998): Terazawa E+, *Anesthesiology* 89, 1296
(1998): Thune P, *Tidsskr Nor Laegeforen* (Norwegian) 118, 3295
(1998): Nikaido S+, *Masui* (Japanese) 47, 330
(1997): Chisholm DG+, *BMJ* 315, 785
(1997): Fujita S+, *Masui* (Japanese) 46, 1118 (2 cases)
(1996): Torricelli R, *Clin Exp Allergy* 26, 112
(1995): Parker F+, *Anaesth Intensive Care* 23, 126
(1994): Okuda T+, *Masui* (Japanese) 43, 1352
(1994): de Groot AC+, *Ned Tijdschr Geneeskd* (Dutch) *138, 1342*
(1994): Russ BR+, *Anaesth Intensive Care* 22, 611
(1994): Visser LE+, *Ned Tijdschr Geneeskd* (Dutch) *138, 778*
(1992): Harukuni I+, *Masui* (Japanese) 41, 455
(1992): Evans RJ, *BMJ* 304, 686
(1992): Peutrell JM, *Anaesthesia* 47, 1013

Dysgeusia (>10%)
(1978): Schaupp H+, *HNO* (German) 26, 335

Gingival bleeding
(1984): Asikainen S+, *J Clin Periodontol* 11, 87
(1982): Ainamo J+, *J Clin Periodontol* 9, 337

Glossitis (1–10%)

Hypersensitivity
(1998): Burlington B, *Ostomy Wound Manage* 44, 84
(1994): Aalto-Korte K+, *Duodecim* (Finnish) 110, 2013
(1989): Okano M+, *Arch Dermatol* 125, 50 (6 cases)
(1988): Bergqvist-Karlsson A, *Contact Dermatitis* 18, 84
(1986): Yaacob H+, *J Oral Med* 41, 145
(1986): Ohtoshi T+, *Clin Allergy* 16, 155
(1971): Wahlberg JE+, *Dermatologica* 143, 376

Oral mucosal reaction
(1982): Skoglund LA+, *Int J Oral Surg* 11, 380 (3 cases)

Stomatitis (1–10%)

Tongue irritation (1–10%)

Tongue pigmentation (>10%)

CHLORMEZANONE

Trade name: Trancopal (Sanofi)
Indications: Anxiety
Category: Antianxiety agent and muscle relaxant
Half-life: 24 hours
Clinically important, potentially serious interactions with: CNS depressants, ethanol

Reactions

Skin

Ankle edema

Edema

Erythema multiforme

Exanthems
(1989): Alanko K+, *Acta Derm Venereol* (Stockh) 69, 223
(1964): Welsh AL, *Med Clin North Am* 48, 459

Fixed eruption
(1998): Leal G, Fortaleza, Brazil (from Internet) (observation)
(1995): Rademacher D+, *Contact Dermatitis* 32, 117
(1992): el-Sayed F+, *Ann Dermatol Venereol* (French) 119, 671
(1991): Lee AY+, *Drug Intell Clin Pharm* 25, 604
(1989): Alanko K+, *Acta Derm Venereol* (Stockh) 69, 223
(1988): McFadden N, *Dermatologica* 176, 106
(1985): Kauppinen K+, *Br J Dermatol* 112, 575
(1985): Verbov J, *Dermatologica* 171, 60 (in combination with acetaminophen)
(1983): Mohamed KN+, *Int J Dermatol* 22, 548
(1974): Kuokkanen K, *Int J Dermatol* 13, 4
(1964): Welsh AL, *Med Clin North Am* 48, 459

Flushing

Pruritus
(1964): Welsh AL, *Med Clin North Am* 48, 459

Rash (sic)
(1991): Lee AY+, *Drug Intell Clin Pharm* 25, 604 (passim)

Stevens–Johnson syndrome
(1995): Roujeau JC+, *N Engl J Med* 333, 1600
(1995): Wolkenstein P+, *Drug Saf* 13, 56

Toxic epidermal necrolysis
(1998): von Boxberg C+, *Dtsch Med Wochenschr* (German) 123, 866 (fatal)
(1996): Blum L+, *J Am Acad Dermatol* 34, 1088
(1995): Roujeau JC+, *N Engl J Med* 333, 1600
(1993): Correia O+, *Dermatology* 186, 32
(1992): Saiag P+, *J Am Acad Dermatol* 26, 567
(1991): Rosenthal E+, *Presse Med* (French) 20, 1459
(1987): Guillaume JC+, *Arch Dermatol* 123, 1166
(1983): Tagami H+, *Arch Dermatol* 119, 910

Urticaria

Other

Acute intermittent porphyria

Dysgeusia
(1976): Rollin H, *Laryngol Rhinol Otol* (Stuttgart) (German) 55, 873

Xerostomia
(1964): Welsh AL, *Med Clin North Am* 48, 459

CHLOROQUINE

Trade name: Aralen (Sanofi)
Other common trade names: *Avloclor; Chlorquin; Emquin; Heliopar; Lagaquin; Malarivon*
Indications: Malaria, rheumatoid arthritis, lupus erythematosus
Category: Antiprotozoal, antimalarial and antirheumatic drug; lupus erythematosus suppressant; polymorphous light eruption, and porphyria cutanea tarda
Half-life: 3–5 days
Clinically important, potentially serious interactions with: antacids, cimetidine, cyclosporine, digoxin, etretinate, methotrexate, methoxsalen, penicillamine, praziquantel

Reactions

Skin

Acute generalized exanthematous pustulosis (AGEP)
(1998): Janier M+, *Dermatology* 196, 271

Angioedema (<1%)
(1993): *Lakartidningen* (Swedish) 90, 54

Bullous pemphigoid
(1999): Millard TP+, *Clin Exp Dermatol* 24, 263

Contact dermatitis
(1984): Kellett JK+, *Contact Dermatitis* 11, 47
(1975): Skog E, *Contact Dermatitis* 1, 187

Ephelides
(1985): Dupre A+, *Arch Dermatol* 121, 1164

Erythema annulare centrifugum
(1982): Koralewski F, *Dermatosen* (German) 30, 125
(1967): Ashurst PJ, *Arch Dermatol* 95, 37

Erythema multiforme (<1%)

Erythroderma
(1990): Simoneaux PW, *Curr Concept Skin Dis* Winter, 15
(1986): Langtry JA+, *Br Med J Clin Res Ed* 292, 1107
(1985): Slagel GA+, *J Am Acad Dermatol* 12, 857

Exanthems (1–5%)
(1991): Ochsendorf FR+, *Hautarzt* (German) 42, 140
(1990): Simoneaux PW, *Curr Concept Skin Dis* Winter, 15
(1973): Rees RB+, *Arch Dermatol* 88, 280 (passim)

Exfoliative dermatitis
(1986): Lavrijsen APM+, *Acta Derm Venereol* (Stockh) 66, 536
(1985): Slagel GA+, *J Am Acad Dermatol* 12, 857
(1980): Koranda FC, *J Am Acad Dermatol* 4, 650 (passim)
(1973): Rees RB+, *Arch Dermatol* 88, 280 (passim)

Fixed eruption (<1%)

Lichenoid eruption
(1990): Simoneaux PW, *Curr Concept Skin Dis* Winter, 15
(1981): Koranda FC, *J Am Acad Dermatol* 4, 650 (passim)
(1979): Krebs A, *Hautarzt* (German) 30, 281
(1973): Rees RB+, *Arch Dermatol* 88, 280 (passim)
(1958): Savage J, *Br J Dermatol* 70, 181
(1948): Alving AS+, *J Clin Invest* 27, 56
Photosensitivity
(1993): *Lakartidningen* (Swedish) 90, 54
(1992): Seideman P+, *Scand J Rheumatol* 21, 101
(1991): Ochsendorf FR+, *Hautarzt* (German) 42, 140
(1989): Ortel B+, *Dermatologica* 178, 39
(1982): van Weelden H, *Arch Dermatol* 118, 290
(1973): Rees RB+, *Arch Dermatol* 88, 280 (passim)
Pigmentation
(1998): Guedira N+, *Rev Rhum Engl Ed* 65, 58
(1991): Ochsendorf FR+, *Hautarzt* (German) 42, 140
(1987): Krebs A, *Schweiz Rundsch Med Prax* (German) 76, 1069
(1982): Levy H, *S Afr Med J* 62, 735
(1981): Koranda FC, *J Am Acad Dermatol* 4, 650 (passim)
(1980): Bentsi-Enchill KO, *Trop Geogr Med* 32, 216
(1975): Marriott P+, *Proc R Soc Med* 68, 535
(1968): Stewart TW+, *Acta Derm Venereol* 48, 47
(1963): Tuffanelli D+, *Arch Dermatol* 88, 419
(1959): Dall JLC+, *BMJ* 1, 1387
Polymorphous light eruption
(1968): Reed WB+, *Arch Dermatol* 98, 327
Pruritus
(2000): Ademowo OG+, *Clin Pharm Ther* 67, 237
(1999): Millard TP+, *Clin Exp Dermatol* 24, 263
(1997): Sowunmi A+, *Trans R Trop Med Hyg* 91, 63
(1997): Adebayo RA+, *Br J Clin Pharmacol* 44, 157
(1996): George AO, *Int J Dermatol* 35, 323
(1995): Osifo NG, *Afr J Med Sci* 24, 67
(1992): Ogunranti JO+, *Eur J Clin Pharmacol* 43, 323
(1991): Ezeamuzie IC+, *J Trop Med Hyg* 94, 184
(1991): Okor RS, *J Clin Pharm Ther* 16, 463
(1991): Mnyika KS, *East Afr Med J* 68, 139
(1991): Mnyika KS+, *J Trop Med Hyg* 94, 27 (47%)
(1991): Ajayi AA+, *Eur J Clin Pharmacol* 41, 383
(1990): Abdulkadir SA+, *Trans Roy Soc Trop Med Hyg* 84, 898
(1990): Simoneaux PW, *Curr Concept Skin Dis* Winter, 15
(1990): Okor RS, *J Clin Pharm Ther* 15, 147
(1989): Hallwood PM+, *Lancet* 2, 397
(1989): Sowunmi A+, *Lancet* 2, 213
(1989): Osifo NG, *Afr J Med Sci* 18, 121
(1989): Soro B+, *Bull Soc Pathol Exot Filiales* (French) 82, 88
(1989): Burnham G+, *Trans R Soc Trop Med Hyg* 83, 527
(1989): Abila B+, *J Trop Med Hyg* 92, 356
(1987): Spencer HC+, *Ann Trop Med Parasitol* 81, 124
(1986): Harries AD+, *Ann Trop Med Parasitol* 80, 479
(1984): Caussade P, *Arch Fr Pediatr* (French) 41, 727
(1984): Osifo NG, *Arch Dermatol* 120, 80
(1984): Bhasin V+, *J Indian Med Assoc* 82, 447
(1982): Spencer HC+, *BMJ* 285, 1703
(1977): Olatunde A, *Afr J Med Sci* 6, 27
(1969): Olatunde IA, *J Nigerian Med Assoc* 6, 23
(1964): Ekpechi OL+, *Arch Dermatol* 120, 80
Psoriasis
(1993): Schopt RE+, *Dermatology* 187, 100
(1992): Vestey JP+, *J Infect* 24, 211
(1991): Damstra RJ+, *Ned Tijdschr Geneeskd* (Dutch) 135, 671
(1990): Okor RS, *J Clin Pharm Ther* 15, 147
(1990): Abdulkadir SA+, *Trans R Soc Trop Med Hyg* 84, 898
(1990): Katugampola G+, *Int J Dermatol* 29, 153
(1989): Mallett R+, *BMJ* 299, 1400
(1988): Nicolas J-F+, *Ann Dermatol Venereol* (French) 115, 289
(1985): Stone OJ, *Int J Dermatol* 24, 539
(1982): Abel EA+, *J Am Acad Dermatol* 15, 2007
(1982): Luzar MJ, *J Rheumatol* 9, 462
(1981): Olsen TG, *Ann Intern Med* 94, 546
(1980): Kuflik EG, *Cutis* 26, 153
(1966): Baker H, *Br J Dermatol* 78, 161
(1957): Cornbleet T+, *Arch Dermatol* 75, 286
Pustular eruption
(1990): Lotem M+, *Acta Derm Venereol* (Stockh) 70, 250
Pustular psoriasis
(1999): Capper N, Mobile, AL (from Internet) (observation)
(1998): Wilairatana P+, *Int J Dermatol* 37, 713
(1997): Wilairatana P+, *Int J Dermatol* 36, 634
(1987): Friedman SJ, *J Am Acad Dermatol* 16, 1256
Stevens–Johnson syndrome
(2000): Madnani N, Bombay, India (from Internet) (observation)
(1989): Ortel B+, *Dermatologica* 178, 39
(1987): Lenox-Smith I, *J Infect* 14, 90 (fatal)
(1986): Bamber MG+, *J Infect* 13, 31 (fatal)
Toxic epidermal necrolysis (<1%)
(1994): Boffa MJ+, *Br J Dermatol* 131, 444
(1988): Phillips-Howard PA+, *Br Med J Clin Res Ed* 296, 1605
(1979): Bazarnaia NS+, *Ter Arkh* (Russian) 51, 99
(1976): Kanwar AJ+, *Indian J Dermatol* 21, 73
(1972): Shul'tsev GP+, *Sov Med* (Russian) 35, 133
Urticaria
(1990): Simoneaux PW, *Curr Concept Skin Dis* Winter, 15
(1980): Koranda FC, *J Am Acad Dermatol* 4, 650 (passim)
(1973): Rees RB+, *Arch Dermatol* 88, 280 (passim)
Vasculitis
Vitiligo
(1997): Selvaag E, *Ann Trop Pediatr* 17, 45
(1996): Selvaag E, *Acta Derm Venereol* 76, 166
(1996): Selvaag E, *Trans R Trop Med Hyg* 90, 683
(1995): Selvaag E+, American Academy of Dermatology Meeting, New Orleans (observation)
(1992): Gonggryp LA+, *Br J Rheumatol* 31, 790
(1980): Bentsi-Enchill KO, *Trop Geogr Med* 32, 216

Hair

Hair – alopecia
Hair – pigmentation (<1%)
(1997): Asch PH+, *Ann Dermatol Venereol* (French) 124, 552
(1992): Bublin JG+, *J Clin Pharm Ther* 17, 297
(1991): Ochsendorf FR+, *Hautarzt* (German) 42, 140
(1981): Koranda FC, *J Am Acad Dermatol* 4, 650 (passim)
(1978): Dubois EL, *Semin Arthritis Rheum* 8, 33
(1976): Sams WM, *Int J Dermatol* 15, 99
(1973): Rees RB+, *Arch Dermatol* 88, 280 (passim)
(1965): Rook A, *Br J Dermatol* 77, 115
Hair – poliosis
(1985): Dupre A+, *Arch Dermatol* 121, 1164
(1968): Pasykowa K+, *Pol Tyg Lek* (Polish) 23, 2014
(1966): Fraga S+, *An Bras Dermatol* (Portuguese) 41, 57

Nails

Nails – discoloration
(1991): Zic JA+, *Arch Dermatol* 127, 1037
Nails – pigmentation
(1981): Koranda FC, *J Am Acad Dermatol* 4, 650 (passim)
(1963): Tuffanelli D+, *Arch Dermatol* 88, 419
Nails – shoreline
(1993): Pavithran K, *Indian J Lepr* 65, 225

Other

Acute intermittent porphyria
(1996): Puri AS+, *Indian Pediatr* 33, 241
Gingival pigmentation
(1992): Veraldi S+, *Cutis* 49, 281
Myalgia
(1998): Guedira N+, *Rev Rhum Engl Ed* 65, 58
Myopathy
(1969): Chapman RS+, *Br J Dermatol* 81, 217
Oral mucosal pigmentation
(1992): Veraldi S+, *Cutis* 49, 281
(1991): Zic JA+, *Arch Dermatol* 127, 1037
(1990): Wollina U+, *Dtsch Z Mund Kiefer Gesichtschir* (German) 14, 104
(1981): Koranda FC, *J Am Acad Dermatol* 4, 650 (passim)
(1980): Bentsi-Enchill KO, *Trop Geogr Med* 32, 216
(1971): Giansanti JS+, *Oral Surg* 31, 66
(1970): Brynolf I, *Sven Tandlak Tidskr* (Swedish) 63, 585
Oral mucosal ulceration
Porphyria
(1980): Gerwel M, *Pol Tyg Lek* (Polish) 35, 1351
(1974): Kordac V+, *Br J Dermatol* 90, 95
(1973): Knutsson F+, *Lakartidningen* (Swedish) 70, 1547
(1962): Cripps DL+, *Arch Dermatol* 86, 575
(1959): Marsden CW, *Br J Dermatol* 71, 219
(1957): Davis MJ+, *Arch Dermatol* 75, 796

(1954): Linden IH+, *Calif Med* 81, 235
Porphyria cutanea tarda
(1985): Handa F+, *Indian J Dermatol* 30, 49
Stomatitis (<1%)
Stomatopyrosis

CHLOROTHIAZIDE

Trade names: Aldochlor (Merck); Diuril (Merck)
Other common trade names: *Azide; Chlothin; Chlotride; Diurazide; Diuret; Saluretil; Saluric*
Indications: Hypertension, edema
Category: Thiazide* diuretic; antihypertensive
Half-life: 1–2 hours
Clinically important, potentially serious interactions with: ACE-inhibitors, allopurinol, amantadine, cyclosporine, digoxin, furosemide, lithium, probenecid, thiazides

Reactions

Skin

Bullous eruption
Erythema multiforme
Exanthems
(1972): Kuokannen K, *Acta Allergol* 27, 407
(1966): Sherlock S+, *Lancet* 1, 1049 (10%)
(1966): Smith JW+, *Ann Intern Med* 65, 629 (1.3%)
(1960): Smirk H+, *BMJ* 1, 515
(1959): Kirkendall WM, *Circulation* 19, 933 (1.1%)
(1958): Rogin JR, *Arch Dermatol* 78, 504
Exfoliative dermatitis
Fixed eruption
(1984): Chan HL, *Int J Dermatol* 23, 607
Lichenoid eruption
(1986): Gonzalez JG+, *J Am Acad Dermatol* 15, 87
(1971): Almeyda J+, *Br J Dermatol* 85, 604
(1959): Harber LC+, *N Engl J Med* 261, 1378
(1959): Harber LC+, *J Invest Dermatol* 33, 83
Lupus erythematosus
(1966): Cohen P+, *JAMA* 197, 817
Photoreactions
Photosensitivity (<1%)
(1994): Enta T, *Can Fam Physicians* 40, 1269
(1993): Iwamoto Y, *Nippon Saikingaku Zasshi* (Japanese) 48, 523
(1984): Horio T, *Int J Dermatol* 23, 376
(1980): Stern RS+, *Arch Dermatol* 116, 1269
(1973): Stern WK, *Acta Derm Venereol* 53, 321
(1970): Zurcher K+, *Dermatologica* 141, 119
(1969): Kalivas J, *JAMA* 209, 1706
(1965): Jung EG+, *Int Arch Allergy Appl Immunol* 27, 313
(1959): Norins AL, *Arch Dermatol* 79, 592
(1959): Harber LC+, *N Engl J Med* 261, 1378
(1959): Harber LC+, *J Invest Dermatol* 33, 83
Pruritus
(1969): Kalivas J, *JAMA* 209, 1706
(1959): Norins AL, *Arch Dermatol* 79, 592
(1958): Rogin JR, *Arch Dermatol* 78, 504
Purpura
(1992): Breathnach SM+, *Adverse Drug Reactions and the Skin*, Blackwell, Oxford 46
(1980): Miescher PA+, *Clin Haematol* 9, 505
(1960): Ball P, *JAMA* 173, 663
(1959): Nordquist P+, *Lancet* 1, 271
(1959): Horowitz HI+, *N Y State J Med* 59, 1117
(1958): Jaffe MO+, *JAMA* 168, 2264
Rash (sic) (<1%)
Stevens–Johnson syndrome
Toxic epidermal necrolysis
Urticaria
(1960): Smirk H+, *BMJ* 1, 515
Vasculitis
(1965): Björnberg A+, *Lancet* 2, 982
(1960): Fitzgerald EW, *Arch Intern Med* 105, 305
(1958): Jaffe MO+, *JAMA* 168, 2264

Hair

Hair – alopecia

Other

Anaphylactoid reaction
Dysgeusia
Oral mucosal lesions
Paresthesias (<1%)
Xanthopsia

***Note:** Chlorothiazide is a sulfonamide and can be absorbed systemically. Sulfonamides can produce severe, possibly fatal, reactions such as toxic epidermal necrolysis and Stevens–Johnson syndrome.

CHLOROTRIANISENE

Trade name: Tace (Aventis)
Other common trade names: *Estregur; Merbentul*
Indications: Inoperable prostate cancer, atrophic vaginitis
Category: Estrogen replacement
Half-life: no data
Clinically important, potentially serious interactions with: anticoagulants, barbiturates, dantrolene, felbamate, phenytoin, rifampin, tricyclic antidepressants

Reactions

Skin

Acne pustulosa
(1964): Sneddon IB+, *Br J Dermatol* 76, 491
Candidiasis
Chloasma (<1%)
Dermatitis (sic)
Edema (>1%)
Erythema
Erythema multiforme
Erythema nodosum
Melasma (<1%)
Peripheral edema (>10%)
Photosensitivity
Rash (sic) (<1%)
Urticaria

Hair

Hair – alopecia
Hair – hirsutism

Other

Acute intermittent porphyria
Gynecomastia (>10%)
Mastodynia (>10%)
Porphyria cutanea tarda
(1970): Roenigk HH+, *Arch Dermatol* 102, 260
(1970): Domonkos AN, *Arch Dermatol* 102, 229
Vaginal candidiasis
Vaginitis

CHLORPHENIRAMINE

Trade names: Aller-Chlor (Rugby), AL-R, Chlo-Amine, Chlorate (Major), Chlor-Pro, Chlor-Trimeton (Schering), Ornade (SmithKline Beecham); Phenetron (Lannett), Rynatan; Telachlor (Major), Teldrin (SmithKline Beecham), Triaminic (Novartis), etc.
Other common trade name: *Chlor-Tripolon*
Indications: Allergic rhinitis, urticaria
Category: Antihistamine, H_1-blocker
Half-life: 20–40 hours
Clinically important, potentially serious interactions with: alcohol, barbiturates, CNS depressants, MAO inhibitors, phenothiazines, tricyclic antidepressants

Reactions

Skin

Angioedema (1–10%)
Contact dermatitis
(1990): Tosti A+, *Contact Dermatitis* 22, 55 (eye-drops)
Dermatitis (1–10%)
Diaphoresis
Photosensitivity (1–10%)

Other

Hypersensitivity
Myalgia (<1%)
Paresthesias (<1%)
Xerostomia (1–10%)

CHLORPROMAZINE

Trade name: Thorazine (SmithKline Beecham)
Other common trade names: *Chloractil; Chlorazin; Chlorpromanyl; Esmino; Largactil; Novo-Chlorpromazine; Ormazine; Propaphenin; Prozin*
Indications: Psychosis, manic-depressive disorders
Category: Phenothiazine antipsychotic and antiemetic
Half-life: initial: 2; terminal: 30 hours
Clinically important, potentially serious interactions with: ACE-inhibitors, alcohol, anticholinergics, beta-blockers, chloroquine, CNS depressants, epinephrine, lithium, MAO inhibitors, meperidine, piperazines, propranolol, tricyclic antidepressants, trazodone, valproic acid, **cigarette smoking**

Note: The prolonged use of chlorpromazine can produce a gray-blue or purplish pigmentation over light-exposed areas. This is a result of either dermal deposits of melanin, a chlorpromazine metabolite, or to a combination of both. Chlorpromazine melanosis is seen more often in women.

Reactions

Skin

Actinic reticuloid
(1982): Amblard P+, *Ann Dermatol Venereol* (French) 109, 225
Angioedema (<1%)
(1958): Hine FR, *Am J Psychiatry* 114, 942
Bullous eruption (<1%)
(1979): Matsuo I+, *Dermatologica* 159, 46
Contact dermatitis
(1955): Lewis GM+, *JAMA* 157, 909
Dermatitis (sic)
Erythema multiforme (<1%)
(1961): Baer RL+, *Year Book of Dermatology*, Chicago, 9–37
Exanthems (>5%)
(1969): Török H, *Dermatol Int* 8, 57
(1968): Raskin A, *J Nerv Ment Dis* 147, 184 (5%)
(1967): Lockey SD, *Med Sci* 18, 43
(1966): Zelickson AS, *JAMA* 198, 341
(1961): Stevanovic DV, *Br J Dermatol* 73, 233
(1957): Bernstein C+, *JAMA* 163, 930 (7–14%)
(1956): Mullins JF+, *JAMA* 162, 946
(1955): Margolis LH+, *Arch Dermatol* 72, 72 (13%)
Exfoliative dermatitis
(1961): Baer RL+, *Year Book of Dermatology*, Chicago, 9–37
Fixed eruption (<1%)
Hypohidrosis (>10%)
Lichenoid eruption
(1979): Matsuo I+, *Dermatologica* 159, 46
Lupus erythematosus
(1996): Matsukawa Y+, *J Int Med Res* 24, 147
(1994): Yung RL+, *Rheum Dis Clin North Am* 20, 61
(1990): Roche-Bayard P, *Chest* 98, 1545
(1985): Pavlidakey GP+, *J Am Acad Dermatol* 13, 109
(1980): Goldman LS+, *Am J Psychiatry* 137, 1613
(1973): Ananth JV+, *Can Med Assoc J* 108, 680
(1972): Dubois EL+, *JAMA* 221, 595
(1963): Shulman LE+, *Arthritis Rheum* 6, 558
Miliaria
(1956): Mullins JF+, *JAMA* 162, 946
Peripheral edema
Photocontact dermatitis
(1962): Calnan CD+, *Trans St. Johns Hosp Derm Soc* 48, 49
Photosensitivity (1–10%)
(1995): Kim TH+, *Photodermatol Photoimmunol Photomed* 11, 170
(1993): Jeanmougin M+, *Ann Dermatol Venereol* (French) 120, 840
(1993): Wolf ME+, *Int J Clin Pharmacol* 31, 365
(1989): Rosen C, *Semin Dermatol* 8, 149
(1989): Hoshino T+, *Arch Dermatol Res* 281, 60
(1986): Lovell CR+, *Contact Dermatitis* 14, 290
(1982): Amblard P+, *Ann Dermatol Venereol* (French) 109, 225
(1979): Matsuo I+, *Dermatologica* 159, 46
(1975): Horio T, *Arch Dermatol* 111, 1469
(1974): Johnson BE, *Proc R Soc Med* 67, 871
(1973): Johnson BE, *Br J Dermatol* 89, 16
(1971): Hägermark O+, *Br J Dermatol* 84, 605
(1969): Kalivas J, *JAMA* 209, 1706 (3%)
(1968): Prien RF+, *Arch Gen Psychiatry* 18, 482 (1–22%)
(1967): Satanove A+, *JAMA* 200, 121
(1967): Lockey SD, *Med Sci* 18, 43
(1961): Stevanovic DV, *Br J Dermatol* 73, 233
(1958): Calnan CD+, *Trans St. Johns Hosp Derm Soc* 44, 26
(1957): Winkelmann NR, *Am J Psychiatry* 113, 961 (3%)
(1957): Epstein JH+, *J Invest Dermatol* 28, 329
(1956): Mullins JF+, *JAMA* 162, 946
(1955): Margolis LH+, *Arch Dermatol* 72, 72
Phototoxic reaction
(1997): Eberlein-Konig B+, *Dermatology* 194, 131
(1979): Matsuo I+, *Dermatologica* 159, 46
(1977): Ljunggren B, *J Invest Dermatol* 69, 383
(1975): Raffle EJ+, *Arch Dermatol* 111, 1364
(1967): Satanove A+, *JAMA* 200, 121
(1964): Greiner AC+, *Can Med Assoc J* 90, 663
Pigmentation (<1%)
(2000): Lal+, *J Psychiatry Neurosci* 25, 281
(1993): Wolf ME+, *Int J Clin Pharmacol* 31, 365 (blue-gray)
(1993): Lal S+, *J Psychiatry Neurosci* 18, 173
(1993): Bloom D+, *Acta Psychiatr Scand* 87, 223
(1988): Benning TL+, *Arch Dermatol* 124, 1541
(1988): Thompson TR+, *Acta Psychiatr Scand* 78, 763
(1975): Robins AH, *S Afr Med J* 49, 1521
(1967): Satanove A+, *JAMA* 200, 209
(1966): Hashimoto K+, *J Invest Dermatol* 47, 296
(1966): Zelickson AS, *JAMA* 198, 341
(1964): Zelickson AS+, *JAMA* 188, 394
(1964): Hays GB+, *Arch Dermatol* 90, 471
(1964): Greiner AC+, *Can Med Assoc J* 90, 663
Pruritus (1–10%)
(1968): Prien RF+, *Arch Gen Psychiatry* 18, 482 (1–22%)
(1957): Bernstein C+, *JAMA* 163, 930 (4%)
Purpura
(1987): Aram H, *J Am Acad Dermatol* 17, 139
(1967): Lockey SD, *Med Sci* 18, 43
(1965): Horowitz HI+, *Semin Hematol* 2, 287
(1957): Shannon J+, *Dermatologica* 114, 101
(1956): Mullins JF+, *JAMA* 162, 946
(1956): Wintrobe MM+, *Arch Intern Med* 98, 559
Pustular eruption
(1994): Burrows NP+, *BMJ* 309, 97

Rash (sic) (1–10%)
Seborrheic dermatitis
(1983): Binder RL+, *Arch Dermatol* 119, 473 (1–5%)
(1981): Kanwar AJ+, *Arch Dermatol* 117, 65 (passim)
(1965): Fellner MJ+, *Int J Dermatol* 19, 392
(1956): Mullins JF+, *JAMA* 162, 946
Toxic epidermal necrolysis (<1%)
(1996): Purcell P+, *Postgrad Med J* 72, 186
(1990): Ward DJ+, *Burns* 16, 97
Urticaria
(1992): Loesche C+, *Contact Dermatitis* 26, 278
(1986): Lovell CR+, *Contact Dermatitis* 14, 290
(1967): Lockey SD, *Med Sci* 18, 43
(1961): Baer RL+, *Year Book of Dermatology*, Chicago, 9–37
(1956): Mullins JF+, *JAMA* 162, 946
Vasculitis
(1987): Aram H, *J Am Acad Dermatol* 17, 139
(1969): Peterkin GAG+, *Practitioner* 202, 117
(1957): Shannon J+, *Dermatologica* 114, 101
Xerosis

Nails

Nails – photo-onycholysis
(1985): Kechijian P, *J Am Acad Dermatol* 12, 552
Nails – pigmentation
(1971): Hägermark O+, *Br J Dermatol* 84, 605
(1966): Zelickson AS, *JAMA* 198, 341
(1965): Satanove A+, *JAMA* 200, 209
(1964): Greiner AC+, *Can Med Assoc J* 90, 663

Other

Anaphylactoid reaction (<1%)
Galactorrhea (1–10%)
Gynecomastia (1–10%)
Injection-site aseptic necrosis
Mastodynia (1–10%)
Oral mucosal eruption
Oral mucosal pigmentation
Oral ulceration
Polyarteritis nodosa
(1960): Meyler L+, *Acta Med Scand* 167, 95
Priapism (<1%)
(1999): Mutlu N+, *Int J Clin Pract* 53, 152
Pseudolymphoma
(1995): Magro CM+, *J Am Acad Dermatol* 32, 419
Tremor
Xerostomia (1–10%)

CHLORPROPAMIDE

Trade name: Diabinese (Pfizer)
Other common trade names: *Apo-Chlorpropamide; Arodoc C; Chlormide; Diabemide; Diabenese; Insogen; Melormin; Tesmel*
Indications: Diabetes
Category: First-generation sulfonylurea* hypoglycemic and antidiuretic
Half-life: 30–42 hours
Clinically important, potentially serious interactions with: androgens, anticoagulants, beta-blockers, chloramphenicol, clofibrate, hydantoins, MAO inhibitors, methyldopa, phenylbutazone, probenecid, rifampin, salicylates, sulfonamides, thiazides, tricyclic antidepressants, warfarin

Reactions

Skin

Angioedema
(1991): Chinchmanian RM+, *Therapie* (French) 46, 163
Bullous eruption (<1%)
Contact dermatitis
(1982): Fisher AA, *Cutis* 29, 551
Cutaneous side effects (sic)
(1967): McKiddie MT+, *Scott Med J* 12, 6 (1.65%)
(1965): Cervantes-Amezcua A+, *JAMA* 193, 759 (1.4%)
(1960): Duncan LJP+, *Pharmacol Rev* 12, 91 (5%)
Edema (<1%)
Erythema multiforme (<1%)
(1980): Kanefsky TM+, *Arch Intern Med* 140, 1543
(1971): Harris EL, *BMJ* 3, 29
(1966): Tullett GL, *BMJ* 1, 148 (fatal)
(1960): Yaffee HS, *Arch Dermatol* 82, 636
(1960): Rothfeld EL+, *JAMA* 172, 54 (passim)
(1959): Greenhouse B, *Ann N Y Acad Sci* 74, 643
(1959): Stewart RC+, *N Engl J Med* 261, 427
Erythema nodosum (<1%)
(1971): Harris EL, *BMJ* 3, 29
(1966): Tullett GL, *BMJ* 1, 148
Exanthems (1–5%)
(1970): Almeyda J+, *Br J Dermatol* 82, 634 (1–5%)
(1960): Rothfeld EL+, *JAMA* 172, 54 (passim)
(1959): Hamff LH+, *Ann N Y Acad Sci* 74, 820
Exfoliative dermatitis
(1971): Harris EL, *BMJ* 3, 29
(1967): Coleman WP, *Med Clin North Am* 51, 1073
(1966): Tullett GL, *BMJ* 1, 148
(1962): Hitselberger JF+, *JAMA* 180, 62
(1960): Rothfeld EL+, *JAMA* 172, 54 (passim)
(1959): Stewart RC+, *N Engl J Med* 261, 427
(1959): Reyes JAG+, *Ann N Y Acad Sci* 74, 1012
Fixed eruption
(1979): Rupp T, *Int J Dermatol* 18, 590
Flushing
(1992): Shelley WB+, *Advanced Dermatologic Diagnosis*, WB Saunders, 582 (passim)
(1983): Fui SNT+, *N Engl J Med* 309, 93 (alcohol flush)
(1983): Jerntorp P+, *Eur J Clin Pharmacol* 24, 237
(1982): Ohlin H+, *Br Med J Clin Res Ed* 285, 838
(1981): Capretti L+, *Br Med J Clin Res Ed* 283, 1361
(1981): Barnett AH+, *Br Med J Clin Res Ed* 283, 939
(1981): Jentorp P+, *Acta Med Scand* Suppl 656, 33
(1981): Medback S+, *BMJ* 283, 937 (alcohol flush)
(1981): Wilkin JK, *Ann Intern Med* 95, 468
(1980): Strakosch CR+, *Lancet* 1, 394
(1979): Leslie RDG+, *Lancet* 1, 997
(1978): Leslie RDG+, *BMJ* 2, 1519 (35%)
(1978): Pyke DA+, *BMJ* 2, 1521
(1971): Harris EL, *BMJ* 3, 29
(1971): Fairman MJ+, *BMJ* 4, 297 (40%)
(1966): Muller SA, *Proc Staff Meet Mayo Clin* 41, 689 (10–30%)
(1962): FitzGerald MG+, *Diabetes* 11, 40
(1962): Larsen JA+, *Proc Soc Exp Biol Med* 109, 120
(1959): Signorelli S, *Ann NY Acad Sci* 74, 900
Granulomas
(1976): Rigberg LA+, *JAMA* 235, 409
Lichenoid eruption
(1990): Franz CB+, *J Am Acad Dermatol* 22, 128
(1984): Barnett JH+, *Cutis* 34, 542
(1971): Almeyda J+, *Br J Dermatol* 85, 604
(1968): Dinsdale RCW+, *BMJ* 1, 100
Lupus erythematosus
(1979): Rupp T, *Int J Dermatol* 18, 590
Photosensitivity (1–10%)
(1973): Feuerman E+, *Dermatologica* 146, 25
(1971): Harris EL, *BMJ* 3, 29
(1962): Hitselberger JF+, *JAMA* 180, 62
Pruritus (<3%)
(1971): Harris EL, *BMJ* 3, 29
(1962): Hitselberger JF+, *JAMA* 180, 62
Purpura
(1977): Cunliffe DJ, *Postgrad Med* 53, 87
(1971): Harris EL, *BMJ* 3, 29
(1965): Horowitz HI+, *Semin Hematol* 2, 287
(1963): FitzPatrick WJ, *Diabetes* 12, 457
(1960): Rothfeld EL+, *JAMA* 172, 54 (passim)
(1959): Haynes WS, *BMJ* 2, 1403
(1959): Yuen H, *Ann N Y Acad Sci* 74, 918
(1959): Grace WJ, *N Engl J Med* 260, 711
Rash (sic) (1–10%)
(1985): Baciewicz AM+, *Diabetes Care* 8, 200
Stevens–Johnson syndrome
(1980): Kanefsky TM+, *Arch Intern Med* 140, 1543

(1966): Coursin DB, *JAMA* 198, 113
(1960): Rothfeld EL+, *JAMA* 172, 54 (passim)
(1960): Yaffee HS, *Arch Dermatol* 82, 636
(1959): Stewart RC+, *N Engl J Med* 261, 427

Toxic epidermal necrolysis
(1989): Stern RS+, *J Am Acad Dermatol* 21, 317
(1966): Tullett GL, *BMJ* 1, 148 (fatal)

Urticaria (1–10%)
(1991): Chinchmanian RM+, *Therapie* (French) 46, 163
(1973): Feuerman E+, *Dermatologica* 146, 25
(1960): Rothfeld EL+, *JAMA* 172, 54 (passim)

Vasculitis
(1983): Batko B, *Wiad Lek* (Polish) 36, 761
(1973): Feuerman E+, *Dermatologica* 146, 25

Hair

Hair – alopecia
(1971): Harris EL, *BMJ* 3, 29

Other

Acute intermittent porphyria

Oral lichenoid eruption
(1988): Zain RB+, *Dent J Malays* 10, 15
(1984): Barnett J+, *Cutis* 34, 542
(1968): Dinsdale RCW+, *BMJ* 1, 100

Paresthesias

Porphyria
(1965): Zarowitz H+, *N Y State J Med* 65, 2385

Porphyria cutanea tarda
(1965): Zarowitz H+, *N Y State J Med* 65, 2385

Tongue ulceration
(1984): Barnett J+, *Cutis* 34, 542

***Note:** Chlorpropamide is a sulfonamide and can be absorbed systemically. Sulfonamides can produce severe, possibly fatal, reactions such as toxic epidermal necrolysis and Stevens–Johnson syndrome.

CHLORTETRACYCLINE

Trade name: Aureomycin (Proter Spa)
Other common trade name: *Aureomicina*
Indications: Various infections due to susceptible organisms
Category: Topical and ophthalmic tetracycline antibiotic
Half-life: no data
Clinically important, potentially serious interactions with: antacids, digoxin

Reactions

Skin

Burning (topical) (ophthalmic)
Edema (topical)
Erythema (topical)
Irritation (topical)
Photosensitivity
(1965): Verhagen AR, *Dermatologica* 130, 439
Pruritus (topical)
Rash (sic) (topical)
Stinging (topical) (ophthalmic)
Xerosis (topical)

Other

Xerostomia (ophthalmic)

CHLORTHALIDONE

Trade names: Combipres (Boehringer Ingelheim); Hygroton (Aventis); Tenoretic (AstraZeneca); Thalitone (Monarch)
Other common trade names: *Higroton; Hydro-Long; Hypertol; Igroton; Thalidone; Uridon*
Indications: Hypertension
Category: Thiazide* diuretic; antihypertensive
Half-life: 35–50 hours
Clinically important, potentially serious interactions with: allopurinol, amphotericin B, antidiabetics, bumetanide, cyclosporine, diazoxide, digoxin, furosemide, lithium, loop diuretics, NSAIDs, probenecid, sulfonylureas

Combipres is chlorthalidone and clonidine

Reactions

Skin

Erythema multiforme
Exanthems
Exfoliative dermatitis
Lupus erythematosus
Necrotizing angiitis
Photosensitivity (1–10%)
(1989): Baker EJ+, *J Am Acad Dermatol* 21, 1026
(1988): Lehmann P+, *Hautarzt* (German) 39, 38
Psoriasis
(1987): Wolf R+, *Cutis* 40, 162
Purpura (<1%)
Rash (sic) (<1%)
Stevens–Johnson syndrome
Toxic epidermal necrolysis
Urticaria (<1%)
(1993): Neaton JD+, *JAMA 279, 713 (passim)*
Vasculitis (<1%)
(1965): Björnberg A+, *Lancet* 2, 982

Hair

Hair – alopecia

Other

Paresthesias (<1%)
Pseudoporphyria
(1989): Baker EJ+, *J Am Acad Dermatol* 21, 1026
Xanthopsia

***Note:** Chlorthalidone is a sulfonamide and can be absorbed systemically. Sulfonamides can produce severe, possibly fatal, reactions such as toxic epidermal necrolysis and Stevens–Johnson syndrome.

CHLORZOXAZONE

Trade names: Paraflex (Ortho-McNeil); Parafon Forte DSC (Ortho-McNeil)
Other common trade names: *Escoflex; Flexaphen; Klorzoxazon; Muscol; Prolax; Remular-S; Solaxin*
Indications: Painful musculoskeletal conditions
Category: Skeletal muscle relaxant
Half-life: 1–2 hours
Clinically important, potentially serious interactions with: alcohol, barbiturates, CNS depressants, disulfiram

Reactions

Skin

Angioedema (1–10%)
Ecchymoses
Erythema multiforme (<1%)
(1979): Lindholm L, *Lakartidningen* (Swedish) 76, 2795
Exanthems

Flushing (1–10%)
Petechiae
Pruritus
Rash (sic) (<1%)
Urticaria (<1%)

Other

Anaphylactoid reaction
Hypersensitivity
Trembling (sic) (1–10%)

CHOLESTYRAMINE

Trade names: Lo-Cholest; Questran (Bristol-Myers Squibb)
Other common trade names: *Chol-Less; Colestrol; Lismol; PMS-Cholestyramine; Prevalite; Quantalan; Questran Lite*
Indications: Pruritus associated with biliary obstruction, primary hypercholesterolemia
Category: Antihyperlipidemic; antipruritic (cholestasis); anti-diarrheal
Half-life: no data
Clinically important, potentially serious interactions with: acetaminophen, amiodarone, anticoagulants, antidiabetics, corticosteroids, digoxin, furosemide, methotrexate, penicillin, piroxicam, propranolol, tetracycline, thiazides, thyroid, tricyclic antidepressants, ursodiol, valproic acid, vancomycin, warfarin

Reactions

Skin

Ecchymoses
Edema
Exanthems
Rash (sic) (<1%)
Urticaria

Other

Dysgeusia
Paresthesias
Tongue irritation (sic) (<1%)

CIDOFOVIR

Trade names: Forvade; Vistide (Gilead)
Indications: Cytomegalovirus retinitis
Category: Antiviral (nucleotide analog)
Indications: Cytomegalovirus (CMV) retinitis in patients with AIDS
Half-life: ~2.6 hours
Clinically important, potentially serious interactions with: aminoglycosides, amphotericin B, foscarnet, nephrotoxic agents, probenecid

Reactions

Skin

Acne (>10%)
Allergic reactions (1–10%)
Chills (24%)
Diaphoresis (1–10%)
Edema
Facial edema
Herpes simplex
Local irritation (sic)
(1998): Zabawski EJ+, *J Am Acad Dermatol* 39, 741
Pallor (1–10%)
Pigmentation (>10%)
Pruritus (1–10%)
Rash (sic) (27%)
Urticaria (1–10%)
Xerosis

Hair

Hair – alopecia (22%)

Other

Aphthous stomatitis
Application site reactions (sic) (39%)
(1998): Zabawski EJ+, *J Am Acad Dermatol* 39, 741
Dysgeusia (1–10%)
Myalgia
Oral candidiasis
Oral ulceration
Paresthesias (>10%)
Stomatitis (1–10%)
Tongue discoloration
Xerostomia

CILOSTAZOL

Synonym: OPC13013
Trade name: Pletal (Otsuka; Pharmacia & Upjohn)
Indications: Peripheral vascular disease, intermittent claudication
Category: Platelet aggregation inhibitor
Half-life: 11–13 hours
Clinically important, potentially serious interactions with: diltiazem, erythromycin, itraconazole, ketoconazole, NSAIDs, omeprazole, SSRIs, **high fat meals, garlic and ginkgo biloba**

Reactions

Skin

Chills (<2%)
Ecchymoses (<2%)
Edema (<2%)
Facial edema (<2%)
Furunculosis (<2%)
Generalized edema
Hypertrophy (sic)
Infection (sic)
Peripheral edema (7–9%)
Pruritus
Purpura (<2%)
Rash (sic) (2%)
Urticaria (<2%)
Xerosis (<2%)

Other

Hyperesthesia (2%)
Myalgia (2–3%)
Paresthesias (2%)
Tongue edema (<2%)
Vaginitis (<2%)

CIMETIDINE

Trade name: Tagamet (SmithKline Beecham)
Other common trade names: *Apo-Cimetidine; Azucimet; Blocan; Cimedine; Cimehexal; Ciuk; Dyspamet; Novocimetine; Nu-Cimet; Peptol; Stomedine; Ulcedine; Zymerol*
Indications: Duodenal ulcer
Category: Histamine H_2-receptor antagonist
Half-life: 2 hours
Clinically important, potentially serious interactions with: beta-blockers, carbamazepine, carmustine, cisapride, fentanyl, fluconazole, indomethacin, isoniazid, itraconazole, ketoconazole, metronidazole, midazolam, moclobemide, morphine, pentazocine, phenytoin, procainamide, propranolol, quinidine, sulfonylureas, tetracyclines, theophylline, tricyclic antidepressants, warfarin, **cigarette smoking**

Reactions

Skin

Acne
Angioedema (<1%)
(1985): Whelan JP, *J Clin Pharmacol* 25, 610
(1982): Sandhu BS+, *Ann Intern Med* 97, 138
(1979): Delaunois L, *N Engl J Med* 300, 1216
Baboon syndrome
(1998): Helmbold P+, *Dermatology* 197, 402
Cutaneous side effects (sic) (0.4%)
(1982): Freston JW, *Ann Intern Med* 97, 728
Erythema annulare centrifugum
(1982): Merrett AC+, *N Z J Med* 12, 107
(1981): Merrett AC+, *BMJ* 283, 698
Erythema multiforme (<1%)
(1987): Talvard O+, *Presse Med* (French) 16, 825
(1983): Guan R+, *Aust N Z J Med* 13, 182
(1982): Wallach D+, *Dermatologica* 165, 197
(1981): Bjaeldager PA, *Ugeskr Laeger* (Danish) 143, 1406
(1978): Ahmed AH+, *Lancet* 2, 433
Erythroderma
Erythrosis-like lesions (sic)
(1979): Angelini G+, *BMJ* 1, 1147
Exanthems
(1986): Peters K, *Contact Dermatitis* 15, 190
(1982): Freston JW, *Ann Intern Med* 97, 728
(1979): Hadfield WA, *Ann Intern Med* 91, 128
Exfoliative dermatitis
(1983): Mitchell GG, *Am J Med* 75, 875
(1980): Yantis PL+, *Dig Dis Sci* 25, 73
Fixed eruption
(1998): Helmbold P+, *Dermatology* 197, 402 (baboon syndrome)
(1995): Inoue A+, *Acta Derm Venereol* 75, 250
Ichthyosis
(1984): Aram H, *Int J Dermatol* 23, 458
Id reaction
(1987): Sander-Jensen K+, *Dermatologica* 174, 103
Lupus erythematosus
(1982): Davidson BL+, *Arch Intern Med* 142, 166 (exacerbation)
(1979): Littlejohn GO+, *Ann Intern Med* 91, 317
Pruritus (<1%)
(1994): Warner DMc+, *J Am Acad Dermatol* 31, 677 (passim)
(1982): Wallach D+, *Dermatologica* 165, 197
(1982): Freston JW, *Ann Intern Med* 97, 728
(1982): Sandhu BS+, *Ann Intern Med* 97, 138
(1981): Taillandier J+, *Nouv Presse Med* (French) 10, 258
(1979): Matthews CNA+, *Br J Dermatol* 101, 57
Psoriasis
(1991): Andersen M, *Ugeskr Laeger* (Danish) 153, 132
(1986): Peters K, *Contact Dermatitis* 15, 190
(1983): Mitchell GG, *Am J Med* 75, 875
(1982): Wallach D+, *Dermatologica* 165, 197
(1980): Yates VM+, *BMJ* 280, 1453
(1979): Rai GS+, *Lancet* 1, 50
Purpura
Pustular psoriasis
(1979): Rai GS+, *Lancet* 1, 50
Rash (sic) (<2%)
(1991): Marshall J+, *Chest* 99, 1016
Seborrheic dermatitis
(1981): Kanwar AJ, *Arch Dermatol* 117, 65
Stevens–Johnson syndrome
(1987): Talvard O+, *Presse Med* (French) 16, 825
(1983): Guan R+, *Aust N Z J Med* 13, 182
(1978): Ahmed AH+, *Lancet* 2, 433
Toxic dermatitis (sic)
(1981): Pasquier P+, *Nouv Presse Med* (French) 10, 2994
Toxic epidermal necrolysis (<1%)
(1998): Tidwell BH+, *Am J Health Syst Pharm* 55, 163
(1983): Dabadie H+, *Gastroenterol Clin Biol* (French) 7, 425
Urticaria
(1985): Goolamali SK, *Postgrad Med J* 61, 925
(1983): Mitchell GG, *Am J Med* 75, 875
(1982): Sandhu BS+, *Ann Intern Med* 97, 138
(1982): Freston JW, *Ann Intern Med* 97, 728
(1981): Brandrup E, *Ugeskr Laeger* (Danish) 143, 1715
(1979): Hadfield WA, *Ann Intern Med* 91, 128
Vasculitis
(1983): Mitchell GG, *Am J Med* 75, 875
(1982): Wallach D+, *Dermatologica* 165, 197
(1981): Dernbach WK+, *JAMA* 246, 331
Xerosis
(1982): Greist MC+, *Arch Dermatol* 118, 253

Hair

Hair – alopecia
(1985): Tullio CJ+, *Clin Pharm* 4, 145
(1983): Khalsa JH+, *Int J Dermatol* 22, 202
(1981): Vircburger MI+, *Lancet* 1, 1160
(1979): Ahmad S, *Ann Intern Med* 91, 930

Other

Anaphylactoid reaction
(1982): Knapp AB+, *Ann Intern Med* 97, 374
Galactorrhea
(1977): Bateson MC+, *Lancet* 2, 247
Gynecomastia (<1%)
(2000): Hugues FC+, *Ann Med Interne (Paris)* (French) 151, 10 (passim)
(1994): Garcia-Rodriguez LA+, *BMJ* 308, 503
(1991): Barth JA, *Zentralbl Gynakol* (German) 113, 667
(1983): Jensen RT+, *N Engl J Med* 308, 883
(1982): Peden NR+, *Br J Clin Pharmacol* 14, 565
(1979): Spence RW+, *Gut* 20, 154
(1977): Della-Fave GF+, *Lancet* 1, 1319
(1976): Hall WH, *N Engl J Med* 841, 295 (letter)
Hypersensitivity
(2000): Evans RD+, *Clin Podiatr Med Surg* 17, 371
(1986): Peters K, *Contact Dermatitis* 15, 190
(1985): Whalen JP, *J Clin Pharmacol* 25, 610
Injection-site pain
Myalgia (<1%)
Myopathy
(1982): Kaplinsky N+, *J Rheumatol* 9, 156
(1980): Feest TG+, *BMJ* 281, 1284
Porphyria
(1985): Singh R+, *J Assoc Physicians India* 33, 187
Pseudolymphoma
(1995): Magro CM+, *J Am Acad Dermatol* 32, 419
Xerostomia

CINOXACIN

Trade name: Cinobac (Oclassen)
Other trade names: *Cerexin; Cinobact; Cinobactin; Gugecin; Nossacin; Noxigram; Uronorm*
Indications: Various urinary tract infections caused by susceptible organisms
Category: Quinoline antibiotic
Half-life: 1.5 hours
Clinically important, potentially serious interactions with: probenecid

Reactions

Skin

Allergic reactions (sic)
Angioedema (<3%)
Edema (<3%)
Erythema multiforme
Photosensitivity
Pruritus (<3%)
Rash (sic)
Stevens–Johnson syndrome
Toxic epidermal necrolysis
Urticaria (<3%)

Other

Anaphylactoid reaction
(1988): Stricker BH+, *BMJ* 297, 1434
Hypersensitivity
(1982): Scavone JM+, *Pharmacotherapy* 2, 266
Dysgeusia (<1%)
Paresthesias (<1%)

CIPROFLOXACIN

Trade names: Ciloxan Ophthalmic (Alcon); Cipro (Bayer)
Other common trade names: *Ciflox; Cimogal; Ciplox; Ciprobay Uro; Cipromycin; Ciproxin; Italnik; Kenzoflex; Uniflox*
Indications: Various infections caused by susceptible organisms
Category: Synthetic fluoroquinolone antibiotic
Half-life: 4 hours
Clinically important, potentially serious interactions with: antacids, anticoagulants, antineoplastics, bismuth subsalicylate, caffeine, calcium salts, cyclosporine, didanosine, foscarnet, glyburide, iron, magnesium salts, sucralfate, theophylline, warfarin, zinc

Ciprofloxacin is chemically related to nalidixic acid

Reactions

Skin

Acne
(1989): Rahm V+, *Scand J Infect Dis* 60, 120
(1988): Campoli-Richards DM+, *Drugs* 35, 373
(1988): Schacht P+, *Infection* 16, S29
Allergic reactions (sic)
(2000): Burke P+, *BMJ* 320, 679
(1999): *Commun Dis Rep CDR Wkly*, 9, 95
Angioedema (<1%)
(1995): Vidal C+, *Postgrad Med J* 71, 318
(1989): Rahm V+, *Scand J Infect Dis* 60, 120
(1989): Schacht P+, *Am J Med* 87, 98S
(1989): Davis H+, *Ann Intern Med* 111, 1041
(1988): Campoli-Richards DM+, *Drugs* 35, 373
(1988): Schacht P+, *Infection* 16, S29
Bullous eruption
(1988): Kaufmann I+, *Z Hautkr* (German) 63, 679
Bullous pemphigoid
(2000): Kimyadi-Asadi A+, *J Am Acad Dermatol* 42, 847
Candidiasis (<1%)
(1997): Litt JZ, Beachwood, OH, personal case (penile) (observation)
(1989): Yangco BG+, *Clin Ther* 11, 503
(1988): Schacht P+, *Infection* 16, S29
Diaphoresis
(1990): Karimi K, *Indiana Med* 83, 266
(1989): Rahm V+, *Scand J Infect Dis* 60, 120
(1988): Campoli-Richards DM+, *Drugs* 35, 373 (0.05%)
(1988): Schacht P+, *Infection* 16, S29
Edema (<1%)
(1995): Shelley ED, Toledo, OH, personal case (observation)
Elastolysis
(1993): Lien YH+, *Am J Kidney* Dis 22, 598
Erythema multiforme
(1994): Win A+, *Int J Dermatol* 33, 512
(1993): Imrie K+, *Am J Hematol* 43, 159
Erythema nodosum (<1%)
Erythroderma (<1%)
(1989): Wurtz RM+, *Lancet* 1, 955
Exanthems
(2000): Litt JZ, Beachwood, OH, personal case (observation)
(1999): Litt JZ, Beachwood, OH, personal case (observation)
(1999): Litt JZ, Beachwood, OH (anecdote from lay person on the Internet)
(1997): Bircher AJ+, *Allergy* 52, 1246
(1996): McCarty JR, Fort Worth, TX (from Internet) (observation)
(1989): Gaut PL+, *Am J Med* 87 (Suppl 5A), 169S
(1988): Campoli-Richards DM+, *Drugs* 35, 373 (0.7%)
Exfoliative dermatitis (<1%)
Fixed eruption
(1998): Maquirriain Gorriz MT+, *Aten Primaria* (Spanish) 21, 585
(1998): Litt JZ, Beachwood, OH, personal case (observation)
(1996): Dhar S+, *Br J Dermatol* 134, 156
(1995): Lozano-Ayllon M+, *Allergy* 50, 598
(1994): Kawada A+, *Contact Dermatitis* 31, 182
(1993): Alonso MD+, *Allergy* 48, 296
(1992): Alonso MD+, *Allergy* 47, 194
Flushing (<1%)
(1988): Campoli-Richards DM+, *Drugs* 35, 373
Hyperpigmentation (<1%)
Livedo reticularis
(1999): Verros CD, Tripolis, Greece (from Internet) (observation) (recurred on rechallenge)
Photosensitivity (<1%)
(2000): Ferguson J+, *J Antimicrob Chemother* 45, 503
(1998): Kimura M+, *Contact Dermatitis* 38, 180
(1997): Ferguson J+, *J Antimicrob Chemother* 40, 93
(1995): Burdge DR+, *Antimicrob Agents Chemother* 39, 793
(1993): Shelley WB+, *Cutis* 52, 27 (observation)
(1993): Shelley WB+, *Cutis* 51, 154 (observation)
(1990): Ferguson J+, *Br J Dermatol* 123, 9
(1989): Rahm V+, *Scand J Infect Dis* 60, 120
(1989): Nedorost ST+, *Arch Dermatol* 125, 433
(1989): Granowitz EV, *J Infect Dis* 160, 910
(1988): Kaufmann I+, *Z Hautkr* (German) 63, 679
(1988): Campoli-Richards DM+, *Drugs* 35, 373
(1988): Schacht P+, *Infection* 16, S29
(1987): Jensen T+, *J Antimicrob Chemother* 20, 585
(1986): Ball P, *J Antimicrob Chemother* 18 (Suppl D), 187
Phototoxic reaction
(2000): Traynor NJ+, *Toxicol Vitr* 14, 275
(1998): Martinez LJ+ *Photochem Photobiol* 67, 399
(1993): Ferguson J+, *Br J Dermatol* 128, 285
Pruritus (<1%)
(1999): Litt JZ, Beachwood, OH, 2 personal cases (observations)
(1989): Rahm V+, *Scand J Infect Dis* 60, 120
(1989): Gaut PL+, *Am J Med* 87 (Suppl 5A), 169S
(1989): Yangco BG+, *Clin Ther* 11, 503
(1989): Schacht P+, *Am J Med* 87, 98S
(1989): Davis H+, *Ann Intern Med* 111, 1041
(1988): Campoli-Richards DM+, *Drugs* 35, 373 (0.3%)
(1988): Thorsteinsson SB+, *Chemotherapy* 34, 256
(1988): Schacht P+, *Infection* 16, S29
(1988): Sanders WE, *Rev Infect Dis* 10, 528
Purpura
(1999): Goldberg EI+, *J Clin Dermatol* 2, 25

(1997): Sapadin A+, New York, American Academy of Dermatology Meeting (SF), Poster #110
(1994): Gamboa F+, *Ann Pharmacol* 29, 84

Rash (sic) (1–10%)
(2000): Johansson A+, *Pediatr Infect Dis J* 19, 449
(2000): Talan DA+, *JAMA* 283, 1583 (4%)
(1995): Chaisson RE, *Infections in Medicine* 12, 48
(1989): Rahm V+, *Scand J Infect Dis* 60, 120
(1989): Fass RJ+, *Am J Med* 87, 164S
(1989): Schacht P+, *Am J Med* 87, 98S
(1989): Modai J, *Am J Med* 87, 243S
(1988): Schacht P+, *Infection* 16, S29
(1988): Sanders WE, *Rev Infect Dis* 10, 528

Stevens–Johnson syndrome (<1%)
(1994): Kamili MA+, *J Assoc Physicians India* 42, 755
(1994): Gohel DR+, *J Assoc Physicians India* 42, 665
(1994): Win A+, *Int J Dermatol* 33, 512
(1994): Bhatia RS, *J Assoc Physicians India* 42, 344

Toxic epidermal necrolysis (<1%)
(1997): Livasy CA+, *Dermatology* 195, 173 (fatal)
(1997): Yerasi AB+, *Ann Pharmacother* 30, 297
(1993): Moshfeghi M+, *Ann Pharmacother* 27, 1467
(1991): Sakellariou G+, *Int J Artif Organs* 14, 634
(1991): Tham TC+, *Lancet* 338, 522

Urticaria (<1%)
(1999): Litt JZ, Beachwood, OH, personal case (observation)
(1994): Guharoy SR, *Vet Hum Toxicol* 36, 540
(1993): Litt JZ, Beachwood, OH, personal case (observation)
(1989): Rahm V+, *Scand J Infect Dis* 60, 120
(1989): Schacht P+, *Am J Med* 87, 98S
(1989): Davis H+, *Ann Intern Med* 111, 1041
(1988): Campoli-Richards DM+, *Drugs* 35, 373 (0.05%)
(1988): Schacht P+, *Infection* 16, S29
(1986): Ball P, *J Antimicrob Chemother* 18 (Suppl D), 187

Vasculitis (<1%)
(2000): Perez Vazquez A+, *An Med Internat* (Spanish) 17, 225
(1999): Goldberg EI+, *J Clin Dermatol* 2, 25
(1997): Reano M+, *Allergy* 52, 599
(1997): Lieu PK+, *Allergy* 52, 593
(1994): Beuselinck B+, *Acta Clin Belg* 49, 173
(1993): Wagh SS+, *Indian J Pediatr* 60, 610
(1992): Stubbings J+, *BMJ* 305, 29
(1991): Kanuga J+, *Ann Allergy* 66, 76
(1989): Choe U+, *N Engl J Med* 320, 257

Other

Anaphylactoid reaction (<1%)
(1999): Corcoy M+, *Rev Esp Anestesiol Reanim* (Spanish) 46, 419
(1999): Erdem G+, *Pediatr Infect Dis J* 18, 563
(1997): Clutterbuck DJ+, *Int J STD AIDS* 8, 707
(1997): Salon EJ+, *Ann Pharmacother* 31, 119
(1995): Assouad M+, *Ann Intern Med* 122, 396
(1993): Soetikno RM+, *Ann Pharmacother* 27, 1404 (in AIDS)
(1994): Beuselinck B+, *Acta Clin Belg* (Dutch; French) 49, 173
(1992): Berger TG+, *J Am Acad Dermatol* 26, 256
(1992): Deamer RL+, *Ann Pharmacother* 26, 1081
(1989): Wurtz RM+, *Lancet* 1, 955
(1989): Davis H+, *Ann Intern Med* 111, 1041

Anosmia

Dysesthesia (<1%)
(1995): Zehnder D+, *BMJ* 311, 1204

Dysgeusia (<1%)
(1988): Schacht P+, *Infection* 16, S29

Gynecomastia (<1%)
(1991): MacGowan AP+, *J Infect* 22, 100

Hypersensitivity
(1992): Deamer RL+, *Ann Pharmacother* 26, 1081
(1991): Bhatia RS, *J Assoc Physicians India* 39, 972

Injection-site pain
(1988): Thorsteinsson SB+, *Chemotherapy* 34, 256
(1987): Thorsteinsson SB+, *Chemotherapy* 33, 448 (with itching and burning)

Lobular panniculitis (erythematous tender nodules of extremities)
(1990): Rodriguez E+, *BMJ* 300, 1468

Oral candidiasis
(1988): Esposito S+, *Infection* 16, S57

Oral mucosal lesions
(1988): Campoli-Richards DM+, *Drugs* 35, 373

Paresthesias
(1989): Rahm V+, *Scand J Infect Dis* 60, 120

Serum sickness
(1994): Guharoy SR, *Vet Hum Toxicol* 36, 540
(1990): Slama TG, *Antimicrob Agents Chemother* 34, 904

Stomatitis
(1989): Rahm V+, *Scand J Infect Dis* 60, 120
(1989): Schacht P+, *Am J Med* 87, 98S
(1988): Schacht P+, *Infection* 16, S29

Tendinitis
(1999): Harrell RM, *South Med J* 92, 622 (passim)
(1998): West MB+, *N Z Med J* 111, 18 (bilateral)
(1998): Blanco Andres C+, *Aten Primaria* (Spanish) 21, 184 (bilateral)
(1997): Carrasco JM+, *Ann Pharmacother* 31, 120

Tendon rupture
(2000): Casparian JM+, *South Med J* 93, 488 (2 cases)
(1998): West MB+, *N Z Med J* 111, 18
(1998): Petersen W+, *Umfallchirurg* (German) 101, 731 (bilateral)
(1997): Poon CC+, *Med J Aust* 166, 665
(1997): Peyrade F+, *Presse Med* (French) 26, 1489
(1997): Shinohara YT+, *J Rheumatol* 24, 238
(1997): Movin T+, *Foot Ankle Int* 18, 297 (2 cases)
(1996): Hugo-Persson M, *Lakartidningen* (Swedish) 93, 1520
(1996): McGarvey WC+, *Foot Ankle Int* 17, 496
(1996): Jagose JT+, *N Z Med J* 109, 471
(1993): Boulay I+, *Ann Med Interne (Paris)* (French) 144, 493
(1992): Lee TW+, *Aust N Z J Med*, 22, 500

Tremor

Vaginitis (<1%)
(1990): Karimi K, *Indiana Med* 83, 266
(1987): Arcieri G+, *Am J Med* 82, 381

Xerostomia
(1989): Rahm V+, *Scand J Infect Dis* 60, 120
(1988): Schacht P+, *Infection* 16, S29
(1988): Campoli-Richards DM+, *Drugs* 35, 373

CISAPRIDE

Trade name: Propulsid (Janssen)
Other common trade names: *Acenalin; Alimix; Enteropride; Kinestase; Prepulsid; Propulsin; Risamol; Sepride; Unamol*
Indications: Gastroesophageal reflux disease (GERD)
Category: Antiemetic; cholinergic enhancer; gastrointestinal emptying adjunct
Half-life: 6–10 hours
Clinically important, potentially serious interactions with: cimetidine, clarithromycin, CNS depressants, diazepam, erythromycin, fluconazole, indinavir, itraconazole, ketoconazole, miconazole, nefazodone, phenothiazines, quinidine, quinolone antibiotics, procainamide, ranitidine, ritonavir, troleandomycin, warfarin

Reactions

Skin

Edema (>1%)
Exanthems
Pruritus (1.2%)
Rash (sic) (>5%)
(1996): White CM+, *Ann Pharmacother* 30, 954
Urticaria

Other

Myalgia (>1%)
Vaginitis (1.2%)
Xerostomia (>5%)

CISPLATIN

Synonym: CDDP
Trade name: Platinol (Bristol-Myers Squibb)
Other common trade names: *Cisplatyl; Platiblastin; Platinex; Platinol-AQ; Platistil; Plasticin*
Indications: Carcinomas, lymphomas
Category: Antineoplastic
Half-life: α phase: 25–49 minutes; β phase: 58–73 hours
Clinically important, potentially serious interactions with: aminoglycosides, amphotericin B, bleomycin, bumetanide, cimetidine, furosemide, loop diuretics, phenytoin, probenecid, vancomycin

Reactions

Skin

Acral erythema
(1998): Vakalis D+, *Br J Dermatol* 139, 750
Angioedema
(1984): Loehrer PJ+, *Ann Intern Med* 100, 704
(1983): Bronner AK+, *J Am Acad Dermatol* 9, 645 (1–5%)
(1981): Weiss RB+, *Ann Intern Med* 94, 66 (1–5%)
(1977): Rozencweig M+, *Ann Intern Med* 86, 803
Contact dermatitis
(1996): Schena D+, *Contact Dermatitis* 34, 220
Diaphoresis
(1983): Bronner AK+, *J Am Acad Dermatol* 9, 645
Erythema
(1983): Bronner AK+, *J Am Acad Dermatol* 9, 645
(1980): Vogl SE+, *Cancer* 45, 11
Exanthems
(1984): Loehrer PJ+, *Ann Intern Med* 100, 704
(1981): Weiss RB+, *Ann Intern Med* 94, 66 (1–5%)
(1980): Vogl SE+, *Cancer* 45, 11
Exfoliative dermatitis
(1994): Lee TC+, *Mayo Clin Proc* 69, 80
Facial edema
(1994): Lee TC+, *Mayo Clin Proc* 69, 80
Flushing
(1998): Kempf W+, *Arch Dermatol* 134, 1343
(1984): Loehrer PJ+, *Ann Intern Med* 100, 704
(1983): Bronner AK+, *J Am Acad Dermatol* 9, 645
(1980): Vogl SE+, *Cancer* 45, 11
Necrosis
(1983): Leyden M+, *Cancer Treat Rep* 67, 199
Pigmentation
(1996): Al-Lamki Z+, *Cancer* 77, 1578
Pruritus
(1994): Lee TC+, *Mayo Clin Proc* 69, 80 (passim)
(1983): Bronner AK+, *J Am Acad Dermatol* 9, 645 (1–5%)
(1981): Weiss RB+, *Ann Intern Med* 94, 66 (1–5%)
Pyoderma (verrucous)
(1982): Person JR+, *Arch Dermatol* 118, 336
Rash (sic)
Raynaud's phenomenon
(1984): Loehrer PJ+, *Ann Intern Med* 100, 704
(1981): Vogelzang NJ+, *Ann Intern Med* 95, 288
Stevens–Johnson syndrome
(1989): Brodsky A+, *J Clin Pharmacol* 29, 821
Urticaria
(1996): Schena D+, *Contact Dermatitis* 34, 220
(1994): Lee TC+, *Mayo Clin Proc* 69, 80 (passim)
(1983): Bronner AK+, *J Am Acad Dermatol* 9, 645 (1–5%)
(1981): Weiss RB+, *Ann Intern Med* 94, 66 (1–5%)
(1980): Vogl SE+, *Cancer* 45, 11

Hair

Hair – alopecia (>10%)
(1996): Planting AS+, *Eur J Cancer* 32A, 2026
(1992): Zaun H+, *Hautarzt* (German) 43, 215
(1989): Umeki S+, *Chemotherapy* 35, 54

Nails

Nails – Beau's lines (transverse nail bands)
(1994): Ben-Dyan D+, *Acta Haematol* 91, 89
Nails – hypomelanosis
(1983): James WD+, *Arch Dermatol* 119, 334

Other

Ageusia
Anaphylactoid reaction (<1%)
(1999): Ozguroglu M+, *Am J Clin Oncol* 22, 172 (intraperitoneal infusion)
(1994): Lee TC+, *Mayo Clin Proc* 69, 80 (passim)
(1983): Bronner AK+, *J Am Acad Dermatol* 9, 645
(1982): Dunagin WG, *Semin Oncol* 9, 14
(1980): Vogl SE+, *Cancer* 45, 11
(1977): Rozencweig M+, *Ann Intern Med* 86, 803
Digital necrosis
(2000): Marie I+, *Br J Dermatol* 142, 833
Extravasation
Gingival pigmentation
(1982): Dunagin WG, *Semin Oncol* 9, 14
Injection-site cellulitis
(1994): Lee TC+, *Mayo Clin Proc* 69, 80 (passim)
(1990): Fields S+, *J Natl Cancer Inst* 82, 1649
(1989): Kerker BJ+, *Semin Dermatol* 8, 173
(1980): Lewis KP+, *Cancer Treat Rep* 64, 1162
Injection-site pain
(1998): Kempf W+, *Arch Dermatol* 134, 1343
Injection-site thrombophlebitis
Oral mucosal lesions (<1%)
(1997): Herlofson BB+, *Eur J Oral Sci* 105, 523
(1990): Al-Sarraf M+, *J Clin Oncol* 8, 1342 (>5%)
Oral ulceration (<1%)
Phlebitis
Porphyria
(1986): Aramburo-Gonzalez P+, *Med Clin (Barc)* (Spanish) 87, 738

CITALOPRAM

Synonym: nitalapram
Trade name: Celexa (Forest)
Indications: Depression; obsessive-compulsive disorder; panic disorder
Category: Antidepressant (SSRI)
Half-life: 33 hours
Clinically important, potentially serious interactions with: alcohol, buspirone, carbamazepine, MAO inhibitors, metoprolol, nefazodone, tramadol

Reactions

Skin

Cellulitis
Dermatitis (sic)
Diaphoresis (11%)
Eczema (sic)
Facial edema
Hot flashes
Hypohidrosis
Photosensitivity
Pigmentation
Pruritus (<10%)
Pruritus ani
Psoriasis
(2000): Elliott P, Logan Central, Australia (from Internet) (observation)
Purpura
Rash (sic) (<10%)
Urticaria
Xerosis

Hair

Hair – alopecia
Hair – hypertrichosis

Other

Dysgeusia
Bruxism
Galactorrhea

Gingival bleeding
Gingivitis
Gynecomastia
Hyperesthesia
Hypesthesia
Mastodynia
Myalgia (>2%)
Paresthesias
Priapism (clitoral)
(1997): BerkM+, *Int Clin Psychopharmacol* 12, 121 (3 cases)
Sialorrhea
Stomatitis
Tremor (<10%)
Xerostomia (20%)

CLADRIBINE

Synonyms: 2-CdA; 2-chlorodeoxyadenosine
Trade name: Leustatin (Ortho)
Indications: Leukemias
Category: Antineoplastic, antimetabolite
Half-life: α phase: 25 minutes; β phase: 6.7 hours
Clinically important, potentially serious interactions with: allopurinol, colchicine, probenecid, sulfinpyrazone

Reactions

Skin

Allergic reactions (sic)
(1997): Robak T+, *J Med* 28, 199
Diaphoresis (1–10%)
Edema (6%)
Erythema (6%)
Exanthems (27–50%)
(1996): Meunier P+, *Acta Derm Venereol* 76, 385 (21%)
Halogenoderma (sic)
(1996): Zevin S+, *Am J Hematol* 53, 209
Petechiae (8%)
Pruritus (6%)
Purpura (10%)
Rash (sic) (27%)
(2000): Grey MR+, *Clin Lab Haematol* 22, 111
Toxic epidermal necrolysis
(1996): Meunier P+, *Acta Derm Venereol* 76, 385
Transient acantholytic dermatosis (sic)
(1997): Cohen PR+, *Acta Derm Venereol* 77, 412

Other

Injection-site edema (9%)
Injection-site erythema (9%)
Injection-site pain (9%)
Injection-site phlebitis (2%)
Injection-site thrombosis (2%)
Myalgia (7%)

CLARITHROMYCIN

Synonym: Cla
Trade name: Biaxin (Abbott)
Other common trade names: *Biaxin HP; Clacine; Clarith; Klacid; Klaricid; Macladin; Veclam*
Indications: Various infections caused by susceptible organisms
Category: Macrolide antibiotic
Half-life: 5–7 hours
Clinically important, potentially serious interactions with: amprenavir, astemizole, benzodiazepines, carbamazepine, cisapride, cyclosporine, digoxin, ergot alkaloids, fluconazole, omeprazole, phenytoin, pimozide, ritonavir, tacrolimus, terfenadine, theophylline, triazolam, warfarin, zidovudine

Reactions

Skin

Exanthems
Fixed eruption
(1988): Rosina P+, *Contact Dermatitis* 38, 105
Pruritus
(1991): Poirier R, *J Antimicrob Chemother* 27 (Suppl A), 109
Psoriasis
(1994): Ellerin P, *The Schoch Letter* 44, 47 (#185) (observation)
Pustular eruption
Rash (sic) (3%)
Stevens–Johnson syndrome (<1%)
Urticaria
Vasculitis
(1998): Gavura SR+, *Ann Pharmacol* 32, 543
(1993): de Vega T+, *Eur J Clin Microbiol Infect Dis* 12, 563

Other

Anaphylactoid reaction (<1%)
Black tongue
(1997): Greco S+, *Ann Pharmacother* 31, 1548
Dysgeusia (3%)
(1997): Saluja A+, *Derm Surg* 23, 539
Glossitis
(1997): Greco S+, *Ann Pharmacother* 31, 1548
Hypersensitivity
(1998): Igea JM+, *Allergy* 53, 107
Oral candidiasis
Parosmia
Pseudolymphoma
(1995): Magro CM+, *J Am Acad Dermatol* 32, 419
Stomatitis
(1997): Greco S+, *Ann Pharmacother* 31, 1548
Tremor (<1%)

CLEMASTINE

Trade name: Tavist (Novartis)
Other common trade names: *Aller-Eze; Antihist-1; Clema; Darvine; Tavegil; Tavegyl*
Indications: Allergic rhinitis, urticaria
Category: H_1-receptor antihistamine
Half-life: 4–6 hours
Clinically important, potentially serious interactions with: alcohol, CNS depressants, doxepin, imipramine, MAO inhibitors, phenothiazines, promazine, protriptyline, tricyclic antidepressants

Reactions

Skin

Angioedema (<1%)
Diaphoresis
Edema (<1%)

Exanthems
(1975): Todd G+, *Curr Med Res Opin* 3, 126
Flushing
(1975): Todd G+, *Curr Med Res Opin* 3, 126
Photosensitivity (<1%)
(1962): Schreiber M+, *Arch Dermatol* 86, 58
Purpura
Rash (sic) (<1%)
Toxic pustuloderma
(1996): Feind-Koopmans A+, *Clin Exp Dermatol* 21, 293
Urticaria
(1984): Savchak VI, *Vestn Dermatol Venerol* (Russian) 1, 47

Other

Anaphylactoid reaction
Hypersensitivity
Myalgia (<1%)
Paresthesias (<1%)
Xerostomia (1–10%)
(1990): Frolund L+, *Allergy* 45, 254

CLIDINIUM

Trade names: Librax (Roche); Quarzan (Roche)
Other common trade names: *Bralix; Diporax; Epirax; Libraxin; Librocol; Nirvaxal; Spasmoten*
Indications: Duodenal and gastric ulcers
Category: Anticholinergic
Half-life: no data
Clinically important, potentially serious interactions with: amantadine, anticholinergics, atenolol, digoxin, tricyclic antidepressants

Librax is clidinium and chlordiazepoxide (See chlordiazepoxide)

Reactions

Skin

Flushing
Hypohidrosis
Urticaria

Other

Ageusia
Anaphylactoid reaction
Dysgeusia
Xerostomia

CLINDAMYCIN

Trade names: Cleocin (Pharmacia & Upjohn); Cleocin-T (Pharmacia & Upjohn); Clindets (Stiefel)
Other common trade names: *Aclinda; BB; Clindacin; Dalacin; Dalacin C; Dalacine; Galecin; Sobelin*
Indications: Various serious infections caused by susceptible organisms
Category: Lincosamide antibiotic and antiprotozoal
Half-life: 2–3 hours
Clinically important, potentially serious interactions with: aminophylline, ampicillin, antacids, barbiturates, chloramphenicol, erythromycin, phenytoin, saquinavir

Reactions

Skin

Acute generalized exanthematous pustulosis
(2000): Schwab RA+, *Cutis* 65, 391
Allergic reactions (sic)
(1996): Garcia R+, *Contact Dermatitis* 35, 116
Contact dermatitis (from topical preparations)
(1995): Vejlstrup E+, *Contact Dermatitis* 32, 110
(1994): Rietschel RL, *Infect Dis Clin North Am* 8, 607
(1992): de Groot AC, *Contact Dermatitis* 8, 428
(1991): Yokayama R+, *Contact Dermatitis* 25, 125
(1983): Conde-Salazar L, *Contact Dermatitis* 9, 225
(1978): Coskey RJ, *Arch Dermatol* 114, 446
(1978): Herstoff JK, *Arch Dermatol* 114, 1402
Eczematous eruption (sic)
(1991): Yokoyama R+, *Contact Dermatitis* 25, 125
Erythema multiforme (<1%)
(1996): Munoz D+, *Contact Dermatitis* 34, 227
(1973): Fulghum DD+, *JAMA* 223, 318
Exanthems
(1999): Mazur N+, *Ann Allergy Asthma Immunol* 82, 443
(1984): Brenner S+, *Harefuah* (Hebrew) 106, 570
(1970): Geddes AM+, *BMJ* 2, 703 (>5%)
Facial edema
(1999): Mazur N+, *Ann Allergy Asthma Immunol* 82, 443
Leukocytoclastic angiitis
(1982): Lamber WC+, *Cutis* 30, 615
Pruritus (<1%)
(1973): Fass RJ+, *Ann Intern Med* 78, 853 (10%)
Pruritus ani
Purpura
Rash (sic) (1–10%)
Rosacea
(1989): de Kort WJ+, *Contact Dermatitis* 20, 72
Stevens–Johnson syndrome (<1%)
(1974): Maulide T+, *Pneumologica* (Lisbon) 5, 79
(1973): Fulghum DD+, *JAMA* 223, 318
(1973): Pickering LK, *JAMA* 223, 1392
Toxic epidermal necrolysis
(1995): Paquet P+, *Br J Dermatol* 132, 665
(1993): Correia O+, *Dermatology* 186, 32
(1992): Saiag P+, *J Am Acad Dermatol* 26, 567
Urticaria (<1%)
(1973): Fulghum DD+, *JAMA* 223, 31
(1972): Meyler L+, *Side Effects of Drugs*, Vol 7, Excerpta Medica, 389
(1970): Newell AC, *Med J Aust* 2, 321
(1969): Lattanzi WE+, *Int Med Dig* 4, 29
Vasculitis
(1982): Lambert WC+, *Cutis* 30, 615
Xerosis (from topical preparations)

Other

Anaphylactoid reaction
(1977): Lochmann O+, *J Hyg Epiderm Microbiol Immunol* 21, 441
Dysgeusia
Hypersensitivity
Injection-site phlebitis (<1%)
Lip edema
(1993): Segars LW+, *Ann Pharmacother* 27, 885
Lymphadenitis
(1997): Southern PM, *Am J Med* 103, 164
Thrombophlebitis

CLOFAZIMINE

Trade name: Lamprene (Novartis)
Other common trade names: *Clofozine; Hansepran; Lampren; Lapren*
Indications: Leprosy
Category: Antileprotic
Half-life: 10 days after a single dose
Clinically important, potentially serious interactions with: dapsone

Reactions

Skin

Acne (<1%)
(1992): Breathnach SM+, *Adverse Drug Reactions and the Skin*, Blackwell, Oxford, 161 (passim)
Acute febrile neutrophilic dermatosis (Sweet's syndrome)
(1994): Tacke J+, *Hautarzt* (German) 45, 184
Ankle edema (<1%)
(1990): Oommen T, *Leprosy Review* 61, 289

Cheilitis (candidal) (<1%)
Discoloration (sic)
(1979): Thomsen K+, *Arch Dermatol* 115, 851
Erythroderma (<1%)
Exanthems
Exfoliative dermatitis
(1985): Pavithran K, *Int J Lepr* 53, 645
Ichthyosis (8–28%)
(1989): Patki AH+, *Indian J Lepr* 61, 92
(1987): Kumar B+, *Indian J Lepr* 59, 63
(1984): Aram H, *Int J Dermatol* 23, 458
(1982): Caver CV, *Cutis* 29, 341
(1979): Thomsen K+, *Arch Dermatol* 115, 851
Pedal edema
(1993): Tyagi PY+, *Int J Lepr Other Mycobact Dis* 61, 636
Photosensitivity (<1%)
(1992): Breathnach SM+, *Adverse Drug Reactions and the Skin*, Blackwell, Oxford, 161 (passim)
Pigmentation (pink to brownish-black) (75–100%)
(1999): *Prescrire Int* 8, 44
(1993): Krop LC+, *N Engl J Med* 329, 1582
(1992): Fitzpatrick JE, *Derm Clinics* 10, 19
(1992): Gallais V+, *Ann Dermatol Venereol* (French) 119, 471
(1991): Garrelts JC, *Ann Pharmacother* 25, 525 (orange-pink)
(1990): Job CK+, *J Am Acad Dermatol* 23, 236
(1989): Patki AH+, *Indian J Lepr* 61, 92 (oral)
(1989): Zhang X+, *J Oral Pathol Med* 18, 471
(1989): Langford A+, *Oral Surg Oral Med Oral Pathol* 67, 301 (oral)
(1988): Mensing H, *Dermatologica* 177, 232
(1987): Kossard S+, *J Am Acad Dermatol* 17, 867 (reddish-blue)
(1987): Kumar B+, *Indian J Lepr* 59, 63
(1983): Moore VJ, *Lepr Rev* 54, 327
(1983): Burte NP+, *Lepr India* 55, 265
(1981): Granstein RD+, *J Am Acad Dermatol* 5, 1 (red)
(1978): Pettit JH, *Int J Lepr Other Mycobact Dis* 46, 227
(1978): Chuaprapaisilp T+, *Br J Dermatol* 99, 303 (deep-red)
(1971): Karat ABA+, *BMJ* 4, 514
(1969): Levy L+, *Int J Lepr* 38, 404
Pruritus (1–5%)
(1992): Breathnach SM+, *Adverse Drug Reactions and the Skin*, Blackwell, Oxford, 161 (passim)
Rash (sic) (1–5%)
(1995): Chaisson RE, *Infections in Medicine* 12, 48
(1992): Breathnach SM+, *Adverse Drug Reactions and the Skin*, Blackwell, Oxford, 161 (passim)
Urticaria
Vitiligo
(1996): Brown-Harrell V+, *Clin Infect Dis* 22, 581
Xerosis (8–28%)
(1992): Breathnach SM+, *Adverse Drug Reactions and the Skin*, Blackwell, Oxford, 161 (passim)

Nails

Nails – discoloration
(1989): Dixit VB+, *Indian J Lepr* 61, 476
(1982): Caver CV, *Cutis* 29, 341
Nails – onycholysis
(1989): Dixit VB+, *Indian J Lepr* 61, 476
Nails – subungual hyperkeratosis
(1989): Dixit VB+, *Indian J Lepr* 61, 476

Other

Chromhidrosis (red sweat) (1–10%)
(1987): Kumar B+, *Indian J Lepr* 59, 63
(1979): Yawalkar SJ+, *Lepr Rev* 50, 135
(1979): Thomsen K+, *Arch Dermatol* 115, 851
Dysgeusia (<1%)

CLOFIBRATE

Trade name: Atromid-S (Wyeth-Ayerst)
Other common trade names: *Abitrate; Claripex; Col; Lipavlon; Novo-Fibrate; Regelan N; Skleromexe*
Indications: Type III hyperlipidemia
Category: Antihyperlipidemic
Half-life: 6–25 hours after a single dose
Clinically important, potentially serious interactions with: anticoagulants, chlorpropamide, furosemide, glyburide, insulin, probenecid, sulfonylureas, warfarin

Reactions

Skin

Dermatitis (sic)
(1988): Murata Y+, *J Am Acad Dermatol* 18, 381
(1972): Inman WHW+, *BMJ* 3, 746
(1972): Krasno LR+, *JAMA* 219, 845
Diaphoresis
Erythema multiforme
(1988): Murata Y+, *J Am Acad Dermatol* 18, 381
Exanthems
(1988): Murata Y+, *J Am Acad Dermatol* 18, 381
(1980): Cumming A, *BMJ* 281, 1529
(1977): Heid E+, *Ann Dermatol Venereol* (French) 104, 494
(1975): Arif MA+, *Lancet* 2, 1202 (7%)
(1971): Five Year Study, *BMJ* 4, 767 (0.8%)
(1965): Hollander W, *Cardiovascular Drug Therapy* 339
Exfoliative dermatitis
(1972): Inman WHW+, *BMJ* 3, 746
Facial dermatitis
(1967): Orgain ES+, *Arch Intern Med* 119, 80
Lupus erythematosus
(1973): Howard EJ+, *JAMA* 226, 1358
Photosensitivity
(1990): Leroy D+, *Photodermatology* 7, 136
(1988): Murata Y+, *J Am Acad Dermatol* 18, 381
(1977): Heid E+, *Ann Dermatol Venereol* (French) 104, 494
(1967): Orgain ES+, *Arch Intern Med* 119, 80
Pruritus (<1%)
Purpura
(1975): Arif MA+, *Lancet* 2, 1202
Rash (sic) (<1%)
Sarcoidosis
(1986): Yamada S+, *J Dermatol* (Tokio) 13, 217
Stevens–Johnson syndrome
(1994): Wong SS, *Acta Derm Venereol* 74, 475
Toxic epidermal necrolysis
Urticaria (<1%)
Vesiculobullous eruption
(1977): Heid E+, *Ann Dermatol Venereol* (French) 104, 494
Xerosis

Hair

Hair – alopecia (<1%)
(1971): Five Year Study, *BMJ* 4, 767 (0.8%)
Hair – dry (<1%)

Other

Dysgeusia
Gynecomastia
Hypogeusia
Myalgia
Myopathy (<1%)
(1976): Rumpf KW+, *Lancet* 1, 249
(1975): Pierides AM+, *Lancet* 2, 1279
(1968): Langer T+, *N Engl J Med* 279, 856
Oral ulceration
(1973): Howard EJ+, *JAMA* 226, 1358
Stomatitis

CLOMIPHENE

Trade names: Clomid (Aventis); Serophene (Serono)
Other common trade names: *Clom 50; Clomifen; Dyneric; Milophene; Omifin; Pergotime; Phenate; Serophene*
Indications: Ovulatory failure
Category: Infertility therapy adjunct; ovulation stimulator
Half-life: 5–7 days
Clinically important, potentially serious interactions with: no data

Reactions

Skin

Acne
Allergic reactions (sic)
Dermatitis (sic) (<1%)
Diaphoresis
Edema
Erythema
Erythema multiforme
Erythema nodosum
(1980): Salvatore MA+, *Arch Dermatol* 116, 557
Exanthems
(1996): Coots NV+, *Cutis* 57, 91
(1966): Johnson JE+, *Pacif Med Surg* 74, 153 (0.8%)
Flushing (10%)
(1966): Johnson JE+, *Pacif Med Surg* 74, 153 (14%)
Hot flashes (>10%)
Melanoma
(1999): Fuller PN, *Am J Obstet Gynecol* 180, 1499
(1995): Rossing MA+, *Melanoma Res* 5, 123
(1992): Kuppens E+, *Melanoma Res* 2, 71
Pruritus
Purpura (palpable)
(1996): Coots NV+, *Cutis* 57, 91
Rash (<1%)
Urticaria
(1969): *Drug and Therapeutic Bulletin* (London), 7, 34

Hair

Hair – alopecia (<1%)
(1969): *Drug and Therapeutic Bulletin* (London), 7, 34 (0.4%)
(1966): Johnson JE+, *Pacif Med Surg* 74, 153 (0.3%)
Hair – hypertrichosis

Other

Gynecomastia (1–10%)
(1978): Check JH+, *Fertility and Sterility* 30, 713
Mastodynia (1–10%)
Myalgia

CLOMIPRAMINE

Trade name: Anafranil (Novartis)
Other common trade names: *Anafranil Retard; Apo-Clomipramine; Clofranil; Clopress; Placil*
Indications: Obsessive-compulsive disorder
Category: Tricyclic antidepressant
Half-life: 21–31 hours
Clinically important, potentially serious interactions with: alcohol, anticholinergics, barbiturates, carbamazepine, cimetidine, clonidine, CNS depressants, epinephrine, fluoxetine, guanethidine, haloperidol, lithium, MAO inhibitors, phenothiazines, phenytoin, SSRIs, tricyclic antidepressants, warfarin

Reactions

Skin

Acne (2%)
Allergic reactions (sic) (<3%)
Cellulitis (2%)
Cheilitis
Chloasma
Contact dermatitis
(1991): Ljunggren B+, *Contact Dermatitis* 24, 259
Dermatitis (sic) (2%)
Diaphoresis (29%)
(1992): Guelfi JD+, *Br J Psychiatry* 160, 519
(1990): McTavish D+, *Drugs* 38, 19 (43%)
Edema (2%)
Erythema
Exanthems
Flushing (8%)
Folliculitis
Photosensitivity (<1%)
(1991): Ljunggren B+, *Contact Dermatitis* 24, 259
(1989): Tunca Z+, *Am J Psychiatry* 146, 552
(1979): Parkes JD+, *Lancet* 2, 1085
Pigmentation (pseudocyanotic)
(1989): Tunca Z+, *Am J Psychiatry* 146, 552
Pruritus (6%)
Psoriasis
Purpura (3%)
Pustular eruption
Rash (sic) (8%)
Seborrhea
Urticaria (1%)
Vasculitis
Xerosis (2%)

Hair

Hair – alopecia (<1%)
Hair – alopecia areata
(1993): Kubota T+, *Acta Neurol Napoli* (Italian) 15, 200
Hair – hypertrichosis

Other

Ageusia
Black tongue
Dysgeusia (8%)
Galactorrhea (<1%)
Gingival bleeding
Gingivitis
Glossitis
Gynecomastia (2%)
Mastodynia (1%)
Myalgia (13%)
Paresthesias
Sialorrhea
Stomatitis
Tongue ulceration
Vaginitis (2%)
Xerostomia (84%)
(1992): Guelfi JD+, *Br J Psychiatry* 160, 519
(1992): DeVeaugh-Geiss J+, *J Am Acad Child Adolesc Psychiatry* 31, 45
(1992): Cohen DJ+, *Psychiatr Clin North Am* 15, 109
(1990): McTavish D+, *Drugs* 38, 19

CLONAZEPAM

Trade name: Klonopin (Roche)
Other common trade names: *Clonex; Iktorivil; Landsen; Lonazep; Rivotril*
Indications: Petit mal and myoclonic seizures
Category: Benzodiazepine anticonvulsant and antipanic
Half-life: 18–50 hours
Clinically important, potentially serious interactions with: alcohol, cimetidine, CNS depressants, ciprofloxacin, clarithromycin, clozapine, digoxin, diltiazem, disulfiram, erythromycin, omeprazole, verapamil

Reactions

Skin

Allergic reactions (sic) (1–10%)
Angioedema
(1976): Pinder RM+, *Drugs* 12, 321
Ankle edema
Dermatitis (sic) (1–10%)
Diaphoresis (>10%)
Erythema multiforme
(1998): Amichai B+, *Clin Exp Dermatology* 23, 206
Exanthems
(1976): Pinder RM+, *Drugs* 12, 321
Facial edema
Hypermelanosis
(1976): Pinder RM+, *Drugs* 12, 321
Pruritus
Pseudo-mycosis fungoides
(1996): Gordon KB+, *J Am Acad Dermatol* 34, 304
Purpura
(1976): Pinder RM+, *Drugs* 12, 321
Rash (sic) (>10%)
Urticaria

Hair

Hair – alopecia
(2000): Mercke Y+, *Ann Clin Psychiatry* 12, 35
Hair – hirsutism

Other

Black tongue
(2000): Heymann WR, *Cutis* 66, 25
Dysgeusia
(2000): Heymann WR, *Cutis* 66, 25
Gingivitis
Injection-site phlebitis
Injection-site thrombosis
Oral mucosal eruption
(1986): Bernard K, *Lijec Vjesn* (Serbo-Croatian-Roman) 108, 235
Oral ulceration
Paresthesias
Pseudolymphoma
(1995): Magro CM+, *J Am Acad Dermatol* 32, 419
Sialopenia (>10%)
Sialorrhea (1–10%)
Xerostomia (>10%)
(2000): Heymann WR, *Cutis* 66, 25

CLONIDINE

Trade names: Catapres (Boehringer Ingelheim); Combipres (Boehringer Ingelheim)
Other common trade names: *Barclyd; Catapres; Catapresan; Daipres; Dixarit; Duraclon; Haemiton; Nu-Clonidine; Sulmidine*
Indications: Hypertension
Category: Alpha$_2$-adrenergic agonist antihypertensive
Half-life: 6–24 hours
Clinically important, potentially serious interactions with: alcohol, barbiturates, beta-blockers, cyclosporine, mirtazepine, tricyclic antidepressants, verapamil

Combipres is clonidine and chlorthalidone

Reactions

Skin

Angioedema (<1%)
(1995): Waldfahrer F+, *HNO* (German) 43, 35
Contact dermatitis (from patch) (20%)
(1999): Polster AM+, *Cutis* 63, 154
(1997): Shelley ED+, *J Geriatr Dermatol* 4, 192
(1995): Corazza M+, *Contact Dermatitis* 32, 246
(1994): Tom GR+, *Ann Pharmacother* 28, 889
(1992): Breathnach SM+, *Adverse Drug Reactions and the Skin*, Blackwell, Oxford, 226 (passim)
(1991): McChesney JA, *West J Med* 154, 736
(1991): Ito MK+, *Am J Med* 91, 42S
(1990): Hogan DJ+, *J Am Acad Dermatol* 22, 811
(1990): Scheper RJ+, *Contact Dermatitis* 23, 81
(1989): Holdiness MR, *Contact Dermatitis* 20, 3
(1989): Fillingim JM+, *Clin Ther* 11, 398
(1988): Horning JR+, *Chest* 93, 941
(1987): Bigby M+, *JAMA* 258, 1819 (letter)
(1987): Maibach HI, *Contact Dermatitis* 16, 1
(1986): Hollifield J, *Am Heart J* 112, 900
(1986): White TM+, *West J Med* 145, 104
(1986): Weber MA, *Am Heart J* 112, 906
(1985): Grattan CEH+, *Contact Dermatitis* 2, 225
(1985): Maibach H, *Contact Dermatitis* 12, 192
(1984): van Ketel WG, *Ned Tijdschr Geneeskd* (Dutch) 128, 34
(1983): Boekhorst JC, *Lancet* 2, 1031
(1983): Groth H+, *Lancet* 2, 850
Depigmentation
(1995): Doe N+, *Arch Intern Med* 155, 2129 (from patch)
Diaphoresis
(1990): Leeman CP, *J Clin Psychiatry* 51, 258
Eczematous eruption (sic)
(1987): Dick JBC+, *Lancet* 1, 516
(1985): Grattan CEH+, *Contact Dermatitis* 12, 225
Edema
Erythema
(1987): Dick JBC+, *Lancet* 1, 516
Exanthems
Herpes simplex
(1987): Wiser TH+, *J Am Acad Dermatol* 17, 143
Hyperpigmentation (from patch)
(1987): Wiser TH+, *J Am Acad Dermatol* 17, 143
Irritation (from patch)
(1999): Dias VC+, *Am J Ther* 6, 19
Lupus erythematosus
(1994): Heilmann G+, *Dtsch Med Wochenschr* (German) 119, 858
(1992): Breathnach SM+, *Adverse Drug Reactions and the Skin*, Blackwell, Oxford, 226 (passim)
(1981): Witman G+, *R I Med J* 64, 147
Pemphigoid (anogenital and cicatricial)
(1980): van Joost T+, *Br J Dermatol* 102, 715
Peripheral edema
Pityriasis rosea
(1998): Reed BR, Denver, CO, 2 cases – in siblings, (from Internet) (observation)
(1992): Breathnach SM+, *Adverse Drug Reactions and the Skin*, Blackwell, Oxford, 226 (passim)

Pruritus (>5%)
(1999): Dias VC+, *Am J Ther* 6, 19
(1987): Dick JBC+, *Lancet* 1, 516
(1984): Weber MA+, *Arch Intern Med* 144, 1211
(1984): Weber MA+, *Lancet* 1, 9
(1983): Boekhorst JC, *Lancet* 2, 1031
Psoriasis
(1981): Wilkin J, *Arch Dermatol* 117, 4
Rash (sic) (1–10%)
(1988): Glassman AH, *JAMA* 259, 2863
Raynaud's phenomenon (<1%)
Ulcer (1–10%)
Urticaria (<1%)

Hair
Hair – alopecia (<1%)

Other
Acute intermittent porphyria
Application-site vesiculation
(1987): Dick JBC+, *Lancet* 1, 516
Dysgeusia (from patch)
Gynecomastia (<1%)
Hyperesthesia (1–10%)
Immune complex disease
(1989): Petersen HH+, *Acta Derm Venereol* (Stockh) 69, 519
Pseudolymphoma
(1997): Shelley WB+, *Lancet* 1223 (at site of patch)
Xerostomia (40%)
(2000): Geyer O+, *Graefes Arch Clin Exp Ophthalmol* 238, 149
(2000): Litt JZ, Beachwood, OH, personal case (observation)
(1999): Dias VC+, *Am J Ther* 6, 19
(1988): Glassman AH, *JAMA* 259, 2863
(1984): Weber MA+, *Arch Intern Med* 144, 1211
(1984): Weber MA+, *Lancet* 1, 9
(1983): Boekhorst JC, *Lancet* 2, 1031

CLOPIDOGREL

Trade name: Plavix (Bristol-Myers Squibb; Sanofi)
Indications: Atherosclerotic events
Category: Oral antiplatelet (thienopyridine derivative)
Half-life: ~8 hours
Clinically important, potentially serious interactions with: anticoagulants, aspirin, fluvastatin, heparin, naproxen, NSAIDs, phenytoin, tamoxifen, tolbutamide, torsemide, warfarin

Reactions

Skin
Allergic reactions (sic) (1–2.5%)
Bullous eruption (1–2.5%)
Eczema (sic) (1–2.5%)
Edema (3–5%)
Exanthems (1–2.5%)
(1999): Smith JG, Mobile, AL (from Internet) (observation) (generalized)
Flu-like syndrome (sic) (7.5%)
Pruritus (3.3%)
(1999): Smith JG, Mobile, AL (from Internet) (observation)
Purpura (5.3%)
Rash (sic) (4.2%)
Thrombocytopenic purpura
(2000): Bennett CL+, *N Engl J Med* 342, 1773 (11 patients)
(2000): SoRelle R, *Circulation* 101, E9036
(2000): Chinnakotla S+, *Transplantation* 70, 550
(1999): Connors JM+, *Transfusion* 39, 56S
(1999): Carwile JM+, *Blood* 94, 1:78
Ulceration (1–2.5%)
Urticaria (1–2.5%)
(1997): Coukell AJ+, *Drugs* 54, 745

Other
Ageusia
(2000): Golka K+, *Lancet* 355, 465
Hypesthesia (1–2.5%)
Paresthesias (1–2.5%)

CLORAZEPATE

Trade name: Tranxene (Abbott)
Other common trade names: *Gen-XENE; Novoclopate; Transene; Tranxal; Tranxen; Tranxilen; Tranxilium*
Indications: Anxiety and panic disorders
Category: Benzodiazepine anxiolytic and sedative-hypnotic; anticonvulsant
Half-life: 48–96 hours
Clinically important, potentially serious interactions with: alcohol, amprenavir, cimetidine, ciprofloxacin, clarithromycin, clozapine, CNS depressants, digoxin, diltiazem, disulfiram, erythromycin, fluconazole, fluoxetine, isoniazid, itraconazole, ketoconazole, miconazole, omeprazole, phenytoin, ritonavir, valproic acid, verapamil

Reactions

Skin
Blistering (sic)
(1979): Herschthal D+, *Arch Dermatol* 115, 499
Dermatitis (sic) (1–10%)
Diaphoresis (>10%)
Exanthems
Photosensitivity
(1989): Torras H+, *J Am Acad Dermatol* 21, 1304
Pruritus
Purpura
Rash (sic) (>10%)
Urticaria
(1981): Bonnetblanc JM+, *Ann Dermatol Venereol* (French) 108, 177
Vasculitis
(1985): Sanchez NP+, *Arch Dermatol* 121, 220

Nails
Nails – photo-onycholysis
(1989): Torras H+, *J Am Acad Dermatol* 21, 1304

Other
Oral ulceration
Paresthesias
Sialopenia (>10%)
Sialorrhea (1–10%)
Tremor
Xerostomia (>10%)

CLOXACILLIN

Trade names: Cloxapen (SmithKline Beecham); Tegopen (Mead Johnson)
Other common trade names: *Alclox; Apo-Cloxi; Ekvacillin; Loxavit; Nu-Cloxi; Orbenin; Orbenine*
Indications: Various infections caused by susceptible organisms
Category: Penicillinase-resistant penicillin antibiotic
Half-life: 0.5–1.1 hours
Clinically important, potentially serious interactions with: anticoagulants, cyclosporine, disulfiram, heparin, oral contraceptives, probenecid

Reactions

Skin
Angioedema
Contact dermatitis
(1996): Gamboa P+, *Contact Dermatitis* 34, 75
Ecchymoses
Erythema multiforme

Exanthems
Exfoliative dermatitis
Hematomas
Jarisch–Herxheimer reaction
Pruritus
Rash (sic) (<1%)
(1979): Puri V+, *Indian Pediatr* 16, 1153
Stevens–Johnson syndrome
Urticaria

Nails

Nails – onycholysis
Nails – shedding
(1984): Daniel CR, *J Am Acad Dermatol* 10, 250
(1969): Eastwood JB+, *Br J Dermatol* 81, 750

Other

Anaphylactoid reaction
Hypersensitivity
Black tongue
Glossitis
Glossodynia
Hypersensitivity
Injection-site pain
Oral candidiasis
Serum sickness (<1%)
Stomatitis
Vaginitis

CLOZAPINE

Trade name: Clozaril (Novartis)
Other common trade names: *Entumin; Entumine; Leponex; Lozapin; Sizopin*
Indications: Schizophrenia
Category: Tricyclic antipsychotic
Half-life: 8–12 hours
Clinically important, potentially serious interactions with: alcohol, benzodiazepines, cimetidine, clarithromycin, CNS depressants, erythromycin, digoxin, MAO inhibitors, neuroleptics, phenytoin, ritonavir, tricyclic antidepressants, valproic acid, warfarin, **cigarette smoking**

Reactions

Skin

Acute generalized exanthematous pustulosis (AGEP)
(1997): Bosonnet S+, *Ann Dermatol Venereol* (French) 124, 547
Dermatitis (sic) (<1%)
Diaphoresis (6%)
(1991): Safferman A+, *Schizophr Bull* 17, 247 (31%)
(1990): Fitton A+, *Drugs* 40, 722
Eczematous eruption (sic) (<1%)
(1994): Shelley WB+, *Cutis* 53, 33 (observation)
Edema (<1%)
Erythema (<1%)
Erythema multiforme (<1%)
Exanthems
Facial erosions
(1994): Shelley WB+, *Cutis* 53, 33 (observation)
Lupus erythematosus
(1994): Wickert WA+, *Postgrad Med J* 70, 940
Pedal edema
(2000): Durst R+, *Isr Med Assoc* 2, 485
Periorbital edema (<1%)
Petechiae (<1%)
(1994): Shelley WB+, *Cutis* 53, 33 (observation)
Photosensitivity
(1995): Howanitz E+, *J Clin Psychiatry* 56, 589
Pruritus (<1%)
Purpura (<1%)
Rash (sic) (2%)
Stevens–Johnson syndrome (<1%)
Urticaria (<1%)
Vasculitis (<1%)

Other

Dysgeusia (<1%)
Glossodynia (1%)
Mastodynia (<1%)
Priapism
(2000): Compton MT+, *Am J Psychiatry* 157, 659
(1994): Barbieri NB+, *Can J Psychiatry* 39, 128
Sialorrhea (31%)
(2000): Wahlbeck K+, *Cochran Database Syst Rev* (2):CD000059
(2000): Miller DD, *J Clin Psychiatry* 61, Suppl 8: 14
(1999): Antonello C+, *J Psychiatry Neurosci* 24, 250
(1999): Campbell M+, *Br J Clin Pharmacol* 47, 13
(1998): Young CR+, *Schizophr Bull* 24, 381
(1997): Spivak B+, *Int Clin Psychopharmacol* 12, 213
(1995): Fritze J+, *Lancet* 346, 1034
(1991): Calabrese JR+, *J Clin Psychopharmacol* 11, 396
(1991): Bourgeois JA+, *Hosp Community Psychiatry* 42, 1174
(1991): Ogle MR+, *Indiana Med* 84, 606
(1991): Kahn N+, *Neurology* 41, 1699
(1991): Copp PJ+, *Br J Psychiatry* 159, 166
(1991): Safferman A+, *Schizophr Bull* 17, 247
(1991): Goumeniouk AD+, *Can J Psychiatry* 36, 234
(1990): Fitton A+, *Drugs* 40, 722
Tremor (1–10%)
Xerostomia (6%)
(1990): Fitton A+, *Drugs* 40, 722
(1991): Safferman A+, *Schizophr Bull* 17, 247 (6%)

CO-TRIMOXAZOLE

Synonyms: sulfamethoxazole-trimethoprim; SMX-TMP; SMZ-TMP; TMP-SMX; TMP-SMZ
Trade names: Bactrim (Roche); Cotrim (Teva); Septra (GlaxoWellcome)
Other common trade names: *Anitrim; Apo-Sulfatrim; Bactelan; Batrizol; Ectaprim; Esteprim; Isobac; Pro-Trin; Roubac; Sulfatrim; Trimzol; Trisulfa*
Indications: Various infections caused by susceptible organisms
Category: Antibacterial and antiprotozoal
Half-life: 6–10 hours
Clinically important, potentially serious interactions with: anticoagulants, cyclosporine, dapsone, oral hypoglycemics, MAO inhibitors, methotrexate, phenytoin, rifampin, sulfones, sulfonylureas, warfarin

Co-trimoxazole is sulfamethoxazole* and trimethoprim

Reactions

Skin

Acute febrile neutrophilic dermatosis (Sweet's syndrome)
(1996): Walker DC+, *J Am Acad Dermatol* 34, 918
(1989): Cobb MW, *J Am Acad Dermatol* 21, 339 (passim)
(1986): Su WPD+, *Cutis* 37, 167
Acute generalized exanthematous pustulosis (AGEP)
(1995): Moreau A+, *Int J Dermatol* 34, 263 (passim)
Angioedema
(1988): Fihn SD+, *Ann Intern Med* 108, 350 (1–5%)
Bullous eruption
(1989): Caumes E+, *Presse Med* (French) 18, 1708
Cutaneous side effects (sic)
(1994): Roudier C+, *Arch Dermatol* 130, 1383 (48% in AIDS patients)
(1971): Koch-Weser J+, *Arch Intern Med* 128, 399.(2.1%)
Dermatitis (sic)
(1989): Atahan IL+, *Br J Radiol* 62, 1107 (at previously irradiated area)
(1984): Shelley WB+, *J Am Acad Dermatol* 11, 53 (at site of previous sunburn)
(1987): Vukelja SJ+, *Cancer Treat Rep* 71, 668 (at previously irradiated area)
(1971): Cotterill JA+, *Br J Dermatol* 84, 366
Erythema multiforme
(1999): Lehman DF+, *J Clin Pharmacol* 39, 533

(1998): Siegfried EC+, *J Am Acad Dermatol* 39, 797 (passim)
(1997): Rieder MJ+, *Pediatr Infect Dis J* 16, 1028 (70% in children with HIV)
(1995): Jick H+, *Pharmacotherapy* 15, 428
(1991): Tilden ME+, *Arch Ophthalmol* 109, 67
(1990): Chan HL+, *Arch Dermatol* 126, 43
(1989): Alanko K+, *Acta Derm Venereol* (Stockh) 69, 223
(1988): Hira SK+, *J Am Acad Dermatol* 19, 451
(1988): Platt R+, *J Infect Dis* 158, 474
(1987): Schöpf E, *Infection* 15 (Suppl 5P), S254
(1987): Penmetcha M, *BMJ* 295, 556
(1985): Heer M+, *Gastroenterology* 88, 1954
(1982): Brettle RP+, *J Infect* 4, 149
(1979): Beck MH+, *Clin Exp Dermatol* 4, 201
(1978): Assaad D+, *Can Med Assoc J* 118, 154
(1978): Azinge NO+, *J Allergy Clin Immunol* 62, 125
(1975): Bernstein LS, *Can Med Assoc J* 112 (Suppl), 96
(1971): Koch-Weser J+, *Arch Intern Med* 128, 399 (0.15%)

Erythema nodosum
(1974): Delaney TJ+, *Br J Dermatol* 90, 205
(1971): Koch-Weser J+, *Arch Intern Med* 128, 399

Erythroderma
(1979): Kennedy C+, *BMJ* 1, 1356

Exanthems
(1999): Iborra C+, *Arch Dermatol* 135, 350
(1998): Blumenthal HL, Beachwood, OH, personal case (observation)
(1998): Litt JZ, Beachwood, OH, personal case (observation)
(1998): Hattori N+, *J Dermatol* 25, 269
(1997): Palau LA+, *Infect Med* 14, 846
(1997): Blumenthal HL, Beachwood, OH, personal case (observation)
(1996): Caumes E, *Rev Mal Respir* (French) 13, 101 (passim)
(1995): Wolkenstein P+, *Arch Dermatol* 131, 544
(1995): Hertl M+, *Br J Dermatol* 132, 215
(1994): Litt JZ, Beachwood, OH, personal case (observation)
(1993): Litt JZ, Beachwood, OH, personal case (observation)
(1993): Malnick SDH+, *Ann Pharmacotherapy* 27, 1139
(1993): Agarwal BR+, *Indian Pediatr* 30, 1026
(1990): Medina I+, *N Engl J Med* 323, 776 (47% in AIDS)
(1988): Sattler FR+, *Ann Intern Med* 109, 280 (44% in AIDS)
(1988): Weinke T+, *Dtsch Med Wochenschr* (German) 113, 1129 (25% in AIDS)
(1988): Fihn SD+, *Ann Intern Med* 108, 350 (1–5%)
(1988): DeRaeve L+, *Br J Dermatol* 119, 521
(1987): Goa KL+, *Drugs* 33, 242 (65% in AIDS)
(1987): Schöpf E, *Infection* 15 (Suppl 5P), S254
(1986): Sonntag MR+, *Schweiz Med Wochenschr* (German) 116, 142
(1985): DeHovitz JA+, *Ann Intern Med* 103, 479
(1985): Maayan S+, *Arch Intern Med* 145, 1607
(1984): Kovacs JA+, *Ann Intern Med* 100, 663 (29% in AIDS)
(1984): Gordon FM+, *Ann Intern Med* 100, 495 (51% in AIDS)
(1983): Mitsuyasu R+, *N Engl J Med* 308, 1535 (69% in AIDS)
(1982): Goetz MB+, *JAMA* 247, 3118
(1980): Fennell RS+, *Clin Pediatr* 19, 124
(1979): Abengowe CU, *Curr Med Res Opin* 5, 749 (3.2%)
(1977): Taylor B+, *BMJ* 2, 552 (12%)
(1976): Gower PE+, *BMJ* 1, 684 (>5%)
(1976): Arndt KA+, *JAMA* 235, 918 (5.9%)
(1975): Sallam MA+, *Curr Med Res Opin* 3, 229 (3.4%)
(1975): Bernstein LS, *Can Med Assoc J* 112 (Suppl), 96 (1.9%)
(1975): Gleckman RA, *JAMA* 233, 427 (0.84%)
(1972): Halpern GM, *BMJ* 1, 691
(1971): Koch-Weser J+, *Arch Intern Med* 128, 399 (1%)

Exfoliative dermatitis
(1990): Ponte CD+, *Drug Intell Clin Pharm* 24, 140 (feet)
(1975): Bernstein LS, *Can Med Assoc J* 112 (Suppl), 96
(1971): Koch-Weser J+, *Arch Intern Med* 128, 399

Fixed eruption
(2000): Ozkaya-Bayazit E+, *Eur J Dermatol* 10, 288
(1999): Mohamed KB, *J Pediatr* 135, 396
(1999): Morelli JG I, *J Pediatr* 134, 365
(1998): Ozkaya-Bayazit E+, *Contact Dermatitis* 39, 87 (trimethoprim)
(1997): Gruber F+, *Clin Exp Dermatol* 22, 144
(1997): Ozkaya-Bayazit E+, *Br J Dermatol* 137, 1028 (linear) (trimethoprim)
(1996): Sharma VK+, *J Dermatol* 23, 530
(1995): Wolkenstein P+, *Arch Dermatol* 131, 544
(1993): Oleaga JM+, *Contact Dermatitis* 29, 155
(1993): Ramam M+, *Indian Pediatr* 30, 110 (in an infant)
(1992): Lim JT+, *Ann Acad Med Singapore* 21, 408
(1991): Thankappen TP+, *Int J Dermatol* 30, 867 (36.3%)
(1991): Smoller BR+, *J Cutan Pathol* 18, 13
(1991): Jain VK+, *Ann Dent* 50, 9 (oral mucous membrane)
(1990): Gaffoor PMA+, *Cutis* 45, 242 (genitalia)
(1989): Gupta R, *Indian J Dermatol* 55, 181 (in an infant)
(1989): Varsano I+, *Dermatologica* 178, 232
(1989): Bharija SC+, *Australas J Dermatol* 30, 43
(1989): Basomba A+, *J Allergy Clin Immunol* 84, 409
(1988): Baird BJ+, *Int J Dermatol* 27, 170 (bullous and generalized)
(1988): Bharija SC+, *Dermatologica* 176, 108 (in an infant)
(1987): Amir J+, *Drug Intell Clin Pharm* 21, 41
(1987): Hughes BR+, *Br J Dermatol* 116, 241
(1987): Van Voorhees A+, *Am J Dermatopathol* 9, 528
(1986): Kanwar AJ+, *Dermatologica* 172, 230
(1985): Gomez B+, *Allergol Immunopathol Madr* (Spanish) 13, 87
(1984): Pandhi RK+, *Sex Transm Dis* 11, 164
(1982): Gibson JR, *BMJ* 284, 1529
(1980): Talbot MD, *Practitioner* 224, 823
(1978): Verbov J, *Arch Dermatol* 114, 963
(1972): Aoyama H+, *Jpn J Dermatol B* 82, 16

Flushing
(1984): Jick SS+, *Lancet* 2, 631

Lichenoid eruption
(1994): Berger TG+, *Arch Dermatol* 130, 609

Linear IgA bullous dermatosis
(1994): Kuechle MK+, *J Am Acad Dermatol* 30, 187

Lupus erythematosus
(1985): Stratton MA, *Clin Pharm* 4, 657
(1975): Grennan DM+, *BMJ* 4, 385

Mucocutaneous syndrome
(1982): Brettle RP+, *J Infect* 4, 149

Photosensitivity
(1994): Shelley WB+, *Cutis* 53, 162 (observation)
(1994): Berger TG+, *Arch Dermatol* 130, 609 (in HIV-infected) (4 cases)
(1987): Schöpf E, *Infection* 15 (Suppl 5P), S254
(1986): Chandler MJ, *J Infect Dis* 153, 1001

Pruritus
(1997): Caumes E+, *Arch Dermatol* 133, 465
(1997): Thaler D, Monona, WI (from Internet) (observation)
(1996): Litt JZ, Beachwood, OH (from Internet) (observation)
(1990): Medina I+, *N Engl J Med* 323, 776 (1–5%)
(1987): Colebunders R+, *Ann Intern Med* 107, 599 (4% in AIDS)
(1986): Sher MR, *J Allergy Clin Immunol* 77, 133
(1984): Kramer BS+, *Cancer* 53, 329
(1975): Gleckman RA, *JAMA* 233, 427 (0.84%)
(1971): Koch-Weser J+, *Arch Intern Med* 128, 399 (0.15%)

Pruritus vulvae
(1981): *Modern Medicine* 49, 111

Psoriasis
(1979): Kennedy C+, *BMJ* 1, 1356

Purpura
(1993): Kaufman DW+, *Blood* 82, 2714
(1989): Saxena SK, *J Assoc Physicians India* 37, 479
(1971): Koch-Weser J+, *Arch Intern Med* 128, 399

Purpuric "gloves and socks syndrome"
(1999): van Rooijen MM+, *Hautarzt* (German) 50, 280

Pustular eruption
(1994): Spencer JM+, *Br J Dermatol* 130, 514
(1990): Guy C+, *Nouv Dermatol* (French) 9, 540
(1989): Grattan CEH, *Dermatologica* 179, 57 (passim)
(1986): Macdonald KJS+, *BMJ* 293, 1279
(1978): Braun-Falco O+, *Hautarzt* (German) 29, 371
(1977): Knudsen L+, *Ugeskr Laeger* (Danish) 139, 1007

Radiation recall
(1990): Leslie MD+, *Br J Radiol* 63, 661
(1987): Vukelja SJ+, *Cancer Treat Rep* 71, 668 (at previously irradiated area)
(1984): Shelley WB+, *J Am Acad Dermatol* 11, 53 (at site of previous sunburn)

Rash (sic) (>10%)
(2000): Talan DA+, *JAMA* 283, 1583 (14%)
(1995): Williams JW+, *JAMA* 273, 1015
(1993): Malnick SD+, *Ann Pharmacother* 27, 1139
(1984): Gordin FM+, *Ann Intern Med* 100, 495
(1978): Lawson DH+, *Am J Med Sci* 275, 53

Allergic reactions (sic)
(1999): ter Hofstede HJ+, *Br Clin Pharmacol* 47, 571
Stevens–Johnson syndrome (1–10%)
(1998): Arola O+, *Lancet* 351, 1102 (trimethoprim)
(1998): Siegfried EC+, *J Am Acad Dermatol* 39, 797 (passim)
(1997): Douglas R+, *Clin Infect Dis* 25, 1480 (2 cases)
(1997): Rieder MJ+, *Pediatr Infect Dis J* 16, 1028 (10% in children with HIV)
(1996): Caumes E, *Rev Mal Respir* (French) 13, 101
(1996): Eastham JH+, *Ann Pharmacother* 30, 606
(1996): McCarty J, Fort Worth, TX (from Internet) (observation)
(1995): Kuper K+, *Ophthalmologe* (German) 92, 823
(1995): Sharma VK+, *Pediatr Dermatol* 12, 178
(1995): Lewis RJ, *Br J Rheumatol* 34, 84
(1995): Wolkenstein P+, *Arch Dermatol* 131, 544
(1994): Shelley WB+, *Cutis* 53, 159 (observation)
(1993): Litt JZ, Beachwood, OH, personal case (observation)
(1990): Chan HL+, *Arch Dermatol* 126, 43
(1988): Platt R+, *J Infect Dis* 158, 474
(1985): Heer M+, *Gastroenterology* 88, 1954
(1982): Brettle RP+, *J Infect* 4, 149
(1979): Beck MH+, *Clin Exp Dermatol* 4, 201
(1978): Azinge NO+, *J Allergy Clin Immunol* 62, 125
(1978): Kikuchi S+, *Lancet* 2, 580
(1978): Thorpe JA+, *Lancet* 1, 276 (fatal)
(1978): Assaad D+, *Can Med Assoc* 118, 154
(1975): Bernstein LS, *Can Med Assoc J* 112 (Suppl), 96
(1970): Shaw DJ+, *Johns Hopkins Med J* 126, 130
Toxic epidermal necrolysis (1–10%)
(2000): Moussala M+, *J Fr Ophtalmol* (French) 23, 229
(1998): Rademaker M+, *New Zealand Adverse Drug Reactions Committee*, April, 1998 (from Internet)
(1998): Siegfried EC+, *J Am Acad Dermatol* 39, 797 (passim)
(1998): Arora VK+, *Indian J Chest Dis Allied Sci* 40, 125
(1996): Caumes E, *Rev Mal Respir* (French) 13, 101
(1996): Wagner FF+, *N Engl J Med* 334, 922
(1996): Rehbein H, Jacksonville, FL (from Internet) (observation)
(1995): Sharma VK+, *Pediatr Dermatol* 12, 178
(1995): Wolkenstein P+, *Arch Dermatol* 131, 544 (7 cases)
(1995): Jick H+, *Pharmacotherapy* 15, 428
(1993): Correia O+, *Dermatology* 186, 32
(1990): Kobza Black A+, *Br J Dermatol* 123, 277
(1990): Ward DJ+, *Burns* 16, 97
(1990): Chan HL+, *Arch Dermatol* 126, 43
(1990): Roujeau JC+, *Arch Dermatol* 126, 37
(1989): Carmichael AJ+, *Lancet* 2, 808
(1989): Whittington RM, *Lancet* 2, 574
(1988): De Raeve L+, *Br J Dermatol* 119, 521 (passim)
(1987): Guillaume JC+, *Arch Dermatol* 123, 1166
(1987): Schöpf E, *Infection* 15 (Suppl 5P), S254
(1986): Miller KD+, *Am J Trop Med Hyg* 33, 451
(1986): Roman O+, *Rev Pediatr Obstet Ginecol Pediatr* (Romanian) 35, 261
(1986): Revuz J, *J Dermatol Paris* 153 (abstract)
(1984): Westly ED+, *Arch Dermatol* 120, 721
(1984): Fong PH+, *Singapore Med J* 25, 184
(1983): Petersen P+, *Ugeskr Laeger* (Danish) 145, 3345
(1982): Ortiz JE+, *Ann Plast Surg* 9, 249
(1978): Assaad D+, *Can Med Assoc J* 118, 154
(1978): Petricevic I+, *Lijec Vjesn* (Serbo-Croatian-Roman) 100, 596
(1978): Anhalt G+, *Plastic Reconstr Surg* 61, 905
(1975): Bernstein LS, *Can Med Assoc J* 112 (Suppl), 96
(1973): Beyvin AJ+, *Anesth Analg Paris* (French) 30, 767
(1972): Chanial G+, *J Med Lyon* (French) 53, 859
(1971): Chanial G+, *Bull Soc Fr Dermatol Syphiligr* (French) 78, 565
Urticaria
(1994): Blumenthal HL, Beachwood, OH, personal case (observation)
(1993): Litt JZ, Beachwood, OH, personal case (observation)
(1991): Greenberger PA, *JAMA* 265, 458
(1987): Schöpf E, *Infection* 15 (Suppl 5P), S254
(1985): Maayan S+, *Arch Intern Med* 145, 1607
(1985): Goolamali SK, *Postgrad Med J* 61, 925
(1984): Kramer BS+, *Cancer* 53, 329
(1981): Abi-Mansur P+, *Am J Gastroenterol* 76, 356
(1971): Koch-Weser J+, *Arch Intern Med* 128, 399
Vasculitis
(1995): Lewis RJ, *Br J Rheumatol* 34, 84
(1989): Verne-Pignatelli J+, *Postgrad Med J* 65, 51
(1987): Schöpf E, *Infection* 15 (Suppl 5P), S254
(1978): Coquin Y+, *Nouv Presse Med* (French) 7, 3145
(1978): Braun-Falco O+, *Hautarzt* (German) 29, 371
(1976): Wåhlin A+, *Lancet* 2, 1415
(1971): Koch-Weser J+, *Arch Intern Med* 128, 399
Vulvovaginitis
(1985): Wong ES+, *Ann Intern Med* 102, 302

Hair

Hair – straight
(1999): Oakley A, Hamilton, New Zealand (from Internet) (observation)

Nails

Nails – loss
(2000): Canning DA, *J Urol* 163, 1386

Other

Anaphylactoid reaction
(1998): Siegfried EC+, *J Am Acad Dermatol* 39, 797 (passim)
(1998): Bijl AM+, *Clin Exp Allergy* 28, 510 (trimethoprim)
(1988): Arnold PA+, *Drug Intell Clin Pharm* 22, 43
(1985): Gossius G+, *Scand J Infect Dis* 16, 373
Aphthous stomatitis
(1981): *J Antimicrob Chemother* 7, 179
Black tongue
(1993): Blumenthal HL, Beachwood, OH, personal case (observation)
Dysgeusia
(1988): Fischl MA+, *JAMA* 259, 1185
Gingival hyperplasia
(1997): Caron F+, *Therapie* (French) 52, 73
Glossitis
Hypersensitivity
(1999): Lehman DF+, *J Clin Pharmacol* 39, 533
(1999): Pakianathan MR+, *AIDS* 13, 1787
(1998): Mohanasundaram J+, *J Indian Med Assoc* 96, 21
(1998): Ryan C+, *WMJ* 97, 23
(1997): Hicks ME+, *Ann Pharmacother* 31, 1259
(1994): Carr A+, *AIDS* 8, 333
(1993): Mehta J+, *J Assoc Physicians India* 41, 235
(1993): Marinac JS+, *Clin Infect Dis* 16, 178
(1993): Martin GJ+, *Clin Infect Dis* 16, 175
(1993): Mathelier-Fusade P+, *Presse Med* (French) 22, 1363
Myalgia
Oral mucosal eruption
(1991): Tilden ME+, *Arch Ophthalmol* 109, 67
(1988): Fihn SD+, *Ann Intern Med* 108, 350 (1–5%)
Oral ulceration
(1987): Hughes WT+, *N Engl J Med* 316, 1627
(1981): Orenstein WA+, *Am J Med Sci* 282, 27
Pseudolymphoma
(1978): Laugier P+, *Z Hautkr* (German) 53, 353
Serum sickness (<1%)
(1988): Platt R+, *J Infect Dis* 158, 474
Stomatitis (<1%)
(1999): Iborra C+, *Arch Dermatol* 135, 350
Tongue ulceration
(1981): *J Antimicrob Chemother* 7, 179
Tremor
(1999): Patterson RG+, *Pharmacotherapy* 19, 1456

***Note:** Co-trimoxazole is a sulfonamide and can be absorbed systemically. Sulfonamides can produce severe, possibly fatal, reactions such as toxic epidermal necrolysis and Stevens–Johnson syndrome.

COCAINE

Trade name: Cocaine
Indications: Topical anesthesia
Category: Topical anesthetic; substance abuse drug
Half-life: 75 minutes
Clinically important, potentially serious interactions with: beta-blockers, digoxin, MAO inhibitors, methyldopa, tricyclic antidepressants

Note: Cocaine is a benzoylmethylecogonine alkaloid derived from the leaves of the *Erythroxylon coca* tree. Street names for cocaine include: coke; flake; snow; toot, etc. Crack cocaine is a highly potent smokable form of cocaine

Reactions

Skin

Angioedema
(1999): Castro-Villamor MA+, *Ann Emerg Med* 34, 296
Bullous eruption
(1985): Tomecki KJ+, *J Am Acad Dermatol* 12, 585
Cutaneous nodules
(1989): Heng MCY+, *J Am Acad Dermatol* 21, 570
Diaphoresis
Formication
Granulomas (foreign body)
(1985): Posner DI+, *J Am Acad Dermatol* 13, 869
Hyperkeratosis (fingers and palms)
(1992): Feeney CM+, *Cutis* 50, 193 (from crack cocaine)
Necrosis
(2000): Carter EL+, *Cutis* 65, 73 (mid-facial)
(1988): Zamora-Quezada JC+, *Ann Intern Med* 108, 564
Scleroderma (reversible)
(1992): Lam M+, *N Engl J Med* 326, 1435
(1991): Bourgeois P+, *Baillieres Clin Rheumatol* 5, 13
(1989): Kerr HD, *South Med J* 82, 1275
Thrombophlebitis
(1987): Heng MC+, *J Am Acad Dermatol* 16, 462
Urticaria
(1999): Castro-Villamor MA+, *Ann Emerg Med* 34, 296
Vasculitis
(1999): Hofbauer GF+, *Br J Dermatol* 141, 600
Warts (snorters' warts)
(1987): Schuster DS, *Arch Dermatol* 123, 571

Other

Ageusia (>10%)
Anosmia (>10%)
Bruxism
(1999): Fazzi M+, *Minerva Stomatol* (Italian) 48, 485
Gingival ulceration
(1999): Fazzi M+, *Minerva Stomatol* (Italian) 48, 485
Injection-site scarring
(1968): Yaffee HS, *Cutis* 4, 286
Nasal septal perforation
(2000): Patel R+, *J Natl Med Assoc* 92, 39
(1986): Schwartz RH+, *Am Fam Physician* 43, 187
Necrosis of palate
(1999): Fazzi M+, *Minerva Stomatol* (Italian) 48, 485
Porphyria
(1987): Dick AD+, *Lancet* 2, 1150
Priapism
(1999): Altman AL+, *J Urol* 161, 1817
(1998): Myrick H+, *Ann Clin Psychiatry* 10, 8 (patient was also taking trazodone)
Tremor (1–10%)

CODEINE

Synonym: methylmorphine
Trade names: Calcidrine; Cheracol; Guaituss AC; Halotussin; Novahistine DH; Nucofed; Robitussin AC; Tussar-2; Tussi-Organidin; and those preparations that include "With Codeine". (Various pharmaceutical companies.)
Other common trade names: *Actacode; Codicept; Codiforton; Paveral; Solcodein; Tricodein*
Indications: Pain, cough suppressant
Category: Opioid (narcotic) analgesic; antitussive
Half-life: 2.5–4 hours
Clinically important, potentially serious interactions with: alcohol, barbiturates, cimetidine, CNS depressants, guanabenz, MAO inhibitors, phenothiazines, ranitidine, tricyclic antidepressants

Reactions

Skin

Acute generalized exanthematous pustulosis (AGEP)
(1995): Lee S+, *Australas J Dermatol* 36, 25
Angioedema
(1992): Breathnach SM+, *Adverse Drug Reactions and the Skin*, Blackwell, Oxford, 211 (passim)
(1960): Schoenfeld MR, *N Y State J Med* 60, 2591
Bullous eruption
(1992): Breathnach SM+, *Adverse Drug Reactions and the Skin*, Blackwell, Oxford, 211 (passim)
Contact dermatitis
(1995): Waclawski ER+, *Contact Dermatitis* 33, 51
(1983): Romaguera C+, *Contact Dermatitis* 9, 170
Diaphoresis
Erythema multiforme (<1%)
(1992): Breathnach SM+, *Adverse Drug Reactions and the Skin*, Blackwell, Oxford, 211 (passim)
(1983): Ponte CD, *Drug Intell Clin Pharm* 17, 128
(1975): Vanderveen TW+, *Am J Hosp Pharm* 32, 1149
(1968): Bianchine JR+, *Am J Med* 7, 390
Erythema nodosum (<1%)
(1992): Breathnach SM+, *Adverse Drug Reactions and the Skin*, Blackwell, Oxford, 211 (passim)
Exanthems
(1985): Hunskaar S+, *Ann Allergy* 54, 240
(1980): Voorhorst R+, *Ann Allergy* 44, 116
(1976): Nishioka K+, *Nippon Rinsho* (Japanese) 34, 3123
(1969): Török H, *Int J Dermatol* 8, 57
(1960): Heijer A, *Acta Derm Venereol* (Stockh) 40, 35
(1934): Scheer M+, *JAMA* 102, 908
Exfoliative dermatitis
(1995): Rodriguez F+, *Contact Dermatitis* 32, 120
Facial edema
Fixed eruption (<1%)
(1996): Gonzalo-Garijo MA+, *Br J Dermatol* 135, 498
(1992): Breathnach SM+, *Adverse Drug Reactions and the Skin*, Blackwell, Oxford, 211 (passim)
(1990): Gaffoor PMA+, *Cutis* 45, 242 (passim)
(1974): Kuokkanen K, *Int J Dermatol* 13, 4
(1969): Török H, *Int J Dermatol* 8, 57
(1960): Heijer A, *Acta Derm Venereol* (Stockh) 40, 35
Flushing
(1983): Shanahan EC+, *Anaesthesia* 38, 40
Pityriasis rosea
(1993): Yosipovitch G+, *Harefuah* (Hebrew) 124, 198; 247
Pruritus (<1%)
(1986): de Groot AC+, *Contact Dermatitis* 14, 209
(1976): von Muhlendahl KE+, *Lancet* 2, 303
(1934): Scheer M+, *JAMA* 102, 908
Radiation recall (sunlight and electronic beam)
(1984): Shelley WB+, *J Am Acad Dermatol* 11, 53
Rash (sic) (1–10%)
(1976): von Muhlendahl KE+, *Lancet* 2, 303
Toxic epidermal necrolysis (<1%)
(1973): Steigleder GK, *Hautarzt* (German) 24, 261
(1972): Monnat A, *Schweiz Med Wochenschr* (French) 102, 1876

Urticaria (1–10%)
(2000): Vidal C+, *Allergy* 55, 416
(1986): Rosenstreich DL, *J Allergy Clin Immunol* 78, 1099
(1986): de Groot AC+, *Contact Dermatitis* 4, 209
(1985): Hunskaar S+, *Ann Allergy* 54, 240
(1976): von Muhlendahl KE+, *Lancet* 2, 303
(1960): Heijer A, *Acta Derm Venereol* (Stockh) 40, 35
(1960): Schoenfeld MR, *N Y State J Med* 60, 2591

Nails

Nails – shoreline
(1985): Shelley WB+, *Cutis* 35, 220

Other

Anaphylactoid reaction
Dysgeusia
Injection-site pain (1–10%)
Oral ulceration
Paresthesias
Trembling (sic) (<1%)
Xerostomia (1–10%)

COLCHICINE

Trade name: ColBenemid (Merck)*
Other common trade names: *Cochiquim; Colchineos; Colgout; Goutnil; Konicine; Kolkicin*
Indications: Gouty arthritis
Category: Uricosuric, antigout anti-inflammatory
Half-life: 20 minutes
Clinically important, potentially serious interactions with: CNS depressants, cyclosporine, erythromycin, NSAIDs

ColBenemid is colchicine and probenecid

Reactions

Skin

Angioedema
Bullous eruption (<1%)
(1957): Ott H+, *Dtsch Med Wochenschr* (German) 82, 1163
Cutaneous side effects (sic) (14%)
(1957): Ott H+, *Dtsch Med Wochenschr* (German) 82, 1163
Erythroderma
(1971): Durkalec J+, *Pol Tyg Lek* (Polish) 26, 1048
Exanthems
Fixed eruption
(1996): Mochida K+, *Dermatology* 192, 61
Flushing
Lichenoid eruption
(1974): Sayag J+, *Bull Soc Fr Dermatol Syphiligr* (French) 81, 94
Necrosis
Photocontact dermatitis
(1992): Foti C+, *Contact Dermatitis* 27, 201
Pruritus (<1%)
(1957): Ott H+, *Dtsch Med Wochenschr* (German) 82, 1163
(1957): Hollander L, *Arch Dermatol* 75, 872
Purpura
Pyoderma
(1957): Ott H+, *Dtsch Med Wochenschr* (German) 82, 1163
Rash (sic) (<1%)
Staphylococcal scalded skin syndrome
(1993): Khuong MA+, *Dermatology* 186, 153
(1967): Halprin KM, *JAMA* 202, 137
Toxic epidermal necrolysis
(1994): Alfandari S+, *Infection* 22, 365
(1990): Roujeau JC+, *Arch Dermatol* 126, 37
Urticaria
(1991): Anderson MH+, *Ann Allergy* 66, 207
Vasculitis
(1993): Barash J+, *Isr J Med Sci* 29, 310
(1964): Sinaly NP, *Ann Intern Med* 60, 470
Vesicular eruption (palms)
(1957): Hollander L, *Arch Dermatol* 75, 872

Hair

Hair – alopecia (1–10%)
(1980): Harms M, *Hautarzt* (German) 31, 161 (20–50%)
(1977): Naidus RM+, *Arch Intern Med* 137, 394
(1970): Wallace S+, *Am J Med* 48, 443
(1967): Spanopoulos GJ, *Practitioner* 198, 426

Other

Anaphylactoid reaction
Hypersensitivity
Injection-site thrombophlebitis
Myopathy (<1%)
(1999): Gruberg L+, *Transplant Proc* 31, 2157
(1998): Duarte J+, *Muscle Nerve* 21, 550
(1997): Ducloux D+, *Nephrol Dial Transplant* 12, 2389
(1997): Sinsawaiwong S+, *J Med Assoc Thai* 80, 667
(1992): Himmelmann F+, *Acta Neuropathologica* 83, 440
Porphyria cutanea tarda
(1971): Kuokkanen K, *Acta Derm Venereol* (Stockh) 51, 318

***Note:** Colchicine, by itself, is generic

COLESEVELAM

Trade name: Welchol (Sankyo Parke Davis)
Indications: Hypercholesterolemia
Category: Antilipemic, bile acid sequestrant
Half-life: no data
Clinically important, potentially serious interactions with: none

Reactions

Skin

Flu-like syndrome (sic)

Other

Myalgia (2%)
Oral ulceration

COLESTIPOL

Trade name: Colestid (Pharmacia & Upjohn)
Other common trade names: *Cholestabyl; Lestid*
Indications: Primary hypercholesterolemia
Category: Antilipidemic
Half-life: no data
Clinically important, potentially serious interactions with: acetaminophen, anticoagulants, carbamazepine, diclofenac, digoxin, furosemide, lovastatin, penicillin, phytonadione, pravastatin, propranolol, tetracycline, simvastatin, ursodiol, vancomycin, vitamin A, vitamin D, warfarin

Reactions

Skin

Dermatitis (sic) (<1%)
Edema
Exanthems (<1%)
Urticaria (<1%)

CORTICOSTEROIDS

Generic names:
Betamethasone
Trade name: Celestone
Cortisone
Trade name: Cortone
Dexamethasone
Trade names: Decadron; Dexameth; Hexadrol
Hydrocortisone
Trade names: Cortef; Solu-Cortef
Methylprednisolone
Trade names: Medrol; Depo-Medrol; Solu-Medrol
Prednisolone
Trade names: Delta-Cortef; Hydeltrasol
Prednisone
Trade names: Deltasone; Meticorten; Orasone
Triamcinolone
Trade names: Aristocort; Aristospan; Kenalog
Category: Anti-inflammatory
Clinically important, potentially serious interactions with: anticholinesterases, anticoagulants, barbiturates, phenytoin, rifampin, salicylates, troleandomycin

Reactions

Skin

Acanthosis nigricans
(1982): Bailin PL+, *Clin Rheum Dis* 8, 493 (passim)
(1980): Gottlieb NL+, *JAMA* 243, 1260
(1968): Brown J+, *Medicine* 47, 33
Acne
(2000): Fung MA+, *Dermatology* 200, 43
(1993): Monk B+, *Clin Exp Dermatol* 18, 148
(1982): Bailin PL+, *Clin Rheum Dis* 8, 493 (passim)
(1953): Smith RC+, *Arch Dermatol* 67, 630
Acute generalized exanthematous pustulosis
(1996): Demitsu T+, *Dermatology* 193, 56
Allergic reactions (sic)
(1999): Alexiou C+, *Laryngorhinootologie* (German) 78, 573
Angioedema
(1980): Ashord RFU+, *Postgrad Med J* 56, 437
Atrophy
(1990): Ford MD+, *Ophthalmic Surg* 21, 215
(1978): Gottlieb NL+, *JAMA* 240, 559
(1975): Kikuchi I+, *Arch Dermatol* 111, 795
(1974): Kikuchi I+, *Arch Dermatol* 109, 558
(1974): Rimbaud P+, *Presse Med* (French) 3, 665
(1972): Di Stefano V+, *Clin Orthop* 87, 254
(1966): Cassidy JT+, *Ann Intern Med* 65, 1008
(1964): Ayres S, *Arch Dermatol* 90, 242
Bacterial infection
Bullous eruption
(1999): Lew DB+, *Pediatr Dermatology* 16, 146
Calcification
(1979): Leigh IM+, *Br J Dermatol* 101, 71
Contact dermatitis
(1997): Murata Y+, *Arch Dermatol* 133, 1053
(1995): Lepoittevin J-P+, *Arch Dermatol* 131, 31
(1993): Hisa T+, *Contact Dermatitis* 28, 174
(1993): Elsner P, *Curr Prob Dermatol* 21, 170
(1993): Fedler R+, *Hautarzt* (German) 44, 91
(1985): Hayakawa R+, *Contact Dermatitis* 12, 213
(1985): Yoshikawa K+, *Contact Dermatitis* 12, 55
Depigmentation
(1974): Rimbaud P+, *Presse Med* (French) 3, 665
(1972): Glick EN, *BMJ* 4, 300
(1972): Bloomfield E, *BMJ* 3, 766
Dermal thinning
(1992): Breathnach SM+, *Adverse Drug Reactions and the Skin*, Blackwell, Oxford, 267 (passim)
(1990): Capewell S+, *BMJ* 300, 1548
Dermatitis (sic)
(2000): Harris A+, *Australas J Dermatol* 41, 124
(1994): Whitmore SE, *Br J Dermatol* 131, 296 (generalized)
Dermatofibromas
(1991): Margolis DJ, *Int J Dermatol* 30, 750
(1991): Cohen PR, *Int J Dermatol* 30, 266
Diaphoresis
(1999): Alexiou C+, *Laryngorhinootologie* (German) 78, 573
Ecchymoses
(1992): Breathnach SM+, *Adverse Drug Reactions and the Skin*, Blackwell, Oxford, 267 (passim)
Eczematous eruption (sic)
(1993): Belsito DV, *Cutis* 52, 291
(1993): Torres V+, *Contact Dermatitis* 29, 106
(1992): Lauerma AI+, *Arch Dermatol* 128, 275
(1988): Lindehof B, *Contact Dermatitis* 18, 309
Erythema (diffuse and widespread)
(1999): Alexiou C+, *Laryngorhinootologie* (German) 78, 573
(1995): Saff DM+, *Arch Dermatol* 131, 742 (localized) (intralesional triamcinolone)
(1993): Räsänen L+, *Br J Dermatol* 128, 407
Erythema multiforme
(1999): Lew DB+, *Pediatr Dermatol* 16, 146
Exanthems
(1995): Whitmore SE, *Contact Dermatitis* 32, 193
(1995): Ijsselmuiden O+, *Acta Derm Venereol* (Stockh) 75, 57 (intraarticular triamcinolone)
(1987): Maucher OM+, *Hautarzt* (German) 38, 577
Facial edema
(1995): Whitmore SE, *Contact Dermatitis* 32, 193
Flushing
(1999): Alexiou C+, *Laryngorhinootologie* (German) 78, 573
Fungal infection
Herpes simplex
Herpes zoster
Hyperpigmentation
(1982): Bailin PL+, *Clin Rheum Dis* 8, 493 (passim)
Kaposi's sarcoma
(1993): Trattner A+, *J Am Acad Dermatol* 29, 890
(1991): Soria C+, *J Am Acad Dermatol* 24, 1027
(1981): Leung F+, *Am J Med* 71, 320
(1981): Ilie B+, *Dermatologica* 163, 455
Leucoderma acquisitum
(1972): Cahn BJ+, *Cutis* 9, 509
Linear atrophy
(1988): Jemec GBE, *J Dermatol Surg Oncol* 14, 88
(1988): Friedman SJ+, *J Am Acad Dermatol* 19, 537
(1987): Gupta A+, *Pediatr Dermatol* 4, 259
(1985): Litt JZ, *Arch Dermatol* 121, 26
(1978): Gupta A+, *Pediatr Dermatol* 4, 259
Linear hypopigmentation
(1999): George WM+, *Cutis* 64, 61 (also perilinear)
(1988): Friedman SJ+, *J Am Acad Dermatol* 19, 537
(1985): Litt JZ, *Arch Dermatol* 121, 26
(1984): McCormack PC+, *Arch Dermatol* 120, 708
(1981): Gottlieb L+, *Arch Dermatol* 117, 605
(1962): Goldman L, *JAMA* 182, 614
Lupus erythematosus
(1973): Hardin JG, *Ann Intern Med* 78, 558
Mycotic infection
Necrosis
(1974): Rimbaud P+, *Presse Med* (French) 3, 665
Perioral dermatitis
(1992): Breathnach SM+, *Adverse Drug Reactions and the Skin*, Blackwell, Oxford, 267 (passim)
Photocontact dermatitis
(1978): Rietchel RL, *Contact Dermatitis* 4, 334
Pigmentation (sic)
(1992): Breathnach SM+, *Adverse Drug Reactions and the Skin*, Blackwell, Oxford, 267 (passim)
Pityriasis rosea
(1981): Leonforte JF, *Dermatologica* 163, 480
Porokeratosis
(1980): Feuerman EJ+, *Acta Derm Venereol* (Stockh) 85, 59
Pruritus
(1999): Alexiou C+, *Laryngorhinootologie* (German) 78, 573
(1999): Lew DB+, *Pediatr Dermatology* 16, 146

(1995): Saff DM+, *Arch Dermatol* 131, 742 (localized) (intralesional triamcinolone)
Pseudoxanthoma elasticum
(1982): Miki Aso+, *J Dermatol* (Tokio) 9, 207
Purpura
(2000): Rosen R, Sydney, Australia, (from Internet) (observation) (from inhaled steroid)
(1990): Capewell S+, *BMJ* 300, 1548
(1982): Bailin PL+, *Clin Rheum Dis* 8, 493 (passim)
(1980): Gottlieb NL+, *JAMA* 243, 1260
Pustular psoriasis
(1982): Bailin PL+, *Clin Rheum Dis* 8, 493 (passim)
Redness of face (sic)
Staphylococcal scalded skin syndrome
(1998): Shirin S+, *Cutis* 62, 223 (in an adult)
Striae
(1982): Bailin PL+, *Clin Rheum Dis* 8, 493 (passim)
(1975): Nikolowski W, *Akt Dermatol* (German) 1, 9
Telangiectases
(1989): Hogan DJ+, *J Am Acad Dermatol* 20, 1129
(1982): Bailin PL+, *Clin Rheum Dis* 8, 493 (passim)
(1972): DiStefano V+, *Clin Orthop* 87, 254
Urticaria
(1995): Whitmore SE, *Contact Dermatitis* 32, 193
(1980): Ashford RF+, *Postgrad Med J* 56, 437
Vasculitis
(1982): Bailin PL+, *Clin Rheum Dis* 8, 493 (passim)
(1969): Rosenberg AL+, *Arthritis Rheum* 12, 317
(1967): Main RA, *Br J Dermatol* 79, 68
Viral infection

Hair

Hair – hirsutism
Hair – hypertrichosis
(1988): Holman GA+, *Pediatrics* 81, 452
(1982): Bailin PL+, *Clin Rheum Dis* 8, 493 (passim)

Other

Anaphylactoid reaction
(2000): Vedamurthy M, Chennai, India (from Internet) (observation) (triamcinolone)
(2000): Alexander J, Tulsa, OK (from Internet) (observation) (triamcinolone)
(1985): Peller JS+, *Ann Allergy* 54, 302
(1960): King RA, *Lancet* 2, 1093
Black tongue
Buffalo hump
(1982): Bailin PL+, *Clin Rheum Dis* 8, 493 (passim)
Hypersensitivity
(2000): Brancaccio RR+, *Cutis* 65, 31 (at injection site)
(1993): Chan AT, *BMJ* 306, 109
Impaired wound healing
(1992): Breathnach SM+, *Adverse Drug Reactions and the Skin*, Blackwell, Oxford, 267 (passim)
Injection-site aseptic necrosis
Injection-site lipoatrophy
(1975): Nikolowski W, *Akt Dermatol* (German) 1, 9
(1974): Kikuchi I+, *Arch Dermatol* 109, 558
(1974): Rimbaud P+, *Presse Med* (French) 3, 665
(1963): Schetman D+, *Arch Dermatol* 88, 820
Moon face
(1982): Bailin PL+, *Clin Rheum Dis* 8, 493 (passim)
Myopathy
(1992): Decramer M+, *Am Rev Resp Dis* 146, 800
(1990): Shee CD, *Respiratory Medicine* 84, 229
(1986): Knox AJ+, *Thorax* 41, 411
(1985): Bowyer SL+, *J Allerg Clin Immunol* 2, 234
(1980): Van Marle W+, *BMJ* 281, 271
Panniculitis
(1988): Saxena AK+, *Cutis* 43, 241

CROMOLYN

Synonyms: cromolyn sodium; disodium cromoglycate
Trade names: Gastrocrom (Medeva); Intal (Aventis)
Other common trade names: *Colimune; Cromlom; Cromoptic; Fivent; Nalcrom; Opticrom; Rynacrom*
Indications: Allergic rhinitis, asthma, mastocytosis
Category: Mast cell stabilizer
Half-life: 80 minutes
Clinically important, potentially serious interactions with: none

Reactions

Skin

Angioedema (1–10%)
(1992): Breathnach SM+, *Adverse Drug Reactions and the Skin*, Blackwell, Oxford, 235 (passim)
(1979): Settipane GA+, *JAMA* 241, 811
(1975): Sheffer AL+, *N Engl J Med* 293, 1220
(1974): Crisp J+, *JAMA* 229, 787
Contact dermatitis
(1997): Camarasa JG+, *Contact Dermatitis* 36, 160 (from eye drops)
(1993): Lewis FM+, *Contact Dermatitis* 28, 246
(1988): Kudo H+, *Contact Dermatitis* 19, 312
Dermatitis (sic) (generalized)
(1979): Settipane GA+, *JAMA* 241, 811
Eczematous eruption (sic)
Edema
Erythema
Exanthems
Exfoliative dermatitis
Facial dermatitis (sic)
(1979): Settipane GA+, *JAMA* 241, 811
(1974): Brogden RN+, *Drugs* 7, 164
Flushing
Photosensitivity
Pruritus
(1975): Sheffer AL+, *N Engl J Med* 293, 1220
Rash (sic) (<1%)
Rosacea
(1979): Mayberry JF+, *BMJ* 2, 1366
Urticaria (<1%)
(1992): Breathnach SM+, *Adverse Drug Reactions and the Skin*, Blackwell, Oxford, 235 (passim)
(1977): Menon MP+, *Scand J Respir Dis* 58, 145
(1975): Sheffer AL+, *N Engl J Med* 293, 1220
Vasculitis
(1978): Rosenberg JL+, *Arch Intern Med* 138, 989

Other

Anaphylactoid reaction (<1%)
(1996): Shearer WT, *Ann Allergy Asthma Immunol* 77, 165
(1996): Ibanez MD+, *Ann Allergy Asthma Immunol* 77, 185
(1992): Breathnach SM+, *Adverse Drug Reactions and the Skin*, Blackwell, Oxford, 235 (passim)
(1983): Ahmad S, *Ann Intern Med* 99, 882
(1975): Sheffer AL+, *N Engl J Med* 293, 1220
Anosmia
(1998): Graedon J+, Newspaper anecdote from *People's Pharmacy* column
Dysgeusia (>10%)
Hypersensitivity (immediate type)
(1987): Skarpass IJK, *Allergy* 42, 318
Myalgia
Myopathy
(1979): Settipane GA+, *JAMA* 241, 811
Paresthesias
Serum sickness
Xerostomia (1–10%)

CYANOCOBALAMIN

Synonym: vitamin B_{12}
Trade names: Berubigen; Crysti-12; Cyanoject (Mayrand); Cyomin (Forest); Ener-B; Nascobal (Schwarz); Rubramin (Bristol-Myers Squibb); Vitamin B_{12}
Other common trade names: *Anacobin; Betolvex; Cobex; Crystamine; Cytamen; Dobetin; Ener-B; Lifaton B12; Redisol; Rubesol-1000; Sytobex; Vicapan N*
Indications: Vitamin B_{12} deficiency, pernicious anemia
Category: Water-soluble nutritional supplement and antianemic
Half-life: 6 days
Clinically important, potentially serious interactions with: chloramphenicol, colchicine, neomycin, omeprazole, phenobarbital, phenytoin, primidone

Reactions

Skin

Acne
- (1991): Sherertz EF, *Cutis* 48, 119
- (1979): Dupre A+, *Cutis* 24, 210
- (1976): Braun-Falco O+, *Münch Med Wochenschr* (German) 118, 155
- (1969): Dugois P+, *Bull Soc Fr Dermatol Syphiligr* (French) 76, 382
- (1969): Dugois P+, *Lyon Med* (French) 221, 1165
- (1967): Puissant A+, *Bull Soc Fr Derm Syphiligr* (French) 74, 813
- (1966): Goldblatt S, *Hautarzt* (German) 17, 106

Allergic reactions (sic)
- (1986): Bigby M+, *JAMA* 256, 3358 (1.79%)

Angioedema
- (1952): Bedford PD, *BMJ* 1, 690

Bullous eruption (<1%)
- (1977): Pevny I+, *Hautarzt* (German) 28, 600

Cheilitis
- (1981): Price ML+, *Contact Dermatitis* 7, 352

Contact dermatitis
- (1994): Rodriguez A+, *Contact Dermatitis* 31, 271
- (1975): Malten KE, *Contact Dermatitis* 1, 325

Eczematous eruption (sic)
- (1977): Pevny I+, *Hautarzt* (German) 28, 600

Exanthems
- (1986): Woodliff HJ, *Med J Aust* 144, 223
- (1977): Pevny I+, *Hautarzt* (German) 28, 600
- (1976): Arndt KA+, *JAMA* 235, 918

Folliculitis
- (1989): Gallastegui C+, *Drug Intell Clin Pharm* 23, 1033

Pruritus (1–10%)
- (1974): Nalivko F+, *Vestn Dermatol Venerol* (Russian) 8, 66

Systemic eczematous contact dermatitis

Urticaria (<1%)
- (1996): Denis R+, *Clin Lab Haematol* 18, 129
- (1986): Woodliff HJ, *Med J Aust* 144, 223
- (1977): Pevny I+, *Hautarzt* (German) 28, 600
- (1974): Nalivko F+, *Vestn Dermatol Venerol* (Russian) 8, 66
- (1971): James J+, *BMJ* 2, 262
- (1969): Meyer de Schmid JJ+, *Bull Soc Fr Dermatol Syphiligr* (French) 76, 670
- (1952): Bedford PD, *BMJ* 1, 690

Other

Anaphylactoid reaction (<1%)
- (1998): Tordjman R+, *Eur J Haematol* 60, 269
- (1984): Sobolevskii AI+, *Vestn Dermatol Venerol* (Russian) April, 66
- (1977): Pevny I+, *Hautarzt* (German) 28, 600
- (1971): James J+, *BMJ* 2, 262
- (1968): Hovding G, *BMJ* 3, 102

Embolia cutis medicamentosa (Nicolau syndrome)
- (1995): Kunzi T+, *Schweiz Rundsch Med Prax* (German) 84, 640

Hypersensitivity
- (1974): Nalivko SN+, *Vestn Dermatol Venerol* (Russian) August, 66

Injection-site aseptic necrosis
- (1995): Kunzi T+, *Schweiz Rundsch Med Prax* (German) 84, 640

Injection-site pain

Paresthesias

Porphyria cutanea tarda
- (1965): DeFeo CP, *Arch Dermatol* 92, 330

CYCLAMATE

Trade name: Sucaryl (Abbott)
Indications: Sweetening
Category: Sulfonamide* sweetener
Half-life: no data
Clinically important, potentially serious interactions with: none

Reactions

Skin

Angioedema
- (1968): Feingold BF, *Ann Allergy* 26, 309

Bullous eruption
- (1968): Feingold BF, *Ann Allergy* 26, 309

Exanthems
- (1965): Boros E, *JAMA* 194, 571

Photosensitivity
- (1981): Fujita M+, *Arch Dermatol* 117, 246 (passim)
- (1972): Jung EG, *Z Haut Geschlechtskr* (German) 47, 329
- (1970): *Nutr Rev* 28, 122
- (1969): Yong JM+, *Lancet* 2, 1273
- (1968): Turk JL+, *Br J Dermatol* 80, 200
- (1968): Feingold BF, *Ann Allergy* 26, 309
- (1966): Kobori T+, *J Asthma Res* 3, 213

Pruritus
- (1968): Feingold BF, *Ann Allergy* 26, 309
- (1967): Lamberg SI, *JAMA* 201, 747
- (1965): Boros E, *JAMA* 194, 571

Urticaria
- (1981): Fujita M+, *Arch Dermatol* 117, 246
- (1968): Feingold BF, *Ann Allergy* 26, 309

Other

Hypersensitivity (nonallergic)
- (1998): Ehlers I+, *Allergy* 53, 1074

Paresthesias
- (1992): Shelley WB+, *Advanced Dermatologic Diagnosis*, WB Saunders, 1039

***Note:** Cyclamate is a sulfonamide and can be absorbed systemically. Sulfonamides can produce severe, possibly fatal, reactions such as toxic epidermal necrolysis and Stevens–Johnson syndrome.

CYCLOBENZAPRINE

Trade name: Flexeril (Merck)
Other common trade names: *Benzamin; Cloben; Cyben; Flexiban; Novo-Cycloprine; Yurelax*
Indications: Muscle spasms
Category: Skeletal muscle relaxant
Half-life: 1–3 days
Clinically important, potentially serious interactions with: alcohol, anticholinergics, bupropion, clonidine, clozapine, CNS depressants, epinephrine, guanethidine, MAO inhibitors, maprotiline, phenothiazines, tricyclic antidepressants

Reactions

Skin

Allergic reactions (sic)

Angioedema (<1%)

Dermatitis (sic) (<1%)

Diaphoresis
- (1984): Heckerling PS+, *Ann Intern Med* 101, 881

Facial edema (<1%)

Flushing
Photosensitivity
Pruritus (<1%)
Purpura
Rash (sic) (<1%)
Urticaria (<1%)

Hair

Hair – alopecia

Other

Ageusia (<1%)
Anaphylactoid reaction (<1%)
Dysgeusia (3%)
Galactorrhea
Gynecomastia
Paresthesias (<1%)
Stomatitis
Tongue edema (<1%)
Tongue pigmentation
Xerostomia (27%)
(1988): Katz WA+, *Clin Ther* 10, 216
(1988): Bennett RM+, *Arthritis Rheum* 31, 1535

CYCLOPHOSPHAMIDE

Synonyms: CPM; CTX; CYT
Trade names: Cytoxan (Bristol-Myers Squibb); Neosar (Pharmacia & Upjohn)
Other common trade names: *Cycloblastin; Cyclostin; Endoxan; Endoxana; Genoxal; Ledoxina; Procytox; Sendoxan*
Indications: Lymphomas
Category: Antineoplastic and immunosuppressant
Half-life: 4–7 hours
Clinically important, potentially serious interactions with: allopurinol, azathioprine, chloramphenicol, cimetidine, digoxin, doxorubicin, phenobarbital, phenytoin, quinolones, thiazides

Reactions

Skin

Acral erythema
(1993): Vukelja SJ+, *Cutis* 52, 89
(1986): Crider MK+, *Arch Dermatol* 122, 1023
Angioedema
(1977): Ross WE+, *Cancer Treat Rep* 61, 495
Condylomata acuminata
(1996): D'Hondt L+, *Acta Gastroenterol Belg* (French) 59, 254
Contact dermatitis
(1967): Maguire HC, *J Invest Dermatol* 48, 39
Dermatitis herpetiformis
(1986): Gottlieb D+, *Med J Aust* 145, 241
Dermatofibromas
(1986): Bargman HB+, *J Am Acad Dermatol* 14, 351
Diaphoresis
Eccrine squamous syringometaplasia
(1997): Valks R+, *Arch Dermatol* 133, 873
Erythema multiforme (<1%)
Erythrodysesthesia syndrome
(1989): Matsuyama JR+, *Drug Intell Clin Pharm* 23, 776
Exanthems
(1992): Hann SK+, *J Dermatol* 20, 94
(1992): Breathnach SM+, *Adverse Drug Reactions and the Skin*, Blackwell, Oxford, 289 (passim)
(1982): Bailin PL+, *Clin Rheum Dis* 8, 493 (passim)
Facial burning
(1994): Kosirog-Glowacki JL+, *Ann Pharmacother* 28, 197
Flushing (1–10%)
(1994): Dhar S+, *Dermatology* 188, 332
Keratoacanthoma
(1972): Lowney ED, *Arch Dermatol* 105, 924
Lymphoma
(1992): Pandya AG+, *Arch Dermatol* 128, 1626 (passim)
(1983): Goslen JB+, *Arch Dermatol* 119, 326
Myxedema
(1971): Coffey VJ, *BMJ* 4, 682
Palmar-plantar erythema
(1990): Pagliuca A+, *Postgrad Med J* 66, 242
Pigmentation (<1%)
(1993): Pai BH, *J Assoc Physicians India* 41, 124
(1992): Babu KG, *J Assoc Physicians India* 40, 211
(1992): Pandya AG+, *Arch Dermatol* 128, 1626 (passim)
(1991): Dutta TK+, *J Assoc Physicians India* 39, 230
(1991): Singal R+, *Pediatr Dermatol* 8, 231
(1981): Nixon DW+, *Cutis* 27, 181
(1975): Shah PC+, *Lancet* 2, 548 (palmar)
(1975): No Author, *Lancet* 2, 128
(1974): Romankiewicz JA, *Am J Hosp Pharm* 31, 1074
(1973): Levantine A+, *Br J Dermatol* 89, 105
(1973): Mani MK+, *J Assoc Physicians India* 21, 799
(1972): Amar Inalsingh CH, *Arch Dermatol* 106, 765 (palmar)
(1972): Harrison BM+, *BMJ* 2, 352
(1966): Solidoro A+, *Cancer Chemotherapy* 50, 265
Polyarteritis nodosa
(1983): Goslen JB+, *Arch Dermatol* 119, 326
Pruritus
(1978): Krutchik AN+, *Arch Intern Med* 138, 1725
Purpura
Rash (sic) (1–10%)
Squamous cell carcinoma
(1992): Pandya AG+, *Arch Dermatol* 128, 1626 (passim)
(1972): Lowney ED, *Arch Dermatol* 105, 924
Stevens–Johnson syndrome
(1996): Assier-Bonnet H+, *Br J Dermatol* 135, 864
(1985): Leititis JU+, *Klin Padiatr* (German) 197, 441
Toxic epidermal necrolysis (<1%)
Ultraviolet light recall
(1993): Williams BJ+, *Clin Exp Dermatol* 18, 452
(1984): Andersen KE+, *Photodermatol* 1, 129
Urticaria
(1992): Breathnach SM+, *Adverse Drug Reactions and the Skin*, Blackwell, Oxford, 289 (passim)
(1987): Grosbois B+, *Rev Med Interne* (French) 8, 208
(1982): Anku V, *Cancer Treat Rep* 66, 2106
(1980): Diaz-Rubio E+, *Rev Clin Esp* (Spanish) 156, 461
(1978): Krutchik AN+, *Arch Intern Med* 138, 1725
(1978): Legha SS+, *Cancer Treat Rep* 62, 180
(1977): Ross WE+, *Cancer Treat Rep* 61, 495
(1976): Lakin JD+, *J Allergy Clin Immunol* 58, 160
Vasculitis
(1989): Green RM+, *Aust N Z J Med* 19, 55

Hair

Hair – alopecia (universal and severe in one-third)
(2000): Tran D+, *Australas J Dermatology* 41, 106
(1996): Infanti L+, *Haematologica* 81, 521
(1992): Pandya AG+, *Arch Dermatol* 128, 1626 (passim)
(1987): Parker R, *Oncol Nurs Forum* 14, 49
(1987): David J+, *Nurs Times* 83, 36
(1985): Middleton J+, *Cancer Treat Rep* 69, 373
(1984): Cline BW, *Cancer Nurs* 7, 221
(1984): Ahmed AR+, *J Am Acad Dermatol* 11, 1115
(1982): Bailin PL+, *Clin Rheum Dis* 8, 493 (passim)
(1980): Maxwell MB, *Am J Nursing* 80, 900
(1979): Holmes W, *ANA Publ* (NP-59), 223
(1972): Harrison BM+, *BMJ* 2, 352
(1966): Herzberg JJ, *Arch Klin Exp Dermatol* (German) 227, 452
(1966): Simister JM, *BMJ* 2, 1138

Nails

Nails – Beau's lines (transverse nail bands)
(1994): Ben-Dyan D+, *Acta Haematol* 91, 89
Nails – dystrophy
(1992): Breathnach SM+, *Adverse Drug Reactions and the Skin*, Blackwell, Oxford, 289 (passim)
Nails – onychodermal band
(1993): Kowal-Vern A+, *Cutis* 52, 43
Nails – pigmentation (<1%)
(1992): Bianchi L+, *Dermatology* 185, 216 (longitudinal)
(1983): Manigand G+, *Sem Hop* (French) 59, 1840

(1982): Bailin PL+, *Clin Rheum Dis* 8, 493 (passim)
(1981): Adam BA, *Singapore Med J* 22, 35
(1980): Sulis E+, *Eur J Cancer* 16, 1517
(1980): Daniel CR+, *Cutis* 25, 595
(1978): Shah PC+, *Br J Dermatol* 98, 675
(1975): Shah PC+, *Lancet* 2, 548
(1975): Markenson AL+, *Lancet* 2, 128 (pigmented banding)
(1973): Mani MK+, *J Assoc Physicians of India* 21, 799
(1972): Amar Inalsingh CH, *Arch Dermatol* 106, 765
(1966): Solidoro A+, *Cancer Chemother* 50, 265

Nails – transverse leukonychia (Meuhrcke's lines)
(1992): Bianchi L+, *Dermatology* 185, 216 (longitudinal)
(1990): Bader-Meunier B+, *Ann Pediatr Paris* (French) 37, 337
(1983): James WD+, *Arch Dermatol* 119, 334

Other

Acute intermittent porphyria

Anaphylactoid reaction (<1%)
(1992): Breathnach SM+, *Adverse Drug Reactions and the Skin*, Blackwell, Oxford, 289 (passim)
(1979): Murti L+, *J Pediatr* 94, 844
(1977): Karchmer RK+, *JAMA* 237, 475

Gingival pigmentation
(1979): Krutchik AN+, *South Med J* 72, 1615
(1972): Harrison BM+, *BMJ* 2, 352

Hypersensitivity
(1996): Popescu NA+, *J Allergy Clin Immunol* 97, 26
(1992): Weiss RB, *Semin Oncol* 19, 458
(1978): Legha SS+, *Cancer Treat Rep* 62, 180

Injection-site pain

Oral mucosal ulceration
(1992): Pandya AG+, *Arch Dermatol* 128, 1626 (passim)
(1982): Bailin PL+, *Clin Rheum Dis* 8, 493 (passim)

Porphyria cutanea tarda
(1988): Manzione NC+, *Gastroenterology* 95, 1119

Scalp burning
(1994): Kosirog-Glowacki JL+, *Ann Pharmacother* 28, 197

Stomatitis (10%)
(1982): Bailin PL+, *Clin Rheum Dis* 8, 493 (passim)
(1975): Carter SK, *Cancer Treat Rev* 2, 295

Tooth discoloration
(1972): Harrison BM+, *BMJ* 2, 352

CYCLOSERINE

Trade name: Seromycin (Dura)
Other common trade names: *Closerin; Closerina; Cyclomycin; Cyclorine; Cycosin; Orientomycin*
Indications: Tuberculosis
Category: Tuberculostatic
Half-life: 10 hours
Clinically important, potentially serious interactions with: alcohol, ethionamide, isoniazid, phenytoin

Reactions

Skin

Allergic reactions (sic)

Dermatitis (sic)
(1972): Levantine A+, *Br J Dermatol* 86, 651
(1971): Nava C, *Med Lav* (Italian) 62, 351

Exanthems
(1985): Holdiness R, *Int J Dermatol* 24, 280
(1973): Mühlberger F, *Schweiz Med Wochenschr* (German) 103, 126
(1969): Agrawal R, *BMJ* 4, 540
(1959): Bereston ES, *J Invest Dermatol* 33, 427

Lichenoid eruption
(1995): Shim JH+, *Dermatology* 191, 142

Pruritus

Rash (sic) (<1%)

Stevens–Johnson syndrome
(1997): Akula SK+, *Int J Tuberc Lung Dis* 1, 187 (in AIDS)

Urticaria
(1959): Bereston ES, *J Invest Dermatol* 33, 427

Other

Oral mucosal lesions

Paresthesias

CYCLOSPORINE

Synonyms: CsA; CyA; cyclosporin A
Trade names: Neoral (Novartis); Sandimmune (Novartis)
Other common trade names: *Ciclosporin; Consupren; Implanta; Sandimmun*
Indications: Prophylaxis of organ rejection in transplants
Category: Immunosuppressant
Half-life: 10–27 hours (adults)
Clinically important, potentially serious interactions with: aminoglycosides, amiodarone, amphotericin B, androgens, cimetidine, clarithromycin, danazol, diltiazem, doxorubicin, erythromycin, etoposide, fluconazole, foscarnet, itraconazole, ketoconazole, lovastatin, nifedipine, NSAIDs, penicillamine, penicillins, pravastatin, rifampin, simvastatin, **grapefruit juice, St John's- wort**

Note: A good discussion of cyclosporine in dermatology can be found in (1989): Gupta AK+, *J Am Acad Dermatol* 21, 1245.

Reactions

Skin

Acne (6%)
(1996): el Shahawy MA+, *Nephron* 72, 679
(1993): Valicenti JMK+, *Arch Dermatol* 129, 794 (passim)
(1986): Bencini PL+, *Br J Dermatol* 114, 396

Angioedema
(1980): Isenberg DA+, *N Engl J Med* 303, 754

Angiomas
(1998): De Felipe I+, *Arch Dermatol* 134, 1487

Ankle edema
(1997): Berthe-Jones J+, *Br J Dermatol* 136, 76

Basal cell carcinoma
(1992): Pakula A+, *J Am Acad Dermatol* 26, 139
(1987): Penn I, *Transplantation* 43, 32

Bullous eruption (1%)
(1990): Petit D+, *J Am Acad Dermatol* 22, 851

Buschke–Lowenstein penile carcinoma
(1993): Piepkorn M+, *J Am Acad Dermatol* 29, 321

Cutaneous neoplasms (sic)
(1995): Kohler LD+, *Hautarzt* (German) 46, 638

Eccrine squamous syringometaplasia
(1997): Valks R+, *Arch Dermatol* 133, 873

Edema
(1997): Shapiro J+, *J Am Acad Dermatol* 36, 114

Epidermal cysts
(1993): Valicenti JMK+, *Arch Dermatol* 129, 794 (passim)
(1993): Richter A+, *Hautarzt* (German) 44, 521
(1992): Schoendorff C+, *Cutis* 50, 36 (epidermoid)
(1986): Bencini PL+, *Dermatologica* 172, 24

Exanthems
(1985): Chapius B+, *N Engl J Med* 312, 1259

Facial edema
(1986): Schmitz-Schumann M, *Prog Allergy* 38, 436

Flushing (>3%)
(2000): Ramsay HM+, *Br J Dermatol* 142, 832
(1992): Shelley WB+, *Advanced Dermatologic Diagnosis*, WB Saunders, 583 (passim)
(1992): Goodman MM+, *J Am Acad Dermatol* 27, 594
(1990): Gupta AK+, *J Am Acad Dermatol* 22, 242
(1986): Kahan BD+, *World J Surg* 10, 348

Folliculitis
(1995): Ojeda-Vargas M+, *Enferm Infecc Microbiol Clin* (Spanish) 13, 637
(1993): Sepp N+, *Br J Dermatol* 128, 213
(1993): Valicenti JMK+, *Arch Dermatol* 129, 794 (passim)
(1993): Richter A+, *Hautarzt* (German) 44, 521

(1986): Bencini PL+, *Dermatologica* 172, 24
Herpes simplex
(1993): Sepp N+, *Br J Dermatol* 128, 213
(1993): Valicenti JMK+, *Arch Dermatol* 129, 794 (passim)
(1986): Bencini PL+, *Dermatologica* 172, 24
Herpes zoster
(1986): Bencini PL+, *Dermatologica* 172, 24
Hidradenitis
(1984): Palestine AG+, *Am J Med* 4:77, 652
Hyperpigmentation
(1997): Oakley A, Hamilton New Zealand (from Internet) (observation)
Hyperkeratosis (follicular spiny)
(1995): Izakovic J+, *Hautarzt* (German) 46, 841
Hypohidrosis
(1990): Gupta AK+, *Arch Dermatol* 126, 339
Ichthyosis
(1986): Bencini PL+, *Dermatologica* 172, 24
Kaposi's sarcoma
(1997): Vella JP+, *N Engl J Med* 336, 1761
(1996): Ozen S+, *Nephrol Dial Transplant* 11, 1162
(1988): Bencini PL+, *Br J Dermatol* 118, 709
(1987): Penn I, *Transplantation* 43, 32
Keratoses
(1995): Yamamoto T+, *J Dermatol* 22, 298
(1993): Piepkorn M+, *J Am Acad Dermatol* 29, 321
(1992): Ross M+, *J Am Acad Dermatol* 26, 128
Keratosis pilaris
(1993): Valicenti JMK+, *Arch Dermatol* 129, 794 (passim)
(1986): Bencini PL+, *Dermatologica* 172, 24
Lichenoid eruption
(1995): Shim JH+, *Dermatology* 191, 142
Lupus erythematosus
(1990): Cooper KD, *Dermatology* 1(2), 3
Lymphocytic infiltration
(1992): Bagot M+, *J Am Acad Dermatol* 26, 283
(1991): Sabourin JC, *Ann Pathol* 11, 208
(1990): Gupta AK+, *J Am Acad Dermatol* 23, 1137
(1990): Gupta AK+, *J Am Acad Dermatol* 22, 242
(1988): Brown MD+, *Arch Dermatol* 124, 1097
Lymphoma
(1993): Masouye I+, *Arch Dermatol* 129, 914
(1992): Zijlmans JM+, *N Engl J Med* 326, 1363
(1992): Koo JY+, *J Am Acad Dermatol* 26, 836
(1991): Tomson CR+, *Nephrol Dial Transplant* 6, 896
(1989): Walker RJ+, *Aust N Z J Med* 19, 154
(1987): Penn I, *Transplantation* 43, 32
(1984): Beveridge T+, *Lancet* 1, 788
(1983): Inglehart JK, *N Engl J Med* 309, 123
Melanoma
(1990): Merot Y+, *Br J Dermatol* 123, 237
Mycosis fungoides
(1990): Fradin MS+, *J Am Acad Dermatol* 23, 1265
Nodular cutaneous T-lymphocyte infiltrate
(1988): Brown MD+, *Arch Dermatol* 124, 1097
Papillomas (facial)
(1993): Valicenti JMK+, *Arch Dermatol* 129, 794
Papulo-vesicular lesions (sic)
(1988): Frosch PJ+, *Hautarzt* (German) 39, 611
Poikiloderma
(1986): Bencini PL+, *Dermatologica* 172, 24
Porokeratosis (superficial actinic)
(1997): Matsushita S+, *J Dermatol* 24, 110
Pruritus (<2%)
(1992): Goodman MM+, *J Am Acad Dermatol* 27, 594
Pseudofolliculitis barbae
(1997): Lear J+, *Br J Dermatol* 136, 132
Psoriasis
(1986): Bencini PL+, *Dermatologica* 172, 24
Purpura (3%)
(1998): Roberts P+, *Transplant Proc* 30, 1512
(1986): Bencini PL+, *Dermatologica* 172, 24
Pustular psoriasis
(1998): Mahendran R+, *Br J Dermatol* 139, 934
(1997): Drugge R, Stamford CT, (from Internet) (observation)
Rash (sic) (10%)
(1992): Goodman MM+, *J Am Acad Dermatol* 27, 594
Raynaud's phenomenon
(1986): Deray G+, *Lancet* 2, 1092
Sebaceous hyperplasia
(1998): Walther T+, *Dtsch Med Wochenschr* 123, 798
(1993): Valicenti JMK+, *Arch Dermatol* 129, 794 (passim)
(1992): Pakula A+, *J Am Acad Dermatol* 26, 139
(1986): Bencini PL+, *Dermatologica* 172, 24
Shivering (sic)
(2000): Lepine EM, Rock Hill, SC (from Internet) (observation)
Squamous cell carcinoma
(1997): van de Kerkhof PC+, *Br J Dermatol* 136, 275
(1996): Cox NH, *Clin Exp Dermatol* 21, 323
(1993): Piepkorn M+, *J Am Acad Dermatol* 29, 321 (penis)
(1990): Fradin MS+, *J Am Acad Dermatol* 23, 1265 (passim)
(1989): Bos JD+, *J Am Acad Dermatol* 21, 1305
(1985): Thompson JF+, *Lancet* 1, 158
(1985): Bencini PL+, *Br J Dermatol* 113, 373
(1985): Price ML+, *N Engl J Med* 313, 1420
(1983): Mortimer PS+, *J R Soc Med* 76, 786
Striae
(1986): Bencini PL+, *Dermatologica* 172, 24
Toxic epidermal necrolysis
(1997): Jarrett P+, *Clin Exp Dermatol* 22, 254
Ulceration (1%)
Urticaria
(1985): Ptachcinski RJ+, *Lancet* 1, 636
Vasculitis
(2000): Gupta MN+, *Ann Rheum Dis* 59, 319
(1994): Henckes M+, *Transpl Int* 7, 292
Verruca vulgaris
(1998): Irimajiri J+, *J Dermatol* 25, 688
Vitiligo
(1986): Bencini PL+, *Dermatologica* 172, 24

Hair

Hair – alopecia (3%)
(1998): Hunt M, *Cosmetic Dermatology* 23
(1987): Keown PA+, *Hospital Practice* 22, 207
Hair – alopecia areata
(1996): Parodi A+, *Br J Dermatol* 135, 657 (universalis)
(1996): Misciali C+, *Arch Dermatol* 132, 843 (universalis)
(1995): Davies MG+, *Br J Dermatol* 132, 835
(1994): Roger D+, *Acta Derm Venereol* 74, 154
Hair – breakage
Hair – growth
(1995): Mannes GP+, *Transpl Int* 8, 247 ("delightful")
(1994): Yamamoto S+, *J Dermatol Sci* 7 Suppl: s47
Hair – hypertrichosis (19%)
(2000): Ionnides D+, *Arch Dermatol* 136, 868
(1997): Ellis CN, *Int J Dermatol* 36 (Supplement), 7 (passim)
(1997): Shapiro J+, *J Am Acad Dermatol* 36, 114
(1997): Brehler R+, *J Am Acad Dermatol* 36, 983 (passim)
(1997): Shupack J+, *J Am Acad Dermatol* 36, 423
(1997): Avci O+, *J Am Acad Dermatol* 36, 796
(1996): Jayamanne DG+, *Nephrol Dial Transplant* 11, 1159 (eyelashes)
(1995): Honeyman JF+, *Int J Dermatol* 34, 583
(1993): Sepp N+, *Br J Dermatol* 128, 213
(1993): Valicenti JMK+, *Arch Dermatol* 129, 794 (passim)
(1992): Humphreys TR+, *J Am Acad Dermatol* 29, 490 (passim)
(1990): Fradin MS+, *J Am Acad Dermatol* 23, 1265
(1988): Penmetcha M+, *Int J Dermatol* 27, 53
(1988): Frosch PJ+, *Hautarzt* (German) 39, 611
(1987): Wysocki GP+, *Clin Exp Dermatol* 12, 191
(1987): Keown PA+, *Hospital Practice* 22, 207
(1986): Kahan BD+, *World J Surg* 10, 348
(1984): Harper JL+, *Br J Dermatol* 110, 469

Nails

Nails – abnormal growth
(1986): Gratwohl A+, *Prog Allergy* 38, 404
Nails – brittle (<2%)
Nails – disorder (sic)
(1994): Wakelin SH+, *Br J Dermatol* 131, 147
Nails – ingrown
(1993): Olujohungbe A+, *Lancet* 342, 1111
Nails – leukonychia
(1986): Bencini PL+, *Dermatologica* 172, 24

Nails – periungual granulation tissue
(1995): Higgins EM+, *Br J Dermatol* 132, 829

Other

Acromegaloid features
(1987): Reznik VM, *Lancet* 1, 1405
Anaphylactoid reaction (<1%)
(1989): Gupta AK+, *J Am Acad Dermatol* 21, 1245
(1985): Chapuis B+, *N Engl J Med* 312, 1259
(1985): Ptachcinski RJ+, *Lancet* 1, 636
(1985): Leunissen KML+, *Lancet* 1, 636
Aphthous stomatitis
(1986): Bencini PL+, *Dermatologica* 172, 24
Breast lumps (sic)
(1980): Rolles K+, *Lancet* 2, 795
Dysesthesia
(2000): Capper N, Mobile, AL (from Internet) (observation)
(1990): Gupta AK+, *J Am Acad Dermatol* 22, 242
Gingival bleeding
(2000): Czech W+, *J Am Acad Dermatol* 42, 653
Gingival hyperplasia (>10%)
(2000): Kirby B+, *Clin Exp Dermatol* 25, 97
(2000): Oettinger-Barak O+, *J Periodontol* 71, 650
(2000): Thomas DW+, *Transplantation* 69, 522
(1999): Spratt H+, *Oral Dis* 5, 27
(1999): Wirnsberger GH+, *Transplantation* 67, 1289
(1998): Nowicki M+, *Ann Transplant* 3, 25
(1998): Cebeci I+, *J Periodontol* 69, 1435
(1998): Nohl F+, *Ther Umsch* (German) 55, 573
(1998): Wirnsberger GH+, *Transplant Proc* 30, 2117
(1998): Kohnle M+, *Transplant Proc* 30, 2122
(1998): Jucgla A+, *Br J Dermatol* 138, 198
(1998): Pilloni A+, *J Periodontol* 69, 791
(1998): Nash MM+, *Transplantation* 65, 1611
(1998): Mattson JS+, *J Am Dent Assoc* 129, 78
(1998): Varga E+, *J Clin Periodontol* 25, 225
(1998): Desai P+, *J Can Dent Assoc* 64, 263
(1997): Silverstein LH+, *Gen Dent* 45, 371
(1997): Ellis CN, *Int J Dermatol* 36 (Supplement), 7 (passim)
(1997): Hall EE, *Curr Opin Peridontology* 4, 59 (passim)
(1997): Cecchin E+, *Ann Intern Med* 126, 409
(1997): Brehler R+, *J Am Acad Dermatol* 36, 983 (passim)
(1997): Gómez E+, *Nephrol Dial Transplant* 12, 2694
(1997): Avci O+, *J Am Acad Dermatol* 36, 796
(1997): Dodd DA, *J Heart Lung Transplant* 16, 579
(1997): Jackson C+, *N Y State Dent J* 63, 46
(1997): Iacopino AM+, *J Periodontol* 68, 73
(1997): Puig JM+, *Transplant Proc* 29, 2379
(1997): Gomez E+, *Nephrol Dial Transplant* 12, 2694
(1996): Cebeci I+, *J Periodontol* 67, 1201
(1996): Somacarrera ML+, *Spec Care Dent* 16, 18
(1996): Darbar UR+, *J Clin Periodontol* 23, 941
(1996): Montebugnoli L+, *J Clin Periodontol* 23, 868
(1996): Boran M+, *Transplant Proc* 28, 2316
(1996): Ashrafi SH+, *Scanning Microsc* 10, 219
(1995): Wahlstrom E+, *N Engl J Med* 332, 753
(1995): Moghadam BKH+, *Cutis* 56, 46 (passim)
(1994): Wong W+, *Lancet* 343, 986
(1993): King GN+, *J Clin Periodontol* 20, 286
(1993): Thomason JM+, *J Clin Periodontol* 20, 37
(1993): Seymour RA+, *J R Coll Surg Edinb* 38, 328
(1993): Seymour RA, *Adverse Drug React Toxicol Rev* 12, 215
(1993): Valicenti JMK+, *Arch Dermatol* 129, 794 (passim)
(1992): Humphreys TR+, *J Am Acad Dermatol* 29, 490 (passim)
(1992): Seymour RA+, *J Clin Periodontol* 19, 1
(1992): Mastrolonardo M+, *Dermatol Clin* (Italian) 4, 246
(1991): Puelacher W+, *Z Stomatol* (German) 88, 7
(1990): Cooper KD, *Dermatology* 1(2), 3
(1989): Ross PJ+, *J Dent Child* 56, 56
(1988): Frosch PJ+, *Hautarzt* (German) 39, 611
(1988): Veraldi S+, *Int J Dermatol* 27, 730
(1987): Reznik VM, *Lancet* 1, 1405
(1987): Keown PA+, *Hospital Practice* 22, 207
(1986): Kahan BD+, *World J Surg* 10, 348
Gingivitis (4%)
Glossitis (atrophic)
(1986): Bencini PL+, *Dermatologica* 172, 24
Gynecomastia (>3%)
(1998): Kollias J+, *Aust N Z J Surg* 68, 679
(1994): Jacobs U+, *Transplant Proc* 26, 3122
(1987): Beris P+, *Schweiz Med Wochenschr* (German) 117, 1751
Hyperesthesia
(1987): Keown PA+, *Hospital Practice* 22, 207
Lingual fungiform papillae hypertrophy (sic)
(1996): Silverberg NB+, *Lancet* 348, 967
Lymphoproliferative disease
(1989): Walker RJ+, *Aust N Z J Med* 19, 154
(1988): Brown MD+, *Arch Dermatol* 124, 1097
Myalgia
(1988): Brown MD+, *Arch Dermatol* 124, 1097 (passim)
Myopathy
(1990): Fernandez-Sola J+, *Lancet* 335, 362
(1989): Chassagne P+, *Lancet* 2, 1104
Oral ulceration
(1986): Bencini PL+, *Dermatologica* 172, 24
Paresthesias (>8%)
(2000): Lepine EM, Rock Hill, SC (from Internet) (observation)
(2000): Baumgaertnet J, LaCrosse, WI (from Internet) (3 observations)
(2000): Thaler D, Monona, WI (from Internet) (observation)
(1997): Ellis CN, *Int J Dermatol* 36 (Supplement), 7 (passim)
(1997): Berthe-Jones J+, *Br J Dermatol* 136, 76
(1997): Shupack J+, *J Am Acad Dermatol* 36, 423
(1992): Goodman MM+, *J Am Acad Dermatol* 27, 594
(1990): Cooper KD, *Dermatology* 1(2), 3
(1988): Bennett WM+, *Ann Rev Med* 37, 215 (passim)
(1987): Dougados M+, *Arthritis Rheum* 30, 83
Pseudolymphoma
(1988): Thestrup-Pedersen K+, *Dermatologica* 177, 376
Stomatitis (7%)
Tremor (>10%)

CYCLOTHIAZIDE

Trade name: Anhydron (Lilly)
Other common trade names: *Doburil; Valmiran*
Indications: Edema, hypertension
Category: Thiazide* diuretic
Half-life: no data
Clinically important, potentially serious interactions with: antidiabetics, bumetanide, cyclophosphamide, diazoxide, digoxin, lithium, methotrexate, thiazides

Reactions

Skin

Exanthems (<1%)
Photosensitivity
Purpura
Rash (sic)
Urticaria
Vasculitis

Other

Paresthesias

***Note:** Cyclothiazide is a sulfonamide and can be absorbed systemically. Sulfonamides can produce severe, possibly fatal, reactions such as toxic epidermal necrolysis and Stevens–Johnson syndrome.

CYPROHEPTADINE

Trade name: Periactin (Merck)
Other common trade names: *Ciplactin; Ciproral; Nuran; Periactine, Periactinol, Peritol; Sigloton*
Indications: Allergic rhinitis, urticaria
Category: H_1-receptor antihistamine and appetite stimulant
Half-life: 1–4 hours
Clinically important, potentially serious interactions with: alcohol, CNS depressants, fluoxetine, MAO inhibitors, phenelzine, SSRIs

Reactions

Skin

Allergic reactions (sic) (<1%)
Angioedema (<1%)
Contact dermatitis
(1995): Li LF+, *Contact Dermatitis* 33, 50
Dermatitis (sic)
Diaphoresis
Edema (<1%)
Erythema
Exanthems
(1964): Gould AH+, *Med Clin North Am* 48, 411
Flushing
Lichenoid eruption
(1971): Baer RL+, in Fitzpatrick, *Dermatology in General Medicine*, McGraw-Hill 1281–1314
Lupus erythematosus
Peripheral edema
Photosensitivity
(1971): Kalivas J, *JAMA* 216, 526
Purpura
Rash (sic) (<1%)
Urticaria
Vasculitis
(1984): Ekenstam E+, *Arch Dermatol* 120, 484

Other

Anaphylactoid reaction
Dysgeusia
(1997): Neufeld-Kaiser W+, *Arch Dermatol* 133, 251
Myalgia (<1%)
Paresthesias (<1%)
Xerostomia (1–10%)
(1990): Kardinal CG+, *Cancer* 65, 2657
(1990): Pontius EB, *J Clin Psychopharmacol* 8, 230

CYTARABINE

Synonyms: arabinosylcytosine; ara-C
Trade names: Cytosar-U (Pharmacia & Upjohn); Tarabine (Pharmacia & Upjohn)
Other common trade names: *Alexan; Arabitin; Arace; Aracytine; Cytarbel; Cytosar; Uducil*
Indications: Leukemias
Category: Antineoplastic; antimetabolite
Half-life: initial: 10–15 minutes
Clinically important, potentially serious interactions with: digoxin, methotrexate, quinolones

Reactions

Skin

Acral erythema
(1999): Azurdia RM+, *Clin Exp Dermatol* 24, 64
(1998): Calista D+, *J Eur Acad Dermatol Venereol* 10, 274
(1997): Arranz FR+, *Arch Dermatol* 133, 499
(1997): Demircay Z+, *Int J Dermatol* 36, 593
(1995): Dechaufour F+, *Ann Dermatol Venereol* (French) 120, 219
(1992): Rongioletti F+, *J Am Acad Dermatol* 26, 284
(1991): Rongioletti F+, *J Cutan Pathol* 18, 453
(1991): Brown J+, *J Am Acad Dermatol* 24, 1023
(1989): Kroll SS+, *Ann Plast Surg* 23, 263
(1989): Alexander J, *Oncol Nurs Forum* 16, 829
(1989): Oksenhendler E+, *Eur J Cancer Clin Oncol* 25, 1181
Acral erythrodysesthesia syndrome
(1993): Waltzer JF+, *Arch Dermatol* 129, 43 (bullous variety)
(1991): Baack BR+, *J Am Acad Dermatol* 24, 457
(1989): Kampmann KK+, *Cancer* 63, 2482 (bullous variety)
(1988): Shall L+, *Br J Dermatol* 119, 249
(1986): Crider MK+, *Arch Dermatol* 122, 1023 (>5%)
(1985): Cardonnier C+, *Ann Intern Med* 97, 783
(1985): Baer MR+, *Ann Intern Med* 102, 556 (bullous variety)
(1985): Peters WG+, *Ann Intern Med* 103, 805 (bullous variety)
(1985): Walker IR+, *Arch Dermatol* 121, 1240 (10–67%, dose-related)
(1985): Levine LE+, *Arch Dermatol* 121, 102
(1983): Herzig RH+, *Blood* 62, 361 (1–5%)
(1982): Burgdorf WHC+, *Ann Intern Med* 97, 61
Actinic keratoses (with pruritus and erythema)
(1989): Kerker BJ+, *Semin Dermatol* 8, 173
Acute febrile neutrophilic dermatosis (Sweet's syndrome)
(1993): Torri O+, *Ann Dermatol Venereol* (French) 120, 884
Allergic edema (sic)
Bullous eruption
(1992): Richards C+, *Oncol Nurs Forum* 19, 1191
Desquamation
(1992): Richards C+, *Oncol Nurs Forum* 19, 1191
Erythema
(1998): Taverna C+, *Schweiz Med Wochenschr* (German) 128, 1117
(1992): Richards C+, *Oncol Nurs Forum* 19, 1191
Erythema and swelling of ears
(1990): Krulder JWM+, *Eur J Cancer* 26, 649
Erythroderma (generalized)
(1988): Benson PM+, *J Assoc Military Derm* XIV, 28 (passim)
Exanthems
(1988): Benson PM+, *J Assoc Military Derm* XIV, 28
(1986): Morant R+, *Schweiz Med Wochenschr* (German) 116, 1415 (60%)
(1983): Herzig RH+, *Blood* 62, 361 (1–5%)
(1983): Shah SS+, *Cancer Treat Rep* 67, 405*
Exfoliative dermatitis
(1989): Williams SF+, *Br J Haematol* 73, 274
Freckles (1–10%)
Herpes zoster
(1973): Stevens DA+, *N Engl J Med* 289, 873
Neutrophilic eccrine hidradenitis
(1997): Jegasothy SM+, Pittsburgh, American Academy of Dermatology Meeting (SF), Gross and Microscopic
(1995): Kanzaki H+, *J Dermatol* 22, 137
(1993): Thorisdottir K+, *J Am Acad Dermatol* 28, 775
(1992): Bernstein EF+, *Br J Dermatol* 127, 529 (recurrent)
(1991): Vion B+, *Dermatologica* 183, 70
(1990): Hurt MA+, *Arch Dermatol* 126, 73
(1989): Bailey DL+, *Pediatr Dermatol* 6, 33
(1989): Kerker BJ+, *Semin Dermatol* 8, 173
(1987): Katsanis E+, *Am J Pediatr Hematol Oncol* 9, 204
(1984): Flynn TC+, *J Am Acad Dermatol* 11, 584
Petechiae
(1998): Taverna C+, *Schweiz Med Wochenschr* (German) 128, 1117
Pruritus (1–10%)
Rash (sic) (>10%)
Seborrheic keratoses (inflammation of) (Leser–Trélat syndrome)
(1999): Williams JV+, *J Am Acad Dermatol* 40, 643
(1979): Kechijian P+, *Ann Intern Med* 91, 868
Syringosquamous metaplasia (sic)
(1990): Bhawan J+, *Am J Dermatopathol* 12, 1
Toxic epidermal necrolysis
(1998): Figueiredo MS+, *Rev Assoc Med Bras* (Portuguese) 44, 53
Ulceration
(1969): Bodey GP+, *Cancer Chemother Rep* 53, 59
Urticaria
Vasculitis*
(1998): Ahmed I+, *Mayo Clin Proc* 73, 239
(1989): Williams SF+, *Br J Haematol* 73, 274
(1989): Kerker BJ+, *Semin Dermatol* 8, 173

Hair

Hair – alopecia (1–10%)
(1988): Benson PM+, *J Assoc Military Derm* XIV, 28 (passim)
(1986): Morant R+, *Schweiz Med Wochenschr* (German) 116, 1415 (100%)
(1970): Upjohn Company, *Clin Pharmacol Ther* 11, 155
(1969): Bodey GP+, *Cancer Chemother Rep* 53, 59

Nails

Nails – Mees' lines
(1982): Jeanmougin M+, *Ann Dermatol Venereol* (French) 109, 169
Nails – transverse leukonychia
(1990): Bader-Meunier B+, *Ann Pediatr Paris* (French) 37, 337

Other

Anal ulceration (>10%)
Anaphylactoid reaction
(1997): Blanca M+, *Allergy* 52, 1009
(1989): Williams SF+, *Br J Haematol* 73, 274
(1980): Rassiga AL+, *Arch Intern Med* 104, 425
Hypersensitivity
(1992): Weiss RB, *Semin Oncol* 19, 458
Injection-site cellulitis (1–10%)
Myalgia (1–10%)
Oral mucosal lesions
(1986): Morant R+, *Schweiz Med Wochenschr* (German) 116, 1415 (1–5%)
(1978): Levine N+, *Cancer Treat Rev* 5, 67
(1974): Levantine A+, *Br J Dermatol* 90, 239 (66%)
(1971): Lang HN+, *Med J Aust* 2, 187
(1968): Howard JP+, *Cancer* 21, 341
Oral ulceration (>10%)
Pseudotumor cerebri
(1999): Fort JA+, *Ann Pharmacother* 33, 576
Thrombophlebitis (>10%)
Stomatitis
(1988): Benson PM+, *J Assoc Military Derm* XIV, 28 (passim)

***Note:** Vasculitis, a part of the cytarabine syndrome, consists of fever, malaise, myalgia, conjunctivitis, arthralgia and a diffuse erythematous maculopapular eruption that occurs from 6 to 12 hours following the administration of the drug.

DACARBAZINE

Synonym: DIC
Trade name: DTIC-Dome (Bayer)
Other common trade names: *Dacatic; D.T.I.C.; Deticene; Detimedac*
Indications: Malignant melanoma, carcinomas
Category: Antineoplastic
Half-life: initial: 20–40 minutes
Clinically important, potentially serious interactions with: aldesleukin, phenytoin

Reactions

Skin

Angioedema
(1981): Wassilew SW+, *Hautarzt* (German) 32 (Suppl 5) 453
Erythema
Exanthems
(1981): Wassilew SW+, *Hautarzt* (German) 32 (Suppl 5) 453
Fixed eruption
(1982): Koehn GG+, *Arch Dermatol* 118, 1018
Flushing (1–10%)
(1982): Dunagin WG, *Semin Oncol* 9, 14
(1978): Levine N+, *Cancer Treat Rev* 5, 67 (100%)
Photosensitivity (<1%)
(1989): Serrano G+, *Photodermatol* 6, 140
(1982): Koehn GG+, *Arch Dermatol* 118, 1018
(1981): Wassilew SW+, *Hautarzt* (German) 32 (Suppl 5) 453
(1981): Yung CW+, *J Am Acad Dermatol* 4, 541
(1981): Bonifazi E+, *Contact Dermatitis* 7, 161
(1980): Beck TM+, *Cancer Treat Rep* 64, 725
(1980): Kunze J+, *Z Hautkr* (German) 55, 100
(1980): Ippen H, *Dtsch Med Wochenschr* (German) 105, 531
(1980): Bolling R+, *Hautarzt* (German) 31, 602
Rash (sic) (1–10%)
Urticaria
(1995): Bourry C+, *Therapie* (French) 50, 588
(1981): Wassilew SW+, *Hautarzt* (German) 32 (Suppl 5) 453
Vasculitis

Hair

Hair – alopecia (1–10%)
(1978): Levine N+, *Cancer Treat Rev* 5, 67

Nails

Nails – pigmentation
(1984): Daniel CR+, *J Am Acad Dermatol* 10, 250

Other

Anaphylactoid reaction (1–10%)
Dysgeusia (1–10%) (metallic taste)
Hypersensitivity
(1992): Weiss RB, *Semin Oncol* 19, 458
Injection-site burning (>10%)
Injection-site cellulitis
(1989): Kerker BJ+, *Semin Dermatol* 8, 173
Injection-site dermatitis
(1987): Dufresne RG, *Cutis* 39, 197
Injection-site necrosis (>10%)
(1987): Dufresne RG, *Cutis* 39, 197
Injection-site pain (>10%)
Injection-site phlebitis
(1989): Kerker BJ+, *Semin Dermatol* 8, 173
Myalgia (1–10%)
Paresthesias (facial)
Stomatitis (<1%)

DACTINOMYCIN

Synonyms: ACT; actinomycin D
Trade name: Cosmegen (Merck)
Other common trade names: *Ac-De; Cosmegen Lyovac; Lyovac*
Indications: Melanonas, sarcomas
Category: Antineoplastic antibiotic
Half-life: 36 hours
Clinically important, potentially serious interactions with: aldesleukin

Reactions

Skin

Acne (>10%)
(1993): Blatt J+, *Med Pediatr Oncol* 21, 373
(1983): Bronner AK+, *J Am Acad Dermatol* 9, 645
(1982): Dunagin WG, *Semin Oncol* 9, 14
(1974): Levantine A+, *Br J Dermatol* 90, 239 (>5%)
(1969): Epstein EH+, *N Engl J Med* 281, 1094
Bullous pemphigoid
(1982): Amer MH+, *Int J Dermatol* 21. 32
Cellulitis
(1989): Kerker BJ+, *Semin Dermatol* 8, 173
Cheilitis
Dermatitis (sic)
(1975): Cassady JR+, *Radiology* 115, 171
Erythema
Erythema, brawny localized
(1997): Coppes MJ+, *Med Pediatr Oncol* 29, 226
Erythema multiforme
Exanthems
Folliculitis
(1981): Henkes J+, *Actas Dermosifiliogr* (Spanish) 72, 469
(1969): Epstein EH+, *N Engl J Med* 281, 1094
Keratoses (reactivation of)
(1989): Kerker BJ+, *Semin Dermatol* 8, 173
Pigmentation
(1995): Kanwar VS+, *Med Pediatr Oncol* 24, 329
(1978): Levine N+, *Cancer Treat Rev* 5, 67 (100%)
(1971): Ma HK+, *J Obstet Gynaecol Br Commonw* 78, 166
Pruritus
(1989): Kerker BJ+, *Semin Dermatol* 8, 173
Pustular eruption
(1983): Bronner AK+, *J Am Acad Dermatol* 9, 645
(1969): Epstein EH+, *N Engl J Med* 281, 1094
Radiation recall (>10%)
(1997): Coppes MJ+, *Med Pediatr Oncol* 29, 226
(1978): Levine N+, *Cancer Treat Rev* 5, 67 (50%)
(1975): Dreizen S+, *Postgrad Med* 58, 150
(1974): Levantine A+, *Br J Dermatol* 90, 239 (>5%)
Serpentine supravenous hyperpigmentation (sic)
(2000): Marcoux D+, *J Am Acad Dermatol* 43, 540 (with vincristine)
Toxic epidermal necrolysis
Urticaria

Hair

Hair – alopecia (>10%)
(1964): Falkson G+, *Br J Dermatol* 76, 309

Other

Anaphylactoid reaction (<1%)
Injection-site extravasation (>10%)
(1997): Coppes MJ+, *Med Pediatr Oncol* 29, 226
Injection-site necrosis (>10%)
(1987): Dufresne RG, *Cutis* 39, 197
Injection-site phlebitis (>10%)
Myalgia
Oral mucosal lesions
(1983): Bronner AK+, *J Am Acad Dermatol* 9, 645 (>5%)
(1975): Dreizen S+, *Postgrad Med* 58, 150
(1972): Cridland MD, *Drugs* 3, 352
Phlebitis
(1989): Kerker BJ+, *Semin Dermatol* 8, 173
Stomatitis (ulcerative) (>5%)

DALTEPARIN

Trade name: Fragmin (Pharmacia & Upjohn)
Other common trade name: *Fragmine*
Indications: Prophylaxis of deep vein thrombosis
Category: Anticoagulant; low molecular weight heparin
Half-life: 4–8 hours
Clinically important, potentially serious interactions with: anticoagulants, aspirin, ketorolac, NSAIDs, platelet inhibitors, salicylates, warfarin

Reactions

Skin

Allergic reactions (sic) (1–10%)
Bullous eruption (1–10%)
(1999): Tong, M, Kota Kinabalu, Maylasia (from Internet) (observation)
Exanthems (<1%)
Pruritus (1–10%)
Rash (sic) (1–10%)

Other

Anaphylactoid reaction (1–10%)
Injection-site hematoma (1–10%)
Injection-site pain (1–10%)
Necrosis

DANAZOL

Trade name: Danocrine (Sanofi)
Other common trade names: *Azol; Bonzol; Cyclomen; D-Zol; Danol; Ladogal; Winobanin; Zoldan-A*
Indications: Endometriosis, fibrocystic breast disease
Category: Synthetic pituitary gonadotropin inhibitor
Half-life: ~4.5 hours
Clinically important, potentially serious interactions with: anticoagulants, carbamazepine, cyclosporine, insulin, lovastatin, oral contraceptives, retinoids

Reactions

Skin

Acne (>10%)
(1982): Madanes AE+, *Ann Intern Med* 96, 625 (20%)
(1980): Hosea SW+, *Ann Intern Med* 93, 809 (8%)
(1979): Greenberg RD, *Cutis* 24, 431
(1977): Spooner JB+, *J Int Med Res* 5 (Suppl 3), 15
Angioedema
(1993): Litt JZ, Beachwood, OH, personal case (observation)
(1988): Guillet G+, *Dermatologica* 177, 370
Diaphoresis (3%)
(1977): Spooner JB+, *J Int Med Res* 5 (Suppl 3), 15
Edema (>10%)
(1977): Spooner JB+, *J Int Med Res* 5 (Suppl 3), 15
Erythema multiforme
(1992): Reynolds NJ+, *Clin Exp Dermatol* 17, 140
(1988): Gately LE+, *Ann Intern Med* 109, 85
Exanthems
(1993): Litt JZ, Beachwood, OH, personal case (observation)
(1989): Ahn YS+, *Ann Intern Med* 111, 723 (6%)
(1982): Madanes AE+, *Ann Intern Med* 96, 625
(1975): *Drug Ther Bull* 13, 94
Flushing
(1988): Henzl MR+, *N Engl J Med* 318, 485 (68%)
(1980): Hosea SW+, *Ann Intern Med* 93, 809 (12%)
(1977): Spooner JB+, *J Int Med Res* 5 (Suppl 3), 15
(1975): *Drug Ther Bull* 13, 94
Guillain–Barré syndrome
(1985): Hory B+, *Am J Med* 79, 111
Lupus erythematosus
(1991): Sassolas B+, *Br J Dermatol* 125, 190
(1988): Guillet G+, *Dermatologica* 177, 370
(1982): Fretwell MD, *Allergy Clin Immunol* 69, 306
Lymphomatoid papulosis
(1985): Wise C+, *Fertil Steril* 44, 702
Petechiae
Photosensitivity (<1%)
Pruritus
(1989): Ahn YS+, *Ann Intern Med* 111, 723 (3.5%)
Purpura
(1990): Taillan B+, *Presse Med* (French) 19, 721
Rash (sic) (3%)
(1977): Spooner JB+, *J Int Med Res* 5 (Suppl 3), 15
Seborrhea
(1989): Ahn YS+, *Ann Intern Med* 111, 723
(1982): Madanes AE+, *Ann Intern Med* 96, 625 (30%)
(1981): Duff P+, *Am J Obstet Gynecol* 141, 349 (passim)
(1977): Spooner JB+, *J Int Med Res* 5 (Suppl 3), 15
Stevens–Johnson syndrome
Urticaria

Hair

Hair – alopecia
(1989): Ahn YS+, *Ann Intern Med* 111, 723 (3.5%)
(1981): Duff P+, *Am J Obstet Gynecol* 141, 349
(1980): Hosea SW+, *Ann Intern Med* 93, 809 (17%)
Hair – hirsutism (>10%)
(1991): Bates GW+, *Clin Obstet Gynecol* 34, 848
(1989): Ahn YS+, *Ann Intern Med* 111, 723 (3.5%)
(1982): Madanes AE+, *Ann Intern Med* 96, 625 (7%)
(1980): Hosea SW+, *Ann Intern Med* 93, 809 (8%)

Other

Acute intermittent porphyria
Bleeding gums
Breast changes (sic)
(1977): Spooner JB+, *J Int Med Res* 5 (Suppl 3), 15
Candidal vaginitis (<1%)
(1977): Spooner JB+, *J Int Med Res* 5 (Suppl 3), 15
Gingivitis
Paresthesias
Vaginal dryness (sic)

DANTROLENE

Trade name: Dantrium (Procter & Gamble)
Other common trade names: *Dantamacrin; Dantrolen*
Indications: Spasticity; malignant hyperthermia
Category: Skeletal muscle relaxant
Half-life: 8.7 hours
Clinically important, potentially serious interactions with: CNS depressants, clindamycin, clofibrate, estrogens, MAO inhibitors, phenothiazines, tolbutamide, verapamil, warfarin

Reactions

Skin

Acne
(1981): Pembroke AC+, *Br J Dermatol* 104, 465
(1980): Dykes MHM, *JAMA* 231, 862
Chills (1–10%)
Dermatitis (sic)
Diaphoresis
Erythema
Exanthems
(1980): Dykes MHM, *JAMA* 231, 862
Photosensitivity
Pruritus
Rash (sic) (>10%)
Urticaria

Hair

Hair – abnormal growth

Other

Anaphylactoid reaction
Dysgeusia
Malignant lymphoma
(1980): Wan HH+, *Postgrad Med J* 56, 261
Myalgia
Thrombophlebitis
Tremor

DAPSONE

Trade name: Dapsone (Jacobus)
Other common trade names: *Avlosulfon; Dapson; Dapson-Fatol; Protogen; Sulfona*
Indications: Leprosy, dermatitis herpetiformis
Category: Antileprotic; dermatitis herpetiformis suppressant
Half-life: 10–50 hours
Clinically important, potentially serious interactions with: amprenavir, didanosine, folic acid antagonists, nelfinavir, probenecid, rifampin, ritonavir, saquinavir, trimethoprim

Reactions

Skin

Bullous eruption (<1%)
(1984): Alarcon GS+, *Arthritis Rheum* 27, 1071
Cyanosis
(1981): Editorial, *Lancet* 2, 184
Dapsone syndrome*
(1998): Kumar RH+, *Indian J Lepr* 70, 271 (17 cases)
(1997): McKenna KE+, *Br J Dermatol* 137, 657
(1994): Hiran S+, *J Assoc Physicians India* 42, 497
(1994): Stephen G+, *J Assoc Physicians India* 42, 72
(1994): Risse L+, *Ann Dermatol Venereol* (French) 121, 242
(1994): Barnard GF+, *Am J Gastroenterol* 89, 2057
(1994): Saito S+, *Clin Exp Dermatol* 19, 152
(1992): Kraus A+, *J Rheumatol* 19, 178
(1991): Ramanan C+, *Indian J Lepr* 63, 226
(1988): Grayson ML+, *Lancet* 1, 531
(1987): Khare AK+, *Indian J Lepr* 59, 106
(1985): Sharma VK+, *Indian J Lepr* 57, 807
(1982): Kromann NP+, *Arch Dermatol* 118, 531
(1981): Tomecki KJ+, *Arch Dermatol* 117, 38
Epidermolysis bullosa
(1992): Kong LN, *Chung Hua Li Tsa Chih* (Chinese) 27, 495
Erythema multiforme (<1%)
(1994): Pertel P+, *Clin Infect Dis* 18, 630
(1993): Stern RS, *Arch Dermatol* 129, 301 (passim)
(1981): Frey HM+, *Ann Intern Med* 94, 777
(1980): Dutta RK, *Lepr India* 52, 306
(1970): Millikan LE+, *Arch Dermatol* 102, 220
(1961): Browne SG+, *BMJ* 1, 550 (passim)
Erythema nodosum
(1993): Stern RS, *Arch Dermatol* 129, 301 (passim)
(1981): Editorial, *Lancet* 2, 184
(1970): Millikan LE+, *Arch Dermatol* 102, 220
Erythroderma
(1989): Patki AH+, *Lepr Rev* 60, 274
Exanthems (1–5%)
(1993): Stern RS, *Arch Dermatol* 129, 301 (passim)
(1986): Lindskov R+, *Dermatologica* 172, 214 (6%)
(1981): Frey HM+, *Ann Intern Med* 94, 777
(1981): Tomecki KJ+, *Arch Dermatol* 117, 38
(1970): Millikan LE+, *Arch Dermatol* 102, 220
(1968): Ramanujam K+, *Lepr India* 40, 6
(1965): Rosenthal AL+, *Arch Intern Med* 115, 73 (1–5%)
(1964): Browne SG, *BMJ* 2, 1041
(1963): Browne SG, *BMJ* 2, 664 (2%)
Exfoliative dermatitis (<1%)
(1993): Stern RS, *Arch Dermatol* 129, 301 (passim)
(1981): Frey HM+, *Ann Intern Med* 94, 777
(1981): Tomecki KJ+, *Arch Dermatol* 117, 38
(1980): Lal S+, *Lepr India* 52, 302
(1971): Browne SG, *BMJ* 2, 558 (passim)
(1970): Millikan LE+, *Arch Dermatol* 102, 220
(1963): Browne SG, *BMJ* 2, 664
(1961): Browne SG+, *BMJ* 1, 550 (passim)
Fixed eruption
(1988): Tham SN+, *Singapore Med J* 29, 300
(1982): Sinha MR, *Lepr India* 54, 152
(1964): Browne SG, *BMJ* 2, 1041 (1–5%)
Lichenoid eruption
Lupus erythematosus (<1%)
(1992): Kraus A+, *J Rheumatol* 19, 178
(1984): Alarcon GS+, *Arthritis Rheum* 27, 1071 (bullous)
(1979): Lang PG, *J Am Acad Dermatol* 1, 479
(1979): Fine RM, *Int J Dermatol* 18, 811
(1974): Vandersteen PR+, *Arch Dermatol* 110, 95
Photosensitivity (<1%)
(1994): Berger TG+, *Arch Dermatol* 130, 609 (in HIV-infected) (4 cases)
(1989): Dhanapaul S, *Lepr Rev* 60, 147
(1988): Fumey SM+, *Z Hautkr* (German) 63, 53
(1987): Joseph MS, *Lepr Rev* 58, 425
(1979): Lang PG, *J Am Acad Dermatol* 1, 479
Pigmentation
(1997): David KP+, *Trans R Soc Trop Med Hyg* 91, 204 ("hyperpigmented dermal macules")
(1977): Sakurai I+, *Int J Lepr Other Mycobact Dis* 45, 343
(1976): Shelley WB+, *Br J Dermatol* 95, 79 (bluish-gray)
(1964): Browne SG, *BMJ* 2, 1041
(1963): Browne SG, *BMJ* 2, 664
(1961): Browne SG+, *BMJ* 1, 550
Pruritus
(1964): Browne SG, *BMJ* 2, 1041
Purpura
(1968): Ramanujam K+, *Lepr India* 40, 6
Rash (sic)
(2000): Chogle A+, *Indian J Gastroenterol* 19, 85
(1996): Beumont MG+, *Am J Med* 100, 611
Scleroderma
(1990): May DG+, *Clin Pharm Ther* 48, 286
Stevens–Johnson syndrome
(1994): Pertel P+, *Clin Infect Dis* 18, 630
(1961): Browne SG+, *BMJ* 1, 550 (passim)
Subcorneal pustular dermatosis
(1983): Halevy S+, *Acta Derm Venereol* (Stockh) 63, 441
Toxic epidermal necrolysis (<1%)
(1993): Stern RS, *Arch Dermatol* 129, 301 (passim)
(1993): Fitzpatrick TB+, *Dermatologic Capsule and Comment* 15, 10 (observation)
(1988): Phillips-Howard PA+, *Br Med J Clin Res Ed* 296, 1605
(1983): Katoch K+, *Lepr India* 55, 133
(1981): Editorial, *Lancet* 2, 184
(1961): Browne SG+, *BMJ* 1, 550
Toxic erythema (sic)
(1993): Stern RS, *Arch Dermatol* 129, 301 (passim)
Urticaria
(1970): Millikan LE+, *Arch Dermatol* 102, 220

Nails

Nails – Beau's lines (transverse nail bands)
(1989): Patki AH+, *Lepr Rev* 60, 274
(1984): Daniel CR+, *J Am Acad Dermatol* 10, 250
(1988): Grayson ML+, *Lancet* 1, 531

Other

Acute intermittent porphyria
Hypersensitivity*
(2000): Chogle A+, *Indian J Gastroenterol* 19, 85
(1998): Pei-Lin Ng P+, *J Am Acad Dermatol* 39, 646
(1998): Siegfried EC+, *J Am Acad Dermatol* 39, 797 (passim)
(1998): Schlienger RG+, *Epilepsia* 39, S3 (passim)
(1996): Prussick R+, *J Am Acad Dermatol* 35, 346
(1995): Bocquet H+, *Ann Dermatol Venereol* (French) 122, 514
(1984): Mohamed KN, *Lepr Rev* 55, 385
Nodular panniculitis
(1986): Uplekar MW+, *Indian J Lepr* 58, 286
Oral mucosal eruption
(1981): Frey HM+, *Ann Intern Med* 94, 777
Oral mucosal fixed eruption

Oral mucosal pigmentation
(1964): Browne SG, *BMJ* 2, 1041
Porphyria cutanea tarda
(1992): Shelley WB+, *Advanced Dermatologic Diagnosis*, WB Saunders, 414 (passim)

***Note:** A hypersensitivity reaction – termed the "sulfone syndrome" or "dapsone syndrome" – may infrequently develop during the first six weeks of treatment. This syndrome consists of exfoliative dermatitis, fever, malaise, nausea, anorexia, hepatitis, jaundice, lymphadenopathy and hemolytic anemia. See (1982): Kromann NP+, *Arch Dermatol* 118, 531

DAUNORUBICIN

Synonyms: daunomycin; DNR; rubidomycin
Trade names: Cerubidine (Bedford); DaunoXome (Nexstar)
Other common trade name: *Daunoxome*
Indications: Acute leukemias
Category: Antineoplastic
Half-life: 14–20 hours
Clinically important, potentially serious interactions with:, aldesleukin, amphotericin B, cyclosporine, quinolones, verapamil

Reactions

Skin

Angioedema
(1983): Bronner AK+, *J Am Acad Dermatol* 9, 645
(1981): Weiss RB+, *Ann Intern Med* 94, 66 (1–5%)
(1978): Levine N+, *Cancer Treat Rev* 5, 67
(1970): Freeman AI, *Cancer Chemother Rep* 54, 475
Chills (<1%)
Contact dermatitis
(1986): Eddy JL+, *Oncol Nurs Forum* 13, 9
(1975): Reich SD+, *Cancer Chemother Rep* 59, 677
Erythema
Exanthems
(1978): Levine N+, *Cancer Treat Rev* 5, 67 (2%)
(1970): Zanoni G+, *Blut* (German) 25, 20
Flushing
Folliculitis
(1997): Fournier S+, *Arch Dermatol* 133, 918 (disseminated)
Hypopigmentation
(1975): Dreizen S+, *Postgrad Med* 58, 150
Neutrophilic eccrine hidradenitis
(1993): Thorisdottir K+, *J Am Acad Dermatol* 28, 775
Pigmentation
(1992): Anderson LL+, *J Am Acad Dermatol* 26, 255
(1984): Kelly TM+, *Arch Dermatol* 120, 262
Pruritus
Rash (sic) (<1%)
Urticaria (<1%)
(1983): Bronner AK+, *J Am Acad Dermatol* 9, 645
(1981): Weiss RB+, *Ann Intern Med* 94, 66 (1–5%)
(1970): Freeman AI, *Cancer Chemother Rep* 54, 475

Hair

Hair – alopecia (>10%)
(1997): Fournier S+, *Arch Dermatol* 133, 918
(1972): Cridland MD, *Drugs* 3, 352
(1972): Jacquillat C+, *BMJ* 4, 468
(1969): Bonadonna G+, *BMJ* 3, 503

Nails

Nails – pigmentation (<1%)
(1983): James WD+, *Arch Dermatol* 119, 334
(1982): Daniel CR+, *Cutis* 30, 348
(1979): Hanada T+, *Nippon Naika Gakkai Zasshi* (Japanese) 68, 1319 (bands)
(1978): de Marinis M+, *Ann Intern Med* 89, 516

Other

Anaphylactoid reaction
Injection-site cellulitis
(1989): Kerker BJ+, *Semin Dermatol* 8, 173
Injection-site necrosis (1–10%)
(1987): Dufresne RG, *Cutis* 39, 197
(1979): Dragon LH+, *Ann Intern Med* 91, 58
Injection-site phlebitis
(1989): Kerker BJ+, *Semin Dermatol* 8, 173
Injection-site ulceration (1–10%)
(1984): Cox RF, *Am J Hosp Pharm* 41, 2410
Oral mucosal lesions
(1983): Bronner AK+, *J Am Acad Dermatol* 9, 645 (>5%)
(1975): Dreizen S+, *Postgrad Med* 58, 75
Stomatitis (>10%)
(1969): Bonadonna G+, *BMJ* 3, 503

DEFEROXAMINE

Trade name: Desferal (Novartis)
Other common trade name: *Desferin*
Indications: Hemochromatosis, acute iron overload
Category: Chelating agent; antidote
Half-life: 6.1 hours
Clinically important, potentially serious interactions with: ascorbic acid, iron salts

Reactions

Skin

Acne
Angioedema
(1984): Romeo MA+, *J Inherited Metab Dis* 7, 121
Dermatitis (sic)
(1988): Venencie PY+, *Ann Dermatol Venereol* (French) 115, 1174
Edema (<1%)
Erythema (<1%)
Erythema multiforme
Exanthems
Flushing (<1%)
Pigmentation
Pruritus (<1%)
(1984): Romeo MA+, *J Inherited Metab Dis* 7, 121
Purpura
Rash (sic) (<1%)
Toxic epidermal necrolysis
Urticaria (<1%)

Other

Anaphylactoid reaction (<1%)
Injection-site erythema
Injection-site inflammation (1–10%)
Injection-site pain (1–10%)
Oral mucosal lesions

DELAVIRDINE

Synonym: U-90152S
Trade name: Rescriptor (Pharmacia & Upjohn)
Indications: HIV-1 infection
Category: Antiretroviral; non-nucleoside reverse transcriptase inhibitor
Half-life: 5.8 hours
Clinically important, potentially serious interactions with: alprazolam, amphetamines, antacids, antiarrhythmics, anticoagulants, astemizole, calcium channel blockers, carbamazepine, cimetidine, cisapride, clarithromycin, dapsone, ergot, famotidine, fluoxetine, indinavir, ketoconazole, lansoprazole, midazolam, omeprazole, phenytoin, quinidine, rifabutin, rifampin, saquinavir, terfenadine, triazolam, warfarin

Reactions

Skin
Allergic reactions (sic) (<2%)
Angioedema (<2%)
Dermatitis (sic) (<2%)
Desquamation (<2%)
Diaphoresis (<2%)
Ecchymoses (<2%)
Edema (<2%)
Epidermal cyst (<2%)
Erythema (<2%)
Erythema multiforme (<2%)
Exanthems (6.6%)
Folliculitis (<2%)
Fungal dermatitis (sic) (<2%)
Lip edema (<2%)
Nodule (sic) (<2%)
Peripheral edema (<2%)
Petechiae (<2%)
Pruritus (<2%)
Purpura (<2%)
Rash (sic) (9.8%)
Seborrhea (<2%)
Stevens–Johnson syndrome (<2%)
Urticaria (<2%)
Vasculitis (<2%)
Vesiculobullous eruption (<2%)
Xerosis (<2%)

Hair
Hair – alopecia (<2%)

Nails
Nails – disorder (sic) (<2%)

Other
Aphthous stomatitis (<2%)
Dysgeusia (<2%)
Gingivitis (<2%)
Gynecomastia (<2%)
Hyperesthesia (<2%)
Hypesthesia (<2%)
Myalgia (<2%)
Oral ulceration (<2%)
Paresthesias (<2%)
Sialorrhea (<2%)
Stomatitis (<2%)
Tingling (<2%)
Tongue edema (<2%)
Vaginal candidiasis (<2%)
Xerostomia (<2%)

DEMECLOCYCLINE

Trade name: Declomycin (Lederle)
Other common trade names: *Ledermicina; Ledermycin; Rynabron*
Indications: Various infections caused by susceptible organisms
Category: Tetracycline antibiotic and antiprotozoal
Half-life: 10–17 hours
Clinically important, potentially serious interactions with: antacids, calcium carbonate, cephalosporins, digoxin, iron salts, oral contraceptives, penicillins, warfarin, zinc salts. Also **food**

Reactions

Skin
Acne
(1969): Weary PE+, *Arch Dermatol* 100, 179
Angioedema
Bullous eruption
Candidiasis
Exanthems
Exfoliative dermatitis (<1%)
Fixed eruption
(1978): Jolly HW+, *Arch Dermatol* 114, 1484
(1970): Savin JA, *Br J Dermatol* 83, 546
(1970): Delaney TJ, *Br J Dermatol* 83, 357
(1968): Sarkany I, *Proc R Soc Med* 61, 891
Lichenoid eruption
(1972): Jones HE+, *Arch Dermatol* 106, 58
Lupus erythematosus
Perianal rash
Photosensitivity (1–10%)
(1984): Kromann N+, *Ugeskr Laeger* (Danish) 146, 515
(1980): Stern RS+, *Arch Dermatol* 116, 1269
(1974): Maibach HI+, *Arch Dermatol* 109, 97 (1.5%) (lichenoid)
(1972): Jones HE+, *Arch Dermatol* 106, 58 (lichenoid)
(1971): Ippen H, *Hautarzt* (German) 22, 549
(1971): Kahn G+, *Arch Dermatol* 103, 94
(1971): Frost P+, *JAMA* 216, 326 (90%)
(1968): Stratigos JD+, *Br J Dermatol* 80, 391
(1967): Kotani Y, *Acta Dermatol Kyoto Engl Ed* (Japanese) 62, 188
(1965): Clendenning WE, *Arch Dermatol* 91, 628 (20%)
(1962): Hicks JH, *South Med J* 55, 357
(1962): de Veber LL, *Can Med Assoc J* 86, 168
(1961): Orentreich N+, *Arch Dermatol* 83, 68
(1961): Shapiro JL+, *JAMA* 176, 596
(1960): Fuhrman DL+, *Arch Dermatol* 82, 244
(1960): Falk MS, *JAMA* 172, 1156
(1960): Morris WE, *JAMA* 172, 1155
(1960): Carey BW, *JAMA* 172, 1196 (1.5%)
Phototoxic reaction
(1968): Blank H+, *Arch Dermatol* 97, 1 (90%)
(1961): Saslaw S, *N Engl J Med* 264, 1301
(1961): Cahn MM+, *Arch Dermatol* 84, 485
Pigmentation
Pruritus (<1%)
Pruritus ani
Purpura
Stevens–Johnson syndrome
Toxic epidermal necrolysis
(1988): Massullo RE+, *J Am Acad Dermatol* 19, 358
Urticaria

Nails
Nails – onycholysis
Nails – photo-onycholysis
(1977): Bethell HJN, *BMJ* 2, 96
(1974): Bettley FR+, *Proc R Soc Med* 67, 600
(1973): Verma KC+, *Indian J Dermatol* 18, 23
(1972): Cabre J+, *Actas Dermosifiliogr* (Spanish) 63, 211
(1962): de Veber LL, *Can Med Assoc J* 86, 168
(1961): Orentreich N+, *Arch Dermatol* 83, 68
Nails – pigmentation (<1%)

Other

Anaphylactoid reaction (<1%)
Glossitis
Mucous membrane pigmentation
Oral mucosal eruption
(1964): Martin WJ, *Med Clin North Am* 48, 255
Paresthesias (<1%)
Porphyria
(1979): Boissonnas A+, *Nouv Presse Med* (French) 8, 210
Pseudotumor cerebri
Tongue pigmentation
Tooth discoloration

DENILEUKIN

Trade name: Ontak (Ligand)
Indications: Cutaneous T-cell lymphoma
Category: Antineoplastic
Half-life: distribution: 2–5 minutes; terminal: 70–80 minutes
Clinically important, potentially serious interactions with: no data

Reactions

Skin

Allergic reactions (1%)
Bullous eruption
Chills (81%)
Diaphoresis (10%)
Ecchymoses
Edema (47%)
Exanthems
Flushing
Infection (48%)
Petechiae
Pruritus (20%)
Purpura
Rash (sic) (34%)
Urticaria
Vesicular eruption

Other

Anaphylactoid reaction (1%)
Hypersensitivity (69%)
Infusion-site reaction (8%)
Myalgia (18%)
Paresthesias (13%)
Phlebitis
Thrombophlebitis

DESIPRAMINE

Trade name: Norpramin (Aventis)
Other common trade names: *Deprexan; Nebril; Nortimil; Pertofran; Pertofrane; Petylyl; PMS-Desipramine*
Indications: Depression
Category: Tricyclic antidepressant and antipanic
Half-life: 7–60 hours
Clinically important, potentially serious interactions with: alcohol, anticholinergics, barbiturates, carbamazepine, cimetidine, clonidine, CNS depressants, diltiazem, epinephrine, fluoxetine, guanethidine, haloperidol, MAO inhibitors, phenytoin, quinidine, SSRIs, verapamil, warfarin

Reactions

Skin

Acne
Allergic reactions (sic) (<1%)
(1987): Joffe RT+, *Can J Psychiatry* 32, 695
(1987): Richter MA+, *Am J Psychiatry* 144, 526
Angioedema
(1963): Mann AM+, *Can Med Assoc J* 88, 1102
Diaphoresis (1–10%)
(1965): Editorial, *JAMA* 194, 82
Ecchymoses
(1968): Rachmilewitz EA+, *Blood* 32, 524
Edema
Erythema
Exanthems
(1988): McLean JD, *Can J Psychiatry* 33, 331
(1988): Biederman J+, *J Clin Psychiatry* 49, 178 (5.8%)
(1987): Joffe RT+, *Can J Psychiatry* 32, 695 (6.2%)
(1987): Ellsworth A+, *Drug Intell Clin Pharm* 21, 510
(1968): Powell WJ+, *JAMA* 206, 642
Exfoliative dermatitis
(1968): Powell WJ+, *JAMA* 206, 642
Flushing
(1965): Editorial, *JAMA* 194, 82
Petechiae
(1968): Rachmilewitz EA+, *Blood* 32, 524
Photosensitivity (1.4%)
(1965): Editorial, *JAMA* 194, 82
Pigmentation (blue-gray) (photosensitive)
(1993): Steele TE+, *J Clin Psychopharmacol* 13, 76
(1993): Narurkar V+, *Arch Dermatol* 129, 474
Pruritus
(1988): Biederman J+, *J Clin Psychiatry* 49, 178
(1987): Ellsworth A+, *Drug Intell Clin Pharm* 21, 510
(1987): Pohl R+, *Am J Psychiatry* 144, 237
(1968): Powell WJ+, *JAMA* 206, 642
Purpura
(1980): Miescher PA+, *Clin Haematol* 9, 505
(1968): Rachmilewitz EA+, *Blood* 32, 524
Rash (sic)
(1965): Editorial, *JAMA* 194, 82
Urticaria
(1991): Bajwa WK+, *J Nerv Ment Dis* 179, 108
(1988): Biederman J+, *J Clin Psychiatry* 49, 178
(1987): Pohl R+, *Am J Psychiatry* 144, 237
Vasculitis
Xerosis

Hair

Hair – alopecia (<1%)
(1991): Warnock JK+, *J Nerv Ment Dis* 179, 441

Other

Black tongue
Bromhidrosis
Dysgeusia (>10%)
Galactorrhea (<1%)
Gynecomastia (<1%)
Hypersensitivity
Mucous membrane desquamation
(1968): Powell WJ+, *JAMA* 206, 642
Paresthesias
Pseudolymphoma
(1995): Magro CM+, *J Am Acad Dermatol* 32, 419
Stomatitis
Xerostomia (>10%)
(1993): Pataki CS+, *J Am Acad Child Adolesc Psychiatry* 32, 1065
(1965): Editorial, *JAMA* 194, 82

DESMOPRESSIN

Trade names: DDAVP (Aventis); Stimate (Centeon)
Other common trade names: *Defirin; Desmospray; Minirin; Minurin; Octostim; Stimate*
Indications: Primary nocturnal enuresis
Category: Antidiuretic; antihemophilic; antihemorrhagic; posterior pituitary hormone
Half-life: 75 minutes
Clinically important, potentially serious interactions with: carbamazepine, chlorpropamide, cisplatin, clofibrate, cyclophosphamide

Reactions

Skin

Allergic reactions (sic)
(1982): Yokota M+, *Endocrinol Jpn* 29, 475
Diaphoresis
(1985): Richardson DW+, *Ann Intern Med* 103, 228
Edema
Flushing (1–10%)
(1985): Richardson DW+, *Ann Intern Med* 103, 228 (1–5%)
Rash (sic)

Other

Injection-site edema
Injection-site erythema
Injection-site pain (1–10%)

DEXCHLORPHENIRAMINE

Trade names: Dexchlor, Poladex, Polaramine (Schering)
Other trade names: *Delamin, Polaramin, Polaronil, Polazit, Trenolone*
Indications: Allergic rhinitis, urticaria
Category: Antihistamine, H_1 blocker
Half-life: 20–24 hours
Clinically important, potentially serious interactions with: CNS depressants, guanabenz, MAO inhibitors, phenothiazines,

Reactions

Skin

Angioedema (<1%)
Chills
Contact dermatitis
(1989): Cusano F+, *Contact Dermatitis* 21, 340
Diaphoresis
Edema (<1%)
Photosensitivity (<1%)
Rash (sic) (<1%)
Urticaria

Other

Anaphylactoid reaction
Myalgia (<1%)
Paresthesias (<1%)
Xerostomia (1–10%)

DEXFENFLURAMINE*

Trade name: Redux (Wyeth)
Other common trade names: *Adifax; Dipondal; Glypolix; Isomeride; Obesine; Siran*
Indications: Obesity
Category: Anorexiant
Half-life: 18 hours
Clinically important, potentially serious interactions with: antidiabetic agents, buspirone, lithium, MAO inhibitors, SSRIs, sumatriptan, trazodone, tricyclic antidepressants, venlafaxine

Reactions

Skin

Allergic reactions (sic) (<1%)
Angioedema
Bullous eruption
Diaphoresis (>1%)
Ecchymoses
Eczema (sic) (<1%)
Edema (<1%)
Erythema multiforme
Exanthems (sic) (<1%)
Pityriasis rosea (<1%)
Pruritus (>1%)
Psoriasis (<1%)
Purpura
Rash (sic) (2.3%)
Stevens–Johnson syndrome
Urticaria (>1%)

Hair

Hair – alopecia (>1%)
Hair – hirsutism (<1%)

Other

Digital necrosis
(1997): Marinella MA+, *N Engl J Med* 337, 1776
Dysgeusia (>1%)
Gynecomastia
Hyperesthesia (<1%)
Hypesthesia
Mastodynia (<1%)
Myalgia (>1%)
Myopathy (<1%)
Oral mucosal lesions
(1990): Turner P, *Drugs* 39, 53 (1–5%)
Oral ulceration (<1%)
Paresthesias (>1%)
Systemic sclerosis
(1999): Korkmaz C+, *Rheumatology* (Oxford) 38, 370
Tongue disorder (sic)
Xerostomia (12.5%)
(1990): Turner P, *Drugs* 39, 53 (12.5%)

***Note:** Dexfenfluramine has been withdrawn in the USA

DEXMEDETOMIDINE

Trade name: Precedex (Abbott)
Indications: Sedation for intensive care unit intubation
Category: Alpha-adrenergic agonist, sedative
Half-life: 2 hours
Clinically important, potentially serious interactions with: anesthetics, anxiolytics, barbiturates, benzodiazepines, hypnotics, opiate agonists, sedatives, skeletal muscle relaxants, tricyclic antidepressants

Reactions

Skin

Diaphoresis (<1%)
Infection (sic) (2%)
Pain (3%)
Photopsia (<1%)
Xerosis

Other

Sialopenia
(1990): Aantaa RE+, *Anesth Analg* 70, 407

DEXTROAMPHETAMINE

Trade names: Adderall (Shire Richwood); Dexedrine (SmithKline Beecham)
Other common trade names: *Dexamphetamine; Dexamphetamini, Dextrostat, Ferndex, Oxydess*
Indications: Narcolepsy, attention deficit disorder (ADD)
Category: Central nervous system stimulant; amphetamine
Half-life: 10–12 hours
Clinically important, potentially serious interactions with: beta-blockers, furazolidone, MAO inhibitors, meperidine, norepinephrine, phenobarbital, phenothiazines, phenytoin, propoxyphene, tricyclic antidepressants

Reactions

Skin

Chills
Diaphoresis (1–10%)
Rash (sic) (<1%)
Toxic epidermal necrolysis
(1975): Giallorenzi AF+, *Oral Surg Oral Med Oral Pathol* 40, 611
Urticaria (<1%)

Other

Dysgeusia
Xerostomia (1–10%)

DEXTROMETHORPHAN

Trade names: Benylin; Cheracol-D; Drixoral; Pertussin; Robitussin; Sucrets; Suppress; Trocal; Vicks Formula 44; etc. (Various pharmaceutical companies.)
Other common trade names: *Balminil; Delsym; Koffex; Triaminic DM*
Indications: Nonproductive cough
Category: Antitussive (nonnarcotic)
Half-life: no data
Clinically important, potentially serious interactions with: amiodarone, fluoxetine, fluvoxamine, MAO inhibitors, paroxetine, quinidine, sertraline

Reactions

Skin

Bullous eruption
(1999): Sahn EE, *Dermatology Times* April, 5 (in an infant with urticaria pigmentosa)
(1996): Cook J+, *Pediatr Dermatol* 13, 410 (in an infant with urticaria pigmentosa)
Fixed eruption
(1991): Smoller BR+, *J Cutan Pathol* 18, 13
(1990): Stubb S+, *Arch Dermatol* 126, 970

Other

Anaphylactoid reaction
(1998): Knowles SR+, *J Allergy Clin Immunol* 102, 316

DIACETYLMORPHINE

(See HEROIN)

DIAZEPAM

Trade names: Diastat (Elan); Dizac; Valium (Roche)
Other common trade names: *Assival; Dialar; Diapax; Diazemuls; Ducene; E-Pam; Meval; Novazam; Solis; Vivol*
Indications: Anxiety
Category: Benzodiazepine anxiolytic and sedative-hypnotic; anticonvulsant
Half-life: 20–70 hours
Clinically important, potentially serious interactions with: alcohol, amprenavir, barbiturates, cimetidine, cisapride, clarithromycin, CNS depressants, digoxin, diltiazem, disulfiram, levodopa, methadone, nelfinavir, omeprazole, phenothiazines, ritonavir, theophylline, tuberculostatics, valproic acid, verapamil, **grapefruit juice, cigarette smoking**

Reactions

Skin

Acne
(1962): Grayson LD, *Gen Pract* 25, 9
Allergic reactions (sic)
(1982): Allin DM, *Curr Med Res Opin* 8, 33
(1977): Padfield A+, *BMJ* 1, 575
Angioedema
(1974): Felix RH+, *Lancet* 1, 1017
Bullous eruption
(1977): Varma AJ+, *Arch Intern Med* 137, 1207
Contact dermatitis
(1995): Kampgen E+, *Contact Dermatitis* 33, 356
(1995): Fisher AA, *Cutis* 55, 327 (systemic)
(1994): Garcia-Bravo B+, *Contact Dermatitis* 30, 40
Dermatitis (sic) (1–10%)
Diaphoresis (>10%)

Eczematous eruption (sic)
(1974): Felix RH+, *Lancet* 1, 1017
Exanthems
(1986): Bigby M+, *JAMA* 256, 3358 (0.04%)
(1981): Adverse Drug Reaction List, *Jpn Med Gaz* (Japanese) 18:6–7, 16
(1976): Arndt KA+, *JAMA* 235, 918 (0.38%)
(1967): Jenner FA+, *Dis Nerv Syst* 28, 245
(1964): Holt KS, *Ann Physiol Med* (Suppl) 16
(1963): Love J, *Dis Nerv Syst* 24, 674
Exfoliative dermatitis
(1967): Satyadas JS+, *J Indian Med Assoc* 3, 49
(1963): Love J, *Dis Nerv Syst* 24, 674
Fixed eruption (<1%)
(1979): Olumide F, *Int J Dermatol* 18, 818
(1966): Jadassohn W+, *Dermatologica* 133, 91
Flushing
(1964): Holt KS, *Ann Physiol Med* (Suppl) 16
Granuloma disciformis (Miescher)
(1969): Clarke DM, *Australas J Dermatol* 10, 194
Melanoma
(1981): Adam S+, *Lancet* 2, 1344
Pellagra
(1982): Stadler R+, *Hautarzt* (German) 33, 276
Pigmentation
(1980): Ferreira JA, *Aesthetic Plast Surg* 4, 343
Pruritus
(1995): Kampgen E+, *Contact Dermatitis* 33, 356
Purpura
(1985): Ambriz-Fernandez R+, *Rev Invest Clin* (Spanish) 37, 347
(1980): Miescher PA+, *Clin Haematol* 9, 505
(1977): Cimo PL+, *Am J Hematol* 2, 65
(1977): Ghosh JS, *BMJ* 1, 902
Rash (sic) (>10%)
(1983): O'Brien JE+, *Curr Ther Res* 34, 825
Urticaria
(1987): Deardon DJ+, *Br J Anaesth* 59, 391
Vasculitis
(1999): Olcina GM+, *Am J Psychiatry* 156, 972

Nails

Nails – parrot-beak nails
(1971): Kandil E, *J Med Liban* 24, 433

Other

Anaphylactoid reaction
(1987): Deardon DJ+, *Br J Anaesth* 59, 391
Gynecomastia
(2000): Hugues FC+, *Ann Med Interne (Paris)* (French) 151, 10 (passim)
(1994): Llop R+, *Ann Pharmacother* 28, 671
(1979): Moerck HJ+, *Lancet* 1, 1344 (letter)
Injection-site phlebitis (>10%)
(1981): Clarke RSJ, *Drugs* 22, 26 (39%)
(1980): Schou-Olesen A+, *Br J Anaesth* 52, 609
Paresthesias
Porphyria
(1979): Stone DR+, *Br J Anaesth* 51, 809
(1978): Mees DE+, *South Med J* 68, 29
Porphyria variegata
Sialorrhea
Tongue, coated
Xerostomia (>10%)

DIAZOXIDE

Trade name: Hyperstat (Schering)
Other common trade names: *Eudimine; Proglicem; Proglycem; Sefulken*
Indications: Hypoglycemia; hypertension
Category: Antihypoglycemic; antihypertensive
Half-life: 20–36 hours
Clinically important, potentially serious interactions with: allopurinol, beta-blockers, colchicine, hydralazine, phenytoin, sulfonylureas, thiazide diuretics, warfarin

Reactions

Skin

Candidiasis
Diaphoresis
Edema
Exanthems
Flushing (<1%)
Herpes (sic)
Leukomelanoderma (sic)
(1967): Saito T+, *Acta Dermatol* (Kyoto) 61, 207
Lichenoid eruption
(1975): Burton JL+, *Br J Dermatol* 93, 707
(1973): Menter MA, *Proc R Soc Med* 66, 326
Photosensitivity
(1967): Saito T+, *Acta Dermatol* (Kyoto) 61, 207
Pruritus
Purpura
Rash (sic) (<1%)
Urticaria
Xerosis
(1975): Burton JL+, *Br J Dermatol* 93, 707

Hair

Hair – alopecia
(1975): Burton JL+, *Br J Dermatol* 93, 707
(1972): Milner RD+, *Arch Dis Child* 47, 537
Hair – hypertrichosis (<1%)
(1989): Rousseau C+, *Dermatologica* 179, 221
(1988): Prigent F+, *Ann Dermatol Venereol* (French) 115, 191
(1987): Turpin G+, *Presse Med* (French) 16, 398
(1983): Schiazza L+, *G Ital Dermatol Venereol* (Italian) 118, 113
(1981): Perez-Mijares R+, *Rev Clin Esp* (Spanish) 162, 225
(1975): Burton JL+, *Br J Dermatol* 93, 707 (>5%)
(1973): Menter MA, *Proc R Soc Med* 66, 326
(1972): Leng JJ+, *Pediatr Clin North Am* 19, 681
(1972): Milner RD+, *Arch Dis Child* 47, 537
(1968): Koblenzer PJ+, *Ann N Y Acad Sci* 150, 373

Other

Ageusia
Cellulitis (<1%)
Dysgeusia
Hypersensitivity
Injection-site pain (<1%)
Injection-site phlebitis (<1%)
Paresthesias
Sialorrhea
Xerostomia

DICLOFENAC

Trade names: Arthrotec (Searle); Voltaren (Novartis)
Other common trade names: *Allvoran; Apo-Diclo; Fenac; Galedol; Liroken; Monoflam; Nu-Diclo; Remethan; Taks; Voltarene; Voltarol*
Indications: Rheumatoid and osteoarthritis
Category: Nonsteroidal anti-inflammatory (NSAID)
Half-life: 1–2 hours
Clinically important, potentially serious interactions with: aminoglycosides, aspirin, anticoagulants, aspirin, cyclosporine, digoxin, diuretics, insulin, lithium, methotrexate, probenecid, salicylates, sulfonylureas, triamterene, warfarin

Arthrotec is diclofenac and misoprostol

Reactions

Skin

Allergic reactions (sic)
(1992): Schiavino D+, *Contact Dermatitis* 26, 357
(1979): Ciucci AG, *Rheum Rehab* 18 (Suppl 2), 116
Angioedema (1–3%)
(2000): Hadar A+, *Harefuah* (Hebrew) 138, 211 (from suppository)
Bullous eruption (1–3%)
(1982): Valsecchi R+, *G Ital Derm Venereol* (Italian) 117, 221
(1981): Gabrielsen TO+, *Acta Derm Venereol* (Stockh) 61, 439
Contact dermatitis
(1998): Ueda K+, *Contact Dermatitis* 39, 323
(1996): Gonzalo MA+, *Dermatology* 193, 59
(1996): Valsecchi R+, *Contact Dermatitis* 34, 150
(1994): Romano A+, *Allergy* 49, 57
(1994): Gebhardt M+, *Contact Dermatitis* 30, 183
Dermatitis (sic) (1–3%)
Dermatitis herpetiformis
(1989): Grob JJ+, *Dermatologica* 178, 58
(1981): Gabrielsen TO+, *Acta Derm Venereol* (Stockh) 61, 439
Dermatomyositis
(1989): Grob JJ+, *Dermatologica* 178, 58
Diaphoresis (<1%)
Eczema (sic) (1–3%)
Edema
Erythema (sic)
(1998): Schaad HJ+, *Ther Umsch* (German) 55, 586 (generalized)
(1992): Barrett PJ+, *Anaesthesia* 47, 83
(1979): Ciucci AG, *Rheum Rehab* 18 (Suppl 2), 116
Erythema multiforme (<1%)
(1999): Emmett SD, Solana Beach, CA (from Internet) (observation)
(1995): Dhar S+, *Dermatology* 191, 76
(1993): Khalil H+, *Arch Intern Med* 153, 1649
(1988): Todd PA+, *Drugs* 35, 244
(1985): Morris BAP+, *Can Med Assoc J* 133, 665
(1982): Seigneuric C+, *Ann Dermatol Venereol* (French) 109, 287
Erythema nodosum (<1%)
Exanthems (1–5%)
(1994): Romano A+, *Allergy* 49, 57
(1992): Breathnach SM+, *Adverse Drug Reactions and the Skin*, Blackwell, Oxford, 188 (passim)
(1988): Todd PA+, *Drugs* 35, 244
(1986): Halevy S+, *Harefuah* (Hebrew) 110, 30
(1985): Morris BAP+, *Can Med Assoc J* 133, 665
(1979): Ciucci AG, *Rheum Rehab* 18 (Suppl 2), 116
Exfoliative dermatitis (<1%)
Flushing (<1%)
Lichenoid eruption
(1999): Fetterman M, Miami, FL (from Internet) (observation)
Linear IgA bullous dermatosis
(1982): Valsecchi R+, *G Ital Derm Venereol* (Italian) 117, 221
(1981): Gabrielsen TO+, *Acta Derm Venereol* (Stockh) 61, 439
Lupus erythematosus
Pemphigus
(1997): Matz H+, *Dermatology* 195, 48
Peripheral edema
Photosensitivity (1–3%)
(1998): Encinas S+, *Chem Res Toxicol* 11, 946
(1997): O'Reilly FM+, American Academy of Dermatology Meeting, Poster #14
(1996): Becker L+, *Acta Derm Venereol* (Stockh) 76, 337
(1992): Le Corre Y+, *Ann Dermatol Venereol* (French) 119, 923 (granuloma annulare type)
(1988): Todd PA+, *Drugs* 35, 244
Pruritus (1–10%)
(1995): Litt JZ, Beachwood, OH, personal case (observation)
(1994): Litt JZ, Beachwood, OH, personal case (observation)
(1992): Breathnach SM+, *Adverse Drug Reactions and the Skin*, Blackwell, Oxford, 188 (passim)
(1988): Todd PA+, *Drugs* 35, 244
(1981): Gabrielsen TO+, *Acta Derm Venereol* (Stockh) 61, 439
(1979): Ciucci AG, *Rheum Rehab* 18 (Suppl 2), 116
Pseudoreactions (sic)
(1991): VanArsdel PP, *JAMA* 266, 3343
Psoriasis
(1999): Fetterman M, Miami, FL (from Internet) (observation)
(1999): Dintiman B, Fairfax, VA (from Internet) (observation)
(1987): Sendagorta E+, *Dermatologica* 175, 300 (pustular)
Purpura (1–3%)
(1988): Todd PA+, *Drugs* 35, 244
(1979): Ciucci AG, *Rheum Rehab* 18 (Suppl 2), 116
Pustular psoriasis
(1999): Dintiman B, Fairfax, VA (from Internet) (observation)
(1999): Fetterman M, Miami, FL (from Internet) (observation)
(1987): Sendagorta E+, *Dermatologica* 175, 300
Rash (sic) (>10%)
(1978): Abrams GJ+, *S Afr Med J* 53, 442
Skin reactions (sic)
(1986): Catalano MA, *Am J Med* 80, 81
Stevens–Johnson syndrome (1–3%) (one fatal case report)
(1988): Todd PA+, *Drugs* 35, 244
(1979): Ciucci AG, *Rheum Rehab* 18 (Suppl 2), 116
Still's disease
(1985): Wouters JM+, *J Rheumatol* 12, 791
Toxic epidermal necrolysis
(1998): Choi KL, Toronto, Canada (from Internet) (observation)
(1993): Correia O+, *Dermatology* 186, 32
(1985): Kamanabroo D+, *Arch Dermatol* 121, 1548
Toxic shock
(1998): Schaad HJ+, *Ther Umsch* (German) 55, 586
Urticaria (1–3%)
(1998): Gala G+, *Allergy* 53, 623
(1995): Litt JZ, Beachwood, OH, personal case (observation)
(1995): Rademaker M, *N Z Med J* 108, 165
(1992): Breathnach SM+, *Adverse Drug Reactions and the Skin*, Blackwell, Oxford, 188 (passim)
(1988): Todd PA+, *Drugs* 35, 244
(1979): Ciucci AG, *Rheum Rehab* 18 (Suppl 2), 116
Vasculitis
(1999): Emmet S, Solana Beach, CA (from Internet) (from ophthalmic solution) (observation)
(1997): Morros R+, *Br J Rheumatol* 36, 503
(1992): Breathnach SM+, *Adverse Drug Reactions and the Skin*, Blackwell, Oxford, 188 (passim)
(1982): Bonafe JL+, *Ann Dermatol Venereol* (French) 109, 283

Hair

Hair – alopecia (1–3%)

Other

Acute intermittent porphyria
Anaphylactoid reaction (1–3%)
(2000): Hadar A+, *Harefuah* (Hebrew) 138, 211 (from suppository)
(2000): Ray M+, *Indian Pediatr* 36, 1067 (fatal)
(1999): Enrique E+, *Allergy* 54, 529
(1996): Levy JH+, *N Engl J Med* 335, 1925
(1993): van der Klauw MM+, *Br J Clin Pharmacol* 35, 400
(1993): Alkhawajah AM+, *Forensic Sci Int* 60, 107
(1992): Australian Adverse Drug Reactions Bulletin 11, 7
Aphthous stomatitis
(1988): Todd PA+, *Drugs* 35, 244
Dysgeusia (1–3%)
Embolia cutis medicamentosa (Nicolau syndrome)
(1999): Forsbach Sanchez G+, *Rev Invest Clin* (Spanish) 51, 71

Hypersensitivity
(2000): del Pozo MD+, *Allergy* 55, 412
(1998): Romano A+, *Ann Allergy Asthma Immunol* 81, 373
Injection-site necrosis
(1989): Tweedie DG, *Anaesthesia* 44, 932
Injection-site pain
(1998): Schaad HJ+, *Ther Umsch* (German) 55, 586
Oral ulceration
Paresthesias (<1%)
Serum sickness
Stomatitis (<1%)
Tongue edema (1–3%)
Xerostomia (1–3%)
(1988): Todd PA+, *Drugs* 35, 244

DICLOXACILLIN

Trade names: Dycill (SmithKline Beecham); Dynapen (Mead Johnson)
Other common trade names: *Brispen; Dichlor-Stapenor; Diclo; Diclocil; Diclocillin; Diclox; Novapen; Pathocil; Posipen*
Indications: Infections due to penicillinase producing staphylococci
Category: Penicillinase-resistant penicillin antibiotic
Half-life: 0.5–1.0 hours
Clinically important, potentially serious interactions with: anticoagulants, cyclosporine, disulfiram, methotrexate, probenecid, tetracyclines, **food**

Reactions

Skin
Angioedema
Bullous eruption
Dermatitis (sic)
Ecchymoses
Erythema multiforme
(1991): Porteous DM+, *Arch Dermatol* 127, 740
Erythema nodosum
Erythroderma
(1985): Shelley WB+, *Cutis* 220, 224
Exanthems (<1%)
Exfoliative dermatitis (<1%)
Hematomas
Jarisch–Herxheimer reaction
Pruritus
(1998): Siegfried EC+, *J Am Acad Dermatol* 39, 797 (passim)
Purpura
Rash (sic) (<1%)
Stevens–Johnson syndrome
(1991): Porteous DM+, *Arch Dermatol* 127, 740
Toxic epidermal necrolysis
Urticaria
(1998): Siegfried EC+, *J Am Acad Dermatol* 39, 797 (passim)
(1985): Green RL+, *JAMA* 254, 531 (postcoital)
Vasculitis
Vesicular eruptions

Nails
Nails – shoreline
(1985): Shelley WB+, *Cutis* 220, 224

Other
Anaphylactoid reaction
(1998): Siegfried EC+, *J Am Acad Dermatol* 39, 797 (passim)
Black tongue
Dysgeusia
Glossitis
Glossodynia
Hypersensitivity (<1%)
Injection-site pain
Myalgia
Oral candidiasis
Serum sickness (<1%)
Stomatitis
Stomatodynia
Vaginitis (<1%)
Xerostomia

DICUMAROL

Synonym: bishydroxycoumarin
Trade name: Dicumarol (Abbott)
Other common trade names: *Apekumarol; Dicumol; Embolin*
Indications: Atrial fibrillation, pulmonary embolism, venous thrombosis
Category: Oral anticoagulant
Half-life: 1–4 days
Clinically important, potentially serious interactions with: several dozen: too numerous to mention here

Reactions

Skin
Acral purpura
(1986): Stone MS+, *J Am Acad Dermatol* 14, 796
Angioedema (<1%)
Bullous eruption
(1986): Stone MS+, *J Am Acad Dermatol* 14, 796 (passim)
Dermatitis (sic)
(1992): Breathnach SM+, *Adverse Drug Reactions and the Skin*, Blackwell, Oxford, 248 (passim)
(1991): Quintavalla R+, *Int Angiol* 10, 103
Ecchymoses
(1988): Cole MS+, *Surgery* 103, 271 (passim)
Exanthems
(1989): Kruis-de Vries MH+, *Dermatologica* 178, 109
(1988): Cole MS+, *Surgery* 103, 271 (passim)
(1978): Kwong P+, *JAMA* 239, 1884
(1968): Schiff BL+, *Arch Dermatol* 98, 136
(1960): Adams CW+, *Circulation* 22, 947
Hemorrhagic skin infarcts
(1989): Geoghegan+, *BMJ* 298, 902
(1988): Cole MS, *Surgery* 103, 271
(1980): Schleicher SM+, *Arch Dermatol* 116, 444
Necrosis
(1992): Sharafuddin MA+, *Arch Dermatol* 128, 105
(1989): Grimaudo V+, *BMJ* 289, 233
(1988): Cole MS+, *Surgery* 103, 271
(1987): Gladson CL+, *Arch Dermatol* 123, 1701a
(1984): Slutzki S+, *Int J Dermatol* 23, 117
(1982): Faraci PA, *Int J Dermatol* 21, 329
(1981): Horn JR+, *Am J Hosp Pharm* 38, 1763
(1976): Kirby JD+, *Br J Dermatol* 94, 97
(1971): Danilov B+, *Rev Med Chir Soc Med Nat Iasi* (Romanian) 75, 479
Pigmentation
(1978): Rebhun J, *Ann Allergy* 40, 44
Pruritus (<1%)
Purplish erythema (feet and toes) (sic)
(1978): Kwong P+, *JAMA* 239, 1884
(1961): Feder W+, *Ann Intern Med* 55, 911
Purpura
(1988): Cole MS+, *Surgery* 103, 271 (passim)
(1965): Selye H+, *Arch Klin Exp Dermatol* (German) 223, 527
Rash (sic)
Urticaria
(1988): Cole MS+, *Surgery* 103, 271 (passim)
(1986): Stone MS+, *J Am Acad Dermatol* 14, 796 (passim)
(1959): Sheps ES+, *Am J Cardiol* 3, 118
Vesicular eruption
(1986): Stone MS+, *J Am Acad Dermatol* 14, 796 (passim)

Hair
Hair – alopecia (1–10%)
(1989): Kruis-de Vries MH+, *Dermatologica* 178, 109 (passim)
(1988): Umlas J+, *Cutis* 42, 63
(1986): Stone MS+, *J Am Acad Dermatol* 14, 796 (passim)
(1969): Baker H+, *Br J Dermatol* 81, 236
(1957): Cornbleet T+, *Arch Dermatol* 75, 440

Other
Hypersensitivity
Oral ulceration
Priapism

DICYCLOMINE

Trade names: Antispaz; Bemote; Bentyl (Aventis); Byclomine; Dibent; Di-Spaz; Neoquess, OrTyl; Spasmoject, etc.
Other common trade names: *Bentylol; Byclomine; Formulex; Lomine; Merbentyl; Notensyl; Panakiron; Spasmoban; Swityl*
Indications: Irritable bowel syndrome
Category: Anticholinergic; antispasmodic
Half-life: initial: 1.8 hours; terminal: 9–10 hours
Clinically important, potentially serious interactions with: alcohol, amantadine, antiarrhythmics, anticholinergics, antihistamines, atenolol, clozapine, digoxin, haloperidol, narcotic analgesics, phenothiazines, tacrine, tricyclic antidepressants

Reactions

Skin
Exanthems
(1987): Castleden CM+, *J Clin Exp Gerontol* 9, 265
(1952): Pakula SF, *Postgrad Med* 11, 123
Flushing
Hypohidrosis (>10%)
Pruritus
(1951): Ausman DC+, *Wisconsin Med J* 50 1089
Rash (sic) (<1%)
(1975): Hennessy WB, *Med J Aust* 2, 421
(1951): Chamberlain DT, *Gastroenterology* 17, 224
Urticaria
Xerosis (>10%)

Other
Ageusia
Anaphylactoid reaction
Dysgeusia
Injection-site reactions (sic) (>10%)
Tremor
Xerostomia (>10%)
(1975): Hennessy WB, *Med J Aust* 2, 421

DIDANOSINE

Trade name: Videx (Bristol-Myers Squibb)
Indications: Advanced HIV infection
Category: Antiretroviral; nucleoside reverse transcriptase inhibitor (NRTI)
Half-life: 1.5 hours
Clinically important, potentially serious interactions with: dapsone, fluoroquinolones, ganciclovir, indinavir, itraconazole, ketoconazole, pentamidine, sulfones, tetracyclines, **food**

Reactions

Skin
Acral erythema
(1993): Pedailles S+, *Ann Dermatol Venereol* (French) 120, 837
Chills
Diaphoresis
Erythema multiforme
(1992): Parneix-Spake A+, *Lancet* 340, 847
Exanthems
Pruritus (9%)
Purpura
Rash (sic) (9%)
Stevens–Johnson syndrome
(1992): Parneix-Spake A+, *Lancet* 340, 847
Urticaria
Vasculitis
(1994): Herranz P+, *Lancet* 344, 680

Hair
Hair – alopecia (<1%)

Other
Anaphylactoid reaction (<1%)
Hypersensitivity (<1%)
Myalgia
Myopathy
Paresthesias
Xerostomia

DIDEOXYCYTIDINE (ddC)

(See ZALCITABINE)

DIETHYLPROPION

Synonym: amfepramone
Trade name: Tenuate (Aventis)
Other common trade names: *Anorex; Linea; Nobesine; Prefamone; Regenon; Tenuate Retard; Tepanil*
Indications: Weight reduction
Category: Anorexiant; CNS stimulant
Half-life: 4–6 hours
Clinically important, potentially serious interactions with: barbiturates, CNS depressants, furazolidone, guanethidine, MAO inhibitors, phenothiazines, sibutramine, sympathomimetics, tricyclic antidepressants

Reactions

Skin
Diaphoresis (<1%)
Ecchymoses
Erythema (<1%)
Erythema multiforme
(1997): Thaler, D, Monona, WI (from Internet) (observation)
Exanthems (<1%)
Flushing (<1%)
Pruritus (<1%)
Purpura (<1%)
Rash (sic)
Scleroderma
(1991): Bourgeois P+, *Baillieres Clin Rheumatol* 5, 13
(1990): Aeschlimann A+, *Scand J Rheumatol* 19, 87
Systemic sclerosis
(1984): Tomlinson, JW+, *J Rheumatol* 11, 254
Urticaria

Hair
Hair – alopecia (<1%)

Other
Dysgeusia
Gynecomastia
Myalgia (<1%)
Tremor
Xerostomia

DIETHYLSTILBESTROL

Synonyms: DES; stilbestrol
Trade name: Diethylstilbestrol (Lilly); Stilphostrol
Other common trade names: *Diethyl Stilbestrol; Distilbene; Honvol; Stilboestrol*
Indications: Metastatic prostate carcinoma, progressive breast cancer
Category: Estrogen; antineoplastic; osteoporosis prophylactic
Half-life: 2–3 days
Clinically important, potentially serious interactions with: anticoagulants, bromocriptine, cimetidine, cyclosporine, felbamate, fluconazole, itraconazole, ketoconazole, phenytoin, propranolol

Reactions

Skin

Acanthosis nigricans
(1974): Banuchi SR+, *Arch Dermatol* 109, 544
(1971): Curth HO, *Birth Defects* 7, 31
Acneform eruption
Angioedema
(1942): Saphir WS+, *JAMA* 119, 557
Bullous eruption
(1971): Kuchera LK, *JAMA* 218, 562
Chloasma (<1%)
Edema
Erythema multiforme
Erythema nodosum
Exanthems
(1984): Lee M+, *J Urol* 131, 767
Exfoliative dermatitis
(1942): Kasselberg LA, *JAMA* 120, 117
Flushing
(1981): Ingle JN+, *N Engl J Med* 304, 16 (3%)
Hyperkeratosis of nipples
(1980): Mold DE+, *Cutis* 26, 95
Lupus erythematosus
(1989): Collins D, *J Rheumatol* 16, 408
Melasma (<1%)
Peripheral edema (>10%)
Pruritus
(1971): Kuchera LK, *JAMA* 218, 562
Purpura
(1984): Lee M+, *J Urol* 131, 767
Rash (sic) (<1%)
Urticaria
(1989): Collins D, *J Rheumatol* 16, 408
(1984): Lee M+, *J Urol* 131, 767

Hair

Hair – alopecia
Hair – hirsutism
(1982): Peress MR+, *Am J Obstet Gynecol* 144, 135

Other

Gynecomastia (>10%)
Mastodynia (>10%)
Periarteritis nodosa
(1967): Keyloun V+, *Vasc Dis* 4, 21
Porphyria cutanea tarda
(1989): Coulson IH+, *Br J Urol* 63, 648
(1978): Weimar VM+, *J Urol* 120, 643
(1972): Reginster JP, *Arch Belg Dermatol Syphiligr* (French) 28, 179
(1970): Roenigk HH+, *Arch Dermatol* 102, 260
(1970): Domonkos AN, *Arch Dermatol* 102, 229
(1969): Degos R+, *Ann Dermatol Syphiligr Paris* (French) 96, 5
(1967): Thivolet J+, *Dermatologica* (French) 135, 455
(1967): Vail JT, *JAMA* 201, 671
(1966): Copeman PW+, *BMJ* 5485, 461
(1966): Levere RD, *Blood* 28, 569
(1965): Becker FT, *Arch Dermatol* 92, 252
(1964): Theologides H+, *Metabolism* 13, 391
(1963): Hurley HJ, *Arch Dermatol* 88, 233
(1963): Walshe M, *Br J Dermatol* 75, 298
Vaginal candidiasis

DIFLUNISAL

Trade name: Dolobid (Merck)
Other common trade names: *Ansal; Apo-Diflunisal; Diflonid; Diflusal; Dolobis; Donobid; Fluniget; Flustar; Nu-Diflunisal*
Indications: Rheumatoid and osteoarthritis
Category: Nonsteroidal anti-inflammatory (NSAID); analgesic
Half-life: 8–12 hours
Clinically important, potentially serious interactions with: acetaminophen, anticoagulants, aspirin, beta-blockers, cyclosporine, digoxin, hydrochlorothiazide, indomethacin, lithium, methotrexate, NSAIDs, phenytoin, probenecid, salicylates, sulfonamides, sulfonylureas, warfarin

Reactions

Skin

Angioedema (<1%)
Bullous eruption
(1989): Street ML+, *J Am Acad Dermatol* 20, 850
Diaphoresis (<1%)
(1986): Muncie HL+, *J Fam Pract* 23, 125
(1979): Papatheodossiou N, *Curr Med Res Opinion* 6, 154
Edema (<1%)
Erythema multiforme (<1%)
(1986): Grom JA+, *Hosp Formul Manage* 21, 353
(1985): Bigby M+, *J Am Acad Dermatol* 12, 866 (5%)
(1985): O'Brien WM+, *J Rheumatol* 12, 13
(1982): Dubois A+, *Presse Med* (French) 11, 606
(1978): Hunter JA+, *BMJ* 2, 1088
Erythroderma
(1989): Street ML+, *J Am Acad Dermatol* 20, 850
(1980): Chan LK+, *BMJ* 280, 84
Exanthems
(1992): Breathnach SM+, *Adverse Drug Reactions and the Skin*, Blackwell, Oxford, 180 (passim)
(1988): Cook DJ+, *Can Med Assoc J* 138, 1029
(1985): Bocanegra TS+, *Curr Res Med Opin* 9, 568 (1.7%)
(1985): Bigby M+, *J Am Acad Dermatol* 12, 866 (5%)
Exfoliative dermatitis (<1%)
(1985): Bigby M+, *J Am Acad Dermatol* 12, 866
Fixed eruption
(1991): Roetzheim RG+, *J Am Acad Dermatol* 24, 1021 (non-pigmenting)
Flushing (<1%)
Lichenoid eruption
(1989): Street ML+, *J Am Acad Dermatol* 20, 850
Peripheral edema
Photosensitivity (<1%)
(1989): Street ML+, *J Am Acad Dermatol* 20, 850
Pruritus (1–10%)
(1992): Breathnach SM+, *Adverse Drug Reactions and the Skin*, Blackwell, Oxford, 180 (passim)
(1986): Hurme M+, *Int J Clin Pharmacol Res* 6, 53
(1985): Bigby M+, *J Am Acad Dermatol* 12, 866 (5%)
Purpura
Rash (sic) (3–9%)
(1987): Masden JJ+, *Curr Ther Res* 42, 319
(1986): Bennett RM, *Clin Ther* 9, 27
(1986): Turner RA+, *Clin Ther* 9, 37
Skin reactions (sic)
(1985): Lee P+, *J Rheumatol* 12, 544
(1983): McQueen EG, *N Z Med J* 96, 95
Stevens–Johnson syndrome (<1%)
(1992): Breathnach SM+, *Adverse Drug Reactions and the Skin*, Blackwell, Oxford, 180 (passim)
(1986): Grom JA+, *Hosp Formul Manage* 21, 353
(1986): Szczeklik A, *Drugs* 32 (Suppl 4), 148
(1985): Bigby M+, *J Am Acad Dermatol* 12, 866
(1982): Dubois A+, *Presse Med* (French) 11, 606
(1979): *Curr Probl* 4, 2
(1978): Hunter JA+, *BMJ* 2, 1088
Toxic epidermal necrolysis (<1%)
(1990): Roujeau JC+, *Arch Dermatol* 126, 37

Urticaria (<1%)
(1995): Arias J+, *Ann Allergy Asthma Immunol* 74, 160
(1992): Breathnach SM+, *Adverse Drug Reactions and the Skin*, Blackwell, Oxford, 180 (passim)
(1987): Morse DR+, *Clin Ther* 9, 500
(1985): Bigby M+, *J Am Acad Dermatol* 12, 866 (5%)
(1983): Griffin JP, *Practitioner* 227, 1283 (passim)
(1980): Chan LK+, *BMJ* 280, 84
Vasculitis (<1%)

Hair

Hair – alopecia
(1978): Bresnihan B+, *Curr Med Res Opinion* 5, 556

Nails

Nails – onycholysis

Other

Anaphylactoid reaction (<1%)
Aphthous stomatitis
Hypersensitivity (<1%)
Oral lichen planus
(1983): Hamburger J+, *BMJ* 287, 1258
Oral ulceration
Paresthesias (<1%)
Pseudoporphyria
(1987): Taylor BJ+, *N Z Med J* 100, 322
Stomatitis (<1%)
Trembling (<1%)
Xerostomia
(1982): Ankri J+, *Clin Ther* 5, 85

DIGOXIN

Trade names: Lanoxicaps (GlaxoWellcome); Lanoxin (GlaxoWellcome)
Other common trade names: *Cardigox; Digacin; Digoxine; Eudigox; Lanicor; Lenoxin; Novo-Digoxin*
Indications: Congestive heart failure, atrial fibrillation
Category: Cardiac glycoside; inotropic; antiarrhythmic
Half-life: 36–48 hours
Clinically important, potentially serious interactions with: ACE-inhibitors, amiodarone, amphotericin B, beta-blockers, bumetanide, calcium preparations, clarithromycin, cyclosporine, diltiazem, doxycycline, erythromycin, ethacrynic acid, furosemide, indomethacin, itraconazole, phenytoin, propafenone, quinidine, quinine, reserpine, rifampin, tetracycline, thiazide diuretics, verapamil, **St John's wort**

Reactions

Skin

Angioedema
Bullous eruption
(1992): Breathnach SM+, *Adverse Drug Reactions and the Skin*, Blackwell, Oxford, 216 (passim)
Diaphoresis
(1980): Lofgren RP, *N Engl J Med* 302, 919
Exanthems (1.6%)
(1994): Shelley WB+, *Cutis* 54, 76 (observation)
(1994): Martin SJ+, *JAMA* 271, 1905 (generalized)
(1992): Breathnach SM+, *Adverse Drug Reactions and the Skin*, Blackwell, Oxford, 216 (passim)
Pruritus
(1994): Martin SJ+, *JAMA* 271, 1905 (generalized)
Psoriasis
(1981): David M+, *J Am Acad Dermatol* 5, 702
Purpura
(1992): Breathnach SM+, *Adverse Drug Reactions and the Skin*, Blackwell, Oxford, 216 (passim)
Rash (sic)
Urticaria
(1994): Shelley WB+, *Cutis* 54, 76 (observation)
(1992): Breathnach SM+, *Adverse Drug Reactions and the Skin*, Blackwell, Oxford, 216 (passim)
Vasculitis
(1972): Brauner GJ+, *Cutis* 10, 441

Hair

Hair – alopecia

Nails

Nails – shedding (finger- and toenails)

Other

Dyschromatopsia (green vision)
Gynecomastia
(200): Hugues FC+, *Ann Med Interne (Paris)* (French) 151, 10 (passim)
Xanthopsia

DIHYDROERGOTAMINE

Trade names: D.H.E. 45 (Novartis); Migranal Nasal Spray (Novartis)
Other trade names: *Dergiflux; Dihydergot; Ergont; Ergovasan; Ikaran; Orstanorm; Seglor; Verladyn; Verteblan*
Indications: Prevention of vascular headaches
Category: Ergot alkaloid
Half-life: 1.3–3.9 hours
Clinically important, potentially serious interactions with: amprenavir, beta-blockers, calcium channel blockers, clarithromycin, epinephrine, erythromycin, heparin, nelfinavir, nitroglycerin, propranolol, ritonavir, troleandomycin

Reactions

Skin

Edema (>10%)
Pruritus

Other

Dysgeusia
Injection-site reaction
Myalgia
Paresthesias (>10%)
Xerostomia (>10%)

DIHYDROTACHYSTEROL

Trade names: DHT (Roxane); Hytakerol (Sanofi-Winthrop)
Other common trade names: *AT 10; Dihydral; Dygratyl; Vitamin D*
Indications: Hypocalcemia associated with hypoparathyroidism
Category: Fat soluble vitamin
Half-life: no data
Clinically important, potentially serious interactions with: MAO inhibitors, thiazide diuretics, verapamil

Reactions

Skin

Exanthems
Livedo reticularis
(1985): Michel B+, *Schweiz Med Wochenschr* (German) 115, 418
Pruritus (1–10%)

Other

Calcification
(1985): Michel B+, *Schweiz Med Wochenschr* (German) 115, 418
Dysgeusia (metallic taste)
Myalgia
Ulcerative necrosis
(1985): Michel B+, *Schweiz Med Wochenschr* (German) 115, 418
Xerostomia

DILTIAZEM

Trade names: Cardizem (Aventis); Cartia-XT; Dilacor XR (Watson); Diltia-XT; Teczem (Aventis); Tiazac (Forest)
Other common trade names: *Alti-Diltiazem; Britiazem; Calcicard; Deltazen; Dilrene; Diltahexal; Nu-Diltiaz; Presoken; Tiamate; Tilazem; Tildiem*
Indications: Angina, essential hypertension
Category: Calcium channel blocker; antianginal, antiarrhythmic and antihypertensive
Half-life: 5–8 hours (for extended-release capsules)
Clinically important, potentially serious interactions with: amiodarone, amprenavir, beta-blockers, carbamazepine, cimetidine, cisapride, cyclosporine, digoxin, fentanyl, nelfinavir, nifedipine, procainamide, quinidine, ranitidine, ritonavir, theophylline, valproic acid

Teczem is diltiazem and enalapril

Reactions

Skin

Acne
(1989): Stern R+, *Arch Intern Med* 149, 829

Acute generalized exanthematous pustulosis (AGEP)
(1998): Knowles S+, *J Am Acad Dermatol* 38, 201 (passim)
(1998): Jan V+, *Dermatology* 197, 274
(1997): Vincente-Calleja JM+, *Br J Dermatol* 137, 837
(1997): Blodgett TP+, *Cutis* 60, 45
(1996): Wolkenstein P+, *Contact Dermatitis* 35, 234
(1995): Wakelin SH+, *Clin Exp Dermatol* 20, 341
(1995): Moreau A+, *Int J Dermatol* 34, 263 (passim)
(1995): Krasovec M+, *Schweiz Rundsch Med Prax* (German) 84, 814
(1993): Janier M+, *Br J Dermatol* 129, 354
(1992): Wittal RA+, *Australas J Dermatol* 33, 11
(1988): Lambert DG+, *Br J Dermatol* 118, 308

Angioedema
(1998): Knowles S+, *J Am Acad Dermatol* 38, 201 (passim)
(1989): Sadick NS+, *J Am Acad Dermatol* 21, 132

Ankle edema
(1994): Litt JZ, Beachwood, OH, personal case (observation)

Capillaritis (Schamberg's)
(1999): Eastern JS, Belleville, NJ, (from Internet) (observation)

Cutaneous side effects (sic)
(1993): Kitamura K+, *J Dermatol* 20, 279 (psoriasiform) (31%)
(1993): Sousa-Basto A+, *Contact Dermatitis* 29, 44

Dermatitis (sic)

Diaphoresis
(1988): Lambert DG+, *Br J Dermatol* 118, 308 (passim)
(1985): Scolnick B+, *Ann Intern Med* 102, 558

Ecchymoses (< 1%)

Edema (1–10%)
(1998): Knowles S+, *J Am Acad Dermatol* 38, 201 (passim)
(1982): Hossack KF, *Am J Cardiol* 49, 567
(1982): McGraw BF, *Drug Intell Clin Pharm* 16, 366

Erythema
(1998): Knowles S+, *J Am Acad Dermatol* 38, 201 (passim)
(1982): McGraw BF, *Drug Intell Clin Pharm* 16, 366

Erythema multiforme (< 1%)
(1998): Knowles S+, *J Am Acad Dermatol* 38, 201 (passim)
(1995): Avila JR+, *Ann Pharmacother* 29, 317
(1993): Sousa-Basto A+, *Contact Dermatitis* 29, 44
(1993): Sanders CJ+, *Lancet* 341, 967
(1993): Kitamura K+, *J Dermatol* 20, 279 (psoriasiform) (31%)
(1992): Wittal RA+, *Australas J Dermatol* 33, 11
(1989): Stern R+, *Arch Intern Med* 149, 829
(1989): Brown FH+, *Ann Dent* 48, 39
(1989): Berbis P+, *Dermatologica* 179, 90

Exanthems
(2000): Heymann WR, *Cutis* 66, 129
(1998): Knowles S+, *J Am Acad Dermatol* 38, 201 (passim)
(1994): Baker BA+, *Ann Pharmacother* 28, 118
(1993): Sousa-Basto A+, *Contact Dermatitis* 29, 44
(1993): Kitamura K+, *J Dermatol* 20, 279 (psoriasiform) (31%)
(1992): Wittal RA+, *Australas J Dermatol* 33, 11 (erythroderma)
(1992): Romano A+, *Ann Allergy* 69, 31
(1990): Wirebaugh SR+, *Drug Intell Clin Pharm* 24, 1046
(1989): Stern R+, *Arch Intern Med* 149, 829
(1989): Jones SK+, *Clin Exp Dermatol* 14, 457
(1988): Wakeel RA+, *BMJ* 296, 1071 (passim)
(1988): Hammentgen R+, *Dtsch Med Wochenschr* (German) 113, 1283
(1988): Lambert DG+, *Br J Dermatol* 118, 308 (passim)
(1986): Gibson RS+, *N Engl J Med* 315, 423 (0.7%)
(1985): Scolnick B+, *Ann Intern Med* 102, 558
(1985): Chaffman M+, *Drugs* 29, 387 (1.3%)

Exfoliative dermatitis (< 1%)
(1998): Knowles S+, *J Am Acad Dermatol* 38, 201 (passim)
(1997): Odeh M, *J Toxicol Clin Toxicol* 35, 101
(1993): Sousa-Basto A+, *Contact Dermatitis* 29, 44
(1989): Stern R+, *Arch Intern Med* 149, 829
(1988): Wakeel RA+, *BMJ* 296, 1071 (passim)
(1986): Lavrijsen APM+, *Acta Derm Venereol* 66, 536 (in a patient with psoriasis)

Flushing (1–10%)
(1992): Shelley WB+, *Advanced Dermatologic Diagnosis*, WB Saunders, 583 (passim)
(1988): Lambert DG+, *Br J Dermatol* 118, 308 (passim)
(1985): Chaffman M+, *Drugs* 29, 387 (0.1–1%)
(1983): Lewis JG, *Drugs* 25, 196
(1982): McGraw BF, *Drug Intell Clin Pharm* 16, 366

Hyperkeratosis (feet)
(1992): Ilia R+, *Int J Cardiol* 35, 115

Lichenoid eruption (photosensitive)
(1988): Lambert DG+, *Br J Dermatol* 118, 308

Lupus erythematosus
(1998): Callen JP, Academy '98 Meeting (4 patients)
(1998): Knowles S+, *J Am Acad Dermatol* 38, 201 (passim)
(1995): Crowson AN+, *N Engl J Med* 333, 1429
(1989): Stern R+, *Arch Intern Med* 149, 829

Parkinsonism

Peeling of palms and soles (sic)
(1985): Scolnick B+, *Ann Intern Med* 102, 558

Periorbital edema
(1993): Friedland S+, *Arch Ophthalmol* 111, 1027

Peripheral edema (5–8%)

Petechiae (< 1%)

Photosensitivity (< 1%)
(1998): Knowles S+, *J Am Acad Dermatol* 38, 201 (passim)
(1997): O'Reilly FM+, American Academy of Dermatology Meeting, Poster #14
(1996): Seggev JS+, *J Allergy Clin Immunol* 97, 852
(1994): Shelley WB+, *Cutis* 53, 161 (observation)
(1992): Wittal RA+, *Australas J Dermatol* 33, 11 (erythroderma)
(1990): Young L+, *Clin Exp Dermatol* 15, 467
(1989): Berbis P+, *Dermatologica* 179, 90
(1988): Lambert DG+, *Br J Dermatol* 118, 308
(1986): Lavrijsen APM+, *Acta Derm Venereol* 66, 536
(1979): Hashimoto M+, *Acta Dermatol* (Kyoto) 74, 181
(1976): Fujiwara N+, *Nippon Rinsho* (Japanese) 34, 3121

Pruritus (< 1%)
(2000): Heymann WR, *Cutis* 66, 129
(1998): Knowles S+, *J Am Acad Dermatol* 38, 201 (passim)
(1994): Baker BA+, *Ann Pharmacother* 28, 118
(1989): Stern R+, *Arch Intern Med* 149, 829
(1986): Gibson RS+, *N Engl J Med* 315, 423 (0.7%)
(1982): McGraw BF, *Drug Intell Clin Pharm* 16, 366

Psoriasis
(1998): Knowles S+, *J Am Acad Dermatol* 38, 201 (passim)
(1993): Kitamura K+, *J Dermatol* 20, 279 (psoriasiform) (31%)

Purpura (< 1%)
(1998): Knowles S+, *J Am Acad Dermatol* 38, 201 (passim)
(1992): Kuo M+, *Ann Pharmacother* 26, 1089

Pustular eruption
(1993): Janier M+, *Br J Dermatol* 129, 354
(1988): Lambert DG+, *Br J Dermatol* 118, 308

Pustular psoriasis
(1989): Stern R+, *Arch Intern Med* 149, 829

Rash (sic) (1.3%)
(1998): Knowles S+, *J Am Acad Dermatol* 38, 201 (passim)
(1989): Stern R+, *Arch Intern Med* 149, 829
(1982): McGraw BF, *Drug Intell Clin Pharm* 16, 366

Skin thickening (sic)
(1998): Knowles S+, *J Am Acad Dermatol* 38, 201 (passim)

(1992): Ilia R+, *Int J Cardiol* 35, 115
Stevens–Johnson syndrome
(1998): Knowles S+, *J Am Acad Dermatol* 38, 201 (passim)
(1993): Sanders CJ+, *Lancet* 341, 967
(1990): Taylor J+, *Clin Pharmacy* 9, 948
(1989): Stern R+, *Arch Intern Med* 149, 829
Subcorneal pustular dermatosis
(1992): Wittal RA+, *Australas J Dermatol* 33, 11
Toxic dermatitis (sic)
(1988): Wakeel RA+, *BMJ* 296, 1071
Toxic epidermal necrolysis
(1998): Knowles S+, *J Am Acad Dermatol* 38, 201 (passim)
(1991): No Author, *Lakartidningen* (Swedish) 88, 3489
(1989): Stern R+, *Arch Intern Med* 149, 829
(1988): Wakeel RA+, *BMJ* 296, 1071 (passim)
Toxic erythema
(1998): Knowles S+, *J Am Acad Dermatol* 38, 201 (passim)
(1988): Wakeel RA+, *BMJ* 296, 1071
Toxic skin eruptions
(1993): Barbaud A+, *Therapie* (French) 48, 499
Ulcerations of legs
(1989): Jones SK+, *Clin Exp Dermatol* 14, 457
(1988): Carmichael AJ+, *BMJ* 297, 562 (vasculitic)
Urticaria (<1%)
(1998): Knowles S+, *J Am Acad Dermatol* 38, 201 (passim)
(1989): Stern R+, *Arch Intern Med* 149, 829
(1989): Sadick NS+, *J Am Acad Dermatol* 21, 132
(1989): Jones SK+, *Clin Exp Dermatol* 14, 457
Vasculitis (<1%)
(1998): Knowles S+, *J Am Acad Dermatol* 38, 201 (passim)
(1992): Wittal RA+, *Australas J Dermatol* 33, 11
(1992): Kuo M+, *Ann Pharmacother* 26, 1089
(1989): Stern R+, *Arch Intern Med* 149, 829
(1988): Sheehan-Dare RA+, *Postgrad Med J* 64, 467
(1988): Sheehan-Dare RA+, *Br J Dermatol* 119, 134

Hair

Hair – alopecia (<1%)
(1998): Knowles S+, *J Am Acad Dermatol* 38, 201 (passim)
(1989): Stern R+, *Arch Intern Med* 149, 829
Hair – hirsutism
(1989): Stern R+, *Arch Intern Med* 149, 829

Nails

Nails – dystrophy
(1989): Stern R+, *Arch Intern Med* 149, 829

Other

Dysgeusia (<1%)
(2000): Zervakis J+, *Physiol Behav* 68, 405
Erythromyalgia
(1989): Stern R+, *Arch Intern Med* 149, 829
Gingival hyperplasia (21%)
(1999): Ellis JS+, *J Periodontol* 70, 63 (74%)
(1998): Knowles S+, *J Am Acad Dermatol* 38, 201 (passim)
(1995): Moghadam BKH+, *Cutis* 56, 46 (passim)
(1993): King GN+, *J Clin Periodontol* 20, 286
(1990): Brown RS+, *Oral Surg* 70, 593
(1987): Giustiniani S+, *Int J Cardiol* 15, 247
Gynecomastia
(1994): Otto C+, *Arch Intern Med* 154, 351
Hypersensitivity
(1998): Knowles S+, *J Am Acad Dermatol* 38, 201 (passim)
Lymphadenopathy
(1985): Scolnick B+, *Ann Intern Med* 102, 558
Parageusia (<1%)
Paresthesias (<1%)
(1982): McGraw BF, *Drug Intell Clin Pharm* 16, 366
Pseudolymphoma
(1995): Magro CM+, *J Am Acad Dermatol* 32, 419
Tremor (<1%)
Xerostomia (<1%)
(1983): Lewis JG, *Drugs* 25, 196
(1981): Pepine CJ+, *Am Heart J* 101, 719

DIMENHYDRINATE

Trade names: Calm-X; Dimetabs; Dramamine; Marmine; Nico-Vert; Tega-Cert; Tega-Vert; Triptone; Vertab; Wehamine, etc. (Various pharmaceutical companies.)
Other common trade names: *Andrumin; Lomarin; Nauseatol; Nausicalm; Travel Tabs; Vomacur; Vomex A; Vomisen*
Indications: Motion sickness, dizziness, nausea, vomiting
Category: H_1-receptor antihistamine and antinauseant
Half-life: no data
Clinically important, potentially serious interactions with: aminoglycoside antibiotics, anticholinergics, CNS depressants, MAO inhibitors, tricyclic antidepressants

Reactions

Skin

Angioedema (<1%)
Diaphoresis
Eczematous eruption (sic)
Edema (<1%)
Exanthems
Fixed eruption (<1%)
(2000): Ozkaya-Bayazit E+, *Eur J Dermatol* 10, 288
(2000): Smith KC, Niagara Falls, Ontario, (from Internet) (observation) (recurrent)
(2000): Saenz de San Pedro B+, *Allergy* 55, 297
(1999): Gallagher W, *The Schoch Letter*, 49, #1, 2
(1998): Smola H+, *Br J Dermatol* 138, 920
(1997): Gonzalo-Garijo MA+, *Br J Dermatol* 135, 661
(1992): Hatzis J+, *Cutis* 50, 50
(1989): Hogan DJ+, *J Am Acad Dermatol* 20, 503
(1982): Schnyder UW+, *Dermatologica* 165, 292
(1960): Kirshbaum BA+, *Am J Med Sci* 240, 512
(1960): Stritzler C+, *J Invest Dermatol* 34, 319
Flushing
Photosensitivity (<1%)
(1976): Horio T, *Arch Dermatol* 112, 1125
Rash (sic) (<1%)
Systemic eczematous contact dermatitis
Urticaria

Other

Acute intermittent porphyria
Anaphylactoid reaction
Injection-site pain (<1%)
Myalgia (<1%)
Paresthesias (<1%)
Xerostomia (1–10%)

DIPHENHYDRAMINE

Trade names: Allermax; Benadryl (Parke-Davis); Benylin (Warner-Lambert); Compoz; Sominex 2; Valdrene, etc.
Other common trade names: *Allerdryl; Allermin; Banophen; Benahist; Dibrondrin; Dolestan; Genahist; Insomnal; Nytol; Resmin; Sediat*
Indications: Allergic rhinitis, urticaria
Category: Antihistamine; antidyskinetic; antiemetic; sedative-hypnotic
Half-life: 2–8 hours
Clinically important, potentially serious interactions with: alcohol, chloral hydrate, CNS depressants, donepezil, glutethimide, levodopa, MAO inhibitors, metoprolol, quinidine, tacrine, tricyclic antidepressants

Reactions

Skin

Allergic reactions (sic)
(1970): Fidel' VG, *Klin Med Mosk* (Russian) 48, 109
Angioedema (<1%)
(1988): Self F+, *J R Soc Med* 81, 544

Contact dermatitis
(1998): Yamada S+, *Contact Dermatitis* 38, 282
(1983): Coskey RJ, *J Am Acad Dermatol* 8, 204
(1976): Horio T, *Arch Dermatol* 112, 1124
(1972): Shelley WB+, *Acta Derm Venereol* (Stockh) 52, 376
Diaphoresis
Eczema (sic)
(1981): Lawrence CM+, *Contact Dermatitis* 7, 276
(1972): Shelley WB+, *Acta Derm Venereol* (Stockh) 52, 376
Edema (<1%)
Exanthems
(1965): Davenport PM+, *Arch Dermatol* 92, 577
Fixed eruption
(1993): Dwyer CM+, *J Am Acad Dermatol* 29, 496
(1973): Csonka GW, *Br J Vener Dis* 49, 316
(1970): Savin JA, *Br J Dermatol* 83, 546
(1961): Welsh AM, *Arch Dermatol* 84, 1004
Livedo reticularis
(1996): Morell A+, *Dermatology* 193, 50
Photosensitivity (<1%)
(2000): Danby FW, Manchester NH (from Internet) (observation)
(1976): Horio T, *Arch Dermatol* 112, 1124
(1974): Emmett EA, *Arch Dermatol* 110, 249
(1962): Schreiber M+, *Arch Dermatol* 86, 58
Pruritus
(1998): Litt JZ, Beachwood, OH, personal case (observation) (following varicella)
(1972): Shelley WB+, *Acta Derm Venereol* (Stockh) 52, 376
(1965): Davenport PM+, *Arch Dermatol* 92, 577
Purpura
(1996): Morell A+, *Dermatology* 193, 50
Rash (sic) (<1%)
Toxic epidermal necrolysis
(1991): Epishin AV+, *Klin Med Mosk* (Russian) 69, 92
(1978): Soskin IaM+, *Akush Ginekol Kruglikova* (Russian) January, 67
(1972): Timperman J+, *Z Rechtsmed* (German) 71, 139
Urticaria
Vasculitis
(1965): Davenport PM+, *Arch Dermatol* 92, 577

Other
Anaphylactoid reaction
(1998): Barranco P+, *Allergy* 53, 814
(1995): Manhart AR+, *J Toxicol Clin Toxicol* 33, 189
(1994): Watanabe T+, *J Toxicol Clin Toxicol* 32, 593
(1980): Sandler BB, *Sov Med* (Russian) (9) 119
Hypersensitivity
Injection-site gangrene
(1989): Ramsdell WM, *J Am Acad Dermatol* 21, 1318
Injection-site necrosis
(1989): Ramsdell WM, *J Am Acad Dermatol* 21, 1318
Myalgia (<1%)
Paresthesias (<1%)
Tremor
Xerostomia (1–10%)

DIPHENOXYLATE

Trade names: Logen; Lomanate; Lomotil (Searle); Lonox (Geneva)
Other common trade names: *Lamocot; Lofene; Low-Quel*
Indications: Diarrhea
Category: Antidiarrheal
Half-life: 2.5 hours
Clinically important, potentially serious interactions with: alcohol, anticholinergics, barbiturates, CNS depressants, digoxin, MAO inhibitors

***Note:** Diphenoxylate is almost always prescribed with atropine sulfate

Reactions

Skin
Angioedema
Diaphoresis (<1%)
Flushing
Pruritus (<1%)
Urticaria (<1%)

Other
Anaphylactoid reaction
Gingivitis
Paresthesias
Xerostomia (3%)

DIPHENYLHYDANTOIN

(See PHENYTOIN)

DIPYRIDAMOLE

Trade names: Aggrenox (Boehringer Ingelheim), Persantine (Boehringer Dupont)
Other common trade names: *Cardoxin; Cleridium; Coronarine; Coroxin; Curantyl N; Lodimol; Novo-Dipiradol; Dipridacot; Persantin*
Indications: Thromboembolic complications following cardiac valve replacement
Category: Platelet aggregation inhibitor and coronary vasodilator
Half-life: 10–12 hours
Clinically important, potentially serious interactions with: adenosine, anticoagulants, aspirin, beta-blockers, heparin, indomethacin, NSAIDs, salicylates, theophylline, valproic acid, warfarin

Aggrenox is dipyridamole and aspirin

Reactions

Skin
Allergic reactions (sic) (<1%)
Angioedema
(1971): Sullivan JM+, *N Engl J Med* 284, 1391
Diaphoresis (0.4%)
Edema (0.3%)
Erythema multiforme
Exanthems
(1971): Sullivan JM+, *N Engl J Med* 284, 1391
Flushing (3.4%)
Pruritus
(1971): Sullivan JM+, *N Engl J Med* 284, 1391
Psoriasis
(1971): Sullivan JM+, *N Engl J Med* 284, 1391
Purpura (1.4%)
(1993): Kaufman DW+, *Blood* 82, 2714
Rash (sic) (2.3%)
(1971): Sullivan JM+, *N Engl J Med* 284, 1391
Stevens–Johnson syndrome
(1971): Sullivan JM+, *N Engl J Med* 284, 1391
Toxic epidermal necrolysis
(1993): Seoane-Leston JM+, *Rev Stomatol Chir Maxillofac* (French) 94, 281
Ulceration (<1%)
Urticaria
(1971): Sullivan JM+, *N Engl J Med* 284, 1391

Other
Anaphylactoid reaction
(1994): Weinmann P+, *Am J Med* 97, 488
Dysgeusia (0.1%)
Gingival bleeding (<1%)
Hypesthesia (0.5%)
Injection-site pain (0.1%)
Injection-site reactions (0.4%)
Mastodynia (0.03%)
Myalgia (0.9%)
Paresthesias (1.3%)

Pseudopolymyalgia rheumatica
(1990): Chassagne P+, *BMJ* 301, 875
Tremor (<1%)

DIRITHROMYCIN

Trade name: Dynabac (Sanofi)
Indications: Various infections caused by susceptible organisms
Category: Macrolide antibiotic
Half-life: 8 hours
Clinically important, potentially serious interactions with: bromocriptine, carbamazepine, cyclosporine, digoxin, estrogens, pimozide, terfenadine

Reactions

Skin
Allergic reactions (sic) (<1%)
Bullous eruption
Diaphoresis (<1%)
Edema (<1%)
Flu-like syndrome (sic) (<1%)
Peripheral edema (<1%)
Pruritus (1.2%)
Rash (sic) (1.4%)
Urticaria (1.2%)

Other
Anaphylactoid reaction
Dysgeusia (<1%)
Myalgia (<1%)
Oral ulceration (<1%)
Paresthesias (<1%)
Tremor (<1%)
Vaginal candidiasis (<1%)
Vaginitis (<1%)
Xerostomia (<1%)

DISOPYRAMIDE

Trade name: Norpace (Searle)
Other common trade names: *Dimodan; Dirythmin SA; Disonorm; Durbis; Isorythm;*
Indications: Ventricular arrhythmias
Category: Antiarrhythmic
Half-life: 4–10 hours
Clinically important, potentially serious interactions with: astemizole, beta-blockers, clarithromycin, digoxin, erythromycin, gatifloxacin, hydantoins, moxifloxacin, procainamide, quinidine, rifampin, sparfloxacin, terfenadine

Reactions

Skin
Angioedema
Dermatitis (sic)
Edema (1–3%)
Erythema nodosum
(1985): Niv Y+, *Harefuah* (Hebrew) 108, 490
Exanthems (1–5%)
(1987): Brogden RN+, *Drugs* 34, 151 (1–2%)
(1973): *Drug Ther Bull* 11, 3
Lupus erythematosus (<1%)
(1985): Epstein A+, *Arthritis Rheum* 28, 158
(1981): Wanner WR+, *Am Heart J* 101, 687,
Photosensitivity
(1987): Brogden RN+, *Drugs* 34, 151
Pruritus (1–3%)
Purpura
(1987): Brogden RN+, *Drugs* 34, 151
Rash (sic) (generalized) (1–3%)
Urticaria
Xerosis

Hair
Hair – alopecia

Other
Gynecomastia (<1%)
Oral mucosal lesions (40%)
(1987): Brogden RN+, *Drugs* 34, 151
Paresthesias (<1%)
Xerostomia (32%)
(1987): Brogden RN+, *Drugs* 34, 151 (40%)

DISULFIRAM

Trade name: Antabuse (Wyeth-Ayerst)
Other common trade names: *Antabus; Busetal; Esperal; Nocbin; Refusal; Tetradin*
Indications: Alcoholism
Category: Deterrent to alcohol consumption
Half-life: no data
Clinically important, potentially serious interactions with: alcohol, anticoagulants, benzodiazepines, chlorzoxazone, hydantoins, isoniazid, MAO inhibitors, metronidazole, phenytoin, theophylline, tricyclic antidepressants, warfarin

Reactions

Skin
Acne
(1967): Hitch JM, *JAMA* 200, 879
(1964): Fegeler F, *Arch Klin Exp Dermatol* (German) 219, 335
(1953): Barefoot SW, *JAMA* 147, 1653
Allergic reactions (sic)
Bullous eruption
(1990): Larbre B+, *Ann Dermatol Venereol* (French) 117, 721
(1979): Webb PK+, *JAMA* 241, 2061
Contact dermatitis (on exposure to rubber)
(1996): Rebandel P+, *Contact Dermatitis* 35, 48
(1995): Fisher AA, *Cutis* 56, 131
(1994): Mathelier-Fusade P+, *Contact Dermatitis* 31, 121
(1992): Baptista A+, *Contact Dermatitis* 26, 140
(1989): Minet A+, *Ann Dermatol Venereol* (French) 116, 543
(1988): Olfson M, *Am J Psychiatry* 145, 651
(1984): van Hecke E+, *Contact Dermatitis* 10, 254
(1982): Fisher AA, *Cutis* 30, 461 (passim)
(1979): Webb PK+, *JAMA* 241, 2061
(1979): *Contact Dermatitis* 5, 199
(1976): Lachapelle JM+, *Nouv Presse Med* (French) 5, 1536
(1975): Lachapelle JM, *Contact Dermatitis* 1, 218
(1974): Kobayasi T+, *Arch Dermatol Forsch* (German) 249, 125
(1970): Gunther WW, *Med J Aust* 1, 1177
(1968): van Ketel WG, *Ned Tijdschr Geneeskd* (Dutch) 112, 406
Dermatitis recall (nickel)
(1993): Gamboa P+, *Contact Dermatitis* 28, 255
(1992): Klein LR+, *J Am Acad Dermatol* 26, 645
(1987): Grondahl-Hansen V+, *Ugeskr Laeger* (Danish) 149, 2401
(1987): Kaaber K+, *Derm Beruf Umwelt* (German) 35, 209
Diaphoresis (<1%) (with alcohol)
Eczematous eruption (sic)
(1994): Mathelier-Fusade P+, *Contact Dermatitis* 31, 121
(1981): Goitre M+, *Contact Dermatitis* 7, 272
Exanthems
(1992): Breathnach SM+, *Adverse Drug Reactions and the Skin*, Blackwell, Oxford, 204 (passim)
(1989): Minet A+, *Ann Dermatol Venereol* (French) 116, 543
Fixed eruption (<1%)
(1961): Welsh AL+, *Arch Dermatol* 84, 1004
(1950): Lewis HM+, *JAMA* 142, 1141

Flushing (< 1%) (with alcohol)
(1992): Shelley WB+, *Advanced Dermatologic Diagnosis*, WB Saunders, 582 (passim)
(1992): Breathnach SM+, *Adverse Drug Reactions and the Skin*, Blackwell, Oxford, 204 (passim)
(1982): Fisher AA, *Cutis* 30, 461 (passim)
(1981): Wilkins JK, *Ann Intern Med* 95, 468
Periarteritis nodosa
(1975): Telerman-Toppet N+, *Acta Clin Belg* (French) 30, 101
Purpura
(1982): Thompson CC+, *J Am Dent Assoc* 105, 465
Pustular eruption
(1990): Larbre R+, *Ann Dermatol Venereol* (French) 117, 721
Rash (sic) (1–10%)
Skin reaction (sic) (from beer-containing shampoo)
(1980): Stoll D+, *JAMA* 244, 2045
Systemic eczematous contact dermatitis (sic)
(1966): Fisher AA, *Ann Allergy* 24, 406
Toxic epidermal necrolysis
(1989): Stern RS+, *J Am Acad Dermatol* 21, 317
Urticaria
(1992): Breathnach SM+, *Adverse Drug Reactions and the Skin*, Blackwell, Oxford, 204 (passim)
(1989): Minet A+, *Ann Dermatol Venereol* (French) 116, 543
(1982): Fisher AA, *Cutis* 30, 461 (passim)
Vasculitis
(1985): Sanchez NP+, *Arch Dermatol* 121, 220
Yellow palms
(1997): Santonastaso M+, *Lancet* 350, 266

Other

Dysgeusia (metallic or garlic aftertaste) (1–10%)
Hypogeusia
Paresthesias
Periarteritis nodosa
(1970): Zanini S+, *Fracastoro* (Italian) 63, 117

DIVALPROEX

(See VALPROIC ACID)

DOBUTAMINE

Trade name: Dobutrex (Lilly)
Other trade names: *Cardiject; Dobril; Dobuject; Dobutamin; Inotrex; Oxiken; Tobrex*
Indications: Cardiac surgery, heart failure
Category: Vasopressor; adrenergic agonist; sympathomimetic
Half-life: 2 minutes
Clinically important, potentially serious interactions with: beta-blockers, digoxin, furazolidone, guanethidine, MAO inhibitors, methyldopa, tricyclic antidepressants

Reactions

Skin

Erythema
(1991): Wu CC+, *Chest* 99, 1547
Pruritus
(1991): Wu CC+, *Chest* 99, 1547
(1986): McCauley CS+, *Ann Intern Med* 105, 966 (scalp)

Other

Dermal cellulitis
(1994): Cernek PK, *Ann Pharmacother* 28, 964
Dermal hypersensitivity (sic)
(1991): Wu CC+, *Chest* 99, 1547
Dermal necrosis
(1979): Hoff JV+, *N Engl J Med* 300, 1280
Injection site pain
Injection-site phlebitis
Paresthesias (1–10%)
Phlebitis

DOCETAXEL

Trade name: Taxotere (Aventis)
Indications: Metastatic breast cancer
Category: Antineoplastic
Half-life: 11–18 hours
Clinically important, potentially serious interactions with: cyclosporine, erythromycin, fluconazole, fluoxetine, itraconazole, ketoconazole, ritonavir, terfenadine, troleandomycin, zileuton

Reactions

Skin

Angioedema
Ankle edema
(1995): Zimmerman GC+, *Arch Dermatol* 131, 202
Edema (1–10%)
(1996): Edmonson JH+, *Am J Clin Oncon* 19, 574
(1993): Schrijvers D+, *Ann Oncol* 4, 610 (20%)
Erythema (0.9%)
(1995): Cortes JE+, *J Clin Oncol* 13, 2643
Erythrodysesthesia syndrome
(1995): Zimmerman GC+, *Arch Dermatol* 131, 202
(1994): Zimmerman GC+, *J Natl Cancer Inst* 86, 557
(1993): Vukelja SJ+, *J Natl Cancer Inst* 85, 1432
Exanthems
(1995): Zimmerman GC+, *Arch Dermatol* 131, 202
(1995): Cortes JE+, *J Clin Oncol* 13, 2643
Fibrosis
(2000): Cleveland MG+, *Cancer* 88, 1078 (generalized cutaneous)
Fixed eruption (erythematous plaque)
(2000): Chu CY+, *Br J Dermatol* 142, 808
Flushing
Peripheral edema (1–10%)
Photo-recall phenomenon
(1995): Zimmerman GC+, *Arch Dermatol* 131, 202
Photosensitivity
(1995): Zimmerman GC+, *Arch Dermatol* 131, 202
Pruritus
(1995): Cortes JE+, *J Clin Oncol* 13, 2643
Rash (sic) (0.9%)
(1996): Edmonson JH+, *Am J Clin Oncon* 19, 574
Scleroderma
(1995): Battafarano DF+, *Cancer* 76,110
Urticaria
Xerosis
(1995): Cortes JE+, *J Clin Oncol* 13, 2643

Hair

Hair – alopecia (80%)
(1995): Lemenager M+, *Lancet* 346, 371

Nails

Nails – Beau's lines (transverse nail bands)
(1999): Correia O+, *Dermatology* 198, 288
Nails – onycholysis
(1999): Correia O+, *Dermatology* 198, 288
(1998): Obermair A+, *Ann Oncol* 9, 230
(1996): Trudeau ME, *Semin Oncol* 22, 17
(1996): Dreyfuss AL+, *J Clin Oncol* 14, 1672
(1995): Zimmerman GC+, *Arch Dermatol* 131, 202
Nails – paronychia
(1999): Correia O+, *Dermatology* 198, 288 (painful)
Nails – pigmentation
(1999): Correia O+, *Dermatology* 198, 288 (orange discoloration)
(1998): Jacob CI+, *Arch Dermatol* 134, 1167 ("nail bed dyschromia")
Nails – subungual hemorrhage
(1999): Correia O+, *Dermatology* 198, 288
Nails – subungual hyperkeratosis
(1999): Correia O+, *Dermatology* 198, 288

Nails – transverse superficial loss of nail plate
(1999): Correia O+, *Dermatology* 198, 288
(1997): Llombart-Cussac A+, *Arch Dermatol* 133, 1466

Other

Dysesthesia (3.9%)
Hypersensitivity (0.9%)
(1996): Hudis CA+, *J Clin Oncol* 14, 58
(1995): Bedikian AY+, *J Clin Oncol* 13, 2895
(1993): Schrijvers D+, *Ann Oncol* 4, 610 (28%)
Infusion-site erythema
(1995): Zimmerman GC+, *Arch Dermatol* 131, 202
Infusion-site extravasation
(2000): Raley J+, *Gynecol Oncol* 78, 259
Infusion-site fixed eruption
(1995): Zimmerman GC+, *Arch Dermatol* 131, 202
Infusion-site hyperpigmentation
(2000): Schrijvers D+, *Br J Dermatol* 142, 1069
(1995): Zimmerman GC+, *Arch Dermatol* 131, 202
Infusion-site inflammation
(1995): Zimmerman GC+, *Arch Dermatol* 131, 202
Myalgia (>10%)
Paresthesias (3.9%)
Stomatitis (42.3%)
(1996): Edmonson JH+, *Am J Clin Oncon* 19, 574

DOCUSATE

Trade names: Colase; Dialose; Diocto; Disonate; DOK; Doxinate; Modane; Regutol; Sulfalax; Surfak, etc. (Various pharmaceutical companies.)
Other common trade names: *Coloxyl; Doxate-S; Hisof; Jamylene; Lambanol; Mollax; Regulex; Regutol; Selax; SoFlax; Softon*
Indications: Constipation
Category: Laxative; stool softener
Onset of action: 12–72 hours
Clinically important, potentially serious interactions with: mineral oil, phenolphthalein

Reactions

Skin

Contact dermatitis
(1998): Lee AY+, *Contact Dermatitis* 38, 355
Diaphoresis
Exanthems (1%)
Rash (sic)

Other

Dysgeusia

DOFETILIDE

Trade name: Tikosyn (Pfizer)
Indications: Conversion of atrial fibrillation and atrial flutter to normal sinus rhythm
Category: Class III antiarrhythmic
Half-life: 10 hours
Clinically important, potentially serious interactions with: aminoglycosides, cimetidine, corticosteroids, erythromycin, haloperidol, ketoconazole, loop diuretics, phenothiazines, protease inhibitors, thiazide diuretics, tricyclic antidepressants, trimethoprim, verapamil, **grapefruit juice**

Reactions

Skin

Angioedema (<2%)
Diaphoresis (>2%)
Edema
Flu-like syndrome (sic) (4%)
Peripheral edema (>2%)
Rash (sic) (3%)

Other

Paresthesias (<2%)

DOLASETRON

Trade name: Anzemet (Aventis)
Indications: Prevention of nausea and vomiting
Category: Antiemetic and antinauseant
Half-life: 7.3 hours
Clinically important, potentially serious interactions with: atenolol, cimetidine, quinidine, rifampin

Reactions

Skin

Chills (>2%)
Diaphoresis
Edema
Facial edema
Flushing
Peripheral edema
Pruritus
Purpura
Rash (sic)
Urticaria

Other

Anaphylactoid reaction
Dysgeusia
Myalgia
Paresthesias
Photophobia
Thrombophlebitis
Twitching (sic)

DONEPEZIL

Synonym: E2020
Trade name: Aricept (Eisai; Pfizer)
Indications: Mild dementia of the Alzheimer's type
Category: Reversible acetylcholinesterase inhibitor for Alzheimer's disease; cholinergic agent
Half-life: 50–70 hours
Clinically important, potentially serious interactions with: bethanechol, benztropine, carbamazepine, cholinesterase inhibitors, ketoconazole, phenytoin, quinidine, succinylcholine

Reactions

Skin

Dermatitis (sic) (<1%)
Diaphoresis (>1%)
Ecchymoses (4%)
Erythema (<1%)
Facial edema (<1%)
Flushing
(1996): Rogers SL+, *Dementia* 7, 293 (3%)
Hyperkeratosis (sic) (<1%)
Neurodermatitis (sic) (<1%)
Periorbital edema (<1%)
Pigmentation (<1%)
Pruritus (>1%)
Purpura (1–10%)
(1998): Bryant CA+, *BMJ 317, 787*
Striae (<1%)

Ulceration (<1%)
Urticaria (>1%)

Hair

Hair – alopecia (<1%)
Hair – hirsutism (<1%)

Other

Dysgeusia (<1%)
Gingivitis (<1%)
Paresthesias (<1%)
Tongue edema (<1%)
Vaginitis (<1%)
Xerostomia (<1%)

DOPAMINE

Trade names: Dopastat; Intropin
Other common trade names: *Cardiosteril; Dopamin; Dopamin AWD; Dopastat; Dynatra; Revimine*
Indications: Hemodynamic imbalances present in shock
Category: Adrenergic agonist; sympathomimetic; vasopressor
Half-life: 2 minutes
Clinically important, potentially serious interactions with: alpha-blockers, beta-blockers, furazolidone, digoxin, guanethidine, MAO inhibitors, methyldopa, phenytoin, procarbazine, tricyclic antidepressants

Reactions

Skin

Exanthems
Piloerection (goose bumps)
Pruritus
Raynaud's phenomenon (<1%)
Urticaria

Hair

Hair – alopecia

Other

Injection-site extravasation
(1998): Chen JL+, *Ann Pharmacother* 32, 545
(1989): Denkler KA+, *Plast Reconstr Surg* 84, 811
Injection-site gangrene
(1977): Boltax RS+, *N Engl J Med* 296, 823
Injection-site necrosis (<1%)
(1992): Breathnach SM+, *Adverse Drug Reactions and the Skin*, Blackwell, Oxford, 233 (passim)
(1982): Pillgram-Larsen J+, *Tidsskr Nor Laegeforen* (Norwegian) 102, 1583
(1976): Green SI+, *N Engl J Med* 294, 114
Injection-site piloerection and vasoconstriction (sic)
(1991): Ross M, *Arch Dermatol* 127, 586
Peripheral ischemia
(1983): Coakley J, *Lancet* 2, 633
Symmetric peripheral gangrene (sic)
(1997): Weinberg JM+, *Arch Dermatol* 133, 249

DORZOLAMIDE

Trade names: Cosopt (Merck); Trusopt (Merck)
Indications: Glaucoma; ocular hypertension
Category: Carbonic anhydrase inhibitor (a sulfonamide)*
Half-life: about 4 months
Clinically important, potentially serious interactions with: salicylates

Cosopt is dorzolamide and timolol

Reactions

Skin

Contact dermatitis
(1998): Aalto-Korte K, *Contact Dermatitis* 39, 206
Edema (eyelid)
(1998): Adamsons IA+, *J Glaucoma* 7, 395
Rash (sic) (<1%)
Stinging (ocular) (33%)
(2000): Stewart WC+, *Am J Ophthalmol* 129, 723
(1998): Adamsons IA+, *J Glaucoma* 7, 395

Other

Dysgeusia (25%)
Ocular burning (33%)

***Note:** Dorzolamide is a sulfonamide and can be absorbed systemically. Sulfonamides can produce severe, possibly fatal, reactions such as toxic epidermal necrolysis and Stevens–Johnson syndrome.

DOXACURIUM

Trade name: Nuromax (GlaxoWellcome)
Indications: Neuromuscular blockade
Category: Skeletal muscle relaxant; neuromuscular blocker
Half-life: 100–200 minutes
Clinically important, potentially serious interactions with: aminoglycosides, beta-blockers, bretylium, calcium channel blockers, carbamazepine, clindamycin, cyclosporine, dantrolene, furosemide, ketamine, lithium, phenytoin, procainamide, quinidine

Reactions

Skin

Rash (sic)
Urticaria (<1%)

DOXAPRAM

Trade name: Dopram (Robins)
Indications: Chronic obstructive pulmonary disease, drug-induced CNS depression
Category: Respiratory stimulant, CNS stimulant
Duration of action: 3.4 hours
Clinically important, potentially serious interactions with: MAO inhibitors, muscle relaxants, sympathomimetics

Reactions

Skin

Diaphoresis (<1%)
Flushing
(1972): *Drug Ther Bull* 10, 43
Pruritus
(1972): *Drug Ther Bull* 10, 43

Other

Injection-site erythema

Injection-site pain
Injection-site phlebitis (<1%)
Oral mucosal lesions
Paresthesias

DOXAZOSIN

Trade name: Cardura (Pfizer)
Other common trade names: *Alfadil; Cardoxan; Cardular; Dedralen; Diblocin; Supressin*
Indications: Hypertension
Category: Alpha-adrenergic blocking agent; antihypertensive
Half-life: 19–22 hours
Clinically important, potentially serious interactions with: ACE-inhibitors, beta-blockers, calcium channel blockers, estrogen, nifedipine, NSAIDs, verapamil

Reactions

Skin

Bruising
(1991): Anon, *Arch Intern Med* 151, 1413
Diaphoresis (1.4%)
(1988): Young JL+, *Drugs* 35, 525
Eczema (sic) (<0.5%)
Edema (4%)
Exanthems (1.7%)
(1988): Young JL+, *Drugs* 35, 525
Facial edema (1%)
Flu-like syndrome (sic) (1.1%)
Flushing (1%)
(1991): Anon, *Arch Intern Med* 151, 1413
Hot flashes (<1%)
Lichen planus
Lupus erythematosus
(1992): Feurle GE, *Dtsch Med Wochenschr* (German) 117, 157
Pallor (<1%)
Peripheral edema
Pruritus (1%)
Purpura (<0.5%)
Rash (sic) (1%)
(1991): Anon, *Arch Intern Med* 151, 1413
Urticaria
(1991): Anon, *Arch Intern Med* 151, 1413
Xerosis (<0.5%)

Hair

Hair – alopecia (<0.5%)
(1991): Anon, *Arch Intern Med* 151, 1413
Hair – growth (sic)
(1991): Anon, *Arch Intern Med* 151, 1413

Other

Dysgeusia (<0.5%)
(1991): Anon, *Arch Intern Med* 151, 1413
Hypesthesia (<1%)
Mastodynia (<1%)
Myalgia (1%)
Paresthesias
Parosmia (<0.05%)
Xerostomia (2%)
(1991): Anon, *Arch Intern Med* 151, 1413

DOXEPIN

Trade names: Sinequan (Pfizer); Zonalon (topical) (Bioglan)
Other common trade names: *Adapin; Alti-Doxepin; Anten; Aponal; Doneurin; Gilex; Mareen; Novo-Doxepin; Sinquan; Triadapin*
Indications: Mental depression, anxiety
Category: Tricyclic antidepressant, antipanic and antipruritic
Half-life: 6–8 hours
Clinically important, potentially serious interactions with: alcohol, amphetamines, anticoagulants, carbamazepine, cimetidine, clonidine, cocaine, diltiazem, disulfiram, epinephrine, fluoxetine, guanethidine, MAO inhibitors, phenothiazines, selegiline, sympathomimetics, verapamil

Reactions

Skin

Ankle edema
(1991): Dalack GW+, *Am J Psychiatry* 148, 1601
Allergic reactions (sic)
Contact dermatitis (from topical)
(1999): Wakelin SH+, *Contact Dermatitis* 40, 214
(1997): Koehn G, *The Schoch Letter* 47, 20 (observation)
(1996): Shelley WB+, *J Am Acad Dermatol* 34, 143
(1996): Taylor JS+, *Arch Dermatol* 132, 515
(1996): Bilbao I+, *Contact Dermatitis* 35, 254
(1996): Rapaport MJ, *Arch Dermatol* 132, 1516
(1996): Smith KC, Niagara Falls, Ontario (from Internet) (observation)
(1996): Shama S, *The Schoch Letter* 46, 36 (observation)
(1995): Greenberg JH, *Contact Dermatitis* 33, 281
(1995): Goldblum O, *The Schoch Letter* 45, 26 (observation)
(1995): Porres J, *The Schoch Letter* 45, 39 (observation)
Diaphoresis (1–10%)
Edema
Erythema
Exanthems
(1970): Pöldinger P+, *Praxis* 59, 1006 (0.4%)
Flushing
(1998): Foster M+, *J Clin Dermatol* Winter, 7
Parkinsonism
Photosensitivity (<1%)
(1985): Walter-Ryan WG+, *JAMA* 254, 357
(1982): *Patient Care* June 15, 208 (list)
Pruritus
(1970): Pöldinger P+, *Praxis* 59, 1006
Purpura
(1972): Nixon DD, *JAMA* 220, 418
Rash (sic)
(1991): Roose SP+, *J Clin Psychiatry* 52, 338
Red, dry skin (sic)
(1991): Kastrup O+, *Dtsch Med Wochenschr* (German) 116, 1748
Toxic dermatitis (sic)
(1995): Vo MY, *Arch Dermatol* 131, 1468
Urticaria
Vasculitis

Hair

Hair – alopecia (<1%)

Other

Aphthous stomatitis
(1980): Ives TJ+, *Am J Hosp Pharm* 37, 1551 (passim)
Application-site burning
Application-site edema
Dysgeusia (>10%)
Galactorrhea (<1%)
Glossalgia
(1980): Ives TJ+, *Am J Hosp Pharm* 37, 1551 (passim)
Glossitis
(1980): Ives TJ+, *Am J Hosp Pharm* 37, 1551
Gynecomastia (<1%)
Paresthesias
Pseudolymphoma
(1995): Magro CM+, *J Am Acad Dermatol* 32, 419

Stomatitis
(1981): Salem RB+, *Drug Intell Clin Pharm* 15, 992
Tremor
Xerostomia (>10%)
(1998): Foster M+, *J Clin Dermatol* Winter, 7 (5%)
(1989): Assalian P+, *Drugs* 38 (Suppl 1) 32
(1989): Lose G+, *J Urol* 142, 1024

DOXERCALCIFEROL

Trade name: Hectorol (Bone Care)
Indications: Secondary hyperparathyroidism
Category: Vitamin D analog (prohormone)
Half-life: 32–37 hours
Clinically important, potentially serious interactions with: magnesium-containing antacids, vitamin D supplements

Reactions

Skin
Edema (34.4%)
Pruritus (8.2%)

DOXORUBICIN

Trade names: Adriamycin (Pharmacia & Upjohn); Doxil (Alza); Rubex (Bristol-Myers Squibb)
Other common trade names: *Adiblastine; Adriablastine; Adriacin; Adriblatina; Farmablastina*
Indications: Carcinomas, leukemias, sarcomas
Category: Anthracycline and antibiotic antineoplastic
Half-life: α phase: 0.6 hours; β phase: 16.7 hours
Clinically important, potentially serious interactions with: cyclophosphamide, cyclosporine, digoxin, interferon alfa, mercaptopurine, quinolones, streptozocin, verapamil

Reactions

Skin
Acral erythrodysesthesia syndrome (hand-foot syndrome)
(1995): Gordon KB+, *Cancer* 75, 2169
(1991): Baack BR+, *J Am Acad Dermatol* 24, 457
(1989): Jones AP+, *Br J Cancer* 59, 814
(1985): Walker IR+, *Arch Dermatol* 121, 1240
(1985): Levine LE+, *Arch Dermatol* 121, 102
(1985): Vogelzang NJ+, *Ann Intern Med* 103, 303
(1984): Lokich JJ+, *Ann Intern Med* 101, 798
(1982): Cordonnier C+, *Ann Intern Med* 97, 783
Allergic reactions (sic) (<1%)
(1979): Fallah-Sohy E+, *JAMA* 241, 1108
Angioedema
(1984): Collins JA, *Drug Intell Clin Pharm* 18, 402
(1983): Bronner AK+, *J Am Acad Dermatol* 9, 645
(1981): Weiss RB+, *Ann Intern Med* 94, 66
(1981): von Eyben FE+, *Cancer* 48, 1535 (passim)
(1979): Maldonado JE, *N Engl J Med* 301, 386
Cellulitis
Contact dermatitis
(1975): Reich SD+, *Cancer Chemother Rep* 59, 677
Dermatitis herpetiformis
(1986): Gottlieb D+, *Med J Aust* 145, 241
Erythema of palms and soles (painful)
(1990): Pagliuca A+, *Postgrad Med J* 66, 242
(1989): Oksenhendler E+, *Eur J Cancer Clin Oncol* 25, 1181
(1988): Shall L+, *Br J Dermatol* 119, 249
(1989): Jones AP+, *Br J Cancer* 59, 814
Exanthems
(1987): Lee M+, *J Urol* 138, 143
(1984): Collins JA, *Drug Intell Clin Pharm* 18, 402
Exfoliative dermatitis
(1975): Manalo FB+, *JAMA* 233, 56
Flushing (1–10%)
(1992): Curran CF, *Arch Dermatol* 128, 1408
(1987): Lee M+, *J Urol* 138, 143
Hyperpigmentation
(1983): Bronner AK+, *J Am Acad Dermatol* 9, 645 (palms and soles)
(1977): Kew MC+, *Lancet* 1, 811
(1974): Pratt CB+, *JAMA* 228, 460 (dermal creases)
Keratoderma
(1975): Manalo FB+, *JAMA* 233, 56
Necrosis (local)
(1998): Bekerecioglu M+, *J Surg Res* 75, 61
(1982): Riegels-Nielsen P+, *Ugeskr-Laeger* (Danish) 144, 1313
(1981): von Eyben FE+, *Cancer* 48, 1535 (passim)
(1976): Rudolph R+, *Cancer* 38, 1087
Pigmentation
(1996): Schulte-Huermann P+, *Dermatology* 191, 65
(1992): Konohana A, *J Dermatol* 19, 250
(1990): Curran CF, *N Z Med J* 103, 517
(1990): Kumar L+, *N Z Med J* 103, 165
(1987): Loureiro C+, *J Clin Oncol* 5, 1705
(1983): Bronner AK+, *J Am Acad Dermatol* 9, 645
(1982): Alagaratnam TT+, *Aust N Z J Surg* 52, 531
(1981): Granstein RD+, *J Am Acad Dermatol* 5, 1 (brown-black)
(1980): Orr LE+, *Arch Dermatol* 116, 273
(1977): Kew MC+, *Lancet* 1, 811
(1976): Rubegni M+, *Nouv Presse Med* (French) 5, 798
(1974): Rothberg H+, *Cancer Chemother Rep* 58, 749
Postirradiation erythema
Pruritus
(1987): Lee M+, *J Urol* 138, 143
(1984): Solimando DA+, *Drug Intell Clin Pharm* 18, 808
Purpura
(1987): Lee M+, *J Urol* 138, 143
(1971): Wang JJ+, *Cancer* 28, 837
Radiation recall (<1%)
(1976): Greco FA+, *Ann Intern Med* 85, 294
(1975): Dreizen S+, *Postgrad Med* 58, 150
(1974): Etcubanas E+, *Cancer Chemother Rep* 58, 757
Rash (sic)
(2000): Israel VP+, *Gynecol Oncol* 78, 143
(1981): Karlin DA+, *Lancet* 2, 534
Raynaud's phenomenon
(1993): von Gunten CF+, *Cancer* 72, 2004
Scrotal skin toxicity (sic)
(2000): Toma S+, *Anticancer Res* 20, 485
Toxic epidermal injury (sic)
(1981): von Eyben FE+, *Cancer* 48, 1535
Urticaria (<1%)
(1986): Wandt H, *Dtsch Med Wochenschr* (German) 111, 356
(1984): Collins JA, *Drug Intell Clin Pharm* 18, 402
(1984): Solimando DA+, *Drug Intell Clin Pharm* 18, 808
(1983): Bronner AK+, *J Am Acad Dermatol* 9, 645
(1981): Weiss RB+, *Ann Intern Med* 94, 66
(1981): von Eyben FE+, *Cancer* 48, 1535 (passim)
(1981): Hatfield AK+, *Cancer Treat Rep* 65, 353
(1978): Souhami J+, *JAMA* 240, 1624
(1974): Pratt CB+, *Am J Dis Child* 127, 534
(1974): Pratt CB+, *JAMA* 228, 460 (passim)

Hair
Hair – alopecia (>10%)
(1995): Bonadonna G+, *JAMA* 273, 542 (96%)
(1994): Bogner JR+, *J Acquir Immune Defic Syndr* 7, 463
(1994): Rodrigeuz R+, *Ann Oncol* 5, 769
(1989): Henderson IC+, *J Clin Oncol* 7, 560 (>5%)
(1988): Giaccone G+, *Cancer Nurs* 11, 170
(1986): Martin-Jiminez M+, *N Engl J Med* 315, 894
(1986): Perez JE+, *Cancer Treat Rep* 70, 1213
(1984): Satterwhite B+, *Cancer* 54, 34
(1984): Wheelock JB+, *Cancer Treat Rep* 68, 1387
(1983): Tigges FJ, *MMW Munch Med Wochenschr* (German) 125, 19
(1983): Howard N+, *Br J Radiol* 56, 963
(1982): Gregory RP+, *Br Med J Clin Res Ed* 284, 1674
(1982): Hunt JM+, *Cancer Nurs* 5, 25
(1981): Tigges FJ, *MMW Munch Med Wochenschr* (German) 123, 737

(1981): Cooke T+, *Br Med J Clin Res Ed* 282, 734
(1981): Anderson JE+, *Br Med J Clin Res* 282, 423
(1981): Hallett N, *Nurs Mirror* 152, 32
(1980): Timothy AR+, *Lancet* 1, 663
(1980): Presser SE, *N Engl J Med* 302, 921
(1979): Lovejoy NC, *Cancer Nurs* 2, 117
(1979): Dean JC+, *N Engl J Med* 301, 1427
(1978): Soukop M+, *Cancer Treat Rep* 62, 489
(1977): Edelstyn GA+, *Lancet* 2, 253
(1975): Manalo FB+, *JAMA* 233, 56
(1974): Cortes EP+, *JAMA* 221, 1132 (100%)
(1974): Blum RH+, *Ann Intern Med* 80, 249 (85–100%)
(1974): Pratt CB+, *Am J Dis Child* 127, 534 (80%)
(1974): Pratt CB+, *JAMA* 228, 460 (passim)
(1971): Wang JJ+, *Cancer* 28, 837
(1971): Middleman E, *Cancer* 25, 844
(1969): Bonadonna G+, *BMJ* 3, 503 (60–100%)

Nails

Nails – Beau's lines (transverse nail bands)
(1994): Ben-Dayan D+, *Acta Haematol* 91, 89
Nails – onycholysis
(1990): Curran CF, *Arch Dermatol* 126, 1244
(1989): Jones AP+, *Br J Cancer* 59, 814
(1985): Kechijian P, *J Am Acad Dermatol* 12, 552
(1980): Runne U+, *Z Haut* (German) 55, 1590
(1975): Manalo FB+, *JAMA* 233, 56
Nails – pigmentation (1–10%)
(1983): Manigand G+, *Sem Hop* (French) 59, 1840
(1982): Sans-Ortiz J+, *Med Clin (Barc)* (Spanish) 79, 49
(1981): Giacobetti R+, *Am J Dis Child* 135, 317
(1980): Sulis E+, *Eur J Cancer* 16, 1517
(1980): Runne U+, *Z Haut* (German) 55, 1590
(1977): Kew MC+, *Lancet* 1, 811
(1974): Pratt CB+, *JAMA* 228, 460 (21%)
Nails – pigmented bands
(1983): James WD+, *Arch Dermatol* 119, 334 (white lines)
(1983): Bronner AK+, *J Am Acad Dermatol* 9, 645
(1981): Giacobetti R+, *Am J Dis Child* 135, 317
(1977): Morris D+, *Cancer Chemother Rep* 61, 499
(1976): Nixon DW, *Arch Intern Med* 113, 1117
(1975): Priestman TJ+, *Lancet* 1, 3337

Other

Anaphylactoid reaction (<1%)
(1984): Collins JA, *Drug Intell Clin Pharm* 18, 402
(1982): Dunagin WG, *Semin Oncol* 9, 14
Injection-site erythema
(1984): Collins JA, *Drug Intell Clin Pharm* 18, 402
(1983): Bronner AK+, *J Am Acad Dermatol* 9, 645
(1982): Dunagin WG, *Semin Oncol* 9, 14
(1981): Weiss RB+, *Ann Intern Med* 94, 66 (>5%)
(1981): von Eyben FE+, *Cancer* 48, 1535 (passim)
(1978): Souhami J+, *JAMA* 240, 1624
(1974): Etcubanas E+, *Cancer Chemother Rep* 58, 757 (>5%)
Injection-site extravasation (>10%)
(1999): Fleming A+, *J Hand Surg [Br]* 24, 390
(1998): Emiroglu M+, *Ann Plast Surg* 41, 103
(1989): Harwood KV+, *Oncol Nurs Forum* 16, 10
(1984): Hankin FM+, *J Pediatr Orthop* 4, 96
(1984): Sonneveld P+, *Cancer Treat Rep* 68, 895
(1983): Pitkanen J+, *J Surg Oncol* 23, 259
(1983): Olver IN+, *Cancer Treat Rep* 67, 407
(1983): Cohen FJ+, *J Hand Surg Am* 8, 43
(1980): Barden GA, *South Med J* 73, 1543
(1978): Bowers DG+, *Plast Reconstr Surg* 61, 86
Injection-site necrosis (>10%)
(1998): Bekerecioglu M+, *J Surg Res* 75, 61
(1987): Dufresne RG, *Cutis* 39, 197
(1983): Bronner AK+, *J Am Acad Dermatol* 9, 645
(1978): Souhami J+, *JAMA* 240, 1624
(1976): Rudolph R+, *Cancer* 38, 1087
Injection-site ulceration (>10%)
(1979): Petro JA+, *Surg Forum* 30, 535
(1979): Zweig JI+, *Cancer Treat Rep* 63, 2101
(1978): Mehta P+, *Clin Pediatr Phila* 17, 663
(1977): Reilly JJ+, *Cancer* 40, 2053

Oral mucosal lesions
(1975): Dreizen S+, *Postgrad Med* 58, 75 (71%)
(1974): Cortes EP+, *JAMA* 221, 1132 (61%)
(1974): Pratt CB+, *Am J Dis Child* 127, 534 (37%)
(1974): Blum RH+, *Ann Intern Med* 80, 249 (79%)
(1971): Wang JJ+, *Cancer* 28, 837
(1971): Middleman E, *Cancer* 25, 844
(1969): Bonadonna G+, *BMJ* 3, 503 (100%)
Oral mucosal pigmentation
(1989): Kerker BJ+, *Semin Dermatol* 8, 173
Oral ulceration
(1974): Pratt CB+, *JAMA* 228, 460 (passim)
Stomatitis (>10%)
(2000): Israel VP+, *Gynecol Oncol* 78, 143
(1994): Bogner JR+, *J Acquir Immune Defic Syndr* 7, 463
(1989): Henderson IC+, *J Clin Oncol* 7, 560 (8.4%)
(1981): von Eyben FE+, *Cancer* 48, 1535 (passim)
(1975): Manalo FB+, *JAMA* 233, 56
(1975): Dreizen S+, *Postgrad Med* 58, 75 (>5%)
(1969): Bonadonna G+, *BMJ* 3, 503 (60–100%)
Tongue pigmentation
(1989): Kerker BJ+, *Semin Dermatol* 8, 173
(1976): Rao SP+, *Cancer Treat Rep* 60, 1402

DOXYCYCLINE

Trade names: Doryx (Warner-Chilcott): Monodox (Oclassen); Vibramycin (Pfizer); Vibra-Tabs (Pfizer)
Other common trade names: *Apo-Dox; Apo-Doxy; Atridox; Azudoxat; Bactidox; Doryx; Doximed; Doxy-100; Doxylin; Doxytec; Vibramycine; Vibravenos*
Indications: Various infections caused by susceptible organisms
Category: Tetracycline antibiotic
Half-life: 12–22 hours
Clinically important, potentially serious interactions with: antacids, barbiturates, bismuth, carbamazepine, digoxin, hydantoins, iron, penicillins, phenytoin, warfarin, zinc, **food.** Also **herbs: barberry, goldenseal, Oregon grape**

Reactions

Skin

Acute generalized exanthematous pustulosis (AGEP)
(1993): Trueb RM+, *Dermatology* 186, 75
Allergic reactions (sic) (0.47%)
(1986): Bigby M+, *JAMA* 256, 3358
Angioedema
(1997): Shapiro LE+, *Arch Dermatol* 133, 1224
Erythema multiforme
(1988): Lewis-Jones MS+, *Clin Exp Dermatol* 13, 245
(1987): Curley RK+, *Clin Exp Dermatol* 12, 124
(1985): Albengres E+, *Therapie* (French) 38, 577
Exanthems
(1987): Bryant SG+, *Pharmacotherapy* 7, 125 (4.4%)
Exfoliative dermatitis
Fixed eruption (<1%)
(1999): Correia O+, *Clin Exp Dermatol* 24, 137 (genital) (cross-reactivity with minocycline)
(1996): Marmelzat J, Los Angeles, CA (from Internet) (observation)
(1989): Alanko K+, *Acta Derm Venereol* (Stockh) 69, 223
(1988): Budde J+, *Aktuel Dermatol* (German) 14, 304
(1987): Jolly HW+, *Arch Dermatol* 114, 1484
(1984): Bargman H, *J Am Acad Dermatol* 11, 900
Lupus erythematosus
Painful eruption of hands (sic)
(1995): Levine N, *Geriatrics* 50, 23
Photosensitivity (<1%)
(1997): Shapiro LE+, *Arch Dermatol* 133, 1224
(1997): Tanaka N+, *Contact Dermatitis* 37, 93
(1997): O'Reilly FM+, American Academy of Dermatology Meeting, Poster #14
(1995): Nowakowski J+, *J Am Acad Dermatol* 32, 223

(1992): Bennett MJ, *J R Army Med Corps* 138, 56
(1987): Edwards R, *N Z Med J* 100, 640
(1980): Möller H+, *Acta Derm Venereol* (Stockh) 60, 495
(1977): Rey M+, *Nouv Presse Med* (French) 6, 3755
(1973): Zuehlke RL, *Arch Dermatol* 108, 837
(1968): Blank H+, *Arch Dermatol* 97, 1 (20%)

Phototoxic reaction
(1999): Litt JZ, Beachwood, OH, personal case (observation)
(1996): McCarty JR, Fort Worth, TX (from Internet) (observation)
(1995): Smith EL+, *Br J Dermatol* 132, 316
(1994): Bjellerup AM+, *Br J Dermatol* 130, 356
(1993): Shea CR+, *J Invest Dermatol* 101, 329
(1993): Layton A+, *Clin Exp Dermatol* 18, 425
(1982): Rosen K+, *Acta Derm Venereol* 62, 246
(1972): Frost P+, *Arch Dermatol* 105, 681

Pigmentation
(1999): Westermann GW+, *J Intern Med* 246, 591
(1980): Möller H+, *Acta Derm Venereol* (Stockh) 60, 495

Pruritus ani

Psoriasis
(1988): Tsankov NK+, *Australas J Dermatol* 29, 111

Purpura

Rash (sic) (<1%)
(1997): Shapiro LE+, *Arch Dermatol* 133, 1224

Seborrhea (sic)
(1997): Rademaker M, New Zealand (from Internet) (observation)

Stevens–Johnson syndrome
(1987): Curley RK+, *Clin Exp Dermatol* 12, 124

Toxic epidermal necrolysis
(1974): Aksnes K, *Tidsskr Nor Laegeforen* (Norwegian) 94, 1254

Urticaria
(1997): Shapiro LE+, *Arch Dermatol* 133, 1224
(1992): Deluze C+, *Allergol Immunopathol Madr* (Spanish) 20, 215
(1989): Alanko K+, *Acta Derm Venereol* (Stockh) 69, 223

Vasculitis
(1981): Rockl H, *Hautarzt* (German) 32, 467

Nails

Nails – discoloration (painful)
(1993): Coffin SE+, *Pediatr Infect Dis J* 12, 702

Nails – onycholysis

Nails – photo-onycholysis
(2000): Yong CK+, *Pediatrics* 106, E13
(1995): Shapero H, *The Schoch Letter* 45 #6, 21 (observation)
(1988): Quirce-Gancedo S+, *Med Clin (Barc)* (Spanish) 90, 636
(1987): Baran R+, *J Am Acad Dermatol* 17, 1012
(1985): Gventer M+, *J Am Podiatr Med Assoc* 75, 658
(1982): Jeanmougin M+, *Ann Dermatol Venereol* (French) 109, 165
(1981): Cavens TR, *Cutis* 27, 53
(1972): Ramelli G+, *Cutis* 10, 155
(1971): Frank SB+, *Arch Dermatol* 103, 520

Other

Anaphylactoid reaction

Anosmia
(1990): Bleasel AF+, *Med J Aust* 152, 440

Dysgeusia

Glossitis

Hypersensitivity

Injection-site phlebitis (<1%)

Paresthesias
(1995): Shapero H, *The Schoch Letter* 45, 21 (observation)
(1994): Blanchard L, *The Schoch Letter* 44, #6 (observation)
(1994): Liss W, *The Schoch Letter* 44, 16, (observation)
(1993): Held J, *The Schoch Letter* 43, 27, (observation)

Phlebitis (<1%)

Pseudotumor cerebri

Serum sickness
(1997): Shapiro LE+, *Arch Dermatol* 133, 1224

Tongue pigmentation

Tooth discoloration (>10%) (in children)
(1998): Lochary ME+, *Pediatr Infect Dis J* 17, 429 (staining of permanent teeth)

Vaginitis
(1995): Nowakowski J+, *J Am Acad Dermatol* 32, 223

DRONABINOL

Synonyms: tetrahydrocannabinol; THC
Trade name: Marinol (Roxane; Unimed)
Indications: Chemotherapy-induced nausea
Category: Antiemetic; appetite stimulant
Half-life: 19–24 hours
Clinically important, potentially serious interactions with: alcohol, amphetamines, barbiturates, benzodiazepines, CNS depressants, cocaine, phenothiazines, sympathomimetics, tricyclic antidepressants

Reactions

Skin

Diaphoresis (<1%)
Flushing (<1%)

Other

Myalgia (<1%)
Paresthesias
Xerostomia (1–10%)

DROPERIDOL

Trade name: Droperidol (AstraZeneca)
Other common trade names: *Dehydrobenzperidol; Droleptan; Inapsin; Sintodian*
Indications: Tranquilizer and antiemetic in surgical procedures
Category: Antiemetic; antipsychotic
Half-life: 2.3 hours
Clinically important, potentially serious interactions with: atropine, CNS depressants, fentanyl, lithium

Reactions

Skin

Chills
Diaphoresis
Shivering (sic)

EDROPHONIUM

Trade names: Enlon (Baxter); Reversol (Organon); Tensilon (ICN)
Indications: Myasthenia gravis diagnosis
Category: Neuromuscular blocking agent; cholinesterase inhibitor; antidote
Half-life: 1.8 hours
Clinically important, potentially serious interactions with: atropine, corticosteroids, digoxin, neostigmine, succinylcholine, tacrine

Reactions

Skin
Diaphoresis (>10%)
Flushing
Rash (sic)
Urticaria

Other
Anaphylactoid reaction
Hypersensitivity (<1%)
Sialorrhea (>10%)
Thrombophlebitis (<1%)

EFAVIRENZ

Trade name: Sustiva (DuPont)
Indications: HIV infection
Category: Antiretroviral non-nucleoside reverse transcriptase inhibitor (NNRTI)
Half-life: 52–76 hours
Clinically important, potentially serious interactions with: astemizole, cisapride, ergot, indinavir, midazolam, nelfinavir, ritonavir, saquinavir, triazolam, warfarin

Reactions

Skin
Eczema (sic) (<2%)
Exanthems (27%)
(1998): Adkins JC+, *Drugs* 56, 1055
Exfoliation (sic) (<2%)
Flushing (<2%)
Folliculitis (<2%)
Hot flashes (<2%)
Peripheral edema (<2%)
Pruritus (<2%)
Rash (sic) (5–20%)
Urticaria (<2%)

Hair
Hair – alopecia (<2%)

Other
Dysgeusia (<2%)
Hypersensitivity
(2000): Bossi P+, *Clin Infect Dis* 30, 227
Hypesthesia (1–2%)
Myalgia (<2%)
Paresthesias (<2%)
Parosmia (<2%)
Thrombophlebitis (<2%)
Tremor (<2%)
Xerostomia (<2%)

EFLORNITHINE

Synonym: DFMO
Trade names: Ornidyl; Vaniqa (Bristol-Myers Squibb)
Indications: Sleeping sickness; hypertrichosis
Category: Ornithine decarboxylase inhibitor
Half-life: IV: 3–3.5 hours; topical: 8 hours
Clinically important, potentially serious interactions with: no data

Reactions

Skin
Acne (24.3%)
Burning skin (4.3%)
Cheilitis (<1%)
Contact dermatitis (<1%)
Erythema (1.3%)
Facial edema (0.3–3%)
Folliculitis (0.5%)
Herpes simplex (<1%)
Irritation (1%)
Lip edema (<1%)
Pruritus (3.8%)
Rash (2.8%)
Rosacea (<1%)
Stinging (7.9%)
Xerosis (1.8%)

Hair
Hair – alopecia (1.5%)
Hair – ingrown (0.3–2%)
Hair – pseudofollicultis barbae (5–15%)

Other
Paresthesias (3.6%)

ENALAPRIL

Trade names: Lexxel (AstraZeneca); Teczem (Aventis); Vasotec (Merck)
Other common trade names: *Amprace; Apo-Enalapril; Enaladil; Enapren; Glioten; Innovace; Pres; Renitec; Reniten; Xanef*
Indications: Hypertension
Category: Angiotensin-converting enzyme (ACE) inhibitor, antihypertensive and vasodilator
Half-life: 11 hours
Clinically important, potentially serious interactions with: alcohol, allopurinol, bumetanide, digoxin, indomethacin, lithium, NSAIDs, phenothiazines, potassium-sparing diuretics, rifampin, salicylates

Lexxel is enalapril and felodipine; Teczem is enalapril and diltiazem; Vaseretic is enalapril and hydrochlorothiazide

Reactions

Skin
Acantholysis (sic)
(1999): Lo Schiavo A+, *Dermatology* 198, 391
Angioedema (<1%)
(1998): *Prescrire Int* 7, 92
(1998): Leuwer A+, *HNO* (German) 46, 56 (9 cases)
(1997): Brown NJ+, *JAMA* 278, 232
(1996): Pillans PI+, *Eur J Clin Pharmacol* 51, 123
(1996): Mullins RJ+, *Med J Aust* 165, 319 (visceral)
(1996): Langauer-Messmer S+, *Postgrad Med J* 72, 383
(1996): Kind B+, *Schweiz Rundsch Med Prax* (German) 85, 567
(1995): Kozel MM+, *Clin Exp Dermatol* 20, 60
(1995): Forslund T+, *J Intern Med* 238, 179
(1995): Juarez-Giminez JC+, *Ann Pharmacother* 29, 317
(1995): Waldfahrer F+, *HNO* (German) 43, 35
(1994): Dupasquier E, *Arch Mal Coeur Vaiss* (French) 87, 1371

(1994): Varma JR+, *J Am Board Fam Pract* 7, 433
(1994): Lehmke J, *Med Klin* (German) 89, 508
(1994): Farraye FA+, *Am J Gastroenterol* 89, 1117
(1994): Nielsen EW+, *Tidsskr Nor Laegeforen* (Norwegian) 114, 804
(1994): Dyer PD, *J Allergy Clin Immunol* 93, 947
(1993): Oike Y+, *Intern Med* 32, 308 (fatal)
(1993): Thompson T+, *Laryngoscope* 103, 10
(1992): Bielory L+, *Allergy Proc* 13, 85
(1992): Diehl KL+, *Dtsch Med Wochenschr* (German) 117, 727
(1992): Dobroschke R+, *Anasthesiol Intensivmed Notfallmed Schmerzther* (German) 27, 510
(1992): Finley CJ+, *Am J Emerg Med* 10, 550
(1992): Hedner T+, *BMJ* 304, 941
(1992): Venable RJ, *J Fam Pract* 34, 201
(1992): Jain M+, *Chest* 102, 871
(1991): Roberts JR+, *Ann Emerg Med* 20, 555
(1991): Candelaria LM+, *J Oral Maxillofac Surg* 49, 1237
(1991): Abidin MR+, *Arch Otolaryngol Head Neck Surg* 117, 1059
(1991): Lanting PJ+, *Ned Tijdschr Geneeskd* (Dutch) 135, 335
(1990): Seidman MD+, *Otolaryngol Head Neck Surg* 102, 727
(1990): DiNardo LJ+, *Trans Pa Acad Ophthalmol Otolaryngol* 42, 998
(1990): Gonnering RS+, *Am J Ophthalmol* 110, 566
(1990): Gannon TH+, *Laryngoscope* 100, 1156
(1990): Chin HL+, *Ann Intern Med* 112, 312
(1990): Orfan N+, *JAMA* 264, 1287
(1990): McAreavey D+, *Drugs* 40, 326 (0.2%)
(1990): Zech J+, *HNO* (German) 38, 143
(1990): Gianos ME+, *Am J Emerg Med* 8, 124
(1989): Giannoccaro PJ+, *Can J. Cardiol* 5, 335 (fatal)
(1989): Huwyler T+, *Schweiz Med Wochenschr* (German) 119, 1253
(1989): Werber JL+, *Otolaryngol Head Neck Surg* 101, 96
(1989): Smith ME+, *Otolaryngol Head Neck Surg* 101, 93
(1989): Barna JS+, *Va Med* 116, 147
(1989): Todd PA+, *Drugs* 37, 141 (<0.1%)
(1988): Schilling H+, *Z Kardiol* 77 (German) (Suppl 3), 47
(1988): Inman WH+, *BMJ* 297, 826
(1988): Slater EE+, *JAMA* 260, 967 (0.1%)
(1988): Wernze H, *Z Kardiol* (German) 77, 61
(1987): Vaillant L+, *Therapie* (French) 42, 411
(1987): Ferner RE+, *BMJ* 294, 1119
(1987): Inman WHW, *BMJ* 294, 578
(1987): Wood SM+, *BMJ* 294, 91
(1986): Marichal JF+, *Therapie* (French) 41, 517

Bullous pemphigoid
(1994): Mullins PD+, *BMJ* 309, 1411
(1993): Smith EP+, *J Am Acad Dermatol* 29, 879

Diaphoresis (<1%)
(1994): Nachbar F+, *Dtsch Med Wochenschr* (German) 119, 321

Erythema
(1993): Carrington PR+, *Cutis* 51, 121

Erythema multiforme (<1%)

Exanthems
(1993): Carrington PR+, *Cutis* 51, 121
(1990): McAreavey D+, *Drugs* 40, 326 (1.4%)
(1990): Ruiz AM+, *Drugs* 39 (Suppl 2) 77 (0.9%)
(1989): Todd PA+, *Drugs* 37, 141
(1988): Warner NJ+, *Drugs* 35 (Suppl 5), 89 (1.4%)
(1986): Gavras H, *Clin Ther* 9, 24
(1986): Todd PA+, *Drugs* 31, 198 (0.5)
(1984): Kubo SH+, *Ann Intern Med* 100, 616
(1983): Barnes JN+, *Lancet* 2, 41

Exfoliative dermatitis (<1%)

Flushing (<1%)
(1989): Healey LA+, *N Engl J Med* 321, 763
(1987): Ferner RE+, *BMJ* (Clin Res) 294, 1119

Herpes zoster (<1%)

Lichenoid eruption
(1995): Roten SV+, *J Am Acad Dermatol* 32, 293
(1993): Kanwar AJ+, *Dermatology* 187, 80 (photosensitive)

Lupus erythematosus
(1990): Schwarz D+, *Lancet* 336, 187

Mycosis fungoides
(1986): Furness PN+, *J Clin Pathol* 39, 902

Pemphigus
(1997): Brenner S+, *J Am Acad Dermatol* 36, 919
(1996): Mitchell DF, Charleston, SC (from Internet) (observation)
(1995): Frangogiannis NG+, *Ann Intern Med* 122, 803 (larynx and esophagus)
(1994): Kuechle MK+, *Mayo Clin Proc* 69, 1166
(1994): Wolf R+, *Dermatology* 189, 1
(1993): Brenner S+, *Clin Dermatol* 11, 501
(1992): Ruocco V+, *Int J Dermatol* 31, 33

Pemphigus foliaceus
(1991): Shelton RM, *J Am Acad Dermatol* 24, 503

Pemphigus vegetans
(1994): Bastiaens MT+, *Int J Dermatol* 33, 168 (3 cases)

Photodermatitis
(1993): Shelley WB+, *Cutis* 52, 81 (observation)

Photosensitivity (<1%)
(1997): O'Reilly FM+, American Academy of Dermatology Meeting, Poster #14
(1993): Kanwar AJ+, *Dermatology* 187, 80

Pruritus (<1%)
(1993): Litt JZ, Beachwood, OH, personal case (observation)
(1990): Heckerling PS, *Ann Intern Med* 112, 879 (vulvovaginal)
(1987): Nugent LW+, *J Clin Pharmacol* 27, 461
(1986): Gavras H, *Clin Ther* 9, 24 (0.75%)

Psoriasis
(1993): Coulter DM+, *N Z Med J* 106, 392
(1990): Wolf R+, *Dermatologica* 181, 51

Purpura
(1989): Grosbois B+, *BMJ* 298, 189 (patient also took quinidine)

Rash (sic) (1.4%)
(1986): Irvin JD+, *Am J Med* 81, 46
(1986): DiBianco R, *Med Toxicol* 1, 122 (passim)
(1984): McFate Smith W+, *J Hypertens* Suppl 2, S113
(1984): Davies RO+, *Am J Med* 77, 23

Stevens–Johnson syndrome (<1%)

Toxic epidermal necrolysis (<1%)

Toxic pustuloderma
(1996): Ferguson JE+, *Clin Exp Dermatol* 21, 54

Urticaria (<1%)
(1996): Pillans PI+, *Eur J Clin Pharmacol* 51, 123
(1993): Carrington PR+, *Cutis* 51, 121
(1988): Slater EE+, *JAMA* 260, 967
(1988): Inman WH+, *BMJ* 297, 826
(1987): Wood SM+, *BMJ* 294, 91

Vasculitis (<1%)
(1993): Carrington PR+, *Cutis* 51, 121
(1991): Ayani I+, *Med Clin (Barc)* (Spanish) 96, 596

Hair

Hair – alopecia (<1%)
(1991): Ahmad S, *Arch Intern Med* 151, 404

Nails

Nails – dystrophy
(1986): Gupta S+, *BMJ* 293, 140

Other

Ageusia
(1984): McFate Smith W+, *J Hypertens* Suppl 2, S113
(1984): Davies RO+, *Am J Med* 77, 23

Anaphylactoid reaction (<1%)
(1989): Todd PA+, *Drugs* 37, 141

Anosmia (<1%)

Dysesthesia (<1%)

Dysgeusia (1–10%)
(2000): Zervakis J+, *Physiol Behav* 68, 405
(1988): Schilling H+, *Z Kardiol* (German) 77 (Suppl 3), 47
(1986): Irvin JD+, *Am J Med* 81, 46
(1986): DiBianco R, *Med Toxicol* 1, 122
(1984): Davies RO+, *Am J Med* 77, 23

Glossitis (<1%)

Glossopyrosis
(1989): Drucker CR+, *Arch Dermatol* 125, 1437

Gynecomastia
(1994): Llop R+, *Ann Pharmacother* 28, 671

Myalgia (<1%)

Oral bleeding (sic)
(1984): Kubo SH+, *Ann Intern Med* 100, 616

Oral mucosal lesions
(1986): Gavras H, *Clin Ther* 9, 24 (0.37%)
(1986): Todd PA+, *Drugs* 31, 198 (0.5)
(1985): Gomez HJ+, *Drugs* 30 (Suppl 1), 13

(1984): Kubo SH+, *Ann Intern Med* 100, 616
Oral mucosal lichenoid eruption
(1989): Firth NA+, *Oral Surg Oral Med Oral Pathol* 67, 41
Oral ulceration
(1982): Viraben R+, *Arch Dermatol* 118, 959
Paresthesias (<1%)
Pseudopolymyalgia
(1989): Leloët X+, *BMJ* 298, 325
Scalded mouth (sic)
(1982): Vlasses PH+, *BMJ* 284, 1672
Stomatitis (<1%)
Tongue edema
(1996): Litt JZ, Beachwood, OH, personal case (observation)
(1990): Zech J+, *HNO* (German) 38, 143
(1986): Marichal JF+, *Therapie* (French) 41, 517
Xerostomia (<1%)

ENOXACIN

Trade name: Penetrex (Aventis)
Other common trade names: *Bactidan; Comprecin; Enoxacine; Enoxen; Enoxor; Gyramid*
Indications: Urinary tract infections
Category: Fluoroquinolone antibiotic
Half-life: 3–6 hours
Clinically important, potentially serious interactions with: antacids, caffeine, cimetidine, cyclosporine, digoxin, famotidine, metoprolol, nizatidine, probenecid, propranolol, ranitidine, sucralfate, theophylline, warfarin

Reactions

Skin
Chills (<1%)
Diaphoresis (<1%)
Edema (<1%)
Erythema multiforme (<1%)
Erythema nodosum
Exanthems
(1988): Henwood JM+, *Drugs* 32, 32 (0.57%)
Exfoliative dermatitis (<1%)
Hyperpigmentation
Photoreactions
(1990): Schauder S, *Z Hautkr* (German) 65, 253
Photosensitivity (<1%)
(1993): Kang JS+, *Photodermatol Photoimmunol Photomed* 9, 159
(1992): Izu R+, *Photodermatol Photoimmunol Photomed* 9, 86
(1990): Schauder S, *Z Hautkr* (German) 65, 253
(1989): Kawabe Y+, *Photodermatology* 6, 57
(1988): Henwood JM+, *Drugs* 32, 32 (0.57%)
Phototoxic reaction
(1998): Martinez LJ+ *Photochem Photobiol* 67, 399
(1994): Fujita H+, *Photodermatol Photoimmunol Photomed* 10, 202
(1990): Schauder S, *Z Hautkr* (German) 65, 253
(1990): Przybilla B+, *Dermatologica* 181, 98
Pruritus (<1%)
Purpura (<1%)
Rash (sic) (<1%)
Stevens–Johnson syndrome (<1%)
Toxic epidermal necrolysis (<1%)
Urticaria (<1%)
(1988): Henwood JM+, *Drugs* 32, 32 (0.57%)

Other
Dysgeusia
Hypersensitivity
Injection-site phlebitis
Myalgia (<1%)
Paresthesias (<1%)
Stomatitis (<1%)
Tendon rupture (<1%)
Tremor (<1%)
Vaginal candidiasis (<1%)
Vaginitis (<1%)
Xerostomia (<1%)

ENOXAPARIN

Trade name: Lovenox (Aventis)
Other common trade names: *Clexan; Clexane 40; Klexane*
Indications: Prevention of deep vein thrombosis
Category: Anticoagulant (heparin, low weight)
Half-life: 4.5 hours
Clinically important, potentially serious interactions with: ketorolac, NSAIDs, oral anticoagulants, platelet inhibitors, warfarin

Reactions

Skin
Cutaneous side effects (sic) (0.2%)
(2000): Enrique E+, *Contact Dermatitis* 42, 43
Ecchymoses (2%)
Edema (3%)
Erythema (1–10%)
(1993): Phillips JK+, *Br J Haematol* 85, 837
Peripheral edema (3%)
Purpura (1–10%)
Urticaria
(1997): Downham TF, Taylor, MI (from Internet) (observation)
Vesicular eruption (<1%)

Other
Anaphylactoid reaction (<1%)
Hypersensitivity
(2000): Romero Ortega MR+, *Aten Primaria* (Spanish) 25, 521
(1998): Mendez J+, *Allergy* 53, 999
(1998): Cabanas R+, *J Investig Allergol Clin Immunol* 8, 383
(1996): Koch P+, *Contact Dermatitis* 34, 156
(1996): Mendez J+, *Allergy* 51, 853
Injection-site erythema
Injection-site infiltrated plaques
(1998): Mendez J+, *Allergy* 53, 999
(1998): Valdes F+, *Allergy* 53, 625
Injection-site-necrosis
(1997): Lefebvre I+, *Ann Dermatol Venereol* (French) 124, 397
(1997): Tonn ME+, *Ann Pharmacother* 31, 323
(1996): Fried M+, *Ann Intern Med* 125, 521
Injection-site pain
Necrosis (<1%)

ENTACAPONE

Trade name: Comtan (Novartis)
Other common trade name: *Comtess*
Indications: Parkinsonism
Category: Antiparkinsonian; reverse COMT inhibitor
Half-life: 2.4 hours
Clinically important, potentially serious interactions with: anxiolytics, apomorphine, barbiturates, benzodiazepines, dobutamine, dopamine, epinephrine, isoproterenol, MAO inhibitors, opiates agonists, phenothiazines, tricyclic antidepressants

Reactions

Skin
Bacterial infection (sic) (1%)
Diaphoresis (2%)
Purpura (2%)

Other
Dysgeusia (1%)
Xerostomia (3%)

EPHEDRINE

Trade names: Ectasule; Efedron; Ephedsol; Marax; Pretz-D; Rynatuss; Vicks Vatronol, etc. (Various pharmaceutical companies.)
Indications: Nasal congestion, acute hypotensive states, asthma
Category: Adrenergic agonist, sympathomimetic bronchodilator
Half-life: 3–6 hours
Clinically important, potentially serious interactions with: atropine, furazolidone, guanethidine, isocarboxazid, MAO inhibitors, methyldopa, phenylpropanolamine, procarbazine, selegiline, theophylline, tranylcypromine, tricyclic antidepressants

Reactions

Skin

Contact dermatitis (following topical application)
(1945): Spencer GA, *Arch Dermatol* 51, 48
(1944): Lewis G, *Arch Dermatol* 49, 379
(1936): Hollander L, *JAMA* February 29, 706
Bullous eruption
(1944): Lewis G, *Arch Dermatol* 49, 379
Dermatitis (sic)
(1993): Villas-Martinez F+, *Contact Dermatitis* 29, 215
(1991): Audicana M+, *Contact Dermatitis* 24, 223
Diaphoresis (1–10%)
Edema
Exanthems
(1933): Abramovitz EW+, *Br J Dermatol* XLV, 236
Exfoliative dermatitis
(1981): Serup J, *Ugeskr Laeger* (Danish) 143, 1660
Fixed eruption
(1997): Garcia Ortiz JC+, *Allergy* 52, 229
(1994): Krivda SJ+, *J Am Acad Dermatol* 31, 291 (non-pigmenting)
(1968): Brownstein MH, *Arch Dermatol* 97, 115
(1960): Englehardt AW, *Hautarzt* (German) 11, 49
Pallor (1–10%)
Purpura
(1933): Abramovitz EW+, *Br J Dermatol* XLV, 236
Urticaria
(1978): Speer F+, *Ann Allergy* 40, 32
(1933): Abramovitz EW+, *Br J Dermatol* XLV, 236
Vasculitis
(1978): Speer F+, *Ann Allergy* 40, 32

Other

Trembling (1–10%)
Tremor (1–10%)
Xerostomia (1–10%)

EPINEPHRINE

Synonym: adrenaline
Trade names: Adrenalin (Parke-Davis); AsthmaHaler; Bronitin; Bronkaid; Epifrin (Allergan); Epipen (CTR Labs); MedihalerEpi; Primatene; Sus-Phrine (Forest)
Other common trade names: *Adrenaline; Ana-Guard; Epi E-Z Pen; Eppy; Eppystabil; Isopto-Epinal; Primatene Mist; S-2; Simplene*
Indications: Cardiac arrest, hay fever, asthma, anaphylaxis
Category: Adrenergic agonist, sympathomimetic bronchodilator
Duration of action: 1–4 hours
Clinically important, potentially serious interactions with: albuterol, alpha-blockers, atenolol, beta-blockers, digoxin, ergotamine, furazolidone, guanethidine, imipramine, MAO inhibitors, methyldopa, metoprolol, propranolol, reserpine, tranylcypromine, tricyclic antidepressants, vasopressors

Reactions

Skin

Contact dermatitis
(1993): Gaspari AA, *Contact Dermatitis* 28, 35
(1980): Romaguera C+, *Contact Dermatitis* 6, 364
(1976): Alani SD+, *Contact Dermatitis* 2, 147
(1970): Gibbs RC, *Arch Dermatol* 101, 92
Diaphoresis (1–10%)
Exanthems
Fixed eruption
Flushing (1–10%)
Necrosis
(1984): Antrum RM+, *Br J Clin Pract* 38, 191
Pallor (<1%)
Pemphigoid (cicatricial)
(1981): Vadot E+, *Bull Soc Ophtalmol Fr* (French) 81, 693
(1977): Norn MS, *Am J Ophthalmol* 83, 138
Urticaria

Hair

Hair – alopecia
(1972): Kass MA+, *Arch Ophthalmol* 88, 429 (eyelashes)

Other

Injection-site necrosis
Injection-site pain
Injection-site urticaria
Trembling (1–10%)
Xerostomia (<1%)

EPIRUBICIN

Trade name: Ellence (Pharmacia & Upjohn)
Indications: Adjuvant therapy in primary breast cancer
Category: Antineoplastic
Half-life: 33 hours
Clinically important, potentially serious interactions with: anticoagulants, cimetidine, immunosuppressives, NSAIDs, platelet inhibitors, salicylates, thrombolytic agents

Reactions

Skin

Cutaneous reactions (sic)
(1999): Ormrod D+, *Drugs Aging* 15, 389
Erythema
Exfoliative dermatitis
Facial flushing
Hot flashes (5–39%)
Photosensitivity
Pigmentation
Pruritus (9%)
Radiation recall
Rash (sic) (1–9%)
Recall phenomenon
(1999): Wilson J+, *Clin Oncol (R Coll Radiol)* 11, 424
Skin changes (sic) (0.7–5%)
Ulceration
Urticaria

Hair

Hair – alopecia (69–95%) (reversible)
(1999): Ormrod D+, *Drugs Aging* 15, 389
(1991): Fountzilas G+, *Tumori* 77, 232 (81%)
(1991): Carmo-Pereira J+, *Cancer Chemother Pharmacol* 27, 394 (95%)
(1986): Kimura K+, *Gan To Kagaku Ryoho* (Japanese) 13, 2440 (71.4%)
(1986): Tominaga T+, *Gan To Kagaku Ryoho* (Japanese) 13, 2187 (66.7%)
(1986): Sakata Y+, *Gan To Kagaku Ryoho* (Japanese) 13, 1887
(1985): Holdener EE+, *Invest New Drugs* 3, 63 (54%)
(1984): Lopez M+, *Invest New Drugs* 2, 315
(1984): Schutte J+, *J Cancer Res Clin Oncol* 107, 38 (88%)
(1980): Bonfante V+, *Recent Results Cancer Res* 74, 192

Nails

Nails – pigmentation

Other

Anaphylactoid reaction
Hypersensitivity
Injection-site extravasation
(1999): Fleming A+, *J Hand Surg [Br]* 24, 390
Injection-site inflammation
Injection-site necrosis
Injection-site reactions (3–20%)
Injection-site ulceration
Myalgia
(1995): Fountzilas G+, *Med Pediatr Oncol* 24, 23 (55%)
Mucositis
(1999): Ormrod D+, *Drugs Aging* 15, 389
Oral ulceration
Phlebitis
Stomatitis
(1995): Fountzilas G+, *Med Pediatr Oncol* 24, 23
(1991): Fountzilas G+, *Tumori* 77, 232 (24%)
(1991): Carmo-Pereira J+, *Cancer Chemother Pharmacol* 27, 394 (35%)
(1986): Kimura K+, *Gan To Kagaku Ruoho* (Japanese) 13, 2440 (12.5%)
(1986): Sakata Y+, *Gan To Kagaku Ryoho* (Japanese) 13, 1887
(1980): Bonfante V+, *Recent Results Cancer Res* 74, 192

EPOETIN ALFA

Synonyms: erythropoietin; EPO
Trade names: Epogen (Amgen); Procrit (Ortho)
Other common trade names: *Epoxitin; Eprex; Erypo*
Indications: Anemia
Category: Colony stimulating factor; growth factor
Half-life: 4–13 hours (in patients with chronic renal failure)
Clinically important, potentially serious interactions with: none

Reactions

Skin

Acne
(1989): Faulds D+, *Drugs* 38, 863
Angioedema (1–5%)
Contact dermatitis
(1993): Hardwick N+, *Contact Dermatitis* 28, 123
Edema (17%)
Exanthems
(1990): Schröder-Kolb B, *Derm Beruf Umwelt* (German) 38, 12 (papular)
Lichenoid eruption
(1997): Puritz E, Smithtown, NY (from Internet) (observation)
Photosensitivity
(1992): Harvey E+, *J Pediatr* 121, 749
Pruritus
(1990): Schröder-Kolb B, *Derm Beruf Umwelt* (German) 38, 12 (papular)
(1989): Faulds D+, *Drugs* 38, 863
Rash (sic) (1–10%)
Urticaria

Hair

Hair – hypertrichosis
(1991): Kleiner MJ+, *Am J Kidney Dis* 18, 689

Other

Anaphylactoid reaction
Hypersensitivity (<1%)
Injection-site pain
(1998): Veys N+, *Clin Nephrol* 49, 41
Injection-site reactions (sic) (7%)
Injection-site thrombophlebitis
Injection-site ulceration
(1997): Siegel DM, New York, NY (from Internet) (observation)
Myalgia
Paresthesias (11%)
Porphyria cutanea tarda
(1992): Harvey E+, *J Pediatr* 121, 749

EPROSARTAN

Trade name: Teveten (Unimed)
Indications: Hypertension
Category: Angiotensin II receptor antagonist, antihypertensive
Half-life: 5–9 hours
Clinically important, potentially serious interactions with: lithium, amiloride, potassium, triamterene, trimethoprim, spironolactone. Also **hawthorn** (*Crataegus laevigata*)

Reactions

Skin

Angioedema
Diaphoresis (<1%)
Eczema (sic) (<1%)
Exanthems (<1%)
Facial edema (<1%)
Furunculosis (<1%)
Herpes simplex (<1%)
Hot flashes (<1%)
Peripheral edema (<1%)
Purpura (<1%)
Pruritus (<1%)
Rash (sic) (<1%)

Other

Gingivitis (<1%)
Myalgia
Paresthesias (<1%)
Tendinitis (<1%)
Tremor (<1%)
Xerostomia (<1%)

EPTIFIBATIDE

Trade name: Integrilin (COR; Key)
Indications: Acute coronary syndrome, unstable angina
Category: Antiplatelet; platelet aggregation inhibitor
Half-life: 2.5 hours
Clinically important, potentially serious interactions with: anticoagulants, clopidogrel, dipyridamole, NSAIDs, ticlopidine

Reactions

Skin

None

Other

Anaphylactoid reaction (<1%)
Injection-site reaction (sic)

ERGOCALCIFEROL

Synonyms: viosterol; vitamin D_2
Trade names: Calciferol (Schwarz); Deltalin (Lilly); Drisdol (Sanofi); Vitamin D
Other common trade names: *Kalciferol; Ostoforte; Radiostol Forte; Sterogyl-15; Vigantol; Vitaminol*
Indications: Rickets, hypoparathyroidism
Category: Fat-soluble nutritional supplement, antihypocalcemic and antihypoparathyroid
Half-life: 19–48 hours
Clinically important, potentially serious interactions with: thiazide diuretics, verapamil

Reactions

Skin

Granulomas (perforating)
(1982): Aliaga A+, *Dermatologica* 164, 62
Pruritus (1–10%)

Other

Dysgeusia) (1–10%) (metallic taste)
Myalgia
Xerostomia

ERYTHROMYCIN

Trade names: E.E.S; E-Mycin; Eramycin; Eryc; Erypar; Ery-Ped; Ery-Tab; Erythrocin; Eryzole*; Ilosone; Ilotycin; PCE; Pediazole*; Robimycin; Wintrocin; Wyamicin S, etc. (Various pharmaceutical companies.)
Other common trade names: *Too numerous to list*
Indications: Various infections caused by susceptible organisms
Category: Bacteriostatic macrolide antibiotic
Half-life: 1.4–2 hours
Clinically important, potentially serious interactions with: anticoagulants, amprenavir, astemizole, bromocriptine, carbamazepine, cisapride, clindamycin, colchicine, cyclosporine, digoxin, dihydroergotamine, ergotamine, lovastatin, methadone, midazolam, nelfinavir, pimozide, ritonavir, terfenadine, theophylline, triazolam, warfarin

***Note:** Eryzole and Pediazole are combinations of erythromycin and sulfisoxazole

Reactions

Skin

Acne
(1969): Weary PE+, *Arch Dermatol* 100, 179
Acute generalized exanthematous pustulosis (AGEP)
(1995): Moreau A+, *Int J Dermatol* 34, 263 (passim)
(1991): Roujeau J-C+, *Arch Dermatol* 127, 1333
Allergic reactions (sic) (<1%)
(1986): Bigby M+, *JAMA* 256, 3358 (2.04%)
(1976): Arndt KA+, *JAMA* 235, 918 (2.3%)
(1967): Nichols JT+, *Oral Surg Oral Med Oral Pathol* 24, 323
Baboon syndrome
(1997): Goossens C+, *Dermatology* 194, 421
Contact dermatitis (systemic)
(1996): Valsecchi R+, *Contact Dermatitis* 34, 428
(1995): Martins C+, *Contact Dermatitis* 33, 360
(1994): Fernandez Redondo V+, *Contact Dermatitis* 30, 311
(1994): Fernandez Redondo V+, *Contact Dermatitis* 30, 43
Eczema (sic)
Erythema multiforme
(1985): Ting HC+, *Int J Dermatol* 24, 587
Exanthems (1–5%)
(1995): Litt JZ, Beachwood, OH, personal case (observation)
(1991): Igea JM+, *Ann Allergy* 66, 216
(1989): Pendleton N+, *Br J Clin Prac* 43, 464
(1979): Hartigan DA+, *Lancet* 2, 411
(1973): Shapera RM+, *JAMA* 226, 531 (3.5%)
Fixed eruption
(1991): Mutalik S, *Int J Dermatol* 30, 751
(1991): Florido-Lopez JF+, *Allergy* 46, 77
(1986): Kanwar AJ+, *Dermatologica* 172, 315
(1984): Pigatto PD, *Acta Derm Venereol* (Stockh) 64, 272
(1976): Naik RPC+, *Dermatologica* 152, 177 (bullous)
Pruritus
Pustular eruption
(1993): Manu Shah R+, *Eur J Dermatol* 3, 576
Rash (sic) (<1%)
(1992): Shirin H+, *Ann Pharmacother* 26, 1522
(1989): Pendleton N+, *Br J Clin Pract* 43, 464
(1983): Furniss LD, *Drug Intell Clin Pharm* 17, 631
Red neck syndrome
(1992): Estrada V+, *Rev Clin Esp* (Spanish) 190, 100
Stevens–Johnson syndrome
(1998): N Z Medicines Adverse Reactions Committee (from Internet) (observation)
(1995): Lestico MR+, *Am J Health Syst Pharm* 52, 1805
(1995): Pandha HS+, *N Z Med J* 108, 13
(1993): Leenutaphong V+, *Int J Dermatol* 32, 428
(1983): Fischer PR+, *Am J Dis Child* 137, 914
Toxic epidermal necrolysis
(1995): Kuper K+, *Ophthalmologe* (German) 92, 823
(1995): Raymond F+, *Arch Pediatr* (French) 2, 494
(1993): Leenutaphong V+, *Int J Dermatol* 32, 428
(1991): Porteous DM+, *Arch Dermatol* 127, 740 (in AIDS)
(1987): Guillaume JC+, *Arch Dermatol* 123, 1166
(1985): Lund-Kofoed ML+, *Contact Dermatitis* 13, 273
(1974): Czaplinska W+, *Pol Tyg Lek* (Polish) 29, 1263
Urticaria
(1998): Siegfried EC+, *J Am Acad Dermatol* 39, 797 (passim)
(1993): Lopez-Serrano C+, *Allergol Immunopathol Madr* (Spanish) 21, 225
(1976): van Ketel WG, *Contact Dermatitis* 2, 363
(1960): Prasard AS, *N Engl J Med* 262, 139
Vasculitis
(1985): Sanchez NP+, *Arch Dermatol* 121 220

Other

Anaphylactoid reaction
(1998): Siegfried EC+, *J Am Acad Dermatol* 39, 797 (passim)
(1996): Jorro G+, *Ann Allergy Asthma Immunol* 77, 456
Enamel hypoplasia (teeth)
(1965): Adno J+, *SA Tydskrif vir Geneeskunde* (English), 1124
Gingival hyperplasia
(1992): Valsecchi R+, *Acta Derm Venereol* (Stockh) 72, 157
Glossodynia
Hypersensitivity (1–10%)
(1999): Gallardo MA+, *Cutis* 64, 129
(1982): Lombardi P+, *Contact Dermatitis* 8, 416
Injection-site phlebitis (1–10%)
Oral candidiasis (1–10%)
Oral ulceration
(1980): Evens RP+, *Drug Intell Clin Pharm* 14, 217
Stomatodynia
Thrombophlebitis
Tooth discoloration
(1965): Adno J+, *SA Tydskrif vir Geneeskunde* (English), 1124

ESMOLOL

Trade name: Brevibloc (Baxter)
Indications: Tachyarrhythmias, tachycardia
Category: Beta-adrenergic blocker; antiarrhythmic class II; antihypertensive
Half-life: 9 minutes
Clinically important, potentially serious interactions with: antidiabetics, calcium channel blockers, clonidine, digoxin, diltiazem, flecainide, MAO inhibitors, morphine, nifedipine, NSAIDs, oral contraceptives, prazosin, sulfonylureas, verapamil

Reactions

Skin

Acne (<1%)
Cold extremities (sic)
Diaphoresis (>10%)
Eczema (<1%)
Edema (<1%)
Erythema (<1%)
Exfoliative dermatitis (<1%)
Facial edema
Flushing (<1%)
Necrosis (<1%)
Pallor (<1%)
Pigmentation (<1%)
Psoriasis (<1%)
Purpura
Rash (sic)
Urticaria

Hair

Hair – alopecia

Other

Dysgeusia
Infusion-site reactions (1–10%)
Injection-site inflammation
(1987): Benfield P+, *Drugs* 33, 392
Injection-site pain (8%)
Paresthesias (<1%)
Thrombophlebitis (<1%)
Xerostomia (<1%)

ESTAZOLAM

Trade name: ProSom (Abbott)
Other common trade names: *Domnamid; Esilgan; Eurodin; Kainever; Nuctalon; Tasedan*
Indications: Insomnia
Category: Benzodiazepine sedative-hypnotic
Half-life: 10–24 hours
Clinically important, potentially serious interactions with: alcohol, CNS depressants, clarithromycin, diltiazem, fluconazole, itraconazole, ketoconazole, levodopa, miconazole, verapamil, **grapefruit juice**

Reactions

Skin

Acne (<1%)
Allergic reactions (sic) (<1%)
Chills (<1%)
Dermatitis (sic) (<1%)
Diaphoresis (1–10%)
Edema (<1%)
Eyelid edema (<1%)
Flushing (1–10%)
Photosensitivity
Pruritus (1–10%)
Purpura (<1%)
Rash (sic) (>10%)
Urticaria (1–10%)
Vaginal pruritus (1–10%)
Xerosis (<1%)

Other

Dysgeusia (1–10%)
Glossitis
Gynecomastia (<1%)
Myalgia (1–10%)
Oral ulceration (<1%)
Paresthesias (1–10%)
Sialopenia (>10%)
Sialorrhea (<1%)
Xerostomia (>10%)

ESTRAMUSTINE

Trade name: Emcyt (Pharmacia & Upjohn)
Other common trade name: *Cellmusin*
Indications: Prostate carcinoma
Category: Antineoplastic, nitrogen mustard
Half-life: 20 hours
Clinically important, potentially serious interactions with: aldesleukin, **dairy products**

Reactions

Skin

Allergic reactions (sic)
Edema (>10%)
Exanthems
(1971): Anderes A+, *Praxis* (German) 60, 1276
Flushing (1%)
Hot flashes (<1%)
Night sweats (<1%)
Pigmentary changes (sic) (<1%)
Pruritus (2%)
(1976): Nagel R+, *Med Klin* (German) 71, 1724
Purpura (3%)
Rash (sic) (1%)
Urticaria
Xerosis (2%)

Hair

Hair – alopecia (<1%)

Other

Gynecomastia (>10%)
Injection-site thrombophlebitis (1–10%)
(1976): Nagel R+, *Med Klin* (German) 71, 1724
Mastodynia (66%)
Thrombophlebitis (3%)

ESTROGENS

Generic:

Chlorotrianisene
Trade name: Tace

Diethylstilbestrol
Trade names: Cyren A; Destrol; Stilphostrol

Estradiol
Trade names: Estrace; Estraderm

Estrogens, conjugated
Trade name: Premarin

Estrogens, esterified
Trade names: Estratab; Menest

Estrone
Trade names: Estroject; Estronol; Gynogen; Theelin, etc.

Estropipate
Trade name: Ogen

Ethinyl estradiol
Trade name: Estinyl

Quinestrol
Trade name: Estrovis

Clinically important, potentially serious interactions with: anticoagulants; barbiturates, carbamazepine, corticosteroids, hydrocortisone, rifampin, tricyclic antidepressants

Reactions

Skin

Acanthosis nigricans
(1974): Banuchi SR+, *Arch Dermatol* 109, 544
Acne
Acute intermittent porphyria
Angioedema
(1942): Saphir WS+, *JAMA* 119, 557
Ankle edema
Bullous eruption
(1971): Kuchera LK, *JAMA* 218, 562
Chloasma (< 1%)
Contact dermatitis
(1981): Ljunggren B, *Contact Dermatitis* 7, 141,
Dermatitis (sic)
(1995): Shelley WB+, *J Am Acad Dermatol* 32, 25
Eczema (sic)
(1995): Shelley WB+, *J Am Acad Dermatol* 32, 25
Edema (< 1%)
Erythema multiforme
Erythema nodosum
(1990): Bartelsmeyer JA+, *Clin Obstet Gynecol* 33, 777
(1980): Salvatore MA+, *Arch Dermatol* 116, 557
Exanthems
(1997): Litt JZ, Beachwood, Ohio, personal case (observation)
(1984): Lee M+, *J Urol* 131, 767
Exfoliative dermatitis
(1942): Kasselberg LA, *JAMA* 120, 117
Fixed eruption (< 1%)
Flushing
(1981): Ingle JN+, *N Engl J Med* 304, 16 (3%)
(1973): Delius L, *Dtsch Med Wochenschr* (German) 98, 1512
Hyperkeratosis of nipples
(1980): Mold DE+, *Cutis* 26, 95
Irritation (sic) (from transdermal system)
Livedo reticularis
Lupus erythematosus
(1989): Colins D, *J Rheumatol* 16, 408
(1986): Barrett C+, *Br J Rheumatol* 25, 300
(1973): Elias PM, *Arch Dermatol* 108, 716
(1971): Laugier P+, *Bull Soc Fr Syphiligr* (French) 78, 623 (SLE-induced)
(1971): Kay DR+, *Arthritis Rheum* 14, 239 (5%) (ANA only)
(1969): Bole CG+, *Lancet* 1, 323
(1968): Hadida E+, *Bull Soc Fr Syphiligr* (French) 75, 616
(1968): Schleicher EM, *Lancet* 1, 821
(1966): Pimstone BL, *S Afr J Obstet Gynecol* 3, 62
Melasma (< 1%)
(1992): Breathnach SM+, *Adverse Drug Reactions and the Skin*, Blackwell, Oxford, 274 (passim)
(1967): Resnic S, *JAMA* 199, 601
Mucha–Habermann disease
(1973): Hollander A+, *Arch Dermatol* 107, 465
Papulovesicular eruption
(1998): Coustou D+, *Ann Dermatol Venereol* (French) 125, 505
Peripheral edema
Photoreactions
Photosensitivity
(1970): Mathison IW+, *Obstet Gynecol Surv* 25, 389
(1968): Erickson LR+, *JAMA* 203, 980
(1965): Daniels F, *Med Clin North Am* 49, 565
Pigmentation
(1999): Oakley A, Auckland, New Zealand (from Internet) (observation) (from topical, over vulva)
(1972): Ippen H+, *Hautarzt* (German) 23, 21 (chloasma)
(1967): Resnic S, *JAMA* 199, 601
Pruritus
(2000): Siepmann M+, *Dtsch Med Wochenschr* (German) 125, 557
(1998): Coustou D+, *Ann Dermatol Venereol* (French) 125, 505
(1995): Shelley WB+, *J Am Acad Dermatol* 32, 25
(1971): Kuchera LK, *JAMA* 218, 562
Purpura
(1984): Lee M+, *J Urol* 131, 767
Rash (sic) (< 1%)
Raynaud's phenomenon
(1998): Fraenkel L+, *Ann Intern Med* 129, 208
Scleroderma
(2000): D'Cruz D, *Toxicol Lett* 112 and 421
Spider nevi
(1992): Breathnach SM+, *Adverse Drug Reactions and the Skin*, Blackwell, Oxford, 274 (passim)
Striae
Telangiectases
(1970): Aram H+, *Acta Derm Venereol* 50, 302
Urticaria
(1995): Shelley WB+, *J Am Acad Dermatol* 32, 25
(1984): Lee M+, *J Urol* 131, 767
(1964): Beall GN, *Medicine* (Baltimore) 43, 131
Vasculitis (cutaneous polyarteritis nodosa)
(1998): Cvancara JL+, *J Am Acad Dermatol* 39, 643

Hair

Hair – alopecia
(1992): Breathnach SM+, *Adverse Drug Reactions and the Skin*, Blackwell, Oxford, 233 (passim)
Hair – hirsutism
(1971): Fusi S+, *Folia Endocrinol* (Italian) 24, 412
Hair – straight
(1994): Litt JZ, Beachwood, Ohio, personal case (observation)

Nails

Nails – onycholysis
(1976): Byrne JP+, *Post Grad Med J* 52, 535

Other

Galactorrhea
Gingival hyperplasia
Gynecomastia (> 10%)
(2000): Felner EI+, *Pediatrics* 105, E55 (in 3 prepubertal boys from an estrogen cream)
(1987): Schmidt KU+, *Dtsch Med Wochenschr* (German) 112, 926
(1984): Gottswinter JM+, *Haarwasser Med Klin* (German) 79, 181
(1978): Gabilove JL+, *Arch Dermatol* 114, 1672
(1969): Goebel M, *Hautarzt* (German) 20, 521
(1969): Degos R+, *Ann Dermatol Syphiligr Paris* (French) 96, 5
(1968): Stewart WM+, *Bull Soc Fr Dermatol Syphiligr* (French) 75, 294
Injection-site pain (1–10%)
Mastodynia (> 10%)
Oral mucosal pigmentation
(1991): Perusse R+, *Cutis* 48, 61
Porphyria
(1994): Siersema PD+, *Eur J Gastroenterol Hepatol* 6, 371
(1989): CoulsonDH+, *Br J Urol* 63, 648

Porphyria cutanea tarda
(1995): Nonaka S+, *Nippon Rinsho* (Japanese) 53, 1427
(1990): Roger D+, *Ann Dermatol Venereol* (French) 117, 127
(1982): Enriquez de Salamanca R+, *Arch Dermatol Res* 274, 179
(1979): Grossman ME+, *Am J Med* 67, 277
(1979): Sweeney GD+, *Can Med Assoc J* 120, 803
(1978): Benedetto AV+, *Cutis* 21, 483
(1976): Byrne JP+, *Post Grad Med J* 52, 535
(1975): Malina L+, *Br J Dermatol* 92, 707
(1975): Haberman HF+, *Can Med Assoc J* 113, 653
(1975): Wanscher B, *Ugeskr Laeger* (Danish) 137, 623
(1973): Palma-Carlos AG+, *Nouv Presse Med* (French) 2, 1996
(1973): Gajdos A+, *Nouv Presse Med* (French) 2, 1131
(1971): Stein KM+, *Obstet Gynecol* 38, 755
(1971): Barth J+, *Dermatol Monatsschr* (German) 157, 160
(1970): Roenigk HH+, *Arch Dermatol* 102, 260
(1969): Duverne+, *Lyon Med* (French) 221, 1097
(1966): Levere RD, *Blood* 28, 569
(1965): Becker FT, *Arch Dermatol* 92, 252
(1964): Theologides H+, *Metabolism* 13, 391
(1963): Hurley HJ, *Arch Dermatol* 88, 233
(1963): Walshe M, *Br J Dermatol* 75, 298
Vaginal candidiasis

ETANERCEPT

Trade name: Enbrel (Immunex; Wyeth-Ayerst)
Indications: Rheumatoid arthritis
Category: Antirheumatic, biologic response modifying; anti-arthritic
Half-life: 98–300 hours
Clinically important, potentially serious interactions with: vaccines

Reactions

Skin

Allergic reactions (sic) (<3%
Erythema
Infection (sic) (<3%)
Malignancies (sic) (<3%)
Pruritus
Rash (sic) (5%)
(2000): *Nurses' Drug Alert*, 24, 4
(1999): Brion PH+, *Ann Int Med* 131, 634
Ulceration

Other

Injection-site reactions (37%)
(2000): Murphy FT+, *Arch Dermatol* 136, 556
(1999): Jarvis B+, *Drugs* 57, 945
(1999): Weinblatt ME+, *N Engl J Med* 340, 253

ETHACRYNIC ACID

Trade name: Edecrin (Merck)
Other common trade names: *Edecril; Edecrina; Hydromedin; Reomax*
Indications: Edema
Category: Loop diuretic
Half-life: 2–4 hours
Clinically important, potentially serious interactions with: ACE-inhibitors, aminoglycosides, amphotericin B, cisplatin, digoxin, gatifloxacin, lithium, moxifloxacin, NSAIDs, salicylates, sparfloxacin, thiazides, warfarin

Reactions

Skin

Allergic reactions (sic)
Chills (<1%)
Exanthems
(1966): Sherlock S+, *Lancet* 1, 1049
Photosensitivity
Purpura (<1%)
Rash (sic) (<1%)
Urticaria
Vasculitis
(1992): Breathnach SM+, *Adverse Drug Reactions and the Skin*, Blackwell, Oxford, 229 (passim)
(1967): Bar-on H+, *Isr J Med Sci* 3, 113

Other

Injection-site pain
Thrombophlebitis (<1%)
Xerostomia

ETHAMBUTOL

Trade name: Myambutol (Dura; Lederle)
Other common trade names: *Apo-Ethambutol; Dexambutol; EMB; Etapiam; Etibi; Stambutol*
Indications: Tuberculosis
Category: Antimycobacterial
Half-life: 3–4 hours
Clinically important, potentially serious interactions with: antacids, kaolin

Reactions

Skin

Acne:
Angioedema
(1985): Holdiness MR, *Int J Dermatol* 24, 280
Bullous eruption
(1985): Holdiness MR, *Int J Dermatol* 24, 280
(1981): Frentz G+, *Acta Derm Venereol* (Stockh) 61, 89
Chills
Contact dermatitis
(1986): Holdiness MR, *Contact Dermatitis* 15, 96
(1986): Holdiness MR, *Contact Dermatitis* 15, 282
Dermatitis (sic)
Diaphoresis
(1985): Holdiness MR, *Int J Dermatol* 24, 280
Erythema multiforme
(1985): Holdiness MR, *Int J Dermatol* 24, 280
(1981): Frentz G+, *Acta Derm Venereol* (Stockh) 61, 89
Exanthems
(1985): Holdiness MR, *Int J Dermatol* 24, 280
(1981): Frentz G+, *Acta Derm Venereol* (Stockh) 61, 89 (1–5%)
(1977): Pasricha JS+, *Arch Dermatol* 113, 1122
Exfoliative dermatitis
(1985): Holdiness MR, *Int J Dermatol* 24, 280
Lichenoid eruption
(1995): Grossman ME+, *J Am Acad Dermatol* 33, 675
(1981): Frentz G+, *Acta Derm Venereol* (Stockh) 61, 89
Lupus erythematosus
(1986): Layer P+, *Dtsch Med Wochenschr* (German) 111,1603
(1977): Djawari D, *Z Hautkr* (German) 53, 180
Photosensitivity
(1994): Berger TG+, *Arch Dermatol* 130, 609 (in HIV-infected)
Pruritus (<1%)
(1985): Holdiness MR, *Int J Dermatol* 24, 280
(1981): Frentz G+, *Acta Derm Venereol* (Stockh) 61, 89
(1969): Council on Drugs, *JAMA* 208, 2463
Purpura
(1972): Levantine A+, *Br J Dermatol* 86, 651
Rash (sic) (<1%)
(1995): Chaisson RE, *Infections in Medicine* 12, 48
(1995): Wong PC+, *Eur Respir J* 8, 866
Stevens–Johnson syndrome
(1979): Surjapranata FJ+, *Paediatr Indones* 19, 195
Toxic epidermal necrolysis
(1985): Heng MCY, *Br J Dermatol* 106, 107
(1981): Pegram PS+, *Arch Intern Med* 141, 1677
Urticaria
(1985): Holdiness MR, *Int J Dermatol* 24, 280
(1981): Frentz G+, *Acta Derm Venereol* (Stockh) 61, 89

Hair

Hair – alopecia
(1985): Holdiness MR, *Int J Dermatol* 24, 280

Other

Anaphylactoid reaction (< 1%)
Dyschromatopsia
Hypersensitivity
(1995): Dhamgaye T+, *Tuber Lung Dis* 76,181
Paresthesias

ETHANOLAMINE

Trade name: Ethamolin (Cypros)
Other common trade name: *Ethanolamine Oleate*
Indications: Bleeding esophageal varices
Category: Sclerosing agent
Half-life: no data
Clinically important, potentially serious interactions with: none

Reactions

Skin

Contact dermatitis
(1995): Kock P, *Contact Dermatitis* 33, 273
(1994): Aranzabal A+, *Contact Dermatitis* 31, 121
(1994): Ortiz-Frutos FJ+, *Contact Dermatitis* 31, 193
(1994): Schnuch A, *Contact Dermatitis* 30, 243

Other

Anaphylactoid reaction (< 1%)
Injection necrosis

ETHCHLORVYNOL

Trade name: Placidyl (Abbott)
Other common trade names: *Arvynol; Nostel*
Indications: Insomnia
Category: Sedative-hypnotic
Half-life: 10–20 hours
Clinically important, potentially serious interactions with: alcohol, anticoagulants, CNS depressants, MAO inhibitors, tricyclic antidepressants

Reactions

Skin

Allergic reactions (sic)
Bullous eruption (from overdose)
(1990): Yell RP, *Am J Emerg Med* 8, 246
(1980): Brodin MD+, *J Cutan Pathol* 7, 326
Diaphoresis
Facial numbness (sic)
Fixed eruption
(1965): Auerbach R, *Arch Dermatol* 92, 184
Pruritus
Purpura
(1972): Jakobson ES, *Ann Intern Med* 77, 73 (fatal)
Rash (sic) (1–10%)
Urticaria

Other

Acute intermittent porphyria
Dysgeusia (> 10%)
Hypersensitivity
Paresthesias
Pressure necrosis
(1990): Chamberlain JM+, *Am J Emerg Med* 8, 467

ETHIONAMIDE

Trade name: Trecator-SC (Wyeth-Ayerst)
Other common trade names: *Ethatyl; Etiocidan: Myobid-250; Tubermin*
Indications: Tuberculosis
Category: Tuberculostatic
Half-life: 2–3 hours
Clinically important, potentially serious interactions with: cycloserine, isoniazid

Reactions

Skin

Acne
(1992): Breathnach SM+, *Adverse Drug Reactions and the Skin*, Blackwell, Oxford, (passim)
(1965): *Drug Ther Bull* 3, 61
(1963): Lees AW, *Am Rev Respir Dis* 88, 347
Allergic reactions (sic)
(1971): *Med Lett* 13, 55 (1%)
Butterfly eruptions on the face (sic)
(1992): Breathnach SM+, *Adverse Drug Reactions and the Skin*, Blackwell, Oxford, (passim)
Eczema (sic) (chiefly involving the forehead)
(1992): Breathnach SM+, *Adverse Drug Reactions and the Skin*, Blackwell, Oxford, 159 (passim)
Exanthems
(1969): Agrawal R, *BMJ* 4, 540
(1965): Carey VCI, *Tubercle* 46, 287
Ichthyosis
(1972): Levantine A+, *Br J Dermatol* 86, 651
Lupus erythematosus
(1973): Desmons MF, *Bull Soc Fr Dermatol Syphiligr* (French) 80, 168
Pellagra
(1987): Schmutz JL+, *Ann Dermatol Venereol* (French) 114, 569
Photosensitivity
(1966): Friedmann ME, *Bull Soc Franc Dermatol Syphiligr* (French) 73, 510
(1966): Baran R, *Hôpital* (French) 54, 445
Purpura
(1992): Breathnach SM+, *Adverse Drug Reactions and the Skin*, Blackwell, Oxford, (passim)
Rash (sic) (< 1%)
Seborrheic dermatitis
(1972): Levantine A+, *Br J Dermatol* 86, 651
Urticaria (1–5%)

Hair

Hair – alopecia (< 1%)
(1992): Breathnach SM+, *Adverse Drug Reactions and the Skin*, Blackwell, Oxford, 159 (passim)
(1966): Baran R, *Hôpital* (French) 54, 445

Other

Dysgeusia (1–10%) (metallic taste)
Gynecomastia (< 1%)
Oral ulceration
Sialorrhea
Stomatitis (< 1%)
(1992): Breathnach SM+, *Adverse Drug Reactions and the Skin*, Blackwell, Oxford, (passim)
Stomatodynia
Xerostomia

ETHOSUXIMIDE

Trade name: Zarontin (Parke-Davis)
Other common trade names: *Emeside; Ethymal; Petnidan; Pyknolepsinum; Simatin; Zarondan*
Indications: Absence (petit mal) seizures
Category: Succinimide anticonvulsant
Half-life: 50–60 hours
Clinically important, potentially serious interactions with: carbamazepine, hydantoins, isoniazid, MAO inhibitors, phenobarbital, pimozide, primidone

Reactions

Skin

Cutaneous side effects (sic) (3.4%)
(1966): Weinstein AW+, *Am J Dis Child* 111, 63
Erythema multiforme (<1%)
(1966): Coursin DB, *JAMA* 198, 113
Exanthems (1–5%)
(1991): Pelekanos J+, *Epilepsia* 32, 554
(1966): Weinstein AW+, *Am J Dis Child* 111, 63 (2.2%)
Exfoliative dermatitis (<1%)
Lupus erythematosus (>10%)
(1996): Wallace SJ, *Drug Saf* 15, 378
(1996): Takeda S+, *Intern Med* 35, 587
(1996): Miyasaka N, *Intern Med 35, 527*
(1994): Riviello JJ+, *J Epilepsy* 7, 23
(1993): Ansell BM, *Lupus* 2, 193
(1993): Drory VE+, *Clin Neuropharmacol* 16, 19 (passim)
(1985): Lovisetto P+, *Recenti Prog Med* (Italian) 76, 84
(1984): Koike K+, *Rinsho Ketsueki* 25, 1635
(1979): Tor J+, *Med Clin (Barc)* (Spanish) 73, 443
(1976): Singsen BH+, *Pediatrics* 57, 529
(1975): Teoh PC+, *Arch Dis Child* 50, 658 (morphea-like)
(1973): Beernink DH+, *J Pediatr* 82, 113
(1970): Alter BP, *J Pediatr* 77, 1093
(1970): Dabbous IA+, *J Pediatr* 76, 617
(1968): Livingston S+, *JAMA* 203, 731
(1968): Monnet P+, *Lyon Med* (French) 220, 467
Periorbital edema
Pruritus
Purpura
(1967): Kontsouliers E, *Lancet* 2, 310
Rash (sic) (<1%)
Raynaud's phenomenon
(1990): Rose CD+, *Arthritis Rheum* 33 (Suppl) R23
(1975): Taaffe A+, *Br Dent J* 138, 172
(1966): Coursin DB, *JAMA* 198, 113
Stevens–Johnson syndrome (>10%)
(1975): Taaffe A+, *Br Dent J* 138, 172
Urticaria (1–5%)
(1966): Weinstein AW+, *Am J Dis Child* 111, 63 (1%)

Hair

Hair – alopecia
Hair – hirsutism

Other

Acute intermittent porphyria
Gingival hyperplasia
Oral ulceration
Tongue edema

ETHOTOIN

Trade name: Peganone (Abbott)
Other common trade name: *Accenon*
Indications: Tonic-clonic (grand mal) seizures
Category: Hydantoin anticonvulsant
Half-life: 3–9 hours
Clinically important, potentially serious interactions with: chloramphenicol, cyclosporine, disulfiram, dopamine, fluconazole, ibuprofen, isoniazid, itraconazole

Reactions

Skin

Bullous eruption
Fixed eruption
Lupus erythematosus
Purpura
(1967): Coleman WP, *Med Clin North Am* 51, 1073
Rash (sic)

Other

Gingival hyperplasia

ETIDRONATE

Trade name: Didronel (MGI; Procter & Gamble)
Other common trade names: *Didronate; Difosfen; Dinol; Diphos; Osteum*
Indications: Paget's disease, osteoporosis
Category: Bone resorption inhibitor; antihypercalcemic
Half-life: 6 hours
Clinically important, potentially serious interactions with: antacids

Reactions

Skin

Angioedema (<1%)
Exanthems:
Pruritus
(1985): Holzmann H+, *Hautarzt* (German) 36, 326
Rash (sic) (<1%)
Stevens–Johnson syndrome
Toxic epidermal necrolysis
(1995): Coakley G+, *Br J Rheumatol* 34, 798
Urticaria

Hair

Hair – alopecia

Other

Ageusia
Dysgeusia (<1%)
Glossitis
Hypersensitivity (<1%)
Paresthesias
Stomatitis

ETODOLAC

Trade name: Lodine (Wyeth-Ayerst)
Other common trade names: *Antilak; Ecridoxan; Edolan; Elderin; Lonine; Tedolan; Utradol; Zedolac*
Indications: Pain
Category: Nonsteroidal anti-inflammatory (NSAID)
Half-life: 7 hours
Clinically important, potentially serious interactions with: aminoglycosides, anticoagulants, aspirin, beta-blockers, cyclosporine, digoxin, lithium, loop diuretics, methotrexate, probenecid, salicylates, warfarin

Reactions

Skin

Angioedema (<1%)
(1991): Astorga-Paulsen G+, *Curr Med Res Opin* 12, 401
Bullous eruption
Dermatitis (sic)
Diaphoresis
Ecchymoses
Edema
Erythema multiforme (<1%)
Exanthems
(1998): Litt JZ, Beachwood, OH, personal case (observation)
(1997): Litt JZ, Beachwood, OH, personal case (observation)
(1990): Schattenkirchner M, *Eur J Rheumatol Inflamm* 10, 56
(1986): Lynch S+, *Drugs* 31, 288 (3%)
Exfoliative dermatitis
Facial edema
(1991): Astorga-Paulsen G+, *Curr Res Med Opin* 12, 401
(1990): Freitas GG, *Curr Med Res Opin* 12, 255
Fixed eruption
(1997): Blumenthal HL, Beachwood, OH, personal case (observation)
Flushing
(1991): Astorga-Paulsen G+, *Curr Med Res Opin* 12, 401
Furunculosis
(1987): Waltham-Weeks CD, *Curr Med Res Opin* 10, 540
Hyperpigmentation
Peeling skin (sic)
Peripheral edema
(1990): Freitas GG, *Curr Med Res Opin* 12, 255
Photosensitivity
(1987): Waltham-Weeks CD, *Curr Med Res Opin* 10, 540
Pruritus (1–10%)
(1998): Litt JZ, Beachwood, OH, personal case (observation)
(1991): Bianchi-Porro G+, *J Intern Med* 229, 5
(1991): Astorga-Paulsen G+, *Curr Res Med Opin* 12, 401
(1991): Karbowski A, *Curr Med Res Opin* 12, 309
(1991): Balfour JA+, *Drugs* 42, 274
(1991): *Med Lett Drug Ther* 33, 79
(1990): Schattenkirchner M, *Eur J Rheumatol Inflamm* 10, 56
(1989): Ciocci A, *Curr Med Res Opin* 11, 471
Purpura
Rash (sic) (>10%)
(1991): Astorga-Paulsen G+, *Curr Med Res Opin* 12, 401
(1991): Balfour JA+, *Drugs* 42, 274
(1991): Anon, *Med Lett Drug Ther* 33, 79
(1989): Williams PI+, *Curr Med Res Opin*
(1989): Ciocci A, *Curr Med Res Opin* 11, 471
Stevens–Johnson syndrome (<1%)
Toxic epidermal necrolysis (<1%)
Urticaria (<1%)
(2000): Mitchell D, Thomasville, GA (from Internet) (observation)
(1996): Thaler D, Monona, WI, personal case (pressure) (observation)
Vasculitis
(1996): Lie JT+, *J Rheumatol* 23, 183 (hypersensitivity)
(1989): Willemin B+, *Ann Méd Int* (French) 140, 529
Vesiculobullous eruption

Hair

Hair – alopecia

Other

Gingival ulceration
Glossitis
Gynecomastia
Parageusia
Paresthesias
Sialorrhea
Stomatitis
Ulcerative stomatitis
Xerostomia

ETOPOSIDE

Synonyms: epipodophyllotoxin; VP-16; VP-16–213
Trade name: VePesid (Bristol-Myers Squibb)
Other common trade names: *Aside; Etopos; Etosid; Lastet; Serozide; Vepeside; VP-TEC*
Indications: Lymphomas, carcinomas
Category: Antineoplastic
Half-life: terminal: 4–15 hours
Clinically important, potentially serious interactions with: calcium antagonists, carmustine, cyclosporine, methotrexate, warfarin

Reactions

Skin

Allergic reactions (sic) (1–2%)
Diaphoresis
Ecchymoses
Eccrine squamous syringometaplasia
(1997): Valks R+, *Arch Dermatol* 133, 873
Erythema
(1994): Portal I+, *Cancer Chemother Pharmacol* 34, 181 (acral)
(1993): Dechaufour F+, *Ann Dermatol Venereol* (French) 120, 219 (acral)
(1993): Vukelja SJ+, *Cutis* 52, 89 (acral)
Erythema multiforme
(1987): Yokel BK+, *J Cutan Pathol* 14, 326
Exanthems
(1992): Beyer J+, *Bone Marrow Transplant* 10, 491
(1992): Breathnach SM+, *Adverse Drug Reactions and the Skin*, Blackwell, Oxford, 301 (passim)
(1987): Yokel BK+, *J Cutan Pathol* 14, 326
(1981): Weiss RB+, *Ann Intern Med* 94, 66
Facial edema
Flushing (<1%)
(1990): Henwood JM+, *Drugs* 39, 438
(1988): Ogle KM+, *Am J Clin Oncol* 11, 663
(1985): Tucci E+, *Chemioterapia* 4, 460
Pigmentation
(1991): Singal R+, *Pediatr Dermatol* 8, 231
Pruritus
Purpura
Radiation recall
(1993): Williams BJ+, *Clin Exp Dermatol* 18, 452 (ultraviolet)
(1992): Breathnach SM+, *Adverse Drug Reactions and the Skin*, Blackwell, Oxford, 301 (passim)
(1987): Yokel BK+, *J Cutan Pathol* 14, 326
Rash (sic)
Stevens–Johnson syndrome
(1992): Breathnach SM+, *Adverse Drug Reactions and the Skin*, Blackwell, Oxford, 301 (passim)
(1987): Yokel BK+, *J Cutan Pathol* 14, 326
(1983): Jameson CH+, *Cancer Treat Rep* 67, 1050
Urticaria

Hair

Hair – alopecia (8–66%)
(1990): Henwood JM+, *Drugs* 39, 438 (100%, dose-dependent)
(1989): Wander HE+, *Cancer Chemother Pharmacol* 24, 261
(1989): Yoshino M+, *Jpn J Clin Oncol* 19, 120 (57%)
(1989): Smit EF+, *Thorax* 44, 631

Nails

Nails – Beau's lines (transverse nail bands)
(1994): Ben-Dayan D+, *Acta Haematol* 91, 89
Nails – onycholysis
(1995): Obermair A+, *Gynecol Oncol* 57, 436

Other

Anaphylactoid reaction (<2%)
(1989): Wander HE+, *Cancer Chemother Pharmacol* 24, 261
(1989): Siddall SJ+, *Lancet* 1, 394
Dysgeusia
Hypersensitivity (<1%)
(1993): Hudson MM+, *J Clin Oncol* 11, 1080
(1992): Weiss RB, *Semin Oncol* 19, 458
(1991): Kellie SJ+, *Cancer* 67, 1070
(1988): Ogle KM+, *Am J Clin Oncol* 11, 663
(1985): Tucci E+, *Chemioterapia* 4, 460
(1984): O'Dwyer PJ+, *Cancer Treat Rep* 68, 959
Injection-site pain
Mucositis (>10%)
Oral mucosal lesions
(1990): Henwood JM+, *Drugs* 39, 438 (1–5%)
Paresthesias
Stomatitis (1–10%)
Thrombophlebitis (<1%)
Tongue edema

FAMCICLOVIR

Trade name: Famvir (SmithKline Beecham)
Indications: Acute herpes zoster, recurrent genital herpes
Category: Antiviral
Half-life: 2–3 hours
Clinically important, potentially serious interactions with: cimetidine, digoxin, probenecid

Reactions

Skin
Dermatitis (sic)
(1996): Sacks SL+, *JAMA* 276, 44
Pruritus (3.7%)

Other
Paresthesias (2.6%)

FAMOTIDINE

Trade name: Pepcid (Merck)
Other common trade names: *Amfamox; Apo-Famotidine; Durater; Famodil; Famoxal; Ganor; Gastro; Motiax; Mylanta AR, Nu-Famotidine; Pepcidine; Pepdul; Sigafam*
Indications: Duodenal ulcer, gastroesophageal reflux disease (GERD)
Category: Histamine H_2-receptor antagonist and anti-ulcer
Half-life: 2.5–3.5 hours
Clinically important, potentially serious interactions with: antacids, cephalosporins, itraconazole, ketoconazole, nifedipine, nisoldipine

Reactions

Skin
Acne (<1%)
Allergic reactions (sic) (<1%)
Angioedema
(1986): Campoli-Richards DM+, *Drugs* 32, 197 (0.05%)
Contact dermatitis
(1994): Guimaraens D+, *Contact Dermatitis* 31, 259
(1990): Monteseirin J+, *Contact Dermatitis* 22, 290
Cutaneous side effects (sic)
(1986): Campoli-Richards DM+, *Drugs* 32, 197 (0.4%)
Dermographism
(1994): Warner DMc+, *J Am Acad Dermatol* 31, 677
Erythema multiforme
(1999): Horiuchi Y+, *Ann Intern Med* 131, 795
Exanthems
Facial edema
Flushing
(1986): Campoli-Richards DM+, *Drugs* 32, 197 (0.2%)
Periorbital edema
Pruritus (<1%)
(1994): Warner DMc+, *J Am Acad Dermatol* 31, 677
(1990): Edge DP, *N Z Med J* 103, 150
Purpura
(1996): Kallal SM+, *West J Med* 164, 446
Rash (sic)
(1989): McCullough AJ+, *Gastroenterology* 97, 860
(1989): Schunack W, *J Int Med Res* 17 (Suppl 1), 9A
Toxic epidermal necrolysis
(1995): Brunner M+, *Br J Dermatol* 133, 814
Urticaria (<1%)
(1994): Warner DMc+, *J Am Acad Dermatol* 31, 677
(1986): Campoli-Richards DM+, *Drugs* 32, 197 (0.1%)
Vasculitis
(1993): Torralba M+, *An Med Interna* (Spanish) 10, 621
(1990): Andreo JA+, *Med Clin (Barc)* (Spanish) 95, 234
Xerosis (<1%)

Hair
Hair – alopecia

Other
Dysgeusia
Gynecomastia
Injection-site pain
Myalgia
Oral mucosal lesions
(1986): Campoli-Richards DM+, *Drugs* 32, 197 (0.15%)
Paresthesias (<1%)
(1997): Litt JZ, Beachwood, OH, personal case (prickly sensation) (observation)
(1997): Litt JZ, Beachwood, OH, personal case (observation)
Xerostomia
(1986): Campoli-Richards DM+, *Drugs* 32, 197 (0.15%)

FELBAMATE

Trade name: Felbatol (Wallace)
Other common trade names: *Felbamyl; Taloxa*
Indications: Partial seizures
Category: Antiepileptic
Half-life: 13–23 hours
Clinically important, potentially serious interactions with: barbiturates, carbamazepine, estrogens, phenytoin, valproic acid

Reactions

Skin
Acne (3.4%)
Bullous eruption (<1%)
Diaphoresis
Edema
Facial edema (3.4%)
Flushing
Lichen planus
Livedo reticularis
Lupus erythematosus
Photosensitivity (<0.01%)
Pruritus (>1%)
Purpura
Pustular eruption
(1994): Shelley WB+, *Cutis* 53, 282 (observation)
Rash (sic) (3.5%)
Stevens–Johnson syndrome
(1994): Jackel RA, *Epilepsia* 35, 98
Toxic epidermal necrolysis
(1995): Travaglini MT+, *Pharmacotherapy* 15, 260
Urticaria (<1%)

Hair
Hair – alopecia

Other
Anaphylactoid reaction (<0.01%)
Dysgeusia (6.1%)
Foetor ex ore (halitosis)
Gingival bleeding
Glossitis
Myalgia (2.6%)
Oral mucosal edema (>1%)
Paresthesias (3.5%)
Thrombophlebitis
Xerostomia (2.6%)

FELODIPINE

Trade names: Lexxel (AstraZeneca); Plendil (Zeneca Merck)
Other common trade names: *AGON SR; Hydac; Modip; Munobal; Penedil; Renedil; Splendil*
Indications: Hypertension
Category: Calcium channel blocker; antihypertensive
Half-life: 11–16 hours
Clinically important, potentially serious interactions with: barbiturates, beta-blockers, carbamazepine, cimetidine, cyclosporine, digoxin, erythromycin, metoprolol, phenobarbital, phenytoin, prazosin, procainamide, quinidine, rifampin, theophylline, **grapefruit juice**

Lexxel is enalapril and felodipine

Reactions

Skin

Ankle edema
(1992): Morgan TO+, *Kidney Int* Suppl 36, S78
(1992): Morgan TO+, *Am J Hypertens* 5, 238
(1991): Dimenas E+, *Eur J Clin Pharmacol* 40, 141
(1991): Liedholm H+, *Drug Intell Clin Pharm* 25, 1007
Diaphoresis
(1988): Saltiel E+, *Drugs* 36, 387
Edema
(1991): *Med Lett Drugs Ther* 33, 115
Erythema (1.5%)
Exanthems
(1993): Litt JZ, Beachwood, OH, personal case (observation)
(1985): Lorimer AR+, *Drugs* 29 (Suppl 2), 154
Facial edema (1.5%)
Flu-like syndrome (sic) (<1%)
Flushing (6%)
(1992): Morgan TO+, *Am J Hypertens* 5, 238
(1991): Dimenas E+, *Eur J Clin Pharmacol* 40, 141
(1991): Liedholm H+, *Drug Intell Clin Pharm* 25, 1007
(1991): *Med Lett Drugs Ther* 33, 115
(1991): Yedinak KC+, *Drug Intell Clin Pharm* 25, 1193
(1991): Frewin DB+, *Eur J Clin Pharmacol* 41, 393
(1988): Saltiel E+, *Drugs* 36, 387 (5–30%; dose-related)
(1987): Elmfeldt D+, *Drugs* 34 (Suppl 3) 132
(1985): Lorimer AR+, *Drugs* 29 (Suppl 2), 154 (25%)
(1985): Aberg H+, *Drugs* 29 (Suppl 2), 117 (44%)
Peripheral edema (22%)
(1991): Frewin DB+, *Eur J Clin Pharmacol* 41, 393
Pruritus (<1%)
Purpura
(1991): Capewell S+, *Eur J Clin Pharmacol* 41, 95
Rash (sic) (1.5%)
Telangiectases (truncal)
(1998): Karonen T+, *Dermatology* 196, 272
Urticaria (1.5%)

Nails

Nails – brittle
(1985): Aberg H+, *Drugs* 29 (Suppl 2), 117 (44%)

Other

Gingival hyperplasia (2–10%)
(1998): Young PC+, *Cutis* 62, 41
Gynecomastia (<1%)
Myalgia (1.5%)
Paresthesias (2.5%)
Xerostomia (<1%)
(1991): Dimenas E+, *Eur J Clin Pharmacol* 40, 141

FENFLURAMINE*

Trade name: Pondimin (Robins)
Other common trade names: *Dima-Fen; Pesos; Ponderal; Ponderax; Ponflural; Wate Down*
Indications: Weight reduction
Category: Anorexiant
Half-life: 11–30 hours
Clinically important, potentially serious interactions with: antidiabetics, barbiturates, clonidine, furazolidone, guanethidine, insulin, MAO inhibitors, phenothiazines, SSRIs, sulfonylureas, tricyclic antidepressants, venlafaxine

Reactions

Skin

Allergic reactions (sic)
Burning (sic)
Diaphoresis (<1%)
Exanthems
Flushing
Pruritus
Rash (sic)
Urticaria

Hair

Hair – alopecia (<1%)

Other

Dysgeusia
Gynecomastia
Myalgia (<1%)
Xerostomia

***Note:** Fenfluramine has been withdrawn in the USA

FENOFIBRATE

Synonyms: procetofene; proctofene
Trade name: Tricor (Abbott)
Other trade name: *Apo-Fenofibrate*
Indications: Hyperlipidemia
Category: Fibric acid cholesterol-lowering agent
Half-life: 20 hours
Clinically important, potentially serious interactions with: anticoagulants, chlorpropamide, cholestyramine, cyclosporine, furosemide, oral anticoagulants, statins

Reactions

Skin

Exanthems
(1990): Balfour JA+, *Drugs* 40, 260
Photoreactions
(1996): Jeanmougin M+, *Ann Dermatol Venereol* (French) 123, 251
Photosensitivity
(1997): Leroy D+, *Photodermatol Photoimmunol Photomed* 13, 93
(1997): Machet L+, *J Am Acad Dermatol* 37, 808
(1996): Diemer S+, *J Dermatol Sci* 13, 172
(1996): Leenutaphong V+ *J Am Acad Dermatol* 35, 775
(1994): Miranda MA+, *Photochem Photobiol* 59, 171
(1993): Jeanmougin M+, *Ann Dermatol Venereol* (French) 120, 549
(1993): Gardeazabal J+, *Photodermatol Photoimmunol Photomed* 9, 156
(1992): Serrano G+, *J Am Acad Dermatol* 27, 204
(1990): Leroy D+, *Photodermatol Photoimmunol Photomed* 7, 136
(1989): Merino MV+, *Actas Dermo-Sif* (Spanish) 80, 703
Phototoxic reaction
(1993): Vargas F+, *Photochem Photobiol* 58, 471
(1990): Merino V+, *Contact Dermatitis* 23, 284
Pruritus (4%)

Rash (sic) (4–8%)
(1989): Blane GF, *Cardiology* 76, 1
(1989): *Am J Med* 83, 26 (2%)
Skin reactions (sic) (1–10%)
(1989): Goldberg AC+, *Clin Ther* 11, 69
Urticaria

Hair

Hair – alopecia
(1990): Gollnick H+, *Z Hautkr* (German) 65, 1128

Other

Muscle tenderness
(1989): *Am J Med* 83, 26 (1%)
Muscle toxicity (sic)
(1989): Muller JP+, *Presse Med* (French) 18, 1033
(1982): Giraud P+, *Rev Rhum Mal Osteartic* (French) 49, 162
Myalgia (<1%)
Myopathy
(1991): Solsona L+, *Med Clin (Barc)* (Spanish) 97, 677
Paresthesias
Polymyositis
(1991): Sauvaget F+, *Rev Med Interne* (French) 12, 52
Vaginitis

FENOPROFEN

Trade name: Nalfon (Dista)
Other common trade names: *Fenoprex; Fenopron; Fepron; Feprona; Nalgesic; Progesic*
Indications: Arthritis
Category: Nonsteroidal anti-inflammatory (NSAID)
Half-life: 2.5–3 hours
Clinically important, potentially serious interactions with: oral anticoagulants, beta-blockers, cyclosporine, lithium, methotrexate, NSAIDs, oral anticoagulants, phenytoin, probenecid, salicylates, sulfonamides, sulfonylureas

Reactions

Skin

Acne
(1974): Wojtulewski JA+, *BMJ* 2, 475
Angioedema (<1%)
Bruising (<1%)
Bullous eruption
Diaphoresis (<0.5%)
Erythema multiforme (<1%)
(1988): Stotts JS+, *J Am Acad Dermatol* 18, 755
Exanthems
(1985): Bigby M+, *J Am Acad Dermatol* 12, 866
(1977): Davis JD+, *Clin Pharmacol Ther* 21, 52
Exfoliative dermatitis (<1%)
Hot flashes (<1%)
Peripheral edema (<1%)
Pruritus (3–9%)
(1992): Breathnach SM+, *Adverse Drug Reactions and the Skin*, Blackwell, Oxford, 186 (passim)
(1985): Bigby M+, *J Am Acad Dermatol* 12, 866
(1977): Davis JD+, *Clin Pharmacol Ther* 21, 52
Purpura (<1%)
(1992): Breathnach SM+, *Adverse Drug Reactions and the Skin*, Blackwell, Oxford, 186 (passim)
(1978): Simpson RE+, *N Engl J Med* 298, 629
Rash (sic) (>10%)
Stevens–Johnson syndrome (<1%)
Toxic epidermal necrolysis (<1%)
(1988): Stotts JS+, *J Am Acad Dermatol* 18, 755
Urticaria (1–3%)
(1992): Breathnach SM+, *Adverse Drug Reactions and the Skin*, Blackwell, Oxford, 186 (passim)
(1985): Bigby M+, *J Am Acad Dermatol* 12, 866
Vesiculobullous eruption
(1992): Breathnach SM+, *Adverse Drug Reactions and the Skin*, Blackwell, Oxford, 186 (passim)

Hair

Hair – alopecia (<1%)

Other

Anaphylactoid reaction
Aphthous stomatitis (<1%)
Dysgeusia (<1%) (metallic taste)
Glossopyrosis (<1%)
Mastodynia (<1%)
Oral ulceration
Stomatitis
Xerostomia (>1%)

FENTANYL

Trade names: Actiq (Abbott); Duragesic (Janssen)
Other common trade names: *Beatryl; Durogesic; Fentanest; Leptanal; Sublimaze*
Indications: Chronic pain
Category: Narcotic agonist analgesic
Half-life: 1.5–6 hours
Clinically important, potentially serious interactions with: amiodarone, cimetidine, CNS depressants, MAO inhibitors, phenothiazines, ranitidine, ritonavir, tricyclic antidepressants

Reactions

Skin

Cold, clammy skin (<1%)
Diaphoresis (>10%)
(1992): Calis KA+, *Clin Pharm* 11, 22
(1992): Friesen RH+, *Anesthesiology* 76, 46
Edema
(1990): Ducker P+, *Z Hautkr* (German) 65, 734
Erythema (at application site) (<1%)
(1992): Mosser KH, *Am Fam Physician* 45, 2289
(1990): Ducker P+, *Z Hautkr* (German) 65, 734
Exanthems
Exfoliative dermatitis
Flushing (3–10%)
Papular eruption (sic) (>1%)
Pruritus (3–10%)
(1999): Herman NL+, *Anesth Analg* 89, 378
(1996): Larijani GE+, *Pharmacotherapy* 16, 958
(1994): Gerwels JW+, *J Dermatol Surg Oncol* 20, 823
(1992): White MJ+, *Can J Anaesth* 39, 594
(1992): Badner NH+, *Can J Anaesth* 39, 330
(1992): Mourisse J+, *Acta Anaesthesiol Scand* 36, 70
(1992): Belzarena SD, *Anesth Analg* 74, 653
(1992): Calis KA+, *Clin Pharm* 11, 22
(1992): Friesen RH+, *Anesthesiology* 76, 46 (facial)
(1992): Sandler ES+, *Pediatrics* 89, 631
(1992): Paech MJ, *Anaesth Intensive Care* 20, 15
(1992): Mosser KH, *Am Fam Physician* 45, 2289
(1992): Varrassi G+, *Anaesthesia* 47, 558
(1989): Jorrot JC+, *Ann Fr Anesth Réanim* (French) 8, 321 (22%)
(1989): Ackerman WE+, *Can J Anaesth* 36, 388
(1988): Davies GG+, *Anesthesiology* 69, 763
(1988): Monk JP+, *Drugs* 36, 286 (40%)
(1986): Shipton EA+, *S Afr Med J* 70, 325 (13%)
Pustules (sic) (<1%)
Rash (sic) (>1%)
(1992): Stoukides CA+, *Clin Pharm* 11, 222
(1992): Sandler ES+, *Pediatrics* 89, 631
Urticaria (<1%)

Other

Anaphylactoid reaction
(1990): Ducker P+, *Z Hautkr* (German) 65, 734

Dysesthesia (<1%)
Dysgeusia (<1%)
Paresthesias (<1%)
Xerostomia (>10%)
(1992): Calis KA+, *Clin Pharm* 11, 22

FEXOFENADINE

Trade name: Allegra (Aventis)
Indications: Allergic rhinitis; pruritus; urticaria
Category: H_1-receptor antagonist; antihistamine (nonsedating)
Half-life: 14.4 hours
Clinically important, potentially serious interactions with: troglitazone

Reactions

Skin
Acne
(1998): Litt JZ, Beachwood, OH, personal case (observation)
Viral infection (sic) (2.5%)

FILGRASTIM

(See GRANULOCYTE COLONY-STIMULATING FACTOR [GCSF])

FINASTERIDE

Trade names: Propecia (Merck); Proscar (Merck)
Other common trade names: *Pro-Cure; Proscar 5*
Indications: Benign prostatic hypertrophy, male-pattern baldness
Category: Androgen hormone inhibitor; antineoplastic; hair growth stimulant
Half-life: 4.8–6 hours
Clinically important, potentially serious interactions with: none

Reactions

Skin
Exanthems
Rash (sic)
(1999): Cather JC+, *Cutis* 64, 167
Urticaria

Hair
Hair – hypotrichosis (sic)
(1998): Panagota PJ, (from Internet) (observation) ("reversal of graying hair")
Hair – patchy hair loss of beard (sic)
(1999): Mitchell D, Thomasville, GA (from Internet) (observation)
(1998): Drayton GE, Los Angeles CA (from Internet) (observation)

Nails
Nails – onychomycosis
(1999): Mitchell D, Thomasville, GA (from Internet) (observation)

Other
Gynecomastia
(2000): Wade MS+, *Australas J Dermatol* 41, 55 (painful and reversible)
(2000): Zimmerman RL+, *Arch Pathol Lab Med* 124 625
(1999): Cather JC+, *Cutis* 64, 167 (passim)
(1999): Miller JA+, *South Med J* 92, 615
(1997): Carlin BI+, *J Urol* 158, 547
(1997): Staiman VR+, *Urology* 50, 929
(1996): Green L+, *New Engl J Med* 335, 823
(1996): Wilton L+, *Br J Urol* 78, 379
(1995): Volpi R+, *Am J Med Sci* 309, 322
Lip swelling
Mastodynia (<1%)
Myopathy (severe)
(1999): Cather JC+, *Cutis* 64, 167

FLAVOXATE

Trade name: Urispas (Alza)
Other common trade names: *Bladderon; Genurin; Harnin; Patricin; Spasuret; Urispadol; Uronid*
Indications: Dysuria, urgency, nocturia
Category: Urinary antispasmodic agent
Half-life: no data*
Clinically important, potentially serious interactions with: amantadine, anticholinergics, atenolol, clozapine, digoxin, haloperidol, phenothiazines, tacrine, tricyclic antidepressants

Reactions

Skin
Exanthems
Rash (sic) (<1%)
(1999): Enomoto U+, *Contact Dermatitis* 40, 337
Urticaria

Other
Hypersensitivity
(1986): Hirohata S+, *Arch Intern Med* 146, 2409
Oral ulceration
(1972): Strouthidis TM+, *Lancet* 1, 72
Xerostomia (>10%)

*Onset of action: 55–60 minutes

FLECAINIDE

Trade name: Tambocor (3M)
Other common trade names: *Almarytm; Apocard; Corflene; Flecaine; Tabco*
Indications: Atrial fibrillation
Category: Antiarrhythmic
Half-life: 7–22 hours
Clinically important, potentially serious interactions with: amiodarone, amprenavir, beta-blockers, cimetidine, digoxin, disopyramide, propranolol, quinidine, quinine, ritonavir, verapamil, **cigarette smoking**

Reactions

Skin
Diaphoresis (<3%)
Edema (3.5%)
Exanthems
(1985): Holmes B+, *Drugs* 27, 301 (1.4%)
Exfoliative dermatitis (<1%)
Flushing (<3%)
Pruritus (<1%)
Psoriasis
(1988): Mancuso G+, *G Ital Dermatol Venerol* (Italian) 123, 171
(1985): Holmes B+, *Drugs* 27, 301
Rash (sic) (<3%)
Urticaria (<1%)

Hair
Hair – alopecia (<1%)

Other
Dysgeusia (<1%) (metallic taste)
Hypesthesia (1–10%)
Myalgia (<1%)

Oral edema
Paresthesias (<1%)
Tongue edema (<1%)
Tremor (5%)
Xerostomia (<1%)

FLUCONAZOLE

Trade name: Diflucan (Pfizer)
Other common trade names: *Biozolene; Flucazol; Flukezol; Fluzone; Fungata; Triflucan*
Indications: Candidiasis
Category: Broad-spectrum bis-triazole antifungal
Half-life: 25–30 hours
Clinically important, potentially serious interactions with: alprazolam, anticoagulants, astemizole, cimetidine, cisapride, cyclosporine, hydantoins, midazolam, phenytoin, rifabutin, sulfonylureas, terfenadine, triazolam, warfarin

Reactions

Skin

Acne
(1998): Drake L, *J Am Acad Dermatol* 38, S87
Angioedema
(1999): Errico MR, Buenos Aires, Argentina (from Internet) (observation)
(1991): Abbott M+, *Lancet* 2, 633
Bullous eruption
(1994): Gupta AK+, *J Am Acad Dermatol* 30, 911
Erythema multiforme
(1994): Gupta AK+, *J Am Acad Dermatol* 30, 911
(1991): Gussenhoven MJE+, *Lancet* 338, 120
Exanthems (1.8%) (in AIDS patients)
(1990): Grant SM+, *Drugs* 39, 877
Exfoliative dermatitis
(1994): Gupta AK+, *J Am Acad Dermatol* 30, 911 (passim)
(1990): Grant SM+, *Drugs* 39, 877
Fixed eruption
(2000): Heikkilä H+, *J Am Acad Dermatol* 42, 883
(1997): Jaffe P, Columbia, SC (from Internet) (observation)
(1997): Danby B, Kingston, Ontario (from Internet) (observation)
(1994): Morgan JM+, *BMJ* 308, 454
Pallor (<1%)
Petechiae
(1995): Mercurio MG+, *J Am Acad Dermatol* 32, 525
Pruritus
(1999): Errico MR, Buenos Aires, Argentina (from Internet) (observation)
(1991): Neuhaus G+, *BMJ* 302, 1341
Purpura
(1990): Agarwal A+, *Ann Intern Med* 113, 899
Rash (sic) (1.8%)
(1998): Scher RK+, *J Am Acad Dermatol* 38, S77
(1995): Powderly WG, *Infections in Medicine*, 257 (passim)
(1994): Gupta AK+, *J Am Acad Dermatol* 30, 911 (1.8%)
Skin hypertrophy (sic)
(1998): Drake L+, *J Am Acad Dermatol* 38, S87
Stevens–Johnson syndrome
(1995): Powderly WG, *Infections in Medicine*, 257 (passim)
(1991): Gussenhoven MJE+, *Lancet* 1, 120
(1990): Sugar AM+, *Rev Infect Dis* 12, S338
Toxic epidermal necrolysis
(1993): Azon-Masoliver A+, *Dermatology* 187, 268
(1990): Grant SM+, *Drugs* 39, 877
Urticaria

Hair

Hair – alopecia
(1996): Goldsmith LA, *Ann Intern Med* 125, 153
(1995): Pappas PG+, *Ann Intern Med* 123, 354
(1993): Weinroth SE+, *Ann Intern Med* 119, 637

Nails

Nail – disorder (sic)
(1998): Drake L,+ *J Am Acad Dermatol* 38, S87
(1998): Ling MR+, *J Am Acad Dermatol* 38, S95
Nail – melanonychia (longitudinal)
(1998): Kar HK, *Int J Dermatol* 37, 719

Other

Anaphylactoid reaction (in patients with AIDS)
Dysgeusia
(1998): Quart AM+, *Infect Med* 15, 379
(1991): Neuhaus G+, *BMJ* 302, 1341
Hypersensitivity (1–4%)
(1997): Craig TJ, *J Am Osteopath Assoc* 97, 584
Oral ulceration
(1998): Ling MR+, *J Am Acad Dermatol* 38, S95
(1991): Abbott M+, *Lancet* 2, 633
Paresthesias
(1991): Neuhaus G+, *BMJ* 302, 1341
Xerostomia
(1998): Quart AM+, *Infect Med* 15, 379

FLUCYTOSINE

Trade name: Ancobon (ICN)
Other common trade names: *5-FC; Alcobon; Ancotil*
Indications: Candidal and cryptococcal infections
Category: Antifungal
Half-life: 3–8 hours
Clinically important, potentially serious interactions with: amphotericin B, carbamazepine, clozapine, cytarabine, zidovudine

Reactions

Skin

Exanthems
(1987): Thyss A+, *Ann Dermatol Venereol* (French) 114, 1131
(1972): Editorial, *N Engl J Med* 286, 777
Parkinsonism (<1%)
Photosensitivity (<1%)
(1987): Thyss A+, *Ann Dermatol Venereol* (French) 114, 1131
(1983): Shelley WB+, *J Am Acad Dermatol* 8, 229
Pruritus
Purpura
Rash (sic) (1–10%)
Urticaria

Other

Anaphylactoid reaction (<1%)
Paresthesias (<1%)
Parkinsonism (<1%)
Xerostomia

FLUDARABINE

Trade name: Fludara (Berlex)
Indications: Chronic lymphocytic leukemia (B-cell)
Category: Purine nucleoside antineoplastic
Half-life: 9 hours
Clinically important, potentially serious interactions with: cytarabine, pentostatin

Reactions

Skin

Chills (>10%)
Edema (>10%)
Exanthems
Paraneoplastic pemphigus
(1995): Bazarbachi A+, *Ann Oncol* 6, 730
Rash (sic) (>10%)
Squamous cell carcinoma
(1997): Davidovitz Y+, *Acta Haematol* 98, 44 (flare-up)

Hair

Hair – alopecia (1–10%)

Other

Dysgeusia (<1%) (metallic taste)
Myalgia (>10%)
Paresthesias (>10%)
Stomatitis (>10%)

FLUMAZENIL

Trade name: Romazicon (Roche)
Other common trade names: *Anexate; Lanexat*
Indications: Benzodiazepine overdose
Category: Benzodiazepine antidote
Half-life: terminal: 41–79 minutes
Clinically important, potentially serious interactions with: cyclic antidepressants

Reactions

Skin

Diaphoresis (3–9%)
Hot flashes (1–10%)
Flushing (1–3%)
Rash (sic)
Urticaria (<1%)

Other

Hypesthesia
Injection-site pain (3–9%)
Injection-site reactions (sic)
Paresthesias (1–10%)
Thick tongue (sic) (<1%)
Thrombophlebitis
Tremor (1–10%)
Xerostomia (1–10%)

FLUOROURACIL

Trade names: Adrucil (Pharmacia & Upjohn); Efudex (ICN); Fluoroplex (Allergan)
Other common trade names: *Efudix; Efurix*
Category: Antineoplastic antimetabolite
Half-life: 8–20 minutes
Clinically important, potentially serious interactions with: aldesleukin, allopurinol, anticoagulants, cimetidine, methotrexate, metronidazole, thiazides

Reactions

Skin

Acral erythema
(1995): Esteve E+, *Ann Med Interne Paris* (French) 146, 192
(1989): Vukelja SJ+, *Ann Intern Med* 111, 688
Actinic keratosis inflammation (sic)
(1999): Nabai H+, *Cutis* 64, 43
(1969): Omura EF+, *JAMA* 208, 150
(1962): Falkson G+, *Br J Dermatol* 74, 229
Angioedema
Bullous eruption
(1970): Bart BJ+, *Arch Dermatol* 102, 457
Contact dermatitis
(1999): Sanchez-Perez J+, *Contact Dermatitis* 41, 106
(1997): Anderson LL+, *J Am Acad Dermatol* 36, 478
(1996): Nadal C+, *Contact Dermatitis* 35, 124 (systemic)
(1977): Goette DK+, *Arch Dermatol* 113, 1058
Dermatitis (sic) (>10%)
Eczematous eruption (sic)
(1977): Bernstein T, *New Engl J Med* 297, 337
Erythema
(1980): Hrushesky WJ, *Cutis* 26, 181
(1962): Falkson G+, *Br J Dermatol* 74, 229
Erythema multiforme
(1980): Ueki H+, *Hautarzt* (German) 31, 207
Erythematous eruption, linear serpentine (sic)
(1998): Pujol RM+, *J Am Acad Dermatol* 39, 839
Exanthems (1–10%)
(1994): Sollitto RB+, *Arch Dermatol* 130, 1194 (sun-exposed areas)
(1994): Leo S+, *J Chemother* 6, 423
Fissuring
Necrosis
(1980): Yaffee HS+, *Cutis* 25, 649 ("ecdysis")
Palmar-plantar erythrodysesthesia syndrome (hand-foot)
(1997): Thaler D, Monona, WI (from Internet) (observation)
(1997): Iurio A+, *Acta Oncol* 36, 653
(1997): Chiara S+, *Eur J Cancer* 33, 967
(1995): Banfield GK+, *J R Soc Med* 88, 356
(1994): Leo S+, *J Chemother* 6, 423
(1993): Beard JS+, *J Am Acad Dermatol* 29, 325
(1991): Jorda E+, *Int J Dermatol* 30, 653
(1989): Vukelja SJ+, *Ann Intern Med* 111, 688
(1989): Curran CF+, *Ann Intern Med* 111, 858
(1988): Guillaume J-C+, *Ann Dermatol Venereol* (French) 115, 1167
(1987): Molina R+, *Proc Am Soc Clin Oncol* 4, 92
(1985): Feldman LD+, *JAMA* 254, 3479
(1985): Atkins JN, *Ann Intern Med* 102, 419
(1984): Lokich JJ+, *Ann Intern Med* 101, 798
Pellagra
(1992): Breathnach SM+, *Adverse Drug Reactions and the Skin*, Blackwell, Oxford, 193 (passim)
Photosensitivity (<1%)
(1999): von Moos R+, *Schweiz Med Wochenschr* (German) 129, 52
(1992): Breathnach SM+, *Adverse Drug Reactions and the Skin*, Blackwell, Oxford, 193 (passim)
(1962): Falkson G+, *Br J Dermatol* 74, 229
Phototoxic reaction
Pigmentation (<1%)
(1997): Miller BH+, *J Am Acad Dermatol* 36, 72
(1995): Allen BJ+, *Int J Dermatol* 34, 219 (reticulate)
(1994): Leo S+, *J Chemother* 6, 423
(1991): Vukelja SJ+, *J Am Acad Dermatol* 25, 905 (serpentine)
(1980): Hrushesky WJ, *Cutis* 26, 181 (sun-exposed areas)
(1977): Goette DK+, *Arch Dermatol* 113, 1058
(1962): Falkson G+, *Br J Dermatol* 74, 229
Pruritus
Radiation recall
(1992): Breathnach SM+, *Adverse Drug Reactions and the Skin*, Blackwell, Oxford, 193 (passim)
Reactivation phenomenon (sic)
(1997): Anderson LL+, *J Am Acad Dermatol* 36, 478
(1993): Prussick R+, *Arch Dermatol* 129, 644
Seborrheic dermatitis
(1962): Falkson G+, *Br J Dermatol* 74, 229
Urticaria
Xerosis (1–10%)

Hair

Hair – alopecia (>10%)
(1992): Breathnach SM+, *Adverse Drug Reactions and the Skin*, Blackwell, Oxford, 193 (passim)
(1962): Falkson G+, *Br J Dermatol* 74, 229

Nails

Nails – onycholysis
Nails – pigmentation (<1%)
(1962): Falkson G+, *Br J Dermatol* 74, 229

Other

Anaphylactoid reaction
(1992): Breathnach SM+, *Adverse Drug Reactions and the Skin*, Blackwell, Oxford, 193 (passim)
Dysgeusia
Ectropion
(1997): Lewis JE, *Int J Dermatol* 36, 79

(1994): Hecker D+, *Cutis* 53, 137
Injection-site burning
(1998): Kraus S+, *J Am Acad Dermatol* 38, 438
(1997): Miller BH+, *J Am Acad Dermatol* 36, 72
Injection-site desquamation
(1998): Kraus S+, *J Am Acad Dermatol* 38, 438
(1997): Miller BH+, *J Am Acad Dermatol* 36, 72
(1997): Swinehart JM+, *Arch Dermatol* 133, 67
(1997): Miller BH+, *J Am Acad Dermatol* 36, 72
(1992): Breathnach SM+, *Adverse Drug Reactions and the Skin*, Blackwell, Oxford, 193 (passim)
Injection-site edema
(1997): Swinehart JM+, *Arch Dermatol* 133, 67
(1997): Miller BH+, *J Am Acad Dermatol* 36, 72
(1992): Breathnach SM+, *Adverse Drug Reactions and the Skin*, Blackwell, Oxford, 193 (passim)
Injection-site erythema
(1998): Kraus S+, *J Am Acad Dermatol* 38, 438
(1997): Swinehart JM+, *Arch Dermatol* 133, 67
(1997): Miller BH+, *J Am Acad Dermatol* 36, 72
(1992): Breathnach SM+, *Adverse Drug Reactions and the Skin*, Blackwell, Oxford, 193 (passim)
Injection-site necrosis
(1998): Kraus S+, *J Am Acad Dermatol* 38, 438
(1997): Swinehart JM+, *Arch Dermatol* 133, 67
Injection-site pain
(1998): Kraus S+, *J Am Acad Dermatol* 38, 438
(1997): Swinehart JM+, *Arch Dermatol* 133, 67
Injection-site ulceration
(1997): Swinehart JM+, *Arch Dermatol* 133, 67
(1997): Miller BH+, *J Am Acad Dermatol* 36, 72
Mucositis (1–10%)
Paresthesias (<1%)
Stomatitis (>10%)

FLUOXETINE

Trade name: Prozac (Dista)
Other common trade names: *Adofen; Apo-Fluoxetine; Dom-Fluoxetine; Fluctin; Fluctine; Fludac; Fluoxac; Fluoxeren; Fluxil; Fontex*
Indications: Depression, obsessive-compulsive disorder
Category: Selective serotonin reuptake inhibitor (SSRI); antidepressant and antiobsessional
Half-life: 2–3 days
Clinically important, potentially serious interactions with: alcohol, alprazolam, carbamazepine, cyproheptadine, diazepam, haloperidol, hydantoins, isocarboxazid, lithium, MAO inhibitors, metoprolol, phenelzine, phenothiazines, phenytoin, pimozide, selegiline, sotalol, terfenadine, tranylcypromine, trazodone, tricyclic antidepressants, tryptophan

Reactions

Skin

Acne (<1%)
Angioedema
(1991): Olfson M+, *J Nerv Mental Dis* 179, 504
Bruising
(1996): Pai VB+, *Ann Pharmacother* 30, 786
Bullous eruption (<1%)
Candidiasis
Cellulitis
Contact dermatitis (<1%)
Cutaneous reaction (sic)
(1998): Beauquier B+, *Encephale* (French) 24, 62
Diaphoresis (8.4%)
(1985): Wernicke JF, *J Clin Psychiatry* 46, 59
Eczema (sic) (<1%)
Erythema multiforme
(1985): Wernicke JF, *J Clin Psychiatry* 46, 59
Erythema nodosum (<1%)
Exanthems (4%)
(1993): Litt JZ, Beachwood, OH, personal case (observation)
(1993): Gupta MA+, *Cutis* 51, 386 (3%), passim
(1993): Gupta RK+, *Med J Aust* 158, 722
(1991): Olfson M+, *J Nerv Mental Dis* 159, 504
(1989): Miller LG+, *Am J Psychiatry* 146, 1616
(1988): Cooper GL, *Br J Psychiatry* 153, 77
(1985): Wernicke JF, *J Clin Psychiatry* 46, 59
Exfoliative dermatitis
Facial edema (<1%)
Flushing (<2%)
Furunculosis (<1%)
Herpes simplex (reactivation)
(1991): Reed SM+, *Am J Psychiatry* 148, 949
Herpes zoster
Hot flashes
Lichenoid eruption
Lupus erythematosus (discoid)
Mycosis fungoides (exacerbation)
(1996): Vermeer MH+, *J Am Acad Dermatol* 35, 635
Peripheral edema (<1%)
Petechiae (<1%)
Photosensitivity
(1998): Pazzagli L+, *Pharm World Sci* 20, 136 (along with alprazolam)
Phototoxic reaction (<1%)
(1995): O'Brien T, *Australas J Dermatology* 36, 103
(1995): Gaufberg E+, *J Clin Psychiatry* 56, 486
Pigmentation (<1%)
Pruritus (2.4%)
(1993): Gupta RK+, *Med J Aust* 158, 722
(1991): Olfson M+, *J Nerv Mental Dis* 159, 504
(1985): Wernicke JF, *J Clin Psychiatry* 46, 59
Pseudo-mycosis fungoides (sic)
(1996): Gordon KB+, *J Am Acad Dermatol* 34, 304
Psoriasis (<1%)
(1992): Hemlock C+, *Ann Pharmacother* 26, 211
Purpura (<1%)
Pustular eruption (<1%)
Rash (sic) (6%)
(1989): Miller LG+, *Am J Psychiatry* 146, 1616
(1987): Zerbe RL, *Int J Obes* 11 (Suppl 3), 191
(1985): Wernicke JF, *J Clin Psychiatry* 46, 59
Seborrhea (<1%)
Stevens–Johnson syndrome
(1998): N Z Medicines Adverse Reactions Committee, (from Internet) (observation)
(1992): Bodokh I+, *Therapie* (French) 47, 441
Subcutaneous nodule (sic)
Toxic epidermal necrolysis
(1992): Bodokh I+, *Therapie* (French) 47, 441
(1991): Rosenthal E+, *Presse Med* (French) 20, 1459
Ulcers (<1%)
Urticaria (4%)
(1994): Blumenthal HL, Beachwood, Ohio, personal case (observation)
(1993): Gupta RK+, *Med J Aust* 158, 722
(1992): Leznoff A+, *J Clin Psychopharmacol* 12, 355
(1991): Olfson M+, *J Nerv Mental Dis* 159, 504
(1989): Miller LG+, *Am J Psychiatry* 146, 1616
Vasculitis
(1999): Fisher A+, *Aust N Z J Med* 29, 375 (focal necrotizing)
(1995): Roger D+, *Dermatology* 191, 164
Xerosis

Hair

Hair – alopecia (<1%)
(1996): Bhatara VS+, *J Clin Psychiatry* 57, 227
(1995): Seifritz E+, *Can J Psychiatry* 40, 362
(1995): Shelley WB+, *Cutis* 55, 144 (observation)
(1994): Shelley WB+, *Cutis* 53, 282 (observation)
(1994): Mareth TR, *J Clin Psychiatry* 55, 163
(1993): Ogilvie AD, *Lancet* 342, 1423
(1991): Jenike MA, *Am J Psychiatry* 148, 392
(1991): Ananth J+, *J Psychiatry* 36, 621
(1991): Gupta S+, *Br J Psychiatry* 159, 737
Hair – hirsutism (<1%)

Other

Ageusia (<1%)
Anaphylactoid reaction (<1%)
Aphthous stomatitis (<1%)
Black tongue
(2000): Heymann WR, *Cutis* 66, 25
Dysgeusia (1.8%)
(2000): Heymann WR, *Cutis* 66, 25
Gingivitis (<1%)
Glossitis (<1%)
Glossodynia
(1994): Shelley WB+, *Cutis* 53, 242 (observation)
Gynecomastia (<1%)
Hyperesthesia (<1%)
Hypersensitivity
(1994): Beer K+, *Arch Dermatol* 130, 803
Hypesthesia (<1%)
Mastodynia (<1%)
Myalgia
Myopathy (<1%)
Oral ulceration (<1%)
Paresthesias
(1996): Bhatara VS+, *J Clin Psychiatry* 57, 227
Parosmia (<1%)
Priapism (<1%)
Pseudolymphoma
(1995): Magro CM+, *J Am Acad Dermatol* 32, 419
(1995): Crowson AN+, *Arch Dermatol* 131, 925
Serum sickness
(1991): Vincent A+, *Am J Psychiatry* 148, 1602
(1989): Miller LG+, *Am J Psychiatry* 146, 1616
Sialorrhea (<1%)
Stomatitis (<1%)
Thrombophlebitis (<1%)
Tongue edema (<1%)
Tongue pigmentation (<1%)
Tremor (2–10%)
Vaginal anesthesia
(1993): King VL+, *Am J Psychiatry* 150, 984
Xerostomia (12%)
(2000): Heymann WR, *Cutis* 66, 25
(1993): Beasley CM+, *Ann Clin Psychiatry* 5, 199
(1985): Wernicke JF, *J Clin Psychiatry* 46, 59

FLUOXYMESTERONE

Trade names: Android-F; Halotensin (Pharmacia & Upjohn)
Other common trade names: *Stenox; Vewon*
Indications: Breast carcinoma, hypogonadism, anemia
Category: Androgen; antineoplastic; antianemic
Half-life: 9.2 hours
Clinically important, potentially serious interactions with: alcohol, anticoagulants, cyclosporine, insulin

Reactions

Skin

Acne (>10%)
(1992): Fryand O+, *Acta Derm Venereol* 72, 148
(1990): Fuchs E+, *J Am Acad Dermatol* 23, 125
(1989): Hartmann AA+, *Monatsschr Kinderheilkd* (German) 137, 466
(1989): Fryand O+, *Tidsskr Nor Laegeforen* (Norwegian) 109, 239
(1989): von Muhlendahl KE+, *Dtsch Med Wochenschr* (German) 114, 712
(1989): Heydenreich G, *Arch Dermatol* 125, 571 (fulminans)
(1989): Scott MJ+, *Cutis* 44, 30
(1988): Traupe H+, *Arch Dermatol* 124, 414 (fulminans)
(1987): Kiraly CL+, *Am J Dermatopathol* 9, 515
(1984): Lamb DR, *Am J Sports Med* 12, 31
(1965): Rook A, *Br J Dermatol* 77, 115
(1965): Kennedy BJ, *J Am Geriatr Soc* 13, 230
Contact dermatitis
(1989): Holdiness MR, *Contact Dermatitis* 20, 3 (from patch)
Edema (>10%)
Exanthems
Flushing (1–5%)
(1965): Kennedy BJ, *J Am Geriatr Soc* 13, 230
Furunculosis
(1989): Scott MJ+, *Cutis* 44, 30
Lichenoid eruption
(1989): Aihara M+, *J Dermatol* (Tokio) 16, 330
Lupus erythematosus
(1978): Robinson HM, *Z Haut* (German) 53, 349
Pruritus
Psoriasis
(1990): O'Driscoll JB+, *Clin Exp Dermatol* 15, 68
Purpura
Seborrhea (sic)
Seborrheic dermatitis
(1989): Scott MJ+, *Cutis* 44, 30
Striae
(1989): Scott MJ+, *Cutis* 44, 30
Urticaria

Hair

Hair – alopecia
(1989): Scott MJ+, *Cutis* 44, 30
(1965): Kennedy BJ, *J Am Geriatr Soc* 13, 230
Hair – hirsutism (1–10%)
(1994): Castillo-Ceballos A+, *Med Clin (Barc)* (Spanish) 102, 78
(1991): Bates GW+, *Clin Obstet Gynecol* 34, 848
(1991): No Author, *Obstet Gynecol* 78, 474
(1991): Parker LU+, *Cleve Clin J Med* 58, 43
(1991): Urman B+, *Obstet Gynecol* 77, 595
(1989): Scott MJ+, *Cutis* 44, 30
(1974): Baron J, *Zentralbl Gynakol* (German) 96, 129
(1971): Fusi S+, *Folia Endocrinol* (Italian) 24, 412
(1965): Kennedy BJ, *J Am Geriatr Soc* 13, 230

Other

Anaphylactoid reaction
Gynecomastia (<1%)
Hypersensitivity (<1%)
Injection-site pain
Mastodynia (>10%)
Paresthesias
Priapism (>10%)
Stomatitis

FLUPHENAZINE

Trade names: Permitil (Schering); Prolixin (Bristol-Myers Squibb)
Other common trade names: *Anatensol; Apo-Fluphenazine; Dapatum D25; Dapotum D; Fludecate; Modecate; Moditen*
Indications: Psychoses
Category: Phenothiazine antipsychotic
Half-life: 84–96 hours
Clinically important, potentially serious interactions with: ACE-inhibitors, alcohol, anticholinergics, barbiturates, beta-blockers, CNS depressants, levodopa, lithium, meperidine, piperazine, propranolol, trazodone, tricyclic antidepressants, valproic acid

Reactions

Skin

Angioedema (<1%)
Contact dermatitis
Dermatitis (sic)
Diaphoresis
Eczema (sic)
Edema
Erythema
Exanthems
Exfoliative dermatitis
Hypohidrosis (>10%)

Lupus erythematosus
(1975): Gallien M+, *Ann Med Psychol* (Paris) (French) 1, 237
Parkinsonism
Peripheral edema
Photosensitivity
Pigmentation (<1%) (blue-gray)
(1987): Krebs A, *Schweiz Rundsch Med Prax* (German) 76, 1069
Pruritus (<1%)
Purpura
Rash (sic) (1–10%)
Seborrhea
Toxic epidermal necrolysis
(1972): Carli-Basset C+, *Sem Hôp* (French) 48, 497
Urticaria
Vitiligo
(1987): Krebs A, *Schweiz Rundsch Med Prax* (German) 76, 1069
(1985): Rampertaap MP, *Mo Med* 82, 24
Xerosis

Other

Anaphylactoid reaction
Galactorrhea (1–10%)
Gynecomastia (1–10%)
Injection-site reaction
Mastodynia (1–10%)
Priapism (<1%)
(1986): Fishbain DA, *Psychosomatics* 27, 538
(1985): Fishbain DA, *Ann Emerg Med* 14, 600
Sialorrhea
(1973): Johnson DAW, *Br J Psychiatry* 123, 519
Trembling (fingers) (sic)
Xerostomia (<1%)

FLURAZEPAM

Trade name: Flurazepam
Other common trade names: *Apo-Flurazepam; Benozil; Dalmadorm; Flunox; Nergart; Novoflupam; Somnol; Som Pam; Valdorm*
Indications: Insomnia
Category: Benzodiazepine hypnotic-sedative
Half-life: 40–114 hours
Clinically important, potentially serious interactions with: alcohol, CNS depressants, carbamazepine, cimetidine, clarithromycin, diltiazem, fluconazole, isoniazid, itraconazole, ketoconazole, miconazole, omeprazole, phenytoin, rifabutin, rifampin, theophylline, valproic acid, verapamil

Reactions

Skin

Dermatitis (sic) (1–10%)
Diaphoresis (>10%)
Exanthems
(1976): Arndt KA+, *JAMA* 235, 918 (0.05%)
Flushing
Pruritus
Purpura
Rash (sic) (>10%)
Urticaria

Other

Acute intermittent porphyria
Dysgeusia (3.4%) (metallic taste)
(1984): Greenblatt DJ+, *J Clin Psychiatry* 45, 192 (3%)
Oral mucosal lesions
(1984): Greenblatt DJ+, *J Clin Psychiatry* 45, 192 (3%)
Paresthesias
Sialopenia (>10%)
Sialorrhea (1–10%)
Xerostomia (>10%)

FLURBIPROFEN

Trade name: Ansaid (Pharmacia & Upjohn)
Other common trade names: *Apo-Flurbiprofen; Cebutid; Flurofen; Flurozin; Froben; Lapole; Nu-Flurprofen*
Indications: Arthritis
Category: Nonsteroidal anti-inflammatory (NSAID)
Half-life: 3–4 hours
Clinically important, potentially serious interactions with: aminoglycosides, anticoagulants, beta-blockers, cyclosporine, heparin, lithium, loop diuretics, methotrexate, probenecid, salicylates, warfarin

Reactions

Skin

Angioedema (<1%)
(1997): Romano A+, *J Intern Med* 241, 81
Burning (ophthalmic)
Contact dermatitis
(2000): Kawada A+, *Contact Dermatitis* 42, 167
Cutaneous side effects (sic) (6%)
(1986): Buson M, *J Int Med Res* 14, 1
(1977): Sheldrake FE+, *Curr Med Res Opin* 5, 106
Dermatitis herpetiformis
(1994): Tousignant J+, *Int J Dermatol* 33, 199
Diaphoresis
Discoloration (sic)
Eczema (sic) (3–9%)
Edema (3–9%)
Erythema multiforme (<1%)
Exanthems
(1997): Romano A+, *J Intern Med* 241, 81
(1977): Cardoe N, *Curr Med Res Opin* 5, 99
(1974): Calin A+, *BMJ* 4, 496 (3%)
Exfoliative dermatitis (<1%)
Fixed eruption
(1993): *Dermatology* 186, 164
Flushing
Furunculosis
Herpes simplex
Herpes zoster
Hot flashes (<1%)
Peripheral edema
Photosensitivity (<1%)
Pruritus (1–5%)
(1977): Cardoe N, *Curr Med Res Opin* 5, 99
Pseudoreactions (sic)
(1991): VanArsdel PP, *JAMA* 266, 3343
Purpura
Rash (sic) (1–3%)
Seborrhea
Stevens–Johnson syndrome (<1%)
Stinging (ophthalmic)
Toxic epidermal necrolysis (<1%)
(1987): Gillaume JC+, *Arch Dermatol* 123, 1166
Ulceration
Urticaria (<1%)
Vasculitis
(1990): Wei M, *Ann Intern Med* 112, 550
Xerosis

Hair

Hair – alopecia (<1%)

Nails

Nails – disorder (sic) (<1%)
Nails – pigmentation

Other

Anaphylactoid reaction (<1%)
Aphthous stomatitis
Dysgeusia (<1%)

Hypersensitivity
(1997): Romano A+, *J Intern Med* 241, 81
Oral lichenoid eruption
(1983): Hamburger J+, *BMJ* 287, 1258
Paresthesias (<1%)
Parosmia (<1%)
Stomatitis
Vulvovaginitis
Xerostomia (<1%)

FLUTAMIDE

Trade name: Eulexin (Schering)
Other common trade names: *Drogenil; Euflex; Eulexine; Flucinom; Fluken; Flulem; Fugerel; Novo-Flutamide*
Indications: Metastatic prostate carcinoma
Category: Antineoplastic (prostate carcinoma); antiandrogen
Half-life: 6 hours
Clinically important, potentially serious interactions with: warfarin

Reactions

Skin
Bullous eruption
Diaphoresis
(1992): Schmeller N, *Internist Berl* (German) 33, 284
Edema (4%)
Erythema
Exanthems
(1999): Fisher BJ, Toronto, Ontario (from Internet) (observation) (generalized)
(1989): Brogden RN+, *Drugs* 38, 185
Flu-like syndrome (sic) (<1%)
Hot flashes (61%)
Lupus erythematosus
(1998): Reid MB+, *J Urol* 159, 2098
Photosensitivity
(1999): Tsien C+, *J Urol* 162, 494
(1998): Vilaplana J+, *Contact Dermatitis* 38, 68
(1998): Yokote R+, *Eur J Dermatol* 8, 427
(1996): Fujimoto M+, *Br J Dermatol* 135, 496
(1991): Moraillon I+, *Photodermatol Photoimmunol Photomed* 8, 264
Rash (sic) (3%)
Toxic epidermal necrolysis
Urticaria

Other
Gynecomastia (9%)
(1997): Staiman VR+, *Urology* 50, 929
(1993): Aso Y+, *Hinyokika Kiyo* (Japanese) 39, 391
Injection-site irritation (3%)
Paresthesias (1–10%)
Pseudoporphyria
(1999): Mantoux F+, *Ann Dermatol Venereol* (French) 126, 150
(1999): Schmutz JL+, *Ann Dermatol Venereol* (French) 126, 374
(1998): Borroni G+, *Br J Dermatol* 138, 711

FLUVASTATIN

Trade name: Lescol (Novartis)
Other common trade names: *Cranoc; Locol*
Indications: Hypercholesterolemia
Category: Antihyperlipidemic; HMG-CoA reductase inhibitor
Half-life: 1.2 hours
Clinically important, potentially serious interactions with: anticoagulants, cimetidine, clofibrate, cyclosporine, digoxin, erythromycin, fenofibrate, gemfibrozil, niacin, omeprazole, ranitidine, rifampin, ritonavir, warfarin

Reactions

Skin
Allergic reactions (sic) (2.6%)
Angioedema
Discoloration (sic)
Erythema multiforme
Flu-like syndrome (sic)
Flushing
Lupus erythematosus
(1998): Sridhar MK+, *Lancet* 352, 114 (fatal)
Photosensitivity
Pruritus
Purpura
Rash (sic) (2.7%)
(1998): N Z Medicines Adverse Reactions Committee, (from Internet) (observation) (2 patients)
Stevens–Johnson syndrome
Toxic epidermal necrolysis
Upper respiratory infection (16%)
Urticaria
Vasculitis
Xerosis

Hair
Hair – alopecia
Hair – changes (sic)

Nails
Nails – changes (sic)

Other
Anaphylactoid reaction
Dysgeusia
Gynecomastia
Myalgia (5–6%)
Paresthesias

FLUVOXAMINE

Trade name: Luvox (Solvay)
Other common trade names: *Apo-Fluvoxamine; Dumirox; Dumyrox; Faverin; Favoxil; Fevarin; Maveral*
Indications: Obsessive-compulsive disorder, depression
Category: Selective serotonin reuptake inhibitor (SSRI); antidepressant
Half-life: 15 hours
Clinically important, potentially serious interactions with: alprazolam, anticoagulants, astemizole, beta-blockers, buspirone, carbamazepine, cimetidine, clozapine, diazepam, diltiazem, lithium, MAO inhibitors, methadone, metoprolol, phenytoin, tacrine, tacrolimus, terfenadine, theophylline, trazodone, triazolam, tricyclic antidepressants

Reactions

Skin
Acne (<1%)
Allergic reactions (sic) (<1%)

Angioedema
(1993): No Author, *Lakartidningen* (Swedish) 90, 54
Bullous eruption
Cutaneous reaction (sic)
(1998): Beauquier B+, *Encephale* (French) 24, 62
Dermatitis (sic) (<1%)
Diaphoresis (7%)
(1986): Benfield P+, *Drugs* 32, 313 (5%)
Ecchymoses (<1%)
Edema (<1%)
Exanthems
Exfoliative dermatitis (<1%)
Furunculosis (<1%)
Photosensitivity (<1%)
(1996): Gillet-Terver MN+, *Australas J Dermatol* 37, 62
(1993): *Lakartidningen* (Swedish) 90, 54
Pigmentation (<1%)
Pruritus
Purpura (<1%)
Rash (sic)
Seborrhea (<1%)
Stevens–Johnson syndrome
Toxic epidermal necrolysis (<1%)
(1993): Wolkenstein P+, *Lancet* 342, 304
Urticaria (<1%)
Xerosis (<1%)

Hair

Hair – alopecia (<1%)
Hair – alopecia areata
(1996): Parameshwar E, *Am J Psychiatry* 153, 581

Other

Ageusia (<1%)
Anaphylactoid reaction
Dysgeusia (3%)
Gingivitis (<1%)
Glossitis (<1%)
Mastodynia (<1%)
Myalgia
Myopathy (<1%)
Oral mucosal lesions
(1986): Benfield P+, *Drugs* 32, 313 (10%)
Paresthesias
Parosmia (<1%)
Priapism
Sialorrhea
Stomatitis (<1%)
Vaginitis (<1%)
Xerostomia (14%)
(1986): Benfield P+, *Drugs* 32, 313 (10%)

FOLIC ACID

Synonyms: folacin; folate; vitamin B_9
Trade name: Folvite (Lederle)
Other common trade names: *Acfol; Apo-Folic; Dalisol; Flodine; Folacin; Folina; Folinsyre; Folitab; Folsan; Lexpec*
Indications: Anemias
Category: Nutritional supplement; water-soluble vitamin
Half-life: no data
Clinically important, potentially serious interactions with: methotrexate, phenytoin, pyrimethamine, triamterene, trimethoprim

Reactions

Skin

Acne
(1964): Fegeler F, *Arch Klin Exp Dermatol* (German) 219, 335
Allergic reactions (sic) (<1%)
Dermatitis (sic)
(1966): Pedersen JT, *Ugeskr Laeger* (Danish) 128, 708
Erythema
(1966): Pedersen JT, *Ugeskr Laeger* (Danish) 128, 708
Exanthems
(1985): Sparling R+, *Clin Lab Haematol* 7, 184
(1964): Fegeler F, *Arch Klin Exp Dermatol* (German) 219, 335
Flushing (<1%)
Pruritus (<1%)
(1966): Pedersen JT, *Ugeskr Laeger* (Danish) 128, 708
(1966): Mathur BP, *Indian J Med Sci* 20, 133
Rash (sic) (<1%)
Urticaria
(1985): Sparling R+, *Clin Lab Haematol* 7, 184

Other

Anaphylactoid reaction
(1966): Woodliff HJ, *Med J Aust* 53, 351

FOSCARNET

Trade name: Foscavir (AstraZeneca)
Other common trade name: *Foscovir*
Indications: Cytomegalovirus retinitis in patients with AIDS
Category: Antiviral; inhibits various viral DNA and RNA polymerases
Half-life: ~3 hours
Clinically important, potentially serious interactions with: aminoglycosides, amphotericin B, ciprofloxacin, cisplatin, cyclosporine, gold, lithium, pentamidine, quinolones, rifampin, vancomycin, zidovudine

Reactions

Skin

Acne
Dermatitis (sic) (<1%)
Diaphoresis (>5%)
Edema (<1%)
Exanthems (>5%)
(1990): Green ST, *J Infection* 21, 227
Facial edema (>5%)
Fixed eruption
(1990): Connolly GM+, *Genitourin Med* 66, 97
Flushing (1–5%)
Herpes simplex (<1%)
Leg edema (<1%)
Penile ulcers
(1997): English JC+, *J Am Acad Dermatol* 37, 1
(1996): Agcaoili DJ+, *Infect Med* 13, 35
(1996): Papini M+, *Ann Dermatol Venereol* (French) 123, 679
(1995): Fitzgerald E+, *Arch Dermatol* 131, 1447
(1993): Schiff TA+, *Int J Dermatol* 32, 526
(1993): Brockmeyer NH+, *Int J Clin Pharmacol Ther Toxicol* 31, 204
(1993): Moyle G+, *AIDS* 7, 140
(1993): Gross AS+, *Clin Infect Dis* 17, 1076
(1993): Bodian AB, *Int J Dermatol* 32, 526
(1992): Katlama C+, *J Acquir Immune Defic Syndr* 5 (Suppl 1), S18
(1992): Evans LM+, *J Am Acad Dermatol* 27, 124
(1991): Chrisp P+, *Drugs* 41, 104
(1990): Lernestedt J-O+, *Lancet* 335, 548
(1990): Moyle G+, *Lancet* 335, 547 (4.7%)
(1990): Fégueux S+, *Lancet* 335, 547
(1990): Gilquin J+, *Lancet* 335, 287
(1990): Van Der Pijl JW+, *Lancet* 335, 286 (30%)
Periorbital edema
Peripheral edema (<1%)
Pigmentation (>5%)
Pruritus (>5%)
Pruritus ani (<1%)
Psoriasis (<1%)
Rash (sic) (generalized) (>5%)
(1991): Blanshard C, *J Infect* 23, 336
(1990): Green ST+, *J Infect* 21, 227
Seborrhea (>5%)

Toxic epidermal necrolysis
(1999): Wharton JR+, *Cutis* 63, 333
(1997): Lauglin CL, Little Rock, Arkansas, American Academy of Dermatology Meeting (SF), Gross and Microscopic
Ulceration (>5%)
Urticaria (<1%)
Vulvar ulceration
(1993): Caumes E+, *J Am Acad Dermatol* 28, 799 (erosion)
(1992): Lacey HB+, *Genitourin Med* 68, 182
Warts (<1%)
Xerosis (<1%)

Hair

Hair – alopecia (<1%)

Other

Dysgeusia (>5%)
Hyperesthesia (<1%)
Hypesthesia
Gynecomastia (<1%)
Injection-site pain (1–10%)
Injection-site thrombophlebitis
(1991): Chrisp P+, *Drugs* 41, 104
Myalgia (>5%)
Oral leukoplakia
Oral ulceration
(1990): Gilquin J+, *Lancet* 335, 287
(1990): Fégueux S+, *Lancet* 335, 547
(1990): Moyle G+, *Lancet* 335, 547
Paresthesias (1–10%)
(1990): Safrin S+, *J Infect Dis* 161, 1078
Stomatitis (<1%)
Thrombophlebitis (<1%)
Tongue ulceration (<1%)
Ulcerative stomatitis (>5%)
Xerostomia

FOSFOMYCIN

Trade name: Monurol (Forest)
Indications: Urinary tract infections
Category: Antibiotic (acute cystitis)
Half-life: 3–9 hours
Clinically important, potentially serious interactions with: metoclopramide, **food**

Reactions

Skin

Angioedema
Exanthems (<1%)
Pruritus (<1%)
Rash (sic) (1.4%)

Other

Anaphylactoid reaction
(1998): Rosales MJ+, *Allergy* 53, 905
Myalgia (<1%)
Paresthesias (<1%)
Vaginitis (7.6%)
Xerostomia (<1%)

FOSINOPRIL

Trade name: Monopril (Bristol-Myers Squibb)
Other common trade names: *Acenor-M; Dynacil; Fosinorm; Fozitec; Staril; Vasopril*
Indications: Hypertension
Category: Angiotensin-converting enzyme (ACE) inhibitor; antihypertensive
Half-life: 11.5 hours
Clinically important, potentially serious interactions with: alcohol, allopurinol, amiloride, bumetanide, digoxin, diuretics, furosemide, indomethacin, insulin, lithium, mercaptopurine, NSAIDs, phenothiazines, salicylates, spironolactone, torsemide

Reactions

Skin

Angioedema (<1%)
(1997): Graumuller S+, *HNO* (German) 45, 1016
Bullous pemphigoid
Diaphoresis (<1%)
Edema (<1%)
Eosinophilic vasculitis
Exfoliative dermatitis
Flu-like syndrome (sic) (<1%)
Flushing
Photosensitivity (<1%)
Pruritus (<1%)
Rash (sic) (<1%)
(1990): Pool JL, *Clin Ther* 12, 520 (0.9%)
Scleroderma
Urticaria (<1%)
Vasculitis

Other

Ageusia (<1%)
Anaphylactoid reaction
Dysgeusia (<1%)
(1992): Murdoch D+, *Drugs* 43, 123
Gynecomastia
Myalgia (<1%)
Paresthesias (<1%)
Tremor (<1%)
Xerostomia (<1%)

FOSPHENYTOIN

Trade name: Cerebyx (Parke-Davis)
Indications: Seizure prophylaxis, status epilepticus
Category: Anticonvulsant
Half-life: 15 minutes
Clinically important, potentially serious interactions with: alcohol, amiodarone, barbiturates, benzodiazepines, carbamazepine, chloramphenicol, cimetidine, CNS depressants, disulfiram, fluconazole, fluoxetine, isoniazid, sulfonamides, valproic acid

Fosphenytoin is a prodrug of phenytoin

Reactions

Skin

Acne (<1%)
Bullous eruption
Chills (sic)
Ecchymoses
Erythema multiforme (<1%)
Exanthems
Exfoliative dermatitis (<1%)
Facial edema
Lupus erythematosus

Pruritus (48.9%)
(1998): Knapp LE+, *J Child Neurol* 13, S15
(1998): Luer MS, *Neurol Res* 20, 178
Rash (sic) (<1%)
Stevens–Johnson syndrome
Toxic epidermal necrolysis

Other

Dysgeusia (3.3%)
Gingival hyperplasia
Hyperesthesia (2.2%)
Hypesthesia
Injection-site pain
Paresthesias (4.4%)
(1998): Luer MS, *Neurol Res* 20, 178
Tongue disorder (sic)
Xerostomia (4.4%)

FURAZOLIDONE

Trade name: Furoxone (Roberts)
Other common trade names: *Furion; Furoxona; Fuxol*
Indications: Various infections caused by susceptible organisms
Category: Nitrofuran antibiotic; antidiarrheal; antiprotozoal
Half-life: no data
Clinically important, potentially serious interactions with: alcohol, anorexiants, antidepressants, dextromethorphan, dopamine, ephedrine, epinephrine, fluoxetine, MAO inhibitors, meperidine, paroxetine, phenylephrine, sertraline, sympathomimetics, trazodone, **tyramine-containing foods***

Reactions

Skin

Contact dermatitis
(1990): de Groot AC+, *Contact Dermatitis* 22, 202
(1980): Goette DK+, *Cutis* 26, 406
(1978): Novak M, *Cesk Dermatol* (Czech) 53, 128
(1974): Bleumink E+, *Hautarzt* (German) 25, 403
Disulfiram-like reaction (with alcohol)(<1%)**
Erythema multiforme
(1986): Fisher AA, *Cutis* 37, 158
(1980): Goette DK+, *Cutis* 26, 406
Exanthems (<1%)
Flushing (with alcohol) (<1%)
Photosensitivity
(1980): Goette DK+, *Cutis* 26, 406
Pruritus
Pruritus ani
Rash (sic) (<1%)
Urticaria (<1%)
(1969): Aaronson CM, *JAMA* 210, 557

Other

Serum sickness
(1978): Wolfe MS+, *Am J Trop Med Hyg* 27, 762

***Note:** Tyramine-containing foods include the following: aged cheeses, avocados, banana skins, bologna and other processed luncheon meats, chicken livers, chocolate, figs, canned pickled herring, meat extracts, pepperoni, raisins, raspberries, soy sauce, vermouth, sherry and red wines

****Note:** The disulfiram-like reaction consists of facial flushing, diaphoresis, tachycardia, and pounding headache

FUROSEMIDE

Trade name: Lasix (Aventis)
Other common trade names: *Apo-Furosemide; Discoid; Dryptal; Edenol; Frusid; Furorese; Furoside; Fusid; Henexal; Lasilix; Novo-Semide; Urex; Uritol*
Indications: Edema
Category: Sulfonamide* loop diuretic; antihypertensive
Half-life: 0.5–1 hour
Clinically important, potentially serious interactions with: ACE-inhibitors, aminoglycoside amphotericin, antibiotics, anticoagulants, cisplatin, clofibrate, digoxin, gatifloxacin, lithium, metformin, moxifloxacin, NSAIDs, phenytoin, salicylates, sparfloxacin, succinylcholine, thiazides

Reactions

Skin

Acute febrile neutrophilic dermatosis (Sweet's syndrome)
(1989): Cobb MW, *J Amer Acad Dermatol* 21, 339
Acute generalized exanthematous pustulosis (AGEP)
(1995): Moreau A+, *Int J Dermatol* 34, 263 (passim)
Bullous eruption (<1%)
(1995): Tamimi NA+, *Nephrol Dial Transplant* 10, 1943
(1993): Landor M+, *Ann Allergy* 70, 196
(1992): Van Olden RW+, *Am J Nephrol* 12, 351 (photosensitive)
(1989): Sfar Z+, *Tunis Med* (French) 67, 805
(1985): Anderson CD+, *Photodermatol* 2, 111
(1982): Hallan H+, *Tidsskr Nor Laegeforen* (Norwegian) 102, 630
(1980): Rees RB+, *J Am Acad Dermatol* 2, 244
(1980): Guin JD, *Cutis* 25, 534
(1977): Heydenreich G+, *Ugeskr Laeger* (Danish) 139, 1847
(1977): Hertzenberg S, *Tidsskr Nor Laegeforen* (Norwegian) 97, 792
(1977): Heydenreich G+, *Acta Med Scand* 202, 61
(1976): Keczkes K+, *BMJ* 2, 236
(1976): Gilchrist B+, *Ann Intern Med* 84, 494
(1976): Burry JN+ *Ann Intern Med* 84, 493
(1976): Coles GA+, *BMJ* 2, 525
(1975): Gilchrist B+, *Ann Intern Med* 83, 480
(1969): Ebringer A+, *Med J Aust* 1, 768
Bullous pemphigoid
(1997): Panayiotou BN+, *Br J Clin Pract* 51, 49 (2 patients)
(1996): Koch CA+, *Cutis* 58, 340
(1995): Siddiqui MA+, *J Am Geriatr Soc* 43, 1183
(1991): Shelley WB+, *Cutis* 48, 367 (passim)
(1986): Ingber A+, *Z Hautarzt* (German)
(1984): Halevy S+, *Harefuah* (Hebrew) 106, 125
(1981): Castel T, *Clin Exp Dermatol* 6, 635
(1980): Neufeld R+, *Cutis* 26, 290
(1976): Fellner J+, *Arch Dermatol* 112, 75
Cutaneous side effects (sic)
(1986): Bigby M+, *JAMA* 256, 3358 (0.05%)
(1976): Arndt KA+, *JAMA* 235, 918 (0.26%)
Diaphoresis
Epidermolysis bullosa
(1976): Kennedy AC, *Br J Dermatol* 94, 495
(1976): Kennedy AC+, *BMJ* 1, 1509
Erythema multiforme (<1%)
(1980): Zugerman C, *Arch Dermatol* 116, 518
(1970): Gibson TP+, *JAMA* 212, 1709
(1969): Ebringer A+, *Med J Aust* 1, 768
Erythema nodosum
(1975): Dargie HJ+, *Meyler's Side Effects of Drugs*, Vol 8, Amsterdam, Excerpta Medica, 483
Exanthems
(1999): Litt JZ, Beachwood, OH, personal case (observation)
(1988): Lin RY, *N Y State J Med* 88, 439
(1979): Naranjo CA+, *Clin Pharmacol Ther* 25, 154 (0.6%)
(1979): Lowe J+, *BMJ* 2, 360 (0.2%)
(1978): Bjoerndal N+, *Ugeskr Laeger* (Danish) 140, 1084
(1977): Greenblatt DJ+, *Am Heart J* 94, 6 (0.2%)
(1970): Gibson TP+, *JAMA* 212, 1709
(1966): Sherlock S+, *Lancet* 1, 1049 (12%)
Exfoliative dermatitis
(1992): Breathnach SM+, *Adverse Drug Reactions and the Skin*, Blackwell, Oxford, 230 (passim)
(1978): Bjoerndal N+, *Ugeskr Laeger* (Danish) 140, 1084

(1975): Dargie HJ+, *Meyler's Side Effects of Drugs*, Vol 8, Amsterdam, Excerpta Medica, 483

Flushing
(1977): Greenblatt DJ+, *Am Heart J* 94, 6

Grinspan's syndrome**
(1990): Lamey PJ+, *Oral Surg Oral Med Oral Path* 70, 184

Lichenoid eruption
(1990): West AJ+, *J Am Acad Dermatol* 23, 689
(1981): Ota J+, *Skin Res* (Japanese) 23, 639

Linear IgA bullous dermatosis
(1999): Cerottini J-P+, *J Am Acad Dermatol* 41, 103

Lupus erythematosus
(1988): Lin RY, *N Y State J Med* 88, 439

Periorbital edema
(1987): Hansbrough JR+, *J Allergy Clin Immunol* 80, 538

Photosensitivity (1–10%)
(1989): Cobb MW, *J Amer Acad Dermatol* 21, 339
(1977): Heydenreich G+, *Acta Med Scand* 202, 61

Phototoxic reaction
(1998): Vargas F+, *J Photochem Photobiol B* 42, 219
(1976): Burry JN, *Br J Dermatol* 94, 495
(1976): Burry JN+ *Ann Intern Med* 84, 493

Porokeratosis (disseminated superficial)
(2000): Kroiss MM+, *Acta Derm Venereol* 80, 52

Pruritus (<1%)
(1993): Litt JZ, Beachwood, OH, personal case (observation)
(1987): Hansbrough JR+, *J Allergy Clin Immunol* 80, 538
(1978): Sibbald RG+, *Can Med Assoc J* 118, 142

Purpura
(1989): Nishioka K+, *J Dermatol* 16, 220 (pigmented)
(1983): Michel M+, *Rev Geriat* (French) 8/10. 505
(1969): Ebringer A+, *Med J Aust* 1, 768

Pustular eruption
(1990): Mothiron C+, *Presse Med* (French) 19, 1504
(1989): Cobb MW, *J Am Acad Dermatol* 21, 339
(1973): Macmillan AL, *Dermatologica* 146, 285

Rash (sic) (<1%)

Stevens–Johnson syndrome
(1991): Chan JC+, *Drug Saf* 6, 230
(1978): Ward B+, *Am J Ophthalmol* 86, 133

Urticaria
(1987): Hansbrough JR+, *J Allergy Clin Immunol* 80, 538
(1967): Milla Santos J, *Summa Med* (Spanish) 10, 3
(1966): Atkins LL, *Geriatrics* 21, 143

Vasculitis
(1990): Bourgain C+, *Presse Med* (French) 19, 1504
(1989): Cobb MW, *J Amer Acad Dermatol* 21, 339
(1988): Lin RY, *N Y State J Med* 88, 439
(1982): de la Chapelle C+, *LARC Med* (French) 2, 760
(1978): Sibbald RG+, *Can Med Assoc J* 118, 142
(1977): Hendricks WM+, *Arch Dermatol* 113, 375 (necrotizing)
(1971): Pathy MS, *Gerontol Clin* 13, 261

Other

Acute intermittent porphyria

Anaphylactoid reaction
(1987): Hansbrough JR+, *J Allergy Clin Immunol* 80, 538

Injection-site erythema (<1%)

Injection-site pain

Paresthesias

Porphyria
(1984): Harber LC+, *J Invest Dermatol* 82, 207

Porphyria cutanea tarda
(1992): Shelley WB+, *Advanced Dermatologic Diagnosis*, WB Saunders, 414 (passim)
(1983): Goldsman CI+, *Cleve Clin Q* 50, 151
(1977): Rufli T+, *Schweiz Med Wochenschr* (German) 107, 1093

Pseudolymphoma
(1995): Magro CM+, *J Am Acad Dermatol* 32, 419

Pseudoporphyria cutanea tarda
(1998): Breier F+, *Dermatology* 197, 271

Thrombophlebitis

Ulcerative stomatitis
(1988): Lin RY, *N Y State J Med* 88, 439

Xanthopsia

Xerostomia
(1967): Milla Santos J, *Summa Med* (Spanish) 10, 3

***Note:** Furosemide is a sulfonamide and can be absorbed systemically. Sulfonamides can produce severe, possibly fatal, reactions such as toxic epidermal necrolysis and Stevens–Johnson syndrome.

****Note:** Grinspan's syndrome is the triad of oral lichen planus, diabetes mellitus, and hypertension

GABAPENTIN

Trade name: Neurontin (Parke-Davis)
Indications: Seizures
Category: Anticonvulsant
Half-life: 5–6 hours
Clinically important, potentially serious interactions with: cimetidine

Reactions

Skin

Acne (>1%)
Acute febrile neutrophilic dermatosis (Sweet's syndrome)
(1999): Smith W, (from Internet) (observation)
Exanthems
Facial edema (<1%)
Peripheral edema (1.7%)
(1998): Rowbotham M+, *JAMA* 280, 1837
Pruritus (1.3%)
Purpura (<1%)
Rash (sic) (>1%)
Stevens–Johnson syndrome
(1998): Gonzalez-Sicilia L+, *Am J Med* 105, 455
Urticaria

Hair

Hair – alopecia
(1997): Picard C+, *Ann Pharmacother* 31, 1260

Other

Foetor ex ore (halitosis)
(1998): Backonja M+, *JAMA* 280, 1831
Gingivitis (<1%)
Glossitis
Myalgia (2%)
Paresthesias (<1%)
Sialorrhea
Stomatitis
Tooth discoloration
Tremor (1–10%)
Xerostomia (1.7%)

GANCICLOVIR

Trade name: Cytovene (Roche)
Other common trade names: *Cymevan; Cymeven; Cymevene; Vitrasert*
Indications: Cytomegalovirus retinitis in immunocompromised patients
Category: Antiviral
Half-life: 2.5–3.6 hours
Clinically important, potentially serious interactions with: amphotericin B, cyclosporine, didanosine, imipenem/cilastin, probenecid, zidovudine, **food**

Reactions

Skin

Acne (<1%)
Bullous eruption (<1%)
Chills (<1%)
Diaphoresis
Edema (<1%)
Exanthems (<1%)
(1987): Chachoua A+, *Ann Intern Med* 107, 133 (4.9%)
(1979): Eyanson S+, *Arch Dermatol* 115, 54 (2%)
Exfoliative dermatitis
Facial edema (<1%)
Fixed eruption (<1%)
Photosensitivity (<1%)
Pigmentation (<1%)
Pruritus (5%)
Psoriasis
Purpura
Rash (sic) (>10%)
Stevens–Johnson syndrome
Urticaria (<1%)

Hair

Hair – alopecia (<1%)
(1990): Faulds D+, *Drugs* 39, 597

Other

Anaphylactoid reaction
Anosmia
Dysgeusia (<1%)
Gingival hypertrophy
Hypesthesia (<1%)
Injection-site edema (<1%)
Injection-site inflammation (2%)
Injection-site pain
(1990): Faulds D+, *Drugs* 39, 597 (4%)
Mastodynia (<1%)
Myalgia (<1%)
Oral ulceration (<1%)
Paresthesias (6–10%)
Phlebitis (2%)
Tongue disorder (sic) (<1%)
Tremor (<1%)
Xerostomia (<1%)

GANIRELIX

Trade name: Antagon (Organon)
Indications: Infertility
Category: Antigonadotropic hormone
Half-life: 16.2 hours
Clinically important, potentially serious interactions with: DHEA

Reactions

Skin

Hot flashes (4–5%)
Pruritus

Other

Injection-site reaction (1.1%)
(2000): Gillies PS+, *Drugs* 59, 107
(2000): Oberye J+, *Hum Reprod* 15, 245

GATIFLOXACIN

Trade name: Tequin (Bristol-Myers Squibb)
Indications: Various infections caused by susceptible organisms
Category: Fluoroquinolone antibiotic
Half-life: 7–14 hours
Clinically important, potentially serious interactions with: antiarrhythmics, antidepressants, antipsychotics, cimetidine, cisapride, digoxin, erythromycin, foscarnet, NSAIDs, phenothiazines, probenecid

Reactions

Skin

Allergic reactions (sic) (0.1–3%)
Angioedema
Burning (sic)
Candidiasis
Cheilitis (<0.1%)
Chills (0.1–3%)
Diaphoresis (0.1–3%)

Ecchymoses (<0.1%)
Edema (<0.1%)
Erythema
Exanthems (<0.1%)
Facial edema (<0.1%)
Peripheral edema (0.1–3%)
Photosensitivity
(2000): Stein GE+, *Inf Med* 17, 564
Pruritus (<0.1%)
Rash (sic) (0.1–3%)
Stevens–Johnson syndrome
Toxic epidermal necrolysis
Urticaria
Vasculitis
Vesiculobullous eruption (<0.1%)

Other
Anaphylactoid reaction
Dysgeusia (0.1–3%)
(2000): Stein GE+, *Inf Med* 17, 564
Foetor ex ore (halitosis) (<1%)
Gingivitis (<0.1%)
Glossitis (0.1–3%)
Hyperesthesia (<0.1%)
Hypersensitivity
Injection-site reactions (5%)
(2000): Gajjar DA+, *Pharmacotherapy* 20, 49S
Mastodynia (<0.1%)
Myalgia (<0.1%)
Oral candidiasis (0.1–3%)
Oral ulceration (0.1–3%)
Paresthesias (0.1–3%)
Parosmia (<0.1%)
Serum sickness
Stomatitis (0.1–3%)
Tendinitis
Tendon rupture
Tongue edema (<0.1%)
Tremor (0.1–3%)
Vaginitis (6%)
(2000): Stein GE+, *Inf Med* 17, 564

GEMCITABINE

Trade name: Gemzar (Lilly)
Indications: Pancreatic carcinoma
Category: Antineoplastic nucleoside analogue
Half-life: 42–94 minutes
Clinically important, potentially serious interactions with: aldesleukin

Reactions

Skin
Allergic reactions (sic) (4%)
Diaphoresis
Edema (13%)
(1995): Tonato M+, *Anticancer Drugs* 6, 27
Erysipeloid rash (sic)
(2000): Brandes A+, *Anticancer Drugs* 11, 15 (confined to areas of lymphedema)
Exanthems
(1996): Chen YM+, *J Clin Oncol* 14, 1743
Flu-like syndrome (sic) (>10%)
Infections (sic) (16%)
Peripheral edema (20%)
(1995): Tonato M+, *Anticancer Drugs* 6, 27
(1994): Abratt RP+, *J Clin Oncol* 12, 1535
Pruritus (13%)
Pruritus ani
(1999): Hejna M+, *N Engl J Med* 340, 655
Petechiae (16%)
Radiation recall
(2000): Burstein HJ, *J Clin Oncol* 18, 693
Rash (sic) (30%)
Vasculitis
(2000): Banach MJ+, *Arch Ophthalmol* 118, 726 (necrotizing)

Hair
Hair – alopecia (15%)
(1995): Tonato M+, *Anticancer Drugs* 6, 27
(1994): Abratt RP+, *J Clin Oncol* 12, 1535

Other
Anaphylactoid reaction
Injection-site reactions (4%)
Lymphedema
(2000): Brandes A+, *Anticancer Drugs* 11, 15 (confined to areas of lymphedema)
Myalgia (>10%)
Paresthesias (10%)
Stomatitis (11%)

GEMFIBROZIL

Trade name: Lopid (Parke-Davis)
Other common trade names: *Bolutol; Decrelip; Fibrocit; Gemlipid; Gen-Fibro; Gevilon Uno; Jezil; Lipur; Nu-Gemfibrozil*
Indications: Hyperlipidemia
Category: Antihyperlipidemic
Half-life: 1.5 hours
Clinically important, potentially serious interactions with: anticoagulants, atorvastatin, bexarotene, chlorpropamide, cyclosporine, fluvastatin, furosemide, glyburide, lovastatin, pravastatin, simvastatin, warfarin

Reactions

Skin
Abscesses
Acanthosis nigricans
Angioedema
Basal cell carcinoma
Dermatitis (sic) (0.4%)
(1988): Todd PA+, *Drugs* 36, 314
Dermatomyositis (<1%)
Eczema (sic) (1.9%)
Erythema multiforme
Exanthems
(1990): Fusella J+, *J Rheumatol* 17, 572
(1988): Todd PA+, *Drugs* 36, 314 (2.1%)
Exfoliative dermatitis (<1%)
Ichthyosis
Lichen planus
Lupus erythematosus
Melanoma
Petechiae
Pruritus (0.8%)
(1988): Todd PA+, *Drugs* 36, 314
Psoriasis
(1989): Frick MH, *Arch Dermatol* 125, 132
(1988): Fisher DA+, *Arch Dermatol* 124, 854
Rash (sic) (1.7%)
Raynaud's phenomenon (<1%)
(1993): Smith GW+, *Br J Rheumatol* 32, 84
Seborrhea
Skin thickening (sic)
Urticaria (0.1%)
(1988): Todd PA+, *Drugs* 36, 314
Vasculitis (<1%)
(1993): Smith GW+, *Br J Rheumatol* 32, 84
Xerosis

Hair
Hair – alopecia
Hair – hirsutism

Nails
Nails – discoloration
(1990): Klein ME, *The Schoch Letter* 40 (#7), 29 (#120) (observation)
Nails – increased growth (sic)

Other
Anaphylactoid reaction
Dysgeusia (<1%)
Hypesthesia (<1%)
Hyperesthesia (<1%)
Myalgia (<1%)
Myopathy
Myositis
Paresthesias (<1%)
Polymyositis
(1990): Fusella J+, *J Rheumatol* 17, 572
Pseudolymphoma
(1995): Magro CM+, *J Am Acad Dermatol* 32, 419

GEMTUZUMAB

Trade name: Mylotarg (Wyeth-Ayerst)
Indications: Acute myeloid leukemia
Category: Antineoplastic monoclonal antibody
Half-life: 45 hours (initial dose)
Clinically important, potentially serious interactions with: no data

Reactions

Skin
Chills (66%)
Ecchymoses (15%)
Herpes simplex (22%)
Infection (sic) (28%)
Peripheral edema (21%)
Petechiae (21%)
Rash (sic) (23%)

Other
Arthralgia (10%)
Local reaction (sic) (25%)
Mucositis (25%)
Stomatitis (32%)

GENTAMICIN

Trade names: Garamycin (Schering); Genoptic, Gentacidin, Jenamicin, Ocumycin
Other common trade names: *Alcomicin; Cidomycin; Diogent; Garatec; Gentalline; Gentalol; I-Gent; Refobacin; Sedanazin*
Indications: Various infections caused by susceptible organisms
Category: Aminoglycoside antibiotic
Half-life: 2–4 hours
Clinically important, potentially serious interactions with: aminoglycosides, amphotericin B, bumetanide, cephalosporins, ethacrynic acid, furosemide, loop diuretics, penicillins, torsemide, vancomycin

Reactions

Skin
Contact dermatitis
(1996): Merlob P+, *Cutis* 57, 429 (neonatal orbital)
(1996): Munoz-Bellido FJ+, *Allergy* 51, 758
(1989): van Ketel WG+, *Contact Dermatitis* 20, 303
(1988): Robinson PM, *J Laryngol Otol* 102, 577
(1970): Lynfield YL, *N Y State J Med* 70, 2235
(1969): Braun W+, *Hautarzt* (German) 20, 108
Eczematous eruption (sic)
(1988): Ghadially R+, *J Am Acad Dermatol* 19, 428
Edema (1–10%)
Erythema (1–10%)
Exanthems
(1990): Flax SH+, *Cutis* 46, 59
(1974): Hewitt WL, *Postgrad Med* 50 (Suppl 7), 55 (0.3%)
(1971): Tümmers H+, *Med Welt* (German) 22, 1404 (1%)
(1969): Braun W+, *Hautarzt* (German) 20, 108
Exfoliative dermatitis
(1989): Guin JD+, *Cutis* 43, 564
Photosensitivity (<1%)
(1990): Flax SH+, *Cutis* 46, 59 (photo recall)
(1966): Hough CE+, *Clin Med Surg* 73, 55
Pruritus (1–10%)
Purpura
(1974): Hewitt WL, *Postgrad Med* 50 (Suppl 7), 55 (0.3%)
Rash (sic)
Urticaria
(1974): Hewitt WL, *Postgrad Med* 50 (Suppl 7), 55 (0.14%)
Toxic epidermal necrolysis
(1984): Sluchenkova LD+, *Pediatriia* (Russian) July, 57
Vasculitis
(1980): Bonnetblanc JM+, *Ann Dermatol Vénéréol* (French) 107, 1089

Hair
Hair – alopecia
(1973): Levantine A+, *Br J Dermatol* 89, 549
(1970): Yoshioka H+, *JAMA* 211, 123

Other
Anaphylactoid reaction
(1983): Fisher AA, *Cutis* 32, 510
Injection-site erythema
(1990): Shen K, *Lancet* 336, 689
Injection-site induration
Injection-site necrosis
(1990): Grob JJ+, *Dermatologica* 180, 258
(1985): Duterque M+, *Ann Dermatol Venereol* (French) 112, 707
(1985): Doutre MS+, *Therapie* (French) 40, 266
(1984): Penso D+, *Presse Méd* (French) 13, 1575
(1984): Taillandier J+, *Presse Méd* (French) 13, 1574
Injection-site pain (<1%)
Paresthesias
Phlebitis
Pseudotumor cerebri (<1%)
Sialorrhea (<1%)
Stomatitis
Thrombophlebitis
Tremor (<1%)

GLIMEPIRIDE

Trade name: Amaryl (Aventis)
Indications: Non-insulin dependent diabetes type II
Category: Second generation sulfonylurea* antidiabetic
Half-life: 5–9 hours
Clinically important, potentially serious interactions with: androgens, anticoagulants, beta-blockers, chloramphenicol, cimetidine, clofibrate, digoxin, fenfluramine, fluconazole, gemfibrozil, MAO inhibitors, methyldopa, miconazole, NSAIDs, phenylbutazone, probenecid, quinidine, salicylates, sulfonamides, thiazides, tricyclic antidepressants

Reactions

Skin
Allergic reactions (sic) (<1%)
Diaphoresis
Edema (<1%)
Erythema (<1%)
Exanthems (<1%)

Peeling (sic)
Photosensitivity (<1%)
Pruritus (<1%)
Psoriasis
(1997): Leal G, Fortaleza, Brazil (from Internet) (observation)
Rash (sic) (<1%)
Urticaria (<1%)

Other

Porphyria cutanea tarda

***Note:** Glimepiride is a sulfonamide and can be absorbed systemically. Sulfonamides can produce severe, possibly fatal, reactions such as toxic epidermal necrolysis and Stevens–Johnson syndrome

GLIPIZIDE

Trade name: Glucotrol (Pfizer)
Other common trade names: *Glibenese; Glipid; Glyde; Melizide; Mindiab; Minidiab; Minodiab*
Indications: Non-insulin dependent diabetes type II
Category: Second generation sulfonylurea* antidiabetic
Half-life: 2–4 hours
Clinically important, potentially serious interactions with: androgens, anticoagulants, captopril, cimetidine, digoxin, enalapril, fluconazole, gemfibrozil, MAO inhibitors, methyldopa, phenylbutazone, probenecid, salicylates, sulfonamides, tricyclic antidepressants, **food**

Reactions

Skin

Eczema (sic)
Edema (<1%)
Erythema (<1%)
Exanthems (<1%)
Flushing (<1%)
Grinspan's syndrome**
(1990): Lamey PJ+, *Oral Surg Oral Med Oral Path* 70, 184
Lichenoid eruption
Peeling (sic)
Photosensitivity (1–10%)
Phototoxic reaction
(2000): Vargas F+, *In Vitr Mol Toxicol* 13, 17
Pruritus (<3%)
Psoriasis (induced)
(1994): Litt JZ, Beachwood, Ohio, 2 personal cases (observation)
Pigmented purpuric dermatosis
(1999): Adams BB+, *J Am Acad Dermatol* 41, 827
Purpura
Rash (sic) (1–10%)
Urticaria (1–10%)

Other

Hypesthesia (<3%)
Myalgia (<3%)
Oral lichen planus
(1990): Lamey PJ+, *Oral Surg Oral Med Oral Path* 70, 184
Paresthesias (<3%)
Porphyria (coproporphyria-like)
(1991): Moder KG+, *Mayo Clin Proc* 66, 312
Porphyria cutanea tarda

***Note:** Glipizide is a sulfonamide and can be absorbed systemically. Sulfonamides can produce severe, possibly fatal, reactions such as toxic epidermal necrolysis and Stevens–Johnson syndrome.

****Note:** Grinspan's syndrome: the triad of oral lichen planus, diabetes mellitus, and hypertension.

GLUCAGON

Trade name: Glucagon Emergency Kit (Lilly)
Indications: Hypoglycemic reactions
Category: Antihypoglycemic; antispasmodic; antidote
Half-life: 3–10 minutes
Clinically important, potentially serious interactions with: beta-blockers, oral anticoagulants, phenytoin

Reactions

Skin

Acute febrile neutrophilic dermatosis (Sweet's syndrome)
(1996): Glass LF+, *J Am Acad Dermatol* 34, 455 (passim)
(1994): Fukutoku M+, *Br J Haematol* 86, 645
(1994): Johnson ML+, *Arch Dermatol* 130, 77
(1993): Paydas S+, *Br J Haematol* 85, 191
(1992): Karp DL, *Ann Intern Med* 117, 875
(1992): Park JW+, *Ann Intern Med* 116, 996
(1991): Cohen PR+, *J Am Acad Dermatol* 25, 734
Angioedema
(1985): Gelfand DW+, *Am J Roentgenol* 144, 405
Epidermolysis bullosa acquisita
(1992): Ward JC+, *Br J Haematol* 81, 27
Erythema multiforme
(1980): Edell SL, *Am J Roentgenol* 134, 385
Erythema nodosum
(1994): Nomiyama J+, *Am J Hematol* 47, 333
Exanthems
(1996): Glass LF+, *J Am Acad Dermatol* 34, 455
(1995): Scott GA, *Am J Dermatopathol* 17, 107
(1994): Sasaki O+, *Intern Med* 33, 641
(1993): Yamashita N+, *J Dermatol* 20, 473
(1993): Peters MS+, *J Cutan Pathol* 20, 465
(1992): Mehregan DR+, *Arch Dermatol* 128, 1055
(1976): Barber SG+, *Lancet* 20, 1138
Folliculitis
(1996): Glass LF+, *J Am Acad Dermatol* 34, 455 (passim)
(1992): Ostlere LS+, *Br J Dermatol* 127, 193
Glucagonoma syndrome (necrolytic migratory erythema)
(1988): Benhamou PY+, *Ann Dermatol Venereol* (French) 115, 717
Pyoderma gangrenosum
(1996): Glass LF+, *J Am Acad Dermatol* 34, 455 (passim)
(1994): Johnson ML+, *Arch Dermatol* 130, 77
(1991): Ross HJ+, *Cancer* 68, 441 (bullous)
Rash (sic)
(1979): Barber SG+, *Ann Intern Med* 91, 213
(1976): Barber SG+, *Lancet* 2, 1138
Urticaria (1–10%)
(1985): Gelfand DW+, *Am J Roentgenol* 144, 405
(1975): Kitabchi AE+, *J Clin Endocrinol Metab* 41, 863
Vasculitis
(1996): Glass LF+, *J Am Acad Dermatol* 34, 455 (passim)
(1995): Vidarsson B+, *Am J Med* 98, 589
(1995): Couderc LJ+, *Respir Med* 89, 237
(1994): Jain KK, *J Am Acad Dermatol* 31, 213
(1994): van Kamp H+, *Br J Haematol* 86, 415
(1994): Johnson ML+, *Arch Dermatol* 130, 77
(1991): Wodzinski MA+, *Br J Haematol* 77, 249
(1990): Welte Z+, *Blood* 75, 1056
(1989): Dreicer R+, *Ann Intern Med* 111, 91

Other

Injection-site cutaneous reaction
(1996): Glass LF+, *J Am Acad Dermatol* 34, 455 (passim)
(1993): Samlaska CP+, *Arch Dermatol* 129, 645
(1992): Mehregan DR+, *Arch Dermatol* 128, 1055

GLYBURIDE

Synonyms: glibenclamide; glybenclamide
Trade names: Diabeta (Aventis); Glucovance (Bristol-Myers Squibb); Glynase (Pharmacia & Upjohn); Micronase (Pharmacia & Upjohn)
Other common trade names: *Albert Glyburide; Daonil; Euglucan; Euglucon; Glimel; Glucal; Hemi-Daonil; Med-Glibe; Miglucan; Norboral*
Indications: Non-insulin dependent diabetes type II
Category: Second generation sulfonylurea* antidiabetic
Half-life: 5–16 hours
Clinically important, potentially serious interactions with: alcohol, beta-blockers, chloramphenicol, clofibrate, dicumarol, fluconazole, gemfibrozil, hydantoins, MAO inhibitors, NSAIDs, oral anticoagulants, phenylbutazone, salicylates, sulfonamides, thiazides, tricyclic antidepressants

Glucovance is glyburide and metformin

Reactions

Skin

Allergic reactions (sic) (0.21%)
(1986): Bigby M+, *JAMA* 256, 3358
Angioedema
Bullous eruption
(1981): Wongpaitoon V+, *Postgrad Med J* 57, 244
Eczema (sic)
Erythema (1–5%)
(1988): Chee Ching S, *Photodermatol* 5, 42
Exanthems (1–5%)
(1971): Editorial, *BMJ* 2, 644
(1970): O'Sullivan DJ+, *BMJ* 2, 572 (0.5–1%)
(1969): Müller R+, *Horm Metab Res* 1, 88
Eyelid edema
(1985): Yitalo P+, *Arzneimittelforsch* (German) 35, 1596
Flushing
(1971): Fairman MJ+, *BMJ* 4, 297
(1971): Wardle EN+, *BMJ* 3, 309
Lichenoid eruption
Linear IgA bullous dermatosis
(1983): Väätäinen N+, *Acta Derm Venereol* (Stockh) 63, 169
Pellagra
(1980): Berova N+, *Dermatol Monatsschr* (German) 174, 50
Peeling (sic)
Pemphigus
(1993): Paterson AJ+, *J Oral Pathol Med* 22, 92
Photosensitivity (1–10%)
(1995): Fujii S+, *Am J Hematol* 50, 223
(1994): Shelley WB+, *Cutis* 53, 287 (observation)
(1994): Shelley WB+, *Cutis* 53, 77 (observation)
(1988): Sun CC, *Photodermatol* 5, 42
(1988): Chee-Ching S, *Photodermatology* 5, 42
(1987): Henrietta G, *Nursing* 17, 56
(1969): Müller R+, *Horm Metab Res* 1, 88
Pruritus (1–10%)
(1988): Chee Ching S, *Photodermatol* 5, 42
(1987): *Physicians Drug Alert* 7, 71
(1970): O'Sullivan DJ+, *BMJ* 2, 572
Psoriasis
(1988): Milner JE, *The Schoch Letter* 38(5), Item 64 (observation)
(1987): Goh CL, *Australas J Dermatol* 28, 30
Purpura
(1986): Dickey W+, *BMJ* 293, 823
(1983): Väätäinen N+, *Acta Derm Venereol* (Stockh) 63, 169
Rash (sic) (1–10%)
Urticaria (1–5%)
(1994): Shelley WB+, *Cutis* 53, 77 (observation)
(1991): Chichmanian RM+, *Therapie* (French) 46, 163
(1986): Kure J, *NC Med J* 47, 149
(1986): Jordan NS+, *Hosp Pharm* 21, 462
(1969): Müller R+, *Horm Metab Res* 1, 88
Vasculitis
(1986): Dickey W+, *BMJ* 293, 823
(1980): Ingelmo M+, *Med Clin (Barc)* (Spanish) 75, 306
(1974): Clarke BF+, *Diabetes* 23, 739
(1970): O'Sullivan DJ+, *BMJ* 2, 572
Vesiculobullous eruption
(1993): Landor M+, *Ann Allergy* 70, 196

Other

Dysgeusia
Hypersensitivity (generalized)
(1974): Clarke BF+, *Diabetes* 23, 739
Myalgia
Paresthesias (<1%)
Porphyria cutanea tarda

***Note:** Glyburide is a sulfonamide and can be absorbed systemically. Sulfonamides can produce severe, possibly fatal, reactions such as toxic epidermal necrolysis and Stevens–Johnson syndrome.

GLYCOPYRROLATE

Trade name: Robinul (Robins; Horizon)
Other trade names: *Gastrodyn; Sroton; Strodin*
Indications: Duodenal ulcer, irritable bowel syndrome
Category: Anticholinergic, antispasmodic
Half-life: no data
Clinically important, potentially serious interactions with: amantadine, digoxin, disopyramide, glutethimide, haloperidol, ketoconazole, levodopa, meperidine, phenothiazines, procainamide, quinidine, tricyclic antidepressants

Reactions

Skin

Allergic reactions (sic)
Anhidrosis
Flushing
Hypohidrosis (>10%)
Photosensitivity (1–10%)
Rash (sic) (<1%)
Urticaria
Xerosis (>10%)

Other

Dysgeusia
Injection-site irritation (>10%)
Xerostomia (>10%)

GOLD and GOLD COMPOUNDS

Generic names:
Auranofin
Trade name: Ridaura (SmithKline Beecham)
Aurothioglucose
Trade name: Solganal (Schering)
Gold sodium thiomalate (sodium aurothiomalate)
Trade name: Myochrysine (Merck)
Other common trade names: *Aureotan; Aurolate; Aurothio; Miocrin; Myocrisine; Shiosol; Tauredon*
Indications: Rheumatoid arthritis
Category: Antiarthritic
Half-life: 5 days
Clinically important, potentially serious interactions with: antimalarials, cytotoxic agents, hydroxychloroquine, immunosuppressants, penicillamine, phenylbutazone

Reactions

Skin

Acne
(1982): Bailin PL+, *Clin Rheum Dis* 8, 493 (passim)

(1977): Hjortshoj A, *Acta Derm Venereol* (Stockh) 57, 165
Angioedema (<1%)
(1989): Herbst WM+, *Hautarzt* (German) 40, 568
Angiofibromatosis
(1989): Herbst WM+, *Hautarzt* (German) 40, 568
Bullous eruption
(1970): Almeyda J+, *Br J Dermatol* 83, 707
(1951): Jaeger H, *Dermatologica* 103, 280
(1940): Wile UJ+, *Arch Dermatol* 42, 1005 (passim)
Bullous pemphigoid
(1983): Wozel G+, *Dermatol Monatsschr* (German) 169, 125
Cheilitis
(1982): Bailin PL+, *Clin Rheum Dis* 8, 493 (passim)
(1974): Penneys NS+, *Arch Dermatol* 109, 372
Contact dermatitis
(2000): Trattner A+, *Contact Dermatitis* 42, 301
(2000): Vamnes JS+, *Contact Dermatitis* 42, 128
(1999): Bruze M+, *Contact Dermatitis* 40, 295
(1999): Fowler JF, *Skin and Allergy News* September, 34 (9.5%)
(1999): Räsänen L+, *Br J Dermatol* 141, 683
(1998): Estlander T+, *Contact Dermatitis* 38, 40
(1998): Wiesner M+, *Contact Dermatitis* 38, 52
(1998): Moller H+, *Am J Contact Dermat* 9, 15
(1997): Silva R+, *Contact Dermatitis* 37, 78
(1997): Moller H+, *Acta Derm Venereol* 77, 370
(1997): Armstrong DK+, *Br J Dermatol* 136, 776
(1997): Kilpikari I, *Contact Dermatitis* 37, 130
(1997): Hostynek JJ, *Food Chem Toxicol* 35, 839
(1997): Fleming C+, *Contact Dermatitis* 37, 298 (lymphomatoid)
(1996): Tan E+, *Australas J Dermatol* 37, 218
(1996): Sabroe RA+, *Contact Dermatitis* 34, 345
(1994): Osawa J+, *Contact Dermatitis* 31, 89
(1994): Webster CG+, *Cutis* 54, 25
(1994): Collet E+, *Ann Dermatol Venereol* (French) 121, 21
(1994): Björkner B+, *Contact Dermatitis* 30, 144
(1994): Bruze M+, *J Am Acad Dermatol* 31, 579
(1993): Aro T+, *Contact Dermatitis* 28, 276
(1993): Hisa T+, *Contact Dermatitis* 28, 174
(1993): Koga T+, *Contact Dermatitis* 28, 303
(1993): Koga T+, *Br J Dermatol* 128, 227
(1990): Wijnands MJ+, *Lancet* 335, 867
(1990): Miller RA+, *J Am Acad Dermatol* 23, 360
(1989): Camarasa JG+, *Med Cutan Ibero Lat Am* (Spanish) 17, 187
(1988): Goh CL, *Contact Dermatitis* 18, 122
(1988): Wicks IP+, *Ann Rheum Dis* 47, 421
(1988): Fowler JF, *Arch Dermatol* 124, 181
(1987): Fisher AA, *J Am Acad Dermatol* 17, 853
(1987): Fisher AA, *Cutis* 39, 473
(1985): Kalamkarian AA+, *Vestn Dermatol Venerol* (Russian) August, 4
(1985): Tosi S+, *Int J Clin Pharmacol Res* 5, 265
(1985): Rapson WS, *Contact Dermatitis* 13, 56
(1985): Silvennoinen-Kassinen S+, *Contact Dermatitis* 11, 156
(1983): Monti M+, *Contact Dermatitis* 9, 150
(1982): Iwatsuki K+, *Arch Dermatol* 118, 608
(1980): Raith L+, *Dermatol Monatsschr* (German) 166, 382
(1978): Budden MG+, *Contact Dermatitis* 4, 172
(1977): Fisher AA, *Cutis* 19, 156
(1977): Rennie N, *BMJ* 1, 446
(1977): Dick D, *BMJ* 1, 51
(1975): Roeleveld CG+, *Contact Dermatitis* 1, 333
(1975): Klaschka F, *Contact Dermatitis* 1, 264
(1973): Petros H+, *Br J Dermatol* 88, 505
(1971): Walzer R+, *Arch Dermatol* 104, 107
(1971): Nava C+, *Med Lav* (Italian) 62, 572
(1971): Rytter M+, *Dermatologica* (German) 142, 209
Cutaneous eruption (sic)
(1998): Pandya AG+, *Arch Dermatol* 134, 1104
Dermatitis (sic)
(2000): ter Borg EJ+, *Arthritis Rheum* 43, 1420
(1999): Räsänen L+, *Br J Dermatol* 141, 683
(1997): Choy EH+, *Br J Rheumatol* 36, 1054
(1996): Bonnetblanc JM, *Presse Med* (French) 25, 1555
(1986): Minghetti G+, *G Ital Dermatol Venereol* (Italian) 121, 425
(1985): Kalamkarian AA+, *Vestn Dermatol Venerol* (Russian) Aug, 4
(1983): Sigler JW, *Am J Med* 75, 59
(1958): Smith RT+, *JAMA* 167, 1197
(1940): Wile UJ+, *Arch Dermatol* 42, 1005 (passim)
Eczematous eruption (sic)
(1994): Lizeaux-Parneix V+, *Ann Dermatol Venereol* (French) 121, 793
(1986): Hofmann C+, *Z Rheumatol* (German) 45, 100
(1976): Rennie JAN, *BMJ* 2, 1294
Erythema annulare centrifugum
(1992): Tsuji T+, *J Am Acad Dermatol* 27, 284
Erythema multiforme
(1982): Bailin PL+, *Clin Rheum Dis* 8, 493 (passim)
(1966): Cameron AJ+, *BMJ* 2, 1125
Erythema nodosum
(1998): Pandya AG+, *Arch Dermatol* 134, 1104 (passim)
(1982): Bailin PL+, *Clin Rheum Dis* 8, 493 (passim)
(1974): Penneys NS+, *Arch Dermatol* 109, 372
(1973): Stone RL+, *Arch Dermatol* 107, 602
Exanthems (>5%)
(1999): Räsänen L+, *Br J Dermatol* 141, 683
(1998): Pandya AG+, *Arch Dermatol* 134, 1104 (passim)
(1996): Bonnetblanc JM, *Presse Med* (French) 25, 1555
(1994): Shelley WB+, *Cutis* 52, 87 (observation)
(1977): Voigt K+, *Hautarzt* (German) 28, 421
(1974): Penneys NS+, *Arch Dermatol* 109, 372
(1972): Walzer RA+, *Arch Dermatol* 106, 231
(1940): Wile UJ+, *Arch Dermatol* 42, 1005 (passim)
Exfoliative dermatitis
(2000): Lancucki J+, *Wiad Lek* (Polish) 21, 1347 (erythroderma)
(1998): Pandya AG+, *Arch Dermatol* 134, 1104 (passim)
(1996): Sigurdsson V+, *J Am Acad Dermatol* 35, 53
(1991): Wilson CL+, *Int J Dermatol* 30, 148
(1989): Ranki A+, *Am J Dermatopathol* 11, 22
(1984): Adachi JD+, *J Rheumatol* 11, 355
(1982): Bailin PL+, *Clin Rheum Dis* 8, 493 (passim)
(1974): Penneys NS+, *Arch Dermatol* 109, 372
(1940): Wile UJ+, *Arch Dermatol* 42, 1005 (passim)
Fixed eruption
Graft-versus-host reaction
(1998): Jappe U+, *Hautarzt* (German) 49, 126 (passim)
Granuloma annulare
(1990): Martin N+, *Arch Dermatol* 126, 1370
(1980): Rothwell RS+, *Arch Dermatol* 116, 863
Herpes zoster
(1981): Fam AG+, *Ann Intern Med* 94, 712
Lichenoid eruption
(1999): Räsänen L+, *Br J Dermatol* 141, 683
(1998): Pandya AG+, *Arch Dermatol* 134, 1104 (passim)
(1997): Choy EH+, *Br J Rheumatol* 36, 1054
(1996): Bonnetblanc JM, *Presse Med* (French) 25, 1555
(1994): Alzieu PH+, *Ann Dermatol Venereol* (French) 121, 798
(1994): Lizeaux-Parneix V+, *Ann Dermatol Venereol* (French) 121, 793
(1971): Almeyda J+, *Br J Dermatol* 85, 604
Lichen planus
(1996): Russell MA+, *N Engl J Med* 334, 603
(1990): Torrelo A+, *Actas Dermo-Sif* (Spanish) 81, 743
(1986): Hofmann C+, *Z Rheumatol* (German) 45, 100
(1986): Ingber A+, *Z Hautkr* (German) 61, 315
(1982): Bailin PL+, *Clin Rheum Dis* 8, 493 (passim)
(1979): Krebs A, *Hautarzt* (German) 30, 281
(1977): Hjorthsoj A, *Acta Derm Venereol* (Stockh) 57, 165
(1974): Penneys NS+, *Arch Dermatol* 109, 372 (32%)
(1974): Delaby MC, *Arch Belg Dermatol* 30, 111
(1937): Hartfall SJ+, *Lancet* 2, 838
Lichen spinulosus
(1932): Throne B+, *Arch Dermatol* 25, 494
Lupus erythematosus
(1988): Balsa A+, *Rev Clin Esp* (Spanish) 182, 505
(1969): Goerz G, *Dtsch Med Wochenschr* (German) 94, 2040
(1967): Kapp W+, *Praxis* (German) 56, 1594
Lymphocytoma cutis
(1992): Kobayashi Y+, *J Am Acad Dermatol* 27, 457
Lymphomatoid eosinophilic reaction (sic)
(1999): Park YM+, *Contact Dermatitis* 40, 216
Pemphigus
(1978): Miyamoto Y+, *Arch Dermatol* 114, 1855
Photosensitivity
(1973): Machtey I, *Harefuah* (Hebrew) 85, 517
(1970): Almeyda J+, *Br J Dermatol* 83, 707
Pigmentation (chrysiasis)
(1998): Pandya AG+, *Arch Dermatol* 134, 1104 (passim)

(1997): Miller ML+, *Cutis* 59, 256
(1996): Fleming CJ+, *J Am Acad Dermatol* 34, 349
(1992): Cremer B+, *Dtsch Med Wochenschr* (German) 117, 558
(1990): Bonet M+, *Clin Rheumatol* 9, 254
(1984): Pelachyk IM+, *J Cutan Pathol* 11, 491
(1984): Fam AG+, *Arthritis Rheum* 27, 119
(1984): Larsen FS+, *Clin Exp Dermatol* 9, 174
(1982): Beckett VL+, *Mayo Clin Proc* 57, 773
(1982): Bailin PL+, *Clin Rheum Dis* 8, 493 (passim)
(1981): Granstein RD+, *J Am Acad Dermatol* 5, 1 (blue-gray)
(1975): Altmeyer P+, *Hautarzt* (German) 26, 330
(1974): Gottlieb NL+, *Arthritis Rheum* 17, 56
(1973): Levantine A+, *Br J Dermatol* 89, 105
(1973): Cox AJ+, *Arch Dermatol* 108, 655
(1971): Franken E, *Dtsch Gesundheitsw* (German) 26, 653
(1965): Bianchi O+, *Arch Argent Dermatol* (Spanish) 15, 464
(1941): Schmidt OEL, *Arch Dermatol* 44, 446
(1928): Hansborg H, *Acta Tuberc Scand* 4, 124

Pityriasis rosea
(1999): Räsänen L+, *Br J Dermatol* 141, 683
(1998): Pandya AG+, *Arch Dermatol* 134, 1104 (passim)
(1994): Lizeaux-Parneix V+, *Ann Dermatol Venereol* (French) 121, 793
(1992): Tsuji T+, *J Am Acad Dermatol* 27, 284
(1986): Hofmann C+, *Z Rheumatol* (German) 45, 100
(1982): Bailin PL+, *Clin Rheum Dis* 8, 493 (passim)
(1977): Maize JC+, *Arch Dermatol* 113, 1457
(1974): Penneys NS+, *Arch Dermatol* 109, 372
(1940): Wile UJ+, *Arch Dermatol* 42, 1005

Pruritus (>10%)
(1998): Pandya AG+, *Arch Dermatol* 134, 1104
(1996): Bonnetblanc JM, *Presse Med* (French) 25, 1555
(1982): Bailin PL+, *Clin Rheum Dis* 8, 493 (passim)
(1975): Gordon MH+, *Ann Intern Med* 82, 47
(1974): Pennys NS+, *Arch Dermatol* 109, 372 (84%)
(1958): Smith RT+, *JAMA* 167, 1197
(1940): Wile UJ+, *Arch Dermatol* 42, 1005 (passim)

Psoriasis
(1991): Smith DL+, *Arch Dermatol* 127, 268

Purpura
(1984): Adachi JD+, *J Rheumatol* 11, 355
(1982): Bailin PL+, *Clin Rheum Dis* 8, 493 (passim)
(1966): Saphir JR+, *JAMA* 195, 782

Pyoderma gangrenosum

Radiation keratosis
(1996): Helm KF+, *Cutis* 57, 435

Rash (sic) (>10%)
(1990): Fremont-Smith P+, *Ann Rheum Dis* 49, 271
(1989): Caspi D+, *Ann Rheum Dis* 48, 730
(1984): Grindulis KA+, *Ann Rheum Dis* 43, 398
(1982): Smith PJ+, *Br Med J (Clin Res Ed)* 285, 595
(1979): Kean WF+, *Arthritis Rheum* 22, 495
(1961): Bayles TB, *Med Clin North Am* 5, 1229
(1956): Bayles TB+, *Ann Rheum Dis* 15, 394

Seborrheic dermatitis
(1982): Bailin PL+, *Clin Rheum Dis* 8, 493 (passim)
(1981): Kanwar AJ+, *Arch Dermatol* 117, 65 (passim)
(1951): Merliss RR+, *Ann Intern Med* 35, 352

Squamous cell carcinoma
(1990): Miller RA+, *J Am Acad Dermatol* 23, 360 (from radioactive gold)
(1973): Holubar K+, *Hautarzt* (German) 24, 489 (from radioactive gold)

Toxic dermatitis (sic)
(1958): Smith RT+, *JAMA* 167, 1197

Toxic epidermal necrolysis
(1998): Pandya AG+, *Arch Dermatol* 134, 1104 (passim)
(1982): Feldman C+, *Rheumatol Rehabil* 21, 222 (with benoxaprofen)
(1982): Braun-Falco O+, *MMM Munch Med Wochenschr* (German) 124, 757 (with benoxaprofen)
(1951): Jaeger H, *Dermatologica* 103, 280

Urticaria (1–10%)
(1998): Pandya AG+, *Arch Dermatol* 134, 1104 (passim)
(1994): Lizeaux-Parneix V+, *Ann Dermatol Venereol* (French) 121, 793
(1982): Bailin PL+, *Clin Rheum Dis* 8, 493 (passim)
(1974): Penneys NS+, *Arch Dermatol* 109, 372
(1970): Almeyda J+, *Br J Dermatol* 83, 707
(1940): Wile UJ+, *Arch Dermatol* 42, 1005 (passim)
(1936): Roche H, *BMJ* 1, 31

Vasculitis
(1984): Hauteville D+, *Rev Rhum Mal Osteoartic* (French) 51, 56
(1982): Bailin PL+, *Clin Rheum Dis* 8, 493 (passim)
(1974): Roenigk HR+, *Arch Dermatol* 109, 253
(1974): Steele DR, *Arch Dermatol* 110, 297

Vitiligo
(1933): Pillsbury DM+, *Arch Dermatol* 27, 36

Xerosis
(1984): Grindulis KA+, *Ann Rheum Dis* 43, 398

Hair

Hair – alopecia (1–10%)
(1998): Pandya AG+, *Arch Dermatol* 134, 1104 (passim)
(1984): Grindulis KA+, *Ann Rheum Dis* 43, 398
(1982): Bailin PL+, *Clin Rheum Dis* 8, 493 (passim)
(1975): Gordon MH+, *Ann Intern Med* 82, 47
(1972): Walzer RA+, *Arch Dermatol* 106, 231

Hair – pigmentation
(1974): Gottlieb NL+, *Arthritis Rheum* 17, 56

Nails

Nails – dystrophy
(1977): Voigt K+, *Hautarzt* (German) 28, 421

Nails – exfoliation
(1938): Boon TH, *BMJ* 1, 780

Nails – lichen planus
(1990): Torrelo A+, *Actas Dermo-Sif* (Spanish) 81, 743

Nails – onycholysis
(1977): Voigt K+, *Hautarzt* (German) 28, 421

Nails – pigmentation
(1984): Fam AG+, *Arthritis Rheum* 27, 119 (gold nails)
(1974): Gottlieb NL+, *Arthritis Rheum* 17, 56

Nails – shedding
(2000): ter Borg EJ+, *Arthritis Rheum* 43, 1420

Other

Acute intermittent porphyria

Anaphylactoid reaction

Aphthous stomatitis
(1989): Caspi D+, *Ann Rheum Dis* 48, 730
(1979): Kean WF+, *Arthritis Rheum* 22, 495
(1976): Kuffer R+, *Rev Stomatol Chir Maxillofac* (French) 77, 747

Burning mouth syndrome
(1994): Laeijendecker R+, *J Am Acad Dermatol* 30, 205

Dysgeusia
(1996): Bonnetblanc JM, *Presse Med* (French) 25, 1555
(1974): Pennys NS+, *Arch Dermatol* 109, 372 (metallic taste)
(1970): Almeyda J+, *Br J Dermatol* 83, 707
(1940): Wile UJ+, *Arch Dermatol* 42, 1005 (passim)

Gingivitis (>10%)
(1976): Adams D+, *J Rheumatol Rehabilitation* 15, 245
(1970): Almeyda J+, *Br J Dermatol* 83, 707

Gingivostomatitis
(1982): Izumi AK, *Arch Dermatol Res* 272, 387 (allergic contact)

Glossitis (>10%)
(1976): Adams D+, *J Rheumatol Rehabilitation* 15, 245
(1975): Gordon MH+, *Ann Intern Med* 82, 47

Hypersensitivity
(1972): Walzer RA+, *Arch Dermatol* 106, 231

Injection-site pain
(1984): Grindulis KA+, *Ann Rheum Dis* 43, 398

Mucocutaneous reaction
(1996): Cheatum DE, *J Rheumatol* 23, 944
(1995): Klinkhoff AV+, *J Rheumatol* 22, 1657

Oral lichenoid eruption
(1990): Vallejo-Irastorza G+, *Av Odontoestomatol* (Spanish) 6, 131

Oral lichen planus
(1994): Lizeaux-Parneix V+, *Ann Dermatol Venereol* (French) 121, 793
(1994): Laeijendecker R+, *J Am Acad Dermatol* 30, 205
(1993): Brown RS+, *Cutis* 51, 183

Oral mucosal eruption
(1968): Bardadin T+, *Reumatologia* (Polish) 6, 287

Oral mucosal pigmentation
(1990): Torrelo A+, *Actas Dermo-Sif* (Spanish) 81, 743
(1984): Sutak J+, *Prakt Zubn Lek* (Czech) 32, 166

Oral ulceration
(1999): Räsänen L+, *Br J Dermatol* 141, 683
(1984): Glenert U, *Oral Surg* 58, 52
(1982): Bailin PL+, *Clin Rheum Dis* 8, 493 (passim)

(1979): Kean WF+, *Arthritis Rheum* 22, 495
(1976): Adams D+, *J Rheumatol Rehabilitation* 15, 245
Pseudolymphoma
(1996): Kalimo K+, *J Cutan Pathol* 23, 328
Stomatitis (>10%)
(1997): Tosti A+, *Semin Cutan Med Surg* 16, 314
(1996): Bonnetblanc JM, *Presse Med* (French) 25, 1555
(1994): Laeijendecker R+, *J Am Acad Dermatol* 30, 205
(1992): Svensson A+, *Ann Rheum Dis* 51, 326
(1989): Caspi D+, *Ann Rheum Dis* 48, 730
(1987): Tumiati B+, *J Rheumatol* 14, 177
(1984): Glenert U, *Oral Surg* 58, 52
(1983): Sigler JW, *Am J Med* 75, 59
(1982): Bailin PL+, *Clin Rheum Dis* 8, 493 (passim)
(1979): Belkahaia C+, *Tunis Med* (French) 57, 234
(1979): Fregert S+, *Contact Dermatitis* 5, 63
(1975): Gordon MH+, *Ann Intern Med* 82, 47
(1971): Myers AR, *Mod Treat* 8, 761
(1970): Schopf E+, *Hautarzt* (German) 21, 422
(1970): Almeyda J+, *Br J Dermatol* 83, 707
(1958): Smith RT+, *JAMA* 167, 1197
Vaginitis
(1978): Webster JC+, *Am J Obstet Gynecol* 131, 700

Note: Adverse reactions can occur months after therapy has been discontinued.

GOSERELIN

Trade name: Zoladex (AstraZeneca)
Other trade name: *Prozoladex*
Indications: Breast and prostate carcinoma, endometriosis
Category: Gonadotropin-releasing analog hormone
Half-life: 5 hours
Clinically important, potentially serious interactions with: no data

Reactions

Skin

Chills
Diaphoresis (1–10%)
Edema (1–10%)
Hot flashes (>10%)
(1993): Bressler LR+, *Ann Pharmacother* 27, 182
Rash (sic) (1–10%)
Urticaria

Other

Anaphylactoid reaction
(1996): Raj SG+, *Am J Med Sci* 312, 187
Gynecomastia (>10%)
Hypersensitivity
(1996): Raj SG+, *Am J Med Sci* 312, 187
Injection-site pain (1–10%)
Mastodynia (1–10%)
Relapsing polychondritis
(1997): Labarthe MP+, *Dermatology* 195, 391

GRANISETRON

Trade name: Kytril (SmithKline Beecham)
Other common trade name: *Kevatril*
Indications: Chemotherapy-related emesis
Category: Antiemetic and antinauseant; serotonin antagonist
Half-life: 3–4 hours; cancer patients: 10–12 hours
Clinically important, potentially serious interactions with: none

Reactions

Skin

Allergic reactions (sic)
Exanthems
Hot flashes (<1%)
Rash (sic)
Urticaria

Hair

Hair – alopecia (3%)

Other

Anaphylactoid reaction
Dysgeusia (2%)
Hypersensitivity

GRANULOCYTE COLONY-STIMULATING FACTOR (GCSF)

Generic name:
Filgrastim (rG-CSF)
Trade name: Neupogen (Amgen)
Sargramostin (rGM-CSF)
Trade names: Leukine (Immunex); Prokine
Other common trade names: *Grasin; Leucogen; Neupogen 30*
Indications: Bone marrow allograft and autograft
Category: Hematopoietic growth factor; neutrophil stimulator
Half-life: filgrastim: 3.5 hours; sargramostin: 2–3 hours
Clinically important, potentially serious interactions with: antineoplastics, corticosteroids, lithium

Reactions

Skin

Acne
(1996): Lee PK+, *J Am Acad Dermatol* 34, 855
Acute febrile neutrophilic dermatosis (Sweet's syndrome)
(1999): Arbetter KR+, *Am J Hematol* 61, 126
(1999): Veres K+, *Orv Hetil* (Hungarian) 140, 1059
(1998): Hasegawa M+, *Eur J Dermatol* 8, 503 (2 patients)
(1998): Chao SC+, *J Formos Med Assoc* 96, 276
(1998): Merkel PA, *Curr Opin Rheumatol* 10, 45
(1996): Prevost-Blank PL+, *J Am Acad Dermatol* 35, 995
(1996): Richard MA+, *J Am Acad Dermatol* 35, 629
(1996): Jain KK, *Cutis* 57, 107
(1996): Shimizu T+, *J Pediatr Hematol Oncol* 18, 282
(1996): Garty BZ+, *Pediatrics* 97, 401
(1996): Petit T+, *Lancet* 347, 690
(1995): Shiga Y+, *Rinsho Ketsueki* (Japanese) 36, 353
(1995): Suzuki Y+, *Br J Dermatol* 133, 483
(1994): Fukutoku M+, *Br J Haematol* 86, 645
(1994): van Kamp H+, *Br J Haematol* 86, 415
(1994): Johnson ML+, *Arch Dermatol* 130, 77
(1993): Paydas S+, *Br J Haematol* 85, 191
(1992): Karp DL, *Ann Intern Med* 117, 875
(1991): Ross HJ+, *Cancer* 68, 441
(1992): Park JW+, *Ann Intern Med* 116, 996
(1990): Morioka N+, *J Am Acad Dermatol* 23, 247
(1989): Groopman JE+, *N Engl J Med* 321, 1449
(1989): Kluin-Nelemans JC+, *Br J Haematol* 73, 419
Diaphoresis
(2000): Khoury H+, *Bone Marrow Transplant* 25, 1197
Erythema
(1990): Farmer KL+, *Arch Dermatol* 126, 1243
(1989): Groopman JE+, *N Engl J Med* 321, 1449
Erythema nodosum
(1994): Nomiyama J+, *Am J Hematol* 47, 333
Exanthems
(1996): Glass LF+, *J Am Acad Dermatol* 34, 455
(1995): Scott GA, *Am J Dermatopathol* 17, 107
(1995): McMullin MF+, *Clin Rheumatol* 14, 204
(1994): Sasaki O+, *Intern Med* 33, 641
(1993): Yamashita N+, *J Dermatol* 20, 473
(1993): Samlaska CP+, *Arch Dermatol* 129, 645
(1991): Cohen PR+, *J Am Acad Dermatol* 25, 734
(1991): Horn TD+, *Arch Dermatol* 127, 49 (>5%)

(1990): Farmer KL+, *Arch Dermatol* 126, 1243
(1990): Lazarus H+, *Proc Am Soc Clin Oncol* 9, 15
(1988): Brandt SJ+, *N Engl J Med* 318, 869 (63%)
Exfoliative dermatitis
(1988): Brandt SJ+, *N Engl J Med* 318, 869 (10%)
Flushing (>10%)
(2000): Khoury H+, *Bone Marrow Transplant* 25, 1197
Folliculitis
(1992): Ostlere LS+, *Br J Dermatol* 127, 193
Linear IgA bullous dermatosis
(1999): Kano Y+, *Eur J Dermatol* 9, 122
Neutrophilic eccrine hidradenitis
(1998): Bachmeyer C+, *Br J Dermatol* 139, 354
Panniculitis, necrotizing
(2000): Dereure O+, *Br J Dermatol* 142, 834
Peripheral edema (1–10%)
Pruritus
(1990): Farmer KL+, *Arch Dermatol* 126, 1243
(1990): Steward WP+, *Int J Cell Cloning* 8, 335
(1989): Steward WP+, *Br J Cancer* 59, 142 (1–5%)
Psoriasis
(1998): Cho SG+, *J Korean Med Sci* 13, 685
(1996): Kavanaugh A, *Am J Med* 101, 567
Pyoderma gangrenosum
(1998): Merkel PA, *Curr Opin Rheumatol* 10, 45
(1991): Ross HJ+, *Cancer* 68, 441
Rash (sic)
Urticaria
Vasculitis
(1999): Andavolu MV+, *Ann Hematol* 78, 79
(1998): Merkel PA, *Curr Opin Rheumatol* 10, 45
(1995): Farhey YD+, *J Rheumatol* 22, 1179
(1995): Vidarsson B+, *Am J Med* 98, 589
(1995): Couderc LJ+, *Respir Med* 89, 237
(1994): Jain KK, *J Am Acad Dermatol* 31, 213
(1994): Johnson ML+, *Arch Dermatol* 130, 77
(1990): Farmer KL+, *Arch Dermatol* 126, 1243
(1989): Kluin-Nelemans JC+, *Br J Haematol* 73, 419

Hair

Hair – alopecia (>10%)
(1990): Lazarus H+, *Proc Am Soc Clin Oncol* 9, 15

Other

Anaphylactoid reaction (<1%)
(2000): Khoury H+, *Bone Marrow Transplant* 25, 1197
(1999): Dupre D+, *Ann Dermatol Venereol* (French) 126, 161
(1999): Keung YK+, *Bone Marrow Transplant* 23, 200
Injection-site bullous eruption
(1990): Farmer KL+, *Arch Dermatol* 126, 1243
Injection-site erythema
(1995): Scott GA, *Am J Dermatopathol* 17, 107
Injection-site lichenoid reaction
(1999): Viallard AM+, *Dermatology* 198, 301
Injection-site nodules
(1990): Farmer KL+, *Arch Dermatol* 126, 1243
Injection-site pain (1–10%)
Injection-site pruritus
(1990): Farmer KL+, *Arch Dermatol* 126, 1243
Injection-site urticaria
(1995): Scott GA, *Am J Dermatopathol* 17, 107
Lymphoproliferative disease
(1994): Kawach Y+, *Leukemia and Lymphoma* 13, 509
(1994): De la Rubia J+, *Bone Marrow Transplantation* 14, 475
Mucositis
(1999): Crawford J+, *Cytokines Cell Mol Ther* 5, 187
Myalgia (>10%)
Oral mucosal lesions
(1990): Lazarus H+, *Proc Am Soc Clin Oncol* 9, 15
Stomatitis (>10%)

GREPAFLOXACIN*

Trade name: Raxar (GlaxoWellcome)
Indications: Various infections caused by susceptible organisms
Category: Fluoroquinolone antibiotic
Half-life: 5–12 hours
Clinically important, potentially serious interactions with: antacids, antidiabetics, caffeine, cimetidine, cisapride, cyclophosphamide, cyclosporine, iron, loop diuretics, NSAIDs, omeprazole, propranolol, tacrine, theophylline, warfarin

Reactions

Skin

Acne (<1%)
Balanitis (<1%)
Cheilitis (<1%)
Diaphoresis (<1%)
Edema (<1%)
Exanthems (<1%)
Exfoliative dermatitis (<1%)
Facial edema (<1%)
Fungal dermatitis (sic) (<1%)
Herpes simplex (<1%)
Peripheral edema (<1%)
Photosensitivity
(1997): Ferguson J+, *J Antimicrob Chemother* 40, 93
(1997): Stahlmann R+, *J Antimicrob Chemother* 40, 83
Phototoxic reactions (2%)
(2000): Traynor NJ+, *Toxicol Vitr* 14, 275
(1998): Lode H, *Infect Med* 15 (Suppl 1), 28
Pruritus (<1%)
Rash (sic) (1.9%)
(1998): Lode H, *Infect Med* 15 (Suppl 1), 28
(1997): Stahlmann R+, *J Antimicrob Chemother* 40, 83
Toxic epidermal necrolysis (<1%)
Urticaria (<1%)
Vesiculobullous eruption (<1%)
Xerosis (<1%)

Hair

Hair – alopecia (<1%)

Other

Ageusia (<1%)
Bromhidrosis (<1%)
Dysgeusia (17%) (metallic taste)
(1998): Lode H, *Infect Med* 15 (Suppl 1), 28
(1998): Chodosh S+, *Antimicrob Agents Chemother* 42, 114
(1997): Stahlmann R+, *J Antimicrob Chemother* 40, 83
Gingivitis (<1%)
Glossitis (<1%)
Hypersensitivity
Hypesthesia (<1%)
Myalgia (<1%)
Oral candidiasis (<1%)
Oral ulceration (<1%)
Paresthesias (<1%)
Parosmia (<1%)
Stomatitis (<1%)
Tendinitis
Tendon rupture
Tongue disorder (sic) (<1%)
Tongue edema (<1%)
Tongue pigmentation (<1%)
Vaginitis (3.3%)
Xerostomia (1.1%)

***Note:** Grepafloxacin has been withdrawn in the USA

GRISEOFULVIN

Trade names: Fulvicin (Schering); Grifulvin V (Ortho); Grisactin (Wyeth-Ayerst); Gris-PEG (Allergan)
Other common trade names: *Fulcin; Fulvina P/G; Grisefuline; Griseostatin; Grisovin; Likudin M; Polygris*
Indications: Fungal infections of the skin, hair and nails
Category: Antifungal
Half-life: 9–24 hours
Clinically important, potentially serious interactions with: alcohol, anticoagulants, barbiturates, cyclosporine, estrogens, oral contraceptives, primidone, salicylates, warfarin

Reactions

Skin

Allergic reactions (sic) (1–5%)
(1971): *Med Lett* 13, 55
Angioedema (<1%)
(1994): Gupta AK+, *J Am Acad Dermatol* 30, 677 (passim)
(1989): Rustin MHA+, *Br J Dermatol* 120, 455
(1961): Goldblatt S, *Arch Dermatol* 83, 936
Angular stomatitis
(1994): Gupta AK+, *J Am Acad Dermatol* 30, 677 (passim)
Bullous eruption (<1%)
(1995): Meffert JJ+, *Cutis* 56, 279
(1960): O'Farrell NM, *Arch Dermatol* 82, 424
Candidiasis
(1972): Bessiere L, *Bull Soc Fr Dermatol Syphiligr* (French) 79, 560
Cold urticaria
(1989): Rustin MHA+, *Br J Dermatol* 120, 455
(1965): Chang T, *JAMA* 193, 848
Erythema multiforme (<1%)
(1994): Gupta AK+, *J Am Acad Dermatol* 30, 677 (passim)
(1990): Almeida L+, *J Am Acad Dermatol* 23, 855
(1989): Rustin MHA+, *Br J Dermatol* 120, 455
(1981): Walinga H+, *Ned Tijdschr Geneeskd* (Dutch) 125, 729
(1961): Sternberg TH+, *Med Clin North Am* 45, 781
Exanthems
(1997): Litt JZ, Beachwood, OH, personal case (observation in a 10-year-old boy)
(1994): Gupta AK+, *J Am Acad Dermatol* 30, 677 (passim)
(1993): Gaudin JL+, *Gastroenterol Clin Biol* 17, 145
(1992): Breathnach SM+, *Adverse Drug Reactions and the Skin*, Blackwell, Oxford, 169 (passim)
(1989): Miyagawa S+, *Am J Med* 87, 100
(1972): Von Pohler M+, *Dermatol Monatsschr* (German) 158, 383
Exfoliative dermatitis
(1989): Rustin MHA+, *Br J Dermatol* 120, 455
(1964): Reaves LE, *J Am Geriatr Soc* 12, 889
Fixed eruption (<1%)
(1994): Gupta AK+, *J Am Acad Dermatol* 30, 677 (passim)
(1989): Rustin MHA+, *Br J Dermatol* 120, 455
(1989): Boudghene-Stambouli O+, *Dermatologica* 179, 92
(1984): Feinstein A+, *J Am Acad Dermatol* 10, 915
(1981): Thyagarajan K+, *Mykosen* (German) 24, 482
(1977): Savage J, *Br J Dermatol* 97, 107
Flushing
(1992): Shelley WB+, *Advanced Dermatologic Diagnosis*, WB Saunders, 582 (passim)
Hemorrhagic eruption (sic)
(1992): Breathnach SM+, *Adverse Drug Reactions and the Skin*, Blackwell, Oxford, 169 (passim)
Herpes zoster
(1969): Chistiakov AM, *Vestn Dermatol Venerol* (Russian) 43, 76
Hypohidrosis
(1986): Duvanel T, *Ann Dermatol Venereol* (French) 113, 471
Jarisch–Herxheimer reaction
(1993): Amita DB+, *Clin Exp Dermatol* 18, 389
Leprosy (exacerbation)
(1982): Shulman DG+, *Arch Dermatol* 118, 909
Lichenoid eruption
(1994): Gupta AK+, *J Am Acad Dermatol* 30, 677 (passim)
(1961): Sternberg TH+, *Med Clin North Am* 45, 781
Lupus erythematosus
(1995): Bonilla-Felix M+, *Pediatr Nephrol* 9, 478
(1994): Gupta AK+, *J Am Acad Dermatol* 30, 677 (passim)
(1990): Okazaki H+, *Ryumachi* (Japanese) 30, 418
(1989): Miyagawa S+, *Am J Med* 87, 100
(1989): Miyagawa S+, *J Am Acad Dermatol* 21, 343
(1985): Madhok R+, *BMJ* 291, 249 (fatal)
(1976): Watsky MS+, *Cutis* 17, 361
(1968): Shinskii GE+, *Sov Med* (Russian) 31, 92
(1966): Lee SL+, *Arch Intern Med* 117, 620
(1966): Anderson W+, *J Med Soc N J* 63, 161
(1963): Steagall RW, *Arch Dermatol* 88, 218
(1962): Alexander S, *Br J Dermatol* 74, 72
Mucocutaneous lymph node syndrome (Kawasaki syndrome)
Petechiae
(1994): Gupta AK+, *J Am Acad Dermatol* 30, 677 (passim)
(1960): Smith NG, *Arch Dermatol* 81, 981
Photosensitivity (1–10%)
(1994): Gupta AK+, *J Am Acad Dermatol* 30, 677 (passim)
(1989): Rustin MHA+, *Br J Dermatol* 120, 455
(1989): Miyagawa S+, *Am J Med* 87, 100
(1989): Kojima K+, *J Dermatol* (Tokio) 15, 76
(1988): Kojima T+, *J Dermatol* 15, 76
(1988): Kawabe Y+, *Photodermatol* 5, 272
(1986): Ljunggren B+, *Photodermatol* 3, 26
(1983): Hawk JLM, *Clin Exp Dermatol* 9, 300
(1977): Martins JE+, *Rev Hosp Clin Fac Med Sao Paulo* (Portuguese) 32, 1
(1976): Jarratt M, *Int J Dermatol* 15, 317
(1972): Gotz H, *Arch Dermatol Forsch* (German) 244, 391
(1969): Kalivas J, *JAMA* 209, 1706
(1967): Tarsitani F+, *Policlinico Prat* (Italian) 74, 329
(1966): Kobori T+, *J Asthma Res* 3, 213
(1965): Chang T, *JAMA* 193, 848
(1961): Lamb JH+, *Arch Dermatol* 83, 568
(1961): Sternberg TH+, *Med Clin North Am* 45, 781
(1960): Quero R, *J Invest Dermatol* 34, 283
Pigmentation
(1968): Vollum DI, *Trans St Johns Hosp Dermatol Soc* 54, 204
(1964): Durand P+, *Minerva Med* (Italian) 55, 2422
Pityriasis rosea
Pruritus (<1%)
(1994): Gupta AK+, *J Am Acad Dermatol* 30, 677 (passim)
(1989): Rustin MHA+, *Br J Dermatol* 120, 455
(1960): Smith NG, *Arch Dermatol* 81, 981
(1960): Quero R, *J Invest Dermatol* 34, 283
Purpura
(1967): Lockey SD, *Med Sci* 18, 43
Rash (sic) (>10%)
Seborrheic dermatitis
(1962): Brodthagen H, *Acta Derm Venereol* (Stockh) 42, 345
Stevens–Johnson syndrome
(1989): Rustin MHA+, *Br J Dermatol* 120, 455
(1981): Walinga H+, *Ned Tijdschr Geneeskd* (Dutch) 125, 729
(1973): Belkin BG+, *Vestn Dermatol Venerol* (Russian) 47, 61
Toxic epidermal necrolysis
(1991): Correia O+, *Ann Fr Anesth Reanim* (French) 10, 493
(1990): Mion G+, *Ann Fr Anesth Reanim* (French) 9, 305 (fatal)
(1989): Mion G+, *Lancet* 2, 1331 (fatal)
(1988): Taylor B+, *J Am Acad Dermatol* 19, 565
Urticaria (>10%)
(1989): Rustin MHA+, *Br J Dermatol* 120, 455
(1984): Feinstein A+, *J Am Acad Dermatol* 10, 915
(1963): Fisher AA, *Arch Dermatol* 87, 660
(1963): Driscoll BJO, *BMJ* 2, 503
(1961): Goldblatt S, *Arch Dermatol* 83, 936
Vasculitis
(1994): Gupta AK+, *J Am Acad Dermatol* 30, 677 (passim)
(1970): Livingood CS+, *Cutis* 6, 1346

Nails

Nails – yellow
(1986): Duvanel T, *Ann Dermatol Venereol* (French) 113, 471
Nails – subungual hemorrhages

Other

Acute intermittent porphyria
(1965): Berman A+, *JAMA* 192, 1005

Anaphylactoid reaction
(1977): Fel'ker Ala+, *Vestn Dermatol Venerol* (Russian) February, 78
Black tongue
(1994): Gupta AK+, *J Am Acad Dermatol* 30, 677 (passim)
Dysgeusia
(1995): Hofmann H+, *Arch Dermatol* 131, 919
(1994): Gupta AK+, *J Am Acad Dermatol* 30, 677 (passim)
(1971): Fogan L, *Ann Intern Med* 74, 795
Glossodynia
(1994): Gupta AK+, *J Am Acad Dermatol* 30, 677 (passim)
Gynecomastia
(1994): Gupta AK+, *J Am Acad Dermatol* 30, 677 (passim)
(1968): Vollum DI, *Trans St Johns Hosp Dermatol Soc* 54, 204
Hypogeusia
(1971): Fogan L, *Ann Intern Med* 74, 795
Oral candidiasis (1–10%)
(1994): Gupta AK+, *J Am Acad Dermatol* 30, 677 (passim)
Paresthesias
(1994): Gupta AK+, *J Am Acad Dermatol* 30, 677 (passim)
Porphyria
(1980): Smith AG+, *Clin Haematol* 9, 399
(1969): Kalivas J, *JAMA* 209, 1706
(1968): Watson CJ+, *Arch Dermatol* 98, 451
(1967): Lochhead AC+, *Br J Dermatol* 79, 96
(1966): Ziprowski L+, *Arch Dermatol* 93, 21
(1965): Berman A+, *JAMA* 192, 1005
(1964): Redeker AG+, *JAMA* 188, 466
(1963): Editorial, *Lancet* 1, 870
(1963): Rimington C+, *Lancet* 2, 318
Porphyria cutanea tarda
(1970): Thiers H+, *Arch Belg Dermatol Syphiligr* (French) 26, 463
Protoporphyria
(1990): Gederaas OA+, *Photodermatol Photoimmunol Photomed* 7, 82
(1983): Poh-Fitzpatrick MB+, *J Clin Invest* 72, 1449
(1970): Perrot H+, *Experientia* (French) 26, 256
Serum sickness
(1994): Gupta AK+, *J Am Acad Dermatol* 30, 677 (passim)
(1989): Rustin MHA+, *Br J Dermatol* 120, 455
Stomatodynia
Xerostomia
(1994): Gupta AK+, *J Am Acad Dermatol* 30, 677 (passim)

GUANABENZ

Trade name: Wytensin (Wyeth-Ayerst)
Other common trade names: *Rexitene; Wytens*
Category: $Alpha_2$ adrenergic agonist, antihypertensive
Half-life: 7–10 hours
Clinically important, potentially serious interactions with: nadalol, propranolol, timolol, tricyclic antidepressants

Reactions

Skin
Edema (<3%)
Hyperhidrosis
Pruritus (<3%)
Rash (sic) (<3%)

Other
Dysgeusia (<3%)
Gynecomastia (<3%)
Sialorrhea
Xerostomia (28%)
(1988): Bork K, *Cutaneous Side Effects of Drugs*, WB Saunders, 307

GUANADREL

Trade name: Hylorel (Medeva)
Indications: Hypertension
Category: Adrenergic blocking agent, antihypertensive
Half-life: 5–45 hours (terminal)
Clinically important, potentially serious interactions with: alpha-blockers, beta-blockers, epinephrine, MAO inhibitors, phenothiazines, tricyclic antidepressants, vasodilators

Reactions

Skin
Peripheral edema (28.6%)

Other
Glossitis (8.4%)
Paresthesias (25.1%)
Xerostomia (1.7%)

GUANETHIDINE

Trade name: Ismelin (Novartis)
Other common trade names: *Apo-Guanethidine; Ismeline*
Indications: Hypertension
Category: $Alpha_2$ adrenergic agonist, antihypertensive
Half-life: 5–10 days
Clinically important, potentially serious interactions with: epinephrine, MAO inhibitors, minoxidil, phenothiazines, tricyclic antidepressants

Reactions

Skin
Dermatitis (sic)
Exanthems
Fixed eruption
(1966): Rastogi SK, *J Indian Med Assoc* 47, 31
Lupus erythematosus
Peripheral edema (>10%)
Purpura
Urticaria
Vasculitis
(1964): Dewar HA+, *BMJ* 2, 609 (polyarteritis nodosa?)

Hair
Hair – alopecia

Other
Glossitis (5%)
Myalgia
Paresthesias (16%)
Priapism
Sialorrhea
Xerostomia (1–10%)

GUANFACINE

Trade name: Tenex (Robins)
Other common trade names: *Entulic; Estulic*
Indications: Hypertension
Category: $Alpha_2$ adrenergic agonist, antihypertensive
Half-life: 10–30 hours
Clinically important, potentially serious interactions with: barbiturates, nadolol, phenytoin, propranolol, timolol, tricyclic antidepressants

Reactions

Skin

Dermatitis (sic) (<3%)
Diaphoresis (<3%)
(1991): Wilson MF+, *J Clin Pharmacol* 31, 318
(1990): Mosqueda-Garcia R, *Am J Med Sci* 299, 73
(1986): Sorkin EM+, *Drugs* 31, 301 (3%)
Edema
Exanthems
Exfoliative dermatitis
Peripheral edema
(1991): Oster JR+, *Arch Intern Med* 151, 1638
Pruritus (<3%)
(1991): Wilson MF+, *J Clin Pharmacol* 31, 318
Purpura (<3%)
Rash (sic)
(1990): Lewin A+, *J Clin Pharmacol* 30, 1081
Urticaria

Hair

Hair – alopecia

Other

Dysgeusia (<3%)
(1988): Cornish LA, *Clin Pharm* 7, 187
Paresthesias (<3%)
Sialorrhea
Xerostomia (47%)
(1991): Wilson MF+, *J Clin Pharmacol* 31, 318
(1990): Lewin A+, *J Clin Pharmacol* 30, 1081
(1990): Mosqueda-Garcia R, *Am J Med Sci* 299, 73
(1988): Board AW+, *Clin Ther* 10, 761
(1988): Cornish LA, *Clin Pharm* 7, 187
(1988): Van Zweiten PA, *Am J Cardiol* 61, 6D

HALOPERIDOL

Trade name: Haldol (Ortho-McNeil)
Other common trade names: *Dozic; Duraperidol; Haloper; Peridol; Seranace; Serenace*
Indications: Psychoses, Tourette's disorder
Category: Phenothiazine, antipsychotic and sedative
Half-life: 20 hours
Clinically important, potentially serious interactions with: alcohol, carbamazepine, CNS depressants, epinephrine, lithium, phenytoin, propranolol, quinidine, tricyclic antidepressants, **cigarette smoking**

Reactions

Skin
Acne
Cellulitis
(1982): Sacks HS, *Hosp Pract Off Ed* 17, 179
Contact dermatitis (<1%)
Diaphoresis
Exanthems
Exfoliative dermatitis
Flushing
(1972): Meyler L+, *Side Effects of Drugs Annual* 7, Excerpta Medica, Amsterdam
Parkinsonism (pseudo)
Photosensitivity (<1%)
(1970): *Med Lett* 12, 104
(1964): Gerle B, *Acta Psychiatr Scand* 40, 65
Pigmentation (<1%)
Pruritus (<1%)
Purpura
Rash (sic) (<1%)
Seborrheic dermatitis
(1984): Binder RL+, *J Clin Psychiatry* 45, 125
(1983): Binder RL+, *Arch Dermatol* 119, 473
Urticaria

Hair
Hair – alopecia (<1%)
(2000): Mercke Y+, *Ann Clin Psychiatry* 12, 35
Hair – alopecia areata
(1994): Kubota T+, *Jpn J Psychiatry Neurol* 48, 579
(1993): Kubota T+, *Acta Neurol Napoli* 15, 200 (3 cases)
Hair – depigmentation
(1964): Simpson GM+, *Clin Pharmacol Ther* 5, 310 (graying and fading)

Other
Galactorrhea (<1%)
Gynecomastia (<1%)
Injection-site hypersensitivity
(1992): Hay J, *J Clin Psychiatry* 53, 256
Injection-site pain and itching
(1990): Hamann GL+, *J Clin Psychiatry* 51, 502
Injection-site reactions
(1995): Maharaj K+, *J Clin Psychiatry* 56, 172
(1992): Reinke M+, *J Clin Psychiatry* 53, 415
(1990): Hamann GL+, *J Clin Psychiatry* 51, 502
Mastodynia
Priapism (<1%)
Sialorrhea
Xerostomia (<1%)

HALOTHANE

Trade name: Fluothane (Wyeth-Ayerst)
Other common trade names: *Halothan; Trothane*
Indications: Induction and maintenance of general anesthesia
Category: Anesthetic
Half-life: no data
Clinically important, potentially serious interactions with: beta-blockers, phenytoin, rifampin, xanthines

Reactions

Skin
Acne
(1987): Guldager H, *Lancet* 1, 1211
(1973): Gomez SW, *Anesth Analg* 52, 861
(1973): Soper LE+, *Anesth Analg* 52, 125
Angioedema
(1988): Slegers-Karsmakers S+, *Anesthesia* 43, 506
Exanthems
(1988): Slegers-Karsmakers S+, *Anesthesia* 43, 506
Sensitivity (sic)
(1979): Bodman R, *Br J Anaesth* 51, 1092 (to vapors)
Urticaria
(1964): Cole WHJ, *Med J Aust* 2, 925

Hair
Hair – alopecia
(1990): Gollnick H+, *Z Haut* (German) 65, 1128

HEPARIN

Trade names: Hep-Flush (Wyeth-Ayerst); Hep-Lock (Elkins-Sinn); Liquaemin (Organon)
Other common trade names: *Calcilean; Calciparin; Caprin; Hepalean; Heparin-Leo; Heparine; Liquemin; Uniparin*
Indications: Venous thrombosis, pulmonary embolism
Category: Anticoagulant
Half-life: 1.5 hours
Clinically important, potentially serious interactions with: ACE-inhibitors, anticoagulants, aspirin, dextran, dipyridamole, ethacrynic acid, hydroxychloroquine, NSAIDs, probenecid, salicylates, valproic acid

Reactions

Skin
Allergic reactions (sic) (1–10%)
(1997): Hermes B+, *Acta Derm Venereol* 77, 35
(1972): Lebeaupin R+, *Anesth Analg* (Paris) (French) 29, 487
Angioedema (<1%)
Baboon syndrome
(1993): Herfs H+, *Hautarzt* (German) 44, 466
Burning (soles) (sic)
(1992): Breathnach SM+, *Adverse Drug Reactions and the Skin*, Blackwell,Oxford, 249 (passim)
Chills
Contact dermatitis
(1996): Boehncke WH+, *Contact Dermatitis* 35, 73
(1996): Koch P+, *Contact Dermatitis* 34, 1256
(1995): Krasovec M+, *Contact Dermatitis* 32, 135
(1992): Valsecchi R+, *Contact Dermatitis* 26, 129
(1988): Young E, *Contact Dermatitis* 19, 152
Ecchymoses
(1985): Tuneu A+, *J Am Acad Dermatol* 12, 1072
(1979): Stavorovsky M+, *Dermatologica* 158, 451
Erythema
Erythematous plaques (sic)
Exanthems
(1996): Warkentin TE, *Br J Haematol* 92, 494
(1994): Greiner D+, *Hautarzt* (German) 45, 569

Fixed eruption
(1995): Mohammed KN, *Dermatology* 190, 91
Hemorrhage
(1992): Breathnach SM+, *Adverse Drug Reactions and the Skin*, Blackwell, Oxford, 249 (passim)
(1986): Levine M+, *Semin Thromb Hemost* 12, 39
Livedo reticularis
(1993): Gross AS+, *Int J Dermatol* 32, 276
Necrosis
(1997): Schechter FG, *N Engl J Med* 336, 589
(1997): Carter RL, *N Engl J Med* 336, 589
(1997): Kumar PD, *N Engl J Med* 336, 588
(1997): McCloskey RV, *N Engl J Med* 336, 588
(1997): Libow LF+, *Cutis* 59, 242
(1996): Whitmore SE+, *Arch Dermatol* 132, 341
(1996): Christiaens GC+, *N Engl J Med* 335, 715
(1995): Balestra B, *Schweiz Med Wochenschr* (German) 125, 361
(1994): Griffin JP, *Adverse Drug React Toxicol Rev* 13, 157
(1994): Leblanc M+, *Nephron* 68, 133
(1994): Yoon TY+, *Ann Dermatol* 6, 74
(1994): Peluso AM+, *Eur J Dermatol* 4, 127
(1993): Yates P+, *Clin Exp Dermatol* 18, 138
(1993): Warkentin TE+, *Am J Med* 95, 662
(1993): Humphries JE, *Acta Haematol* 90, 52
(1992): Calzavara-Pinton PG+, *EJD* 2, 171
(1992): Thomas D+, *Chest* 102, 1578
(1992): Soundararajan R+, *Am J Med* 93, 467
(1991): Ritchie AJ+, *Ulster Med J* 60, 248
(1991): Humphries JE+, *Am J Kidney Dis* 17, 233
(1990): Adcock DM+, *Semin Thromb Hemost* 16, 283
(1990): Fowlie J+, *Postgrad Med J* 66, 573
(1990): Bircher AJ+, *Br J Dermatol* 123, 507 (passim)
(1989): Rongioletti F+, *Dermatologica* 178, 47
(1989): Vinti H+, *Presse Med* (French) 18, 128
(1989): Armengol R+, *Med Clin (Barc)* (Spanish) 93, 699
(1989): Diem E, *Hautarzt* (German) 40, 239
(1988): Hartman AR+, *J Vasc Surg* 7, 781
(1988): Cohen GR+, *Obstet Gynecol* 73, 498
(1987): Jones BF+, *Australas J Dermatol* 28, 117
(1987): Alegre A+, *Med Clin (Barc)* (Spanish) 88, 170
(1987): Jones BF+, *Australas J Dermatol* 28, 117
(1986): Lim KB+, *Singapore Med J* 27, 356
(1985): Barthelemy H+, *Ann Dermatol Venereol* (French) 112, 245
(1985): Tuneu A+, *J Am Acad Dermatol* 12, 1072
(1984): Monreal M+, *Lancet* 2, 820
(1984): Nodel'son SE+, *Ter Arkh* (Russian) 56, 118
(1984): Mathieu A+, *Ann Dermatol Venereol* (French) 111, 733
(1984): Hasegawa GR, *Drug Intell Clin Pharm* 18, 313
(1984): Ulrick PJ+, *Med J Aust* 140, 287
(1983): Jehn U+, *Dtsch Med Wochenschr* (German) 108, 1148
(1983): Levine LE+, *Arch Dermatol* 119, 400
(1982): Isaacs P+, *Br Med J Clin Res Ed* 284, 201
(1982): No Author, *Am J Hosp Pharm* 39, 412
(1982): Shelley WB+, *J Am Acad Dermatol* 7, 674
(1981): Jackson AM+, *Br Med J Clin Res Ed* 283, 1087
(1981): Kelly RA+, *JAMA* 246, 1582
(1981): Berkessy S+, *Orv Hetil* (Hungarian) 122, 3075
(1980): Hall JC+, *JAMA* 244, 1831
(1979): White PW+, *Ann Surg* 190, 595
Peripheral edema
(1993): Phillips JK+, *Br J Haematol* 84, 349
Petechiae
(1979): Stavorovsky M+, *Dermatologica* 158, 451
Pruritus (<1%)
Purpura (>10%)
Rash (sic)
Scleroderma
(1985): Barthelemy H+, *Ann Dermatol Venereol* (French) 112, 245
Skin lesions (sic)
(1996): Warkentin TE, *Br J Haematology* 92, 494
Toxic dermatitis (sic)
(1996): Gallais V+, *Presse Med* (French) 25, 1040
Toxic epidermal necrolysis
(1991): Lemziakov TG+, *Vrach Delo* (Ukrainian) November, 113
(1985): Leung A, *JAMA* 253, 201
Urticaria (<1%)
(1992): Breathnach SM+, *Adverse Drug Reactions and the Skin*, Blackwell, Oxford, 249 (passim)
(1990): Bircher AJ+, *Br J Dermatol* 123, 507 (passim)
(1975): Hancock BW+, *BMJ* 3, 746
(1964): Zinn WJ, *Am J Cardiol* 14, 36
(1962): Rajka G+, *Acta Derm Venereol* (Stockh) 42, 27
Vasculitis
(1989): Guillet G+, *J Am Acad Dermatol* 20, 1130
(1989): Korstanje MJ+, *Contact Dermatitis* 20, 283
(1982): Kearsley JH+, *Aust N Z J Med* 12, 288
(1979): Ranft K+, *Med Welt* (German) 30, 1489
(1979): Stavorovsky M+, *Dermatologica* 158, 451

Hair

Hair – alopecia
(1980): Jaques LB, *Pharmacol Rev* 31, 99
(1969): Baker H+, *Br J Dermatol* 81, 236

Nails

Nails – discoloration of lunulae

Other

Anaphylactoid reaction
(1992): Breathnach SM+, *Adverse Drug Reactions and the Skin*, Blackwell, Oxford, 249 (passim)
(1990): Bircher AJ+, *Br J Dermatol* 123, 507 (passim)
Gingival bleeding (>10%)
Hypersensitivity
(2000): Koch P+, *J Am Acad Dermatol* 42, 612
(1995): Sanders MN+, *Int J Dermatol* 34, 443
(1994): Patriarca G+, *Allergy* 49, 292
(1993): Dupin N+, *Ann Dermatol Venereol* (French) 120, 845
(1993): O'Donnell BF+, *Br J Dermatol* 129, 634
(1992): de Kort WJ+, *Ned Tijdschr Geneeskd* (Dutch) 136, 2379
(1992): Manoharan A, *Eur J Haematol* 48, 234
(1991): Rivers JK+, *Aust N Z J Surg* 61, 865
(1989): Korstanje MJ+, *Contact Dermatitis* 20, 383
(1989): Patrizi A+, *Contact Dermatitis* 20, 309
(1973): Curry N+, *Arch Intern Med* 132, 744
Injection-site eczematous patches (<1%)
(2000): Koch P+, *J Am Acad Dermatol* 42, 612
(1995): Mathelier-Fusade P+, *Presse Med* (French) 24, 323
(1990): Bircher AJ+, *Br J Dermatol* 123, 507
(1993): Phillips JK+, *Br J Haematol* 84, 349 (erythema)
Injection-site hematoma
Injection-site induration
(1993): Phillips JK+, *Br J Haematol* 84, 349
(1989): Klein GF+, *J Am Acad Dermatol* 21, 703
(1989): Guillet G+, *J Am Acad Dermatol* 20, 1130
(1987): Mayou SC+, *Br J Dermatol* 117, 664
Injection-site necrosis (<1%)
(1995): Mar AW+, *Australas J Dermatol* 36, 201
(1988): Cohen GR+, *Obstet and Gyn* 72, 498
(1984): Hasegawa GR, *Drug Intell Clin Pharm* 18, 313
(1980): Hall JC+, *JAMA* 244, 1831
Injection-site plaques
(2000): Koch P+, *J Am Acad Dermatol* 42, 612
(1990): Bircher AJ+, *Br J Dermatol* 123, 507
Injection-site urticaria
(1995): Mathelier-Fusade P+, *Presse Med* (French) 24, 323
Priapism

HEROIN

Trade name: Heroin
Indications: Recreational drug
Category: Diacetylmorphine; a semisynthetic narcotic; substance abuse drug
Half-life: no data
Clinically important, potentially serious interactions with: no data

Reactions

Skin

Abscesses
(1990): Rasokat H, *Z Haut* (German) 65, 351
(1987): Muller F+, *Infection* 15, 201
(1987): Podzamczer D+, *J Am Acad Dermatol* 16, 386
(1984): O'Sullivan M+, *Ir Med J* 77, 68
(1980): Espiritu MB+, *Laryngoscope* 90, 1111 (neck)
(1979): Webb D+, *West J Med* 130, 200
(1971): Young AW+, *Arch Dermatol* 104, 80
Acanthosis nigricans
(1973): Young AW+, *Am Fam Physician* 7, 79
(1971): Young AW+, *Arch Dermatol* 104, 80
Acne
(1973): Young AW+, *Am Fam Physician* 7, 79
Angioedema
(1973): Young AW, *N Y State J Med* 73, 1681
Blistering (arms)
(1995): Mielke-Ibrahim R+, *Dtsch Med Wochenschr* (German) 120, 55
Bullous impetigo
(1973): Young AW, *N Y State J Med* 73, 1681
Candidiasis
(1987): Bielsa I+, *Int J Dermatol* 26, 314 (systemic)
(1987): Puig L+, *Int J Dermatol* 26, 257
(1985): Calandra T+, *Eur J Clin Microbiol* 4, 340 (disseminated)
Cellulitis
(1988): O'Rourke MG+, *Med J Aust* 148, 54
(1984): Alguire PC, *Cutis* 34, 93 (necrotizing of the scrotum)
(1975): Lewis RJ+, *JAMA* 232, 54
Contact dermatitis
(1973): Young AW+, *Am Fam Physician* 7, 79
Cutaneous side effects (sic) (85%)
Ecthyma
(1990): Rasokat H, *Z Haut* (German) 65, 351
Ecthyma gangrenosum
(1977): Mandell IN+, *Arch Dermatol* 113, 199
Edema
(1990): Rasokat H, *Z Haut* (German) 65, 351
(1973): Young AW+, *Am Fam Physician* 7, 79
(1973): McCabe WP+, *Plast Reconstr Surg* 52, 538
(1973): Young AW, *N Y State J Med* 73, 1681 (eyelids)
(1971): Young AW+, *Arch Dermatol* 104, 80
(1971): Weidman AJ+, *N Y State J Med* 71, 2643 (eyelids)
Exanthems
(1973): Young AW, *N Y State J Med* 73, 1681
(1970): Vollum DI, *BMJ* 2, 647
Excoriations
(1990): Rasokat H, *Z Haut* (German) 65, 351
Fixed eruption
(1983): Westerhof W+, *Br J Dermatol* 109, 605 (tongue)
(1973): Young AW, *N Y State J Med* 73, 1681
Folliculitis (candidal)
(1987): Cristobal-Rodriguez P+, *Med Cutan Ibero Lat Am* (Spanish) 15, 411
(1986): Darcis JM+, *Am J Dermatopathol* 8, 501 (with septicemia)
(1986): Leclerc G+, *Int J Dermatol* 25, 100
(1985): Calandra T+, *Eur J Clin Microbiol* 4, 340
Kaposi's sarcoma
(1986): Schofer H+, *Hautarzt* (German) 37, 159
Necrolytic migratory erythema
(1994): Bencini PL+, *Dermatology* 189, 72
Necrosis
(1990): Rasokat H, *Z Haut* (German) 65, 351
(1972): Dunne JH+, *Arch Dermatol* 105, 544
Necrotizing fasciitis
(1990): Rasokat H, *Z Haut* (German) 65, 351
Pemphigus
(1989): Civatte J, *Dermatol Monatsschr* (German) 175, 1
Pemphigus erythematosus
(1978): Fellner MJ+, *Int J Dermatol* 17, 308
Pemphigus vegetans
(1998): Downie JB+, *J Am Acad Dermatol* 39, 872
Perforating collagenosis
(1989): Bank DE+, *J Am Acad Dermatol* 21, 371
Photosensitivity
(1973): Young AW, *N Y State J Med* 73, 1681
(1971): Young AW+, *Arch Dermatol* 104, 80
Pigmentation
(1990): Rasokat H, *Z Haut* (German) 65, 351
(1973): Young AW+, *Am Fam Physician* 7, 79
(1973): Young AW, *N Y State J Med* 73, 1681 (photolocalized)
(1971): Young AW+, *Arch Dermatol* 104, 80 (photolocalized)
Polyarteritis nodosa
(1982): Ojeda E+, *Rev Clin Esp* (Spanish) 167, 275
Pruritus
(1990): Rasokat H, *Z Haut* (German) 65, 351
(1973): Young AW+, *Am Fam Physician* 7, 79
(1973): Young AW, *N Y State J Med* 73, 1681
(1971): Young AW+, *Arch Dermatol* 104, 80
(1970): Vollum DI, *BMJ* 2, 647
(1967): Minkin W+, *N Engl J Med* 277, 473
Purpura
(1973): Young AW+, *Am Fam Physician* 7, 79
Pustular eruption
(1993): Badillet G+, *Ann Dermatol Venereol* (French) 110, 691 (candidal)
(1992): Gallais V+, *Presse Med* (French) 21, 677 (candidal)
(1990): Altes J+, *Enferm Infecc Microbiol Clin* (Spanish) 8, 464
(1985): Cabre L+, *Med Clin (Barc)* (Spanish) 84, 542 (candidal)
(1984): Pinilla-Moraza J+, *Med Clin (Barc)* (Spanish) 83, 557
Toxic epidermal necrolysis
(1990): Llibre LM+, *Med Clin (Barc)* (Spanish) 94, 799
(1974): Lewis RJ, *JAMA* 230, 375
Ulceration
(1990): Rasokat H, *Z Haut* (German) 65, 351
(1990): Abidin MR+, *Ann Plast Surg* 24, 268
(1973): McCabe WP+, *Plast Reconstr Surg* 52, 538
(1971): Young AW+, *Arch Dermatol* 104, 80
Urticaria
(1990): Shaikh WA, *Allergy* 45, 555
(1973): Young AW, *N Y State J Med* 73, 1681
(1973): Young AW+, *Am Fam Physician* 7, 79
Vasculitis
(1984): Rosman JB+, *Neth J Med* 27, 50
(1979): Redmond WJ, *Arch Dermatol* 115, 111

Other

Dental decay
(1999): Fazzi M+, *Minerva Stomatol* (Italian) 48, 485
Hypersensitivity
(1990): Rasokat H, *Z Haut* (German) 65, 351
Injection-site scarring
(1990): Rasokat H, *Z Haut* (German) 65, 351
Injection-site ulceration
(1995): Hatton MQ+, *Clin Oncol R Coll Radiol* 7, 268
(1982): White WB+, *Cutis* 29, 63 (penis)
(1973): Bennett RG+, *Arch Dermatol* 107, 121
Myopathy
(1990): Shoji S, *Nippon Rinsho* (Japanese) 48, 1517
Necrotizing vasculitis (tongue)
(1995): Jurgensen O+, *Schweiz Monatsschr Zahnmed* (German; French) 105, 54
Oral mucosal ulceration (tongue)
(1983): Westerhof W+, *Br J Dermatol* 109, 605
Serum sickness
(1971): Weidman AJ+, *N Y State J Med* 71, 2643
Sweat gland necrosis
(1986): Rocamora A+, *J Dermatol* 13, 49
Tongue pigmentation (fixed eruption)
(1983): Westerhof W+, *Br J Dermatol* 109, 605

HYDRALAZINE

Trade names: Apresazide (Novartis); Apresoline (Novartis); Ser-Ap-Es (Novartis)
Other common trade names: *Alphapress; Apdormin; Apresolin; Novo-Hylazin; Nu-Hydral; Solesorin; Stable*
Indications: Hypertension
Category: Vasodilator; antihypertensive
Half-life: 3–7 hours
Clinically important, potentially serious interactions with: beta-blockers, diuretics, indomethacin, MAO inhibitors, metoprolol, NSAIDs, propranolol

Apresazide is hydralazine and hydrochlorothiazide; Ser-Ap-Es is hydralazine, reserpine and hydrochlorothiazide

Reactions

Skin

Acute febrile neutrophilic dermatosis (Sweet's syndrome)
(1995): Gilmour E+, *Br J Dermatol* 133, 490
(1991): Juanola X+, *J Rheumatol* 18, 948
(1990): Ramsay-Goldman R+, *J Rheumatol* 17, 682
(1987): Servitje O+, *Arch Dermatol* 123, 1436
(1986): Sequeira W+, *Am J Med* 81, 558
Allergic reactions (sic)
(1986): Bigby M+, *JAMA* 236, 3358
Angioedema (<1%)
Bullous eruption
(1988): Dodd HJ+, *Br J Dermatol* 119 (Suppl 33), 27
Chills
Diaphoresis
Edema (<1%)
Erythema nodosum
(1984): Peterson LL, *J Am Acad Dermatol* 10, 379
Exanthems
(1984): Schapel GJ, *Med J Aust* 141, 765
(1984): Peterson LL, *J Am Acad Dermatol* 10, 379
(1981): Finlay AY+, *BMJ* 282, 1703
(1967): Alarcon-Segovia D+, *Medicine* (Baltimore) 46, 1
Fixed eruption (<1%)
(1986): Sehgal VN+, *Int J Dermatol* 25, 394
Flushing (>10%)
(1967): Alarcon-Segovia D+, *Medicine* (Baltimore) 46, 1
Lupus erythematosus
(1998): Hari CK+, *J Laryngol Otol* 112, 875
(1997): Yung R+, *Arthritis Rheum* 40, 1436
(1996): Miyasaka N, *Intern Med* 35, 587
(1996): Pirmohamed M, *Hum Exp Toxicol* 15, 361
(1994): Nassberger L+, *Scand J Rheumatol* 23, 206
(1994): Cohen MG, *J Rheumatol* 21, 578
(1994): Hofstra AH, *Drug Metab Rev* 26, 485
(1992): Skaer TL, *Clin Ther* 14, 496
(1992): Yonga GO, *East Afr Med J* 69, 649
(1992): Rubin RL, *Clin Biochem* 25, 223
(1991): Alarcon-Segovia D+, *Baillieres Clin Rheumatol* 5, 1
(1991): Hess EV, *Curr Opin Rheumatol* 3, 809
(1991): Juanola X+, *J Rheumatol* 18, 948
(1990): Nassberger L+, *Clin Exp Immunol* 81, 380
(1990): Ramsay-Goldman R+, *J Rheumatol* 17, 682
(1990): Richards FM+, *Am J Med* 88, 56N
(1990): Mulder H, *Eur J Clin Pharmacol* 38, 303
(1989): Sim E, *Complement Inflamm* 6, 119
(1989): Mitchell JA+, *Clin Exp Immunol* 78, 354
(1989): Speirs C+, *Lancet* 1, 922
(1989): Fleming MG+, *Int J Dermatol* 28, 321 (bullous)
(1989): Palsson L+, *Clin Pharmacol Ther* 46, 177
(1989): Yemini M+, *Eur J Obstet Gynecol Reprod Biol* 30, 193
(1988): Sturman SG+, *Lancet* 2, 1304 (fatal)
(1988): Uetrecht JP, *Chem Res Toxicol* 1, 133
(1988): Chong WK+, *BMJ* 297, 660
(1988): Dodd HJ+, *Br J Dermatol* 119 (Suppl 33), 27
(1988): Jiang M, *Chung Kuo I Hsueh Yuan Hsueh Pao* (Chinese) 10, 379
(1987): Craft JE+, *Arthritis Rheum* 30, 689
(1987): Martinez-Vea A+, *Am J Nephrol* 7, 71
(1987): Servitje O+, *Arch Dermatol* 123, 1436
(1987): Andersson OK, *Eur J Clin Pharmacol* 31, 741
(1986): Asherson RA+, *Ann Rheum Dis* 45, 771
(1986): Innes A+, *Br J Rheumatol* 25, 225
(1986): Sequeira W+, *Am J Med* 81, 558
(1985): Stratton MA, *Clin Pharm* 4, 657
(1985): Lovisetto P+, *Recenti Prog Med* (Italian) 76, 110
(1985): Doherty M+, *Br Med J Clin Res Ed* 290, 675
(1985): Cush JJ+, *Am J Med Sci* 290, 36
(1985): Totoritis MC+, *Postgrad Med* 78, 149
(1985): Kale SA, *Postgrad Med* 77, 231
(1985): Epstein A+, *Arthritis Rheum* 28, 158
(1984): Christophidis N, *Lancet* 2, 868
(1984): No Author, *Lancet* 2, 441
(1984): Sim E+, *Lancet* 2, 422
(1984): Brand C+, *Lancet* 1, 462
(1984): Shapiro KS+, *Am J Kidney Dis* 3, 270
(1984): Ramsay LE+, *Br Med J Clin Res Ed* 289, 1310
(1984): Timbrell JA+, *Eur J Clin Pharmacol* 27, 555
(1984): French WJ, *Ala J Med Sci* 21, 427
(1984): Weiser GA+, *Arch Intern Med* 144, 2271
(1984): Naparstek Y+, *Arthritis Rheum* 27, 822
(1984): Wollina U, *Z Gesamte Inn Med* (German) 39, 69
(1984): Peterson LL, *J Am Acad Dermatol* 10, 379
(1984): Cameron HA+, *BMJ* 289, 410 (6.7%)
(1983): Shoenfeld Y+, *Br Med J Clin Res Ed* 286, 224
(1983): Macleod WN, *Scott Med J* 28, 181
(1982): Freestone S+, *Br Med J Clin Res Ed* 285, 1536
(1982): Harmon CE+, *Clin Rheum Dis* 8, 121
(1982): Ramsay LE+, *Br Med J Clin Res Ed* 284, 1711
(1982): Aylward PE+, *Aust N Z J Med* 12, 546
(1982): Ohe A+, *Osaka City Med J* 28, 149
(1982): Hess EV, *Arthritis Rheum* 25, 857
(1982): Mansilla-Tinoco R+, *BMJ* 284, 936
(1981): Reidenberg MM, *Arthritis Rheum* 24, 1004
(1981): Dubroff LM+, *Arthritis Rheum* 24, 1082
(1981): Sinclair AJ+, *Hum Toxicol* 1, 65
(1981): Neville E+, *Postgrad Med* 57, 378
(1981): Perry HM, *Arthritis Rheum* 24, 1093
(1981): Chisholm JC, *J Natl Med Assoc* 73, 278
(1980): Batchelor JR+, *Lancet* 1, 1107
(1980): Weinstein A, *Prog Clin Immunol* 4, 1
(1980): Harland SJ+, *BMJ* 281, 273
(1979): Ryan PF+, *Lancet* 2, 1248
(1979): Kissin MW+, *BMJ* 2, 1330
(1978): Jones WN+, *Ariz Med* 35, 16
(1978): Anderson B+, *JAMA* 239, 1392
(1978): Weinstein J, *Am J Med* 65, 553
(1976): Hess EV+, *Arthritis Rheum* 19, 122
(1976): Demay-Wechsler P, *Rev Stomatol Chir Maxillofac* (French) 77, 727
(1976): Berkowitz HS, *S Afr Med J* 50, 797
(1975): Lee SL+, *Semin Arthritis Rheum* 5, 83
(1975): Irias JJ, *Am J Dis Child* 129, 862
(1975): Johansson M+, *Lakartidningen* (Swedish) 72, 153
(1974): Blumenkrantz N+, *Acta Med Scand* 195, 443
(1973): Perry HM, *Am J Med* 54, 58 (12%)
(1973): Almeyda J+, *Br J Dermatol* 88, 313 (13%)
(1971): Alkalay I+, *Ann Allergy* 29, 35
(1967): Alarcon-Segovia D+, *Medicine* (Baltimore) 46, 1
(1966): White AB, *J Am Geriatr Soc*, 14, 361
(1963): Shulman LE+, *Arthritis Rheum* 6, 558 (1–3%)
Photosensitivity
(1967): Alarcon-Segovia D+, *Medicine* (Baltimore) 46, 1
Pruritus
(1984): Peterson LL, *J Am Acad Dermatol* 10, 379
Purpura
(1984): Peterson LL, *J Am Acad Dermatol* 10, 379
(1980): Petty R+, *BMJ* 280, 482
(1967): Alarcon-Segovia D+, *Medicine* (Baltimore) 46, 1
Pyoderma gangrenosum
(1984): Peterson LL, *J Am Acad Dermatol* 10, 379
Rash (sic) (<1%)
Sjøgren's syndrome
(1988): Darwaza A+, *Int J Oral Maxillopfac* 17, 92
Systemic eczematous contact dermatitis
(1964): van Ketel WG, *Acta Derm Venereol* (Stockh) 44, 49
Ulceration
(1980): Petty R+, *BMJ* 280, 482
(1980): Brooks AP+, *BMJ* 280, 482

Urticaria
Vasculitis
(1998): Merkel PA, *Curr Opin Rheumatol* 10, 45
(1993): Reynolds NJ+, *Br J Dermatol* 129, 82
(1982): Kincaid-Smith P+, *Lancet* 2, 348
(1981): Peacock A+, *BMJ* 282, 1121
(1981): Finlay AY+, *Br Med J Clin Res Ed* 282, 1703
(1980): Brooks AP+, *BMJ* 280, 482
(1980): Bernstein RM+, *BMJ* 280, 156

Other

Hypersensitivity
Myalgia
Oral ulceration
(1984): Peterson LL, *J Am Acad Dermatol* 10, 379
(1980): Brooks AP+, *BMJ* 280, 482
Orogenital ulceration
(1984): Peterson LL, *J Am Acad Dermatol* 10, 379
(1981): Neville E+, *Postgrad Med* 57, 378
Paresthesias
Relapsing polychondritis
(1983): Dahlqvist A+, *Acta Otolaryngol Stockh* 96, 355
Tremor

HYDROCHLOROTHIAZIDE

Trade names: Aldactazide; Aldoril; Apresazide; Avalide; Capozide; Dyazide; Esidrix; E-Zide; Hydro-Chlor; Hydro-D; Hydro-Par; HydroDIURIL; Maxzide; Microzide; Oretic; Prinizide; Ser-Ap-Es. (Various pharmaceutical companies.)
Other common trade names: *Apo-Hydro; Clothia; Dichlotride; Diu-Melsin; Diuchlor H; Esidrex; Hydrosaluric; Urozide*
Indications: Edema
Category: Thiazide diuretic*; antihypertensive
Half-life: 5.6–14.8 hours
Clinically important, potentially serious interactions with: allopurinol, amantadine, antidiabetics, bumetanide, diazoxide, digoxin, insulin, lithium, loop diuretics, methotrexate, NSAIDs, sulfonylureas, tetracyclines

Aldactazide is spironolactone and hydrochlorothiazide; Aldoril is methyldopa and hydrochlorothiazide; Avalide is irbesartan and hydrochlorothiazide; Capozide is captopril and hydrochlorothiazide; Dyazide is triamterene and hydrochlorothiazide; Maxzide is triamterene and hydrochlorothiazide; Moduretic is amiloride and hydrochlorothiazide; Prinizide is lisinopril and hydrochlorothiazide; Ser-Ap-Es is reserpine, hydralazine and hydrochlorothiazide

Reactions

Skin

Actinic reticuloid
(1985): Robinson HN+, *Arch Dermatol* 121, 522
Bullous eruption (<1%)
Dermatitis (sic)
(1984): Fisher RS+, *J Am Acad Dermatol* 11, 146
(1960): Smirk H+, *BMJ* 1, 515
Diaphoresis
(1979): Fan WJ+, *Pediatrics* 64, 698
Erythema annulare centrifugum
(1988): Goette DK+, *Int J Dermatol* 27, 129
(1973): Rekant SI+, *Arch Dermatol* 107, 424
Erythema multiforme (<1%)
(1985): Ting HC+, *Int J Dermatol* 24, 587
Exanthems
(1960): Smirk H+, *BMJ* 1, 515
Exfoliative dermatitis
Fixed eruption
(1985): Kauppinen K+, *Br J Dermatol* 112, 575
Lichenoid eruption
(1986): Halevy S+, *Ann Allergy* 56, 402
(1971): Almeyda J+, *Br J Dermatol* 85, 604
(1959): Harber LC+, *N Engl J Med* 261, 1378
(1959): Harber LC+, *J Invest Dermatol* 33, 83
Lupus erythematosus
(1998): Callen JP, Academy '98 Meeting (5 patients)
(1996): Litt JZ, Beachwood, OH, personal case (observation)
(1995): Rich MW+, *J Rheumatol* 22, 1001
(1993): Goodrich AL+, *J Am Acad Dermatol* 28, 1001
(1991): Wollenberg A+, *Hautarzt* (German) 42, 709
(1989): Parodi A+, *Photodermatology* 6, 100
(1989): Alanko K+, *Acta Derm Venereol* (Stockh) 69, 223
(1989): Fine RM, *Int J Dermatol* 28, 375 (Comment)
(1988): Darken M+, *J Am Acad Dermatol* 18, 38
(1985): Reed BR+, *Ann Intern Med* 103, 49
(1977): Weiss RB, *W V Med J* 73, 101
Photoreactions
(1994): Bielan B, *Dermatol Nurs* 6, 30
(1985): Reed BR+, *Ann Intern Med* 103, 49
(1965): Fellner MJ+, *Med Clin North Am* 49, 709
(1959): Harber LC+, *J Invest Dermatol* 33, 83
(1959): Harber LC+, *N Engl J Med* 261, 1378
Photosensitivity (<1%)
(1994): Shelley WB+, *Cutis* 53, 287 (observation)
(1994): Shelley WB+, *Cutis* 53, 77 (observation)
(1987): Addo HA+, *Br J Dermatol* 116, 749
(1985): Reed BR+, *Ann Intern Med* 103, 49
(1985): Robinson HN+, *Arch Dermatol* 121, 522
(1984): Ophir O+, *Harefuah* (Hebrew) 107, 14
(1983): White IR, *Contact Dermatitis* 9, 237
(1982): No Author, *Ugeskr Laeger* (Danish) 144, 1101
(1981): Journet M, *Union Med Can* 110, 356
(1980): Okrasinski H, *Lakartidningen* (Swedish) 77, 2718
(1980): Torinuki W, *J Dermatol* (Tokio) 7, 293
(1969): Kalivas J, *JAMA* 209, 1706
(1965): Jung EG+, *Int Arch Allergy Appl Immunol* 27, 313
(1959): Norins AL, *Arch Dermatol* 79, 592
(1959): Harber LC+, *J Invest Dermatol* 33, 83
(1959): Harber LC+, *N Engl J Med* 261, 1378
Phototoxic reaction
(1989): Diffey BL, *Arch Dermatol* 125, 1355
(1987): Addo HA+, *Br J Dermatol* 116, 749
(1982): Rosen K+, *Acta Derm Venereol* (Stockh) 62, 246
Porokeratosis (Mibelli)
(1984): Inamoto N+, *J Am Acad Dermatol* 11, 359
Pruritus (<1%)
(1992): Shelley WB+, *Cutis* 49, 391 (observation)
(1969): Kalivas J, *JAMA* 209, 1706
Purpura
(1980): Miescher PA+, *Clin Haematol* 9, 505
(1971): Eisner EW+, *JAMA* 215, 480
(1966): Smith JW+, *Ann Intern Med* 65, 629
(1963): Bettman JW, *Arch Intern Med* 112, 840
(1960): Ball P, *JAMA* 173, 663
(1960): Gesink MH+, *JAMA* 172, 556
Rash (sic)
(1976): Weisburst M+, *South Med J* 69, 126
Stevens–Johnson syndrome
(1978): Assaad D+, *Can Med Assoc* 118, 154
Systemic eczematous contact dermatitis
Toxic epidermal necrolysis
(1978): Assaad D+, *Can Med Assoc J* 118, 154
(1973): Björnberg A, *Acta Derm Venereol* (Stockh) 53, 149
Urticaria
(1960): Smirk H+, *BMJ* 1, 515
Vasculitis
(1989): Grunwald MH+, *Isr J Med Sci* 25, 572
(1965): Björnberg A+, *Lancet* 2, 982

Other

Dysgeusia
(2000): Zervakis J+, *Physiol Behav* 68, 405
Oral lichenoid eruption (erosive)
(1990): Espana A+, *Med Clin (Barc)* (Spanish) 94, 559
Paresthesias
Pseudoporphyria
(1990): Motley RJ, *BMJ* 300, 1468
Xanthopsia
Xerostomia

***Note:** Hydrochlorothiazide is a sulfonamide and can be absorbed systemically. Sulfonamides can produce severe, possibly fatal, reactions such as toxic epidermal necrolysis and Stevens–Johnson syndrome

HYDROCODONE*

Trade names: Bacomine, Ban-Tuss HC, Codamine, Duratuss, Hycodan, Hycomine, Hycophen, Hydromine, Hydrophen, Lorcet, Lortab, Morcomine, Propachem, Ru-Tuss, Tussgen, Tussionex, Tussogest, Vicodin, Vicoprofen, Zydone, etc. (Various pharmaceutical companies.)
Indications: Acute pain; coughing
Category: Narcotic analgesic and antitussive
Half-life: 3.8 hours
Clinically important, potentially serious interactions with: ACE-inhibitors, anticoagulants, aspirin, cimetidine, CNS depressants, lithium, MAO inhibitors, methotrexate, opiate agonists, tricyclic antidepressants

Reactions

Skin

Diaphoresis
Edema
Erythema multiforme
Exanthems
(2000): Litt JZ, Beachwood, OH, personal case (observation)
Flushing
Hot flashes
Pruritus (1–10%)
(2000): Litt JZ, Beachwood, OH, personal case (observation)
(1999): Litt JZ, Beachwood, OH, personal case (observation)
(1999): Sorkin MJ, Denver CO, (from Internet) (observation)
Rash (sic) (>10%)
Stevens–Johnson syndrome
Toxic epidermal necrolysis
Urticaria (>10%)

Other

Xerostomia

***Note:** Hydrocodone is included in many combination drugs. Other medications that can be included in these preparations include: phenylpropanolamine, phenylephrine, pyrilamine, pseudoephedrine, acetaminophen, ibuprofen, and others.

HYDROFLUMETHIAZIDE

Trade name: Diucardin (Wyeth-Ayerst)
Other common trade names: *Diademil; Hydravern; Hydrenox; Leodrine; Rivosil; Rontyl*
Indications: Hypertension, edema
Category: Thiazide* diuretic; antihypertensive
Duration of action: 12–24 hours
Clinically important, potentially serious interactions with: allopurinol, antidiabetics, diazoxide, digoxin, furosemide, lithium, loop diuretics, methyldopa, sulfonylureas

Reactions

Skin

Photosensitivity (<1%)
Purpura
Rash (sic) (<1%)
Urticaria
Vasculitis

Other

Dysgeusia
Paresthesias (<1%)
Xanthopsia

***Note:** Hydroflumethiazide is a sulfonamide and can be absorbed systemically. Sulfonamides can produce severe, possibly fatal, reactions such as toxic epidermal necrolysis and Stevens–Johnson syndrome.

HYDROMORPHONE

Trade name: Dilaudid (Knoll)
Other common trade names: *Dilaudid HP; HydroStat IR; Palladone*
Indications: Pain
Category: Narcotic analgesic; antitussive
Half-life: 1–3 hours
Clinically important, potentially serious interactions with: barbiturates, CNS depressants, cimetidine, MAO inhibitors, phenothiazines, ranitidine, tricyclic antidepressants

Reactions

Skin

Diaphoresis
Exanthems
(1992): de Cuyper C+, *Contact Dermatitis* 27, 220 (generalized)
Flushing (1–10%)
Pruritus (<1%)
(1992): Chaplan SR+, *Anesthesiology* 77, 1090 (11.5%)
Rash (sic) (<1%)
Urticaria (<1%)

Hair

Hair – alopecia

Other

Dysgeusia
Injection-site reactions
Paresthesias
Xerostomia (1–10%)

HYDROXYCHLOROQUINE

Trade name: Plaquenil (Sanofi)
Other common trade names: *Ercoquin; Oxiklorin; Plaquinol; Quensyl; Toremonil; Yuma*
Indications: Malaria, lupus erythematosus, rheumatoid arthritis
Category: Antimalarial, anti-lupus and antirheumatic
Half-life: elimination in blood: 50 days
Clinically important, potentially serious interactions with: cyclosporine, digoxin, penicillamine

Reactions

Skin

Acute generalized exanthematous pustulosis (AGEP)
(1996): Assier-Bonnet H+, *Dermatology* 193, 70
(1995): Bonnetblanc JM+, *Ann Dermatol Venereol* (French) 122, 604
(1995): Moreau A+, *Int J Dermatol* 34, 263 (passim)
(1993): Assier H+, *Ann Dermatol Venereol* (French) 120, 848
Angioedema (<1%)
Bullous eruption
(1995): Kutz DC+, *Arthritis Rheum* 38, 440
Contact dermatitis
(1999): Meier H+, *Hautarzt* (German) 50, 665
Dermatomyositis
(1994): Bloom BJ+, *J Rheumatology* 21, 2171
Erythema annulare centrifugum
(1985): Hudson LD, *J Am Acad Dermatol* 36, 129
(1982): Koralewski F, *Dermatosen* (German) 30, 125
(1967): Ashurst PJ, *Arch Dermatol* 95, 37
Erythema multiforme (<1%)
(1997): Rudolph R, Wyomissing, PA (from Internet) (observation)
Erythema nodosum
(1996): Jarrett P+, *Br J Dermatol* 134, 373 (chronic)
Erythroderma
(1990): Simoneaux PW, *Curr Concept Skin Dis* Winter, 15
(1985): Slagel GA+, *J Am Acad Dermatol* 12, 857
Exanthems (1–5%)
(1995): Blumenthal HL, Beachwood, OH, personal case (observation)

(1991): Ochsendorf FR+, *Hautarzt* (German) 42, 140
(1990): Simoneaux PW, *Curr Concept Skin Dis* Winter, 15
Exfoliative dermatitis
(1995): Blumenthal HL, Beachwood, OH, personal case (observation)
(1986): Lavrijsen APM+, *Acta Derm Venereol* (Stockh) 66, 536
(1985): Slagel GA+, *J Am Acad Dermatol* 12, 857
(1980): Koranda FC, *J Am Acad Dermatol* 4, 650 (passim)
Fixed eruption (<1%)
Lichenoid eruption
(1990): Simoneaux PW, *Curr Concept Skin Dis* Winter, 15
(1980): Koranda FC, *J Am Acad Dermatol* 4, 650 (passim)
(1958): Savage J, *Br J Dermatol* 70, 181
(1948): Alving AS+, *J Clin Invest* 27, 56
Photosensitivity
(2000): Ainsworth GE, Salina, KS (from Internet) (observation)
(1991): Ochsendorf FR+, *Hautarzt* (German) 42, 140
(1982): van Weelden H, *Arch Dermatol* 118, 290
(1981): Journet M, *Union Med Can* (French) 110, 356
Pigmentation (1–10%)
(1991): Ochsendorf FR+, *Hautarzt* (German), 42, 140
(1982): Levy H, *S Afr Med J* 2, 735
(1980): Koranda FC, *J Am Acad Dermatol* 4, 650 (passim)
(1963): Tuffanelli D+, *Arch Dermatol* 88, 419
(1959): Dall JLC+, *BMJ* 1, 1387
Polymorphous light eruption
(1968): Reed WB+, *Arch Dermatol* 98, 327
Pruritus (>10%)
(1999): Holme SA+, *Acta Derm Venereol* (Stockh) 79, 333
(1995): Blumenthal HL, Beachwood, OH, personal case (observation)
(1994): Fain O+, *Rev Med Interne* (French) 15, 433
(1991): Mnyika KS+, *J Trop Med Hyg* 94, 27 (47% incidence)
(1990): Abdulkadir SA+, *Trans Roy Soc Trop Med Hyg* 84, 898
(1990): Simoneaux PW, *Curr Concept Skin Dis* Winter, 15
(1984): Osifo NG, *Arch Dermatol* 120, 80
(1982): Spencer HC+, *BMJ* 285, 1703
(1969): Olatunde IA, *J Nigerian Med Assoc* 6, 23
(1964): Ekpechi OL+, *Arch Dermatol* 120, 80
Psoriasis (exacerbation)
(1993): Potter B, *Cutis* 52, 229 (passim)
(1988): Nicolas J-F+, *Ann Dermatol Venereol* (French) 115, 289
(1985): Gray RG, *J Rheumatol* 12, 391
(1982): Abel EA+, *J Am Acad Dermatol* 15, 2007
(1982): Luzar MJ, *J Rheumatol* 9, 462
(1981): Olsen TG, *Ann Intern Med* 94, 546
(1966): Baker H, *Br J Dermatol* 78, 161
(1957): Cornbleet T+, *Arch Dermatol* 75, 286
Purpura
Pustular eruption
(1990): Lotem M+, *Acta Derm Venereol* (Stockh) 70, 250
Pustular psoriasis
(1996): Vine JE+, *J Dermatol* 23, 357
(1987): Friedman SJ, *J Am Acad Dermatol* 16, 1256
Rash (sic) (1–10%)
Toxic epidermal necrolysis (<1%)
Urticaria
(1990): Simoneaux PW, *Curr Concept Skin Dis* Winter, 15
(1980): Koranda FC, *J Am Acad Dermatol* 4, 650 (passim)
Vasculitis

Hair

Hair – alopecia
Hair – discoloration
(1999): Lecocq P+, *Presse Med* (French) 28, 741
Hair – pigmentation (bleaching) (1–10%)
(1991): Ochsendorf FR+, *Hautarzt* (German) 42, 140
(1985): Dupré A+, *Arch Dermatol* 121, 1164
(1980): Koranda FC, *J Am Acad Dermatol* 4, 650 (passim)
(1978): Dubois EL, *Semin Arthritis Rheum* 8, 33
(1976): Sams WM, *Int J Dermatol* 15, 99
(1965): Rook A, *Br J Dermatol* 77, 115

Nails

Nails – discoloration
(1991): Zic JA+, *Arch Dermatol* 127, 1037
Nails – pigmentation
(1980): Koranda FC, *J Am Acad Dermatol* 4, 650 (passim)
(1963): Tuffanelli D+, *Arch Dermatol* 88, 419

Other

Dysgeusia
(1996): Weber JC+, *Presse Med* (French) 25, 213
Gingival pigmentation
(1992): Veraldi S+, *Cutis* 49, 281
Lymphoproliferative disease
(1980): Schechter SL+, *Arthritis Rheum* 23, 256
Myopathy
(1998): Richards AJ, *J Rheumatol* 25, 1642
(1969): Chapman RS+, *Br J Dermatol* 81, 217
Oral mucosal pigmentation
(1992): Veraldi S+, *Cutis* 49, 281
(1991): Zic JA+, *Arch Dermatol* 127, 1037
(1980): Koranda FC, *J Am Acad Dermatol* 4, 650 (passim)
(1971): Giansanti JS+, *Oral Surg* 31, 66
Oral mucosal ulceration
Porphyria
(1993): Potter B, *Cutis* 52, 229 (passim)
(1976): Baler GR, *Cutis* 17, 96
(1974): Kordac V+, *Br J Dermatol* 90, 95
(1962): Cripps DL+, *Arch Dermatol* 86, 575
(1959): Marsden CW, *Br J Dermatol* 71, 219
(1957): Davis MJ+, *Arch Dermatol* 75, 796
(1954): Linden IH+, *Calif Med* 81, 235
Stomatopyrosis

HYDROXYUREA

Trade names: Droxia (Bristol-Myers Squibb); Hydrea (Bristol-Myers Squibb)
Other common trade names: *Droxia; Litalir; Onco-Carbide*
Indications: Leukemia, malignant tumors
Category: Antineoplastic
Half-life: 3–4 hours
Clinically important, potentially serious interactions with: cytarabine, fluorouracil

Reactions

Skin

Acral erythema
(1993): Brincker H+, *Cancer Chemother Pharmacol* 32, 496 (edema and soreness)
(1992): Parodi A+, *G Ital Dermatol Venereol* (Italian) 127, 361 (fingers and toes)
(1991): Baack BR+, *J Am Acad Dermatol* 24, 457
(1989): Kampmann KK+, *Cancer* 63, 2482 (passim)
(1984): Sigal M+, *Ann Dermatol Venereol* (French) 111, 895 (band-like)
(1983): Silver FS+, *Ann Intern Med* 98, 675
Atrophy
(1997): Ena P+, *J Geriatr Dermatol* 5, 310
Baboon syndrome
(1999): Chowdhury MM+, *Clin Exp Dermatol* 24, 336
Band-like erythema
(1984): Sigal M+, *Ann Dermatol Venereol* (French) 111, 895 (fingers and toes)
Collodion-like skin
(1996): Gauthier O+, *Ann Dermatol Venereol (French)* 123, 727
Cutaneous side effects (sic)
(1998): Radaelli F+, *Am J Hematol* 58, 82
(1975): Kennedy BJ+, *Arch Dermatol* 111, 183 (35%)
(1973): Moschella SL+, *Arch Dermatol* 107, 363 (7%)
Dermatitis (sic) (dry, scaly)
(1984): Sigal M+, *Ann Dermatol Venereol* (French) 111, 895
(1975): Kennedy BJ+, *Arch Dermatol* 111, 183
Dermatomyositis
(2000): Kirby B+, *Clin Exp Dermatol* 25, 256
(1998): Suehiro M+, *Br J Dermatol* 139, 748
(1998): Velez A+, *Clin Exp Dermatol* 23, 94
(1997): Ena P+, *J Geriatr Dermatol* 5, 310
(1996): Bahadoran P+, *Br J Dermatol* 134, 1161
(1995): Senet P+, *Br J Dermatol* 133, 455
(1995): Weber L+, *Hautarzt* 46, 717

(1994): Kelly RI+, *Australas J Dermatol* 35, 61
(1994): Perrot JL+, *Ann Dermatol Venereol* (French) 121, 499
(1989): Richard M+, *J Am Acad Dermatol* 21, 797
(1984): Sigal M+, *Ann Dermatol Venereol* (French) 111, 895

Erythema multiforme (<1%)

Exanthems (1–10%)
(1992): Breathnach SM+, *Adverse Drug Reactions and the Skin*, Blackwell, Oxford, 303 (passim)

Facial erythema (<1%)
(1975): Kennedy BJ+, *Arch Dermatol* 111, 183

Fixed eruption (<1%)
(1991): Boyd AS+, *J Am Acad Dermatol* 25, 518
(1976): Moschella SL, *Int J Dermatol* 15, 373
(1972): Hunter GA+, *Aust J Dermatol* 13, 93
(1969): Moschella SL+, *Arch Dermatol* 107, 363

Ichthyosis
(1997): Ena P+, *J Geriatr Dermatol* 5, 310

Keratoderma (palmar and plantar)
(1997): Ena P+, *J Geriatr Dermatol* 5, 310 (plantar)
(1992): Parodi A+, *G Ital Dermatol Venereol* (Italian) 127, 361
(1992): Breathnach SM+, *Adverse Drug Reactions and the Skin*, Blackwell, Oxford, 303 (passim)
(1989): Richard M+, *J Am Acad Dermatol* 21, 797 (passim)
(1984): Sigal M+, *Ann Dermatol Venereol* (French) 111, 895

Keratoses
(1998): Salmon-Her V+, *Dermatology* 196, 274
(1995): Grange F+, *Ann Dermatol Venereol* (French) 122, 16

Lichenoid eruption
(1997): Daoud MS+, *J Am Acad Dermatol* 36, 178
(1997): Ena P+, *J Geriatr Dermatol* 5, 310

Lichen planus
(1998): Bohn J+, *J Eur Acad Dermatol Venereol* 10, 187 (ulcerative)
(1991): Renfro L+, *J Am Acad Dermatol* 24, 143 (ulcerative)
(1975): Kennedy BJ+, *Arch Dermatol* 111, 183 (atrophic)

Lupus erythematosus
(1994): Layton AM+, *Br J Dermatol* 131, 581
(1994): Layton AM+, *Br J Dermatol* 130, 687

Photosensitivity
(1992): Breathnach SM+, *Adverse Drug Reactions and the Skin*, Blackwell, Oxford, 303 (passim)

Pigmentation (1–10%)
(1995): Weber L+, *Hautarzt* (German) 46, 717
(1993): Brincker H+, *Cancer Chemother Pharmacol* 32, 496
(1993): Gropper CA+, *Int J Dermatol* 32, 731
(1990): Majumdar G+, *BMJ* 300, 1468
(1989): Richard M+, *J Am Acad Dermatol* 21, 797 (passim)
(1989): Layton AM+, *Br J Dermatol* 121, 647
(1984): Sigal M+, *Ann Dermatol Venereol* (French) 111, 895 (band-like)
(1982): Jeanmougin M+, *Ann Dermatol Venereol* (French) 109, 169
(1975): Kennedy BJ+, *Arch Dermatol* 111, 183
(1972): Dahl MH+, *BMJ* 4, 585 (yellow-gray-brown)
(1966): Kennedy BJ+, *JAMA* 195, 162

Poikiloderma
(1997): Daoud MS+, *J Am Acad Dermatol* 36, 178

Pruritus (<1%)
(1995): Weber L+, *Hautarzt* 46, 717
(1992): Vosburgh E, *Am J Hematol* 41, 70
(1975): Kennedy BJ+, *Arch Dermatol* 111, 183

Purpura
(1973): Moschella SL+, *Arch Dermatol* 107, 363
(1973): Roe LD+, *Arch Dermatol* 108, 426

Radiation recall (sic)
(1974): Levantine A+, *Br J Dermatol* 90, 239
(1964): Sears ME, *Cancer Chemother Rep* 40, 31

Rash (sic)

Squamous cell carcinoma
(2000): Bateman B, reported by *Skin and Allergy News*, August, 3 (observation)

Telangiectases
(1997): Daoud MS+, *J Am Acad Dermatol* 36, 178
(1995): Weber L+, *Hautarzt* (German) 46, 717

Tumors
(1998): Salmon-Her V+, *Dermatology* 196, 274
(1998): Best PJ+, *Mayo Clin Proc* 73, 961 (multiple malignant)
(1998): De Simone C+, *Eur J Dermatol* 8, 114 (multiple squamous cell)
(1993): Papi M+, *J Am Acad Dermatol* 28, 485 (on light-exposed areas)
(1992): Stasi R+, *Eur J Haematol* 48, 121

Ulceration
(2000): Tarumoto T+, *Jpn J Clin Oncol* 30, 159 (heels)
(1999): Kato N+, *J Dermatol* 26, 56
(1999): Stagno F+, *Blood* 94, 1479
(1999): Sirieix M-E+, *Arch Dermatol* 135, 818
(1998): Liebschutz S+, *Rev Med Interne* (French) 19, 360 (malleolar)
(1998): Disla E+, *Ann Intern Med* 129, 252
(1998): Kennedy BJ, *Ann Intern Med* 129, 252
(1998): Reichenberger F, *Schweiz Rundsch Med Praxis* (German) 87, 1370
(1998): Ruiz-Arguelles GL+, *Mayo Clin Proc* 73, 1125
(1998): Suehiro M+, *Br J Dermatol* 139, 748 (large leg ulcer)
(1998): Radaelli F+, *Am J Hematol* 58, 82 (hands)
(1998): Weinlich G+, *J Am Acad Dermatol* 39, 372 (painful) (legs) (2 cases)
(1998): Best PJ+, *Ann Intern Med* 128, 29 (leg)
(1998): Kido M+, *Br J Dermatol* 139, 1124
(1997): Ena P+, *J Geriatr Dermatol* 5, 310 (malleolar squamous cell)
(1997): Cox C+, *Ann Plastic Surg* 39, 546 (ankle)
(1997): Glazier DB+, WOUNDS 9, 169
(1997): Best PJ+, *Ann Int Med* 128, 29
(1996): Callot-Mellot C+, *Arch Dermatol* 132, 1395
(1996): Esteve E+, *Ann Dermatol Venereol* (French) 123, 271
(1996): Iwama H+, *Gan To Kagaku Ryoho* (Japanese) 23, 937
(1995): Masuoka H+, *Rinsho Ketsueki* (Japanese) 36, 156
(1993): Nguyen TV+, *Cutis* 52, 217 (painful legs ulcers)
(1986): Montefusco E+, *Tumori* (Italian) 72, 317 (legs) (17 cases)
(1985): Stahl RL+, *Am J Med* 78, 869
(1984): Sigal M+, *Ann Dermatol Venereol* (French) 111, 895

Urticaria

Vasculitis
(1997): Reed BR, Denver, CO (from Internet) (observation)
(1992): Breathnach SM+, *Adverse Drug Reactions and the Skin*, Blackwell, Oxford, 303 (passim)
(1989): Richard M+, *J Am Acad Dermatol* 21, 797 (passim)
(1976): Moschella SL, *Int J Dermatol* 15, 373
(1973): Roe LD+, *Arch Dermatol* 108, 426
(1973): Moschella SL+, *Arch Dermatol* 107, 363

Xerosis (1–10%)
(1995): Weber L+, *Hautarzt* (German) 46, 717
(1989): Richard M+, *J Am Acad Dermatol* 21, 797 (passim)
(1984): Sigal M+, *Ann Dermatol Venereol* (French) 111, 895
(1975): Kennedy BJ+, *Arch Dermatol* 111, 183

Hair

Hair – alopecia (1–10%)
(1992): Breathnach SM+, *Adverse Drug Reactions and the Skin*, Blackwell, Oxford, 303 (passim)
(1989): Layton AM+, *Br J Dermatol* 121, 647
(1989): Richard M+, *J Am Acad Dermatol* 21, 797 (passim)
(1976): Bergstresser PR+, *Arch Dermatol* 112, 977
(1975): Kennedy BJ+, *Arch Dermatol* 111, 183

Nails

Nails – atrophic
(1984): Sigal M+, *Ann Dermatol Venereol* (French) 111, 895
(1984): Daniel CR+, *J Am Acad Dermatol* 10, 250
(1975): Kennedy BJ+, *Arch Dermatol* 111, 183

Nails – dystrophy
(1992): Breathnach SM+, *Adverse Drug Reactions and the Skin*, Blackwell, Oxford, 303 (passim)
(1989): Richard M+, *J Am Acad Dermatol* 21, 797 (passim)

Nails – onycholysis
(1992): Breathnach SM+, *Adverse Drug Reactions and the Skin*, Blackwell, Oxford, 303 (passim)
(1989): Richard M+, *J Am Acad Dermatol* 21, 797 (passim)

Nails – pigmentation
(1999): Hernández-Martin A+, *J Am Acad Dermatol* 40, 333
(1997): Ena P+, *J Geriatr Dermatol* 5, 310
(1996): Kwong YL, *J Am Acad Dermatol* 35, 275
(1995): Delmas-Marsalet B+, *Nouv Rev Fr Hematol* (French) 37, 205
(1989): Baran R+, *J Am Acad Dermatol* 21, 1165

Nails – pigmented bands
(1999): Hernández-Martin A+, *J Am Acad Dermatol* 40, 333
(1997): Cakir B+, *Int J Dermatol* 36, 234
(1994): Pirard C+, *Ann Dermatol Venereol* (French) 121, 106 (longitudinal)
(1993): Gropper CA+, *Int J Dermatol* 32, 731
(1992): Kelsey PR, *Clin Lab Haematol* 14, 337

(1991): Vomvouras S+, *J Am Acad Dermatol* 24, 1016
(1984): Sigal M+, *Ann Dermatol Venereol* (French) 111, 895
(1982): Jeanmougin M+, *Ann Dermatol Venereol* 109, 169

Other

Myositis
(1998): Ikeda K+, *Rinsho Ketsueki* (Japanese) 39, 676
Oral mucosal lesions
(1976): Bergstresser PR+, *Arch Dermatol* 112, 977
(1975): Kennedy BJ+, *Arch Dermatol* 111, 183
Oral ulceration
(1997): Norhaya MR+, *Singapore Med J* 38, 283
(1989): Richard M+, *J Am Acad Dermatol* 21, 797 (passim)
Stomatitis (>10%)
(1993): Brincker H+, *Cancer Chemother Pharmacol* 32, 496
(1992): Breathnach SM+, *Adverse Drug Reactions and the Skin*, Blackwell, Oxford, 303 (passim)
(1989): Richard M+, *J Am Acad Dermatol* 21, 797 (passim)
Tongue pigmentation
(1997): Ena P+, *J Geriatr Dermatol* 5, 310
(1993): Gropper CA+, *Int J Dermatol* 32, 731

HYDROXYZINE

Trade names: Atarax (Pfizer); Marax (Pfizer); Vistaril (Pfizer)
Other common trade names: *AH3 N; Anaxanil; Bobsule; Iremofar; Masmoran; Multipax; Otarex; Paxistil; Quiess; Rezine; Vamate*
Indications: Anxiety and tension, pruritus
Category: Antihistamine, anxiolytic and antiemetic
Half-life: 3–7 hours
Clinically important, potentially serious interactions with: anticholinergics, CNS depressants

Reactions

Skin

Angioedema (<1%)
(1971): *Drug Ther Bull* 9, 84
(1964): Welsh AL, *Med Clin North Am* 48, 459
(1958): Cohen AE+, *J Allergy* 29, 542
Contact dermatitis
(1997): Menne T, *Am J Contact Dermat* 8, 1
Diaphoresis
Edema (<1%)
Erythema multiforme (<1%)
(1959): Wright W, *JAMA* 171, 1642
Exanthems
(1964): Welsh AL, *Med Clin North Am* 48, 459
(1959): Wright W, *JAMA* 171, 1642
(1958): Cohen AE+, *J Allergy* 29, 542
Fixed eruption
(1997): Cohen HA+, *Ann Pharmacother* 31, 327 (penis)
(1996): Cohen HA+, *Cutis* 57, 431 (scrotum)
Flushing
(1998): Foster M+, *J Clin Dermatol* Winter, 7
Photosensitivity (<1%)
Purpura
Rash (sic) (<1%)
Urticaria
(1964): Welsh AL, *Med Clin North Am* 48, 459
(1959): Wright W, *JAMA* 171, 1642

Other

Hypersensitivity
(1978): Massoud N, *J Pediatr* 93, 308
Injection-site necrosis
(1995): Tokodi G+, *J Am Osteopath Assoc* 95, 609
Myalgia (<1%)
Priapism
(1994): Thavundayil JX+, *Neuropsychobiology* 30, 4
Xerostomia (1–10%)
(1998): Foster M+, *J Clin Dermatol* Winter, 7 (12.5%)
(1990): Kalivas J+, *J Allergy Clin Immunol* 86, 1014

IBUPROFEN

Trade names: Advil (Wyeth); Genpril; Haltran; Medipren; Midol 220; Motrin (McNeil); Nuprin; Pamprin; Profen; Rufen; Trendar; Uni-Proc, etc. (Various pharmaceutical companies.)
Other common trade names: *Act-3; Actiprofen; Anco; Apsifen; Brufen; Ebufac; Lidifen; Proflex; Tabalom; Urem*
Indications: Arthritis; pain
Category: Nonsteroidal anti-inflammatory (NSAID); antipyretic
Half-life: 2–4 hours
Clinically important, potentially serious interactions with: anticoagulants, beta-blockers, digoxin, furosemide, lithium, loop diuretics, methotrexate, NSAIDs, phenytoin, probenecid, salicylates, warfarin

Reactions

Skin

Angioedema (<1%)
(1994): Halpern SM, *Arch Dermatol* 130, 259 (passim)
(1987): Shelley ED+, *J Am Acad Dermatol* 17, 1057
(1985): Bigby M+, *J Am Acad Dermatol* 12, 866
(1984): Stern RS+, *JAMA* 252, 1433
(1982): Bailin PL+, *Clinics in Rheumatic Diseases*, WB Saunders 8, 493 (passim)

Bullous eruption (<1%)
(1994): Halpern SM, *Arch Dermatol* 130, 259 (passim)
(1988): Laing VB+, *J Am Acad Dermatol* 19, 91
(1984): Stern R+, *JAMA* 252, 1433

Bullous pemphigoid
(1993): Fellner MJ, *Clin Dermatol* 11, 515
(1981): Pompeova L, *Cesk Dermatol* (Czech) 56, 256

Contact dermatitis (<1%)
(1993): Ophaswongse S+, *Contact Dermatitis* 29, 57
(1986): Veronesi S+, *Contact Dermatitis* 15, 103
(1985): Valsecchi R+, *Contact Dermatitis* 12, 286

Dermatitis herpetiformis
(1994): Tousignant J+, *Int J Dermatol* 33, 199

Diaphoresis
(1974): Regalado RG+, *J Int Med Res* 2, 115

Eczematous eruption (sic)
(1986): Veronesi S+, *Contact Dermatitis* 15, 103

Edema (<1%)

Erythema multiforme (<1%)
(1995): Lesko SM+, *JAMA* 273, 929
(1994): Halpern SM, *Arch Dermatol* 130, 259 (passim)
(1992): Breathnach SM+, *Adverse Drug Reactions and the Skin*, Blackwell, Oxford, 186 (passim)
(1985): Bigby M+, *J Am Acad Dermatol* 12, 866
(1985): O'Brien WM+, *J Rheumatol* 12, 13
(1984): Stern R+, *JAMA* 252, 1433
(1978): Sternlieb P+, *N Y State J Med* 78, 1239

Erythema nodosum
(1994): Halpern SM, *Arch Dermatol* 130, 259 (passim)

Exanthems
(1994): Litt JZ, Beachwood, OH, personal case (observation)
(1994): Halpern SM, *Arch Dermatol* 130, 259 (passim)
(1985): Bigby M+, *J Am Acad Dermatol* 12, 866
(1980): Shoenfeld Y+, *JAMA* 244, 547
(1979): Finch WR+, *JAMA* 241, 2616
(1978): Sonnenblick M+, *BMJ* 1, 619
(1975): Blechman WJ+, *JAMA* 233, 336 (3.4%)
(1974): Regalado RG+, *J Int Med Res* 2, 115 (0.86%)
(1973): Mills SB+, *BMJ* 4, 82 (>5%)

Fixed eruption (<1%)
(1996): Eichwald M, Redding CA (observation)
(1994): Shelley WB+, *Cutis* 53, 282 (observation)
(1992): Breathnach SM+, *Adverse Drug Reactions and the Skin*, Blackwell, Oxford, 186 (passim)
(1991): Kuligowski ME+, *Contact Dermatitis* 25, 259
(1990): Bharija SC+, *Dermatologica* 181, 237
(1985): Bigby M+, *J Am Acad Dermatol* 12, 866
(1984): Stern R+, *JAMA* 252, 1433
(1984): Kanwar AJ+, *J Dermatol* 11, 383

Flushing

Hot flashes (<1%)

Livedo reticularis
(1979): Finch WR+, *JAMA* 241, 2616

Lupus erythematosus
(1996): Vigouroux C+, *Rev Med Interne* (French) 14, 856
(1985): O'Brien WM+, *J Rheumatol* 12, 13
(1980): Bar-Sela S+, *J Rheumatol* 7, 379
(1978): Pereyo-Torrellas N, *Arch Dermatol* 114, 1097
(1978): Sonnenblick M+, *BMJ* 1, 619 (exacerbation)

Pemphigoid
(1988): Laing VB+, *J Am Acad Dermatol* 19, 91

Periorbital edema
(1979): Finch WR+, *JAMA* 241, 2616

Photoreactions
(1982): Bailin PL+, *Clinics in Rheumatic Diseases*, WB Saunders 8, 493

Photosensitivity
(1994): Halpern SM, *Arch Dermatol* 130, 259 (passim)
(1994): Berger TG+, *Arch Dermatol* 130, 609 (in HIV-infected) (5 cases)
(1992): Bergner T+, *J Am Acad Dermatol* 26, 114
(1990): Bergner T+, *J Allergy Clin Immunol* 85, 177
(1985): Bigby M+, *J Am Acad Dermatol* 12, 866

Pruritus (1–5%)
(1994): Halpern SM, *Arch Dermatol* 130, 259 (passim)
(1992): Breathnach SM+, *Adverse Drug Reactions and the Skin*, Blackwell, Oxford, 186 (passim)
(1985): Bigby M+, *J Am Acad Dermatol* 12, 866 (1–5%)
(1979): Finch WR+, *JAMA* 241, 2616
(1975): Blechman WJ+, *JAMA* 233, 336 (1.8%)

Psoriasis (palms)
(1986): Ben-Chetrit E+, *Cutis* 38, 45 (exacerbation)
(1985): Bigby M+, *J Am Acad Dermatol* 12, 866

Purpura
(1969): Ward T, *BMJ* 4, 430

Rash (sic) (>10%)
(1974): Regalado RG+, *J Int Med Res* 2, 115

Stevens–Johnson syndrome (<1%)
(1994): Halpern SM, *Arch Dermatol* 130, 259 (passim)
(1978): Sternlieb P+, *N Y State J Med* 78, 1239

Toxic epidermal necrolysis (<1%)
(1994): Halpern SM, *Arch Dermatol* 130, 259 (passim)
(1980): Sternlieb P+, *Ann Intern Med* 92, 570

Urticaria (>10%)
(1994): Halpern SM, *Arch Dermatol* 130, 259 (passim)
(1993): Litt JZ, Beachwood, Ohio, personal case (observation)
(1987): Shelley ED+, *J Am Acad Dermatol* 17, 1057
(1985): Bigby M+, *J Am Acad Dermatol* 12, 866
(1984): Stern RS+, *JAMA* 252, 1433
(1982): Bailin PL+, *Clinics in Rheumatic Diseases*, WB Saunders 8, 493 (passim)
(1975): Blechman WJ+, *JAMA* 233, 336 (0.2%)

Vasculitis
(1996): Peters F+, *J Rheumatol* 23, 2008
(1994): Halpern SM, *Arch Dermatol* 130, 259 (passim)
(1992): Breathnach SM+, *Adverse Drug Reactions and the Skin*, Blackwell, Oxford, 186 (passim)
(1982): Labbe A+, *Ann Dermatol Venereol* (French) 109, 995
(1985): Bigby M+, *J Am Acad Dermatol* 12, 866
(1984): Stern R+, *JAMA* 252, 1433
(1978): Pereyo-Torrellas N, *Arch Dermatol* 114, 1097

Vesiculobullous eruption
(1992): Breathnach SM+, *Adverse Drug Reactions and the Skin*, Blackwell, Oxford, 186 (passim)
(1988): Laing VB+, *J Am Acad Dermatol* 19, 91 (passim)

Hair

Hair – alopecia (<1%)
(1985): O'Brien WM+, *J Rheumatol* 12, 13
(1979): Meyer HC, *JAMA* 242, 142

Hair – disorders (sic)
(1994): Halpern SM, *Arch Dermatol* 130, 259 (passim)

Nails

Nails – disorder (sic)
(1994): Halpern SM, *Arch Dermatol* 130, 259 (passim)

Nails – onycholysis
(1982): Bailin PL+, *Clinics In Rheumatic Diseases*, WB Saunders 8, 493

Other

Anaphylactoid reaction (<1%)
(2000): Takahama H+, *J Dermatol* 27, 337
(1998): Menendez R+, *Ann Allergy Asthma Immunol* 80, 225
(1985): O'Brien WM+, *J Rheumatol* 12, 13
(1979): Finch WR+, *JAMA* 241, 2616
Aphthous stomatitis
Gingival ulceration (<1%)
Gynecomastia (<1%)
Hypersensitivity
(1981): Ruppert GB+, *South Med J* 74, 241
Impaired wound healing
(1988): Proper SA+, *J Am Acad Dermatol* 18, 1173
Myopathy
(1987): Ross NS+, *JAMA* 257, 62
Oral lichenoid eruption
(1983): Hamburger J+, *BMJ* 287, 1258
Oral mucosal lesions
(1974): Regalado RG+, *J Int Med Res* 2, 115
Oral ulceration
(1974): Regalado RG+, *J Int Med Res* 2, 115
Paresthesias
Pseudoporphyria
(1992): Petersen CS+, *Ugeskr Laeger* (Danish) 154, 1713
Serum sickness
(1995): Lesko SM+, *JAMA* 273, 929
Stomatitis
Xerostomia (<1%)

IBUTILIDE

Trade name: Corvert (Pharmacia & Upjohn)
Indications: Atrial fibrillation and flutter
Category: Antiarrhythmic class III
Half-life: 2–12 hours
Clinically important, potentially serious interactions with: amiodarone, antiarrhythmics, bretylium, digoxin, disopyramide, erythromycin, gatifloxacin, maprotiline, moxifloxacin, phenothiazines, procainamide, quinidine, sotalol, sparfloxacin, tricyclic antidepressants

Reactions

Skin

Bullous eruption
Contact dermatitis
(1998): Dodds ES+, *Pharmacotherapy* 18, 880 (bullous)

IDARUBICIN

Synonyms: 4-demethoxydaunorubicin; 4-DMDR
Trade name: Idamycin (Pharmacia & Upjohn)
Other common trade name: *Zavedos*
Indications: Acute myeloid leukemia
Category: Antineoplastic antibiotic
Half-life: 14–35 hours (oral)
Clinically important, potentially serious interactions with: aldesleukin, probenecid, sulfinpyrazone

Reactions

Skin

Acral erythema
(1993): Cohen PR, *Cutis* 51, 175
Bullous eruption (palms and soles)
Erythematous streaking (sic) (>10%)
Exanthems (<1%)
Radiation recall
(1995): Gabel C+, *Gynecol Oncol* 57, 266
Rash (sic) (>10%)
(1998): Stuart NS+, *Cancer Chemother Pharmacol* 21, 351
(1997): Maloney DG+, *J Clin Oncol* 15, 3266
Urticaria (>10%)
(1997): Maloney DG+, *J Clin Oncol* 15, 3266

Hair

Hair – alopecia (77%)
(1988): Gillies H+, *Cancer Chemother Pharmacol* 21, 261
(1993): Ogawa M+, *Gan To Kaguku Ryoho* (Japanese) 20, 897
(1993): Ogawa M+, *Gan To Kaguku Ryoho* (Japanese) 20, 907
(1991): Hollingshead LM+, *Drugs* 42, 690
(1986): Lopez M+, *Invest New Drugs* 4, 39
(1986): Dodion P+, *Invest New Drugs* 4, 31

Nails

Nails – pigmentary changes
(1997): Borecky Derrick J+, *Cutis* 59, 203

Other

Extravasation-site necrosis (>10%)
Injection-site urticaria
Mucositis (50%)
(1986): Dodion P+, *Invest New Drugs* 4, 31
Stomatitis (>10%)

IFOSFAMIDE

Trade name: Ifex (Bristol-Myers Squibb)
Other common trade names: *Holoxan; Ifoxan; Mitoxana; Tronoxal*
Indications: Cancers, sarcomas, leukemias, lymphomas
Category: Antineoplastic; nitrogen mustard
Half-life: 4–15 hours
Clinically important, potentially serious interactions with: anticoagulants, chloral hydrate, cisplatin, NSAIDs, phenobarbital, phenytoin, vancomycin

Reactions

Skin

Allergic reactions (sic) (1–10%)
Dermatitis (sic) (1–10%)
Pigmentation (1–10%)
(1994): Yule SM+, *Cancer* 73, 240
(1993): Teresi ME+, *Cancer* 71, 2873

Hair

Hair – alopecia (50–83%)
(1988): Negretti E+, *Tumori* (Italian) 74, 163 (100%)
(1971): Kunz W+, *Schweiz Med Wochenschr (German)* 101, 1151

Nails

Nails – ridging (1–10%)
(1994): Ben Dayan D+, *Acta Haematol* 91, 89

Other

Anaphylactoid reaction
Oral mucosal lesions
Phlebitis (2%)
Sialorrhea (<1%)
Stomatitis (<1%)

IMIPENEM/CILASTATIN

Synonym: imipemide
Trade name: Primaxin (Merck)
Other common trade names: *Tenacid; Tienam; Tienam 500; Zienam*
Indications: Various infections caused by susceptible organisms
Category: Carbapenem antibiotic
Half-life: 1 hour
Clinically important, potentially serious interactions with: beta-lactam antibiotics, cyclosporine, ganciclovir, probenecid, theophylline

Reactions

Skin

Acute generalized exanthematous pustulosis (AGEP)
(1989): Escallier F+, *Ann Dermatol Venereol* (French) 116, 407
Allergic reactions (sic) (1–3%)
(1994): Pleasants RA+, *Chest* 106, 1124 (in patients with cystic fibrosis)
Angioedema (0.2%)
(1987): Clissold SP+, *Drugs* 33, 183
Candidiasis (0.2%)
Diaphoresis (0.2%)
Erythema multiforme (0.2%)
(1987): Clissold SP+, *Drugs* 33, 183
Exanthems (<1%)
(1989): Escallier F+, *Ann Dermatol Venereol* (French) 116, 407
(1987): Clissold SP+, *Drugs* 33, 183
(1985): Calandra GB+, *Am J Med* 78, 73 (1–5%)
Flushing (0.2%)
Pruritus (0.3%)
(1991): Machado ARL+, *J Allergy Clin Immunol* 87, 754
(1989): Escallier F+, *Ann Dermatol Venereol* (French) 116, 407
(1987): Clissold SP+, *Drugs* 33, 183
Pruritus vulvae (0.2%)
Pustular eruption
(1994): Spencer JM+, *Br J Dermatol* 130, 514
Rash (sic) (4%)
(1994): Grayson ML+, *Clin Infect Dis* 18, 683
Toxic epidermal necrolysis (0.2%)
Urticaria (0.2%)
(1991): Hantson P+, *BMJ* 302, 294
(1989): Escallier F+, *Ann Dermatol Venereol* (French) 116, 407
(1987): Clissold SP+, *Drugs* 33, 183
Vasculitis
(1997): Reiner MR+, *J Am Podiatr Med Assoc* 87, 245

Other

Dysgeusia (0.2%)
Glossitis (0.2%)
Hypersensitivity
(1988): Donowitz GR+, *N Engl J Med* 318, 490
Injection-site erythema (0.4%)
Injection-site pain (0.2%)
(1991): *Drug Ther Bull* 29, 43
(1985): Calandra GB+, *Am J Med* 78, 73 (0.7%)
Injection-site phlebitis
(1991): *Drug Ther Bull* 29, 43
(1988): Gould IM+, *Drugs Exp Clin Res* 14, 555
(1987): Clissold SP+, *Drugs* 33, 183 (2%)
(1985): Calandra GB+, *Am J Med* 78, 73 (3.8%)
Oral mucosal lesions
Paresthesias (0.2%)
Phlebitis (3%)
Sialorrhea (0.2%)
Thrombophlebitis (3.1%)

IMIPRAMINE

Trade name: Tofranil (Novartis)
Other common trade names: *Apo-Imipramine; Imidol; Imipramin; Impril; Novo-Pramine; Primonil; Pryleugan*
Indications: Depression
Category: Tricyclic antidepressant
Half-life: 6–18 hours
Clinically important, potentially serious interactions with: alcohol, carbamazepine, cimetidine, clonidine, CNS depressants, dicumarol, epinephrine, fluoxetine, guanethidine, indinavir, lithium, MAO inhibitors, phenothiazines, quinidine, rifampin, ritonavir, SSRIs, sympathomimetics, warfarin

Reactions

Skin

Acne
Allergic reactions (sic)
Angioedema (<1%)
(1971): Almeyda J, *Br J Dermatol* 84, 298
Ankle edema
Bullous eruption
(1977): Varma AJ+, *Arch Intern Med* 137, 1207 (passim)
Diaphoresis (1–10%)
(1990): Leeman CP, *J Clin Psychiatry* 51, 258
(1989): Butt MM, *J Clin Psychiatry* 50, 146
(1971): Almeyda J, *Br J Dermatol* 84, 298
(1962): Busfield BL+, *J Nerv Ment Dis* 134, 339 (25%)
(1961): Kiloh LG+, *BMJ* 1, 168
(1959): Mann AM+, *Can Psychiatr Assoc J* 4, 38
Edema
(1961): Kiloh LG+, *BMJ* 1, 168
Erythema
Exanthems (1–5%)
(1992): Breathnach SM+, *Adverse Drug Reactions and the Skin*, Blackwell, Oxford, 197 (passim)
(1988): Warnock JK+, *Am J Psychiatry* 145, 425 (6%)
(1985): Walter-Ryan WG+, *JAMA* 254, 357
(1971): Almeyda J, *Br J Dermatol* 84, 298
(1968): Powell WJ+, *JAMA* 206, 642
(1959): Mann AM+, *Can Psychiatr Assoc J* 4, 38
Exfoliative dermatitis
(1992): Breathnach SM+, *Adverse Drug Reactions and the Skin*, Blackwell, Oxford, 197 (passim)
(1971): Almeyda J, *Br J Dermatol* 84, 298
(1968): Powell WJ+, *JAMA* 206, 642
(1959): Mann AM+, *Can Psychiatr Assoc J* 4, 38
Fixed eruption (<1%)
(1978): Sehgal VN+, *Int J Dermatol* 17, 78
Flushing
(1961): Kiloh LG+, *BMJ* 1, 168
Lichen planus
(1971): Almeyda J, *Br J Dermatol* 84, 298
Lupus erythematosus
(1971): Almeyda J, *Br J Dermatol* 84, 298
Parkinsonism (1–10%)
Petechiae
Photoreactions
Photosensitivity (<1%)
(1985): Walter-Ryan WG+, *JAMA* 354, 357
(1971): Almeyda J, *Br J Dermatol* 84, 298
(1960): Gesensway D+, *Am J Psychiatry* 116, 1027
Pigmentation
(1999): Ming ME+, *J Am Acad Dermatol* 40, 159 (4 cases)
(1991): Hashimoto K+, *J Am Acad Dermatol* 25, 357 (slate-gray)
(1990): Goldberg NC, *Dermatology Perspectives* 6, 8
(1988): Warnock JK+, *Am J Psychiatry* 145, 425
(1970): Hare PJ, *Br J Dermatol* 83, 420 ("visage mauve")
Pruritus
(1988): Warnock JK+, *Am J Psychiatry* 145, 425 (3%)
(1987): Pohl R+, *Am J Psychiatry* 144, 237
(1971): Almeyda J, *Br J Dermatol* 84, 298
(1968): Powell WJ+, *JAMA* 206, 642

(1961): Kiloh LG+, *BMJ* 1, 168
(1959): Mann AM+, *Can Psychiatr Assoc J* 4, 38
Purpura
(1988): Warnock JK+, *Am J Psychiatry* 145, 425
(1971): Almeyda J, *Br J Dermatol* 84, 298
(1971): Kosakova M, *Cesk Dermatol* (Czech) 46, 158
Rash (sic)
Urticaria
(1992): Breathnach SM+, *Adverse Drug Reactions and the Skin*, Blackwell, Oxford, 197 (passim)
(1987): Pohl R+, *Am J Psychiatry* 144, 237
(1985): Burnett GB+, *South Med J* 78, 71
(1971): Almeyda J, *Br J Dermatol* 84, 298
(1961): Kiloh LG+, *BMJ* 1, 168
(1959): Mann AM+, *Can Psychiatr Assoc J* 4, 38
Vasculitis
(1992): Breathnach SM+, *Adverse Drug Reactions and the Skin*, Blackwell, Oxford, 197 (passim)
Xerosis

Hair

Hair – alopecia (<1%)
(1994): Friedman M, *J Fam Pract* 39, 114
(1991): Warnock JK+, *J Nerv Ment Dis* 179, 441
Hair – alopecia areata
(1987): Baral J+, *Int J Dermatol* 26, 198

Nails

Nails – parrot beak nails
(1971): Kandil E, *J Med Liban* (French) 24, 433

Other

Black tongue
Dysgeusia (>10%) (metallic taste)
(1961): Kiloh LG+, *BMJ* 1, 168
Galactorrhea (<1%)
(1964): Klein JJ+, *N Engl J Med* 271, 510
Glossitis
(1992): Breathnach SM+, *Adverse Drug Reactions and the Skin*, Blackwell, Oxford, 197 (passim)
(1959): Delay J+, *Can Psychiatr Assoc J* 4, 100
Glossodynia
Gynecomastia (<1%)
(1964): Klein JJ+, *N Engl J Med* 271, 510
Hypogeusia
Mucous membrane desquamation
(1968): Powell WJ+, *JAMA* 206, 642
Oral mucosal lesions
(1971): Almeyda J, *Br J Dermatol* 84, 298
(1964): Pollack B+, *Am J Psychiatry* 121, 384
(1962): Busfield BL+, *J Nerv Ment Dis* 134, 339 (21%)
Oral ulceration
Paresthesias
Stomatitis
(1992): Breathnach SM+, *Adverse Drug Reactions and the Skin*, Blackwell, Oxford, 197 (passim)
(1964): Pollack B+, *Am J Psychiatry* 121, 384
Tremor
Vaginitis
Xerostomia (>10%)
(1971): Almeyda J, *Br J Dermatol* 84, 298
(1962): Busfield BL+, *J Nerv Ment Dis* 134, 339 (21%)
(1961): Kiloh LG+, *BMJ* 1, 168
(1959): Mann AM+, *Can Psychiatr Assoc J* 4, 38

INAMRINONE

Trade name: Inocor (Sanofi)
Other trade names: *Amcoral; Cartonic; Vestistol*
Indications: Congestive heart failure
Category: Positive inotropic agent
Half-life: 4.6 hours
Clinically important, potentially serious interactions with: disopyramide, diuretics, furosemide

Reactions

Skin

None

Other

Hypersensitivity
Injection-site burning (0.2%)

INDAPAMIDE

Trade name: Lozol (Aventis)
Other common trade names: *Dapa-tabs; Fludex; Ipamix; Lozide; Naplin; Natrilix; Pamid*
Indications: Edema
Category: Oral antihypertensive sulfonamide* diuretic
Half-life: 14–18 hours
Clinically important, potentially serious interactions with: amiodarone, antidiabetics, beta-blockers, cyclosporine, diazoxide, digoxin, furosemide, insulin, lithium, loop diuretics, NSAIDs, sulfonylureas

Reactions

Skin

Angioedema
(1994): Gales BJ+, *Am J Hosp Pharm* 51, 118
(1992): Spinler SA+, *Cutis* 50, 200
(1987): Stricker BHC+, *Br Med J Clin Res Ed* 295, 1313
Bullous eruption
Diaphoresis
Erythema multiforme
(1994): Gales BJ+, *Am J Hosp Pharm* 51, 118
(1987): Stricker BHC+, *Br Med J Clin Res Ed* 295, 1313
Exanthems
(1987): Stricker BHC+, *Br Med J Clin Res Ed* 295, 1313
Fixed eruption
(1998): De Barrio M+, *J Investig Allergol Clin Immunol* 8, 253
Flushing (<5%)
(1985): Chaignon M+, *Arch Mal Coeur Vaiss* (French) 78, 67
Necrotizing angiitis
Peripheral edema (<5%)
Photosensitivity (<1%)
Pruritus (<5%)
(1985): Kirsten R+, *Z Kardiol* (German) 74, 66
(1982): Brennan L+, *Clin Ther* 5, 121
Purpura
Rash (sic) (<5%)
(1988): Kandela D+, *BMJ* 296, 573
(1985): Kirsten R+, *Z Kardiol* (German) 74, 66
(1983): Slotkoff L, *Am Heart J* 106, 233
(1982): Brennan L+, *Clin Ther* 5, 121
Stevens–Johnson syndrome
(1992): Spinler SA+, *Cutis* 50, 200
Toxic epidermal necrolysis
(1993): Partanen J+, *Arch Dermatol* 129, 793
(1990): Black RJ+, *Br Med J Clin Res Ed* 301, 1280
(1987): Stricker BHC+, *Br Med J Clin Res Ed* 295, 1313
Urticaria (<5%)
(1987): Stricker BHC+, *Br Med J Clin Res Ed* 295, 1313
Vasculitis (<5%)

Other

Anaphylactoid reaction
Paresthesias (<5%)
Xanthopsia
Xerostomia (<5%)
(1985): Kirsten R+, *Z Kardiol* (German) 74, 66
(1982): Brennan L+, *Clin Ther* 5, 121

***Note:** Indapamide is a sulfonamide and can be absorbed systemically. Sulfonamides can produce severe, possibly fatal, reactions such as toxic epidermal necrolysis and Stevens–Johnson syndrome.

INDINAVIR

Trade name: Crixivan (Merck)
Indications: HIV infection
Category: Antiretroviralviral; protease inhibitor*
Half-life: ~1.8 hours
Clinically important, potentially serious interactions with: alprazolam, amprenavir, astemizole, atorvastatin, benzodiazepines, cerivastatin, chlordiazepoxide, cisapride, clonazepam, clorazepate, delavirdine, diazepam, didanosine, itraconazole, ketoconazole, lovastatin, midazolam, nelfinavir, rifabutin, rifampin, simvastatin, terfenadine, triazolam, **grapefruit juice, St John's wort**

Reactions

Skin

Allergic reactions (sic)
(1998): Rijnders B+, *Clin Infect Dis* 26, 523
Buffalo hump
(2000): Calista D+, *Eur J Dermatol* 10, 292
Buffalo neck
(1999): Milpied-Homsi B+, *Ann Dermatol Venereol* (French) 126, 254
Cheilitis
(2000): Calista D+, *Eur J Dermatol* 10, 292 (51.7%)
Contact dermatitis (<2%)
Dermatitis (sic) (<2%)
Diaphoresis (<2%)
Erythema multiforme
Exanthem
(1999): Fung HB+, *Pharmacotherapy* 19, 1328
Eyelid edema (<2%)
Flushing (<2%)
Folliculitis (<2%)
Herpes simplex (<2%)
Herpes zoster (<2%)
Pigmentation
Pruritus
(2000): Calista D+, *Eur J Dermatol* 10, 292 (11.9%)
(1999): Gajewski LK+, *Ann Pharmacother* 33, 17 (86%)
Pyogenic granuloma
(1998): Bouscarat F+, *N Engl J Med* 338, 1776 (great toes)
Rash (sic)
(1999): Gajewski LK+, *Ann Pharmacother* 33, 17 (67%)
Seborrhea (<2%)
Stevens–Johnson syndrome
(1998): Teira R+, *Scand J Infect Dis* 30, 634
Striae
(1999): Darvay A+, *J Am Acad Dermatol* 41, 467
Urticaria (<2%)
Xerosis
(2000): Calista D+, *Eur J Dermatol* 10, 292 (11.9%)

Hair

Hair – alopecia
(2000): Calista D+, *Eur J Dermatol* 10, 292 (11.9%)
(1999): Bouscarat F+, *N Engl J Med* 341, 618
(1998): d'Arminio Monforte A+, *AIDS* 12, 328

Nails

Nails – ingrown
(2000): Miot HA, Sao Paulo, Brasil (from Internet) (observation)
(2000): Heim M+, *Haemophilia* 6, 191
Nails – paronychia
(2000): Dauden E+, *Br J Dermatol* 142, 1063 (toes and finger)
(1998): Bouscarat F+, *N Engl J Med* 338, 1776 (great toes)
Nails – pyogenic granulomas
(2000): Calista D+, *Eur J Dermatol* 10, 292 (5.9%)

Other

Aphthous stomatitis (<2%)
Bromhidrosis (<2%)
Bruxism (<2%)
Dysesthesia (<2%)
Dysgeusia (2.6%)
Foetor ex ore (halitosis) (<2%)
Gingivitis (<2%)
Gynecomastia
(1998): Toma E+, *AIDS* 12, 681
(1998): Lui A+, *Clin Infect Dis* 26, 1482
(1998): Caeiro JP+, *Clin Infect Dis* 27, 1539
Hypesthesia (<2%)
Lipodystrophy
(2000): Calista D+, *Eur J Dermatol* 10, 292 (14.3%)
(2000): Hartmann M+, *Hautarzt* (German) *51, 159*
(1999): Hermieu JF+, *Prog Urol* (French) 9, 537
(1999): Krautheim A, *Schweiz Rundsch Med Prax* (German) 88, 285
(1998): Viraben R+, *AIDS* 12, F37
(1998): Miller KD+, *Lancet* 351, 871
(1997): Herry I+, *Clin Infect Dis* 25, 937 (breast hypertrophy)
Lipomatosis
(2000): Calista D+, *Eur J Dermatol* 10, 292
(1997): Hengel RL+, *Lancet* 350, 1596 (benign symmetric)
Myalgia (<2%)
Paresthesias (<2%)
Porphyria (acute)
(1999): Fox PA+, *AIDS* 16, 322
Xerostomia (0.5%)

***Note:** Protease inhibitors cause dyslipidemia which includes elevated triglycerides and cholesterol and redistribution of body fat centrally to produce the so-called "protease paunch," breast enlargement, facial atrophy, and "buffalo hump."

INDOMETHACIN

Synonym: indometacin
Trade name: Indocin (Merck)
Other common trade names: *Amuno; Apo-Indomethacin; Durametacin; Imbrilon; Indochron; Indocid; Indolar SR; Indotec; Nu-Indo; Rhodacine; Vonum*
Indications: Arthritis
Category: Nonsteroidal anti-inflammatory (NSAID); antipyretic
Half-life: 4.5 hours
Clinically important, potentially serious interactions with: ACE-inhibitors, aminoglycosides, anticoagulants, aspirin, beta-blockers, cyclosporine, digoxin, diuretics, heparin, lithium, methotrexate, NSAIDs, probenecid, salicylates, triamterene

Reactions

Skin

Angioedema (<1%)
(1981): Juhlin L, *Br J Dermatol* 104, 369
(1966): Rothermich ND, *JAMA* 195, 531 (0.5%)
Bullous eruption (<1%)
(1986): Harrington CI+, *Br J Dermatol* 114, 265
(1969): Duperrat B+, *Bull Soc Franc Dermatol Syphiligr* (French) 76, 26
Contact dermatitis
(1999): Pulido Z+, *Contact Dermatitis* 41, 112
(1998): Ueda K+, *Contact Dermatitis* 39, 323
(1993): Ophaswongse S+, *Contact Dermatitis* 29, 57
(1993): Goday-Bujan JJ+, *Contact Dermatitis* 28, 111

(1987): Beller U+, *Contact Dermatitis* 17, 121
Cutaneous side effects (sic)
(1986): Bigby M+, *JAMA* 256, 3358 (0.21%)
Dermatitis herpetiformis (exacerbation)
(1986): Harrington CI+, *Br J Dermatol* 114, 265
(1985): Griffiths CEM+, *Br J Dermatol* 112, 443
Diaphoresis (<1%)
Ecchymoses (<1%)
Eczematous eruption (sic)
(1987): Beller U+, *Contact Dermatitis* 17, 121
Edema (3–9%)
(1978): Castles JJ+, *Arch Intern Med* 138, 362 (5.6%)
Erythema multiforme (<1%)
(1985): Ting HC+, *Int J Dermatol* 24, 58
Erythema nodosum (<1%)
(1982): Elizaga FV, *Ann Intern Med* 96, 383
Exanthems
(1978): Castles JJ+, *Arch Intern Med* 138, 362 (5.6%)
(1976): Arndt KA+, *JAMA* 235, 918 (0.4%)
(1975): Pasquariello G+, *Curr Med Res Opin* 3, 109 (1.8%)
(1973): Thorne N, *Practitioner* 211, 606
(1970): Almeyda J+, *Br J Dermatol* 83, 707
(1967): Boardman PL+, *Ann Rheum Dis* 26, 127 (1.7%)
(1967): *Clin Pharmacol Ther* 8, 11 (11%)
Exfoliative dermatitis (<1%)
(1983): O'Sullivan M+, *Br J Rheumatol* 22, 47
Fixed eruption
(1976): Mackie BS, *Arch Dermatol* 112, 122
Flushing (>1%)
Generalized eruption (sic)
(1966): Kern AB, *Arch Dermatol* 93, 239
Granulomas (plasma cell)
(1975): Shelley WB+, *Acta Derm Venereol* (Stockh) 55, 489
Hot flashes (<1%)
Lichen planus
(1983): Hamburger J+, *BMJ* 287, 1258
Pemphigus
Periorbital edema
(1970): Almeyda J+, *Br J Dermatol* 83, 707
(1966): Rothermich NO, *JAMA* 195, 531
Peripheral edema
Petechiae (>1%)
Photoreactions
(1984): Stern RS+, *JAMA* 252, 1433
Pruritus (1–10%)
(1973): Thorne N, *Practitioner* 211, 606
(1970): Almeyda J+, *Br J Dermatol* 83, 707
(1967): *Clin Pharmacol Ther* 8, 11 (5%)
Psoriasis
(1993): Shelley WB+, *Cutis* 51, 415 (observation)
(1989): Lazarova AZ+, *Clin Exp Dermatol* 14, 260 (from topical application)
(1987): Sendagorta E+, *Dermatologica* 175, 300
(1987): Powles AV+, *Br J Dermatol* 117, 799
(1986): Abel EA+, *J Am Acad Dermatol* 15, 1007
(1981): Katayama H+, *J Dermatol* (Tokio) 8, 323
(1980): Katayama H+, *Nippon Hifuka Gakkai Zasshi* (Japanese) 90, 1027
Purpura (<1%)
(1984): Camba L+, *Acta Hematol* 71, 350
(1974): Cuthbert MF, *Curr Med Res Opin* 2, 600
(1973): Thorne N, *Practitioner* 211, 606
(1970): Almeyda J+, *Br J Dermatol* 83, 707
(1968): Bartoletti L+, *Riv Crit Clin Med* (Italian) 68, 279
Pustular psoriasis
(1987): Sendagorta E+, *Dermatologica* 175, 300
Rash (sic) (>10%)
(1967): Boardman PL+, *Ann Rheum Dis* 26, 127
Reiter's syndrome (exacerbation)
(1989): Allegue F+, *Med Cutan Ibero Lat Am* (Spanish) 17, 113
Stevens–Johnson syndrome (<1%)
Toxic epidermal necrolysis (<1%)
(1996): Lear JT+, *Postgrad Med J* 72, 186
(1990): Roujeau JC+, *Arch Dermatol* 126, 37
(1989): Roth DE+, *Med Clin North Am* 73, 1275
(1986): Johnson VB+, *La Pharm* 45, 4
(1985): Heng MCY, *Br J Dermatol* 113, 597
(1983): O'Sullivan M+, *Br J Rheumatol* 22, 47
Urticaria
(1995): Gebhardt M+, *Z Rheumatol* (German) 54, 405
(1992): Shelley WB+, *Cutis* 50, 87 (observation)
(1985): O'Brien WM+, *J Rheumatol* 12, 13
(1981): Juhlin L, *Br J Dermatol* 104, 369
(1974): Mathews JI+, *Ann Intern Med* 80, 771
(1973): Thorne N, *Practitioner* 211, 606
(1970): Almeyda J+, *Br J Dermatol* 83, 707
Urticaria pigmentosa
(1968): Vissian L+, *Bull Soc Franc Dermatol Syphiligr* (French) 75, 591
Vasculitis (<1%)
(1988): Gamboa PM+, *Allergol Immunopathol Madr* (Spanish) 16, 53
(1985): O'Brien WM+, *J Rheumatol* 12, 13
(1985): Bigby M, *J Am Acad Dermatol* 12, 866
(1971): Marsh FP+, *Ann Rheum Dis* 30, 501
(1970): Almeyda J+, *Br J Dermatol* 83, 707

Hair

Hair – alopecia (<1%)

Nails

Nails – onycholysis

Other

Ageusia
(1967): Boardman PL+, *Ann Rheum Dis* 26, 127
Anaphylactoid reaction (<1%)
Aphthous stomatitis
Gynecomastia (<1%)
Hypersensitivity (<1%)
Oral lichenoid eruption
(1983): Hamburger J+, *BMJ* 287, 1258
Oral mucosal lesions
(1967): Boardman PL+, *Ann Rheum Dis* 26, 127 (0.5%)
(1967): *Clin Pharmacol Ther* 8, 11 (7%)
Oral ulceration
(1983): Hamburger J+, *BMJ* 287, 1258
(1975): Guggenheimer J+, *J Am Dent Assoc* 90, 632
(1967): Boardman PL+, *Ann Rheum Dis* 26, 127
Paresthesias (<1%)
Serum sickness
(1985): Ferraccioli G+, *Acta Haematol* 73, 45
Temporal arteritis
(1985): O'Brien WM+, *J Rheumatol* 12, 13
(1967): Easterbrook WM+, *Can Med Assoc J* 97, 296
Tongue edema
(1967): Boardman PL+, *Ann Rheum Dis* 26, 127
Ulcerative stomatitis (<1%)
(1982): Bailin PL+, *Clin Rheum Dis* 8, 493 (passim)
Xerostomia

INFLIXIMAB

Trade name: Remicade (Centocor)
Indications: Crohn's disease
Category: Monoclonal antibody; tumor necrosis factor alpha blocker
Half-life: 9.5 days
Clinically important, potentially serious interactions with: no data

Reactions

Skin

Candidiasis (5%)
Chills (5–9%)
Edema
(1999): Lichenstein GR+, *Biologics in Clinical Practice Symposium*, Orlando, FL, May 19
Infections (sic) (21%)
Lupus erythematosus (<1%)
Pruritus (5%)
(1999): Lichenstein GR+, *Biologics in Clinical Practice Symposium*, Orlando, FL, May 19

Rash (sic) (6%)
(1999): Lichenstein GR+, *Biologics in Clinical Practice Symposium*, Orlando, FL, May 19
Urticaria
(1999): Lichenstein GR+, *Biologics in Clinical Practice Symposium*, Orlando, FL, May 19

Other

Hypersensitivity
(1999): Lichenstein GR+, *Biologics in Clinical Practice Symposium*, Orlando, FL, May 19
Infusion reactions (sic) (16%)
Myalgia (5%)
(1999): Lichenstein GR+, *Biologics in Clinical Practice Symposium*, Orlando, FL, May 19
Paresthesias (1–4%)

INH

(See ISONIAZID)

INSULIN

Trade names: Humulin (Lilly); Iletin Lente (Lilly); Novolin R (Bristol-Myers Squibb); NPH (Lilly); Protamine (Lilly); Velosulin (Novo Nordisk), etc.
Other common trade names: *Humalog; Huminsulin; Humulin; Insuman; Velosuline Humaine; Monotard, etc.*
Indications: Diabetes
Category: Hypoglycemic
Duration of action: 5–28 hours
Clinically important, potentially serious interactions with: alcohol, beta-blockers, clofibrate, corticosteroids, diltiazem, dobutamine, epinephrine, fenfluramine, guanethidine, MAO inhibitors, niacin, oral contraceptives, phenylbutazone, salicylates, sulfinpyrazone, tetracyclines, thiazide diuretics, thyroid hormone, **cigarette smoking**

Note: About 25% of patients with insulin allergy have a concomitant history of penicillin allergy.

Reactions

Skin

Allergic reactions (sic)
(1985): Bruni B+, *Diabetes Care* 8, 201
(1984): Grammer LC+, *JAMA* 251, 1459
(1982): Carveth-Johnson AO+, *Lancet* 2, 1287
(1981): Hasche H+, *Dtsch Med Wochenschr* (German) 106, 1451
(1980): Jegasothy BV, *Int J Dermatol* 19, 139 (immediate and delayed) (10–56%)
(1969): Aubert J+, *Rev Fr Allergol* (French) 9, 40
Angioedema
(1983): Grammer LC+, *J Allergy Clin Immunol* 71, 250
(1981): Kahn CB, *Handbook of Diabetes Mellitus* Garland STPM, 75
(1979): Lynfield Y+, *Arch Dermatol* 115, 591 (passim)
(1978): Galloway JA+, *Med Clin North Am* 62, 663
(1976): Lamkin N+, *J Allergy Clin Immunol* 58, 213
(1952): Dolger H, *Med Clin North Am* 36, 783
Bullous eruption
(1974): Haroon TS, *Scott Med J* 19, 257
Contact dermatitis
(1994): Goldfine AB+, *Curr Ther Endocrinol Metab* 5, 461
(1989): Geldof BA+, *Contact Dermatitis* 20, 384
Diaphoresis (1–10%)
Edema (1–10%)
(1981): Galloway JA+, *Diabetes Mellitus* Bowie 5, 117
(1979): Lawrence JR+, *BMJ* 2, 445
Exanthems
(1978): Galloway JA+, *Med Clin North Am* 62, 663
Flushing
(1961): Hanauer L+, *Diabetes* 10, 105
Granulomas (zinc)
(1989): Jordaan HF+, *Clin Exp Dermatol* 14, 227
Hyperkeratotic verrucous papules
(1989): Jordaan HF+, *Clin Exp Dermatol* 14, 277
(1986): Fleming MG+, *Arch Dermatol* 122, 1054 (resembling acanthosis nigricans)
(1969): Erickson L+, *JAMA* 209, 934
Keloid formation
(1970): Jelinek JE, *Year Book of Dermatology*, Chicago 5–35
Necrosis
(1974): Rohan P+, *Arch Dermatol Forsch* 250, (German) 121
Pallor (1–10%)
Pigmentation
(1970): Jelinek JE, *Year Book of Dermatology*, Chicago 5–35
Pigskin appearance (sic)
(1925): Lawrence RD, *Lancet* 1, 1125
Pruritus (1–10%)
(1981): Knick B, *MMW Munch Med Wochenschr* (German) 123, 1197
(1925): Lawrence RD, *Lancet* 1, 1125
(1922): Banting FG+, *J Metab Res* 2, 547
Purpura
(1976): Lamkin N+, *J Allergy Clin Immunol* 58, 213
(1956): Constam GR, *Diabetes* 5, 121
Urticaria (1–10%)
(1996): Rowland-Payne CM+, *Br J Dermatol* 134, 184
(1995): Chng HH+, *Allergy* 50, 984
(1988): Plantin P+, *Ann Dermatol Venereol* (French) 115, 813
(1983): Grammer LC+, *J Allergy Clin Immunol* 71, 250
(1982): Patterson R+, *JAMA* 248, 2637 (passim)
(1982): Mirouze J+, *Nouv Presse Med* (French) 11, 3121
(1981): Kahn CB, *Handbook of Diabetes Mellitus* Garland STPM, 75
(1979): Lynfield Y+, *Arch Dermatol* 115, 591 (passim)
(1979): Levy WJ+, *Cleve Clin Q* 46, 155
(1978): Galloway JA+, *Med Clin North Am* 62, 663
(1978): Reisner C+, *BMJ* 2, 56
(1976): Lamkin N+, *J Allergy Clin Immunol* 58, 213
(1962): Arkins JA+, *J Allergy* 33, 69
(1952): Dolger H, *Med Clin North Am* 36, 783
(1925): Lawrence RD, *Lancet* 1, 1125
(1922): Banting FG+, *J Metab Res* 2, 547
Vasculitis
(1983): Grammer LC+, *J Allergy Clin Immunol* 71, 250
Xanthomatosis
(1975): Vermeer BJ+, *Dermatologica* 151, 43

Other

Allergic reactions (local) (sic)
(1989): Zinman B, *N Engl J Med* 321, 363
(1988): Plantin P+, *Ann Dermatol Venereol* (French) 115, 813 (>5%)
(1981): Kahn CB, *Handbook of Diabetes Mellitus* Garland STPM, 75
(1979): Borsey DQ+, *Postgrad Med J* 55, 199
(1961): Hanauer L+, *Diabetes* 10, 105
(1939): Kern RA+, *JAMA* 113, 198
Anaphylactoid reaction (1–10%)
(1983): Grammer LC+, *J Allergy Clin Immunol* 71, 250
(1982): Patterson R+, *JAMA* 248, 2637 (passim)
(1981): Kahn CB, *Handbook of Diabetes Mellitus* Garland STPM, 75
(1979): Lynfield Y+, *Arch Dermatol* 115, 591 (passim)
(1978): Galloway JA+, *Med Clin North Am* 62, 663
(1976): Lamkin N+, *J Allergy Clin Immunol* 58, 213
(1952): Dolger H, *Med Clin North Am* 36, 783
(1925): Lawrence RD, *Lancet* 1, 1125
Dermal atrophy
(1978): Oakley WG+, *Diabetes and its Management*, Blackwell, 103
Dermal reactions (sic) (50%)
(1982): Patterson R+, *JAMA* 248, 2637 (passim)
Hypersensitivity
(1983): Berman BA+, *Cutis* 32, 320
(1982): deShazo RD+, *J Allergy Clin Immunol* 69, 229
(1974): Federlin K, *Dtsch Med Wochenschr* (German) 99, 535
Hypertrophic lipodystrophy
(1983): Johnson DA+, *Cutis* 32, 273
Injection-site calcification
(1995): Ullman HR+, *J Comput Assist Tomogr* 19, 657
Injection-site cancer (sic)
(1976): Sampson WI, *JAMA* 235, 374

Injection-site induration
(1983): White WB+, *Am J Med* 74, 909
(1981): Galloway JA+, *Diabetes Mellitus* Bowie 5, 117
(1979): Feinglos MN+, *Lancet* 1, 122 (due to zinc)
(1979): Lynfield Y+, *Arch Dermatol* 115, 591 (with erythema)
(1978): Galloway JA+, *Med Clin North Am* 62, 663
Injection-site pruritus
(1988): Plantin P+, *Ann Dermatol Venereol* (French) 115, 813
(1979): Lynfield Y+, *Arch Dermatol* 115, 591
Lipoatrophy (1–10%)
(1998): Murao S+, *Intern Med* 37, 1031
(1996): Logwin S+, *Diabetes Care* 19, 255
(1993): Chantelau E+, *Exp Clin Endocrinol* 101, 194
(1992): Igea JM+, *Allergol Immunopathol Madr* (Spanish) 20, 173
(1989): Gyimesi A+, *Orv Hetil* (Hungarian) 130, 2751
(1989): Zinman B, *N Engl J Med* 321, 363
(1988): McNally PG+, *Postgrad Med J* 64, 850
(1988): Perrot H, *Ann Dermatol Venereol* (French) 115, 523
(1983): Blickle JF+, *Presse Med* (French) 12, 2534
(1982): Levandoski LA+, *Diabetes Care* 5, 6
(1981): Jones GR+, *BMJ* 282, 190
(1981): Kahn CB, *Handbook of Diabetes Mellitus* Garland STPM, 75
(1980): Reeves WG+, *BMJ* 280, 1500
(1979): Asherov J+, *Diabete Metab* 5, 1
(1978): Talantov VV, *Sov Med* (Russian) June, 104
(1978): Aw TC+, *Singapore Med J* 19, 227
(1978): Oakley WG+, *Diabetes and its Management*, Blackwell, 103
(1978): Galloway JA+, *Med Clin North Am* 62, 663
(1977): Kumar O+, *Diabetes* 26, 296
(1976): Maaz E, *Z Gesamte Inn Med* (German) 31, 941
(1976): Whitley TH+, *JAMA* 235, 839
(1975): Jablonska S+, *Acta Derm Venereol* 55, 135
(1974): Teuscher A, *Diabetologia* 10, 211
(1974): Talantov VV, *Sov Med* (Russian) 37, 80
(1972): Bloom A, *BMJ* 4, 366
Lipodystrophy
(1990): Kohli V+, *Indian Pediatr* 27, 1120
(1988): Field LM, *J Am Acad Dermatol* 19, 570
(1988): Verbenko EV+, *Sov Med* (Russian) 3, 104
(1987): Goldman JM+, *Am J Med* 83, 195
(1985): Valenta LJ+, *Ann Intern Med* 102, 790
(1984): De Mattia G+, *Clin Ter* (Italian) 111, 169
(1984): Tebuev AM, *Pediatriia* (Russian) December 59
(1984): Campbell IW+, *Postgrad Med J* 60, 439
(1982): Levandoski LA+, *Diabetes Care* 5, 6
(1981): Libman E+, *Med Pregl* (Serbo-Croatian-Roman) 34, 49
(1981): Pisarskaia IV+, *Med Sestra* (Russian) 40, 54
(1979): Welk DS, *Nursing* 9, 42
(1978): da Cruz-Borges RC+, *Rev Bras Enferm* (Portuguese) 31, 252
(1974): Mehnert H, *Dtsch Med Wochenschr* (German) 99, 1274
(1973): Watson D+, *Med J Aust* 1, 248
(1972): Mehnert H, *Med Klin* (German) 67, 1384
(1971): Sapelkina LV+, *Pediatriia* (Russian) 50, 18
(1969): Todorovic M, *Med Pregl* (Serbo-Croatian-Cyrillic) 22, 177
(1968): Gleize J+, *Diabete* (French) 16, 281
(1968): Thosteson GC, *Mich Med* 67, 609
(1967): Jablonska S+, *Pol Tyg Lek* (Polish) 22, 977
(1967): Hintz R, *Pol Tyg Lek* (Polish) 22, 828
(1967): Hintz R, *Pol Tyg Lek* (Polish) 22, 902
(1965): Aubertin E+, *J Med Bord* (French) 142, 605
Lipohypertrophy (1–10%)
(1996): Hauner H+, *Exp Clin Endocrinol Diabetes* 104, 106
(1990): Schiazza L+, *J Am Acad Dermatol* 22, 148
(1989): Zinman B, *N Engl J Med* 321, 363
(1988): McNally PG+, *Postgrad Med J* 64, 850
(1987): Samadaei A+, *J Am Acad Dermatol* 17, 506
(1984): Young RJ+, *Diabetes Care* 7, 479
(1983): Johnson DA+, *Cutis* 32, 273
(1982): Mier A+, *BMJ* 285, 1539
(1969): Erickson L+, *JAMA* 209, 934
Panniculitis
(1988): Verbenko EV+, *Vestn Dermatol Venerol* (Russian) 1, 63
Paresthesias (1–10%)
Tremor (1–10%)
Tumors (nodules)
(1981): Galloway JA+, *Diabetes Mellitus*, Bowie 5, 117
(1978): Oakley WG+, *Diabetes and its Management*, Blackwell, 103
(1960): Oakley WG, *Br Med Bull* 16, 247

INTERFERONS, ALFA-2

Synonyms: IFLrA; IFN; rLFN-A; INF; INF-alpha-2;
Trade names: Alferon N (Interferon); Infergen (Amgen); Intron A (Schering); Rebetron (Schering); Roferon-A (Roche)
Other common trade names: *Roceron-A; Green-Alpha; Introna; Introne; Laroferon*
Indications: Chronic hepatitis C virus infection
Category: Biologic response modulator and antineoplastic
Half-life: 2 hours
Clinically important, potentially serious interactions with: cimetidine, theophylline, vinblastine

Rebetron is interferon and ribavirin

Nota Bene: Many of the adverse reactions depend on the nature of the disease being treated. Either hairy cell leukemia [L] or AIDS-related Kaposi's sarcoma [K].

Reactions

Skin

Acne (1%)
Acrocyanosis
(1998): Campo-Voegeli A+, *Dermatology* 196, 361
Behçet's disease
(1995): Segawa F+, *J Rheumatol* 22, 1183
Bullous eruption
(1995): Chang LW+, *Cutis* 56, 144
(1993): Parodi A+, *Dermatology* 186, 155
(1993): Andry P+, *Ann Dermatol Venereol* (French) 120, 843
Candidiasis (1%)
Chills
(2000): Cornejo P+, *Arch Dermatol* 136, 429
Contact dermatitis
(1995): Chang LW+, *Cutis* 56, 144
Cutaneous malignancy
(1991): Wagner RF+, *Arch Dermatol* 127, 272
Cutaneous necrosis
(1997): de Ledinghen V+, *Gastroenterol Clin Biol* 21, 523
(1995): Trautinger F+, *N Engl J Med* 333, 1222
(1991): Cnudde F+, *Int J Dermatol* 30, 147
(1989): Rasokat H+, *Dtsch Med Wochenschr* (German) 114, 458
Cutaneous reaction (sic)
(1996): Azagury M+, *Eur J Cancer* 32A, 1821 (severe)
Cutaneous vascular lesions (sic)
(1989): Dreno B+, *Ann Intern Med* 111, 95
Dermatitis herpetiformis
(1995): Dmochowski M+, *Postepy Dermatol* 12, 7
Dermatologic toxicity (sic)
(1993): Miglino M+, *Haematologica* 78, 411
Diaphoresis (22%) [L]; (7%) [K]
(1999): Angulo MP+, *Pediatr Cardiol* 20, 293 [L]
Discoloration (sic) (<1%)
Ecchymoses [L]
Eczematous eruption (sic)
(1999): Sookoian S+, *Arch Dermatol* 135, 999 (with ribavirin) [K]
(1989): Detmar U+, *Contact Dermatitis* 20, 149
Edema (11%) [L]
Erythema
(1999): Sookoian S+, *Arch Dermatol* 135, 999 (with ribavirin) (malar) [K]
Exanthems
(1994): Toyofuku K+, *J Dermatol* 21, 732
(1994): Sollitto RB+, *Arch Dermatol* 130, 1194
(1986): Quesada JR+, *Lancet* 1, 1466
Flu-like syndrome (sic) (>10%)
Fungal infection (sic) (<1%)
Herpes simplex (1%)
(1995): Chang LW+, *Cutis* 56, 144
(1992): Breathnach SM+, *Adverse Drug Reactions and the Skin*, Blackwell, Oxford, 322 (passim)
Hot flashes (sic) (1%)
Kaposi's sarcoma
(1993): Ariad S+, *South Afr Med J* 83, 430

Keratoses
(1994): Sollitto RB+, *Arch Dermatol* 130, 1194
Lichen myxedematosus
(1998): Rongioletti F+, *J Am Acad Dermatol* 38, 760
Lichen planus
(1999): Herstoff JK, Newport RI, (from Internet) (observation)
(1999): Sookoian S+, *Arch Dermatol* 135, 999 (with ribavirin) [K]
(1998): Dalekos GN+, *Eur J Gastroenterol Hepatol* 10, 933
(1995): Chang LW+, *Cutis* 56, 144
(1995): Hyrailles V+, *Gastroenterol Clin Biol* (French) 19, 833
(1995): Fornaciari G+, *J Clin Gastroenterol* 20, 346
(1993): Protzer U+, *Gastroenterology* 104, 903
(1993): Heintges T+, *J Hepatol* 18, 129
(1993): Boccia S+, *Gastroenterology* 105, 1921
Linear IgA bullous dermatosis
(1993): Parodi A+, *Dermatology* 187, 155
(1990): Guillaume JC+, *Ann Dermatol Venereol* (French) 117, 899
Lupus erythematosus
(1998): Garcia-Porrua C+, *Clin Exp Rheumatol* 16, 107
(1994): Flores A+, *Br J Rheumatol* 33, 787
(1994): Sanchez Roman J+, *Med Clin (Barc)* (Spanish) 102, 198
(1994): Fritzler MJ, *Lupus* 3, 455
(1992): Mehta ND+, *Am J Hematol* 41, 141
(1992): Tolaymat A+, *J Pediatr* 120, 429
(1991): Hess EV, *Curr Opin Rheumatol* 3, 809
(1991): Schilling JP+, *Cancer* 68, 1536
Melanoma
(1988): Bork K+, *Dermatologica* 177, 249 (exacerbation)
Necrosis
(1998): Sickler JB+, *Am J Gastroenterol* 93, 463
(1995): Chang LW+, *Cutis* 56, 144
Nodules (painful)
(1995): Chang LW+, *Cutis* 56, 144
Pemphigus
(1995): Kirsner RS+, *Br J Dermatol* 132, 474
(1994): Niizeki H+, *Dermatology* 189 (Suppl), 129
Photosensitivity (<1%)
(1994): Sollitto RB+, *Arch Dermatol* 130, 1194
Pruritus (13%) [L]; (5%) [K]
(1994): Czarnetzki BM+, *J Am Acad Dermatol* 30, 500
(1992): Breathnach SM+, *Adverse Drug Reactions and the Skin*, Blackwell, Oxford, 322 (passim)
Psoriasis
(2000): Taylor C+, *Postgrad Med J* 76, 365
(1996): Wolfer LU+, *Hautarzt* (German) 47, 124
(1995): Wolfe JT+, *J Am Acad Dermatol* 32, 887
(1995): Chang LW+, *Cutis* 56, 144
(1994): Matsuoka H+, *Rinsho Ketsueki* (Japanese) 35, 309
(1993): Georgetson MJ+, *Am J Gastroenterol* 88, 756
(1993): Cleveland MG+, *J Am Acad Dermatol* 29, 788
(1993): Garcia-Lora E+, *Dermatology* 187, 280
(1993): Pauluzzi P+, *Acta Derm Venereol* 73, 395
(1991): Funk J+, *Br J Dermatol* 125, 463
(1990): Kusec R+, *Dermatologica* 181, 170
(1990): Kowalzick L+, *Arch Dermatol* 126, 1515 (at injection site)
(1990): Fierlbeck G+, *Arch Dermatol* 126, 351 (at injection site)
(1990): Jucgla A+, *Arch Dermatol* 127, 910 (exacerbation)
(1989): Harrison P, *J Invest Dermatol* 93, 555
(1989): Hartmann F+, *Dtsch Med Wochenschr* (German) 114, 96 (exacerbation)
(1986): Quesada JR+, *Lancet* 1, 1466 (exacerbation)
Purpura
Rash (sic) (44%) [L]; (11%) [K]
(1999): Sookoian S+, *Arch Dermatol* 135, 999 (with ribavirin) [K]
Raynaud's phenomenon
(1996): Creutzig A+, *Ann Intern Med* 125, 423
(1994): Arslan M+, *J Intern Med* 235, 503
Reiter's syndrome (incomplete)
(1993): Cleveland MG+, *J Am Acad Dermatol* 29, 788
Sarcoidosis
(1999): Pietropaoli A+, *Chest* 116, 569
(1993): Blum L+, *Rev Med Interne* (Paris) (French) 14, 1161
Seborrheic dermatitis
(1986): Quesada JR+, *Lancet* 1, 1466
Sjøgren's syndrome
(1994): Lunel F, *Gastroenterol Clin Biol* (French) 19, 442
Telangiectases
(1989): Dreno B+, *Ann Intern Med* 111, 95
Ulceration
(1992): Orlow SJ+, *Arch Dermatol* 128, 566
Urticaria (<3%) [K]
(1994): Czarnetzki BM+, *J Am Acad Dermatol* 30, 500
(1992): Breathnach SM+, *Adverse Drug Reactions and the Skin*, Blackwell, Oxford, 322 (passim)
Vasculitis
(1998): Gordon AC+, *J Infect* 36, 229
(1996): Pateron D+, *Clin Exp Rheumatol* 14, 79
(1995): Chang LW+, *Cutis* 56, 144
(1992): Liet JM+, *Rev Med Interne* (French) 13, 169
(1983): Sangster G+, *Eur J Cancer Clin Oncol* 19, 1647
Vitiligo
(1997): Nouri K+, *Cutis* 60, 289
(1996): Le Gal F-A+, *J Am Acad Dermatol* 35, 650
(1996): Simsek H+, *Dermatology* 193, 65
(1995): Bernstein D+, *Am J Gastroenterol* 90, 1176
(1994): Scheibenbogen C+, *Eur J Cancer* 30A, 1209
Xerosis (17%) [L]; (22%) [K]

Hair

Hair – alopecia (1–10%)
(1997): Brehler R+, *J Am Acad Dermatol* 36, 983 (passim)
(1995): Chang LW+, *Cutis* 56, 144
(1994): Czarnetzki BM+, *J Am Acad Dermatol* 30, 500
(1992): Tosti A+, *Dermatology* 184, 124
(1989): Olsen EA+, *J Am Acad Dermatol* 20, 395
(1987): Werter MJBP, *Ned Tijdschr Geneeskd* (Dutch) 131, 2081
Hair – alopecia areata
(1999): Kernland KH+, *Dermatology* 198, 418
Hair – discoloration
(1996): Fleming CJ+, *Br J Dermatol* 135, 337
(1995): Bernstein D+, *Am J Gastroenterol* 90, 1176 (canities)
Hair – hypertrichosis
(1996): Ariyoshi K+, *Am J Hematol* 53, 50 (eyebrows)
(1990): Berglund EF+, *South Med J* 83, 363
(1984): Foon KA+, *N Engl J Med* 19, 1259 (eyelashes)

Other

Anosmia
(1998): Maruyama S+, *Am J Gastroenterol* 93, 122
Aphthous stomatitis
(1998): Dalekos GN+, *Eur J Gastroenterol Hepatol* 10, 933
Chills
(2000): Shenefelt PD+, *Arch Dermatol* 136, 837
Dysgeusia (25%) (metallic taste) [K]
(1995): Chang LW+, *Cutis* 56, 144
Halo dermatitis
(1999): Krischer J+, *J Am Acad Dermatol* 40, 105
Hypesthesia
Injection-site alopecia
(1999): Lang AM+, *Arch Dermatol* 135, 1127
Injection-site erythema
(1995): Chang LW+, *Cutis* 56, 144
Injection-site induration
(1997): Siegel M, New York, NY (from Internet) (observation)
(1995): Chang LW+, *Cutis* 56, 144
Injection-site necrosis
(1998): Krainick U+, *J Interferon Cytokine Res* 18, 823
(1997): Weinberg JM+, *Acta Derm Venereol* (Stockh) 77, 146
(1996): Kontochristopoulos G+, *J Hepatol* 25, 271
(1996): Konohana A+, *J Am Acad Dermatol* 35, 788
(1995): Shinohara K, *N Engl J Med* 333, 1222
(1994): Akiyama Y+, *Jpn J Dermatol* (Japanese) 104, 436
(1994): Tone T+, *Jpn J Dermatol* 104, 1047
(1993): Oeda E+, *Am J Hematol* 44, 213
(1993): Christian B+, *Presse Med* (French) 22, 783
(1993): Mihara K+, *Miyazakiikaishi* (Japanese) 17, 40
(1993): Nagai A+, *Int J Hematol* 58, 129
(1992): Orlow SJ+, *Arch Dermatol* 128, 566
(1991): Cnudde F+, *Int J Dermatol* 30, 147
(1989): Rasokat H+, *Dtsch Med Wochenschr* (German) 114, 158
Injection-site pruritus
(1989): Detmar U+, *Contact Dermatitis* 20, 149

Injection-site vasculitis
(1997): Christian MM+, *J Am Acad Dermatol* 37, 118
Lymphoma, malignant
(1994): Arico M+, *Blood* 83, 869
Myalgia (71%) [L]; (69%) [K]
(2000): Shenefelt PD+, *Arch Dermatol* 136, 837
(1999): Spieth K+, *Arch Dermatol* 135, 1035
(1997): Brehler R+, *J Am Acad Dermatol* 36, 983 (passim)
(1984): Foon KA+, *N Engl J Med* 19, 1259 (passim)
Myopathy
(1998): Dippel E, *Arch Dermatol* 134, 880 (4 patients)
Oral lichen planus
(1997): Schlesinger TE+, *J Am Acad Dermatol* 36, 1023 (erosive)
(1997): Kutting B+, *Br J Dermatol* 137, 836
(1995): Chang LW+, *Cutis* 56, 144
(1994): Papini M+, *Int J Dermatol* 33, 221
(1994): Perreard M+, *Gastroenterol Clin Biol* (French) 18, 1051
(1993): Sassigneux P+, *Gastroenterol Clin Biol* (French) 17, 764
Paresthesias (12%) [L]; (8%) [K]
Sialopenia
Stomatitis (1–10%)
Xerostomia (>10%)

INTERLEUKIN-2

(See ALDESLEUKIN)

IPODATE

Trade names: Bilivist (Berlex); Oragrafin (Bristol-Myers Squibb)
Indications: Cholecystography
Category: Cholecystographic contrast medium
Half-life: no data
Clinically important, potentially serious interactions with: no data

Reactions

Skin
Allergic reactions (sic)
(1986): Bigby M+, *JAMA* 256, 3358 (2.78%)
Exanthems
Pruritus
Purpura
(1966): Stacher A, *Wien Klin Wochenschr* (German) 75, 820
Rash (sic)
Urticaria

Other
Anaphylactoid reaction
Hypersensitivity
Serum sickness

IPRATROPIUM

Trade names: Atrovent (Boehringer Ingelheim); Combivent (Boehringer Ingelheim)
Other common trade names: *Alti-Ipratropium; Novo-Ipramide*
Indications: Bronchospasm
Category: Aerosol bronchodilator; anticholinergic
Half-life: 2 hours
Clinically important, potentially serious interactions with: albuterol, anticholinergics, cromolyn, dronabinol

Combivent is albuterol and ipratropium

Reactions

Skin
Contact dermatitis
(1988): Eedy DJ+, *Postgrad Med J* 64, 306
Exanthems
Flushing (<1%)
Miliaria profunda
(1990): Saurat JH+, *Pediatr Dermatol* 7, 325
Pruritus (<1%)
Rash (sic) (1.2%)
Urticaria (<1%)

Hair
Hair – alopecia (<1%)

Other
Anaphylactoid reaction
(1993): Bone WD+, *Chest* 103, 981
Dysgeusia (1%) (metallic taste)
(1980): Pakes GE+, *Drugs* 20, 237
Oral mucosal lesions (1–5%)
(1980): Pakes GE+, *Drugs* 20, 237
Oral mucosal ulceration (<1%)
(1987): High AS, *BMJ* 294, 375
(1986): Spencer PA, *BMJ* 292, 380
Paresthesias (<1%)
Stomatitis (<1%)
Trembling (1–10%)
Xerostomia (3.2%)
(1980): Pakes GE+, *Drugs* 20, 237

IRBESARTAN

Trade names: Avalide (Bristol-Myers Squibb); Avapro (Bristol-Myers Squibb; Sanofi)
Indications: Hypertension
Category: Angiotensin II receptor antagonist; antihypertensive
Half-life: 11–15 hours
Clinically important, potentially serious interactions with: amiloride, lithium, nifedipine, potassium, spironolactone, tolbutamide

Avalide is irbesartan and hydrochlorothiazide (a sulfonamide)*

Reactions

Skin
Chills (<1%)
Dermatitis (sic) (<1%)
Ecchymoses (<1%)
Edema (1–10%)
Erythema (<1%)
Facial edema (<1%)
Flushing (<1%)
Pruritus (<1%)
Rash (sic) (1–10%)
Urticaria (<1%)

Other

Oral lesions (<1%)
Paresthesias (<1%)
Tremor (<1%)

***Note:** Avalide contains a sulfonamide which can be absorbed systemically. Sulfonamides can produce severe, possibly fatal, reactions such as toxic epidermal necrolysis and Stevens–Johnson syndrome.

IRINOTECAN

Synonyms: Camptothecin-11; CPT-11
Trade name: Camptosar (Pharmacia & Upjohn)
Indications: Metastatic colorectal carcinoma
Category: Antineoplastic
Half-life: 6–10 hours
Clinically important, potentially serious interactions with: anticoagulants, immunosuppressives, laxatives, NSAIDs, platelet inhibitors, prochlorperazine, salicylates, thrombolytic agents, vaccines

Reactions

Skin

Allergic reactions (sic)
(1997): Verschraegen CF+, *J Clin Oncol* 15, 625 (9%)
Chills (13.8%)
Diaphoresis (16%)
Edema (10.2%)
Flushing (11%)
Pigmentation
Rash (sic) (12.8%)
(1997): Verschraegen CF+, *J Clin Oncol* 15, 625 (21%)

Hair

Hair – alopecia (60.5%)
(1999): Takahashi Y+, *Gan To Kagaku Ryoho* (Japanese) 26, 1193
(1998): Berg D, *Oncol Nurs Forum* 25, 535
(1997): Verschraegen CF+, *J Clin Oncol* 15, 625 (48%)
(1996): Rougier P+, *Semin Oncol* 23, 34
(1995): Catimel G+, *Ann Oncol* 6, 133
(1995): Abigerges D+, *J Clin Oncol* 13, 210 (53%)
(1994): de Forni M+, *Cancer Res* 54, 4347
(1994): Sakata Y+, *Gan To Kagaku Ryoho* (Japanese) 21, 1039 (40%)
(1994): Taguchi T+, *Gan To Kagaku Ryoho* (Japanese) 21, 1017 (30%)
(1994): Taguchi T+, *Gan To Kagaku Ryoho* (Japanese) 21, 83 (61%)
(1992): Fukuoka M+, *J Clin Oncol* 10, 16 (4%)
(1991): Takeuchi S+, *Gan To Kagaku Ryoho* (Japanese) 18, 1681 (33%)
(1991): Negoro S+, *Gan To Kagaku Ryoho* (Japanese) 18, 1013
(1991): Takeuchi S+, *Gan To Kagaku Ryoho* (Japanese) 18, 579 (33%)
(1990): Taguchi T+, *Gan To Kagaku Ryoho* (Japanese) 17, 115

Other

Dysgeusia (metallic taste)
Mucositis (2%)
Oral ulceration
Sialorrhea
Stomatitis (12%)
(2000): Adjei AA+, *J Clin Oncol* 18, 1116
(1997): Verschraegen CF+, *J Clin Oncol* 15, 625 (14%)
Thrombophlebitis (1–10%)

ISOCARBOXAZID

Trade name: Marplan (Roche)
Other common trade name: *Enerzer*
Indications: Depression
Category: Monoamine oxidase (MAO) inhibitor; antidepressant and antipanic
Half-life: no data
Clinically important, potentially serious interactions with: amphetamines, barbiturates, dextroamphetamine, disulfiram, dopamine, ephedrine, fluoxetine, levodopa, meperidine, reserpine, sulfonamides, sympathomimetics, tricyclic antidepressants, **tyramine-containing foods***

Reactions

Skin

Diaphoresis
(1962): Busfield BL+, *J Nerv Ment Dis* 134, 339 (30%)
Exanthems (7%)
(1962): Busfield BL+, *J Nerv Ment Dis* 134, 339
Peripheral edema (1–10%)
Photosensitivity (4%)
(1962): Busfield BL+, *J Nerv Ment Dis* 134, 339
Pruritus (4%)
(1962): Busfield BL+, *J Nerv Ment Dis* 134, 339
Rash (sic)
Telangiectases

Other

Black tongue
Xerostomia (1–10%)
(1962): Busfield BL+, *J Nerv Ment Dis* 134, 339 (11%)

***Note:** Tyramine-containing foods include the following: aged cheeses, avocados, banana skins, bologna and other processed luncheon meats, chicken livers, chocolate, figs, canned pickled herring, meat extracts, pepperoni, raisins, raspberries, soy sauce, vermouth, sherry and red wines.

ISOETHARINE

Trade names: Arm-a-Med; Beta-2; Bronkometer (Sanofi); Bronkomed; *Bronkosol (Sanofi); Dey-Lute*
Other trade names: *Asthmalitan; Numotac*
Indications: Bronchial asthma
Category: Adrenergic agonist; bronchodilator; sympathomimetic
Half-life: no data
Clinically important, potentially serious interactions with: digoxin, epinephrine

Reactions

Skin

None

Other

Anaphylactoid reaction
(1982): Twarog FJ+, *JAMA* 248, 2030
Trembling (1–10%)
Tremor
Xerostomia (1–10%)

ISONIAZID

Synonym: INH
Trade names: Rifamate (Aventis); Rifater (Aventis)
Other common trade names: *Cemidon; Diazid; Isotamine; Isozid; Nicotibine; Nicozid; PMS-Isoniazid; Tibinide*
Indications: Tuberculosis
Category: Tuberculostatic
Half-life: 1–4 hours
Clinically important, potentially serious interactions with: alcohol, anticoagulants, benzodiazepines, carbamazepine, cycloserine, disulfiram, hydantoins, ketoconazole, meperidine, phenytoin, rifampin, valproic acid

Reactions

Skin

Acne
(1988): Oliwiecki S+, *Clin Exp Dermatol* 13, 283
(1988): Yamanaka M+, *Kekkaku* (Japanese) 63, 11
(1982): Rosin MA+, *Southern Med J* 75, 81 (passim)
(1974): Cohen LK+, *Arch Dermatol* 109, 377
(1969): Lantis SH, *J Am Med Wom Assoc* 24, 305
(1959): Bereston ES, *J Invest Dermatol* 33, 427

Acute generalized exanthematous pustulosis (AGEP)
(1995): Moreau A+, *Int J Dermatol* 34, 263 (passim)

Angioedema (<1%)
(1989): Yagi S+, *Kekkaku* (Japanese) 64, 407
(1959): Bereston ES, *J Invest Dermatol* 33, 427

Bullous eruption
(1999): Scheid P+, *Allergy* 54, 294

Contact dermatitis
(1993): Meseguer J+, *Contact Dermatitis* 28, 110 (systemic)
(1986): Holdiness MR, *Contact Dermatitis* 15, 282
(1978): Ippen H, *Derm Beruf Umwelt* (German) 26, 57

Cutaneous side effects (sic)
(1985): Holdiness MR, *Int J Dermatol* 24, 280 (2%)

Cutis laxa
(1985): Koch SE+, *Pediatr Dermatol* 2, 282

Dermatomyositis
(1975): Fayolle J+, *Lyon Med* (French) 233, 135

Erythema multiforme (<1%)
(1988): Hira SK+, *J Am Acad Dermatol* 19, 451 (in AIDS patients)
(1976): Bomb BS+, *Tubercle* 57, 229

Exanthems
(1982): Rosin MA+, *Southern Med J* 75, 81 (passim)
(1979): Byrd RB+, *JAMA* 241, 1239 (0.9%)
(1963): Honeycutt WM+, *Arch Dermatol* 88, 190
(1959): Bereston ES, *J Invest Dermatol* 33, 427

Exfoliative dermatitis
(1985): Holdiness MR, *Int J Dermatol* 24, 280
(1982): Rosin MA+, *Southern Med J* 75, 81
(1969): Agrawal R, *BMJ* 4, 540
(1963): Abrahams I+, *Arch Dermatol* 87, 96
(1963): Honeycutt WM+, *Arch Dermatol* 88, 190

Flushing
(1953): Witbind E+, *Dis Chest* 23, 16 (>5%)

Herpes zoster
(1959): Bereston ES, *J Invest Dermatol* 33, 427

Keratoacanthoma
(1966): Randazzo SD, *G Ital Dermatol Minerva Dermatol* (Italian) 107, 1195

Lichenoid eruption
(1974): Haldar B, *Indian J Dermatol* 19, 71

Lupus erythematosus
(1994): Yung RL+, *Rheum Dis Clin North Am* 20, 61
(1992): Skaer TL, *Clin Ther* 14, 496
(1992): Salazar-Pama M+, *Ann Rheum Dis* 51, 1085
(1992): Rubin RL+, *J Clin Invest* 90, 165
(1992): Hofstra AH+, *Drug Metab Dispos* 20, 205
(1991): Gatenby PA, *Autoimmunity* 11, 61
(1990): Guleria R+, *Indian J Chest Dis Allied Sci* 32, 55
(1989): Ueda Y+, *Kekkaku* (Japanese) 64, 613
(1988): Jiang M, *Chung Kuo I Hsueh Ko Hsueh Yuan Hseuh Pao* (Chinese) 10, 379
(1988): Umeki S, *Kekkaku* (Japanese) 63, 713
(1986): Layer P+, *Dtsch Med Wochenschr* (German) 111, 1603
(1985): Stratton MA, *Clin Pharm* 4, 657
(1985): Lovisetto P+, *Recenti Prog Med* (Ital) 76, 110
(1985): Cush JJ+, *Am J Med Sci* 290, 36
(1985): Kale SA, *Postgrad Med* 77, 231
(1985): Holdiness MR, *Int J Dermatol* 24, 280
(1984): No Author, *Lancet* 2, 441
(1984): Sim E+, *Lancet* 2, 422
(1983): Escolar-Castellon F+, *Rev Clin Esp* (Spanish) 169, 209
(1982): Harmon CE+, *Clin Rheum Dis* 8, 121
(1982): Grunwald M+, *Dermatologica* 165, 172
(1981): Reidenberg MM, *Arthritis Rheum* 24, 1004
(1980): Weinstein A, *Prog Clin Immunol* 4, 1
(1980): Agarwal MB+, *J Postgrad Med* 26, 263
(1977): Dandavino R+, *Ann Med Interne Paris* (French) 128, 39
(1977): Seedat YK+, *S Afr Med J* 51, 335
(1976): Cohmen G, *Med Klin* (German) 71, 789
(1976): Dutt AK+, *Indian J Chest Dis Allied Sci* 18, 146
(1975): Laroche C+, *Sem Hop* (French) 51, 2515
(1974): McEwen J, *Lancet* 2, 1570
(1974): Harpey JP, *Ann Allergy* 33, 256
(1974): No Author, *Va Med Mon* 101, 299 (passim)
(1974): *Med Lett Drugs Ther* 16, 34
(1973): Alarcon-Segovia D, *Chest* 63, 299
(1973): Blomgren SE, *Semin Hematol* 10, 345
(1973): Godeau P+, *Ann Med Interne Paris* (French) 124, 181
(1973): Durand JP+, *Cah Med* (French) 14, 9
(1973): Bar-On H, *Harefuah* (Hebrew) 84, 25
(1972): Gaultier Cl+, *Ann Pédiatr Paris* (French) 19, 459
(1972): Greenberg JH+, *JAMA* 222, 191
(1972): Goldman AL+, *Chest* 62, 71
(1972): Dorfmann H+, *Nouv Presse Med* (French) 1, 2907
(1971): Delepierre F+, *Rev Tuberc Pneumol Paris* (French) 35, 397
(1970): Trad J+, *Sem Hop* (French) 46, 3013
(1970): No Author, *BMJ* 2, 192
(1969): Alarcon-Segovia D, *Mayo Clin Proc* 44, 664
(1967): Auquier L+, *Bull Mem Soc Med Hop Paris* (French) 118, 372
(1967): Siegel M+, *Arthritis Rheum* 10, 407
(1967): Hothersall TE+, *Scott Med J* 13, 245
(1967): Masel MA, *Med J Aust* 54, 738
(1963): Zingale SB+, *Arch Intern Med* 112, 63

Pellagra
(1999): Muratake T+, *Am J Psychiatry* 156, 660
(1987): Schmutz JL+, *Ann Derm Venereol* (French) 114, 569
(1983): Jorgensen J, *Int J Dermatol* 22, 44
(1981): Meyrick Thomas RH+, *BMJ* 283, 287
(1977): Comaish JS+, *Arch Dermatol* 113, 986
(1977): Harrington CI, *Practitioner* 218, 716
(1976): Comaish JS+, *Arch Dermatol* 112, 70
(1974): Schlenzka K+, *Dermatol Monatsschr* (German) 160, 848
(1974): Forstrom L+, *Arch Dermatol* 110, 635
(1974): Cohen LK+, *Arch Dermatol* 109, 377
(1972): Jansen CT+, *Duodecim* 88, 928
(1972): Harber LC+, *J Invest Dermatol* 58, 327
(1972): Bjornstad RT, *Tidsskr Nor Laegeforen* (Norwegian) 92, 640
(1969): Polano MK+, *Arch Belg Dermatol Syphiligr* (Dutch) 25, 345
(1967): Di Lorenzo PA, *Acta Derm Venereol* (Stockh) 47, 318
(1964): Aspinall DL, *BMJ* 2, 1177
(1959): Bereston ES, *J Invest Dermatol* 33, 427
(1958): Haynes WS, *East Afr Med J* 35, 171
(1956): Harrison RJ+, *BMJ* 2, 853
(1955): Wood MM, *Br J Tuberc Dis Chest* 49, 20
(1952): McConnell RB+, *Lancet* 2, 959

Photosensitivity
(1998): Lee AY+, *Photodermatol Photoimmunol Photomed* 14, 77 (lichenoid) (2 patients)
(1987): Schmutz JL+, *Ann Dermatol Venereol* (French) 114, 569
(1972): Kauppinen K, *Acta Derm Venereol* (Stockh) 52 (Suppl) 68
(1969): Kalivas J, *JAMA* 209, 1706

Pruritus
(1953): Witbind E+, *Dis Chest* 23, 16 (>5%)

Purpura
(1992): Breathnach SM+, *Adverse Drug Reactions and the Skin*, Blackwell, Oxford, 159 (passim)
(1982): Rosin MA+, *Southern Med J* 75, 81 (passim)
(1980): Miescher PA+, *Clin Haematol* 9, 505
(1979): Byrd RB+, *JAMA* 241, 1239

(1965): Horowitz HI+, *Semin Hematol* 2, 287
(1964): Duncan JT, *Am Rev Respir Dis* 89, 103
(1959): Bereston ES, *J Invest Dermatol* 33, 427

Pustular eruption
(1993): Webster GF, *Clin Dermatol* 11, 541
(1985): Yamasaki R+, *Br J Dermatol* 112, 504 (subcorneal)

Rash (sic) (<1%)
(2000): Gordin F+, *JAMA* 283, 1445

Stevens–Johnson syndrome
(1976): Bomb BS+, *Tubercle* 57, 229
(1965): Ingle VN+, *Indian Pediatr* 2, 305

Striae
(1967): Hofer W, *Z Haut Geschlechtskr* (German) 42, 603

Systemic eczematous contact dermatitis
(1993): Meseguer J+, *Contact Dermatitis* 28, 110

Toxic epidermal necrolysis (<1%)
(1990): Nanda A+, *Arch Dermatol* 126, 125
(1983): Katoch K+, *Lepr India* 55, 133
(1976): Mital OP+, *Indian J Tuberc* 23, 32
(1974): Faye I+, *Bull Soc Med Afr Noire Lang Fr* (French) 19, 185 (fatal)
(1973): Sehgal VN+, *Indian J Chest Dis* 15, 57
(1967): Lowney ED+, *Arch Dermatol* 95, 359

Urticaria (1–5%)
(1992): Breathnach SM+, *Adverse Drug Reactions and the Skin*, Blackwell, Oxford, 159 (passim)
(1982): Rosin MA+, *Southern Med J* 75, 81 (passim)
(1959): Bereston ES, *J Invest Dermatol* 33, 427
(1953): Cormia FE+, *Arch Dermatol* 68, 536 (4%)

Vasculitis
(1982): Rosin MA+, *Southern Med J* 75, 81 (passim)
(1963): Honeycutt WM+, *Arch Dermatol* 88, 190

Hair

Hair – alopecia
(1996): FitzGerald JM+, *Lancet* 347, 472
(1978): Krivokhizh VN+, *Vestn Dermatol Venerol* (Russian) 3, 63

Nails

Nails – onycholysis

Other

Acute intermittent porphyria

Gynecomastia

Hypersensitivity
(1992): Dukes CS+, *Trop Geogr Med* 44, 308
(1969): Rykowska Z, *Gruzlica* (Polish) 37, 777

Injection-site irritation

Myopathy
(1989): Cronkright PJ+, *Ann Intern Med* 110, 945

Oral mucosal lesions
(1973): Parish LC+, *Int J Dermatol* 12, 324
(1971): *Med Lett* 13, 55 (1–5%)

Oral mucosal ulceration

Paresthesias
(1982): Porter IH, *Handbook of Clinical Neurology* 44, 648

Serum sickness
(1981): Simelaro J+, *J Am Osteopath Assoc* 80, 348

Xerostomia

ISOPROTERENOL

Trade names: Aerolone; Arm-a-Med; Isuprel (Sanofi); Medihaler-ISO (3M); Norisodrine (Abbott)
Other common trade names: *Isopro; Isuprel Mistometer; Isuprel Nebulimetro; Saventrine; Vapo-Iso*
Indications: Bronchospasm, ventricular arrhythmias
Category: Adrenergic bronchodilator; sympathomimetic
Half-life: 2.5–5 minutes
Clinically important, potentially serious interactions with: beta-blockers, digoxin, general anesthetics, sympathomimetics, tricyclic antidepressants

Reactions

Skin

Diaphoresis (1–10%)

Edema

Flushing (1–10%)

Pruritus

Rash (sic)

Urticaria

Other

Oral mucosal lesions
(1969): Warth J+, *JAMA* 209, 417

Saliva discoloration (sic) (pinkish-red) (>10%)

Trembling

Tremor

Xerostomia (>10%)

ISOSORBIDE DINITRATE

Synonyms: ISD; ISDN
Trade names: Dilatrate-SR (Schwarz); Isordil (Wyeth-Ayerst); Sorbitrate (AstraZeneca)
Other common trade names: *Apo-ISDN; Cedocard; Coradur*
Indications: Angina pectoris
Category: Antianginal; vasodilator
Half-life: 4 hours (oral)
Clinically important, potentially serious interactions with: alcohol, antihypertensives, sildenafil, vasodilators

Reactions

Skin

Ankle edema
(1981): Rodger JC, *BMJ* 283, 1365

Diaphoresis

Edema (<1%)

Flushing (>10%)
(1981): Rodger JC, *BMJ* 283, 1365 (passim)

Pallor

Peripheral edema

Other

Xerostomia

ISOSORBIDE MONONITRATE

Synonym: ISMN
Trade names: Imdur (Key); Ismo (Wyeth-Ayerst); Monoket (Schwarz)
Indications: Angina pectoris
Category: Antianginal; vasodilator
Half-life: ~4 hours
Clinically important, potentially serious interactions with: alcohol, aspirin, calcium channel blockers, ergot alkaloids, sildenafil

Reactions

Skin

Ankle edema
(1981): Rodger JC, *BMJ* 283, 1365
Diaphoresis
Edema (<1%)
Flushing (>10%)
(1981): Rodger JC, *BMJ* 283, 1365 (passim)
Pruritus (<1%)
Rash (sic) (<1%)

Other

Hypesthesia (<1%)
Tooth disorder (sic) (<1%)

ISOSORBIDE

Trade name: Ismotic
Indications: Acute angle-closure glaucoma
Category: Osmotic diuretic
Half-life: 5–9.5 hours
Clinically important, potentially serious interactions with: alcohol, aspirin, calcium channel blockers, ergot alkaloids

Reactions

Skin

Rash (sic) (<1%)

ISOTRETINOIN

Synonym: 13-*cis*-retinoic acid
Trade name: Accutane (Roche)
Other common trade names: *Isotrex; Roaccutane; Roaccutan; Roacutan; Roacuttan*
Indications: Cystic acne
Category: Retinoid; inhibits sebaceous gland function
Half-life: 10–20 hours
Clinically important, potentially serious interactions with: acitretin, carbamazepine, dexamethasone, etretinate, fish oil supplements, minocycline, tetracycline, vitamin A

Reactions

Skin

Acne (fulminans)
(1997): Tan BB+, *Clin Exp Dermatol* 22, 26
(1996): Faverge B+, *Arch Pediatr* (French) 3, 188
(1993): Bottomley WW+, *Acta Derm Venereol* (Stockh) 73, 74
(1993): Lepagney ML+, *Ann Dermatol Venereol* (French) 120, 917
(1992): Jenkinson HA, *Br J Dermatol* 127, 62
(1992): Hagler J+, *Int J Dermatol* 31, 199
(1992): Choi EH+, *J Dermatol* 19, 378
(1991): Elias LM+, *J Dermatol* 18, 366
(1991): Joly P+, *Ann Dermatol Venereol* (French) 118, 369
(1989): Rotoli M+, *G Ital Dermatol Venereol* (Italian) 124, 120
(1988): Blanc D+, *Dermatologica* 177, 16
(1985): Kellett JK+, *BMJ* 290, 820
(1984): Darley CR+, *J R Soc Med* 77, 328
Bruising (sic)
(1993): Green C, *Br J Dermatol* 128, 465
Cheilitis (>90%)
(1999): Graham BS+, *Arch Dermatol* 349
(1997): Berger R, *The Schoch Letter* 47, 5
(1997): Goulden V+, *Br J Dermatol* 137, 106
(1988): Shalita AR+, *Cutis* 42, 10
(1976): Peck GL+, *Lancet* 2, 1172
Desquamation (palms and soles) (5%)
(1988): Shalita AR+, *Cutis* 42, 10
Diaphoresis
(1988): Rees JL+, *Br J Dermatol* 119, 79
Edema (subcutaneous, recurrent)
(1999): Graham BS+, *Arch Dermatol* 135, 349
(1999): Choquet-Kastylevsky G+, *Therapie* (French) 54, 263
Eruptive xanthoma
(1983): Shalita AR+, *J Am Acad Dermatol* 9, 629
(1980): Dicken CH+, *Arch Dermatol* 116, 951
Erythema multiforme
(1988): Bigby M+, *J Am Acad Dermatol* 18, 543
Erythema nodosum
(1997): Tan BB+, *Clin Exp Dermatol* 22, 26
(1988): Bigby M+, *J Am Acad Dermatol* 18, 543
(1985): Kellett JK+, *BMJ* 290, 820
Exanthems
(1993): Litt JZ, Beachwood, Ohio, personal case, non-pruritic (observation)
(1988): Bigby M+, *J Am Acad Dermatol* 18, 543
Facial cellulitis
(1994): Boffa MJ+, *J Am Acad Dermatol* 31, 800
Facial edema (1–10%)
Facial scarring
(1994): Katz BE+, *J Am Acad Dermatol* 30, 852
Fixed eruption
(1988): Bigby M+, *J Am Acad Dermatol* 18, 543
Flushing
(1998): Gass M, (from Internet) (2 observations)
(1998): Frederickson K, (from Internet) (observation)
Folliculitis
(1990): Hughes BR+, *Br J Dermatol* 122, 683
Fragility
(2000): *Prescrire Int* 7, 178 (from wax epilation)
(1997): Woollons A+, *Br J Dermatol* 137, 389
(1997): Litt JZ, Beachwood, OH (lips from wax epilation), 2 personal cases (observations)
(1995): Holmes SC+, *Br J Dermatol* 132, 165
Granulation tissue
(1991): Rodland O+, *Tidsskr Nor Laegeforen* (Norwegian) 111, 2630
(1985): Miller RA+, *J Am Acad Dermatol* 5, 888
(1984): Robertson DB+, *Br J Dermatol* 111, 689
Herpes (sic)
(1990): Joly P+, *Ann Dermatol Venereol* (French) 117, 860
Hyperpigmentation
(1988): Bigby M+, *J Am Acad Dermatol* 18, 543
Keloid formation
(1999): Ginarte M+, *Int J Dermatol* 38, 228
(1997): Bernestein LJ+, *Arch Dermatol* 133, 111
(1994): Katz BE+, *J Am Acad Dermatol* 30, 852
(1988): Zachariae H, *Br J Dermatol* 118, 703
Keratolysis exfoliativa
Leucoderma
(1988): Bigby M+, *J Am Acad Dermatol* 18, 543
Melasma
(1998): Thaler D, Monona, WI (from Internet) (3 observations)
(1997): Verros CD, Tripolis, Greece (from Internet) (observation)
Miliaria
(1986): Gupta AK+, *Cutis* 38, 275
Nummular eczema
(1987): Bettoli V+, *J Am Acad Dermatol* 16, 617
Pallor (1–10%)
Peeling (1–10%)
Pemphigus
(1995): Georgala S+, *Acta Derm Venereol* 75, 413

Photosensitivity (>10%)
(1991): Auffret N+, *J Am Acad Dermatol* 23, 321
(1986): Ferguson J+, *Br J Dermatol* 115, 275
(1986): Wong RC+, *J Am Acad Dermatol* 14, 1095
(1985): Diffey BL+, *J Am Acad Dermatol* 12, 119
(1983): McCormack LS+, *J Am Acad Dermatol* 9, 273
Pityriasis rosea
(1984): Helfman RJ+, *Cutis* 33, 297
Pruritus (1–5%)
(1994): Yee KC+, *Dermatology* 189, 117
(1988): Shalita AR+, *Cutis* 42, 10
(1976): Peck GL+, *Lancet* 2, 1172
Pyoderma gangrenosum
(1997): Gangaram HP+, *Br J Dermatol* 136, 636
Pyogenic granuloma
(1992): Hagler J+, *Int J Dermatol* 31, 199 (fatal)
(1988): Blanc D+, *Dermatologica* 177, 16
(1984): Robertson DB+, *Br J Dermatol* 111, 689
(1983): Campbell JP+, *J Am Acad Dermatol* 9, 708
(1983): Exner JH+, *Arch Dermatol* 119, 808
(1983): Spear KL+, *Mayo Clin Proc* 58, 509
(1983): Valentic JP+, *Arch Dermatol* 119, 871
Rash (sic)
Sebaceous casts (sic)
(2000): Agarwal S+, *Br J Dermatol* 143, 228 (nasolabial follicular)
Telangiectases
(1994): Thompson D, *The Schoch Letter* 44, 47 (#186) (observation)
Toxic epidermal necrolysis
(1994): Rosen T, *Arch Dermatol* 130, 260
Urticaria
(2000): Madnani N, Bombay, India (from Internet) (observation)
(1988): Bigby M+, *J Am Acad Dermatol* 18, 543
Varicosities
(1994): Thompson D, *The Schoch Letter* 44, 47 (#186) (observation)
Vasculitis
(1990): Aractingi S+, *Lancet* 335, 362
(1989): Reynolds P+, *Lancet* 2, 1216
(1989): Dwyer JM+, *Lancet* 2, 494
(1987): Epstein EH, *Arch Dermatol* 123, 1124
Xerosis (>10%)
(1997): Berger R, *The Schoch Letter* 47, 5
(1988): Shalita AR+, *Cutis* 42, 10
(1976): Peck GL+, *Lancet* 2, 1172

Hair

Hair – alopecia (16%)
(2000): Dintiman BJ, Fairfax, VA (from Internet) (4 observations)
(2000): Frederickson KS, Novalo, CA (from Internet) (observation)
(2000): Rehbein HM, Jacksonville, FL (from Internet) (2 observations)
(1998): Thaler D, Monona, WI (from Internet) (observation)
(1998): Litt JZ, Beachwood OH, personal case (observation)
(1997): Berger R, *The Schoch Letter* 47, 5 (diffuse)
(1997): Thaler D, Monona, WI (from Internet) (observation)
(1994): Shelley WB+, *Cutis* 53, 237 (observation)
Hair – hirsutism
Hair – pili torti (curly hair)
(1996): van der Pijl JW+, *Lancet* 348, 622
(1990): Bunker CB+, *Clin Exp Dermatol* 15, 143
(1985): Hays SB+, *Cutis* 25, 466
Hair – trichotillomania
(1990): Mahr G, *Psychosomatics* 31, 235

Nails

Nails – growth
(1994): Litt JZ, Beachwood, OH, personal case (observation)
Nails – median canaliform dystrophy
(1997): Dharmagunawardena B+, *Br J Dermatol*
(1992): Bottomley WW+, *Br J Dermatol* 127, 447
(1988): Bigby M+, *J Am Acad Dermatol* 18, 543
Nails – onycholysis
(1988): Bigby M+, *J Am Acad Dermatol* 18, 543
Nails – paronychia
(1998): Lepine EM, Rock Hill, SC (from Internet) (observation)
(1988): Bigby M+, *J Am Acad Dermatol* 18, 543
(1986): DeRaeve L+, *Dermatologica* 172, 278
(1984): Blumental G, *J Am Acad Dermatol* 10, 677
Nails – periungual hemorrhage
(1997): Leal G, Fortaleza, Brazil (from Internet) (observation)

Other

Ageusia
(1996): Halpern SM+, *Br J Dermatol* 134, 378. br
Cellulitis (1–10%)
Dysgeusia
(1990): Heise E+, *Eur Arch Otorhinolaryngol* 247, 382
Dysosmia
(1990): Heise E+, *Eur Arch Otorhinolaryngol* 247, 382
Galactorrhea
(1985): Larsen GK, *Arch Dermatol* 121, 450
Gynecomastia
(1994): Shelley WB+, *Cutis* 54, 149 (passim)
(1992): Fluckiger R, *Schweiz Rundsch Med Prax* (German) 81, 1370
Mucosal denudation of lips
(1999): Graham BS+, *Arch Dermatol* 349
Myalgia (>10%)
Myopathy
(1996): Fiallo P+, *Arch Dermatol* 132, 1521
(1986): Hodak E, *BMJ* 293. 425
Pseudoporphyria
(1993): Riordan CA+, *Clin Exp Dermatol* 18, 69
Pseudotumor cerebri
(1998): Sorkin MJ, Denver, CO (from Internet) (observation of 4 cases)
(1995): Lee AG, *Cutis* 55, 165
(1988): Roytman M+, *Cutis* 42, 399
Xerostomia (>10%)
(1992): Breathnach SM+, *Adverse Drug Reactions and the Skin*, Blackwell, Oxford, 259 (passim)

ISOXSUPRINE

Trade names: Vasodilan (Bristol-Myers Squibb); Voxsuprine
Other trade names: *Duvadilan; Isoxine; Sincen; Vasolan; Vasosuprina; Xuprin*
Indications: Peripheral vascular disease, Raynaud's phenomenon
Category: Peripheral vasodilator
Half-life: no data
Clinically important, potentially serious interactions with: none

Reactions

Skin

Allergic dermatitis (sic)
(1978): Horowitz JJ+, *Am J Obstet Gynecol* 131, 225

ISRADIPINE

Trade name: DynaCirc (Novartis)
Other common trade names: *Dynacirc SRO; Lomir; Lomir SRO; Prescal; Vascal*
Indications: Hypertension
Category: Calcium channel blocker; antihypertensive
Half-life: 8 hours
Clinically important, potentially serious interactions with: azole antifungals, barbiturates, beta-blockers, calcium salts, carbamazepine, cyclosporine, digoxin, fentanyl, propranolol, quinidine, rifampin, theophylline

Reactions

Skin

Diaphoresis (<1%)
Edema (7.2%)
(1992): Madias NE+, *Am J Hypertens* 5, 141
(1992): Lopez LM+, *Ann Pharmacother* 26, 789
(1991): Galloe AM+, *J Intern Med* 229, 447
(1991): Eisner GM+, *Am J Hypertens* 4, 154S

(1991): Schachter M, *J Clin Pharm Ther* 16, 79
(1990): Vidt DG, *Cleve Clin J Med* 57, 677

Exanthems
(1993): Blumenthal HL, Beachwood, OH, personal case (observation)
(1990): Fitton A+, *Drugs* 40, 31 (1.5%)

Flushing (2.6%)
(1992): Lopez LM+, *Ann Pharmacother* 26, 789
(1991): Galloe AM+, *J Intern Med* 229, 447
(1991): Schachter M, *J Clin Pharm Ther* 16, 79
(1990): Fitton A+, *Drugs* 40, 31 (10–15%)
(1990): Zubair M+, *Drugs* 40 (Suppl 2), 26 (7.8%)
(1990): Welzel D+, *Drugs* 40 (Suppl 2), 60
(1990): Vidt DG, *Cleve Clin J Med* 57, 677

Peripheral edema

Pruritus (<1%)
(1990): Zubair M+, *Drugs* 40 (Suppl 2), 26 (5.9%)

Rash (sic) (1.5%)

Urticaria (<1%)

Other

Gingival hyperplasia (<1%)

Oral mucosal lesions
(1990): Zubair M+, *Drugs* 40 (Suppl 2), 26 (5.9%)

Paresthesias (<1%)

Xerostomia (<1%)

ITRACONAZOLE

Trade name: Sporanox (Janssen)
Other common trade names: *Isox; Itranax; Sopronox; Sporacid; Sporal; Sporanox 15 D*
Indications: Onychomycosis, deep mycoses
Category: Antifungal
Half-life: 21 hours
Clinically important, potentially serious interactions with: alprazolam, amprenavir, anticoagulants, astemizole, atorvastatin, buspirone, busulfan, calcium channel blockers, cerivastatin, cisapride, cyclosporine, digoxin, felodipine, lovastatin, midazolam, nelfinavir, phenytoin, rifampin, ritonavir, sildenafil, simvastatin, sulfonylureas, tacrolimus, terfenadine, triazolam, vinblastine, vincristine, warfarin

Reactions

Skin

Acute generalized exanthematous pustulosis (AGEP)
(1997): Park YM+, *J Am Acad Dermatol* 36, 794
(1995): Heymann WR+, *J Am Acad Dermatol* 33, 130

Angioedema
(1996): Foong H, Malaysia (from Internet) (observation)

Cutaneous side effects (sic)
(1999): Gupta AK+, *Dermatology* 199, 248
(1997): Gupta AK+, *J Am Acad Dermatol* 36, 789

Edema (3.5%)
(1998): N Z Medicines Adverse Reactions Committee, (peripheral) (from Internet) (observation)
(1996): Tailor SA+, *Arch Dermatol* 132, 350 (peripheral) (with nifedipine)
(1994): Gupta AK+, *J Am Acad Dermatol* 30, 911
(1994): Rosen T, *Arch Dermatol* 130, 260
(1992): *Med Lett Drugs Ther* 34, 14
(1991): Diaz M+, *Chest* 100, 682
(1991): Sharkey PK+, *Antimicrob Agents Chemother* 35, 707
(1990): Sharkey PK+, *J Am Acad Dermatol* 23, 577
(1990): Tucker RM+, *J Antimicrob Chemother* 26, 561
(1990): Denning DW+, *J Am Acad Dermatol* 23, 602 (2%)

Eruption (sic)
(2000): Goto Y+, *Acta Derm Venereol* 80, 72

Erythema multiforme
(1998): Rademaker M+, *New Zealand Adverse Drug Reactions Committee*, April, 1998 (from Internet)

Exanthems
(1999): Burrow WH, Jackson, MS, (from Internet) (2 cases) (observation)
(1999): Valentine MC, Everett, WA (from Internet) (2 cases) (observation)
(1998): Litt JZ, Beachwood, OH, personal case (observation)
(1997): Danby FW, Kingston, Ontario, 2 cases (from Internet) (observation)
(1997): Blumenthal HL, Beachwood, Ohio, personal case (observation)
(1996): Degreef H, *Cutis* 58, 90
(1994): Litt JZ, Beachwood, OH, 2 personal cases (observation)
(1991): Smith DE+, *AIDS* 5, 1367
(1990): Roseeuw D+, *Clin Exp Dermatol* 15, 101 (2.6%)
(1990): Tucker RM+, *J Am Acad Dermatol* 23, 593 (3%)

Facial dermatitis (papular, id-like)
(1996): Thaler D, Monona, WI (2 cases) (from Internet) (observation)

Fixed eruption
(1997): Perry S, *The Schoch Letter* 47, 19
(1994): Litt JZ, Beachwood, OH, personal case (observation)

Peripheral edema (4%)

Photoreactions
(1996): Moreland A, *The Schoch Letter* 46, 19 (observation)

Phototoxic reaction
(1999): Gass M, Davis, CA (from Internet) (observation)
(1995): Epstein E Jr, *The Schoch Letter* 45, 28 (observation)
(1994): Milstein H, *The Schoch Letter* 44, 5 (observation)

Pruritus (2.5%)
(1997): Gupta AK+, *J Am Acad Dermatol* 36, 789
(1994): Gupta AK+, *J Am Acad Dermatol* 30, 911 (0.7%)
(1992): Lavrijsen AP+, *Lancet* 340, 251
(1992): Cleary JD+, *Ann Pharmacother* 26, 502
(1991): De Beule K+, *Curr Ther Res* 49, 814
(1990): Tucker RM+, *J Antimicrob Chemother* 26, 561
(1989): Grant SM+, *Drugs* 39, 877 (0.6%)

Purpura
(1997): Kramer KE+, *J Am Acad Dermatol* 37, 994

Rash (sic) (8.6%)
(1996): Odom R+, *J Am Acad Dermatol* 35, 110 (severe)
(1994): Gupta AK+, *J Am Acad Dermatol* 30, 911 (1.1%)
(1990): Tucker RM+, *J Am Acad Dermatol* 23, 593
(1990): Tucker RM+, *J Antimicrob Chemother* 26, 561
(1990): Sharkey PK+, *J Am Acad Dermatol* 23, 577

Skin eruptions (sic)
(1992): Cleary JD+, *Ann Pharmacother* 26, 502

Stevens–Johnson syndrome

Urticaria
(1999): Valentine MC, Everett, WA (from Internet) (observation)
(1997): :Billon S, *The Schoch Letter* 47, 32 (observation)
(1996): Thaler D, Monona, WI (from Internet) (observation)
(1994): Litt JZ, Beachwood, OH, personal case (observation)
(1993): Litt JZ, Beachwood, OH, personal case (observation)
(1992): Piepponen T+, *J Antimicrob Chemother* 29, 195

Vasculitis
(1996): Odom R+, *J Am Acad Dermatol* 35, 110

Hair

Hair – alopecia
(1995): Litt JZ, Beachwood, OH, personal case (observation)
(1992): de Gans J+, *AIDS* 6, 185
(1986): Moller Heilesen A, *BMJ* 293, 823

Nails

Nails – beading
(1994): Donker PD+, *Clin Exp Dermatol* 19, 404

Nails – onychocryptosis
(1995): Arenas R+, *Int J Dermatol* 34, 138

Other

Anaphylactoid reaction

Gynecomastia (<1%)
(1994): Gupta AK+, *J Am Acad Dermatol* 30, 911

Myalgia (1%)

Serum sickness
(1998): Park H+, *Ann Pharmacother* 32, 1249

Xerostomia
(1990): Tucker RM+, *J Antimicrob Chemother* 26, 561
(1990): Tucker RM+, *J Am Acad Dermatol* 23, 593

IVERMECTIN

Trade name: Stromectol (Merck)
Indications: Various infections caused by susceptible helmintic organisms
Category: Antihelmintic antibiotic
Half-life: 16–35 hours
Clinically important, potentially serious interactions with: no data

Reactions

Skin

Bullous eruption
(1993): Burnham GM, *Trans R Soc Trop Med Hyg* 87, 313
Burning
(1999): Editorial, *Arch Dermatol* 135, 705
Dermatitis (sic)
(1999): Editorial, *Arch Dermatol* 135, 705
Edema
(1998): Jaramillo-Ayerbe F+, *Arch Dermatol* 134, 143
(1995): Darge K+, *Trop Med Parasitol* 46, 206 (arms and legs) (10%)
(1993): Burnham GM, *Trans R Soc Trop Med Hyg* 87, 313
(1992): Collins RC+, *Am J Trop Med Hyg* 47, 156 (facial) (31.8%)
(1992): Chijioke CP+, *Trans R Soc Trop Med Hyg* 86, 284
(1992): Zea-Flores R+, *Trans R Soc Trop Med Hyg* 86, 663 (53%)
(1991): Bryan RT+, *Lancet* 337, 304
(1991): Guderian RH+, *Lancet* 337, 188 (leg)
Exanthems
(1993): Burnham GM, *Trans R Soc Trop Med Hyg* 87, 313
(1991): Whitworth JAG+, *Lancet* 337, 625 (1–5%)
(1990): Ette EI+, *Drug Intell Clin Pharm* 24, 426 (34%)
Facial edema (1.2%)
(1998): Jaramillo-Ayerbe F+, *Arch Dermatol* 134, 143
(1993): Burnham GM, *Trans R Soc Trop Med Hyg* 87, 313
Peripheral edema
Pruritus (2.8%–27.5%)
(1998): Jaramillo-Ayerbe F+, *Arch Dermatol* 134, 143
(1995): Darge K+, *Trop Med Parasitol* 46, 206
(1993): Kar SK+, *Acta Trop* 55, 21
(1993): Burnham GM, *Trans R Soc Trop Med Hyg* 87, 313
(1992): Chijioke CP+, *Trans R Soc Trop Med Hyg* 86, 284 (71.2%)
(1992): Collins RC+, *Am J Trop Med Hyg* 47, 156 (34%)
(1991): Whitworth JAG+, *Lancet* 337, 625 (8%)
(1991): Bryan RT+, *Lancet* 337, 304
(1990): Ette EI+, *Drug Intell Clin Pharm* 24, 426 (9.6%)
(1989): Guderian RH+, *Eur J Epidemiol* 5, 294 (4%)
Pustular eruption
Rash (sic) (0.9%)
(1998): Jaramillo-Ayerbe F+, *Arch Dermatol* 134, 143
(1993): Kar SK+, *Acta Trop* 55, 21
(1991): Bryan RT+, *Lancet* 337, 304 (93%)
(1991): Whitworth JAG+, *Lancet* 337, 625 (8%)
(1991): Guderian RH+, *Lancet* 337, 188
(1989): Guderian RH+, *Eur J Epidemiol* 5, 294 (4%)
Urticaria (0.9–22.7%)

Other

Myalgia
(1995): Darge K+, *Trop Med Parasitol* 46, 206 (20%)
(1993): Kar SK+, *Acta Trop* 55, 21
Tremor

KANAMYCIN

Trade name: Kantrex (Apothecon)
Other common trade names: *Kanamicina; Kanamycine; Kanamytrex; Kanescin; Kannasyn; Randikan*
Indications: Various infections caused by susceptible organisms
Category: Aminoglycoside antibiotic
Half-life: 2–4 hours
Clinically important, potentially serious interactions with: aminoglycosides, amphotericin B, bumetanide, cephalosporins, digoxin, diuretics, ethacrynic acid, furosemide, loop diuretics, methotrexate, penicillins, torsemide

Reactions

Skin

Burning
Edema (>10%)
Erythema (<1%)
Exanthems
Photosensitivity (<1%)
Pruritus (1–10%)
Rash (sic) (1–10%)
Systemic eczematous contact dermatitis
(1986): Holdiness MR, *Contact Dermatitis* 15, 282
Urticaria

Other

Hypersensitivity
Injection-site irritation
Injection-site pain (<1%)
Paresthesias
Phlebitis
Pseudotumor cerebri
Sialorrhea (<1%)
Tremor

KETAMINE

Trade name: Ketalar (Parke-Davis)
Other common trade names: *Calypsol; Ketalin; Ketanest; Ketolar; Petar*
Indications: Induction of anesthesia
Category: Anesthetic; sedative hypnotic
Half-life: 2–3 hours
Clinically important, potentially serious interactions with: antidepressants, barbiturates, hydroxyzine, narcotics, thyroid

Reactions

Skin

Erythema
Exanthems
Rash (sic) (1–10%)

Other

Injection-site erythema
Injection-site pain (1–10%)
Sialorrhea (<1%)
Tremor (>10%)

KETOCONAZOLE

Trade name: Nizoral (Janssen)
Other common trade names: *Aquarius; Fungarest; Fungoral; Ketoderm; Ketoisidin; Nazoltec*
Indications: Fungal infections
Category: Imidazole antifungal
Half-life: initial: 2 hours; terminal: 8 hours
Clinically important, potentially serious interactions with: alcohol, alprazolam, anticoagulants, astemizole, chlordiazepoxide, cimetidine, cisapride, cyclosporine, digoxin, isoniazid, midazolam, lovastatin, omeprazole, phenytoin, ranitidine, rifampin, simvastatin, terfenadine, theophylline, triazolam, warfarin

Reactions

Skin

Allergic reactions (sic)
(1983): van Ketel WG, *Contact Dermatitis* 9, 313
Angioedema
(1994): Gupta AK+, *J Am Acad Dermatol* 30, 677 (passim)
(1994): Gonzalez-Delgado P+, *Ann Allergy* 73, 326
(1983): van Dijke CPH+, *BMJ* 287, 1673
Chills (1–3%)
Contact dermatitis
(1993): Valsecchi R+, *Contact Dermatitis* 29, 162
(1993): Lodi A+, *Contact Dermatitis* 29, 97
(1992): Santucci B+, *Contact Dermatitis* 27, 274
Eczema (generalized)
(1989): Garcia-Bravo B+, *Contact Dermatitis* 21, 346
Exanthems
(1985): Bradsher RW+, *Ann Intern Med* 103, 872 (2%)
(1985): Study Group, *Ann Intern Med* 103, 861 (9.7%)
(1984): Kahana M+, *Arch Dermatol* 120, 837
(1984): Ford GP+, *Br J Dermatol* 111, 603 (5%)
(1983): Dismukes WE+, *Ann Intern Med* 98, 13 (4%)
(1983): Rand R+, *Arch Dermatol* 119, 97
(1982): Heel RC+, *Drugs* 23, 1 (0.7%)
Exfoliative dermatitis
(1984): Parent D+, *Ann Dermatol Venereol* (French) 111,339
(1983): Rand R+, *Arch Dermatol* 119, 97
Fixed eruption
(1994): Gupta AK+, *J Am Acad Dermatol* 30, 677 (passim)
(1988): Bharija SC+, *Int J Dermatol* 27, 278
Jarisch–Herxheimer reaction
Photosensitivity
(1988): Mohamed KN, *Clin Exp Dermatol* 13, 54
Pigmentation
(1992): Gallais V+, *Ann Dermatol Venereol* (French) 119, 471
(1990): Poizot-Martin I+, *Int Conf AIDS* 6, 357
(1985): Tucker WS+, *JAMA* 253, 2413
Pruritus (1.5%)
(1994): Gupta AK+, *J Am Acad Dermatol* 30, 677 (passim)
(1988): Mohamed KN, *Clin Exp Dermatol* 13, 54 (passim)
(1985): Study Group, *Ann Intern Med* 103, 861 (9.7%)
(1983): Rand R+, *Arch Dermatol* 119, 97 (1.5%)
(1982): Heel RC+, *Drugs* 23, 1 (1.7%)
Purpura
(1994): Gupta AK+, *J Am Acad Dermatol* 30, 677 (passim)
(1982): Heel RC+, *Drugs* 23, 1
Rash (sic) (1–3%)
(1994): Gupta AK+, *J Am Acad Dermatol* 30, 677 (passim)
Urticaria (1–3%)
(1994): Gupta AK+, *J Am Acad Dermatol* 30, 677 (passim)
(1985): Bradsher RW+, *Ann Intern Med* 103, 872 (2%)
Vasculitis
(1982): Heel RC+, *Drugs* 23, 1
Xerosis
(1994): Gupta AK+, *J Am Acad Dermatol* 30, 677 (passim)
(1985): Study Group, *Ann Intern Med* 103, 861

Hair

Hair – alopecia
(1994): Gupta AK+, *J Am Acad Dermatol* 30, 677 (passim)

(1990): Venturoli S+, *J Clin Endocrinol Metab* 71, 335
(1985): Study Group, *Ann Intern Med* 103, 861 (3.7%)
(1982): Heel RC+, *Drugs* 23, 1 (0.2%)
Hair – trichoptilosis
(1993): Aljabre SH, *Int J Dermatol* 32, 150

Nails

Nails – pigmentation
(1985): Dreessen K, *Z Hautkr* (German) 60, 679 (black longitudinal bands)

Other

Anaphylactoid reaction
(1994): Gupta AK+, *J Am Acad Dermatol* 30, 677 (passim)
(1983): van Dijke CPH+, *BMJ* 287, 1673
Gingival bleeding
(1994): Gupta AK+, *J Am Acad Dermatol* 30, 677 (passim)
(1983): Dismukes WE+, *Ann Intern Med* 98, 13
Gingival hyperplasia
(1988): Veraldi S+, *Int J Dermatol* 27, 730
Gynecomastia (1–3%)
(1994): Gupta AK+, *J Am Acad Dermatol* 30, 677 (passim)
(1993): Thompson DF+, *Pharmacotherapy* 13, 37
(1982): Moncada B, *J Am Acad Dermatol* 7, 557
(1981): DeFelice R+, *Antimicrob Agents Chemo* 19, 1073
Hypersensitivity
(1994): Gonzalez-Delgado P+, *Ann Allergy* 73, 326
(1992): Verschueren GL+, *Contact Dermatitis* 26, 47
(1989): Garcia-Bravo B+, *Contact Dermatitis* 21, 346
Myopathy
(1991): Garty BZ+, *Am J Dis Child* 145, 970
Oral hyperpigmentation
(1991): Poizot-Martin I+, *Presse Med* (French) 20, 632
(1989): Langford A+, *Oral Surg Oral Med Oral Pathol* 67, 301 (in HIV-infected patients)
Oral lichenoid eruption
(1993): Ficarra G+, *Oral Surg Oral Med Oral Pathol* 76, 460
(1986): Markitziu A+, *Mykosen* (German) 29, 317
Oral mucosal lesions
(1994): Gupta AK+, *J Am Acad Dermatol* 30, 677 (passim)
(1985): Study Group, *Ann Intern Med* 103, 861 (1–5%)
(1983): Dismukes WE+, *Ann Intern Med* 98, 13 (2%)
Paresthesias
(1994): Gupta AK+, *J Am Acad Dermatol* 30, 677 (passim)
Tongue pigmentation
(1982): Heel RC+, *Drugs* 23, 1

KETOPROFEN

Trade names: Orudis (Wyeth-Ayerst); Oruvail (Wyeth-Ayerst)
Other common trade names: *Alrheumat; Alrheumun; Aneol; Bi-Profenid; Gabrilen Retard; Keduril; Novo-Keto; Rhodis; Rhovail*
Indications: Arthritis
Category: Nonsteroidal anti-inflammatory (NSAID); analgesic
Half-life: 1.5–4 hours
Clinically important, potentially serious interactions with: aminoglycosides, anticoagulants, aspirin, cyclosporine, lithium, methotrexate, probenecid, salicylates

Reactions

Skin

Allergic reactions (sic) (<1%)
Angioedema (<1%)
(1978): Frith P+, *Lancet* 2, 847
Bullous eruption (<1%)
Contact dermatitis
(1998): Baudot S+, *Therapie* (French) 53, 137
(1997): *Lakartidningen* (Swedish) 94, 2664
(1996): Pigatto P+, *Am J Contact Dermat* 7, 220
(1996): Jeanmougin M+, *Ann Dermatol Venereol* (French) 123, 251
(1995): Navarro LA+, *Contact Dermatitis* 32, 181
(1995): Gebhardt M+, *Z Rheumatol* (German) 54, 405
(1994): Mastrolonardo M+, *Contact Dermatitis* 30, 110
(1994): Oh VM, *BMJ* 309, 512
(1993): Ophaswongse S+, *Contact Dermatitis* 29, 57
(1990): Mozzanica N+, *Contact Dermatitis* 23, 336
(1990): Tosti A+, *Contact Dermatitis* 23, 112
(1990): Valsecchi R+, *Contact Dermatitis* 21, 345
(1989): Romaguera C+, *Contact Dermatitis* 20, 310
(1989): Lanzarini M+, *Contact Dermatitis* 21, 51
(1987): Mozzanica N, *Contact Dermatitis* 17, 325
(1985): Camarasa JG, *Contact Dermatitis* 12, 121
(1983): Valsecchi R+, *Contact Dermatitis* 9, 163
(1983): Angelini G+, *Contact Dermatitis* 9, 234
Cutaneous side effects (sic)
(1989): Le-Loet X, *Scand J Rheumatol* Suppl 83, 21 (0.7%)
Diaphoresis (<1%)
(1989): Roth DE+, *Med Clin North Am* 73, 1275
Eczematous eruption (sic) (<1%)
(1990): Tosti A+, *Contact Dermatitis* 23, 112
(1987): Mozzanica N, *Contact Dermatitis* 17, 325
Erythema multiforme (<1%)
Exanthems
(1975): Hingorani K+, *Curr Med Res Opin* 3, 407
Exfoliative dermatitis (<1%)
Facial edema (<1%)
Hot flashes (<1%)
Peripheral edema (1–3%)
Photocontact dermatitis
(1998): Le Coz CJ+, *Contact Dermatitis* 38, 245
(1997): Bastien M+, *Ann Dermatol Venereol* (French) 124, 523 (5 cases)
(1996): Jeanmougin M+, *Ann Dermatol Venereol* (French) 123, 251
(1995): Nabeya R+, *Contact Dermatitis* 32, 52
(1993): Ophaswongse S+, *Contact Dermatitis* 29, 57 (phototoxic and photoallergic)
(1992): Serrano G+, *J Am Acad Dermatol* 27, 204 (passim)
(1987): Cusano F+, *Contact Dermatitis* 27, 50
(1990): Mozzanica N+, *Contact Dermatitis* 23, 336
(1987): Cusano F+, *Contact Dermatitis* 17, 108
(1985): Alomar A, *Contact Dermatitis* 12, 112
Photosensitivity (<1%)
(1998): Baudot S+, *Therapie* (French) 53, 137
(1997): Mirande-Romero A+, *Contact Dermatitis* 37, 242 (connubial)
(1997): Leroy D+, *Photodermatol Photoimmunol Photomed* 13, 93
(1990): Black AK+, *Br J Dermatol* 123, 277 (observation)
(1989): Roth DE+, *Med Clin North Am* 73, 1275
(1985): Alomar A, *Contact Dermatitis* 12, 112
Pigmentation (<1%)
Pruritus (1–10%)
(1975): Hingorani K+, *Curr Med Res Opin* 3, 407
Psoriasis
(1992): Shelley WB+, *Cutis* 51, 23 (observation)
Purpura (<1%)
(1989): Roth DE+, *Med Clin North Am* 73, 1275
Rash (sic) (>10%)
Stevens–Johnson syndrome (<1%)
Toxic epidermal necrolysis (<1%)
(1995): Tijhuis GJ+, *Dermatology* 190, 176
Urticaria (<1%)
(1978): Frith P+, *Lancet* 2, 847

Hair

Hair – alopecia (<1%)
(1989): Roth DE+, *Med Clin North Am* 73, 1275

Nails

Nails – onycholysis (<1%)
(1989): Roth DE+, *Med Clin North Am* 73, 1275

Other

Acute intermittent porphyria
Anaphylactoid reaction (<1%)
(1985): O'Brien WM+, *J Rheumatol* 12, 13
(1978): Frith P+, *Lancet* 2, 847
Aphthous stomatitis
Dysgeusia (<1%)
Gynecomastia (<1%)
Myalgia (<1%)
Oral mucosal lesions
(1975): Hingorani K+, *Curr Med Res Opin* 3, 407

Paresthesias (<1%)
Pseudoporphyria
(1992): Breathnach SM+, *Adverse Drug Reactions and the Skin*, Blackwell, Oxford, (passim)
(1987): Taylor BJ+, *N Z Med J* 100, 322
Sialorrhea (<1%)
Stomatitis (<1%)
Xerostomia (<1%)

KETOROLAC

Trade names: Acular (Allergan); Toradol (Roche)
Other common trade names: *Dolac; Kelac; Ketonic; Nodine; Topadol; Torolac; Torvin*
Indications: Pain
Category: Nonsteroidal anti-inflammatory (NSAID)
Half-life: 2–8 hours
Clinically important, potentially serious interactions with: aminoglycosides, anticoagulants, beta-blockers, cyclosporine, heparin, lithium, methotrexate, NSAIDs, probenecid, salicylates

Reactions

Skin

Allergic reactions (sic)
Angioedema
(1994): Shapiro N, *J Oral Maxillofac Surg* 52, 626
Cutaneous side effects (sic) (0.7%)
(1990): Buckley MMT+, *Drugs* 39, 86
Dermatitis (sic) (3–9%)
Diaphoresis (1–10%)
(1990): Buckley MMT+, *Drugs* 39, 86
Edema (3–9%)
Exanthems (3–9%)
(1990): Buckley MMT+, *Drugs* 39, 86
Excoriated papules
(1994): Shelley WB+, *Cutis* 53, 235 (observation)
Exfoliative dermatitis (<1%)
Flushing (<1%)
Pruritus (3–9%)
Purpura (>1%)
(1994): Shelley WB+, *Cutis* 54, 149 (palpable) (observation)
Rash (sic) (>1%)
Stevens–Johnson syndrome (<1%)
Toxic epidermal necrolysis (<1%)
Urticaria
(1990): Buckley MMT+, *Drugs* 39, 86

Other

Anaphylactoid reaction (<1%)
Aphthous stomatitis (<1%)
(1990): Buckley MMT+, *Drugs* 39, 86
Dysgeusia
Hypersensitivity
Injection-site pain (1–10%)
Myalgia
Paresthesias
Stinging (from topical)
(2000): Shiuey Y+, *Ophthalmology* 107, 1512
Stomatitis (>1%)
Tongue edema (<1%)
Xerostomia
(1990): Buckley MMT+, *Drugs* 39, 86

KETOTIFEN

Trade name: Zaditor (CIBA Vision)
Indications: Allergic conjunctivitis
Category: Ophthalmic antihistamine H_1-blocker
Half-life: 22 hours
Clinically important, potentially serious interactions with: none

Reactions

Skin

Allergic reactions (sic) (1–10%)
Burning (1–10%)
Photosensitivity
Pityriasis rosea
(1985): Wolf R+, *Dermatologica* 171–355
Pruritus (1–10%)
Rash (sic) (1–10%)
Stinging (1–10%)

Other

Xerophthalmia (1–10%)

LABETALOL

Trade names: Normodyne (Schering); Normozide; Trandate (Faro)
Other common trade names: *Abetol; Amipress; Hybloc; Ipolab; Labrocol; Presolol; Salmagne*
Indications: Hypertension
Category: Alpha-adrenergic and beta-adrenergic blocker; antihypertensive
Half-life: 3–8 hours
Clinically important, potentially serious interactions with: calcium channel blockers, cimetidine, clonidine, diltiazem, diuretics, flecainide, indomethacin, insulin, MAO inhibitors, nifedipine, nitroglycerin, oral contraceptives, prazosin, terazosin, tricyclic antidepressants, verapamil

Note: Cutaneous side-effects of beta-receptor blockaders are clinically polymorphous. They apparently appear after several months of continuous therapy. Atypical psoriasiform, lichen planus-like, and eczematous chronic rashes are mainly observed. (1983): Hödl St, *Z Hautkr* (German) 1:58, 17.

Normozide is labetalol and hydrochlorothiazide

Reactions

Skin

Angioedema
  (1986): Ferree CE, *Ann Intern Med* 104, 729
Contact dermatitis
  (1990): Bause GS+, *Contact Dermatitis* 23, 51
Cutaneous side effects (sic) (5.5%)
  (1982): Waal-Manning HJ+, *Br J Clin Pharmacol* 13 (Suppl 1), 65S
  (1978): No Author, *BMJ* 1, 987
Diaphoresis (<1%)
Eczematous eruption (sic)
Edema (<2%)
Exanthems
  (1989): Goa KL+, *Drugs* 37, 583
  (1984): Prichard BNC, *Drugs* 28 (Suppl 2), 51 (1–5%)
  (1978): Finlay AY+, *BMJ* 1, 987
  (1978): Branford WA+, *Practitioner* 221, 765
Exfoliative dermatitis
Facial edema
Flushing
  (1978): Harris C, *Curr Med Res Opin* 5, 618 (19%)
Lichenoid eruption
  (1982): Bertani E+, *G Ital Dermatol Venereol* (Italian) 117, 229
  (1980): Staughton R+, *Lancet* 2, 581
  (1978): Finlay AY+, *BMJ* 1, 987
  (1978): Branford WA+, *Practitioner* 221, 765
  (1978): Savage RL+, *BMJ* 1, 987
Lichen planus (bullous)
  (1978): Gange RW+, *BMJ* 1, 816
Lupus erythematosus
  (1984): Prichard BNC, *Drugs* 28 (Suppl 2), 51
  (1981): Brown RC+, *Postgrad Med J* 57, 189
  (1979): Griffiths ID+, *BMJ* 2, 496
Peripheral edema
Pigmentation (slate-gray)
  (1978): Branford WA+, *Practitioner* 221, 765
Pityriasis rubra pilaris
  (1978): Branford WA+, *Practitioner* 221, 765
  (1978): Finlay AY+, *BMJ* 1, 987
Pruritus (1–10%)
  (1984): Prichard BNC, *Drugs* 28 (Suppl 2), 51 (1–5%)
  (1978): Finlay AY+, *BMJ* 1, 987
  (1978): Harris C, *Curr Med Res Opin* 5, 618 (7.5%)
Psoriasis (exacerbation)
  (1987): Savola J+, *BMJ* 295, 637 (induction)
  (1986): Czernielewski J+, *Lancet* 1, 808
  (1984): Arntzen N+, *Acta Derm Venereol* (Stockh) 64, 346
Purpura
  (1978): Harris C, *Curr Med Res Opin* 5, 618
Rash (sic) (<1%)
Raynaud's phenomenon (<1%)
Urticaria
  (1986): Ferree CE, *Ann Intern Med* 104, 729
Xerosis

Hair

Hair – alopecia (reversible)
  (1978): Finlay AY+, *BMJ* 1, 987

Other

Anaphylactoid reaction
  (1990): Bause GS+, *Contact Dermatitis* 23, 51
  (1986): Ferree CE, *Ann Intern Med* 104, 729
Dysgeusia (1–10%)
  (2000): Zervakis J+, *Physiol Behav* 68, 405
Hypersensitivity
Hypesthesia (1%)
Myopathy
  (1989): Willis J+, *Ann Neurology* 26, 456
  (1981): Teicher A+, *BMJ* 282, 1824
  (1977): Bolli P+, *N Z Med J* 86, 557
  (1976): Andersson O+, *Br J Clin Pharmacol* 3, 757
Paresthesias (7%)
  (1984): Prichard BNC, *Drugs* 28 (Suppl 2), 51 (scalp) (6%)
  (1977): Bailey RR, *Lancet* 2, 720 (tingling of scalp)
Peyronie's disease
  (1979): Kristensen BO, *Acta Med Scand* 206, 511
Priapism
Scalp tingling
  (1979): Coulter DM, *N Z Med J* 90, 397
  (1977): Bailey RR, *Lancet* 2, 720
  (1977): Hua AS+, *Lancet* 2, 295
Xerostomia

LAMIVUDINE

Synonym: 3TC
Trade names: Epivir (GlaxoWellcome); Combivir (GlaxoWellcome)
Indications: HIV progression
Category: Antiretroviral, nucleoside reverse transcriptase inhibitor (NRTI)
Half-life: 5–7 hours
Clinically important, potentially serious interactions with: co-trimoxazole, zidovudine

Combivir is lamivudine and zidovudine

Reactions

Skin

Angioedema
  (1996): Kainer MA+, *Lancet* 348, 1519
Buffalo hump
  (2000): Carr A+, *AIDS* 14, F25
Chills (1–10%)
Contact dermatitis
  (2000): Smith KJ+, *Cutis* 65, 227
Exanthems
Pruritus
  (2000): Smith KJ+, *Cutis* 65, 227
Rash (sic) (9%)
Urticaria
  (1996): Kainer MA+, *Lancet* 348, 1519

Hair

Hair – alopecia
  (1994): Fong IW, *Lancet* 344, 1702

Nails

Nails – paronychia
  (1998): Zerboni R+, *Lancet* 351, 1256

Other

Myalgia (8%)
Paresthesias (>10%)

LAMOTRIGINE

Synonyms: BW-430C; LTG
Trade name: Lamictal (GlaxoWellcome)
Indications: Epilepsy
Category: Anticonvulsant
Half-life: 24 hours
Clinically important, potentially serious interactions with: acetaminophen, carbamazepine, phenobarbital, phenytoin, primidone, valproic acid

Reactions

Skin

Acne (1.3%)
Angioedema (1–10%)
Diaphoresis (<1%)
Ecchymoses (<1%)
Eczema (sic) (<1%)
Erythema (<1%)
Erythema multiforme
Exanthems (1–10%)
(1997): Hyson C+, *Can J Neurol Sci* 24, 245
(1996): Dooley J+, *Neurology* 46, 240 (7%)
(1996): Li LM+, *Arq Neuropsiquiatr* 54, 47
(1995): Brodie MJ, *Can J Neurol Sci* 23, S6 (<5%)
(1995): Tavernor SJ+, *Seizure* 4, 67
(1995): Fitton A+, *Drugs* 50, 691
(1995): Makin AJ+, *BMJ* 311, 292
(1994): Tavernor SJ+, *Epilepsia* 35, 72
Facial edema (<1%)
Flu-like syndrome (sic) (7%)
Flushing (<1%)
Hot flashes (1–10%)
Lupus erythematosus
(1997): Mackay FJ+, *Epilepsia* 38, 881
Petechiae (<1%)
Photosensitivity
(1999): Bozikas V+, *Am J Psychiatry* 156, 2015
Pruritus (3.1%)
Rash (sic) (10%)
(2000): Husain AM+, *South Med J* 93, 335
(2000): Jurynczyk J+, *Neurol Neurochir Pol* (Polish) 34, 43
(2000): Messenheimer JA+, *Drug Saf* 22, 303
(2000): Messenheimer JA+, *Epilepsia* 41, 488
(2000): Besag FM+, *Seizure* 9, 282
(1999): Faught E+, *Epilepsia* 40, 1135
(1999): Guberman AH+, *Epilepsia* 40, 985
(1999): Matsuo F, *Epilepsia* 40, S30
(1998): Messenheimer JA, *Can J Neurol Sci* 25, S14
(1998): Buzan RD+, *J Clin Psychiatry* 59, 87 (re-challenged)
(1997): Mackay FJ+, *Epilepsia* 38, 881
Stevens–Johnson syndrome (1–10%)
(1999): Guberman AH+, *Epilepsia* 40, 985
(1999): Rzany B+, *Lancet* 353, 2190
(1999): Borowitz SM, *Pediatric Pharmacotherapy* 5, 3
(1999): Bocquet H+, *Ann Dermatol Venereol* (French) 126, 46
(1998): Zachariae CO+, *Ugeskr Laeger* (Danish) 160, 6656
(1998): Schlienger RG+, *Epilepsia* 39, S22
(1998): *Drugs and Therapy Perspectives* 11, 11
(1997): Mackay FJ+, *Epilepsia* 38, 881
(1997): Sachs B+, *Dermatology* 195, 60
(1996): Dooley J+, *Neurology* 46, 240 (7%)
(1995): Campistol J+, *Rev Neurol* (Spanish) 23, 1236
(1995): Duval X+, *Lancet* 345, 1301
Toxic epidermal necrolysis
(1999): Rzany B+, *Lancet* 353, 2190
(1999): *Actas Dermosifiliogr* (Spanish) 90, 612
(1999): Borowitz SM, *Pediatric Pharmacotherapy* 5, 3
(1999): Bocquet H+, *Ann Dermatol Venereol* (French) 126, 46
(1998): Page RL+, *Pharmacotherapy* 18, 392 (fatal)
(1998): Zachariae CO+, *Ugeskr Laeger* (Danish) 160, 6656
(1998): *Drugs and Therapy Perspectives* 11, 11
(1998): Schlienger RG+, *Epilepsia* 39, S22
(1997): Vukelic D+, *Dermatology* 195, 307
(1997): Fogh K+, *Seizure* 6, 63
(1997): Chaffin JJ+, *Ann Pharmacother* 31, 720 (suspected)
(1996): Sullivan JR+, *Australas J Dermatol* 37, 208
(1996): Wadelius M+, *Lancet* 348, 1041
(1996): Sachs B+, *Lancet* 348, 1597
(1995): Sterker M+, *Int J Clin Pharmacol Ther* 33, 595
(1995): Duval X+, *Lancet* 345, 1301
Urticaria (<1%)
Xerosis (<1%)

Hair

Hair – alopecia (1.3%)
Hair – hirsutism (<1%)

Other

Anaphylactoid reaction
(1999): Borowitz SM, *Pediatric Pharmacotherapy* 5, 3
Dysgeusia (<1%)
Foetor ex ore (halitosis) (<1%)
Gingival hyperplasia (<1%)
Gingivitis (<1%)
Hypersensitivity (1–10%)
(2000): Schaub N+, *Allergy* 55, 191
(1999): Guberman AH+, *Epilepsia* 40, 985
(1999): Knowles SR+, *Drug Safety* 21, 489
(1999): Mylonakis E+, *Ann Pharmacol* 33, 557
(1999): Borowitz SM, *Pediatric Pharmacotherapy* 5, 3
(1999): Brown TS+, *Pediatr Dermatology* 16, 46
(1998): Iannetti P+, *Epilepsia* 39, 502
(1998): Chapman MS+, *Br J Dermatol* 138, 710
(1998): Tugendhaft P+, *J Am Acad Dermatol* 38, 785 (phenytoin-like)
(1997): Jones D+, *J Am Acad Dermatol* 36, 1016 (phenytoin-like)
Hypesthesia (<1%)
Myalgia (>1%)
Oral ulceration (<1%)
Paresthesias (>1%)
Photosensitivity
(1999): Borowitz SM, *Pediatric Pharmacotherapy* 5, 3
Porphyria
(1996): Gregersen H+, *Ugeskr Laeger* (Danish) 158, 4091
Pseudolymphoma
(1998): Pathak P+, *Neurology* 50, 1509
Sialorrhea (<1%)
Stomatitis (<1%)
Tic disorder
(2000): Sotero de Menezes MA+, *Epilepsia* 41, 862
Tremor
(2000): Messenheimer JA+, *Drug Saf* 22, 303
Vaginal candidiasis (<1%)
Vaginitis (4.1%)
Xerostomia (1%)

LANSOPRAZOLE

Trade name: Prevacid (TAP)
Indications: Active duodenal ulcer
Category: Gastric acid secretion (proton pump) inhibitor
Half-life: 2 hours
Clinically important, potentially serious interactions with: digoxin, ketoconazole, itraconazole, nifedipine, sucralfate, theophylline

Reactions

Skin

Acne (<1%)
Acute generalized exanthematous pustulosis (AGEP)
(1997): Dewerdt S+, *Acta Derm Venereol* (Stockh) 77, 250
Candidiasis (<1%)
Edema (<1%)
Diaphoresis
(2000): Natsch S+, *Ann Pharmacother* 34, 474

Erythroderma
(1999): Cockayne SE+, *Br J Dermatol* 141, 173
Exanthems
(1996): Litt JZ, Beachwood, OH, personal case (observation)
(1996): Blumenthal HL, Beachwood, OH, personal case (observation)
Facial edema
(2000): Natsch S+, *Ann Pharmacother* 34, 474
Lichenoid eruption
(2000): Bong JL+, *BMJ* 320, 283
Pruritus (3–10%)
(2000): Natsch S+, *Ann Pharmacother* 34, 474
Rash (sic) (3–10%)
Urticaria (<1%)
(2000): Natsch S+, *Ann Pharmacother* 34, 474
(2000): Gerson LB+, *Aliment Pharmacol* 14, 397 (1%)

Hair

Hair – alopecia (<1%)
(2000): Litt JZ, Beachwood, OH, personal case (observation)

Other

Anaphylactoid reaction
(2000): Natsch S+, *Ann Pharmacother* 34, 474
Black tongue
(1997): Greco S+, *Ann Pharmacother* 31, 1548
Dysgeusia (<1%)
Foetor ex ore (halitosis) (<1%)
Glossitis
(1997): Greco S+, *Ann Pharmacother* 31, 1548
Gynecomastia (<1%)
(2000): Comas A+, *Med Clin (Barc)* (Spanish) 114, 397
Hypersensitivity
(1999): Baudot S, *Therapie* (French) 54, 491
Mastodynia (<1%)
Myalgia (<1%)
(1998): Smith JD+, *Ann Pharmacother* 32, 196 (with eosinophilia)
Paresthesias (<1%)
Stomatitis (<1%)
(1997): Greco S+, *Ann Pharmacother* 31, 1548
Xerostomia (<1%)

LATANOPROST

Trade name: Xalatan (Pharmacia & Upjohn)
Indications: Glaucoma
Category: Prostaglandin ophthalmic; anti-glaucoma
Half-life: 17 minutes
Clinically important, potentially serious interactions with: none

Reactions

Skin

Allergic reactions (sic) (1.1%)
Blepharitis (0.4%)
Ecchymoses (0.2%
Eczema (sic) (0.7%)
Eyelid burning (1.1%)
Eyelid edema (1–4%)
Eyelid erythema (1–4%)
Eyelid pain (0.4%)
Eyelid pigmentation
(2000): Kook MS+, *Am J Ophthalmol* 129, 804
Eyelid pruritus (1.7%)
Eyelid stinging (0.4%)
Facial rash
(1997): Rowe JA+, *Am J Ophthalmol* 124, 683
Pruritus (0.2%)
(1997): Crowe MA, Puyallup, WA (from Internet) (observation)
Rash (sic) (1–10%)

Hair

Hair – eyelash hyperpigmentation
(1998): Reynolds A+, *Eye* 12, 741
(1997): Johnstone MA, *Am J Ophthalmol* 124, 544
(1997): Wand M, *Arch Ophthalmol* 115, 1206
Hair – hypertrichosis
(1997): Johnstone MA, *Am J Ophthalmol* 124, 544

Other

Gynecomastia (0.2%)
Iris pigmentation increased
(2000): Camras CB+, *J Glaucoma* 9, 95
(2000): Alm A+, *Acta Ophthalmol Scand* 78, 71
Myalgia (1–10%)

LEFLUNOMIDE

Trade name: Arava (Aventis)
Indications: Rheumatoid arthritis
Category: Immunosuppressant; antimetabolite
Half-life: 14–15 days
Clinically important, potentially serious interactions with: methotrexate, rifampin

Reactions

Skin

Acne (1–10%)
Allergic reactions (sic) (2%)
(1999): Goldenberg MM, *Clin Ther* 21, 1837
(1997): Silva Junior HT+, *Am J Med Sci* 313, 289
(1995): Mladenovic V+, *Arthritis Rheum* 38, 1595
Bullous eruption
(2000): Lepine G, Rock Hill, SC, (from Internet) (observation) (occurred 6 months after starting drug)
Dermatitis (sic) (1–10%)
Diaphoresis (1–10%)
Eczema (sic) (2%)
Herpes infection (sic) (1–10%)
Infection (sic) (4%)
Nodule (1–10%)
Peripheral edema (1–10%)
Pigmentation (1–10%)
Purpura (1–10%)
Pruritus (4%)
Rash (sic) (10%)
(1999): Goldenberg MM, *Clin Ther* 21, 1837
(1999): Smolen JS+, *Lancet* 353, 259
(1997): Silva Junior HT+, *Am J Med Sci* 313, 289
(1995): Mladenovic V+, *Arthritis Rheum* 38, 1595
Stevens–Johnson syndrome
Subcutaneous nodule (sic) (1–10%)
Toxic epidermal necrolysis
Ulcer (1–10%)
Urticaria (<1%)
Vasculitis (1–10%)
Xerosis (2%)

Hair

Hair – alopecia (10%)
(1999): Goldenberg MM, *Clin Ther* 21, 1837
(1999): Smolen JS+, *Lancet* 353, 259 (8%)
(1997): Silva Junior HT+, *Am J Med Sci* 313, 289
(1995): Mladenovic V+, *Arthritis Rheum* 38, 1595
Hair – discoloration (1–10%)

Nails

Nails – disorder (sic) (1–10%)

Other

Anaphylactoid reaction (<1%)
Dysgeusia (1–10%)
Gingivitis (1–10%)
Myalgia (1–10%)
Oral candidiasis (3%)
Oral ulceration (3%)

Paresthesias (2%)
Stomatitis (3%)
Tendon rupture (1–10%)
Tooth disorder (sic) (1–10%)
Vaginal candidiasis (1–10%)
Xerostomia (1–10%)

LETROZOLE

Trade name: Femara (Novartis)
Indications: Breast cancer
Category: Nonsteroidal aromatase inhibitor; antineoplastic
Half-life: ~2 days
Clinically important, potentially serious interactions with: none

Reactions

Skin
Diaphoresis (<5%)
Exanthems (5%)
Hot flashes (6%)
Pruritus (2%)
Psoriasis (5%)
Rash (sic) (1–10%)
Vesicular eruption (5%)

Hair
Hair – alopecia (<5%)

LEUCOVORIN

Synonyms: citrovorum factor; folinic acid
Trade name: Leucovorin
Other trade names: *Antrex; Citrec; Lederfolin; Refolinin; Rescufolin; Rescuvolin*
Indications: Overdose of methotrexate
Category: Antidote; methotrexate toxicity prophylactic agent
Half-life: 15 minutes
Clinically important, potentially serious interactions with: barbiturates, fluorouracil, hydantoins, methotrexate, phenobarbital, primidone

Reactions

Skin
Erythema (<1%)
Pruritus (<1%)
Rash (sic) (<1%)
Urticaria (<1%)

Other
Anaphylactoid reaction (<1%)
Hypersensitivity

LEUPROLIDE

Synonym: leuprorelin acetate
Trade name: Lupron (TAP)
Other common trade names: *Carcinil; Enantone; Lucrin; Procren Depot; Procrin; Tapros*
Indications: Prostate carcinoma, endometriosis
Category: Gonadotropin-releasing hormone
Half-life: 3–4 hours
Clinically important, potentially serious interactions with: none

Reactions

Skin
Acne
Dermatitis (sic) (5%)
Diaphoresis
Ecchymoses (<5%)
Edema (1–10%)
Exanthems
Diaphoresis
Flushing
(1989): Crawford ED+, *N Engl J Med* 321, 419 (61%)
Hot flashes
(1993): Bressler LR+, *Ann Pharmacother* 27, 182
Lupus erythematosus
(1994): Fritzler MJ, *Lupus* 3, 455
Peripheral edema (12%)
(1989): Crawford ED+, *N Engl J Med* 321, 419 (4%)
Pigmentation (<5%)
Photosensitivity
Pruritus (<5%)
Purpura (<1%)
Rash (sic) (1–10%)
Urticaria
Xerosis (<5%)

Hair
Hair – alopecia (<5%)
Hair – growth (sic) (<1%)

Other
Dysgeusia (<5%)
Injection-site inflammation
(1989): Crawford ED+, *N Engl J Med* 321, 419 (2.1%)
Injection-site pruritus
(1989): Crawford ED+, *N Engl J Med* 321, 419 (2.1%)
Gynecomastia (7%)
Mastodynia (7%)
Myalgia (3%)
Paresthesias (<5%)
Thrombophlebitis (2%)
Vaginitis

LEVAMISOLE

Trade name: Ergamisol (Janssen)
Other common trade names: *Ascaridil; Decaris; Detrax 40; Ketrax; Solaskil; Termizole*
Indications: Susceptible helmintic organism infections, colorectal carcinoma
Category: Antineoplastic adjunct, immune modulator and anthelmintic
Half-life: 2–6 hours
Clinically important, potentially serious interactions with: alcohol, disulfiram, phenytoin, warfarin

Reactions

Skin

Angioedema (< 1%)
(1978): Multiple Authors, *Lancet* 2, 1007
Cutaneous side effects (sic)
(1978): Multiple Authors, *Lancet* 2, 1007 (20%)
Dermatitis (sic) (1–10%)
Edema (1–10%)
Erythema annulare
(1989): Lioté F+, *Rev Rhum Mal Ostéoartic* (French) 56, 11
Erythema multiforme
(1979): Hodinka L+, *Int Arch Allergy Appl Immunol* 58, 362
Exanthems
(1989): Lioté F+, *Rev Rhum Mal Ostéoartic* (French) 56, 11
(1980): Miller B+, *Arthritis Rheum* 23, 172 (> 10%)
(1978): Multiple Authors, *J Rheumatol* 5 (Suppl 4), 5
(1978): Secher L+, *Acta Derm Venereol* 58, 372
(1978): Symoens J+, *Cancer Treat Rep* 62, 1721 (2.6%)
(1978): Pinals RS, *J Rheumatol* 5 (Suppl 4), 71 (>5%)
(1976): Rosenthal M+, *N Engl J Med* 295, 1204
Exfoliative dermatitis
Fixed eruption
(1994): Clavère P+, *Ann Dermatol Venereol* (French) 121, 238 (pigmented)
(1991): Thankappen TP+, *Int J Dermatol* 30, 867 (0.88%)
Hemorrhagic eruption (sic)
(1982): Papageorgiou P+, *J Clin Lab Immunol* 8, 121
Infection (sic) (1–10%)
Lichenoid eruption
(1980): Kirby JD+, *J R Soc Med* 73, 208
(1978): Multiple Authors, *Lancet* 2, 1007
(1978): Pinals RS, *J Rheumatol* 5 (Suppl 4), 71
Pemphigus
(1980): Mashkilleison NA, *Vestn Dermatol Venerol* (Russian) October 46
Pruritus (< 1%)
(1992): Breathnach SM+, *Adverse Drug Reactions and the Skin*, Blackwell, Oxford, 178 (passim)
(1989): Lioté F+, *Rev Rhum Mal Ostéoartic* (French) 56, 11
(1980): Kirby JD+, *J R Soc Med* 73, 208
(1978): Pinals RS, *J Rheumatol* 5 (Suppl 4), 71
(1978): Secher L+, *Acta Derm Venereol* 58, 372
Psoriasis
(1980): Kirby JD+, *J R Soc Med* 73, 208 (passim)
Purpura
Rash (sic)
(1980): Husain Z+, *J Rheumatol* 7, 825
(1980): Kinsella PL+, *J Rheumatol* 7, 288
(1980): Miller B+, *Arthritis Rheum* 23, 172
(1979): Scherak O+, *Wien Klin Wochenschr* (German) 91, 758
(1978): Secher L+, *Acta Derm Venereol* 58, 372
(1978): Symoens J+, *Cancer Treat Rep* 62, 1721
(1978): Pinals RS, *J Rheumatol* 5 (Suppl 4), 71
(1977): Parkinson DR+, *Lancet* 2, 1129
Stevens–Johnson syndrome (< 1%)
Urticaria (< 1%)
(1992): Breathnach SM+, *Adverse Drug Reactions and the Skin*, Blackwell, Oxford, 178 (passim)
(1989): Lioté F+, *Rev Rhum Mal Ostéoartic* 56 (French) 11
(1979): Hodinka L+, *Int Arch Allergy Appl Immunol* 58, 362
(1978): Pinals RS, *J Rheumatol* 5 (Suppl 4), 71
Vasculitis
(1989): Lioté F+, *Rev Rhum Mal Ostéoartic* (French) 56, 11
(1983): Ferlazzo B+, *Boll Ist Sieroter Milan* (Italian) 62, 107
(1980): Huskisson EC, *Agents Actions* Suppl 7, 55
(1978): Scheinberg MA+, *BMJ* 1, 408
(1978): Multiple Authors, *Lancet* 2, 1007
(1978): MacFarlane DG+, *BMJ* 1, 407
Xerosis
(1980): Kirby JD+, *J R Soc Med* 73, 208

Hair

Hair – alopecia (1–10%)
(1980): Kirby JD+, *J R Soc Med* 73, 208

Other

Anaphylactoid reaction
Dysgeusia) (1–10%) (metallic taste)
(1977): Runge LA+, *Arthritis Rheum* 20, 1445
(1977): Veys EM+, Willoughby DA+, *Perspectives in Inflammation*, Lancaster, England, MTP Press, W3 FU966 v3
Erosive lichen planus
(1980): Kirby JD+, *J R Soc Med* 73, 208 (passim)
Myalgia (1–10%)
Oral mucosal lesions
(1989): Lioté F+, *Rev Rhum Mal Ostéoartic* (French) 56, 11 (2.1%)
(1980): Miller B+, *Arthritis Rheum* 23, 172 (> 10%)
(1978): Symoens J+, *Cancer Treat Rep* 62, 1721 (0.3%)
(1978): Multiple Authors, *J Rheumatol* 5 (Suppl 4), 5 (2.3%)
(1978): Multiple Authors, *Lancet* 2, 1007 (5.9%)
Oral ulceration
(1978): Symoens J+, *Cancer Treat Rep* 62, 1721
Paresthesias (1–10%)
Parosmia (< 1%)
Stomatitis (1–10%)
(1980): Kinsella PL+, *J Rheumatol* 7, 288
(1978): Multiple Authors, *Lancet* 2, 1007 (6%)

LEVETIRACETAM

Trade name: Keppra (UCB Pharma)
Indications: Partial onset seizures
Category: Anticonvulsant
Half-life: 7 hours
Clinically important, potentially serious interactions with: alcohol

Reactions

Skin

Ecchymoses (< 1%)
Flu syndrome (sic)
(2000): Cereghino JJ+, *Neurology* 55, 236
Fungal infection (> 1%)
Infection (13%)
(2000): Cereghino JJ+, *Neurology* 55, 236
Rash (sic) (> 1%)

Other

Gingivitis (> 1%)
Paresthesias (2%)

LEVOBUNOLOL

Trade names: AKBeta; Betagan (Allergan)
Other common trade names: *AK-Beta; Bunolgan; Gotensin; Vistagan; Vistagen*
Indications: Glaucoma, ocular hypertension
Category: Ophthalmic beta adrenergic blocker
Half-life: no data*
Clinically important, potentially serious interactions with: antidiabetic agents, beta-blockers, cimetidine, epinephrine, quinidine, tacrine, verapamil

Reactions

Skin

Burning eyes
Contact dermatitis
(1999): Erdmann S+, *Contact Dermatitis* 41, 44
(1995): Koch P, *Contact Dermatitis* 33, 140
(1995): Zucchelli V+, *Contact Dermatitis* 33, 66
(1995): di Lernia V+, *Contact Dermatitis* 33, 57
(1993): van der Meeren HL+, *Contact Dermatitis* 28, 41
(1989): Schultheiss E, *Derm Beruf Umwelt* (German) 37, 185
Erythema
Lichen planus
(1995): Beckman KA+, *Am J Ophthalmol* 120, 530
Pruritus (<1%)
Rash (sic) (<1%)
Stinging eyes
Urticaria

Hair

Hair – alopecia (1–10%)

Other

Hypersensitivity

*Peak effect: 1–7 days

LEVODOPA

Synonym: L-dopa
Trade names: Atamet (Athena); Sinemet (DuPont)
Other common trade names: *Brocadopa; Dopaflex; Doparl; Eldopal; Levodopa-Woelm*
Indications: Parkinsonism
Category: Antidyskinetic; antiparkinsonian
Half-life: 1–3 hours
Clinically important, potentially serious interactions with: antacids, anticholinergics, benzodiazepines, hydantoins, MAO inhibitors, papaverine, phenytoin, pyridoxine, tricyclic antidepressants

Sinemet is carbidopa and levodopa

Reactions

Skin

Diaphoresis
(1995): Sage JI+, *Ann Neurol* 37, 120
Exanthems
(1976): Arndt KA+, *JAMA* 235, 918
(1970): Schwarz GA+, *Med Clin North Am* 54, 773
Flushing
Hot flashes
Leukoplakia
Lupus erythematosus
(1985): Stratton MA, *Clin Pharm* 4, 657
(1979): Massarotti G+, *BMJ* 2, 553
Melanoma
(1997): Pfützner W+, *J Am Acad Dermatol* 37, 332
(1996): Kleinhans M+, *Hautarzt* (German) 47, 432
(1993): Weiner WJ+, *Neurology* 43, 674
(1992): Haider SA+, *Br J Ophthalmol* 76, 246
(1992): Sandyk R, *Int J Neurosci* 63, 137
(1989): Kande'l EI, *Zh Nevropatol Psikhiatr* (Russian) 89, 126
(1987): Morpurgo G+, *Eur J Cancer Clin Oncol* 23, 1213
(1985): Przybilla B+, *Acta Derm Venereol* (Stockh) 65, 556
(1985): Kochar AS, *Am J Med* 79, 119
(1985): Rampen FHJ, *J Neurol Neurosurg Psychiatry* 48, 585
(1984): Abramson DH+, *JAMA* 252, 1011
(1984): Rosin MA+, *Cutis* 33, 572
(1982): Van Rens GH+, *Ophthalmology* 89, 1464
(1980): Bernstein JE+, *Arch Dermatol* 116, 1041
(1980): Warner TF+, *J Cutan Pathol* 7, 50
(1979): Fermaglich J+, *JAMA* 241, 883
(1979): Botteri A+, *Lakartidningen (Swedish)* 76, 316
(1978): Fermaglich J, *Neurology* 28, 404
(1978): Sober AJ+, *JAMA* 240, 554
(1977): Fermaglich J+, *J Neurology* 215, 221
(1975): Pelfrene AF, *Nouv Presse Med* (French) 4, 1365
(1974): Happle R, *Fortschr* (German) 92, 1065
(1974): Liebermann AN+, *Neurology* 24, 340
(1973): Robinson E+, *Arch Pathol* 95, 213
(1972): Skibba JL+, *Arch Pathol* 93, 556
Pemphigus
(1986): Pisani M+, *G Ital Dermatol Venereol* (Italian) 121, 39
Purpura
(1976): Wanamaker WM+, *JAMA* 235, 2217
Rash (sic)
(1984): Goetz CG, *Clin Neuropharmacol* 7, 107
(1983): Goetz CG, *N Engl J Med* 309, 1387
Urticaria

Hair

Hair – alopecia
(1971): Marshall A+, *BMJ* 1, 407
Hair – repigmentation
(1989): Reynolds NJ+, *Clin Exp Dermatol* 14, 317
(1973): Grainger KM, *Lancet* 1, 97

Nails

Nails – increased growth
(1984): Danial CR+, *J Am Acad Dermatol* 10, 250
(1973): Miller E, *N Engl J Med* 288, 916

Other

Ageusia
Black cartilage
(1986): Connolly CE+, *Lancet* 1, 690
Bruxism
Chromhidrosis (1–10%)
Dysgeusia
Glossopyrosis
Paresthesias
Phlebitis
Priapism
Sialorrhea
Xerostomia (1–10%)

LEVOFLOXACIN

Trade name: Levaquin (Ortho-McNeil)
Indications: Various infections caused by susceptible organisms
Category: Fluoroquinolone antibiotic
Half-life: 6–8 hours
Clinically important, potentially serious interactions with: antacids, caffeine, cimetidine, cyclosporine, digoxin, iron salts, NSAIDs, probenecid, sucralfate, theophylline; warfarin, zinc salts

Reactions

Skin

Candidiasis (0.3%)
Diaphoresis (0.1%)
Edema (0.1%)
Erythema
(1992): Kanzaki H+, *Jpn J Antibiot* (Japanese) 45, 576

Erythema multiforme
Erythema nodosum (<3%)
Photosensitivity (<0.1%)
(2000): Boccumini LE+, *Ann Pharmacol* 34, 453
Pruritus (1.6%)
Purpura (<0.5%)
Rash (sic) (1.7%)
Stevens–Johnson syndrome
Toxic epidermal necrolysis
Urticaria (<0.5%)

Other

Anaphylactoid reaction
Dysgeusia (0.2%)
Injection-site reaction
Myalgia (<0.5%)
Paresthesias
Tendinitis
(2000): Casado Burgos E+, *Med Clin (Barc)* (Spanish) 114, 319
(1999): Lewis JR+, *Ann Pharmacother* 33, 792 (achilles, bilateral)
Tendon rupture (many reports)
Tremor
Vaginitis (1.8%)
Xerostomia (<1%)

LEVOTHYROXINE

Synonyms: L-thyroxine sodium; T_4
Trade names: Eltroxin; Levo-T; Levothyroid (Forest); Levoxyl (Jones); Synthroid (Knoll)
Other common trade names: *Berlthyrox; Droxine; Eferox; Levo-T; Levothyrox; Thevier*
Indications: Hypothyroidism
Category: Synthetic thyroid hormone
Half-life: 6–7 days
Clinically important, potentially serious interactions with: cholestyramine, colestipol, digitalis, iron, oral anticoagulants, phenytoin, propranolol, sympathomimetics, theophylline, tricyclic antidepressants, warfarin

Reactions

Skin

Acne
Allergic reactions (sic)
Angioedema
(1991): Levesque H+, *Lancet* 338, 393
(1990): Pandya AG+, *Arch Dermatol* 126, 1238
Dermatitis herpetiformis
(1974): From E+, *Br J Dermatol* 91, 221
Diaphoresis (<1%)
Flushing
Nevi
(1976): Tofahrn J+, *Z Hautkr* (German) 51, 617 (eruption)
Pruritus
(1990): Pandya AG+, *Arch Dermatol* 126, 1238
Rash (sic)
Urticaria
(1994): Magner J+, *Thyroid* 4, 341 (from the blue dye)
(1990): Pandya AG+, *Arch Dermatol* 126, 1238
(1966): Romanski B+, *Pol Med Sci Hist* 9, 92
Xerosis

Hair

Hair – alopecia (<1%)

Other

Diaphoresis
Hypersensitivity
Myalgia (<1%)
Pseudotumor cerebri (in infants)
Tremor

LIDOCAINE

Synonym: lignocaine
Trade names: Anestacon (PolyMedica); ELA-Max (Ferndale); EMLA (AstraZeneca); Xylocaine (AstraZeneca)
Other common trade names: *Dentipatch; DermaFlex; Dilocaine; Lidodan; Lidoject-2; Octocaine; Xylocard*
Indications: Ventricular arrhythmias, topical anesthesia
Category: Anesthetic; antiarrhythmic
Half-life: terminal: 1.5–2 hours
Clinically important, potentially serious interactions with: amprenavir, antiarrhythmics, anticonvulsants, beta-blockers, cimetidine, MAO inhibitors, phenytoin, procainamide, propranolol, succinylcholine, tricyclic antidepressants

Reactions

Skin

Angioedema
(1987): Bricker SR+, *Anaesthesia* 42, 323
(1961): Rajka G, *Allergie Asthma* (German) 7, 237
(1961): Noble DS+, *Lancet* 2, 1436
Bullous eruption
Contact dermatitis
(1996): Bassett IB+, *Australas J Dermatol* 37, 155
(1995): Thakur BK+, *J Allergy Clin Immunol* 95, 776
(1994): Hardwick N+, *Contact Dermatitis* 30, 245
(1993): Handfield-Jones SE+, *Clin Exp Dermatol* 18, 342
(1993): Duggan M+, *Contact Dermatitis* 28, 190
(1990): Black RJ+, *Contact Dermatitis* 23, 117
(1989): Budde J+, *Derm Beruf Umwelt* (German) 37, 181
(1986): Curley KR, *Arch Dermatol* 122, 924
(1985): Fernandes-de-Corres L+, *Contact Dermatitis* 12, 114
(1983): Nurse DS+, *Contact Dermatitis* 9, 513
(1979): Kernekamp AS+, *Contact Dermatitis* 5, 403
(1979): Fregert S+, *Contact Dermatitis* 5, 185
(1977): Turner TW, *Contact Dermatitis* 3, 210
Eczema (sic)
(1990): Huwyler T+, *Schweiz Monatsschr Zahnmed* (German) 100, 751
(1986): Curley KR, *Arch Dermatol* 122, 924
(1961): Rajka G, *Allergie Asthma* (German) 7, 237
Edema (<1%)
Erythema multiforme
(1987): Arrowsmith JB+, *Ann Intern Med* 107, 693
Exanthems
Exfoliative dermatitis
(1987): Arrowsmith JB+, *Ann Intern Med* 107, 693
(1975): Hoffmann H+, *Arch Dermatol* 111, 266
Fixed eruption
(1996): Kawada A+, *Contact Dermatitis* 35, 375
(1997): Garcia JC+, *J Investig Allergol Clin Immunol* 7, 127
Lupus erythematosus
(1988): Oliphant LD+, *Chest* 94, 427
Pigmentation
(1987): Curley RK+, *Br Dent J* 162, 113
Pruritus (<1%)
(1961): Rajka G, *Allergie Asthma* (German) 7, 237
Purpura
Rash (<1%)
Shivering (1–10%)
Stevens–Johnson syndrome
(1987): Arrowsmith JB+, *Ann Intern Med* 107, 693
Urticaria
(1980): Chin TM+, *Int J Dermatol* 19, 147
(1969): Aldrete JA+, *JAMA* 207, 356
(1961): Rajka G, *Allergie Asthma* (German) 7, 237

Other

Acute intermittent porphyria
Anaphylactoid reaction
(1999): Bircher AJ+, *Aust Dent J* 44, 64
(1984): Metzner HH+, *Dermatol Monatsschr* (German) 170, 648
(1980): Agathos M, *Contact Dermatitis* 6, 236
(1975): Tannenbaum H+, *J Allergy Clin Immunol* 56, 226

Embolia cutis medicamentosa (Nicolau syndrome)
(1990): Wand A+, *Aktuel Dermatol* (German) 16, 128
Hypersensitivity
(1996): Bircher AJ+, *Contact Dermatitis* 34, 387
(1996): Whalen JD+, *Arch Dermatol* 132, 1256
(1975): Ravindranathan N, *Br Dent J* 138, 101
Injection-site pain
Injection-site phlebitis
Paresthesias (<1%)
Stomatitis
(1987): Arrowsmith JB+, *Ann Intern Med* 107, 693
Tremor

LINCOMYCIN

Trade name: Lincocin (Pharmacia & Upjohn)
Other common trade names: *Albiotic; Cillimicina; Cillimycin; Lincocine; Princol; Zumalin*
Indications: Various infections caused by susceptible organisms
Category: Macrolide antibiotic
Half-life: 2–11.5 hours
Clinically important, potentially serious interactions with: antacids, neuromuscular blocking agents

Reactions

Skin
Allergic reactions (sic)
(1971): *Med Lett* 13, 55 (1–5%)
Angioedema
Contact dermatitis
(1991): Vilaplana J+, *Contact Dermatitis* 24, 225
(1985): Conde-Salazar L+, *Contact Dermatitis* 12, 59 (erythema multiforme-like)
Erythema multiforme
Exanthems
Exfoliative dermatitis
Photosensitivity
Pruritus
(1965): Kanee B, *Can Med Assoc J* 93, 220
Pruritus ani (<1%)
Purpura
(1973): Raff M, *Ann Intern Med* 78, 779
Rash (sic) (<1%)
Stevens–Johnson syndrome (<1%)
(1973): Pickering LK+, *JAMA* 223, 1392
Urticaria (<1%)
Vesiculobullous eruption

Other
Anaphylactoid reaction
Glossitis (<1%)
Injection-site erythema
(1990): Shen K, *Lancet* 336, 689
Oral mucosal lesions
Serum sickness
Stomatitis (<1%)
Vaginitis (<1%)

LINEZOLID

Trade name: Zyvox (Pharmacia & Upjohn)
Indications: Various infections caused by susceptible organisms
Category: Oxazolidinone antibiotic
Half-life: 4–5 hours
Clinically important, potentially serious interactions with: dextromethorphan, meperidine, trazodone, tricyclic antidepressants, SSRIs, venlafaxine, **tyramine-containing foods***

Reactions

Skin
Fungal infections (0.1–2%)
Pruritus
Rash (sic) (2%)

Other
Candidal vaginitis (1–2%)
Dysgeusia (1–2%)
Oral candidiasis (<1%)
Tongue pigmentation (<1%)

***Note:** Tyramine-containing foods include the following: aged cheeses, avocados, banana skins, bologna and other processed luncheon meats, chicken livers, chocolate, figs, canned pickled herring, meat extracts, pepperoni, raisins, raspberries, soy sauce, vermouth, sherry and red wines.

LIOTHYRONINE

Synonym: T_3 sodium
Trade names: Cytomel (Jones); Triostat (Jones)
Other common trade names: *Cynomel; T3; Tertroxin; Thyronine; Trijodthyronin BC N*
Indications: Hypothyroidism
Category: Synthetic thyroid hormone
Half-life: 16–49 hours
Clinically important, potentially serious interactions with: anticoagulants, antidiabetics, beta-blockers, cholestyramine, colestipol, digoxin, iron, metoprolol, phenytoin, theophylline

Reactions

Skin
Allergic reactions (sic)
Diaphoresis (<1%)
Rash (sic)
Urticaria
(1994): Magner J+, *Thyroid* 4, 341 (from the blue dye)
(1990): Pandya AG+, *Arch Dermatol* 126, 1238
(1966): Romanski B+, *Pol Med Sci Hist* 9, 92
Xerosis

Hair
Hair – alopecia (<1%)

Other
Hypersensitivity
Myalgia (<1%)
Phlebitis (1%)
Pseudotumor cerebri
Tremor

LISINOPRIL

Trade names: Prinivil (Merck); Prinizide (Merck); Zestoretic (AstraZeneca); Zestril (AstraZeneca)
Other common trade names: *Acerbon; Alapril; Apo-Lisinopril; Carace; Coric; Prinil; Tensopril; Vivatec*
Indications: Hypertension
Category: Angiotensin-converting enzyme (ACE) inhibitor; antihypertensive
Half-life: 12 hours
Clinically important, potentially serious interactions with: alcohol, allopurinol, amiloride, bumetanide, digoxin, diuretics, furosemide, indomethacin, insulin, lithium, mercaptopurine, NSAIDs, phenothiazines, salicylates, spironolactone, torsemide, triamterene

Prinizide is lisinopril and hydrochlorothiazide; Zestoretic is lisinopril and hydrochlorothiazide

Reactions

Skin

Angioedema
(1999): Guo X+, *J Okla State Med Assoc* 92, 71
(1999): Neutel JM+, *Am J Ther* 6, 161
(1999): Maestre ML+, *Rev Esp Anestesiol Reanim* (Spanish) 46, 88
(1997): Brown NJ+, *JAMA* 278, 232
(1997): Pavletic AJ, *J Am Board Fam Pract* 10, 370
(1996): Pillans PI+, *Eur J Clin Pharmacol* 51, 123
(1995): Kuo DC+, *J Emerg Med* 13, 327 (uvular)
(1995): Bauwens LJ+, *Ned Tijdschr Geneeskd* (Dutch) 139, 674
(1995): Frontera Y+, *J Am Dent Assoc* 126, 217
(1994): Krikorian RK+, *Chest* 106, 1922
(1993): Soo Hoo GW+, *West J Med* 158, 412
(1992): Shelley WB+, *Cutis* 49, 391 (tongue) (observation)
(1992): McElligott S+, *Ann Intern Med* 116, 426
(1990): Laher MS, *Drugs* 39 (Suppl 2), 55
(1990): McAreavey D+, *Drugs* 40, 326 (0.4%)
(1990): Orfan N+, *JAMA* 264, 1287
(1988): Lancaster SG+, *Drugs* 35, 646 (0.6%)
(1987): Rush JE+, *J Cardiovasc Pharmacol* 9, s99
Bullous eruption
(1988): Barlow RJ+, *Clin Exp Dermatol* 13, 117
Diaphoresis (<1%)
Edema (1%)
Erythema (1%)
Exanthems
(1990): Laher MS, *Drugs* 39 (Suppl 2), 55
(1990): McAreavey D+, *Drugs* 40, 326 (3.2%)
(1988): Lancaster SG+, *Drugs* 35, 646 (3.2%)
(1988): Barlow RJ+, *Clin Exp Dermatol* 13, 117
Facial edema (<1%)
Flushing (<1%)
(1997): Litt JZ, Beachwood, OH, personal case (observation)
(1990): Laher MS, *Drugs* 39 (Suppl 2), 55
(1989): Healy LA+, *N Engl J Med* 321, 763
Lichenoid eruption
(1992): Shelley WB+, *Cutis* 50, 182 (observation)
Lupus erythematosus
Pemphigus
Peripheral edema (<1%)
(1988): Uretsky BF+, *Am Heart J* 116, 480
Photosensitivity (<1%)
Pruritus (1.2%)
(2000): Kalikhman ZM, (from Internet) (observation)
Purpura
(1993): Sztern B+, *Presse Med* (French) 22, 967
(1988): Barlow RJ+, *Clin Exp Dermatol* 13, 117
Rash (sic) (1.5%)
(1999): Horiuchi Y+, *J Dermatol* 26, 128
(1989): Giles TD+, *J Am Coll Cardiol* 13, 1240
(1988): Uretsky BF+, *Am Heart J* 116, 480
(1987): Rush JE+, *J Cardiovasc Pharmacol* 9, s99
(1987): Bolzano K+, *J Cardiovasc Pharmacol* 9, s43
Rosacea
(1999): Oakley A, Hamilton, New Zealand (from Internet) (observation)
Stevens–Johnson syndrome
Telangiectasia
(1999): Oakley A, Hamilton, New Zealand (from Internet) (observation)
Toxic epidermal necrolysis
Ulceration (ischemic skin ulcer) (sic)
(1987): Rush JE+, *J Cardiovasc Pharmacol* 9, s99
Urticaria (<1%)
(1996): Pillans PI+, *Eur J Clin Pharmacol* 51, 123
(1989): Cameron HA+, *J Human Hypertension* 3, 177
Vasculitis (<1%)
(1988): Barlow RJ+, *Clin Exp Dermatol* 13, 117

Hair

Hair – alopecia (<1%)

Other

Anaphylactoid reaction (<1%)
Dysesthesia (<1%)
Dysgeusia
(1988): Uretsky BF+, *Am Heart J* 116, 480
Mastodynia (<1%)
Myalgia (0.5%)
Paresthesias (0.8%)
Tremor
Xerostomia (<1%)

LITHIUM

Trade names: Eskalith (SmithKline Beecham); Lithobid (Solvay); Lithonate (Solvay); Lithotabs (Solvay)
Other common trade names: *Carbolith; Duralith; Hynorex Retard; Lithicarb; Lithizine; Priadel; Teralithe*
Indications: Manic-depressive states
Category: Antidepressants, antipsychotic and antimanic
Half-life: 18–24 hours
Clinically important, potentially serious interactions with: ACE-inhibitors, acetazolamide, caffeine, captopril, CNS depressants, carbamazepine, chlorpromazine, clozapine, fluoxetine, haloperidol, indomethacin, iodide salts, ketorolac, loop diuretics, MAO inhibitors, methyldopa, NSAIDs, phenothiazines, phenylbutazones, piroxicam, theophyllines, thiazides, tricyclic antidepressants, valsartan, verapamil

Note: An excellent review of the cutaneous conditions associated with lithium can be found in (1983): Sarantidis D+, *Br J Psychiatry* 143, 42

Reactions

Skin

Acanthosis nigricans
(1979): Arnold HL+, *J Am Acad Dermatol* 1, 93
Acne
(1991): Srebrnik A+, *Cutis* 48, 65
(1986): Remmer HI+, *J Clin Psychiatry* 47, 48
(1985): Albrecht G, *Hautarzt* (German) 36, 77 (passim)
(1984): Lambert D+, *Ann Med Interne Paris* (French) 135, 637
(1983): Sarantidis D+, *Br J Psychiatry* 143, 42 (11%)
(1982): Lambert D+, *Ann Dermatol Venereol* (French) 109, 19
(1982): Heng MCY, *Arch Dermatol* 118, 246
(1982): Heng MCY, *Br J Dermatol* 106, 107
(1982): Deandrea D+, *J Clin Psychopharmacol* 2, 199
(1980): Vestergaard P+, *Acta Psychiatrica Scand* 62, 193
(1978): Oei TT+, *Ned Tijdschr Geneeskd* (Dutch) 122, 1302
(1977): Reiffers J+, *Dermatologica* 155, 155
(1977): Okrasinski H, *Dermatologica* 154, 251
(1975): Yoder FW, *Arch Dermatol* 111, 396
(1971): Kusumi Y, *Dis Nerv Syst* 32, 853
Angioedema
(1985): Berova N+, *Dermatol Venerol* (Sofia) (Bulgarian) 24, 23
(1982): Lambert D+, *Ann Dermatol Venereol* (French) 109, 19
Angular cheilitis
(1983): Sarantidis D+, *Br J Psychiatry* 143, 42 (1%)

Atopic dermatitis
(1983): Sarantidis D+, *Br J Psychiatry* 143, 42 (3%)
Bullous eruption
(1987): McWhirter JD+, *Arch Dermatol* 123, 1122
Cutaneous side effects (sic)
(1985): Berova N+, *Dermatol Venerol* (Sofia) (Bulgarian) 24, 23 (23%)
(1983): Sarantidis D+, *Br J Psychiatry* 143, 42 (up to one-third)
(1982): Lambert D+, *Ann Dermatol Venereol* (French) 109, 19
Darier's disease
(1995): Rubin MB, *J Am Acad Dermatol* 32, 674
(1990): Milton GP, *J Am Acad Dermatol* 23, 926 (exacerbation)
(1986): Clark RD Jr+, *Psychosomatics* 27, 800 (exacerbation)
Dermatitis (sic)
(1980): Aldoroty N+, *Am J Psychiatry* 137, 870
(1973): Ruiz-Maldonado R+, *JAMA* 224, 1534
(1973): Kurtin SB, *JAMA* 223, 802
(1972): Posey RE, *JAMA* 221, 1517
Dermatitis herpetiformis
(1985): Albrecht G, *Hautarzt* (German) 36, 77 (passim)
(1983): Sarantidis D+, *Br J Psychiatry* 143, 42
(1982): Heng MCY, *Arch Dermatol* 118, 246
Discoloration of fingers and toes (sic) (<1%)
Eczema (sic)
(1980): Vestergaard P+, *Acta Psychiatrica Scand* 62, 193
Edema
(1984): Lambert D+, *Ann Med Interne Paris* (French) 135, 637
(1975): Baldessarini RJ+, *Ann Intern Med* 83, 527
(1970): Demers R+, *JAMA* 214, 1845 (pretibial)
Erythema
(1996): Wakelin SH+, *Clin Exp Dermatol* 21, 296
Erythema multiforme
(1991): Balldin J+, *J Am Acad Dermatol* 24, 1015
Exanthems
(1985): Albrecht G, *Hautarzt* (German) 36, 77 (passim)
(1983): Sarantidis D+, *Br J Psychiatry* 143, 42
(1982): Lambert D+, *Ann Dermatol Venereol* (French) 109, 19
(1982): Deandrea D+, *J Clin Psychopharmacol* 2, 199
(1980): Meinhold JM+, *J Clin Psychiatry* 41, 395
(1975): Baldessarini RJ+, *Ann Intern Med* 83, 527
(1970): No Author, *Ann Intern Med* 73, 291
(1968): Callaway CL+, *Am J Psychiatry* 124, 1124
Exfoliative dermatitis
(1985): Albrecht G, *Hautarzt* (German) 36, 77 (passim)
(1983): Sarantidis D+, *Br J Psychiatry* 143, 42 (1%)
(1979): Kuhnley EJ+, *Am J Psychiatry* 136, 1340
Follicular keratosis (sic)
(1996): Wakelin SH+, *Clin Exp Dermatol* 21, 296
(1982): Lambert D+, *Ann Dermatol Venereol* (French) 109, 19
(1977): Reiffers J+, *Dermatologica* 155, 155
Folliculitis
(1985): Hogan DJ+, *J Am Acad Dermatol* 13, 245 (passim)
(1983): Sarantidis D+, *Br J Psychiatry* 143, 42
(1973): Rifkin A+, *Am J Psychiatry* 130, 1018
(1973): Kurtin SB, *JAMA* 223, 803
Hidradenitis suppurativa
(1997): Marinella MA, *Acta Derm Venereol* 77, 483
(1996): Blumenthal HL, Beachwood, OH, personal case (observation)
(1995): Gupta AK+, *J Amer Acad Dermatol* 32, 382
(1981): Stamm T+, *Psychiatr Prax* (German) 8, 152
Hyperplasia (verrucous)
(1984): Frenk E, *Z Hautkr* (German), 2, 97
Ichthyosis
(1983): Sarantidis D+, *Br J Psychiatry* 143, 42 (1%)
(1977): Reiffers J+, *Dermatologica* 155, 155
Linear IgA bullous dermatosis
(1996): Tranvan A+, *J Am Acad Dermatol* 35, 865
(1987): McWhirter JD+, *Arch Dermatol* 123, 1122
Keratoderma
(1991): Labelle A+, *J Clin Psychopharmacol* 11, 149
Keratosis pilaris
(1985): Albrecht G, *Hautarzt* (German) 36, 77 (passim)
(1973): Rifkin A+, *Am J Psychiatry* 130, 1018
Lichen planus
(1994): Thompson DF+, *Pharmacotherapy* 14, 561
Lichen simplex chronicus
(1984): Shukla S+, *Am J Psychiatry* 141, 909

Linear IgA bullous dermatosis
(1987): McWhirter JD+, *Arch Dermatol* 123, 1122
Lupus erythematosus
(1985): Stratton MA, *Clin Pharm* 4, 657
(1982): Shukla VR+, *JAMA* 248, 921
(1981): Hess EV, *Arthritis Rheum* 24, 6
Morphea
(1982): Lambert D+, *Ann Dermatol Venereol* (French) 109, 19
Myxedema
(1981): Kvetny J+, *Ugeskr Laeger* (Danish) 143, 1323
(1979): Medley ES+, *J Fam Pract* 8, 855
(1978): Perrild H+, *BMJ* 1, 1108
(1973): Pousset G+, *Ann Endocrinol Paris* (French) 34, 549
(1973): Pousset G+, *Ann Endocrinol Paris* (French) 34, 454
(1972): Vestergaard PA+, *Lancet* 2, 427
(1972): Wiener JD, *JAMA* 220, 587
(1972): Brandrup FO, *Ugeskr Laeger* (Danish) 134 2710
(1972): Vestergaard PA+, *Ugeskr Laeger* (Danish) 134, 1282
(1971): Luby ED+, *JAMA* 218, 1298
Papular eruption (elbows)
(1973): Kurtin SB, *JAMA* 223, 802
(1972): Posey RE, *JAMA* 221, 1517
Parkinsonism
(2000): Muthane UB+, *J Neurol Sci* 176, 78
Port-wine stain
(1987): Leung AK, *J Natl Med Assoc* 79, 877
Prurigo nodularis
(1983): Sarantidis D+, *Br J Psychiatry* 143, 42 (1%)
Pruritus (<1%)
(1985): Berova N+, *Dermatol Venerol* (Sofia) (Bulgarian) 24, 23 (1–5%)
(1984): Lambert D+, *Ann Med Interne Paris* (French) 135, 637
(1983): Sarantidis D+, *Br J Psychiatry* 143, 42
(1982): Lambert D+, *Ann Dermatol Venereol* (French) 109, 19
(1980): Vestergaard P+, *Acta Psychiatrica Scand* 62, 193
(1977): Reiffers J+, *Dermatologica* 155, 155
(1970): No Author, *Ann Intern Med* 73, 291
(1968): Callaway CL+, *Am J Psychiatry* 124, 1124
Psoriasis
(1996): Ockenfels HM+, *Arch Dermatol Res* 288, 173
(1994): Dorevitch A, *Harefuah* (Hebrew) 127, 228
(1993): Hermle L+, *Nervenarzt* (German) 64, 208
(1992): Rudolph RI, *J Am Acad Dermatol* 26, 135
(1992): Abel EA, *Semin Dermatol* 11, 269
(1992): Hemlock C+, *Ann Pharmacother* 26, 211
(1989): Sasaki T+, *J Dermatol* (Tokio) 16, 59 (exacerbation)
(1988): Koo E+, *Orv Hetil* (Hungarian) 129, 1699
(1988): Zirilli G+, *Minerva Psichiatr* (Italian) 29, 43
(1987): Gupta MA+, *Gen Hosp Psychiatry* 9, 157
(1986): Segui-Montesinos J+, *Med Clin (Barc)* (Spanish) 86, 261
(1986): Holy B+, *Acta Univ Carol Med Praha* (Czech) 32, 217
(1986): Pande AC+, *J Clin Psychiatry* 47, 330 (exacerbation)
(1986): Abel EA+, *J Am Acad Dermatol* 15, 1007 (exacerbation)
(1986): Ghadirian AM+, *J Clin Psychiatry* 47, 212
(1985): Albrecht G, *Hautarzt* (German) 36, 77 (passim)
(1984): Fox BJ+, *J Assoc Military Dermatol* 10, 35 (exacerbation)
(1984): Alvarez WA+, *Int J Psychosom* 31, 21
(1984): Lin HN+, *Taiwan I Hsueh Hui Tsa Chih* (Chinese) 83, 1064
(1984): Farber EM+, *J Am Acad Dermatol* 10, 511
(1984): Lambert D+, *Ann Med Interne Paris* (French) 135, 637
(1983): Hollander A, *Hautarzt* (German) 34, 487
(1983): Sarantidis D+, *Br J Psychiatry* 143, 42 (2%)
(1982): Lambert D+, *Ann Dermatol Venereol* (French) 109, 19 (exacerbation)
(1982): Heng MCY, *Arch Dermatol* 118, 246 (exacerbation)
(1982): Heng MCY, *Br J Dermatol* 106, 107 (exacerbation)
(1982): Deandrea D+, *J Clin Psychopharmacol* 2, 199
(1982): Pincelli C+, *G Ital Dermatol Venereol* (Italian) 117, 113
(1981): No Author, *Drug Ther Bull* 19, 68
(1980): Bakris GL+, *Int J Psychiatry Med* 10, 327
(1980): Thiers B, *J Am Acad Dermatol* 3, 101
(1979): Umbert P+, *Actas Dermosifiliogr* (Spanish) 70, 623
(1979): Skoven I+, *Arch Dermatol* 115, 1185 (exacerbation)
(1979): Lazarus GS+, *Arch Dermatol* 115, 1183
(1979): Evans DL+, *Am J Psychiatry* 136, 1326
(1978): Mobacken H+, *Br J Dermatol* 98, 597
(1978): Robak OH, *Tidsskr Nor Laegeforen* (Norwegian) 98, 566
(1978): Thormann J, *Ugeskr Laeger* (Danish) 140, 721
(1977): No Author, *Lakartidningen* (Swedish) 74, 2109

(1977): Skott AH+, *Br J Psychiatry* 131, 223
(1977): Skott AH+, *Br J Dermatol* 96, 445 (exacerbation)
(1977): Reiffers J+, *Dermatologica* 155, 155 (exacerbation)
(1976): Bakker JB+, *Psychosomatics* 17, 143 (exacerbation)
(1972): Carter TN, *Psychosomatics* 13, 325

Purpura
(1984): Lambert D+, *Ann Med Interne Paris* (French) 135, 637
(1982): Lambert D+, *Ann Dermatol Venereol* (French) 109, 19

Pustular eruption
(1993): Webster GF, *Clin Dermatol* 11, 541
(1982): White SW, *J Am Acad Dermatol* 7, 660 (palms and soles)

Pustular psoriasis
(1979): Skoven I+, *Arch Dermatol* 115, 1185
(1979): Evans DL+, *Am J Psychiatry* 136, 10
(1978): Lowe NJ+, *Arch Dermatol* 114, 1788

Rash (sic) (1–10%)
(1980): Bone S+, *Am J Psychiatry* 137:1, 103

Seborrheic dermatitis
(1984): Lambert D+, *Ann Med Interne Paris* (French) 135, 637
(1983): Sarantidis D+, *Br J Psychiatry* 143, 42
(1982): Lambert D+, *Ann Dermatol Venereol* (French) 109, 19

Subcorneal pustular dermatosis (Sneddon–Wilkinson)
(1988): Sterling GB+, *Cutis* 41, 165

Telangiectases
(1983): Brinkmann W+, *Z Hautkr* (German) 9, 681

Tinea versicolor
(1997): Fearfield LA+, *Clin Exp Dermatol* 22, 57

Toxicoderma
(1985): Lambert D, *Dermatologica* (French) 171, 209

Ulceration (lower extremities)
(1984): Lambert D+, *Ann Med Interne Paris* (French) 135, 637
(1975): Baldessarini RJ+, *Ann Intern Med* 83, 527
(1971): Kusumi Y, *Dis Nerv Syst* 32, 853
(1970): No Author, *Ann Intern Med* 73, 291
(1968): Callaway CL+, *Am J Psychiatry* 124, 1124

Urticaria
(1985): Berova N+, *Dermatol Venerol* (Sofia) (Bulgarian) 24, 23
(1984): Lambert D+, *Ann Med Interne Paris* (French) 135, 637
(1982): Lambert D+, *Ann Dermatol Venereol* (French) 109, 19

Vasculitis
(1994): Blumenthal HL, Beachwood, OH, personal case (observation)
(1984): Lambert D+, *Ann Med Interne Paris* (French) 135, 637
(1982): Lambert D+, *Ann Dermatol Venereol* (French) 109, 19
(1970): *Ann Intern Med* 73, 291

Verrucous lesions (sic)
(1984): Frenk E, *Z Hautkr* (German) 59, 97

Warts
(1982): White SW, *Int J Dermatol* 21, 107

Xerosis
(1975): Hoxtell E+, *Arch Dermatol* 111, 1073

Hair

Hair – alopecia
(2000): Mercke Y+, *Ann Clin Psychiatry* 12, 35 (12–19%)
(1999): van dem Bent PM+, *Ned Tijdschr Geneeskd* (Dutch) *143, 990*
(1998): Litt JZ, Beachwood, OH, personal case (observation)
(1996): McKinney PA+, *Ann Clin Psychiatry* 8, 183 (10%)
(1991): Wagner KD+, *Psychosomatics* 32, 355
(1986): Ghadirian AM+, *J Clin Psychiatry* 47, 212
(1985): Albrecht G, *Hautarzt* (German) 36, 77 (passim)
(1984): Mortimer PS+, *Int J Dermatol* 23, 603
(1984): Lambert D+, *Ann Med Interne Paris* (French) 135, 637
(1983): Shader RI, *J Clin Psychopharmacol* 3, 122
(1983): Yassa R+, *Can J Psychiatry* 28, 132
(1983): Orwin A, *Br J Dermatol* 108, 503 (12%)
(1982): Lambert D+, *Ann Dermatol Venereol* (French) 109, 19
(1982): Muniz CE+, *Psychosomatics* 23, 312
(1982): Dawber R+, *Br J Dermatol* 107, 125
(1982): No Author, *Psychosomatics* 23, 563

Hair – alopecia areata
(1988): Silvestri A+, *Gen Hosp Psychiatry* 10, 46
(1983): Sarantidis D+, *Br J Psychiatry* 143, 42 (2%)
(1980): Vestergaard P+, *Acta Psychiatr Scand* 62, 193

Hair – brittle
(1970): No Author, *Ann Intern Med* 73, 291

Hair – changes in texture
(1985): McCreadle RG+, *Acta Psychiatr Scand* 72, 387

Nails

Nails – Beau's lines (transverse nail bands)
(1988): Don PC+, *Cutis* 41, 20

Nails – dystrophy
(1988): Don PC+, *Cutis* 41, 20
(1982): Lambert D+, *Ann Dermatol Venereol* (French) 109, 19

Nails – onychomadesis
(1988): Don PC+, *Cutis* 41, 20

Nails – psoriasis
(1992): Rudolph RI, *J Am Acad Dermatol* 26, 135

Other

Dysgeusia (>10%)

Geographic tongue
(1992): Patki AH, *Int J Dermatol* 31, 386

Gingival hyperplasia
(1968): Callaway CL+, *Am J Psychiatry* 124, 1124

Glossodynia

Lichenoid stomatitis
(1995): Menni S+, *Ann Dermatol Venereol* (French) 122, 91
(1991): Srebrnik A+, *Cutis* 48, 65
(1985): Hogan DJ+, *J Am Acad Dermatol* 13, 245

Oral ulceration
(1985): Bar Nathan EA+, *Am J Psychiatry* 142, 1126
(1985): Hogan DJ+, *J Am Acad Dermatol* 13, 245

Pseudolymphoma
(1995): Magro CM+, *J Am Acad Dermatol* 32, 419

Pseudotumor cerebri (<1%)

Sialorrhea

Stomatitis
(1985): Bar Nathan EA+, *Am J Psychiatry* 142, 1126
(1978): Muniz CE+, *JAMA* 239, 2759

Stomatodynia
(1985): Bar Nathan EA+, *Am J Psychiatry* 142, 1126

Tremor

Vaginal ulceration
(1991): Srebrnik A+, *Cutis* 48, 65

Xerostomia (<1%)
(1980): Bone S+, *Am J Psychiatry* 137:1, 103

LOMEFLOXACIN

Trade name: Maxaquin (Unimed)
Other common trade names: *Logiflox; Ontop*
Indications: Various infections caused by susceptible organisms
Category: Broad-spectrum fluoroquinolone antibacterial
Half-life: 4–6 hours
Clinically important, potentially serious interactions with: azlocillin, betaxolol, caffeine, cimetidine, cyclosporine, didanosine, iron salts, metoprolol, probenecid, theophylline, warfarin, zinc salts

Reactions

Skin

Allergic reactions (sic) (<1%)

Ankle edema

Chills (<1%)

Diaphoresis (<1%)
(1992): Crome P+, *Am J Med* 92 (Suppl 4A), 126S
(1992): Iravani A, *Am J Med* 92, 75S

Eczema (sic)

Edema (<1%)

Exanthems

Exfoliation (sic) (<1%)

Facial edema (<1%)

Flu-like syndrome (sic) (<1%)

Flushing (<1%)

Genital pruritus (sic)
(1992): Iravani A, *Am J Med* 92, 75S

Photosensitivity (2.4%)
(2000): Ferguson J+, *J Antimicrob Chemother* 45, 503
(1998): Arata J+, *Antimicrob Agents Chemother* 42, 3141

(1998): Kimura M+, *Contact Dermatitis* 38, 180
(1996): Young AR+, *J Photochem Photobiol B* 32, 165
(1994): Lowe NJ+, *Clin Pharmacol Ther* 56, 587
(1994): Poh-Fitzpatrick MB, *Arch Dermatol* 130, 261
(1994): Correia O+, *Arch Dermatol* 130, 808 (bullous)
(1994): Cohen JB+, *Arch Dermatol* 130, 805 (following tanning bed)
(1993): Tozawa K+, *Hinyokika Kiyo* (Japanese) 39, 801
(1992): Crome P+, *Am J Med* 92 (Suppl 4A), 126S
(1992): Rizk E, *Am J Med* 92, 130S (2.4%)
(1992): Kurumaji Y+, *Contact Dermatitis* 26, 5
(1992): Iravani A, *Am J Med* 92, 75S
(1990): LeBel M+, *Antimicrob Agents Chemother* 34, 1254

Phototoxic reaction
(2000): Traynor NJ+, *Toxicol Vitr* 14, 275
(1998): Martinez LJ+ *Photochem Photobiol* 67, 399

Pruritus (<1%)
(1992): Klimberg IW+, *Am J Med* 92, 121S
(1992): Gotfried MH+, *Am J Med* 92, 108S
(1992): Kemper P+, *Am J Med* 92, 98S
(1992): Mouton Y+, *Am J Med* 92, 87S
(1992): Cox CE, *Am J Med* 92, 82S
(1991): Wadworth AN+, *Drugs* 42, 1018

Purpura (<1%)

Pustular eruption
(1992): Mouton Y+, *Am J Med* 92, 87S

Rash (sic) (<1%)
(1992): Crome P+, *Am J Med* 92 (Suppl 4A), 126S
(1992): Gotfried MH+, *Am J Med* 92, 108S
(1992): Mouton Y+, *Am J Med* 92, 87S
(1992): Iravani A, *Am J Med* 92, 75S
(1991): Wadworth AN+, *Drugs* 42, 1018

Stevens–Johnson syndrome

Toxicoderma (sic)
(1991): Wadworth AN+, *Drugs* 42, 1018

Urticaria (<1%)
(1991): Wadworth AN+, *Drugs* 42, 1018

Vasculitis

Other

Dysgeusia (<1%)

Hypersensitivity
(1991): Wadworth AN+, *Drugs* 42, 1018

Myalgia (<1%)

Paresthesias (<1%)
(1992): Crome P+, *Am J Med* 92 (Suppl 4A), 126S

Tendon rupture (many reports)

Tongue pigmentation (<1%)

Tremor

Vaginal candidiasis

Vaginitis (<1%)

Xerostomia (<1%)
(1992): Mant TG, *Am J Med* 92, 26S

LOMUSTINE

Synonym: CCNU
Trade name: CeeNU (Bristol-Myers Squibb)
Other common trade names: *Belustine; CCNU; Cecenu; Lomeblastin; Lucostine; Lundbeck*
Indications: Brain tumors, lymphomas, melanoma
Category: Nitrosurea alkylating antineoplastic
Half-life: 16–72 hours
Clinically important, potentially serious interactions with: cimetidine, phenobarbital

Reactions

Skin

Acral erythema
(1989): Oksenhendler E+, *Eur J Cancer Clin Oncol* 25, 1181

Flushing
(1992): Breathnach SM+, *Adverse Drug Reactions and the Skin*, Blackwell, Oxford 290

Neutrophilic eccrine hidradenitis
(1996): Shear NH+, *J Am Acad Dermatol* 35, 819

Rash (sic) (1–10%)

Hair

Hair – alopecia (<1%)

Other

Stomatitis (1–10%)

LOPERAMIDE

Trade name: Imodium (McNeil)
Other common trade names: *Brek; Diar-Aid; Diarr-Eze; Diarstop-L; Imossel; Lop-Dia; Loperhoe; Maalox Anti-Diarrheal; Stopit; Vancotil*
Indications: Diarrhea
Category: Antidiarrheal
Half-life: 9–14 hours
Clinically important, potentially serious interactions with: CNS depressants, erythromycin, phenothiazines, tricyclic antidepressants

Reactions

Skin

Erythema nodosum

Exanthems

Pruritus

Rash (sic)

Urticaria

Hair

Hair – alopecia
(1993): Litt JZ, Beachwood, OH, personal case (observation)

Other

Gingivitis
(1990): DuPont HL+, *Am J Med* 88, 20S

Hypersensitivity

Oral mucosal lesions (1.1%)
(1990): DuPont HL+, *Am J Med* 88, 20S

Xerostomia
(1990): DuPont HL+, *Am J Med* 88, 20S

LORACARBEF

Trade name: Lorabid (Lilly)
Other common trade name: *Carbac*
Indications: Various infections caused by susceptible organisms
Category: Beta-lactam antibiotic (carbacephem)
Half-life: 60 minutes
Clinically important, potentially serious interactions with: aminoglycosides, anticoagulants, cimetidine, cyclosporine, furosemide, omeprazole, probenecid, ranitidine

Reactions

Skin

Candidiasis

Erythema multiforme (<1%)

Pruritus (<1%)

Rash (sic) (1.2%)

Stevens–Johnson syndrome (<1%)

Urticaria (<1%)

Other

Candidal vaginitis (1.3%)

Serum sickness (<1%)

LORATADINE

Trade names: Claritin (Schering); Claritin-D (Schering)
Other common trade names: *Civeran; Claratyne; Claritine; Lisino; Lorastine; Velodan; Zeos*
Indications: Allergic rhinitis, urticaria
Category: H_1-receptor antihistamine and antiasthmatic
Half-life: 3–20 hours
Clinically important, potentially serious interactions with: alcohol, amprenavir, azole antifungals, cimetidine, CNS depressants, erythromycin, ketoconazole, MAO inhibitors, nelfinavir, procarbazine, ritonavir, tricyclic antidepressants

Reactions

Skin
Angioedema (>2%)
(1989): Clissold SP+, *Drugs* 37, 42
Dermatitis (sic) (>2%)
Diaphoresis (>2%)
Erythema multiforme (>2%)
Exanthems
Flushing (>2%)
Peripheral edema (>2%)
Photosensitivity (>2%)
Pruritus (>2%)
(1989): Barenholtz HA+, *Drug Intell Clin Pharm* 23, 445
Purpura (>2%)
Rash (sic) (>2%)
Urticaria (>2%)
(1992): Boner AL+, *Allergy* 47, 98
(1989): Clissold SP+, *Drugs* 37, 42
Xerosis (>2%)

Hair
Hair – alopecia (>2%)
Hair – dry (sic) (>2%)

Other
Anaphylactoid reaction (>2%)
Dysgeusia (>2%)
Gynecomastia (>2%)
Hypesthesia (>2%)
Mastodynia (1–10%)
Myalgia (>2%)
Paresthesias (>2%)
Sialorrhea (>2%)
Stomatitis (>2%)
Vaginitis (>2%)
Xerostomia (>10%)
(1992): Olson OT+, *Arzneimittelforschung* (German) 42, 1227
(1992): Monroe EW+, *Arzneimittelforschung* (German) 42, 1119
(1990): Irander K+, *Allergy* 45, 86
(1990): Del Carpio J+, *J Allergy Clin Immunology* 84, 741
(1990): Simons FE, *Clin Exp Allergy* 20, 19
(1989): Barenholtz HA+, *Drug Intell Clin Pharm* 23, 445
(1989): Bruttman G+, *J Allergy Clin Immunology* 83, 411
(1988): Gutkowski A+, *J Allergy Clin Immunology* 81, 902

LORAZEPAM

Trade name: Ativan (Wyeth-Ayerst)
Other common trade names: *Apo-Lorazepam; Durazolam; Laubeel; Merlit; Nu-Loraz; Punktyl; Tavor; Temesta; Titus*
Indications: Anxiety, depression
Category: Benzodiazepine anxiolytic; anticonvulsant; antiemetic
Half-life: 10–20 hours
Clinically important, potentially serious interactions with: alcohol, CNS depressants, clarithromycin, digoxin, fluconazole, itraconazole, ketoconazole, levodopa, loxapine, MAO inhibitors, miconazole, morphine, theophylline, tricyclic antidepressants, verapamil

Reactions

Skin
Dermatitis (sic) (1–10%)
Diaphoresis (>10%)
Erythema multiforme
(1991): Porteous DM+, *Arch Dermatol* 127, 741
Exanthems
Fixed eruption
(1988): Jafferany M+, *Dermatologica* 177, 386
Pruritus
Purpura
Rash (sic) (>10%)
Stevens–Johnson syndrome
(1991): Porteous DM+, *Arch Dermatol* 127, 741
Urticaria

Hair
Hair – alopecia
Hair – hirsutism

Other
Gingival lichenoid reaction
(1986): Colvard MD+, *Periodont Case Rep* 8, 69
Injection-site pain (>10%)
(1981): Ameer B+, *Drugs* 21, 161 (7–52%)
Injection-site phlebitis (>10%)
(1981): Clarke RSJ, *Drugs* 22, 26 (15%)
Paresthesias
Pseudolymphoma
(1995): Magro CM+, *J Am Acad Dermatol* 32, 419
Sialopenia (>10%)
Sialorrhea (<1%)
(1978): Dodson ME+, *Br J Anaesth* 50, 1059
Tremor (1–10%)
Xerostomia (>10%)

LOSARTAN

Synonyms: DuP 753; MK 594
Trade names: Cozaar (Merck); Hyzaar (Merck)
Indications: Hypertension
Category: Angiotensin II receptor antagonist; antihypertensive
Half-life: 2 hours
Clinically important, potentially serious interactions with: cimetidine, fluconazole, ketoconazole, lithium, phenobarbital, rifampin

Hyzaar is losartan and hydrochlorothiazide

Reactions

Skin
Angioedema (<1%)
(1999): Rupprecht R+, *Allergy* 54, 81
(1999): Rivera JO, *Ann Pharmacother* 33, 933
(1998): van Rijnsoever EW+, *Arch Intern Med* 158, 2063
(1996): Boxer M, *J Allergy Clin Immunol* 98, 471
(1996): *Med Sci Bull* 18, 6
(1995): Acker CG+, *N Engl J Med* 333, 1572

Dermatitis (sic) (<1%)
Diaphoresis (<1%)
Ecchymoses (<1%)
Edema (<1%)
Erythema (<1%)
Exanthems
Facial edema (<1%)
Flushing (<1%)
(1995): Ahmad S, *JAMA* 274, 1266
Photosensitivity (<1%)
Pruritus (<1%)
Purpura
(1998): Bosch X, *Arch Intern Med* 158, 191
Rash (<1%)
Urticaria (<1%)
Xerosis (<1%)

Hair

Hair – alopecia (<1%)

Other

Ageusia
(1996): Schlienger RG+, *Lancet* 347, 471
Anaphylactoid reaction (<1%)
Aphthous stomatitis
(1998): Goffin E+, *Clin Nephrol* 50, 197
Dysgeusia (<1%)
(1998): Heeringa M+, *Ann Intern Med* 129, 72
Hypesthesia (<1%)
Myalgia (1%)
Paresthesias (<1%)
(1995): Ahmad S, *JAMA* 274, 1266
Pseudolymphoma
(1999): Goldstein E, Toronto, ON (from Internet) (observation)
(1997): Viraben R+, *Lancet* 350, 1366
Tremor (<1%)
Xerostomia (<1%)

LOVASTATIN

Trade name: Mevacor (Merck)
Other common trade names: *Apo-Lovastatin; Lovalip; Mevinacor; Mevinolin; Nergadan; Rovacor; Taucor*
Indications: Hypercholesterolemia
Category: Antihyperlipidemic; HMG-CoA reductase inhibitor
Half-life: 1–2 hours
Clinically important, potentially serious interactions with: anticoagulants, amprenavir, clarithromycin, clofibrate, cyclosporine, danazol, diltiazem, erythromycin, fluconazole, fluvoxamine, gemfibrozil, indinavir, isradipine, itraconazole, ketoconazole, levothyroxine, miconazole, nefazodone, nelfinavir, niacin, ritonavir, saquinavir, verapamil, warfarin

Reactions

Skin

Erythema
Erythema multiforme
Exanthems
(1988): Henwood JM+, *Drugs* 36, 429 (5%)
(1988): Tobert JA+, *Am J Cardiol* 62 (Suppl), 28J (0.3%)
(1987): Havel RJ+, *Ann Intern Med* 107, 609 (1%)
Lupus erythematosus
(1993): Ahmad S, *Heart Dis Stroke* 2, 262
(1991): Ahmad S, *Arch Intern Med* 151, 1667
Pruritus (5.2%)
(1988): Tobert JA+, *Am J Cardiol* 62 (Suppl), 28J
Purpura
(1999): Stein EA+, *JAMA* 281, 137
Rash (sic) (5.2%)
(1993): Merck Laboratories, *The Lovastatin Study Groups I through IV*, 153, 1079
(1993): Krasovec M+, *Dermatology* 186, 248
Stevens–Johnson syndrome
(1998): Downs JR+, *JAMA* 279, 1615
Toxic epidermal necrolysis
Urticaria
Vasculitis

Hair

Hair – alopecia (>1%)

Other

Dysgeusia (0.8%)
Gynecomastia (1–10%)
(1999): Stein EA+, *JAMA* 281, 137
Hypersensitivity
Hyposmia
(1992): Weber R+, *Laryngorhinootologie* (German) 71, 483
Myalgia (2.4%)
Myopathy (1–10%)
(1990): Kogan AD+, *Postgrad Med J* 66, 294
(1989): Vaher VMG+, *Lancet* 2, 1098
Paresthesias (>1%)
Stomatitis
Xerostomia (>1%)

LOXAPINE

Trade name: Loxitane (Watson)
Other common trade names: *Desconex; Loxapac*
Indications: Psychoses
Category: Tricyclic antipsychotic, anxiolytic and antidepressant
Half-life: 12–19 hours (terminal)
Clinically important, potentially serious interactions with: alcohol, benzodiazepines, bromocriptine, carbamazepine, CNS depressants, guanabenz, lorazepam, MAO inhibitors, propranolol, trazodone, tricyclic antidepressants, **cigarette smoking**

Reactions

Skin

Cutaneous side effects (sic)
Dermatitis (sic)
(1992): Breathnach SM+, *Adverse Drug Reactions and the Skin*, Blackwell, Oxford, 203 (passim)
Diaphoresis
Exanthems
Facial edema
Parkinsonism
Photosensitivity (<1%)
(1991): Anon, *Drug Ther Bull* 29, 41
Pigmentation (<1%)
Pruritus (<1%)
(1992): Breathnach SM+, *Adverse Drug Reactions and the Skin*, Blackwell, Oxford, 203 (passim)
Purpura
Rash (sic) (1–10%)
Seborrhea
(1992): Breathnach SM+, *Adverse Drug Reactions and the Skin*, Blackwell, Oxford, 203 (passim)
Urticaria

Hair

Hair – alopecia

Other

Galactorrhea (<1%)
Gynecomastia (1–10%)
Myopathy
(1984): Thase ME+, *J Clin Psychopharmacol* 4, 46
Paresthesias
Priapism (<1%)
Xerostomia (>10%)

MAPROTILINE

Trade name: Ludiomil (Novartis)
Other common trade names: *Delgian; Maprostad; Melodil; Mirpan; Nono-Maprotiline; Psymion; Retinyl*
Indications: Depression, anxiety
Category: Tetracyclic antidepressant
Half-life: 27–58 hours
Clinically important, potentially serious interactions with: alcohol, anticholinergics, benzodiazepines, CNS depressants, guanethidine, MAO inhibitors, phenothiazines, propranolol, sympathomimetics, thyroid

Reactions

Skin

Acne
(1988): Warnock JK+, *Am J Psychiatry* 145, 425
(1985): Oakley AM+, *Aust N Z J Med* 15, 256
(1982): Ponte CD, *Am J Psychiatry* 139, 141
Diaphoresis
(1977): Pinder RM+, *Drugs* 13, 321 (3–8%)
Edema
Erythema
Erythema multiforme
(1990): Zukervar P+, *J Toxicol Clin Exp* 10, 169
Exanthems (1–5%)
(1988): Warnock JK+, *Am J Psychiatry* 145, 425
(1977): Pinder RM+, *Drugs* 13, 321 (3–9%)
(1976): Johnson NM+, *Lancet* 2, 1357 (4%)
Flushing
Ichthyosis
(1991): Niederauer HH+, *Hautarzt* (German) 42, 455
Parkinsonism
Petechiae
Photosensitivity
(1989): KochP+, *Derm Beruf Umwelt* (German) 37, 203
(1988): Warnock JK+, *Am J Psychiatry* 145, 425
Pruritus
Purpura
(1988): Warnock JK+, *Am J Psychiatry* 145, 425
Rash (sic) (>10%)
Stevens–Johnson syndrome
(1990): Zukervar P+, *J Toxicol Clin Exp* 10, 169
Urticaria
(1988): Warnock JK+, *Am J Psychiatry* 145, 425
(1976): Johnson NM+, *Lancet* 2, 1357 (4%)
Vasculitis
(1985): Oakley AM+, *Aust N Z J Med* 15, 256

Hair

Hair – alopecia
(2000): Mercke Y+, *Ann Clin Psychiatry* 12, 35
(1991): Niederauer HH+, *Hautarzt* (German) 42, 455

Other

Black tongue
Dysgeusia
Galactorrhea
Gynecomastia (<1%)
Sialorrhea
Stomatitis
Tremor
Xerostomia (22%)
(1977): Pinder RM+, *Drugs* 13, 321 (30–40%)

MARIHUANA

Trade name: Marihuana (Marijuana)
Indications: Nausea and vomiting, substance abuse drug
Category: Hallucinogen
Half-life: no data
Clinically important, potentially serious interactions with: no data

Note: Marihuana is the popular name for the dried flowering leaves of the hemp plant, *Cannabis sativa*. It contains tetrahydrocannabinols. It is also known as "pot," "grass," "hashish," etc.

Reactions

Skin

Allergic reactions (sic)
(2000): Perez JA, *J Emerg Med* 18, 260
Exanthems
Pruritus
Urticaria

Other

Anaphylactoid reaction
(1971): Liskow B+, *Ann Intern Med* 75, 571

MAZINDOL

Trade names: Mazanor (Wyeth-Ayerst); Sanorex (Novartis)
Other common trade names: *Diestet; Liofindol; Solucaps; Teronac*
Indications: Obesity
Category: Anorexiant (appetite suppressant)
Half-life: 10 hours
Clinically important, potentially serious interactions with: barbiturates, guanethidine, MAO inhibitors, tricyclic antidepressants

Reactions

Skin

Diaphoresis
Edema
Exanthems
Rash (sic)
Urticaria

Other

Dysgeusia
Paresthesias
Xerostomia

MEBENDAZOLE

Trade name: Vermox (McNeil)
Other common trade names: *Amycil; Bantenol; Helminzole; Lomper; Mebensole; Mindol; Nemasol; Pantelmin; Revapole; Toloxim; Vermicol*
Indications: Parasitic worm infestations
Category: Anthelmintic
Half-life: 1–12 hours
Clinically important, potentially serious interactions with: carbamazepine, phenytoin

Reactions

Skin

Allergic reactions (sic)
(1979): Kern P+, *Tropenmed Parasitol* 30, 65 (2 in 7 patients)
Angioedema (<1%)
Exanthems
Pruritus (<1%)

Rash (sic) (<1%)
Stevens–Johnson syndrome
(2000): Ajonuma LC+, *Trop Doc* 30, 57
Urticaria

Hair

Hair – alopecia
(1992): Breathnach SM+, *Adverse Drug Reactions and the Skin*, Blackwell, Oxford, 177 (passim)

Other

Xerostomia

MECHLORETHAMINE

Synonyms: mustine, nitrogen mustard
Trade name: Mustargen (Merck)
Other common trade names: *Mustine; Mustine Hydrochloride Boots*
Indications: Hodgkin's disease, mycosis fungoides
Category: Antineoplastic
Half-life: <1 minute
Clinically important, potentially serious interactions with: aldesleukin, succinylcholine

Reactions

Skin

Acanthosis nigricans
(1988): Schweitzer WJ+, *J Am Acad Dermatol* 19, 951
Allergic dermatitis (sic)
(1999): Estève E+, *Arch Dermatol* 135, 1349
Angioedema
(1981): Wilson KS+, *Ann Intern Med* 94, 823
Bullous eruption
(1990): Goday JJ+, *Contact Dermatitis* 22, 306
(1981): Weiss RB+, *Ann Intern Med* 94, 66
Cellulitis
(1981): Wilson KS+, *Ann Intern Med* 94, 823
Contact dermatitis
(1991): Sheehan MP+, *J Pediatr* 119, 317
(1988): Ramsay DL+, *J Am Acad Dermatol* 19, 684
(1986): Mauduit G+, *Br J Dermatol* 115, 82
(1985): Arrazola JM+, *Int J Dermatol* 24, 608
(1985): Zachariae H, *Int J Clin Pharmacol Res* 5, 193
(1984): Ramsay DL+, *Arch Dermatol* 120, 1585
(1984): Vonderheid EC, *Int J Dermatol* 23, 180
(1983): Bronner AK+, *J Am Acad Dermatol* 9, 645
(1983): Nusbaum BP+, *Arch Dermatol* 119, 117
(1983): Price NM+, *Cancer* 52, 2214
(1982): Price NM+, *Arch Dermatol* 118, 234
(1981): Shelley WB, *Acta Derm Venereol* 61, 161
(1981): Halprin KM+, *Br J Dermatol* 105, 71
(1979): Handler RM+, *Int J Dermatol* 18, 758
(1978): Volden G+, *BMJ* 2, 865
(1978): du Vivier A+, *BMJ* 2, 1300
(1977): Sanchez-Yus E+, *Actas Dermosifiliogr* (Spanish) 68, 39
(1977): Volden G+, *Tidsskr Nor Laegeforen* (Norwegian) 97, 1671
(1977): Price NM+, *Br J Dermatol* 97, 547
(1976): Pariser DM+, *Arch Dermatol* 112, 1113
(1976): Grunnet E, *Br J Dermatol* 94, 101
(1975): Mitchell JC+, *Contact Dermatitis* 1, 363
(1975): Constantine VS+, *Arch Dermatol* 111, 484
(1971): Mandy S+, *Arch Dermatol* 103, 272
(1970): Van Scott EJ+, *Arch Dermatol* 102, 507
Epidermal cysts
(1991): Smith SP+, *J Am Acad Dermatol* 25, 940
Erythema multiforme (<1%)
(1967): Brauer MJ+, *Arch Intern Med* 120, 499
Exanthems (<1%)
Fungal infection (sic)
(1981): Shelley WB, *Acta Derm Venereol* 61, 164
Herpes zoster (>10%)
Hyperpigmentation
(1984): Vonderheid EC, *Int J Dermatol* 23, 180
(1983): Bronner AK+, *J Am Acad Dermatol* 9, 645
(1982): Price NM+, *Arch Dermatol* 118, 234
(1977): Price NM, *Arch Dermatol* 113, 1387
(1975): O'Doherty CS, *Lancet* 2, 365
(1973): Flaxman BA+, *J Invest Dermatol* 60, 321
(1970): Van Scott EJ+, *Arch Dermatol* 102, 507
(1970): Epstein E Jr+, *Arch Dermatol* 102, 504
Pruritus
(1981): Wilson KS+, *Ann Intern Med* 94, 823
(1981): Weiss RB+, *Ann Intern Med* 94, 66
Purpura
(1981): Weiss RB+, *Ann Intern Med* 94, 66
Rash (sic) (<1%)
Squamous cell carcinoma
(1991): Smith SP+, *J Am Acad Dermatol* 25, 940
(1982): Lee LA+, *J Am Acad Dermatol* 7, 590
(1978): du Vivier A+, *Br J Dermatol* 99, 61
Stevens–Johnson syndrome
(1997): Newman JM+, *J Am Acad Dermatol* 36, 112
Urticaria
(1981): Wilson KS+, *Ann Intern Med* 94, 823
(1981): Weiss RB+, *Ann Intern Med* 94, 66
(1973): Daughters D+, *Arch Dermatol* 107, 429
Xerosis
(1984): Vonderheid EC, *Int J Dermatol* 23, 180

Hair

Hair – alopecia (1–10%)

Other

Anaphylactoid reaction (1–10%)
(1983): Bronner AK+, *J Am Acad Dermatol* 9, 645
(1977): Sanchez-Yus E+, *Actas Dermosifiliogr* (Spanish) 68, 39
(1976): Grunnet E, *Br J Dermatol* 94, 101
(1973): Daughters D+, *Arch Dermatol* 107, 429
Dysgeusia (1–10%) (metallic taste)
Hypersensitivity (1–10%)
(1972): Zackheim HS+, *Arch Dermatol* 105, 702
Injection-site extravasation (1–10%)
Injection-site thrombophlebitis (1–10%)
(1989): Kerker BJ+, *Semin Dermatol* 8, 173
(1981): Wilson KS+, *Ann Intern Med* 94, 823

MECLIZINE

Trade name: Antivert (Pfizer)
Other common trade names: *Antrizine; Bonamine; Bonine; Dizmiss; Dramamine II; Dramine; Meni-D; Nico-Vert; Peremesin; Postadoxin; Postafen; Suprimal; Vergon*
Indications: Motion sickness
Category: Antiemetic and antivertigo; antihistamine H_1 blocker
Half-life: 6 hours
Clinically important, potentially serious interactions with: alcohol, anticholinergics, CNS depressants, neuroleptics

Reactions

Skin

Angioedema (<1%)
Exanthems
Photosensitivity (<1%)
Rash (sic) (<1%)
Urticaria

Other

Myalgia (<1%)
Paresthesias (<1%)
Tremor
Xerostomia (1–10%)

MECLOFENAMATE

Trade name: Meclofenamate
Other common trade names: *Kyroxan; Melvon; Movens*
Indications: Arthritis
Category: Nonsteroidal anti-inflammatory (NSAID)
Half-life: 2 hours
Clinically important, potentially serious interactions with: aminoglycosides, anticoagulants, cyclosporine, lithium, methotrexate, salicylates, warfarin

Reactions

Skin

Angioedema (<1%)
(1984): Stern RS+, *JAMA* 252, 1433
Bullous eruption
Edema (>1%)
Erythema multiforme (<1%)
(1985): Bigby M+, *J Am Acad Dermatol* 12, 866
(1984): Stern RS+, *JAMA* 252, 1433
(1983): Harrington T, *J Rheumatol* 10, 169
Erythema nodosum (<1%)
Erythroderma
(1985): Bigby M+, *J Am Acad Dermatol* 12, 866
Exanthems (1–5%)
(1992): Breathnach SM+, *Adverse Drug Reactions and the Skin*, Blackwell, Oxford, 190 (passim)
(1985): Bigby M+, *J Am Acad Dermatol* 12, 866 (3–9%)
(1984): Stern RS+, *JAMA* 252, 1433
(1978): Dresner AJ, *Curr Ther Res* 23, 107
Exfoliative dermatitis (<1%)
(1992): Breathnach SM+, *Adverse Drug Reactions and the Skin*, Blackwell, Oxford, 190 (passim)
(1984): Stern RS+, *JAMA* 252, 1433
Fixed eruption (<1%)
(1992): Breathnach SM+, *Adverse Drug Reactions and the Skin*, Blackwell, Oxford, 190 (passim)
(1985): Bigby M+, *J Am Acad Dermatol* 12, 866
(1984): Stern RS+, *JAMA* 252, 1433
Hot flashes (<1%)
Lupus erythematosus
Peripheral edema
Photosensitivity
(1985): Bigby M+, *J Am Acad Dermatol* 12, 866
(1984): Stern RS+, *JAMA* 252, 1433
Pruritus (1–10%)
(1992): Breathnach SM+, *Adverse Drug Reactions and the Skin*, Blackwell, Oxford, 190 (passim)
(1985): Bigby M+, *J Am Acad Dermatol* 12, 866
(1984): Stern RS+, *JAMA* 252, 1433
Psoriasis (exacerbation)
(1983): Meyerhoff JO, *N Engl J Med* 309, 496
Purpura (>1%)
(1992): Breathnach SM+, *Adverse Drug Reactions and the Skin*, Blackwell, Oxford, 190 (passim)
(1985): Bigby M+, *J Am Acad Dermatol* 12, 866
(1984): Stern RS+, *JAMA* 252, 1433
(1981): Rodriguez J, *Drug Intell Clin Pharm* 15, 999
Rash (sic) (3–9%)
(1984): Stern RS+, *JAMA* 252, 1433
Stevens–Johnson syndrome (<1%)
Toxic epidermal necrolysis (<1%)
Urticaria (>1%)
(1985): Bigby M+, *J Am Acad Dermatol* 12, 866
(1984): Stern RS+, *JAMA* 252, 1433
Vasculitis
(1992): Breathnach SM+, *Adverse Drug Reactions and the Skin*, Blackwell, Oxford, 190 (passim)
(1985): Bigby M+, *J Am Acad Dermatol* 12, 866
(1984): Stern RS+, *JAMA* 252, 1433
Vesiculobullous eruption
(1992): Breathnach SM+, *Adverse Drug Reactions and the Skin*, Blackwell, Oxford, 190 (passim)
(1984): Stern RS+, *JAMA* 252, 1433

Hair

Hair – alopecia (<1%)

Other

Aphthous stomatitis
(1996): Fetterman M, Hialeah, FL (from Internet) (observation)
Dysgeusia (<1%)
Hypersensitivity
(1993): Fernandez-Rivas M+, *Ann Allergy* 71, 515
Oral ulceration
Paresthesias (<1%)
Porphyria
Serum sickness
Stomatitis (1–3%)
Xerostomia

MEDROXYPROGESTERONE

Trade names: Amen (Carnrick); Curretab (Solvay); Cycrin (ESI Lederle); Depo-Provera (Pharmacia & Upjohn); Premphase (Wyeth-Ayerst); Prempro (Wyeth-Ayerst); Provera (Pharmacia & Upjohn)
Other common trade names: *Alti-MPA; Aragest 5; Clinofem; Curretab; Gestapuran;Novo-Medrone; Perlutex; Progevera; Ralovera*
Indications: Secondary amenorrhea, renal or endometrial carcinoma
Category: Progestin; contraceptive; antineoplastic
Half-life: 30 days
Clinically important, potentially serious interactions with: aminoglutethimide, bromocriptine, phenytoin, rifampin

Reactions

Skin

Acne (1–5%)
(1974): Pochi PE, *Arch Dermatol* 109, 556
Allergic reactions (sic) (<1%)
Angioedema
Ankle edema
Chloasma (1–10%)
Diaphoresis (<1%)
(1990): Willemse PHB+, *Eur J Cancer* 26, 337 (31%)
Edema (>10%)
Erythema nodosum
(1974): Berant N, *Harefuah* (Hebrew) 87, 19
Exanthems
Flushing
(1990): Willemse PHB+, *Eur J Cancer* 26, 337 (12%)
Hemorrhagic eruption (sic)
Hot flashes
Melasma (1–10%)
Mucha–Habermann disease
(1973): Hollander A+, *Arch Dermatol* 107, 465
Photosensitivity
Pigmented purpuric eruption
(2000): Tsao H+, *J Am Acad Dermatol* 43, 308
Pruritus (1–10%)
Rash (sic) (1–5%)
Scleroderma (<1%)
Striae
(2000): Gupta M, *Br J Fam Plann* 26, 104
Urticaria
Xerosis (<1%)

Hair

Hair – alopecia (1–5%)
Hair – hirsutism (<1%)
(1984): Delanoe D+, *Lancet* 1, 276

Other

Anaphylactoid reaction (<1%)
Bromhidrosis (<1%)
Galactorrhea (<1%)
(1998): Cromwell P+, *J Adolesc Health* 23, 61

Gynecomastia (< 1%)
Injection-site pain (> 10%)
Mastodynia (1–5%)
Paresthesias (< 1%)
Thrombophlebitis (1–10%)
Vaginitis (1–5%)

MEFENAMIC ACID

Trade name: Ponstel (Parke-Davis)
Other common trade names: *Dysman; Lysalgo; Mefac; Mefic; Parkemed; Ponstan; Ponstyl*
Indications: Pain, dysmenorrhea
Category: Nonsteroidal anti-inflammatory (NSAID)
Half-life: 3.5 hours
Clinically important, potentially serious interactions with: aminoglycosides, anticoagulants, cyclosporine, lithium, methotrexate, salicylates

Reactions

Skin

Angioedema (< 1%)
Bullous pemphigoid
(1986): Shepherd AN+, *Postgrad Med J* 62, 67
Diaphoresis
Edema
Erythema multiforme (< 1%)
(1990): Sowden JM+, *Clin Exp Dermatol* 15, 387
(1985): Ting HC+, *Int J Dermatol* 24, 587
Exanthems
(1992): Breathnach SM+, *Adverse Drug Reactions and the Skin*, Blackwell, Oxford, 190 (passim)
Exfoliative dermatitis
(1992): Breathnach SM+, *Adverse Drug Reactions and the Skin*, Blackwell, Oxford, 190 (passim)
Facial edema
Fixed eruption
(1992): Long CC+, *Br J Dermatol* 126, 409
(1991): Mohamed KN, *Aust N Z J Med* 21, 291
(1990): Sowden JM+, *Clin Exp Dermatol* 15, 387
(1986): Watson A+, *Australas J Dermatol* 27, 6
(1986): Wilson CL+, *BMJ* 293, 1243
Hot flashes (< 1%)
Photosensitivity
(1997): O'Reilly FM+, American Academy of Dermatology Meeting, Poster #14
Pruritus (1–10%)
Purpura
Rash (sic) (> 10%)
Stevens–Johnson syndrome (< 1%)
(1991): Chan JC+, *Drug Safety* 6, 230
Toxic epidermal necrolysis (< 1%)
(1991): Sakellariou G+, *Int J Artif Organs* 14, 634
(1990): Black AK+, *Br J Dermatol* 123, 277 (observation)
Urticaria (< 1%)
(1992): Breathnach SM+, *Adverse Drug Reactions and the Skin*, Blackwell, Oxford, 190 (passim)
Vasculitis
(1980): Malik S+, *Lancet* 2, 746

Other

Anaphylactoid reaction
(1985): O'Brien WM+, *J Rheumatol* 12, 13
Glossitis
Oral ulceration
Pseudoporphyria
(1998): O'Hagan AH+, *Br J Dermatol* 139, 1131
Sialorrhea
Xerostomia

MEFLOQUINE

Trade name: Lariam (Roche)
Other common trade names: *Laricam; Mephaquin; Mephaquine*
Indications: Malaria
Category: Antimalarial
Half-life: 21–22 days
Clinically important, potentially serious interactions with: beta-blockers, chloroquine, quinidine, quinine, valproic acid

Reactions

Skin

Erythema
(1992): Breathnach SM+, *Adverse Drug Reactions and the Skin*, Blackwell, Oxford 176 (passim)
Erythema multiforme
Exanthems
(1999): Smith HR+, *Clin Exp Dermatol* 24, 249 (30%)
Exfoliative dermatitis
(1993): Martin GJ+, *Clin Infect Dis* 16, 341
Facial dermatitis
(1991): Shlim DR, *JAMA* 266, 2560
Pruritus
(1999): Smith HR+, *Clin Exp Dermatol* 24, 249 (4–10%)
(1989): Sowunmi A+, *Lancet* 2, 313; 397
Psoriasis
(1998): Potasman I+, *J Travel Med* 5, 156
Rash (sic) (1–10%)
Stevens–Johnson syndrome
(1999): Smith HR+, *Clin Exp Dermatol* 24, 249
(1991): Van den Enden E+, *Lancet* 337, 683
Toxic epidermal necrolysis
(1999): Smith HR+, *Clin Exp Dermatol* 24, 249 (fatal)
(1997): McBride SR+, *Lancet* 349, 101
Urticaria
(1999): Smith HR+, *Clin Exp Dermatol* 24, 249
Vasculitis
(1999): Smith HR+, *Clin Exp Dermatol* 24, 249
(1995): White AC+, *Ann Intern Med* 123, 894
(1993): Scerri L+, *Int J Dermatol* 32, 517

Hair

Hair – alopecia (< 1%)

Other

Myalgia (1–10%)

MELOXICAM

Trade name: Mobic (Boehringer Ingelheim)
Indications: Osteoarthritis
Category: Nonsteroidal anti-inflammatory (NSAID)
Half-life: 15–20 hours
Clinically important, potentially serious interactions with: alcohol, anticoagulants, antiplatelet drugs, aspirin, corticosteroids, hydralazine, lithium, thiazide diuretics

Reactions

Skin

Allergic reactions (sic) (<2%)
Angioedema (<2%)
(2000): Quaratino D+, *Ann Allergy Asthma Immunol* 84, 613
Bullous eruption (<2%)
Erythema multiforme (<2%)
(1999): Nikas SN+, *Am J Med* 107, 532
Exanthems (<2%)
(2000): Quaratino D+, *Ann Allergy Asthma Immunol* 84, 613
Edema (2–5%)

Facial edema
(2000): Quaratino D+, *Ann Allergy Asthma Immunol* 84, 613
Hot flashes (<2%)
Photosensitivity (<2%)
Pruritus (<2%)
Purpura (<2%)
Rash (sic) (1–3%)
Skin disorders (sic)
(1996): Huskisson EC+, *Br J Rheumatol* 35, 29 (18%)
Stevens–Johnson syndrome (<2%)
Toxic epidermal necrolysis (<2%)
Urticaria (<2%)
(2000): Quaratino D+, *Ann Allergy Asthma Immunol* 84, 613
Vasculitis (<2%)

Other

Anaphylactoid reaction (<2%)
Dysgeusia (<2%)
Paresthesias (<2%)
Tremor (<2%)
Ulcerative stomatitis (<2%)
Xerostomia (<2%)

MELPHALAN

Trade name: Alkeran (GlaxoWellcome)
Indications: Multiple myeloma, carcinomas
Category: Antineoplastic; nitrogen mustard
Half-life: 90 minutes
Clinically important, potentially serious interactions with: cyclosporine

Reactions

Skin

Angioedema
(1983): Bronner AK+, *J Am Acad Dermatol* 9, 645
(1981): Weiss RB+, *Ann Intern Med* 94, 66
Eccrine squamous syringometaplasia
(1997): Valks R+, *Arch Dermatol* 133, 873
Edema
Exanthems
(1981): Weiss RB+, *Ann Intern Med* 94, 66
(1981): Harvey HA+, *Ann Intern Med* 94, 542
(1978): Levine N+, *Cancer Treat Rev* 5, 67
(1969): Hoogstraten B+, *JAMA* 209, 251 (4%)
Petechiae
Pruritus (1–10%)
(1983): Bronner AK+, *J Am Acad Dermatol* 9, 645
Purpura
Rash (sic) (1–10%)
Urticaria
(1983): Bronner AK+, *J Am Acad Dermatol* 9, 645
(1981): Harvey HA+, *Ann Intern Med* 94, 542
(1981): Weiss RB+, *Ann Intern Med* 94, 66
Vasculitis (1–10%)
(1986): Hannedouche T+, *Ann Med Intern Paris* (French) 137, 57
Vesiculation (1–10%)

Hair

Hair – alopecia (1–10%)
(1992): Zaun H+, *Hautarzt* (German) 43, 215
(1978): Levine N+, *Cancer Treat Rev* 5, 67

Nails

Nails – Beau's lines (transverse nail bands)
(1992): Zaun H+, *Hautarzt* (German) 43, 215
(1983): James WD+, *Arch Dermatol* 119, 334
(1982): Jeanmougin M+, *Ann Dermatol Venereol* (French) 109, 169
(1977): Malacarne P+, *Arch Dermatol Res* 25, 81

Other

Anaphylactoid reaction
(1983): Bronner AK+, *J Am Acad Dermatol* 9, 645
(1982): Dunagin WG, *Semin Oncol* 9, 14
Hypersensitivity (1–10%)
(1992): Weiss RB, *Semin Oncol* 19, 458
Perfusion-edema
(1995): Vrouenraets BC+, *Melanoma Res* 5, 425
Perfusion-erythema
(1995): Vrouenraets BC+, *Melanoma Res* 5, 425
Oral mucosal lesions
Oral ulceration
Scleroderma (localized)
(1998): Landau M+, *J Am Acad Dermatol* 39, 1011 (2 cases)
Stomatitis (1–10%)

MEPACRINE

(See QUINACRINE)

MEPERIDINE

Trade names: Demerol (Sanofi); Mepergan (Wyeth-Ayerst)
Other common trade names: *Dolantin; Dolestine; Dolosal; Opistan; Pethidine; Petidin*
Indications: Pain
Category: Narcotic agonist analgesic
Half-life: 3–4 hours
Clinically important, potentially serious interactions with: acyclovir, alcohol, cimetidine, CNS depressants, fluoxetine, furazolidone, isocarboxazid, isoniazid, MAO inhibitors, phenelzine, phenothiazines, phenytoin, ranitidine, ritonavir, selegiline, tranylcypromine, tricyclic antidepressants

Reactions

Skin

Angioedema
(1960): Schoenfeld MR, *N Y State J Med* 60, 2591
Diaphoresis
Flushing
Herpes (sic)
(1986): Acalovschi I, *Anaesthesia* 41, 1271
Necrotizing angiitis
(1971): Halpern M+, *Am J Roentgenol Radium Ther Nucl Med* 111, 663
Pruritus
(1993): Riley RH, *Anaesth Intensive Care* 21, 474
(1984): Saissy JM, *Ann Fr Anesth Reanim* (French) 3, 402
(1960): Schoenfeld MR, *N Y State J Med* 60, 2591
Rash (sic) (<1%)
Toxic epidermal necrolysis
(1967): Caldwell IW+, *Br J Dermatol* 79, 287
Urticaria (<1%)
(2000): Anibarro B+, *Allergy* 55, 305

Other

Cold microabscesses
(1978): Waisbren BA, *JAMA* 239, 1395
Embolia cutis medicamentosa (Nicolau syndrome)
(1995): Faucher L+, *Pediatr Dermatol* 12, 187
Injection-site erythema
(1993): Kundrotas L+, *Gastrointest Endosc* 39, 109
(1960): Schoenfeld MR, *N Y State J Med* 60, 2591
Injection-site pain (1–10%)
Injection-site scarring
(1994): Danielsen AG+, *Ugeskr Laeger* (Danish) 156, 162
Injection-site ulceration
(1994): Danielsen AG+, *Ugeskr Laeger* (Danish) 156, 162
Myopathy
(1968): Aberfeld DC+, *Arch Neurol* 19, 384
Tremor
Xerostomia (1–10%)

MEPHENYTOIN

Trade name: Mesantoin (Novartis)
Other common trade names: *Epilan-Gerot; Epilanex*
Indications: Partial seizures
Category: Hydantoin anticonvulsant
Half-life: 7 hours (for the active metabolite: 95–144 hours)
Clinically important, potentially serious interactions with: chloramphenicol, cyclosporine, disulfiram, dopamine, fluconazole, isoniazid, itraconazole

Reactions

Skin

Acne
(1951): Frankel AZ+, *Ohio State Med J* 47, 1013
Angioedema
(1951): Frankel AZ+, *Ohio State Med J* 47, 1013
Bullous eruption
(1948): Ruskin DB, *JAMA* 137, 1031
Cutaneous side effects (sic)
(1951): Frankel AZ+, *Ohio State Med J* 47, 1013 (10%)
Dermatomyositis
(1977): Zangemeister WH+, *Fortschr Neurol Psychiatr Grenzgeb* (German) 45, 501
Edema
Erythema multiforme
(1979): Pollack MA+, *Ann Neurol* 5, 262
(1951): Frankel AZ+, *Ohio State Med J* 47, 1013
(1951): Lindermayr W, *Hautarzt* (German) 2, 313
Exanthems
(1972): Levantine A+, *Br J Dermatol* 87, 646 (8–10%)
(1954): Dreyer R, *Dtsch Med Wochenschr* (German) 79, 1215
(1952): McArthur P, *Lancet* 1, 592 (5%)
(1951): Frankel AZ+, *Ohio State Med J* 47, 1013 (8.85%)
(1951): Lindermayr W, *Hautarzt* (German) 2, 313
Exfoliative dermatitis
(1951): Frankel AZ+, *Ohio State Med J* 47, 1013
Lupus erythematosus
(1989): Vivino FB+, *Arthritis Rheum* 32, 560
(1977): Zangemeister WH+, *Fortschr Neurol Psychiatr Grenzgeb* (German) 45, 501
(1976): Singsen BH+, *Pediatrics* 57, 529
(1968): Cochran M+, *Proc R Soc Med* 61, 656
(1967): Losada M+, *Rev Med Chil* (Spanish) 95, 380 (generalized)
(1965): Schütz E+, *Med Klin* (German) 60, 537
(1963): Jacobs JC, *Pediatrics* 32, 257
(1957): Lindquist T, *Acta Med Scand* 158, 131
(1957): Ruppli H+, *Schweiz Med Wochenschr* (German) 88, 1555
(1955): Capalbo EE+, *Rev Soc Argent Hemat* (Spanish) 5, 19
Pigmentation
(1964): Krebs A, *Schweiz Med Wochenschr* (German) 94, 748
(1964): Kuske H+, *Dermatologica* 129, 121
(1951): Hunter H+, *JAMA* 147, 744
(1954): Dreyer R, *Dtsch Med Wochenschr* (German) 79, 1215 (addison-like)
Pruritus
(1954): Dreyer R, *Dtsch Med Wochenschr* (German) 79, 1215
Purpura
(1955): Capalbo EE+, *Rev Soc Argent Hemat* (Spanish) 5, 19
Scleroderma
(1990): May DG+, *Clin Pharmacol Ther* 28, 286
Stevens–Johnson syndrome
(1951): Frankel AZ+, *Ohio State Med J* 47, 1013
Toxic epidermal necrolysis
(1979): Pollack MA+, *Ann Neurol* 5, 262
(1976): Babala J+, *Acta Paediatr Acad Sci Hung* 17, 9
(1976): Nozickova M+, *Cesk Dermatol* (Czech) 51, 375
(1962): Walker J, *Med Proc* 8, 208
Urticaria
(1972): Levantine A+, *Br J Dermatol* 87, 646
(1951): Frankel AZ+, *Ohio State Med J* 47, 1013
(1951): Lindermayr W, *Hautarzt* (German) 2, 313

Hair

Hair – alopecia

Other

Gingival hyperplasia
Oral mucosal eruption
(1954): Dreyer R, *Dtsch Med Wochenschr* (German) 79, 1215
Polyarteritis nodosa
(1951): Frankel AZ+, *Ohio State Med J* 47, 1013
Stomatitis
(1996): Meloni G+, *Lancet* 347, 1691

MEPHOBARBITAL

Trade name: Mebaral (Sanofi)
Other common trade name: *Prominal*
Indications: Epilepsy, anxiety
Category: Long-acting barbiturate; anticonvulsant, sedative
Half-life: 34 hours
Clinically important, potentially serious interactions with: benzodiazepines, chloramphenicol, CNS depressants, methylphenidate, phenobarbital, propoxyphene, valproic acid

Reactions

Skin

Angioedema (<1%)
Exanthems
Exfoliative dermatitis (<1%)
Purpura
Rash (sic) (<1%)
Stevens–Johnson syndrome (<1%)
Urticaria

Other

Serum sickness
Thrombophlebitis (<1%)

MEPROBAMATE

Trade names: Equanil (Wyeth-Ayerst); Miltown (Wallace)
Other common trade names: *Harmonin; Meditran; Meditrara; Meprate; Meprospan; Miltaun; Neuramate; Praol; Probamyl; Urbilat; Visanon*
Indications: Anxiety; insomnia
Category: Anxiolytic
Half-life: 10 hours
Clinically important, potentially serious interactions with: alcohol, CNS depressants, MAO inhibitors, tricyclic antidepressants

Reactions

Skin

Allergic reactions (sic)
(1955): Selling LS, *JAMA* 157, 1594 (1.1%)
Angioedema (<1%)
(1964): Welsh AL, *Med Clin North Am* 48, 459
(1958): Hollister LE, *Ann Intern Med* 49, 17
(1957): Bernstein C+, *JAMA* 163, 930
(1955): Selling LS, *JAMA* 157, 1594
Bullous eruption (<1%)
(1977): Varma AJ+, *Arch Intern Med* 137, 1208 (passim)
(1974): Tay C, *Asian J Med* 10, 223
Cutaneous side effects (sic)
(1972): Kauppinen K, *Acta Derm Venereol* (Stockh) 52 (Suppl), 68 (2%)
(1968): Montgomery DC+, *Can Med Assoc J* 99, 712 (2%)
Dermatitis (sic) (<1%)
Ecchymoses
Eczematous eruption (sic)
(1981): Edwards JG, *Drugs* 22, 495 (passim)

Erythema multiforme (<1%)
(1972): Kauppinen K, *Acta Derm Venereol* (Stockh) 52, 68
(1959): Wright W, *JAMA* 171, 1642
Erythema nodosum (<1%)
Exanthems
(1981): Edwards JG, *Drugs* 22, 495 (passim)
(1972): Kauppinen K, *Acta Derm Venereol* (Stockh) 52 (Suppl), 68
(1969): Savin JA, *Proc R Soc Med* 62, 349
(1967): Lockey SD, *Med Sci* 18, 43
(1966): Smith JW+, *Ann Intern Med* 65, 629 (2%)
(1965): Fellner MJ+, *Med Clin North Am* 49, 709
(1964): Welsh AL, *Med Clin North Am* 48, 459
(1959): Wright W, *JAMA* 171, 1642
(1958): Marcussen PV, *Acta Derm Venereol* (Stockh) 38, 398
(1957): Falk MS, *Arch Dermatol* 75, 437
(1956): Friedman HT+, *JAMA* 162, 628
Exfoliative dermatitis
Fixed eruption (<1%)
(1985): Kauppinen K+, *Br J Dermatol* 112, 575
(1984): Boyle J+, *BMJ* 289, 802
(1981): Edwards JG, *Drugs* 22, 495 (passim)
(1972): Kauppinen K, *Acta Derm Venereol* (Stockh) 52 (Suppl), 68
(1965): Gore HC+, *Arch Dermatol* 91, 627
Lupus erythematosus
(1957): Bernstein C+, *JAMA* 163, 930
Pemphigus
(1980): Godard W+, *Ann Dermatol Venereol* (French) 107, 1213
Pemphigus foliaceus
(1980): Godard W+, *Ann Dermatol Venereol* (French) 107, 1213
Peripheral edema (<1%)
Petechiae
(1956): Carmel WJ+, *N Engl J Med* 255, 770
Photosensitivity
(1957): Bernstein C+, *JAMA* 163, 930
Pityriasis rosea
(1959): Wright W, *JAMA* 171, 1642
Pruritus (<1%)
(1970): Savin JA, *Br J Dermatol* 83, 546
(1969): Savin JA, *Proc R Soc Med* 62, 349
(1964): Welsh AL, *Med Clin North Am* 48, 459
(1957): Falk MS, *Arch Dermatol* 75, 437
(1956): Friedman HT+, *JAMA* 162, 628
(1956): Carmel WJ+, *N Engl J Med* 255, 770
Purpura (<1%)
(1993): Pang BK+, *Ann Acad Med Singapore* 22, 870
(1985): Ambriz-Fernandez R+, *Rev Invest Clin* (Spanish) 37, 347
(1981): Edwards JG, *Drugs* 22, 495 (passim)
(1970): Savin JA, *Br J Dermatol* 83, 546
(1969): Savin JA, *Proc R Soc Med* 62, 349
(1969): Peterkin GAG+, *Practitioner* 202, 117
(1967): Lockey SD, *Med Sci* 18, 43
(1967): Peterson WC+, *Arch Dermatol* 95, 40
(1957): Bernstein C+, *JAMA* 163, 930
(1957): Falk MS, *Arch Dermatol* 75, 437
(1957): Levan NE, *Arch Dermatol* 75, 437
(1956): Friedman HT+, *JAMA* 162, 628
(1956): Carmel WJ Jr+, *N Engl J Med* 255, 770
Rash (sic) (1–10%)
Stevens–Johnson syndrome (<1%)
(1972): Kauppinen K, *Acta Derm Venereol* (Stockh) 52 (Suppl), 68
(1959): Wright W, *JAMA* 171, 1642
Toxic epidermal necrolysis (<1%)
(1969): Sander-Jensen K, *Tidsskr Nor Laegeforen* (Norwegian) 89, 398
Toxic erythema
(1974): Felix RH+, *Lancet* 1, 1017
Urticaria
(1981): Edwards JG, *Drugs* 22, 495 (passim)
(1972): Kauppinen K, *Acta Derm Venereol* (Stockh) 52 (Suppl), 68
(1967): Lockey SD, *Med Sci* 18, 43
(1966): Smith JW+, *Ann Intern Med* 65, 629 (2%)
(1964): Welsh AL, *Med Clin North Am* 48, 459
(1959): Wright W, *JAMA* 171, 1642
(1958): Hollister LE, *Ann Intern Med* 49, 17
(1957): Bernstein C+, *JAMA* 163, 930
(1956): Friedman HT+, *JAMA* 162, 628
(1955): Selling LS, *JAMA* 157, 1594
Vasculitis
(1964): Welsh AL, *Med Clin North Am* 48, 459
(1962): Schwank R, *Cesk Dermatol* 37, 6
(1959): Wright W, *JAMA* 171, 1642
(1958): von Marcussen P, *Acta Derm Venereol* (Stockh) 38 398
(1957): Falk MS, *Arch Dermatol* 75, 437
(1957): Bernstein C+, *JAMA* 163, 930
(1957): Levan NE, *Arch Dermatol* 75, 437
(1956): Carmel WJ+, *N Engl J Med* 255, 770

Other

Acute intermittent porphyria
(1967): de Matteis F, *Pharmacol Rev* 19, 523
Anaphylactoid reaction
(1974): Felix RH+, *Lancet* 1, 1017
Gynecomastia
Hypersensitivity
Oral mucosal eruption
(1959): Wright W, *JAMA* 171, 1642
Oral ulceration
Paresthesias
Polyarteritis nodosa
(1962): Schwank R, *Cesk Dermatol* 37, 6
Porphyria
(1984): Magnus IA, *BMJ* 288, 1474
Stomatitis (<1%)
(1959): Brachfeld J+, *JAMA* 169, 1321
Xerostomia

MERCAPTOPURINE

Synonyms: 6-mercaptopurine; 6-MP
Trade name: Purinethol (GlaxoWellcome)
Other common trade names: *Classen; Ismipur; Leukerin; Puri-Nethol*
Indications: Leukemias
Category: Antineoplastic; antimetabolite; immunosuppressant
Half-life: triphasic: 45 minutes; 2.5 hours; 10 hours
Clinically important, potentially serious interactions with: allopurinol, anticoagulants, doxorubicin, methotrexate

Reactions

Skin

Acral erythema
(1991): Baack BR+, *J Am Acad Dermatol* 24, 457
Dermatitis (sic)
(1968): Moore GE+, *Cancer Chemother Abstr* 52, 655 (2%)
Edema
Exanthems
(1989): Present DH+, *Ann Intern Med* 111, 641 (0.5%)
Herpes zoster
(1999): Korelitz BI+, *Am J Gastroenterology* 94, 424
Lichenoid eruption
(1973): Beylot C+, *Bull Soc Fr Dermatol Syphiligr* (French) 80, 190
Lupus erythematosus
(1966): Lee SL+, *Arch Intern Med* 117, 620
Palmar-plantar erythema
(1986): Cox GJ+, *Arch Dermatol* 122, 1413
Pellagra
(1987): Schmutz JL+, *Ann Dermatol Venereol* (French) 114, 569
(1960): Ludwig GD+, *Clin Res* 8, 212
Petechiae
Photosensitivity
(1987): Schmutz JL+, *Ann Dermatol Venereol* (French) 114, 569
(1960): Ludwig GD+, *Clin Res* 8, 212
Pigmentation (1–10%)
Pruritus
Purpura
Radiation recall
(1975): Dreizen S+, *Postgrad Med* 58, 150
Rash (sic) (1–10%)

Toxic epidermal necrolysis
(1969): Amerio PL+, *G Ital Dermatol Venereol* (Italian) 110, 514
Urticaria
(1985): Sparling R+, *Clin Lab Haematol* 7, 184

Hair

Hair – alopecia

Nails

Nails – loss (sic)

Other

Glossitis (<1%)
Lobular panniculitis
(1997): Andersen JM+, *Pharmacotherapy* 17, 173
Mucositis (1–10%)
Oral mucosal lesions
(1983): Bronner AK+, *J Am Acad Dermatol* 9, 645 (1–5%)
(1968): Moore GE+, *Cancer Chemother Abstr* 52, 655 (2%)
Serum sickness
(1997): Andersen JM+, *Pharmacotherapy* 17, 173
Stomatitis (1–10%)
Vasculitis
(1997): Andersen JM+, *Pharmacotherapy* 17, 173

MESALAMINE

Synonyms: 5-aminosalicylic acid; 5-ASA; fisalamine; mesalazine
Trade names: Asacol (Procter & Gamble); Pentasa (Roberts); Rowasa (Solvay)
Other common trade names: *Asacolitin; Claversal; Mesalazine; Mesasal; Pentasa SR; Quintasa; Salofalk; Tidocol*
Indications: Ulcerative colitis
Category: Anti-inflammatory; bowel-disease suppressant
Half-life: 0.5–1.5 hours
Clinically important, potentially serious interactions with: digoxin

Reactions

Skin

Acne (1.2%)
Allergic reactions (sic) (<1%)
(1990): Boulain T+, *Gastroenterol Clin Biol* (French) 14, 288
(1989): Brogden RN+, *Drugs* 38, 500
Diaphoresis (3%)
Ecchymoses
Eczema (sic)
Edema (1.2%)
Erythema
(1990): Boulain T+, *Gastroenterol Clin Biol* 14, 288 (rectal)
Erythema nodosum
Exanthems
(1991): LeGros V+, *BMJ* 302, 970
(1988): Fardy JM+, *J Clin Gastroenterol* 10, 635
(1988): Gron I+, *Ugeskr Laeger* (Danish) 150, 32
Facial edema
(1990): Boulain T+, *Gastroenterol Clin Biol* 14, 288 (rectal application)
Folliculitis
(1996): Lizasoain J+, *Am J Gastroenterol* 91, 819
Kawasaki-like syndrome (sic) (<1%)
Lichen planus
(1991): Alstead EM+, *J Clin Gastroenterol* 13, 335
Lupus erythematosus
(1997): Timsit MA+, *Rev Rhum Engl Ed* 64, 586
(1992): Pent MT+, *BMJ* 305, 159
Mucocutaneous lymph node syndrome (Kawasaki syndrome)
(1991): Waanders H+, *Am J Gastroenterol* 86, 219
Peripheral edema (0.61%)
Photosensitivity
(1999): Horiuchi Y+, *Am J Gastroenterol* 94, 3386
Pruritus (1.2%)
Psoriasis
Pyoderma gangrenosum
Rash (sic) (3%)
(1992): Hautekeete ML+, *Gastroenterology* 103, 1925
(1991): Lesur G+, *Gastroenterol Clin Biol* (French) 15, 457
Urticaria
Vasculitis
(1994): Lim AG+, *BMJ* 308, 113
Xerosis

Hair

Hair – alopecia (0.86%)
(1997): Timsit MA+, *Rev Rhum Engl Ed* 64, 586
(1995): Netzer P, *Schweiz Med Wochenschr* (German) 125, 2438
(1991): Hadjigogos K, *Ital J Gastroenterol* (Italian) 23, 257
(1989): Brogden RN+, *Drugs* 38, 500
(1982): Kutty PK+, *Ann Intern Med* 97, 785

Nails

Nails – disorder (sic)

Other

Dysgeusia
Hypersensitivity (<1%)
(1996): Aparicio J+, *Am J Gastroenterol* 91, 620
(1992): Hautekeete ML+, *Gastroenterology* 103, 1925
Myalgia (3%)
Oral candidiasis
Oral lichenoid eruption
(1991): Alstead EM+, *J Clin Gastroenterol* 13, 335
Oral ulceration
Paresthesias

MESNA

Trade name: Mesnex (Bristol-Myers Squibb)
Other common trade names: *Mexan; Uromitexan*
Indications: Hemorrhagic cystitis induced by ifosfamide
Category: Hemorrhagic cystitis prophylactic
Half-life: 24 minutes
Clinically important, potentially serious interactions with: warfarin

Reactions

Skin

Allergic reactions (sic)
(1991): D'Cruz D+, *Lancet* 338, 705
Angioedema
(1998): Leal G, Fortaleza, Brazil (from Internet) (observation)
(1992): Zonzits E+, *Arch Dermatol* 128, 80
(1992): Breathnach SM+, *Adverse Drug Reactions and the Skin*, Blackwell, Oxford 289
Erythema
(1992): Breathnach SM+, *Adverse Drug Reactions and the Skin*, Blackwell, Oxford 289
Exanthems
(1998): Leal G, Fortaleza, Brazil (from Internet) (observation)
(1992): Zonzits E+, *Arch Dermatol* 128, 80
(1992): Breathnach SM+, *Adverse Drug Reactions and the Skin*, Blackwell, Oxford 289
Fixed eruption
(1998): Leal G, Fortaleza, Brazil (from Internet) (observation) 2 patients
(1992): Zonzits E+, *Arch Dermatol* 128, 80
Flushing
(1992): Breathnach SM+, *Adverse Drug Reactions and the Skin*, Blackwell, Oxford 289
Pruritus (<1%)
Rash (sic) (<1%)
Urticaria
(1998): Leal G, Fortaleza, Brazil (from Internet) (observation)
(1992): Zonzits E+, *Arch Dermatol* 128, 80
(1992): Breathnach SM+, *Adverse Drug Reactions and the Skin*, Blackwell, Oxford 289
(1988): Pratt CB+, *Drug Intell Clin Pharm* 22, 913

Other

Dysgeusia (>17%)
Oral mucosal lesions
(1988): Pralt CB+, *Drug Intell Clin Pharm* 22, 913
Oral mucosal ulceration
(1992): Breathnach SM+, *Adverse Drug Reactions and the Skin*, Blackwell, Oxford 289

MESORIDAZINE

Trade name: Serentil (Boehringer Ingelheim)
Other common trade name: *Mesorin*
Indications: Schizophrenia
Category: Phenothiazine antipsychotic
Half-life: 24–48 hours
Clinically important, potentially serious interactions with: alcohol, barbiturates, chloroquine, CNS depressants, levodopa, lithium, MAO inhibitors, piperazine, propranolol, trazodone, tricyclic antidepressants, **cigarette smoking**

Reactions

Skin

Angioedema
Contact dermatitis
Eczema (sic)
Edema
Erythema
Exfoliative dermatitis
Flushing
Hypohidrosis (>10%)
Lupus erythematosus
Peripheral edema
Photosensitivity (1–10%)
Pigmentation (blue-gray) (<1%)
Pruritus
Rash (sic) (1–10%)
Seborrhea
Urticaria
Xerosis

Hair

Hair – alopecia

Other

Anaphylactoid reaction
Galactorrhea (<1%)
Gynecomastia
Hypertrophic papillae of tongue
Mastodynia (1–10%)
Paresthesias
Priapism (<1%)
Sialorrhea
Tremor
Xerostomia

METAXALONE

Trade name: Skelaxin (Carnrick)
Indications: Muscle spasm
Category: Skeletal muscle relaxant
Half-life: 2–3 hours
Clinically important, potentially serious interactions with: alcohol, CNS depressants

Reactions

Skin

Allergic dermatitis (sic) (<1%)
Fixed eruption
(2000): Mostow EN, Akron, OH (from Internet) (observation)
Pruritus
Rash (sic)
Urticaria

Other

Anaphylactoid reaction (<1%)

METFORMIN

Trade names: Glucophage (Bristol-Myers Squibb); Glucovance (Bristol-Myers Squibb)
Other common trade names: *Apo-Metformin; Diabex; Diaformin; Diformin; Gen-Metformin; Glucomet; Metforal; Metomin; Novo-Metformin*
Indications: Diabetes
Category: Antidiabetic
Half-life: 6.2 hours
Clinically important, potentially serious interactions with: alcohol, amiloride, cimetidine, digoxin, furosemide, morphine, nifedipine, procainamide, quinidine, quinine, ranitidine, triamterene, trimethoprim, vancomycin

Glucovance is metformin and glyburide

Reactions

Skin

Eczema (sic)
(1970): Lawson AAH+, *Lancet* 2, 437
Erythema (transient)
(1966): Beurey J+, *Ann Dermatol Syphiligr* (French) 93,13
(1966): Berger W+, *Schweiz Med Wochenschr* (German) 96, 1335
(1964): Puchegger R+, *Wien Klin Wochenschr* (German) 76, 335
Exanthems
Grinspan's syndrome*
(1990): Lamey PJ+, *Oral Surg Oral Med Oral Pathol* 70, 184
Lichenoid eruption
(1970): Lawson AAH+, Lancet 2, 437
Photosensitivity (1–10%)
Pruritus
(1964): Puchegger R+, *Wien Klin Wochenschr* (German) 76, 335
Purpura
(1966): Berger W+, *Schweiz Med Wochenschr* (German) 96, 1335
Rash (sic) (1–10%)
Urticaria (1–10%)
(1966): Beurey J+, *Ann Dermatol Syphiligr* (French) 93,13
(1966): Berger W+, *Schweiz Med Wochenschr* (German) 96, 1335
(1964): Puchegger R+, *Wien Klin Wochenschr* (German) 76, 335
Vasculitis
(1986): Klapholz L+, *BMJ* 293, 483

Hair

Hair – alopecia
(1999): Smith JG, Mobile, AL (from Internet) (2 observations)
(1998): Klein AD, Statesboro, GA (from Internet) (observation)

Other

Dysgeusia (3%) (metallic taste)

*__Note:__ Grinspan's syndrome: the triad of oral lichen planus, diabetes mellitus, and hypertension

METHADONE

Trade name: Dolophine (Roxane)
Other common trade names: *Eptadone; L-Polamidon; Mephenon; Metadon; Methadose; Physeptone*
Indications: Pain, narcotic addiction
Category: Narcotic analgesic; antitussive; suppressant (narcotic abstinence syndrome)
Half-life: 15–25 hours
Clinically important, potentially serious interactions with: barbiturates, cimetidine, CNS depressants, hydantoins, MAO inhibitors, phenothiazines, phenytoin, rifampin, tricyclic antidepressants

Reactions

Skin

Angioedema
Cellulitis
(1988): Naschitz JE+, *Harefuah* (Hebrew) 115, 271
Diaphoresis
(1973): Kreek MJ, *JAMA* 223, 665 (48%)
Edema (face)
Exanthems
Flushing
Pruritus (<1%)
Purpura
Rash (sic) (<1%)
Urticaria (<1%)

Other

Injection-site burning
Injection-site induration
Injection-site pain (1–10%)
Xerostomia (1–10%)

METHAMPHETAMINE

Trade name: Desoxyn (Abbott)
Indications: Attention deficit disorder, obesity
Category: Central nervous system stimulant
Half-life: 4–5 hours
Clinically important, potentially serious interactions with: antipsychotics, barbiturates, furazolidone, guanethidine, MAO inhibitors, tricyclic antidepressants

Reactions

Skin

Acaraphobia
(1971): Yaffee NS, *Arch Dermatol* 104, 687
Delusions of parasitosis
(1999): Gregg LJ, Tulsa, OK, (from Internet) (4 observations)
Diaphoresis (1–10%)
Lichenoid eruption
(1994): Deloach-Banta LJ, *Cutis* 53, 97
Pigmentation
(1971): Yaffee NS, *Arch Dermatol* 104, 687
Rash (sic) (<1%)
Urticaria (<1%)

Other

Dysgeusia
Polyarteritis nodosa
(1973): Koff RS+, *N Engl J Med* 288, 946
(1970): Citron BP+, *N Engl J Med* 283, 1003
Tremor
Xerostomia (1–10%)

METHANTHELINE

Trade name: Banthine (SCS)
Other common trade name: *Vagantin*
Indications: Duodenal ulcer
Category: Gastrointestinal anticholinergic and antispasmodic
Half-life: no data
Clinically important, potentially serious interactions with: amantadine, anticholinergics, atenolol, clozapine, digoxin, haloperidol, phenothiazines, tricyclic antidepressants

Reactions

Skin

Exanthems
Exfoliative dermatitis
Flushing
Hypohidrosis
Urticaria
Xerosis

Other

Ageusia
Anaphylactoid reaction
Dysgeusia
Sialopenia
Xerostomia

METHAZOLAMIDE

Trade name: Methazolamide
Indications: Glaucoma
Category: Carbonic anhydrase inhibitor; sulfonamide diuretic
Half-life: ~14 hours
Clinically important, potentially serious interactions with: cyclosporine, diflunisal, digoxin, ephedrine, phenytoin, quinidine, salicylates

Reactions

Skin

Exanthems (<1%)
(1998): Litt JZ, Beachwood, OH, personal case (observation)
(1993): Gandham SB+, *Arch Ophthalmol* 111, 370
Photosensitivity
Pruritus
Purpura
Rash (sic)
Stevens–Johnson syndrome
(1998): Cotter JB, *Arch Ophthalmol* 116, 117
(1997): Shirato S+, *Arch Ophthalmol* 115, 550
(1995): Flach AJ+, *Ophthalmology* 102, 1677
Toxic epidermal necrolysis
Urticaria
(1993): Gandham SB+, *Arch Ophthalmol* 111, 370
Vasculitis

Other

Anosmia (<1%)
Dysgeusia (>10%) (metallic taste)
Hypersensitivity (<1%)

Paresthesias (<1%)
Trembling
Xerostomia (<1%)

METHENAMINE

Trade names: Hiprex; Mandelamine (Warner Chilcott); Prosed (Star); Urex (3M); Urised (PolyMedica); Uroqid
Other common trade names: *Dehydral; Haiprex; Hip-Rex; Hipeksal; Hippramine; Reflux; Urasal; Urotractan*
Indications: Urinary tract infections
Category: Urinary tract antibacterial
Half-life: 3–6 hours
Clinically important, potentially serious interactions with: acetazolamide, carbonic anhydrase inhibitors, sulfonamides

Reactions

Skin

Edema
Erythema multiforme (<1%)
Exanthems
(1976): Arndt KA+, *JAMA* 235, 918 (0.6%)
(1968): *Med Lett* 10, 58
Fixed eruption (<1%)
(1961): Welsh AL, *Arch Dermatol* 84, 1004
Photosensitivity
(1994): Selvaag E+, *Photodermatol Photoimmunol Photomed* 10, 259
Pruritus (<1%)
Rash (sic) (3.5%)
Systemic eczematous contact dermatitis
Urticaria

Other

Stomatitis

METHICILLIN

Trade name: Staphcillin (Mead Johnson)
Other common trade names: *Estafcilina; Lucoperin; Mechicillin*
Indications: Various infections caused by susceptible organisms
Category: Penicillinase-resistant penicillin antibiotic
Half-life: 30 minutes
Clinically important, potentially serious interactions with: anticoagulants, atenolol, cyclosporine, disulfiram, methotrexate, oral contraceptives, probenecid, tetracyclines

Reactions

Skin

Angioedema
Bullous eruption
(1976): Schiffer CA+, *Ann Intern Med* 85, 338
Ecchymoses
Erythema multiforme
(1969): Kaminska M+, *Pediatr Pol* (Polish) 44, 873
Erythema nodosum
Exanthems
(1980): Fields DA, *West J Med* 133, 521
(1978): Kancir LM+, *Arch Intern Med* 138, 909 (29%)
Exfoliative dermatitis
(1966): Hadida E+, *Bull Soc Fr Dermatol Syphiligr* (French) 73, 497
Hematomas
Jarisch–Herxheimer reaction
Pruritus
Purpura
Pustular psoriasis
(1966): Hadida E+, *Bull Soc Fr Dermatol Syphiligr* (French) 73, 497
Rash (sic) (1–10%)
Stevens–Johnson syndrome
Toxic epidermal necrolysis
Urticaria
Vasculitis

Other

Anaphylactoid reaction
Black tongue
Dysgeusia
Glossitis
Glossodynia
Hypersensitivity
Injection-site pain
Oral candidiasis
Phlebitis (<1%)
Serum sickness (<1%)
Stomatitis
Stomatodynia
Vaginitis
Xerostomia

METHIMAZOLE

Synonym: thiamazole
Trade name: Tapazole (Jones)
Other common trade names: *Strumazol; Thacapzol; Thiamazol; Thyrozol; Unimazole*
Indications: Hyperthyroidism
Category: Antithyroid agent
Half-life: 4–13 hours
Clinically important, potentially serious interactions with: amiodarone, anticoagulants, beta-blockers, digoxin, iodine, lithium, metoprolol, potassium iodide, propranolol, theophylline

Reactions

Skin

Cutaneous side effects (sic) (28% in high dosages)
(1972): Wiberg JJ+, *Ann Intern Med* 77, 414 (1–5%)
Edema (<1%)
Erythema nodosum
Exanthems
(1986): Shiroozu A+, *J Clin Endocrinol Metab* 63, 125 (5–15%)
(1972): Wiberg JJ+, *Ann Intern Med* 77, 414 (1–5%)
(1970): Amrhein JA+, *J Pediatr* 76, 54
(1951): Bartels EC+, *J Clin Endocrinol Metab* 11, 1057 (6%)
Exfoliative dermatitis
Fixed eruption
(1984): Chan HL, *Int J Dermatol* 23, 607
Lupus erythematosus (1–10%)
(1995): Kawachi Y+, *Clin Exp Dermatol* 20, 345
(1994): Sato-Matsumura KC+, *J Dermatol* 21, 501
(1987): Sakata S+, *Jpn J Med* 26, 373
(1981): Searles RP+, *J Rheumatol* 8, 498
(1981): Takuwa N+, *Endocrinol Jpn* 28, 663
(1973): Hung W+, *J Pediatr* 82, 852
(1970): Librik L+, *J Pediatr* 76, 64
Pigmentation
Pruritus (3–5%)
(1986): Shiroozu A+, *J Clin Endocrinol Metab* 63, 125 (2–3%)
(1972): Wiberg JJ+, *Ann Intern Med* 77, 414 (1–5%)
Purpura
(1972): Wiberg JJ+, *Ann Intern Med* 77, 414 (1%)
Rash (sic) (>10%)
Urticaria
(1972): Wiberg JJ+, *Ann Intern Med* 77, 414 (>5%)
(1970): Amrhein JA+, *J Pediatr* 76, 54
Vasculitis
(1995): Kawachi Y+, *Clin Exp Dermatol* 20, 345

Hair

Hair – alopecia (<1%)

Other

Ageusia (1–10%)
Aplasia cutis congenita
(1995): Vogt T+, *Br J Dermatol* 133, 994
(1992): Martinez-Frias ML+, *Lancet* 339, 742
(1985): Milham S, *Teratology* 32, 321
(1984): Bachrach LK+, *Can Med Assoc J* 130, 1264
Dysgeusia
Oral ulceration
Myalgia
Paresthesias (<1%)
Polyarteritis nodosa
Scalp defects (sic)
(1985): Milham S, *Teratology* 32, 321
Serum sickness
(1983): Van Kuyk M+, *Acta Clin Belg* (French) 38, 68
Sialadenitis

METHOCARBAMOL

Trade name: Robaxin (Robins)
Other common trade names: *Carbametin; Carxin; Delaxin; Lumirelax; Marbaxin; Miowas; Ortoton; Robinax; Robomol; Trolar*
Indications: Muscle spasm, tetanus
Category: Skeletal muscle relaxant
Half-life: 1–2 hours
Clinically important, potentially serious interactions with: CNS depressants

Reactions

Skin

Allergic reactions (sic) (1–10%)
Exanthems
Flushing (1–10%)
Pruritus
Rash (sic)
Urticaria

Other

Anaphylactoid reaction
Dysgeusia
Injection-site pain (<1%)
Thrombophlebitis (<1%)

METHOHEXITAL

Trade name: Brevital (Jones)
Other common trade names: *Brietal; Brietal Sodium; Brevimytal*
Indications: General anesthesia
Category: General anesthetic; barbiturate
Half-life: 4–8 minutes
Clinically important, potentially serious interactions with: CNS depressants, narcotic analgesics, propranolol

Reactions

Skin

Angioedema
(1972): Driggs RL+, *J Oral Surg* 30, 906
(1972): Reichert EF+, *J Oral Surg* 30, 910
Erythema
Exanthems
(1972): Driggs RL+, *J Oral Surg* 30, 906
Rash (sic)
Urticaria
(1972): Reichert EF+, *J Oral Surg* 30, 910
(1972): Driggs RL+, *J Oral Surg* 30, 906

Other

Anaphylactoid reaction
Injection-site edema
Injection-site pain (18%)
Injection-site phlebitis
(1981): Clark RSJ, *Drugs* 27, 26
Sialorrhea
Thrombophlebitis (<1%)
Tremor

METHOTREXATE

Synonyms: amethopterin; MTX
Trade name: Rheumatrex (Lederle)
Other common trade names: *Farmitrexat; Lantarel; Ledertrexate; Maxtrex; Metex; Texate*
Indications: Carcinomas, leukemias, lymphomas, psoriasis, rheumatoid arthritis
Category: Anti-inflammatory, antiarthritic, antineoplastic and antimetabolite
Half-life: 3–10 hours
Clinically important, potentially serious interactions with: alcohol, aminoglycosides, amiodarone, cephalothin, chloroquine, cisplatin, colchicine, cyclosporine, diclofenac, digoxin, etretinate, ibuprofen, indomethacin, ketoprofen, magnesium trisalicylate, naproxen, NSAIDs, penicillins, phenylbutazone, probenecid, retinoids, salicylates, sulfamethoxazole, sulfapyridine, sulindac, trimethoprim, vincristine

Reactions

Skin

Acne
Acral erythema
(1996): Hellier I+, *Arch Dermatol* 132, 590 (bullous variety)
(1989): Kampmann KK+, *Cancer* 63, 2482
(1983): Doyle LA+, *Ann Intern Med* 98, 611
Acute inflammation (sic) (reactivation)
(1969): Möller H, *J Invest Dermatol* 52, 437
Allergic reactions (sic)
(2000): Postovsky S+, *Med Pediatr Oncol* 35, 131
Bullous eruption
(1987): Chang JC, *Arch Dermatol* 123, 990
(1983): Reed KM+, *J Am Acad Dermatol* 8, 677
Burning (palms and soles)
(1978): McDonald CJ+, *Cancer Treat Rep* 62, 1009
Candidiasis
(1970): Baker H, *Br J Dermatol* 82, 65
Capillaritis
(1978): McDonald CJ+, *Cancer Treat Rep* 62, 1009
(1976): Jacobs SA+, *J Clin Invest* 57, 534
Carcinoma (sic)
(1971): Craig LR+, *Arch Dermatol* 103, 505
Cutaneous necrolysis (sic)
(1970): Baker H, *Br J Dermatol* 82, 65
Cutaneous side effects (sic)
(1997): Kasteler JS+, *J Am Acad Dermatol* 36, 67 (passim)
(1996): Furuya T+, *Rymachi* (Japanese) 36, 746
Dermatitis (sic)
(1996): Giordano N+, *Clin Exp Rheumatol* 14, 450
Ecchymoses
(1998): Roenigk HH+, *J Am Acad Dermatol* 38, 478
Eccrine squamous syringometaplasia
(1997): Valks R+, *Arch Dermatol* 133, 873
Epidermal necrosis (sic)
(1987): Harrison PV, *Br J Dermatol* 116, 867
(1983): Reed KM+, *J Am Acad Dermatol* 8, 677
(1982): Lawrence CM+, *Br J Dermatol* 107, 24
Erosion of psoriatic plaques (sic)
(1996): Pearce HP+, *J Am Acad Dermatol* 35, 835
(1988): Kaplan DL+, *Int J Dermatol* 27, 59
(1988): Shupack JL+, *JAMA* 259, 3594
(1987): Ng HW+, *BMJ* 295, 752

(1984): Lawrence CM+, *J Am Acad Dermatol* 11, 1059
(1983): Reed KM+, *J Am Acad Dermatol* 8, 677
(1969): McDonald CJ+, *Arch Dermatol* 100, 655

Erosions
(1996): Zackheim HS+, *J Am Acad Dermatol* 34, 626

Erythema (>10%)

Erythema multiforme
(1989): Taylor SW+, *Gynecol Oncol* 33, 376
(1978): Moe PJ+, *Acta Paediatr Scand* (French) 67, 265

Erythematous papules (sic)
(1999): Goerttler E+, *J Am Acad Dermatol* 40, 702 (4 cases)

Erythroderma
(1996): Zackheim HS+, *J Am Acad Dermatol* 34, 626

Exanthems (15%)
(1979): Stoller RG+, *Cancer Res* 39, 908
(1971): Hansen HH+, *Br J Cancer* 25, 298

Folliculitis
(1970): Baker H, *Br J Dermatol* 82, 65

Furunculosis
(1996): Zackheim HS+, *J Am Acad Dermatol* 34, 626

Herpes simplex
(1996): Vonderheid EC+, *J Am Acad Dermatol* 34, 470

Melanoma
(1984): Wemmer U, *Z Hautkr* (German) 59, 665

Nodules
(1998): Williams FM+, *J Am Acad Dermatol* 39, 359
(1996): Muzaffer MA+, *J Pediatr* 128, 698
(1996): Smith MD, *J Rheumatol* 23, 2004
(1995): Berris B+, *J Rheumatol* 22, 2359
(1995): Das SK+, *J Assoc Physicians India* 43, 651
(1994): Smith MD, *J Rheumatol* 22, 1439
(1994): Abu-Shakra M+, *J Rheumatol* 21, 934
(1994): Karam NE+ *J Rheumatol* 21, 1960
(1992): Kerstens PJSM+, *J Rheumatol* 19, 867
(1988): Segal R+, *Arthritis Rheum* 31, 1182

Photosensitivity (5%)
(1996): Zackheim HS+, *J Am Acad Dermatol* 34, 626
(1994): Oliver F, *The Schoch Letter* 44, 6 (observation)
(1969): Roenigk HH Jr+, *Arch Dermatol* 99, 86
(1969): Möller H, *J Invest Dermatol* 52, 437
(1965): Vogler WR+, *Arch Intern Med* 115, 285

Pigmentation (1–10%)

Pruritus (1–5%)
(1998): Roenigk HH+, *J Am Acad Dermatol* 38, 478

Purpura

Radiation recall
(1995): Guzzo C+, *Photodermatol Photoimmunol Photomed* 11, 55 (sunburn)

Radiodermatitis (reactivation)

Rash (sic) (1–3%)
(1995): Copur S+, *Anticancer Drugs* 6, 154

Scabies (reactivation)
(1975): Burrows D, *Br J Dermatol* 93, 219

Squamous cell carcinoma
(1989): Jensen DB+, *Acta Derm Venereol* (Stockh) 69, 274
(1971): Harris CC, *Arch Dermatol* 103, 501

Stevens–Johnson syndrome
(1993): Cuthbert RJ+, *Ulster Med J* 62, 95
(1978): Moe PJ+, *Acta Paediatr Scand* (French) 67, 265

Sunburn (reactivation)
(1998): Roenigk HH+, *J Am Acad Dermatol* 38, 478
(1987): Westwick TJ+, *Cutis* 39, 49
(1986): Mallory SB+, *Pediatrics* 78, 514
(1981): Korossy KS+, *Arch Dermatol* 117, 310

Telangiectases

Toxic epidermal necrolysis (<1%)
(1997): Primka EJ+, *J Am Acad Dermatol* 36, 815 (fatal)
(1970): Baker H, *Br J Dermatol* 82, 65
(1967): Lyell A, *Br J Dermatol* 79, 367

Ulceration
(1998): Ben-Amitai D+, *Ann Pharmacother* 32, 651
(1998): Roenigk HH+, *J Am Acad Dermatol* 38, 478 (of psoriatic lesions)
(1970): Baker H, *Br J Dermatol* 82, 65

Urticaria
(1998): Roenigk HH+, *J Am Acad Dermatol* 38, 478
(1995): al-Lamki Z+, *Med Pediatr Oncol* 24, 137
(1983): Bronner AK+, *J Am Acad Dermatol* 9, 645

Vasculitis (>10%)
(2000): Borcea A+, *Br J Dermatol* 143, 203 (urticarial)
(1998): Halevy S+, *J Eur Acad Dermatol Venereol* 10, 81
(1997): Torner O+, *Clin Rheumatol* 16, 108
(1995): Blanco R+, *Arthritis Rheum* 39, 1016
(1989): Fondevila CG+, *Br J Haematol* 72, 591
(1989): Jeurissen MEC+, *Clin Rheumatol* 8, 417
(1986): Navarro M+, *Ann Intern Med* 105, 471
(1984): Marks CR+, *Ann Intern Med* 100, 916

Hair

Hair – alopecia (1–3%)
(1998): Roenigk HH+, *J Am Acad Dermatol* 38, 478
(1998): Zieglschmid ME+, *J Am Acad Dermatol* 38, 130
(1997): Kasteler JS+, *J Am Acad Dermatol* 36, 67 (passim)
(1996): Zackheim HS+, *J Am Acad Dermatol* 34, 626
(1995): Zieglschmid-Adams ME+, *J Am Acad Dermatol* 32, 754
(1989): Fehlauer CS+, *J Rheumatol* 16, 307
(1988): Weinblatt ME+, *Arthritis Rheum* 31 (Suppl), s115
(1982): Bachman DM, *Arthritis Rheum* 25, s65
(1982): Bertino JR, *Med Pediatr Oncol* 10, 401
(1971): Hansen HH+, *Br J Cancer* 25, 298
(1969): Roenigk HH Jr+, *Arch Dermatol* 99, 86 (6%)

Hair – pigmented bands
(1983): Wheeland RG+, *Cancer* 51, 1356

Nails

Nails – discoloration

Nails – onycholysis
(1987): Chang JC, *Arch Dermatol* 123, 990

Nails – paronychia
(1983): Wantzin GL+, *Arch Dermatol* 119, 623

Nails – pigmentation
(1981): Nixon DW+, *Cutis* 27, 181

Other

Anaphylactoid reaction (1–10%)
(1996): Alkins SA+, *Cancer* 77, 2123
(1995): Lobelle C+, *Pediatr Hematol Oncol* 12, 213
(1979): Gluck-Kuyt I+, *Cancer Treat Rep* 63, 797
(1978): Goldberg NH+, *Cancer* 41, 52

Dysgeusia
(1988): Duhra P+, *Clin Exp Dermatol* 13, 126

Hodgkin's disease (nodular sclerosing)
(2000): Moseley AC+, *J Rheumatol* 27, 810

Gingivitis (>10%)

Glossitis (>10%)

Gynecomastia
(1995): Thomas E+, *J Rheumatol* 22, 2189
(1995): Finger DR+, *J Rheumatol* 22, 796
(1983): Del Paine DW+, *Arthritis Rheum* 26, 691

Malignant lymphoma
(1997): Kamel OW, *Arch Dermatol* 133, 903
(1996): Viraben R+, *Br J Dermatol* 135, 116
(1994): Zimmer-Galler I+, *Mayo Clin Proc* 69, 258
(1993): Kamel OW+, *N Engl J Med* 328, 1317

Myalgia

Oral mucositis
(1997): Plevova P+, *J Natl Cancer Inst* 89, 326
(1996): Rask C+, *Pediatr Hematol Oncol* 13, 359
(1996): Moe PJ, *Pediatr Hematol Oncol* 13, 313
(1996): Zackheim HS+, *J Am Acad Dermatol* 34, 626
(1979): Oliff A+, *Cancer Chemother Pharmacol* 2, 225

Oral ulceration
(1986): Barrett AP, *J Periodontol* 57, 318

Peyronie's disease
(1992): Phelan MJI, *Br J Rheumatol* 31, 425

Porphyria cutanea tarda
(1983): Malina L+, *Z Hautkr* (German) 58, 241

Pseudolymphoma
(1997): Flipo RM+, *J Rheumatol* 24, 809
(1995): Delaporte E+, *Ann Dermatol Venereol* (French) 122, 521 (20 cases)

Stomatitis (3–10%)
(1998): Roenigk HH+, *J Am Acad Dermatol* 38, 478 (ulcerative)
(1998): Zieglschmid ME+, *J Am Acad Dermatol* 38, 130
(1997): Kasteler JS+, *J Am Acad Dermatol* 36, 67 (passim)

(1996): Vonderheid EC+, *J Am Acad Dermatol* 34, 470
(1995): Zieglschmid-Adams ME+, *J Am Acad Dermatol* 32, 754
(1994): Montecucco C+, *Arthritis Rheum* 37, 777
(1978): Moe PJ+, *Acta Paediatr Scand* (French) 67, 265

METHOXSALEN

Trade names: 8-MOP (ICN); Oxsoralen (ICN)
Other common trade names: *Geroxalen; Meladinine; Oxsoralon; Puvasoralen; Ultra-MOP*
Indications: Psoriasis; vitiligo
Category: Repigmenting agent and antipsoriatic
Half-life: 1.1 hours
Clinically important, potentially serious interactions with: chloroquine, griseofulvin, isotretinoin, nalidixic acid, phenothiazines, sulfonamides, tetracyclines, thiazides

Reactions

Skin

Acne
(1978): Nielsen EB+, *Acta Derm Venereol* (Stockh) 58, 374
Basal cell carcinoma
(1996): Stern RS+, *J Pediatr* 129, 915
(1995): Gritiyarangsan P+, *Photodermatol Photoimmunol Photomed* 11, 174
Bowen's disease
(1979): Tam DW+, *Arch Dermatol* 115, 203
Bullous eruption (with UVA)
(1982): Stüttgen G, *Int J Dermatol* 21, 198
(1979): Abel EA+, *Arch Dermatol* 115, 988
(1977): Melski JW+, *J Invest Dermatol* 68, 328
(1976): Thomsen K+, *Br J Dermatol* 95, 568
Bullous pemphigoid
(1996): Perl S+, *Dermatology* 193, 245
Burning (1–10%)
(1982): Stüttgen G, *Int J Dermatol* 21, 198 (passim)
Burns
(1996): Geary P, *Burns* 22, 636
(1991): Boucaud C+, *Presse Med* (French) 20, 1945
Cancer (sic)
(1995): Halder RM+, *Arch Dermatol* 131, 734
(1984): Halprin KM+, *Natl Cancer Inst Monogr* 66, 185
(1979): Stern RS+, *N Engl J Med* 301, 555
(1979): Spellman CW, *N Engl J Med* 301, 554
(1979): Morgan RW, *N Engl J Med* 301, 554
(1976): Moller R+, *Arch Dermatol* 112, 1613 (multiple basal cell carcinomas)
Cheilitis (1–10%)
Contact dermatitis
(1994): Korffmacher H+, *Contact Dermatitis* 30, 283
(1991): Takashima A+, *Br J Dermatol* 124, 37
(1980): Weissmann I+, *Br J Dermatol* 102, 113
(1979): Saihan EM, *BMJ* 2, 20
Eczematous eruption (sic)
(1979): Saihan EM, *BMJ* 2, 20
Edema (1–10%)
Erythema (1–10%)
Exanthems
(1986): Gisslen P+, *Photodermatol* 3, 308
Exfoliative dermatitis
Freckles (1–10%)
(1995): Gritiyarangsan P+, *Photodermatol Photoimmunol Photomed* 11, 174
(1995): Pierard GE+, *Dermatology* 190, 338
(1984): Kietzmann E+, *Dermatologica* 168, 306
(1983): Kietzmann H+, *Ann Dermatol Venereol* (French) 110, 63
(1983): Kanerva L+, *Dermatologica* 166, 281
Granuloma annulare
(1979): Dorval JC+, *Ann Dermatol Venereol* (French) 106, 79
Herpes simplex
(1982): Stüttgen G, *Int J Dermatol* 21, 198
Herpes zoster
(1982): Stüttgen G, *Int J Dermatol* 21, 198
(1977): Roenigk HH+, *Arch Dermatol* 113, 1667
Hypopigmentation (1–10%)
Lupus erythematosus
(1985): Bruze M+, *Acta Derm Venereol* (Stockh) 65, 31
(1979): Eyanson S+, *Arch Dermatol* 115, 54
(1978): Millns J+, *Arch Dermatol* 114, 1177
Miliaria
Pemphigoid
(1978): Robinson JK, *Br J Dermatol* 99, 709
Photoreactions
(1992): Jeanmougin M+, *Ann Dermatol Venereol* (French) 119, 277
(1978): Plewig G+, *Arch Derm Res* 261, 201
(1968): Fulton JE+, *Arch Derm* 98, 445
Photocontact dermatitis
(1998): Clark SM+, *Contact Dermatitis* 38, 289
(1991): Takashima A+, *Br J Dermatol* 124, 37
(1990): Cox NH+, *Clin Exp Dermatol* 15, 75
Photosensitivity
(1991): Boucaud C+, *Presse Med* (French) 20, 1945
(1989): Cox NH+, *Photodermatol* 6, 96
Phototoxic reaction
(1997): Morison WL+, *J Am Acad Dermatol* 36, 183
(1993): Calzavara-Pinton PG+, *J Am Acad Dermatol* 28, 657
(1989): Morison WL, *Arch Dermatol* 125, 433 (topical)
(1985): Berakha GJ+, *Ann Plast Surg* 14, 458
(1984): Meffert H+, *Photodermatol* 1, 191
(1979): de Koning GA+, *Hautarzt* (German) 30, 27
(1979): Swanbeck G+, *Clin Pharmacol Ther* 25, 478
Pigmentation
(1989): Weiss E+, *Int J Dermatol* 28, 188
(1987): Bruce DR+, *J Am Acad Dermatol* 16, 1087
(1986): MacDonald KJS+, *Br J Dermatol* 114, 395
Porokeratosis (actinic)
(1988): Beiteke U+, *Photodermatology* 5, 274
(1985): Hazen PG+, *J Am Acad Dermatol* 12, 1077
(1980): Reymond JL, *Acta Derm Venereol* (Stockh) 60, 539
Prurigo
(1982): Stüttgen G, *Int J Dermatol* 21, 198 (passim)
Pruritus (>10%)
(1982): Stüttgen G, *Int J Dermatol* 21, 198 (passim)
Purpura
(1981): Barriere H+, *Nouv Presse Med* (French) 10, 337
Rash (sic) (1–10%)
Scleroderma
(1976): Duperrat B+, *Bull Soc Franc Dermatol Syphiligr* (French) 83, 79
Seborrheic dermatitis
(1983): Tegner E, *Acta Derm Venereol* (Stockh) Suppl 107, 5
Skin pain
(1987): Norris PG+, *Clin Exp Dermatol* 12, 403
(1983): Tegner E, *Acta Derm Venereol* (Stockh) Suppl 107, 5
Squamous cell carcinoma
(1998): Stern RS+, *Arch Dermatol* 134, 1582 (with UVA)
(1986): Kahn JR+, *Clin Exp Dermatol* 11, 398
(1979): Verdich J, *Arch Dermatol* 115, 1338
(1979): Tam DW+, *Arch Dermatol* 115, 203
Tumors (sic)
(1988): Gupta AK+, *J Am Acad Dermatol* 19, 67
(1987): Henseler T+, *J Am Acad Dermatol* 16, 108
Urticaria
(1994): Bech-Thomsen N+, *J Am Acad Dermatol* 31, 1063
Vasculitis
(1981): Barriere H+, *Presse Med* (French) 10, 37
Vitiligo
(1983): Tegner E, *Acta Derm Venereol* (Stockh) Suppl 107, 5
(1976): Duperrat B+, *Bull Soc Franc Dermatol Syphiligr* (French) 83, 79
Xerosis
Warts
(1982): Stüttgen G, *Int J Dermatol* 21, 198

Hair

Hair – hypertrichosis
(1983): Rampen FHJ, *Br J Dermatol* 109, 657
(1967): Singh G+, *Br J Dermatol* 79, 501
(1959): Elliot JA, *J Invest Dermatol* 32, 311

Nails
Nails – photo-onycholysis
(1990): Baran R+, *Ann Dermatol Venereol* (French) 117, 367
(1984): Balato N+, *Photodermatol* 1, 202
(1978): Rau RC+, *Arch Dermatol* 114, 448
(1977): Vella-Briffa D+, *BMJ* 2, 1150
(1977): Zala L+, *Dermatologica* 154, 203
Nails – pigmentation
(1990): Trattner A+, *Int J Dermatol* 29, 310
(1989): Weiss E+, *Int J Dermatol* 28, 188
(1986): MacDonald KJS+, *Br J Dermatol* 114, 395
(1982): Naik RPC+, *Int J Dermatol* 21, 275
(1979): Naik RP+, *Br J Dermatol* 100, 229

Other
Lymphoproliferative disease
(1989): Aschinoff R+, *J Am Acad Dermatol* 21, 1134

METHSUXIMIDE

Trade name: Celontin (Parke-Davis)
Other common trade name: *Petinutin*
Indications: Absence (petit-mal) seizures
Category: Succinimide anticonvulsant
Half-life: 2–4 hours
Clinically important, potentially serious interactions with:
phenytoin, primidone, valproic acid

Reactions

Skin
Acanthosis nigricans
(1972): Petko E+, *Arch Dermatol* 106, 918
Erythema multiforme
Exanthems
(1972): Petko E+, *Arch Dermatol* 106, 918
Exfoliative dermatitis (<1%)
Lupus erythematosus (>10%)
Periorbital edema
Pruritus
Purpura
Rash (sic)
Stevens–Johnson syndrome (>10%)
Urticaria (<1%)

Hair
Hair – alopecia
Hair – hirsutism

Other
Gingival hyperplasia
Oral ulceration

METHYCLOTHIAZIDE

Trade names: Aquatensen (Wallace); Enduron (Abbott)
Other common trade names: *Enduron-M; Thiazidil; Urimor*
Indications: Hypertension
Category: Thiazide* diuretic; antihypertensive
Half-life: no data
Clinically important, potentially serious interactions with:
allopurinol, digoxin, lithium, methyldopa

Reactions

Skin
Erythema multiforme
Exanthems
Photosensitivity (<1%)
Purpura
Rash (sic) (<1%)
Stevens–Johnson syndrome
Urticaria

Other
Anaphylactoid reaction
Dysgeusia
Paresthesias (<1%)

***Note:** Methyclothiazide is a sulfonamide and can be absorbed systemically. Sulfonamides can produce severe, possibly fatal, reactions such as toxic epidermal necrolysis and Stevens–Johnson syndrome.

METHYLDOPA

Trade names: Aldoclor (Merck); Aldomet (Merck); Aldoril (Merck)
Other common trade names: *Amodopa; Densul; Dopamet; Equibar; Hydopa; Medimet; Nu-Medopa; Polinal; Presinol; Prodopa*
Indications: Hypertension
Category: Alpha-adrenergic inhibitor; antihypertensive
Half-life: 1.7 hours
Clinically important, potentially serious interactions with:
barbiturates, beta-blockers, haloperidol, iron, levodopa, lithium, MAO inhibitors, phenothiazines, tolbutamide, tricyclic antidepressants

Aldoril is methyldopa and hydrochlorothiazide

Reactions

Skin
Ankle edema
(1969): Varadi DP+, *Arch Intern Med* 124, 13
Cheilitis
(1973): Almeyda J+, *Br J Dermatol* 88, 313
Eczematous eruption (sic)
(1974): Church R, *Br J Dermatol* 91, 373
(1969): Peterkin GAG, *Practitioner* 202, 117 (keratotic – palms and soles)
(1965): Dollery CT, *Prog in Cardiovasc Dis* 8, 278
Edema
Erythema multiforme (<1%)
(1985): Ting HC+, *Int J Dermatol* 24, 587
(1975): Böttiger LE+, *Acta Med Scand* 198, 229
Erythema nodosum
(1978): Furhoff AK, *Acta Med Scand* 203, 425
Exanthems
(1986): Gidseg G, *South Med J* 79, 389
(1978): Furhoff AK, *Acta Med Scand* 203, 425
(1971): Perry HM+, *J Lab Clin Med* 78, 905 (3%)
Fixed eruption
(1974): Burry JN+, *Br J Dermatol* 91, 475
Granulomas
(1974): Wells JD+, *Ann Intern Med* 81, 701
Lichenoid eruption
(1986): Gonzalez JG+, *J Am Acad Dermatol* 15, 87
(1982): Brooks SL, *J Oral Med* 37, 42
(1982): Wiesenfeld D+, *Oral Surg Oral Med Oral Pathol* 54, 527
(1980): *Med J Aust* 2, 130
(1976): Burry JN, *Arch Dermatol* 112, 880 (ulcerative)
(1974): Holt PJA+, *BMJ* 3, 234
(1973): Almeyda J+, *Br J Dermatol* 88, 313
(1971): Almeyda J+, *Br J Dermatol* 85, 604
(1971): Stevenson CJ, *Br J Dermatol* 85, 600
Lichen planus
(1994): Thompson DF+, *Pharmacotherapy* 14, 561
(1979): Krebs A, *Hautarzt* (German) 30, 281
(1974): Burry JN+, *Br J Dermatol* 91, 475
Lupus erythematosus (<1%)
(1995): Sakurai Y+, *Nippon Naika Gakkai Zasshi* (Japanese) 84, 2069
(1992): Skaer TL, *Clin Ther* 14, 496
(1989): Nordstrom DM+, *Arthritis Rheum* 32, 205
(1985): Stratton MA, *Clin Pharm* 4, 657
(1985): Cush JJ+, *Am J Med Sci* 290, 36
(1983): Homberg JC+, *J Pharmacol* (French) 14, 61
(1982): Dupont A+, *BMJ* 2, 693

(1981): Harrington TM+, *Chest* 79, 696
(1977): Schubothe H+, *Immun Infekt* (German) 5, 142
(1974): Gustavsen WR, *Tidsskr Nor Laegeforen* (Norwegian) 94, 22
(1972): Dorfmann H+, *Nouv Presse Med* (French) 1, 2907
(1967): Sherman JD+, *Arch Intern Med* 120, 321

Papulo-vesicular eruption
(1977): Heid E+, *Ann Dermatol Venereol* (French) 104, 494

Parkinsonism

Peripheral edema (>10%)

Petechiae
(1978): Furhoff AK, *Acta Med Scand* 203, 425

Photosensitivity
(1988): Vaillant L+, *Arch Dermatol* 124, 326
(1973): Almeyda J+, *Br J Dermatol* 88, 313

Pigmentation
(1986): Brody HJ+, *Cutis* 38, 187
(1973): Almeyda J+, *Br J Dermatol* 88, 313
(1969): Varadi DP+, *Arch Intern Med* 124, 13

Pruritus
(1973): Almeyda J+, *Br J Dermatol* 88, 313

Purpura
(1971): Menohitharajah SM+, *BMJ* 1, 494

Rash (sic) (<1%)

Seborrheic dermatitis
(1974): Church R, *Br J Dermatol* 91, 373
(1974): Burry JN+, *Br J Dermatol* 91, 475
(1973): Church R, *Br J Dermatol* 89, 10

Stevens–Johnson syndrome
(1985): Ting HC+, *Int J Dermatol* 24, 587

Toxic epidermal necrolysis

Urticaria
(1986): Gidseg G, *S Med J* 79, 389
(1978): Furhoff AK, *Acta Med Scand* 203, 425

Vasculitis
(1989): Matteson EL+, *Arthritis Rheum* 32, 356

Hair

Hair – alopecia

Other

Acute intermittent porphyria

Black tongue (<1%)
(1986): Brody HJ+, *Cutis* 38, 137

Galactorrhea
(1963): Pettinger WA+, *BMJ* 1, 1460

Glossodynia

Gynecomastia (<1%)

Hypersensitivity
(1993): Wolf R+, *Ann Allergy* 71, 166

Myalgia

Oral lichenoid eruption
(1988): Zain RB+, *Dent J Malays* 10, 15
(1982): Brooks SL, *J Oral Med* 37, 42

Oral mucosal eruption
(1973): Almeyda J+, *Br J Dermatol* 88, 313

Oral ulceration
(1990): Espana A+, *Med Clin (Barc)* (Spanish) 94, 559 (lichenoid)
(1980): McLellan GH+, *Clin Prevent Dent* 2, 18
(1978): Hay KD+, *Br Dent J* 145, 195
(1974): Burry JN+, *Br J Dermatol* 91, 475
(1971): Stevenson CJ, *Br J Dermatol* 85, 600
(1967): Mackie BS, *Br J Dermatol* 79, 106 (LIP)

Paresthesias (<1%)

Xerostomia (1–10%)
(1969): Varadi DP+, *Arch Intern Med* 124, 13

METHYLPHENIDATE

Trade names: Methylin (Mallinckrodt); Ritalin (Novartis)
Other common trade names: *Centedrin; Rilatine; Rubifen*
Indications: Attention deficit disorder; narcolepsy
Category: Central nervous system stimulant
Half-life: 2–4 hours
Clinically important, potentially serious interactions with: caffeine, CNS stimulants, guanethidine, MAO inhibitors, phenobarbital, phenytoin, primidone, tricyclic antidepressants, warfarin

Reactions

Skin

Angioedema
(1977): Sverd J+, *Pediatrics* 59, 115
(1972): Rothschild CJ+, *Can Med Assoc J* 106, 1064

Delusions of parasitosis
(1999): Eisner J, (from Internet) (observation)

Diaphoresis

Edema (eyelids)
(1972): Rothschild CJ+, *Can Med Assoc J* 106, 1064

Eosinophilic syndrome
(1978): Wolf J+, *Ann Intern Med* 89, 224

Erythema multiforme

Exanthems
(1977): Sverd J+, *Pediatrics* 59, 115

Exfoliative dermatitis
(1977): Sverd J+, *Pediatrics* 59, 115
(1968): Weil AJ, *Ann Allergy* 26, 402

Fixed eruption
(1992): Cohen HA+, *Ann Pharmacother* 26, 1378 (scrotum)

Photosensitivity
(1977): Sverd J+, *Pediatrics* 59, 115

Pruritus

Purpura
(1978): Wolf J+, *Ann Intern Med* 89, 224

Rash (sic) (<1%)

Urticaria
(1977): Sverd J+, *Pediatrics* 59, 115

Vasculitis
(1977): Sverd J+, *Pediatrics* 59, 115

Hair

Hair – alopecia

Other

Bruxism
(2000): Gara L+, *J Child Adolesc Psychopharmacol* 10, 39 (with valproic acid)

Hypersensitivity (1–10%)
(1990): Calis KA+, *Clin Pharm* 9, 632

Injection-site abscess
(1976): Elenbaas RM+, *JACEP* 5, 977

Tourette's syndrome

Xerostomia
(1993): Pataki CS+, *J Am Acad Child Adolesc Psychiatry* 32, 1065

METHYLTESTOSTERONE

Trade names: Android (ICN); Estratest (Solvay); Metandren; Oreton (ICN); Testred (ICN); Virilon (Star)
Other common trade names: *Androral; Enarmon; Teston; Testotonic "B"; Testovis; Viromone*
Indications: Hypogonadism; impotence; metastatic breast cancer
Category: Androgen; antineoplastic
Half-life: 2.5–3.5 hours
Clinically important, potentially serious interactions with: anticoagulants, cyclosporine, imipramine

Reactions

Skin

Acanthosis nigricans
(1987): Shuttleworth D+, *Clin Exp Dermatol* 12, 288
Acne (>10%)
(1992): Fryand O+, *Acta Derm Venereol* 72, 148
(1990): Fuchs E+, *J Am Acad Dermatol* 23, 125
(1989): Hartmann AA+, *Monatsschr Kinderheilkd* (German) 137, 466
(1989): Fryand O+, *Tidsskr Nor Laegeforen* (Norwegian) 109, 239
(1989): von Muhlendahl KE+, *Dtsch Med Wochenschr* (German) 114, 712
(1989): Heydenreich G, *Arch Dermatol* 125, 571 (fulminans)
(1989): Scott MJ+, *Cutis* 44, 30
(1988): Traupe H+, *Arch Dermatol* 124, 414 (fulminans)
(1987): Kiraly CL+, *Am J Dermatopathol* 9, 515
(1984): Lamb DR, *Am J Sports Med* 12, 31
(1965): Rook A, *Br J Dermatol* 77, 115
(1965): Kennedy BJ, *J Am Geriatr Soc* 13, 230
Contact dermatitis
(1989): Holdiness MR, *Contact Dermatitis* 20, 3 (from patch)
Edema (>10%)
Exanthems
Flushing (1–5%)
(1965): Kennedy BJ, *J Am Geriatr Soc* 13, 230
Furunculosis
(1989): Scott MJ+, *Cutis* 44, 30
Lichenoid eruption
(1989): Aihara M+, *J Dermatol* (Tokio) 16, 330
Lupus erythematosus
(1978): Robinson HM, *Z Haut* (German) 53, 349
Pruritus
Psoriasis
(1990): O'Driscoll JB+, *Clin Exp Dermatol* 15, 68
Purpura
Seborrhea
Seborrheic dermatitis
(1989): Scott MJ+, *Cutis* 44, 30
Striae
(1989): Scott MJ+, *Cutis* 44, 30
Urticaria

Hair

Hair – alopecia
(1989): Scott MJ+, *Cutis* 44, 30
(1965): Kennedy BJ, *J Am Geriatr Soc* 13, 230
Hair – hirsutism (1–10%) (in females)
(1994): Castillo-Ceballos A+, *Med Clin (Barc)* (Spanish) 102, 78
(1991): Bates GW+, *Clin Obstet Gynecol* 34, 848
(1991): No Author, *Obstet Gynecol* 78, 474
(1991): Parker LU+, *Cleve Clin J Med* 58, 43
(1991): Urman B+, *Obstet Gynecol* 77, 595
(1989): Scott MJ+, *Cutis* 44, 30
(1974): Baron J, *Zentralbl Gynakol* (German) 96, 129
(1971): Fusi S+, *Folia Endocrinol* (Italian) 24, 412
(1965): Kennedy BJ, *J Am Geriatr Soc* 13, 230

Other

Anaphylactoid reaction
Gynecomastia (<1%)
Hypersensitivity (<1%)
Injection-site pain
Mastodynia (>10%)
Paresthesias
Priapism (>10%)
Stomatitis

METHYSERGIDE

Trade name: Sansert (Novartis)
Other common trade names: *Deseril; Desernil; Deserril; Deseryl*
Indications: Vascular (migraine) headaches
Category: Vascular headache prophylactic; ergot alkaloid
Half-life: 10 hours
Clinically important, potentially serious interactions with: beta-blockers, clarithromycin, ergot alkaloids, erythromycin, nicotine, troleandomycin

Reactions

Skin

Collagenosis (sic)
(1973): Anker N, *Ugeskr Laeger* (Danish) 135, 2225
Exanthems
Flushing
(1964): Graham JR, *N Engl J Med* 270, 67 (0.8%)
Hypermelanosis
(1964): Graham JR, *N Engl J Med* 270, 67
Lupus erythematosus
(1968): Racouchot J+, *Bull Soc Franc Dermatol Syphiligr* (French) 75, 513
(1968): Racouchot J+, *Lyon Med* (French) 220, 1766
Orange-peel skin (sic)
(1964): Graham JR, *N Engl J Med* 270, 67 (1%)
Peripheral edema (1–10%)
Pruritus
Rash (sic) (1–10%)
Raynaud's phenomenon
Scleroderma
(1984): Garcia de Quesada FJ+, *Med Clin (Barc)* (Spanish) 82, 604
(1980): Graham JR, *Trans Am Clin Climatol Assoc* 92, 122
(1978): Goldberg NC+, *Arch Dermatol* 114, 550
Skin reactions (sic)
(1991): Mylecharane EJ, *J Neurol* 238, S45
Telangiectases
Urticaria

Hair

Hair – alopecia
(1991): Mylecharane EJ, *J Neurol* 238, S45
(1974): Sadjadpour K, *JAMA* 229, 639
(1964): Graham JR, *N Engl J Med* 270, 67 (1%)
(1964): Leyton N, *Lancet* 1, 830 (0.4%)

Other

Hyperesthesia (<1%)
Myalgia
Paresthesias

METOCLOPRAMIDE

Trade name: Reglan (Robins)
Other common trade names: *Apo-Metoclop; Duraclamid; Emex; Gastrocil; Gastronerton; Maxeran; Maxolon; Mygdalon; Primperan*
Indications: Gastroesophageal reflux
Category: Dopaminergic blocking agent; peristaltic stimulant; antiemetic
Half-life: 4–6 hours
Clinically important, potentially serious interactions with: alcohol, CNS depressants, cyclosporine, digoxin, levodopa, opiate analgesics, procainamide, quinidine, succinylcholine, tacrine

Reactions

Skin

Allergic reactions (sic)
(1986): Bigby M+, *JAMA* 256, 3358
Angioedema
(1983): Pinder RM+, *Drugs* 25, 451
(1976): Pinder RM+, *Drugs* 12, 81
Exanthems
(1983): Pinder RM+, *Drugs* 25, 451
(1976): Pinder RM+, *Drugs* 12, 81
(1976): Arndt KA+, *JAMA* 235, 918 (0.4%)
Flushing
Parkinsonism
Rash (sic) (1–10%)
Urticaria
(1983): Pinder RM+, *Drugs* 25, 451
(1976): Pinder RM+, *Drugs* 12, 81

Other

Blue tongue
(1989): Alroe C+, *Med J Aust* 150, 724
Galactorrhea
Gynecomastia
(1997): Madani S+, *J Clin Gastroenterol* 24, 79
Mastodynia (1–10%)
Paresthesias
(1997): du Bois A+, *Oncology* 54, 7
Porphyria
(1997): Gorchein A, *Lancet* 350, 1104
(1981): Doss M+, *Lancet* 2, 91
Xerostomia (1–10%)

METOLAZONE

Trade names: Mykrox (Medeva); Zaroxolyn (Medeva)
Other common trade names: *Barolyn; Diondel; Metenix 5; Normelan; Xuret*
Indications: Hypertension, edema
Category: Sulfonamide* diuretic; antihypertensive
Half-life: 6–20 hours
Clinically important, potentially serious interactions with: ACE-inhibitors, antidiabetics, beta-blockers, bumetanide, cyclosporine, diazoxide, digoxin, furosemide, lithium, methotrexate, NSAIDs, sulfonylureas

Reactions

Skin

Chills (1–10%)
Edema (<2%)
Exanthems
Exfoliative dermatitis
Necrotizing angiitis
Photosensitivity (<2%)
Pruritus (<2%)
Purpura (<1%)
Rash (sic) (<2%)
Stevens–Johnson syndrome
Toxic epidermal necrolysis
(1991): Lacy JA, *Nutr Clin Pract* 6, 18
Urticaria (<2%)
Vasculitis
(1991): Cox NH+, *Postgrad Med J* 67, 860
(1982): Weinrauch LA+, *Cutis* 30, 83
Xerosis (<2%)

Other

Anaphylactoid reaction (<2%)
Dysgeusia (<2%)
Paresthesias (<2%)
Xanthopsia (<2%)
Xerostomia (<2%)

***Note:** Metolazone is a sulfonamide and can be absorbed systemically. Sulfonamides can produce severe, possibly fatal, reactions such as toxic epidermal necrolysis and Stevens–Johnson syndrome.

METOPROLOL

Trade names: Lopressor (Novartis); Toprol XL (AstraZeneca)
Other common trade names: *Beloc-Zoc; Betaloc; Betazok; Kenaprol; Mycol; Prolaken; Ritmolol; Seloken-Zok; Selozok*
Indications: Hypertension; angina pectoris
Category: Beta-adrenergic blocker; antihypertensive
Half-life: 3–4 hours
Clinically important, potentially serious interactions with: barbiturates, calcium channel blockers, cimetidine, clonidine, diltiazem, diphenhydramine, flecainide, fluoxetine, hydralazine, lidocaine, nifedipine, NSAIDs, oral contraceptives, prazosin, propafenone, quinidine, rifampin, salicylates, sulfonylureas, terazosin, verapamil

Note: Cutaneous side-effects of beta-receptor blockaders are clinically polymorphous. They apparently appear after several months of continuous therapy. Atypical psoriasiform, lichen planus-like, and eczematous chronic rashes are mainly observed. (1983): Hödl St, *Z Hautkr* (German) 58, 17.

Lopressor HCT is metoprolol and hydrochlorothiazide

Reactions

Skin

Angioedema
(1994): Krikorian RK+, *Chest* 106, 1922
Diaphoresis
Eczematous eruption (sic)
(1981): Neumann HAM+, *Dermatologica* 162, 330
(1979): Neumann HAM+, *Lancet* 2, 745
Edema
Erythema multiforme
Exanthems
(1986): Benfield P+, *Drugs* 31, 376 (1.5%)
Exfoliative dermatitis
Gangrene (feet)
(1979): Gokal R+, *BMJ* 19, 837
Hyperkeratosis (palms and soles)
Lichenoid eruption
(1988): Kardaun SH+, *Br J Dermatol* 118, 545
(1983): Hödl St, *Z Hautkr* (German) 58, 17
(1978): Savage RL+, *BMJ* 1, 987
Lupus erythematosus
(1981): Paladini G, *Int J Tissue React* 3, 95
Peripheral edema (1%)
Pigmentation
Pityriasis rubra pilaris
(1978): Finlay AY+, *BMJ* 1, 987
Prurigo
(1983): Hödl St, *Z Hautkr* (German) 58, 17
Pruritus (1–5%)
(1994): Shelley WB+, *Cutis* 53, 39 (scalp) (observation)
(1986): Benfield P+, *Drugs* 31, 376

Purpura
Psoriasis (induction and aggravation of)
(1993): Litt JZ, Beachwood, OH, personal case (observation)
(1988): Heng MCY+, *Int J Dermatol* 27, 619 (pustular, generalized)
(1987): Altomare GF+, *G Ital Dermatol Venereol* (Italian) 122, 531
(1986): Czernielewski J+, *Lancet* 1, 808
(1986): Abel EA+, *J Am Acad Dermatol* 15, 1007
(1984): Arntzen N+, *Acta Derm Venereol* (Stockh) 64, 346
(1981): Neumann HAM+, *Dermatologica* 162, 330
(1979): Neumann HAM+, *Lancet* 2, 745
Rash (sic)(<5%)
Raynaud's phenomenon (<1%)
(1984): Eliasson K+, *Acta Med Scand* 215, 333
(1976): Marshall AJ+, *BMJ* 1, 1498
Scleroderma
(1980): Graham JR, *Trans Am Clin Climatol Assoc* 92, 122
Toxic epidermal necrolysis
Urticaria
Xerosis

Hair
Hair – alopecia
(1981): Graeber CW+, *Cutis* 28, 633

Nails
Nails – bluish
Nails – dystrophy
Nails – onycholysis
Nails – transverse depression (sic)
(1981): Graeber CW+, *Cutis* 28, 633

Other
Dysgeusia
Oculo-mucocutaneous syndrome
(1982): Cocco G+, *Curr Ther Res* 31, 362
Oral lichenoid eruption
Paresthesias
Peyronie's disease
(1981): Neumann HAM+, *Dermatologica* 162, 330
(1981): Paladini G, *Int J Tissue React* 3, 95
(1981): Jones HA+, *Med J Aust* 2, 514
(1979): Pryor JP+, *Lancet* 1, 331
(1977): Yudkin JS, *Lancet* 2, 1355
Polymyalgia
(1991): Snyder S, *Ann Intern Med* 114, 96
Scalp tingling
(1979): Coulter DM, *N Z Med J* 90, 397

METRONIDAZOLE

Trade names: Flagyl (Searle); Metrocream (Galderma); Metrogel (Galderma); Metrolotion (Galderma); Noritate (Dermik); Protostat; Satric
Other common trade names: *Arilin; Ariline; Asuzol; Clont; Fossyol; Milezzol; Nida Gel; Novo-Nidazol; Otrozol; Rozagel; Rozex; Trikacide; Zadstat*
Indications: Various infections caused by susceptible organisms, rosacea
Category: Antiprotozoal, anthelmintic and antibiotic
Half-life: 6–12 hours
Clinically important, potentially serious interactions with: alcohol, anticoagulants, astemizole, barbiturates, cimetidine, disulfiram, fluorouracil, phenobarbital, phenytoin, terfenadine, warfarin

Reactions

Skin
Acute generalized exanthematous pustulosis (AGEP)
(1999): Watsky KL, *Arch Dermatol* 135, 93
(1994): Manders SM+, *Cutis* 54, 194 (with cefazolin)
Angioedema
(1978): Shevliakov LV, *Vestn Dermatol Venerol* (Russian) February, 49
Candidiasis (exacerbation)
(1977): Maize JC+, *Arch Dermatol* 113, 1457 (passim)
Contact dermatitis
(1997): Vincenzi C+, *Contact Dermatitis* 36, 116
Erythema
Exanthems
(1995): Litt JZ, Beachwood, OH, personal case (observation)
(1977): Swami B+, *Curr Med Res Opin* 5, 152 (1–5%)
(1969): *Med Lett* 11, 27 (1–5%)
Fixed eruption
(1998): Thami GP+, *Dermatology* 196, 368
(1990): Gaffoor PMA+, *Cutis* 45, 242
(1990): Kanwar AJ+, *Dermatologica* 180, 277
(1990): Mishra D+, *Int J Dermatol* 29, 740
(1987): Shelley WB+, *Cutis* 39, 393
(1977): Naik RPC+, *Dermatologica* 155, 59
Flushing
(1992): Shelley WB+, *Advanced Dermatologic Diagnosis*, WB Saunders, 582 (passim)
(1977): Maize JC+, *Arch Dermatol* 113, 1457 (passim)
Pityriasis rosea
(1977): Maize JC+, *Arch Dermatol* 113, 1457
Pruritus (1–5%)
(1977): Maize JC+, *Arch Dermatol* 113, 1457 (passim)
(1977): Swami B+, *Curr Med Res Opin* 5, 152 (10%)
(1963): Foster SA+, *Am J Obstet Gynecol* 87, 1013
Rash (sic)
Toxic epidermal necrolysis
(1981): Titov RL, *Klin Med Mosk* (Russian) 59, 85
Urticaria
(1997): Blumenthal HL, Beachwood, OH, personal case (observation)
(1977): Maize JC+, *Arch Dermatol* 113, 1457 (passim)
(1963): Foster SA+, *Am J Obstet Gynecol* 87, 1013

Other
Acute intermittent porphyria
Disulfiram-type reaction
Dysgeusia (<1%) (metallic taste)
(1997): Palop Larrea V+, *Aten Primaria* (Spanish) 20, 524
Glossitis
(1987): Shelley WB+, *Cutis* 39, 393
Gynecomastia
(1985): Fagan TC+, *JAMA* 254, 3217
Hypersensitivity (<1%)
Injection-site vasculitis
Oral mucosal eruption
(1969): *Med Lett* 11, 27
Oral ulceration
Paresthesias
Serum sickness
(1983): Weart CW+, *South Med J* 76, 410
Stomatitis
(1987): Shelley WB+, *Cutis* 39, 393
Thrombophlebitis (<1%)
Tongue furry (<1%)
(1987): Shelley WB+, *Cutis* 39, 393
(1977): Maize JC+, *Arch Dermatol* 113, 1457 (passim)
Vaginal candidiasis (<1%)
Xerostomia (<1%)

MEXILETINE

Trade name: Mexitil (Boehringer Ingelheim)
Other common trade names: *Mexihexal; Mexilen; Mexitec*
Indications: Ventricular arrhythmias
Category: Antiarrhythmic (class I-b)
Half-life: 10–12 hours
Clinically important, potentially serious interactions with: allopurinol, atropine, caffeine, cimetidine, metoclopramide, phenytoin, rifampin, theophylline

Reactions

Skin
Diaphoresis (<1%)
Edema (3.8%)

Exanthems
(1997): Higa K+, *Pain* 73, 97
(1996): Nagayama H+, *J Dermatol* 23, 899
(1992): Habot B+, *Harefuah* (Hebrew) 123, 462
(1991): Kikuchi K+, *Contact Dermatitis* 25, 70
(1988): Kardaun SH+, *Br J Dermatol* 118, 545
(1984): Ribera Pibernat M+, *Med Clin (Barc)* (Spanish) 83, 825
(1979): Habeler G+, *Dtsch Med Wochenschr* (German) 104, 1244
Exfoliative dermatitis (<1%)
Hot flashes (<1%)
Lupus erythematosus (<1%)
Pruritus
(1997): Higa K+, *Pain* 73, 97
Purpura
Rash (sic) (3.8%)
Stevens–Johnson syndrome (<1%)
Urticaria
(1994): Yamazaki S+, *Br J Dermatol* 130, 538
(1988): Kardaun SH+, *Br J Dermatol* 118, 545
Xerosis (<1%)

Hair

Hair – alopecia (<1%)

Other

Dysgeusia (<1%)
(2000): Zervakis J+, *Physiol Behav* 68, 405
Paresthesias (3.8%)
Salivary changes (sic) (<1%)
Trembling (1–10%)
Tremor (12.6%)
Xerostomia (2.8%)

MEZLOCILLIN

Trade name: Mezlin (Bayer)
Other common trade name: *Baypen*
Indications: Various infections caused by susceptible organisms
Category: Beta-lactamase-sensitive penicillin antibiotic
Half-life: 0.8–1.0 hours
Clinically important, potentially serious interactions with:
cyclosporine, heparin, methotrexate, probenecid, tetracycline

Reactions

Skin

Allergic reactions (sic)
(1994): Pleasants RA+, *Chest* 106, 1124 (in patients with cystic fibrosis)
Angioedema
Bullous eruption
Contact dermatitis
(1992): Keller K+, *Contact Dermatitis* 27, 348
Ecchymoses
Erythema multiforme
Erythema nodosum
Exanthems
Exfoliative dermatitis (<1%)
Hematomas
Jarisch–Herxheimer reaction
Pruritus
Rash (sic) (<1%)
Stevens–Johnson syndrome
Toxic epidermal necrolysis
Urticaria
Vasculitis

Other

Anaphylactoid reaction
Black tongue
Dysgeusia
Glossitis
Glossodynia
Hypersensitivity
(1992): Keller K+, *Contact Dermatitis* 27, 348
Injection-site pain
Oral candidiasis
Phlebitis
Serum sickness (<1%)
Stomatitis
Stomatodynia
Thrombophlebitis
Vaginitis
Xerostomia

MIBEFRADIL*

Trade name: Posicor (Roche)
Indications: Hypertension, angina
Category: Calcium channel ion influx inhibitor
Half-life: 17–25 hours
Clinically important, potentially serious interactions with:
astemizole, cisapride, cyclosporine, diltiazem, lovastatin, metoprolol, propranolol, quinidine, simvastatin, terfenadine, tricyclic antidepressants, verapamil

Reactions

Skin

Allergic reactions (sic) (>1%)
Angioedema (<1%)
Diaphoresis (<1%)
Exfoliative dermatitis (<1%)
Flushing (>1%)
Leg edema (4%)
(1997): Kobrin I+, *Am J Cardiol* 80, 40C
(1997): Massie BM+, *Am J Cardiol* 80, 27C
Pedal edema (5.1%)
(1997): Kobrin I+, *Am J Cardiol* 80, 40C
Peripheral edema
Rash (sic) (<1%)

Other

Paresthesias (<1%)

***Note:** Mibefradil has been withdrawn in the USA

MICONAZOLE

Trade names: Monistat (Ortho); Monistat-Derm (Ortho)
Other common trade names: *Aflorix; Aloid; Daktarin; Florid; Funcort; Fungoid Tincture, Micotef; Miracol; Monazole-7; Zole, etc.*
Indications: Fungal infections
Category: Imidazole antifungal
Half-life: initial: 40 minutes; terminal: 24 hours
Clinically important, potentially serious interactions with:
amphotericin B, anticoagulants, astemizole, carbamazepine, cisapride, cyclosporine, isoniazid, phenytoin, rifampin, sulfonylureas, terfenadine, warfarin

Reactions

Skin

Angioedema
(1983): Stevens DA, *Drugs* 26, 347 (2.4%)
Bullous eruption
(1983): Stevens DA, *Drugs* 26, 347
Chills (>5%)
Contact dermatitis
(1996): Fernandez L+, *Contact Dermatitis* 34, 217
(1995): Goday JJ+, *Contact Dermatitis* 32, 370
(1991): Baes H, *Contact Dermatitis* 24, 89

(1988): Perret CM+, *Contact Dermatitis* 19, 75
(1988): Raulin C+, *Contact Dermatitis* 18, 76
(1984): Aldridge RD+, *Contact Dermatitis* 10, 58
(1983): Frenzel UH+, *Contact Dermatitis* 9, 74
(1982): Foged EK+, *Contact Dermatitis* 8, 284
(1979): Wade TR+, *Contact Dermatitis* 5, 168
(1977): Samsoen M+, *Contact Dermatitis* 3, 351
(1975): Degreef H+, *Contact Dermatitis* 1, 269

Erythema
Exanthems
(1987): Verhagen C+, *Eur J Haematol* 38, 225 (28%)
(1983): Stevens DA, *Drugs* 26, 347 (2.4%)
(1980): Heel RC+, *Drugs* 19, 7 (3–8%)
(1977): Fischer TJ+, *J Pediatr* 91, 815 (10%)
(1977): Sung JP+, *N Engl J Med* 297, 786 (87%)
Flushing (<1%)
(1983): Stevens DA, *Drugs* 26, 347
(1980): Heel RC+, *Drugs* 19, 7 (1–2%)
Pruritus (21%)
(1983): Stevens DA, *Drugs* 26, 347 (36%)
(1980): Heel RC+, *Drugs* 19, 7 (2–21%)
(1977): Fischer TJ+, *J Pediatr* 91, 815 (21%)
Purpura
(1980): Heel RC+, *Drugs* 19, 7 (3–8%)
Rash (sic) (9%)
Urticaria
(1983): Stevens DA, *Drugs* 26, 347 (2.4%)
Xanthomas
(1978): Barr RJ+, *Arch Dermatol* 114, 1544 (eruptive)

Other

Anaphylactoid reaction
Injection-site pain (>10%)
(1980): Heel RC+, *Drugs* 19, 7 (0.5–2%)
Phlebitis (>5%)
(1983): Stevens DA, *Drugs* 26, 347 (35%)
(1980): Heel RC+, *Drugs* 19, 7 (6–28%)
(1977): Fischer TJ+, *J Pediatr* 91, 815 (79%)

MIDAZOLAM

Trade name: Versed (Roche)
Other common trade name: *Dormicum*
Indications: Preoperative sedation
Category: Benzodiazepine, sedative-hypnotic; anesthetic
Half-life: 1–4 hours
Clinically important, potentially serious interactions with: alcohol, amprenavir, barbiturates, cimetidine, clarithromycin, CNS depressants, diltiazem, fluvoxamine, itraconazole, narcotics, nelfinavir, propofol, ritonavir, theophylline, valproic acid, verapamil

Reactions

Skin

Angioedema
(1992): Yakel DL+, *Crit Care Med* 20, 307
Exanthems
Peripheral edema (<1%)
Pruritus (<1%)
(1989): Yates A+, *Anaesthesia* 44, 449
Rash (sic) (<1%)
Urticaria (<1%)

Other

Anaphylactoid reaction (<1%)
Dysgeusia (<1%) (acid taste)
Injection-site pain (>10%)
(1984): Dundee JW+, *Drugs* 28, 519 (26%)
Injection-site reactions (>10%)
Localized flare reaction
(1993): Kundrotas L+, *Gastrointest Endosc* 39, 109
Paresthesias
Sialorrhea (<1%)

MIFEPRISTONE

Synonym: RU-486
Trade name: Mifeprex (Danco)
Indications: Medical termination of intrauterine pregnancy
Category: Abortifacient; glucocorticoid antagonist
Half-life: ~20 hours
Clinically important, potentially serious interactions with*: carbamazepine, dexamethasone, erythromycin, itraconazole, ketoconazole, phenobarbital, phenytoin, rifampin, **grapefruit juice, St. John's wort**

Reactions

Skin

Chills (3%)
Viral infections (4%)

Other

Vaginal bleeding (~100%)
Vaginitis (3%)

***Note:** Although specific drug or food interactions have not been studied, on the basis of mifepristone's metabolism of CYP 3A4, it is possible that these drugs and products may inhibit its metabolism (increasing serum levels of mifepristone)

MIGLITOL

Trade name: Glyset (Pharmacia & Upjohn)
Indications: Non-insulin dependent diabetes type II
Category: Antidiabetic (alpha-glucosidase inhibitor)
Half-life: ~2 hours
Clinically important, potentially serious interactions with: corticosteroids, digestive enzymes, digoxin, diuretics, propranolol, ranitidine, thyroid

Reactions

Skin

Rash (sic) (1–10%)

MINOCYCLINE

Trade names: Dynacin (Medicis); Minocin (Lederle)
Other common trade names: *Alti-Minocycline; Apo-Minocycline; Mestacine; Minoclir 50; Minogalen; Minomycin; Mynocine; Syn-Minocycline*
Indications: Various infections caused by susceptible organisms
Category: Tetracycline antibiotic
Half-life: 11–23 hours
Clinically important, potentially serious interactions with: antacids, anticoagulants, carbamazepine, corticosteroids, digoxin, insulin, iron salts, isotretinoin, oral contraceptives, penicillins, phenytoin, retinoids, vitamin A, warfarin, **herbals such as goldenseal, barberry, and Oregon grape**

Reactions

Skin

Acute febrile neutrophilic dermatosis (Sweet's syndrome)
(1992): Thibault M-J+, *J Am Acad Dermatol* 27, 801
(1991): Mensing H+, *Dermatologica* 182, 43
Acute generalized exanthematous pustulosis (AGEP)
(1997): Yamamoto T+, *Acta Derm Venereol* (Stockh) 77, 168 (in a patient with pustular psoriasis)
Angioedema
(1997): Shapiro LE+, *Arch Dermatol* 133, 1224

(1994): Levy SB, Chapel Hill, NC, personal case, reproducible (observation)
(1993): Litt JZ, Beachwood, OH, personal case (observation)

Candidiasis

Cellulitis
(1994): Kaufmann D+, *Arch Intern Med* 154, 1983
(1989): Andreano JM+, *J Am Acad Dermatol* 20, 934

Eosinophilic pustular folliculitis (Ofuji's disease)
(1989): Andreano JM+, *J Am Acad Dermatol* 20, 934

Erythema multiforme
(1987): Shoji A+, *Arch Dermatol* 123, 18

Erythema nodosum
(1990): Bridges AJ+, *J Am Acad Dermatol* 22, 959

Exanthems
(1996): Knowles SR+, *Arch Dermatol* 132, 934
(1995): Litt JZ, Beachwood, OH, 2 personal cases, mother and daughter (observation)
(1995): Karofsky PS+, *Arch Pediatr Adolesc Med* 149, 217
(1994): Kaufmann D+, *Arch Intern Med* 154, 1983
(1975): Brogden RN+, *Drugs* 9, 251
(1973): Shelley WB+, *JAMA* 224, 125

Exfoliative dermatitis (<1%)
(1997): MacNeil M+, *J Am Acad Dermatol* 36, 347
(1996): Knowles SR+, *Arch Dermatol* 132, 934
(1989): Davies MG+, *BMJ* 298, 1523

Fixed eruption (<1%)
(1994): Chu P+, *J Am Acad Dermatol* 30, 802 (pigmentation)
(1984): Bargman H, *J Am Acad Dermatol* 11, 900
(1983): LePaw MI, *J Am Acad Dermatol* 8, 263
(1978): Jolly HW+, *Arch Dermatol* 114, 1484
(1977): Shimizu Y+, *Jpn J Dermatol* 4, 73

Folliculitis
(1994): Kaufmann D+, *Arch Intern Med* 154, 1983 (pustular)
(1989): Andreano JM+, *J Am Acad Dermatol* 20, 934

Lichenoid eruption
(1993): Litt JZ, Beachwood, OH, personal case (observation)

Livedo reticularis
(2000): Schlienger RG+, *Dermatology* 200, 223

Lupus erythematosus
(2000): Dunphy J+, *Br J Dermatol* 142, 461
(2000): Schlienger RG+, *Dermatology* 200, 223 (57 cases)
(1999): Sturkenboom MC+, *Arch Intern Med* 159, 493
(1999): Dadamessi I+, *Rev Med Interne* (French) 20, 930
(1999): Piette AM+, *Rev Med Interne* (French) 20, 869
(1999): Angulo JM+, *J Rheumatol* 26, 1420
(1999): Elkayam O+, *Semin Arthritis Rheum* 28, 392
(1999): Katz R, *Skin and Allergy News*, May, 13
(1999): Tournigand C+, *Lupus* 8, 773
(1999): Thaler D, Monona, WI (from Internet) (observation)
(1998): Blumenthal HL, Beachwood, OH, personal case (observation)
(1998): Akin E+, *Pediatrics* 101, 926
(1998): Angulo JM+, *Semin Arthritis Rheum* 28, 187
(1998): Knights SE+, *Clin Exp Dermatol* 16, 587
(1997): Singer SJ+, *JAMA* 277, 295
(1997): Hoefnagel JJ+, *Ned Tijdschr Geneeskd* 141, 1424
(1997): Wilde JL+, *Arch Dermatol* 133, 1344
(1997): Golstein PE+, *Am J Gastroenterol* 92, 143
(1997): Crosson J+, *J Am Acad Dermatol* 36, 867
(1997): Farver DK, *Ann Pharmacother* 31, 1160
(1997): Pointud P, *J Rheumatol* 24, 1851
(1997): Emery P+, *J Rheumatol* 24, 1850
(1996): Knowles SR+, *Arch Dermatol* 132, 934
(1996): Hewack J, *Gastroenterology* 110, A1211
(1996): Gough A+, *BMJ* 312, 169 (18 cases)
(1996): Masson C+, *J Rheumatol* 23, 2160
(1995): Gendi NS+, *Br J Rheumatol* 34, 584
(1995): Bulgen DY, *Br J Rheumatol* 34, 398
(1995): Gordon P+, *Br J Dermatol* 132, 120
(1994): Byrne PA+, *Br J Rheumatol* 33, 674
(1994): Quilty B+, *Br J Rheumatol* 33, 1197
(1994): Inoue CN+, *Eur J Pediatr* 153, 540
(1992): Matsuura T+, *Lancet* 340, 1553
(1984): Alston LL, *The Schoch Letter* 34, #8, Item 110

Nodules (facial, blue-gray)
(1998): Dawe RS+, *Arch Dermatol* 134, 861

Petechiae
(2000): Warshaw E, Minneapolis, MN *The Schoch Letter* 50, February #16

Photosensitivity (1–10%)
(1996): Goulden V+, *Br J Dermatol* 134, 693
(1996): Uhlemann J, St. Charles, MO (from Internet) (observation)
(1996): Wegman A, Sydney, Australia (from Internet) (observation)
(1996): Carrington PR, Little Rock, AR (from Internet) (observation) (from tanning bed)
(1994): Litt JZ, Beachwood, OH, personal case (observation)
(1990): Black AK+, *Br J Dermatol* 123, 277 (observation)
(1985): Basler RSW, *Arch Dermatol* 121. 606
(1972): Frost P+, *Arch Dermatol* 105, 681

Pigmentation
(2000): Ozog DM+, *Arch Dermatol* 136, 1133 (7 cases; all with pemphigus or pemphigoid)
(2000): Mouton RW, Poster Exhibit at University of Vienna clinical dermatology meeting (bluish)
(2000): Joseph WS+, *J Am Podiatr Med Assoc* 90, 268
(1999): Gregg LJ, Tulsa, OK (from Internet) (observation)
(1999): Frederickson K, Novalo, CA (from Internet) (observation)
(1999): Pepper, M, Madison, WI, *The Schoch Letter* 49, 25 (linear purple streaks of back)
(1999): Frederickson K, Novato, CA (from Internet) (observation)
(1999): Koester GA, Edmond, OK (from Internet) (observation)
(1999): Aylesworth RJ, Rhinelander, WI (from Internet) (observation)
(1999): Drayton GE, Los Angeles, CA (from Internet) (observation)
(1999): Lycka BAS, Edmonton, Alberta (from Internet) (observation)
(1999): Johnston AM+, *N Engl J Med* 340, 1597
(1998): Morrow GL+, *Am J Ophthalmol* 125, 396
(1998): Greve B+, *Lasers Surg Med* 22, 223
(1998): Karrer S+, *Hautarzt* (German) 49, 219
(1998): Eisen D+, *Drug Saf* 18, 431
(1998): Wood B+, *Br J Dermatol* 139, 562
(1998): Wasel NR+, *J Cutan Med Surg* 3, 105
(1998): Patel K+, *Br J Dermatol* 185, 560
(1997): Houck HE+, *Arch Dermatol* 133, 15
(1997): Hoefnagel JJ+, *Ned Tijdschr Geneeskd* 141, 1424
(1997): Smith KC, Niagara Falls, Ontario (from Internet) (observation)
(1997): Rademaker M, New Zealand (eyelids) (from Internet) (observation)
(1996): Collins P+, *Br J Dermatol* 135, 317
(1996): Knoell AG+, *Arch Dermatol* 132, 1251
(1996): Tsao H+, *Arch Dermatol* 132, 1250
(1996): Hardman CM+, *Clin Exp Dermatol* 21, 244
(1996): Fleming CJ+, *Br J Dermatol* 134, 784
(1996): Goulden V+, *Br J Dermatol* 134, 693
(1995): Poskitt L+, *Br J Dermatol* 132, 784
(1995): Meyer AJ+, *Arch Dermatol* 131, 1447
(1995): Hung PH+, *J Fam Pract* 41, 183
(1994): Miralles ES+, *J Dermatol* 21, 965
(1994): Siller GM+, *J Am Acad Dermatol* 30, 350
(1993): Okada N+, *Br J Dermatol* 129, 403
(1993): Dwyer CM+, *Br J Dermatol* 129, 158
(1993): Schofield JK+, *Br J Gen Pract* 43, 173
(1993): Pepine M+, *J Am Acad Dermatol* 28, 295
(1992): Altman DA+, *J Cutan Pathol* 19, 340
(1992): Fakhfakh AC+, *Ann Dermatol Venereol* (French) 119, 975
(1992): Ridgway HB+, *Arch Dermatol* 128, 565 ("pseudo-mongolian")
(1991): Leffell D, *J Am Acad Dermatol* 24, 501
(1991): Eedy DJ+, *Clin Exp Dermatol* 15, 55
(1990): Black AK+, *Br J Dermatol* 123, 277 (observation)
(1990): Bamberger N+, *Ann Dermatol Venereol* (French) 117, 299
(1990): Bridges AJ+, *J Am Acad Dermatol* 22, 959
(1989): Okada N+, *Br J Dermatol* 121, 247
(1989): Cataldo E+, *J Mass Dent Soc* 38, 5
(1987): Zijdenbos AM+, *Ned Tijdschr Geneeskd* (Dutch) 131, 999
(1987): Argenyi ZB+, *J Cutaneous Pathol* 14, 176
(1987): Angeloni VL+, *Cutis* 40, 229
(1986): Shum DT+, *Arch Dermatol* 122, 18
(1986): Prigent F+, *Ann Dermatol Venereol* (French) 113, 227
(1996): Korbol M+, *J Am Podiatr Med Assoc* 76, 87
(1985): Basler RSW+, *J Am Acad Dermatol* 12, 577
(1985): Basler RSW, *Arch Dermatol* 121. 606
(1985): Gordon G, *Arch Dermatol* 121, 618
(1985): Liu TTT+, *Cutis* 35, 254
(1985): Butler JM+, *Clin Exp Dermatol* 10, 432
(1984): Wolfe ID+, *Cutis* 33, 457
(1983): Verret JL+, *Ann Dermatol Venereol* (French) 110, 777
(1983): White SW+, *Arch Dermatol* 119, 1

(1982): Ridgway HA, *Br J Dermatol* 107, 95
(1981): Leroy JP+, *Ann Dermatol Venereol* (French) 108, 871
(1980): Fenske NA+, *J Am Acad Dermatol* 3, 308
(1980): McGrae JD+, *Arch Dermatol* 116, 1262
(1980): Simons JJ+, *J Am Acad Dermatol* 3, 244
(1975): Brogden RN+, *Drugs* 9, 251

Pigmentation at sites of cutaneous inflammation
(1992): Altman DA+, *J Cutaneous Pathol* 19, 340 (in patients with bullous pemphigoid)
(1991): Eady DJ+, *Clin Exp Dermatol* 16, 55
(1991): Leffell DJ, *J Am Acad Dermatol* 24, 501
(1988): Serwatka LM, *J Assoc Military Derm* 14, 10
(1980): Fenske NA+, *JAMA* 244, 1103

Pruritus (<1%)
(1996): Montemarano AD+, *J Am Acad Dermatol* 34, 253
(1996): Goulden V+, *Br J Dermatol* 134, 693
(1973): Shelley WB+, *JAMA* 224, 125

Purpura
(2000): Warshaw E, Minneapolis, MN *The Schoch Letter* 50, February #16
(1995): Karofsky PS+, *Arch Pediatr Adolesc Med* 149, 217

Pustular eruption (generalized)
(1999): Antunes A+, *Ann Dermatol Venereol* 126, 518

Rash (sic) (<1%)
(2000): Schlienger RG+, *Dermatology* 200, 223
(1997): Shapiro LE+, *Arch Dermatol* 133, 1224
(1995): Karofsky PS+, *Arch Pediatr Adolesc Med* 149, 217
(1994): Kaufmann D+, *Arch Intern Med* 154, 1983
(1994): Sitbon O+, *Arch Intern Med* 154, 1633

Raynaud's phenomenon
(1996): Hewack J, *Gastroenterology* 110, A1211

Stevens–Johnson syndrome
(1996): Knowles SR+, *Arch Dermatol* 132, 934
(1987): Shoji A+, *Arch Dermatol* 123, 18

Urticaria
(1997): Shapiro LE+, *Arch Dermatol* 133, 1224
(1996): Knowles SR+, *Arch Dermatol* 132, 934
(1996): Goulden V+, *Br J Dermatol* 134, 693
(1996): Ottuso P, Vero Beach, Florida, *The Schoch Letter* 46, 37 (from generic)
(1995): Wallis M, *The Schoch Letter* 45, 38 (from generic)
(1994): Litt JZ, Beachwood, OH, personal case (observation)
(1993): Litt JZ, Beachwood, OH, 2 personal cases (observation)
(1990): Puyana J+, *Allergy* 45, 313
(1975): Brogden RN+, *Drugs* 9, 251

Vasculitis
(1999): Elkayam O+, *Semin Arthritis Rheum* 28, 392
(1999): Schrodt BJ+, *South Med J* 92, 502
(1999): Schrodt BJ, *Skin and Allergy News* April, 22 (2 cases)
(1998): Merkel PA, *Curr Opin Rheumatol* 10, 45

Nails

Nails – onycholysis

Nails – photo onycholysis
(1987): Baran R+, *J Am Acad Dermatol* 17, 1012 (passim)
(1981): Kestel JL, *Cutis* 28, 53

Nails – pigmentation (<1%)
(1998): Morrow GL+, *Am J Ophthalmol* 125, 396
(1995): Hung PH+, *J Fam Pract* 41, 183
(1994): Mallon E+, *Br J Dermatol* 130, 794
(1989): Berger RS+, *J Am Acad Dermatol* 21, 1300 (3–5%)
(1988): Mooney E+, *J Dermatol Surg Oncol* 14, 1011
(1987): Angeloni VL+, *Cutis* 40, 229
(1985): Liu TTT+, *Cutis* 35, 254
(1984): Wolfe ID+, *Cutis* 33, 457
(1982): Litt JZ, *Diagnosis* 4, 23

Hair

Hair – alopecia
(2000): Schlienger RG+, *Dermatology* 200, 223

Other

Anaphylactoid reaction (<1%)
(1996): Okano M+, *Acta Derm Venereol* (Stockh) 76, 164

Black tongue
(1995): Katz J+, *Arch Dermatol* 131, 620
(1975): Brogden RN+, *Drugs* 9, 251

Galactorrhea (black)
(1996): Hunt MJ+, *Br J Dermatol* 134, 943
(1985): Basler RSW+, *Arch Dermatol* 121, 417

Gingival pigmentation
(1989): Berger RS+, *J Am Acad Dermatol* 21, 1300 (8%)

Glossitis

Gynecomastia
(1995): Davies JP+, *Br J Clin Pract* 49, 179

Hypersensitivity*
(1999): Lupton JR+, *Cutis* 64, 91 (infectious-mononucleosis-like)
(1999): Piette AM+, *Rev Med Interne* (French) 20, 869
(1999): Clayton BD+, *Arch Dermatol* 135, 139
(1999): Antunes A+, *Ann Dermatol Venereol* 126, 518
(1998): Dutz J, Vancouver, Canada (from Internet) (observation)
(1998): Schlienger RG+, *Epilepsia* 39, S3 (passim)
(1997): Hoefnagel JJ+, *Ned Tijdschr Geneeskd* (Dutch) 141, 1424
(1997): Shapiro LE+, *Arch Dermatol* 133, 1224
(1997): MacNeil M+, *J Am Acad Dermatol* 36, 347
(1995): Parneix-Spake A+, *Arch Dermatol* 131, 490
(1994): Sitbon O+, *Arch Intern Med* 154, 1633
(1973): Shelley WB+, *JAMA* 224, 125

Myalgia
(1998): Matteson EL+, *J Rheumatol* 25, 1653

Oral pigmentation
(1998): Cockings JM+, *Aust Dent J* 43, 14
(1998): Patel K+, *Br J Dermatol* 185, 560
(1997): Eisen D, *Lancet* 349, 379
(1997): Smith KC, Niagara Falls, Ontario (from Internet) (observation) (blue on lips)
(1995): Odell EW+, *Oral Surg Oral Med Oral Pathol Oral Radiol Endod* 79, 459
(1994): Siller GM+, *J Am Acad Dermatol* 30, 350
(1994): Chu P+, *J Am Acad Dermatol* 30, 802
(1989): Regezi JA+, *Oral Pathology*, WB Saunders, 166
(1989): Berger RS+, *J Am Acad Dermatol* 21, 1300 (7%)
(1986): Beehner ME+, *J Oral Maxillofac Surg* 44, 582
(1985): Salman RA+, *J Oral Med* 40, 154
(1984): Fendrich P+, *Oral Surg Oral Med Oral Pathol 58*, 288

Oral ulceration
(2000): Schlienger RG+, *Dermatology* 200, 223

Paresthesias (<1%)
(1994): Blanchard L, *Schoch Letter* 44, #6 (observation)

Polyarteritis nodosa
(1999): Schrodt BJ+, *Pediatrics* 103, 503

Pseudo-mongolian spot (sic)
(1992): Ridgway HB+, *Arch Dermatol* 128, 565

Pseudotumor cerebri
(2000): Frederickson KS, Novato, CA, (from Internet) (observation)
(1998): Chiu AM+, *Am J Ophthalmol* 126, 116
(1990): Shelley WB, *The Schoch Letter* 40, 27
(1990): Delaney RA+, *Mil Med* 156, A5
(1980): Beran RG, *Med J Aust* 1, 323

Serum sickness
(1999): Elkayam O+, *Semin Arthritis Rheum* 28, 392
(1998): Martinez JA+, *Med Clin (Barc)* (Spanish) 111, 198
(1997): Hoefnagel JJ+, *Ned Tijdschr Geneeskd* (Dutch) 141, 1424
(1997): Shapiro LE+, *Arch Dermatol* 133, 1224
(1997): Blumenthal HL, Beachwood, OH, personal case (observation)
(1997): Zabawski E, Dallas TX (from Internet) (observation)
(1996): Levenson T+, *Allergy Asthma Proc* 17, 79
(1996): Harel L+, *Ann Pharmacother* 30, 481
(1990): Puyana J+, *Allergy* 45, 313

Tongue discoloration
(2000): Tanzi E+, *Arch Dermatol* 136, 427
(1995): Katz J+, *Arch Dermatol* 131, 620
(1995): Meyerson M+, *Oral Surg Oral Med Oral Pathol Oral Radiol Endod* 79, 180

Tooth discoloration (>10%) (primarily in children)
(2000): McKenna BE+, *Dent Update* 26, 160 (in an adult)
(2000): Bark JP, Lexington, KY (from Internet) (observation)
(2000): Thaler D, Monona, WI (from Internet) (observation)
(1999): Cheek CC+, *J Esthet Dent* 11, 43
(1998): Dodd MA+, *Ann Pharmacother* 32, 887 (68-year-old woman)
(1998): Morrow GL+, *Am J Ophthalmol* 125, 396
(1998): Patel K+, *Br J Dermatol* 185, 560 (in an adult)
(1997): Bowles WK+, *J Esthet Dent* 9, 30
(1997): Smith KC, Niagara Falls, Ontario (from Internet) (observation)

(1995): Hung PH+, *J Fam Pract* 41, 183
(1994): Hofmann H, *Hautarzt* (German) 45, 803
(1991): Allegue F+, *Actas Dermo-Sif* (Spanish) 82, 43
(1989): Berger RS+, *J Am Acad Dermatol* 21, 1300 (3–5%)
(1989): Regezi JA+, *Oral Pathology*, WB Saunders, 166
(1989): Rosen T+, *J Am Acad Dermatol* 21, 569
(1988): Cale AE+, *J Periodontol* 59, 112
(1985): Poliak SC+, *JAMA* 254, 2930
(1984): Wolfe ID+, *Cutis* 33, 457
(1980): Caro I, *J Am Acad Dermatol* 3, 317

***Note:** The antiepileptic drug hypersensitivity syndrome is a severe, occasionally fatal, disorder characterized by any or all of the following: pruritic exanthem, toxic epidermal necrolysis, Stevens–Johnson syndrome, exfoliative dermatitis, fever, hepatic abnormalities, eosinophilia, and renal failure.

MINOXIDIL

Trade names: Minoxidil (Par); Rogaine (topical) (Pharmacia & Upjohn)
Other common trade names: *Alopexy; Apo-Gain; Hairgaine; Lonolox; Loonoten; Minoximen; Regaine*
Indications: Hypertension, androgenetic alopecia
Category: Antihypertensive; vasodilator
Half-life: 4.2 hours
Clinically important, potentially serious interactions with: diazoxide, guanethidine

Note: For topical reaction patterns, I have added a bracket [T]

Reactions

Skin

Acne
(1985): Baral J, *J Am Acad Dermatol* 13, 1051 (scalp comedones)
Ankle edema
Allergic reactions (sic) [T]
Bullous eruption (<1%)
(1981): DiSantis DJ+, *Arch Intern Med* 141, 1515
(1978): Rosenthal T+, *Arch Intern Med* 138, 1856
Contact dermatitis (7.4%) [T]
(1995): Ebner H+, *Contact Dermatitis* 32, 316
(1992): Veraldi S+, *Contact Dermatitis* 26, 211
(1992): Ruas E+, *Contact Dermatitis* 26, 57
(1991): Wilson C+, *J Am Acad Dermatol* 24, 661
(1988): Alomar A+, *Contact Dermatitis* 18, 51
(1988): van Joost T, *Ned Tijdschr Geneeskd* (Dutch) 132, 1141
(1987): Valsecchi R+, *Contact Dermatitis* 17, 58
(1985): Tosti A+, *Contact Dermatitis* 13, 275
(1985): Degreef H+, *Contact Dermatitis* 13, 194
Eczematous eruption (sic)
(1992): Ruas E+, *Contact Dermatitis* 26, 57
(1987): van der Willigen AH+, *Contact Dermatitis* 17, 44
Edema (>10%) [T]
(1977): Nawar T+, *Can Med Assoc J* 117, 1178
Erythema [T]
Erythema multiforme
(1981): DiSantis DJ+, *Arch Intern Med* 141, 1515
Erythroderma
(1988): Ackerman BH+, *Drug Intell Clin Pharm* 22, 703
Exanthems
(1988): Ackerman BH+, *Drug Intell Clin Pharm* 22, 703
(1981): DiSantis DJ+, *Arch Intern Med* 141, 1515
(1981): Campese VM, *Drugs* 22, 257
(1977): Nawar T+, *Can Med Assoc J* 117, 1178
Folliculitis [T]
(1996): Duvic M+, *J Am Acad Dermatol* 35, 74
Flushing [T]
Lupus erythematosus
(1987): Tunkel AR+, *Arch Intern Med* 147, 599
(1981): Mitas JA, *Arthritis Rheum* 24, 570
Peripheral edema (7%)
Pigmentation
Pruritus [T]
(1996): Duvic M+, *J Am Acad Dermatol* 35, 74
(1990): Colamarino R+, *Ann Intern Med* 113, 256
(1977): Nawar T+, *Can Med Assoc J* 117, 1178
Pyogenic granuloma
(1989): Baran R, *Dermatologica* 179, 76 (explosive, of the scalp)
Rash (sic) (<1%)
Seborrhea [T]
Stevens–Johnson syndrome (<1%)
(1981): DiSantis DJ+, *Arch Intern Med* 141, 1515
Sunburn (<1%)
Urticaria
Xerosis

Hair

Hair – alopecia [T]
(1987): Olsen EA, *J Am Acad Dermatol* 16, 145
(1983): Ingles RM+, *Int J Dermatol* 22, 120
Hair – discoloration
(1989): Rebora A+, *J Am Acad Dermatol* 21, 1314
(1983): Ingles RM+, *Int J Dermatol* 22, 120 (red)
Hair – hirsutism (in women)
(1981): Campese VM, *Drugs* 22, 257 (100%)
(1973): Pettinger WA+, *N Engl J Med* 289, 167
Hair – hypertrichosis (80%)
(1997): Peluso AM+, *Br J Dermatol* 136, 118
(1995): Veyrac G+, *Therapie* (French) 50, 474 (in an infant)
(1994): Gonzalez M+, *Clin Exp Dermatol* 19, 157 (topical application)
(1990): Miwa LJ+, *Drug Intell Clin Pharm* 24, 365
(1989): Rousseau C+, *Dermatologica* 179, 221
(1988): Toriumi DN+, *Arch Otolaryngol Head Neck Surg* 114, 918
(1985): Lorette G+, *Ann Dermatol Venereol* (French) 112, 527
(1985): Bencini PL+, *G Ital Dermatol Venereol* (Italian) 120, 137
(1984): Henkes J+, *Med Clin (Barc)* (Spanish) 83, 89
(1983): Wilkin JK+, *Cutis* 31, 61
(1983): Ingles RM+, *Int J Dermatol* 22, 120
(1981): Campese VM, *Drugs* 22, 257 (100%)
(1981): Nielsen PG, *Lakartidningen* (Swedish) 78, 1891
(1980): Ryckmanns F, *Hautarzt* (German) 31, 205
(1980): Feldman HA+, *Curr Ther Res* 27, 205
(1979): Burton JL+, *Br J Dermatol* 101, 593
(1979): Pierard GE+, *Dermatologica* (French) 158, 17.5
(1977): Earhart RN+, *South Med J* 70, 442
(1977): Nawar T+, *Can Med Assoc J* 117, 1178

Other

Anosmia
(1993): Litt JZ, Beachwood, OH, personal case (observation)
Dysgeusia [T]
(1993): Litt JZ, Beachwood, OH, personal case (observation)
Gynecomastia
Mastodynia (<1%)
Paresthesias
Polymyalgia
(1990): Colamarino R+, *Ann Intern Med* 113, 256
Tendinitis [T]

MIRTAZAPINE

Trade name: Remeron (Organon)
Indications: Depression
Category: Tetracyclic antidepressant; alpha-2 antagonist
Half-life: 20–40 hours
Clinically important, potentially serious interactions with: alcohol, benzodiazepines, clonidine, CNS depressants, diazepam, MAO inhibitors

Reactions

Skin

Acne
Rash (sic) (1–10%)
Cellulitis
Chills
Diaphoresis
(1999): Leinonen E+, *Int Clin Psychopharmacol* 14, 329

Edema (1–10%)
Exfoliative dermatitis
Facial edema
Flu-like syndrome (sic) (1–10%)
Herpes simplex
Peripheral edema (1–10%)
Petechiae
Photosensitivity
Pruritus
Rash (sic)
Seborrhea
Ulcer
Xerosis

Other

Ageusia
Aphthous stomatitis
Dysgeusia
Glossitis (1–10%)
Gynecomastia
Hypesthesia
Mastodynia
Myalgia (1–10%)
Oral candidiasis
Paresthesias
Parosmia
Phlebitis
Sialorrhea
Stomatitis
Tendon rupture
Tongue discoloration
Tongue edema
Tremor (1–10%)
Vaginitis
Xerostomia (25%)
(1995): Montgomery SA, *Int Clin Psychopharmacol* 10, 37

MISOPROSTOL

Trade names: Arthrotec (Searle); Cytotec (Searle)
Other common trade name: *Symbol*
Indications: Prevention of NSAID-induced ulcer
Category: Synthetic prostaglandin E_1 analogue; anti-ulcer agent
Half-life: 20–40 minutes
Clinically important, potentially serious interactions with: none

Arthrotec is diclofenac and misoprostol

Reactions

Skin

Dermatitis (sic)
Diaphoresis
Shivering
(1999): Lumbiganon P+, *Br J Obstet Gynaecol* 106, 304
Exanthems
(1987): Monk JP+, *Drugs* 33, 1
Rash (sic)

Hair

Hair – alopecia

Other

Anaphylactoid reaction
Gingivitis
Gynecomastia
(1994): Garcia-Rodriguez LA+, *BMJ* 308, 503

MITHRAMYCIN

(See PLICAMYCIN)

MITOMYCIN

Synonyms: mitomycin-C; MTC
Trade name: Mutamycin (Bristol-Myers Squibb)
Other common trade names: *Ametycine; Mitomycin; Mitomycin-C; Mitomycine*
Indications: Carcinomas
Category: Antineoplastic antibiotic
Half-life: 23–78 minutes
Clinically important, potentially serious interactions with: carbamazepine, chloramphenicol, clozapine, doxorubicin, zidovudine

Reactions

Skin

Angioedema
Bullous eruption
(1984): Ritch PS+, *Cancer* 54, 32
Contact dermatitis
(1997): Gomez Torrrijos E+, *Allergy* 52, 687
(1993): Wahlberg JE+, *Lakartidningen* (Swedish) 90, 158
(1992): Vidal C+, *Dermatology* 184, 208
(1981): Nissenkorn I+, *J Urol* 126, 596
Dermatitis (sic)
(1990): Colver GB+, *Br J Dermatol* 122, 217
(1987): Sala F+, *G Ital Dermatol Venereol* (Italian) 122, 265
(1984): Neild VJ+, *J R Soc Med* 77, 610
(1975): Med Lett 17, 62
Edema
Erythema
Erythema multiforme
(1984): Spencer HJ, *J Surg Oncol* 26, 47
Exanthems
(1995): Echechipia S+, *Contact Dermatitis* 33, 432
(1987): Sala F+, *G Ital Dermatol Venereol* (Italian) 122, 265
Exfoliative dermatitis
(1987): Sala F+, *G Ital Dermatol Venereol* (Italian) 122, 265
(1985): Bencini PL+, *Int J Dermatol* 24, 472
Palmar desquamation
(1981): Nissenkorn I+, *J Urol* 126, 596
Photosensitivity
(1981): Fuller B+, *Ann Intern Med* 94, 542
Pigmentation
(1989): Kerker BJ+, *Semin Dermatol* 8, 173
Pityriasis rosea
(1987): Sala F+, *G Ital Dermatol Venereol* (Italian) 122, 265
Pruritus (<1%)
Purpura
Rash (sic) (<1%)
(1981): Nissenkorn I+, *J Urol* 126, 596 (generalized)
Ulceration
(1992): Ellsworth-Wolk J, *Oncol Nurs Forum* 19, 1554
Urticaria
(1981): Weiss RB+, *Ann Intern Med* 94, 66

Hair

Hair – alopecia (1–10%)
(1975): *Med Lett* 17, 62

Nails

Nails – pigmented bands (purple) (1–10%)

Other

Injection-site cellulitis (>10%)
Injection-site necrosis (>10%)
(1987): Dufresne RG, *Cutis* 39, 197
(1987): Aizawa H+, *Acta Derm Venereol* (Stockh) 67, 364
(1987): Sala F+, *G Ital Dermatol Venereol* (Italian) 122, 265

Injection-site thrombophlebitis
Oral mucosal lesions
(1987): Sala F+, *G Ital Dermatol Venereol* (Italian) 122, 265
(1983): Bronner AK+, *J Am Acad Dermatol* 9, 645
(1978): Levine N+, *Cancer Treat Rev* 5, 67 (2–8%)
(1975): *Med Lett* 17, 62
Oral ulceration (1–10%)
(1984): Spencer HJ, *J Surg Oncol* 26, 47
Paresthesias (1–10%)
Stomatitis (>10%)
Thrombophlebitis (<1%)

MITOTANE

Synonym: o,p'-DDD
Trade name: Lysodren (Bristol-Myers Squibb)
Other common trade name: *Opeprim*
Indications: Inoperable adrenocortical carcinoma
Category: Antiadrenal; antineoplastic
Half-life: 18–159 days
Clinically important, potentially serious interactions with: barbiturates, CNS depressants, phenytoin, spironolactone, warfarin

Reactions

Skin

Acral erythema
(1991): Baack BR+, *J Am Acad Dermatol* 24, 457
(1974): Zühlke RL, *Dermatologica* 148, 90
Angioedema (<1%)
Cutaneous side effects (sic)
(1973): Lubitz JA+, *JAMA* 223, 1109 (13%)
(1966): Hutter AM+, *Am J Med* 41, 581 (17%)
Erythema multiforme
(1978): Levine N+, *Cancer Treat Rev* 5, 67
(1966): Hutter AM+, *Am J Med* 41, 581
Exanthems
(1973): Lubitz JA+, *JAMA* 223, 1109 (9%)
(1966): Hutter AM+, *Am J Med* 41, 581 (16%)
Flushing (1–10%)
Pigmentation
(1973): Lubitz JA+, *JAMA* 223, 1109
(1966): Hutter AM+, *Am J Med* 41, 581 (16%)
Pruritus
(1974): Zühlke RL, *Dermatologica* 148, 90
Rash (sic) (15%)
Urticaria
(1966): Hutter AM+, *Am J Med* 41, 581
Vasculitis (<1%)

Hair

Hair – alopecia
(1973): Lubitz JA+, *JAMA* 223, 1109
(1966): Hutter AM+, *Am J Med* 41, 581 (16%)

Other

Myalgia (1–10%)
Tremor (<1%)

MODAFINIL

Trade name: Provigil (Cephalon)
Other trade name: *Alertec*
Indications: Narcolepsy
Category: Central nervous system stimulant, analeptic
Half-life: ~15 hours
Clinically important, potentially serious interactions with: anticonvulsants, barbiturates, carbamazepine, diazepam, itraconazole, ketoconazole, MAO inhibitors, oral contraceptives, phenobarbital, phenytoin, rifampin, warfarin

Reactions

Skin

Allergic reactions (>1%)
Chills (2%)
Diaphoresis (>1%)
Ecchymoses (>1%)
Edema, generalized (>1%)
Erythema
Herpes simplex (1%)
Hot flashes
Pruritus (>1%)
Psoriasis (>1%)
Rash (sic) (>1%)
Xerosis (1%)

Other

Dysgeusia (>1%)
Gingivitis (1%)
Myalgia (>1%)
Oral ulceration (1%)
Paresthesias (3%)
Sialorrhea
Tooth disorder (sic) (>1%)
Tremor (1%)
Xerostomia (5%)

MOEXIPRIL

Trade names: Uniretic (Schwarz); Univasc (Schwarz)
Indications: Hypertension
Category: Angiotensin converting enzyme (ACE) inhibitor; antihypertensive
Half-life: 1 hour
Clinically important, potentially serious interactions with: alcohol, allopurinol, bumetanide, digoxin, diuretics, indomethacin, lithium, probenecid, salicylates

Uniretic is moexipril and hydrochlorothiazide

Reactions

Skin

Angioedema (<1%)
Diaphoresis (<1%)
Exanthems (1.6%)
Flushing (1.6%)
(1995): Drayer JIM+, *Am J Ther* 2, 525
Pemphigus (<1%)
Peripheral edema (1–10%)
(1995): Drayer JIM+, *Am J Ther* 2, 525
Photosensitivity (<1%)
Pruritus (1–10%)
Rash (sic) (1.6%)
Skin reactions (sic)
(1994): White WB+, *J Human Hypertens* 8, 917
Urticaria (<1%)

Hair
Hair – alopecia (1–10%)

Other
Anaphylactoid reaction (<1%)
Dysgeusia (<1%)
Myalgia (1.3%)
Xerostomia (<1%)

MOLINDONE

Trade name: Moban (Endo)
Indications: Schizophrenia
Category: Antipsychotic
Half-life: 1.5 hours
Clinically important, potentially serious interactions with: alcohol, anticonvulsants, antihypertensives, chloroquine, CNS depressants, lithium, MAO inhibitors, maprotiline, propranolol, trazodone, tricyclic antidepressants, **cigarette smoking**

Reactions

Skin
Allergic reactions (sic)
Edema
Hypohidrosis (<1%)
Peripheral edema
Photosensitivity (<1%)
Pigmentation (<1%)
Pruritus (<1%)
Rash (sic) (<1%)

Other
Galactorrhea (<1%)
Gynecomastia (1–10%)
Sialorrhea
Xerostomia (>10%)

MONTELUKAST

Trade name: Singulair (Merck)
Indications: Asthma
Category: Antiasthmatic (leukotriene receptor antagonist)
Half-life: 2.7–5.5 hours
Clinically important, potentially serious interactions with: phenobarbital, rifampin

Reactions

Skin
Allergic granulomatous angiitis (Churg–Strauss syndrome)
(2000): Wechsler ME+, *Chest* 117. 708
(2000): Price D, *Drugs* 59, 35 (passim)
(2000): Villena V+, *Eur Resp J* 15, 626
Angioedema
(1998): Condrys P, Webster, NY (from Internet) (observation)
Erythema nodosum
(2000): Dellaripa PF+, *Mayo Clin Proc* 75, 643
Flu-like syndrome (sic) (1–10%)
Peripheral edema
(2000): Geller M, *Ann Intern Med* 132, 924
Rash (sic) (1.6%)
Urticaria (1.6%)
(1998): Knorr B+, *JAMA* 279, 1181
(1998): Jaffe P, Columbia, SC (from Internet) (observation)

MORICIZINE

Trade name: Ethmozine (Roberts)
Indications: Ventricular arrhythmias
Category: Antiarrhythmic, class I
Half-life: 3–4 hours
Clinically important, potentially serious interactions with: anticoagulants, cimetidine, digoxin, diltiazem, theophylline

Reactions

Skin
Diaphoresis (2–5%)
Exanthems (<1%)
Periorbital edema (1–10%)
Pruritus (<2%)
Rash (sic) (<1%)
Urticaria (<2%)
Xerosis (<2%)

Other
Dysgeusia (<2%)
Hypesthesia (2–5%)
Oral mucosal lesions
(1990): Fitton A+, *Drugs* 40, 138
Paresthesias (2–5%)
Thrombophlebitis (<2%)
Tongue edema (<2%)
Xerostomia (2–5%)
(1990): Fitton A+, *Drugs* 40, 138 (2%)
(1990): Carnes CA+, *Drug Intell Clin Pharm* 24, 745 (2–5%)

MORPHINE

Trade names: Astramorph; Duramorph; Infumorph; Kadian; MS Contin; MSIR Oral; MS/L; MS/S; OMS Oral; Oramorph SR; RMS; Roxanol, etc. (Various pharmaceutical houses.)
Other trade names: *Anamorph; Astramorph; Contalgin; Epimorph; Morphine-HP; MOS; MS-IR; MST Continus; Moscontin; Sevredol; Statex*
Indications: Severe pain; acute myocardial infarction
Category: Narcotic analgesic
Half-life: 2–4 hours
Clinically important, potentially serious interactions with: CNS depressants, dextroamphetamine, MAO inhibitors, opiate antagonists, tricyclic antidepressants

Reactions

Skin
Diaphoresis
Edema
Exanthems
(1977): Voorhorst R+, *Ned Tijdschr Geneeskd* (Dutch) *121, 737*
Flushing
Hypesthesia
Pallor
Peripheral edema
Pruritus (<1%)
(2000): Gunter JB+, *Paediatr Anaesth* 10, 167
(2000): Yeh HM+, *Anesth Analg* 91, 172
(1998): Thangaturai D+, *Anaesthesia* 43, 1055 (62%)
(1988): Gustafson LL+, *Drugs* 35, 597 (5–10%)
(1986): Attia J+, *Anesthesiology* 65, 590 (20%)
Rash (sic)

Other
Gynecomastia
Injection-site pain (>10%)
Trembling (1–10%)
Xerostomia (>10%)
(1989): White JD+, *BMJ* 298, 1222 (75%)

MOXIFLOXACIN

Trade name: Avelox (Bayer)
Indications: Various infections caused by susceptible organisms
Category: Fluoroquinolone antibiotic
Half-life: 12 hours
Clinically important, potentially serious interactions with: antacids, antiarrhythmics, astemizole, bepridil, cimetidine, cisapride, claithromycin, digoxin, diltiazem, disopyramide, diuretics, erythromycin, foscarnet, NSAIDs, phenothiazines, probenecid, tricyclic antidepressants, verapamil

Reactions

Skin

Allergic reactions (sic)
Burning
Candidiasis (<1%)
Chills (<1%)
Diaphoresis (<1%)
Edema
Peripheral edema (<1%)
Photosensitivity (<1%)
(2000): Stein GE+, *Inf Med* 17, 564
(2000): Balfour JA+, *Drugs* 59, 115
(2000): Traynor NJ+, *Toxicol Vitr* 14, 275
Pruritus (<1%)
Rash (sic) (<1%)
Urticaria (<1%)
Xerosis (<1%)

Other

Dysgeusia (>1%)
(2000): Stein GE+, *Inf Med* 17, 564
Glossitis (<1%)
Myalgia (<1%)
Paresthesias (<1%)
Stomatitis (<1%)
Tendinitis
Tendon rupture
Tremor (<1%)
Vaginitis (<1%)
(2000): Stein GE+, *Inf Med* 17, 564
Xerostomia (<1%)

MYCOPHENOLATE

Synonym: mycophenolate mofetil
Trade name: CellCept (Roche)
Indications: Prophylaxis of organ rejection
Category: Immunosuppressant
Half-life: 18 hours
Clinically important, potentially serious interactions with: acyclovir, antacids, azathioprine, cholestyramine, ganciclovir, probenecid

Reactions

Skin

Acne (>10%)
Carcinoma (non-melanoma) (4%)
Diaphoresis
Edema (12.2%)
Infection (sic) (12–20%)
Peripheral edema (28.6%
Pruritus
Rash (sic) (7.7%)

Hair

Hair – alopecia

Other

Gingival hyperplasia
Gingivitis
Myalgia
Oral candidiasis (10.1%)
Paresthesias
Thrombophlebitis (1–10%)
Tremor (11%)

NABUMETONE

Trade name: Relafen (SmithKline Beecham)
Other common trade names: *Arthaxan; Consolan; Nabuser; Prodac; Relif; Relifex; Unimetone*
Indications: Arthritis
Category: Nonsteroidal anti-inflammatory (NSAID)
Half-life: 22.5–30 hours
Clinically important, potentially serious interactions with: aminoglycosides, anticoagulants, cyclosporine, diuretics, heparin, lithium, methotrexate, probenecid, salicylates, warfarin

Reactions

Skin

Acne (<1%)
Angioedema (<1%)
(1990): Jenner PN, *Drugs* 40 (Suppl 5), 80
Bullous eruption (<1%)
Cutaneous side effects (sic)
(1991): Riccieri V+, *Clin Ter* (Italian) 137, 185
Diaphoresis (1–3%)
Edema (3–9%)
(1990): Munzel P+, *Drugs* 40 (Suppl 5), 62
Erythema
(1990): Alianti M+, *Clin Ter* (Italian) 133, 299
Erythema multiforme (<1%)
Exanthems (1.2%)
(1999): Litt JZ, Beachwood, OH, personal case (observation)
(1988): Friedel HA+, *Drugs* 35, 504
Hot flashes (<1%)
Parkinsonism
Photosensitivity (<1%)
(1998): Litt JZ, Beachwood, OH, personal case (observation)
(1994): Shelley WB+, *Cutis* 54, 70 (observation)
(1993): Litt JZ, Beachwood, OH, personal case (observation)
(1989): Kaidbey KH+, *Arch Dermatol* 125, 783
(1988): Friedel HA+, *Drugs* 35, 504
Phototoxic reaction
(1989): Kaidbey KH+, *Arch Dermatol* 125, 783 and 824
Pruritus (3–9%)
(1999): Litt JZ, Beachwood, OH, personal case (observation)
(1988): Friedel HA+, *Drugs* 35, 504
Rash (sic) (3–9%)
(1988): Friedel HA+, *Drugs* 35, 504
(1987): Mullen BJ, *Am J Med* 83, 70
(1987): Jackson RE+, *Am J Med* 83, 115
(1987): Jenner PN+, *Am J Med* 83, 110
Skin reactions (sic)
(1990): Fletcher AP, *Drugs* 40 (Suppl 5) 43
Stevens–Johnson syndrome (<1%)
(1997): Sienkiewicz G, Johnson City, NY (from Internet) (observation)
Toxic epidermal necrolysis (<1%)
Urticaria (<1%)
Vasculitis (necrotizing)
(1990): Willkins RF, *Drugs* 40 (Suppl 5) 34
Xerosis
(1987): Mullen BJ, *Am J Med* 83, 70

Hair

Hair – alopecia (<1%)
(1987): Mullen BJ, *Am J Med* 83, 70

Other

Anaphylactoid reaction (<1%)
Gingivitis (<1%)
Glossitis (<1%)
Myalgia
Oral ulceration
(1989): Lussier A+, *J Clin Pharmacol* 29, 225
Paresthesias (<1%)
Porphyria cutanea tarda (<1%)
Pseudoporphyria
(2000): Antony F+, *Br J Dermatol* 142, 1067
(1999): Aylesworth R, Rhinelander, WI (from Internet) (observation)
(1999): Krischer J+, *J Am Acad Dermatol* 40, 492
(1999): Magro CM+, *J Cutan Pathol* 26, 42
(1998): Varma S+, *Br J Dermatol* 138, 549
Sialorrhea
Stomatitis (1–3%)
Xerostomia (1–3%)

NADOLOL

Trade name: Corzide (Bristol-Myers Squibb)
Other common trade names: *Apo-Nadolol; Farmagard; Nadic; Solgol; Syn-Nadolol*
Indications: Hypertension, angina pectoris
Category: Beta-adrenergic blocker; antihypertensive; antianginal
Half-life: 10–24 hours
Clinically important, potentially serious interactions with: albuterol, calcium channel blockers, clonidine, diltiazem, epinephrine, flecainide, insulin, lidocaine, nifedipine, NSAIDs, oral contraceptives, prazosin, propranolol, salicylates, sulfonylureas, terazosin, verapamil

Corzide is nadolol and bendroflumethiazide*

Note: Cutaneous side-effects of beta-receptor blockaders are clinically polymorphous. They apparently appear after several months of continuous therapy. Atypical psoriasiform, lichen planus-like, and eczematous chronic rashes are mainly observed. (1983): Hödl St, *Z Hautkr* (German) 58, 17.

Reactions

Skin

Bullous pemphigoid
(1984): Stage AH+, *Am J Obstet Gynecol* 150, 169
Diaphoresis (<1%)
(1980): Heel RC+, *Drugs* 20, 1 (0.6%)
Eczematous eruption (sic)
Edema (1–5%)
Erythema multiforme
Exanthems
(1980): Heel RC+, *Drugs* 20, 1 (0.4%)
Exfoliative dermatitis
Facial edema (<1%)
Hyperkeratosis (palms and soles)
Infiltrative dermatitis of the scalp (sic)
(1985): Shelley ED+, *Cutis* 35, 148
Lichenoid eruption
(1978): Savage RL+, *BMJ* 1, 987
Lupus erythematosus
Pityriasis rubra pilaris
(1978): Finlay AY+, *BMJ* 1, 987
Pruritus (1–5%)
Psoriasis
(1988): Heng MCY+, *Int J Dermatol* 27, 619
(1988): Gold MH+, *J Am Acad Dermatol* 19, 837 (aggravation of)
(1986): Czernielewski J+, *Lancet* 1, 808
(1984): Arntzen N+, *Acta Derm Venereol* (Stockh) 64, 346
Pustular eruption
(1991): Bernard P+, *Dermatologica* 182, 115
Rash (sic) (1–5%)
Raynaud's phenomenon (2%)
(1984): Eliasson K+, *Acta Med Scand* 215, 333
(1976): Marshall AJ+, *BMJ* 1, 1498
Toxic epidermal necrolysis
Urticaria
Xerosis

Hair

Hair – alopecia
(1985): Shelley ED+, *Cutis* 35, 148

Nails

Nails – bluish
Nails – dystrophy

Nails – onycholysis

Other

Dysgeusia
Numbness (fingers and toes) (>5%)
Oculo-mucocutaneous syndrome
(1982): Cocco G+, *Curr Ther Res* 31, 362
Oral lichenoid eruption
Oral mucosal eruption
(1980): Heel RC+, *Drugs* 20, 1 (0.6%)
Paresthesias (>5%)
Peyronie's disease
(1979): Pryor JP+, *Lancet* 1, 331
Xerostomia (<1%)
(1980): Heel RC+, *Drugs* 20, 1

***Note:** Bendroflumethiazide is a sulfonamide and can be absorbed systemically. Sulfonamides can produce severe, possibly fatal, reactions such as toxic epidermal necrolysis and Stevens–Johnson syndrome.

NAFARELIN

Trade name: Synarel (Searle)
Other common trade name: *Synarela*
Indications: Endometriosis
Category: Posterior pituitary hormone; gonadotropin inhibitor
Half-life: ~3 hours
Clinically important, potentially serious interactions with: no data

Reactions

Skin

Acne (>10%)
Chloasma (<1%)
Edema (1–10%)
Exanthems (<1%)
Flushing
(1990): Chrisp P+, *Drugs* 39, 523 (90%)
(1988): Henzl MR+, *N Engl J Med* 318, 485 (90%)
Hot flashes (>10%)
Pruritus (1–10%)
Rash (sic) (1–10%)
Seborrhea (1–10%)
Urticaria (1–10%)

Hair

Hair – hirsutism (1–10%)

Other

Gynecomastia (<1%)
Hypersensitivity (0.2%)
Mastodynia
Myalgia (>10%)
Paresthesias (<1%)
Vaginitis

NAFCILLIN

Trade name: Nafcil (Apothecon)
Other common trade name: *Vigopen*
Indications: Various infections caused by susceptible organisms
Category: Penicillinase-resistant penicillin antibiotic
Half-life: 0.5–1.5 hours
Clinically important, potentially serious interactions with: anticoagulants, atenolol, cyclosporine, disulfiram, heparin, methotrexate, probenecid, tetracycline

Reactions

Skin

Allergic reactions (sic)
(1994): Pleasants RA+, *Chest* 106, 1124 (in patients with cystic fibrosis)
Angioedema
Bullous eruption
Ecchymoses
Erythema multiforme
Exanthems
(1978): Kancir LM+, *Arch Intern Med* 138, 909 (10%)
Exfoliative dermatitis
Hematomas
Jarisch–Herxheimer reaction
Pruritus
Rash (sic) (<1%)
Stevens–Johnson syndrome
Toxic epidermal necrolysis
Urticaria
Vasculitis

Other

Anaphylactoid reaction
Black tongue
Dysgeusia
Glossitis
Glossodynia
Hypersensitivity (<1%)
Injection-site necrosis
(1987): Dufresne RG, *Cutis* 39, 197
(1980): Tilden SJ+, *Am J Dis Child* 134, 1046
Injection-site pain
Oral candidiasis
Serum sickness
Stomatitis
Stomatodynia
Thrombophlebitis (<1%)
Vaginitis
Xerostomia

NALIDIXIC ACID

Trade name: NegGram (Sanofi)
Other common trade names: *Betaxina; Granexin; Mytacin; Nalidixin; Negram; Nogram; Youdix*
Indications: Various urinary tract infections caused by susceptible organisms
Category: Urinary tract anti-infective; quinolone antibiotic
Half-life: 6–7 hours
Clinically important, potentially serious interactions with: anticoagulants, warfarin

Reactions

Skin

Angioedema (<1%)
Bullous eruption (<1%)
(1981): Wolf A, *Z Hautkr* (German) 56, 109

(1970): Brehm G+, *Med Welt* (German) 11, 423
(1969): Puissant A+, *Bull Soc Fr Dermatol Syphiligr* (French) 76, 84
(1969): Birkett DA, *Br J Dermatol* 81, 342
(1968): Baes H, *Dermatologica* 136, 61
(1966): Burry JN+, *Med J Aust* 2, 243

Erythema multiforme (<1%)
(1971): Alexander S+, *Br J Dermatol* 84, 429

Exanthems (>5%)
(1971): Alexander S+, *Br J Dermatol* 84, 429
(1969): Atlas E+, *Ann Intern Med* 70, 713 (7%)
(1963): Barlow AM, *BMJ* 2, 1308 (3.5%)
(1963): Lishman IV+, *Br J Urol* 35, 116
(1962): Buchbinder M+, *Antimicrob Agents Chemother* 2, 308

Exfoliative dermatitis
(1971): Alexander S+, *Br J Dermatol* 84, 429

Lupus erythematosus
(1979): Rubinstein A, *N Engl J Med* 301, 1288
(1971): Alexander S+, *Br J Dermatol* 84, 429

Photoreactions
(1972): Jung EG, *Z Haut Geschlechtskr* (German) 47, 329

Photosensitivity (<1%)
(1997): O'Reilly FM+, American Academy of Dermatology Meeting, Poster #14
(1993): Wainwright NJ+, *Drug Saf* 9, 437
(1990): Bilsland D+, *Br J Dermatol* 123, 548
(1986): Ljunggren B+, *Photodermatol* 3, 26
(1985): Epstein JH+, *Drugs* 30, 42
(1982): Rosen K+, *Acta Derm Venereol* (Stockh) 62, 246
(1981): Closas J+, *Rev Clin Esp* (Spanish) 162, 219
(1981): Boisvert A+, *Drug Intell Clin Pharm* 15, 126
(1980): Stern RS+, *Arch Dermatol* 116, 1269
(1978): Fiocchi A+, *Minerva Pediatr* (Italian) 30, 585
(1974): Ramsay CA+, *Br J Dermatol* 91, 523
(1973): Ramsay CA, *Proc R Soc Med* 66, 747
(1971): Alexander S+, *Br J Dermatol* 84, 429
(1970): Luscombe HA, *Arch Dermatol* 101, 122
(1970): Neering KEHP, *Dermatologica* 141, 361
(1970): Thivolet J+, *Bull Soc Fr Dermatol Syphiligr* (French) 77, 286
(1970): No Author, *Tidsskr Nor Laegeforen* (Norwegian) 90, 2100
(1969): Garrett MH, *Med J Aust* 1, 83
(1968): Baes H, *Dermatologica* 136, 61
(1967): Haven E+, *Arch Belg Dermatol Syphiligr* (French) 23, 421
(1966): Mathew FH, *Med J Aust* 53, 243
(1965): Elmes PC, *Prescrib J* 5, 12
(1965): Cahal DA, *BMJ* 1, 130
(1965): Susskind W+, *BMJ* 1, 316

Phototoxic bullous eruption
(1978): Brauer GJ, *Am J Med* 58, 576
(1977): Hertzenberg S, *Tidsskr Nor Laegeforen* (Norwegian) 97, 792
(1976): Frodin T+, *Lakartidningen* (Swedish) 73, 3763
(1976): van Dijk E, *Ned Tijdschr Geneeskd* (Dutch) 120, 592
(1976): Klaasen CH+, *Ned Tijdschr Geneeskd* (Dutch) 120, 247
(1975): Brauner GJ, *Am J Med* 58, 576
(1974): Burry JN, *Arch Dermatol* 109, 263
(1974): Ramsay CA+, *Br J Dermatol* 91, 523
(1973): Louis P+, *Hautarzt* (German) 24, 445
(1969): Birkett DA, *Br J Dermatol* 81, 342
(1968): Baes H, *Dermatologica* 136, 61
(1966): Burry JN+, *Med J Aust* 2, 243
(1964): Zelickson AS, *JAMA* 190, 556

Pruritus (<1%)
(1971): Alexander S+, *Br J Dermatol* 84, 429
(1969): Atlas E+, *Ann Intern Med* 70, 713

Purpura
(1971): Alexander S+, *Br J Dermatol* 84, 429

Rash (sic) (<1%)

Toxic epidermal necrolysis
(1971): Alexander S+, *Br J Dermatol* 84, 429

Urticaria (<1%)
(1985): Goolamali SK, *Postgrad Med J* 61, 925
(1971): Alexander S+, *Br J Dermatol* 84, 429
(1966): Beaty HN+, *Ann Intern Med* 65, 641

Hair

Hair – alopecia
(1971): Alexander S+, *Br J Dermatol* 84, 429

Other

Acute intermittent porphyria

Anaphylactoid reaction

Paresthesias

Porphyria cutanea tarda
(1992): Shelley WB+, *Advanced Dermatologic Diagnosis*, WB Saunders, 414 (passim)
(1983): Goldsman CI+, *Cleve Clin Q* 50, 151

Pseudoporphyria
(1990): Bilsland D+, *Br J Dermatol* 123, 547
(1984): Harber LC+, *J Invest Dermatol* 82, 207

Pseudotumor cerebri
(1998): Ryiaz A+, *J Indian Med Assoc* 96, 308

NALOXONE

Trade name: Narcan (Endo)
Other common trade names: *Nalpin; Narcanti; Narcotan; Zynox*
Indications: Narcotic overdose
Category: Opioid (narcotic) antagonist
Half-life: 1–1.5 hours
Clinically important, potentially serious interactions with: narcotic analgesics

Reactions

Skin

Angioedema
(1982): Smitz S+, *Ann Intern Med* 97, 788

Diaphoresis (1–10%)

Exanthems

Pruritus
(1982): Smitz S+, *Ann Intern Med* 97, 788

Rash (sic) (1–10%)

Urticaria
(1982): Smitz S+, *Ann Intern Med* 97, 788

NAPROXEN

Trade name: Naprosyn (Roche)
Other common trade names: *Aleve; Anaprox; Apranax; Dymenalgit; Flanax; Laraflex; Naprelan; Naprogesic; Napron X; Naprosyne; Naxen; Novo-Naprox; Nu-Naprox; Supradol; Synflex; Velsay*
Indications: Pain, arthritis
Category: Nonsteroidal anti-inflammatory (NSAID)
Half-life: 13 hours
Clinically important, potentially serious interactions with: beta-blockers, cyclosporine, furosemide, heparin, hydantoins, lithium, methotrexate, oral anticoagulants, probenecid, salicylates, sulfonamides, sulfonylureas, warfarin

Reactions

Skin

Angioedema (<1%)
(1984): Stern RS+, *JAMA* 252, 1433

Bullous eruption
(1996): Gonzalo-Garijo MA+, *Allergol Immunopathol Madr* (Spanish) 24, 89
(1990): Suarez SM+, *Arthritis Rheum* 33, 903
(1989): Rivers JK+, *Med J Aust* 151, 167
(1984): Stern RS+, *JAMA* 252, 1433

Cutaneous side effects (sic)
(1985): Bigby M+, *J Am Acad Dermatol* 12, 866 (up to 5%)
(1990): Todd PA+, *Drugs* 40, 91 (up to 9%)
(1974): Cuthbert MF, *Curr Med Res Opin* 2, 600 (5%)

Diaphoresis (<3%)
(1990): Todd PA+, *Drugs* 40, 91 (<3%)
(1985): Bigby M+, *J Am Acad Dermatol* 12, 866

(1982): Bailin PL+, *Clin Rheum Dis* 8, 493 (passim)
Ecchymoses (3–9%)
Edema (3–9%)
(1978): Castles JJ+, *Arch Intern Med* 138, 362 (1–5%)
Erythema multiforme (<1%)
(1985): Bigby M+, *J Am Acad Dermatol* 12, 866
(1984): Stern RS+, *JAMA* 252, 1433
Erythema nodosum
(1990): Todd PA+, *Drugs* 40, 91
Exanthems (>5%)
(1994): Shelley WB+, *Cutis* 55, 21 (observation)
(1990): Todd PA+, *Drugs* 40, 91
(1985): Bigby M+, *J Am Acad Dermatol* 12, 866 (1–5%)
(1984): Stern RS+, *JAMA* 252, 1433
(1979): Brogden RN+, *Drugs* 18, 241
(1978): Castles JJ+, *Arch Intern Med* 138, 362 (5.3%)
(1976): Dyer HR, *Ann Intern Med* 84, 221
(1975): Brigden RN+, *Drugs* 9, 326
(1975): Bowers DE+, *Ann Intern Med* 83, 470 (14%)
Exfoliative dermatitis
Fixed eruption
(2000): Ozkaya-Bayazit E+, *Eur J Dermatol* 10, 288
(1998): Leal G, Fortaleza, Brazil (from Internet) (observation)
(1996): Gonzalo-Garijo MA+, *Allergol Immunopathol Madr* (Spanish) 24, 89
(1996): Enta T, *Can Fam Physician* 42, 1099
(1991): Shelley WB+, *Cutis* 48, 368 (observation)
(1990): Black AK+, *Br J Dermatol* 123, 277 (observation)
(1990): Todd PA+, *Drugs* 40, 91
(1987): Habbema L+, *Dermatologica* 174, 184
(1985): Bigby M+, *J Am Acad Dermatol* 12, 866
(1984): Stern RS+, *JAMA* 252, 1433
Hot flashes (<1%)
Lichenoid eruption
(1996): Shelley WB+, *Cutis* 60, 20
(1990): Todd PA+, *Drugs* 40, 91
(1985): Bigby M+, *J Am Acad Dermatol* 12, 866
Lichen planus
(1999): *Acta Derm Venereol* (Stockh) 79, 329 (bullous)
(1984): Heymann WR+, *J Am Acad Dermatol* 10, 299
Lupus erythematosus
(1992): Parodi A+, *JAMA* 268, 51
Peripheral edema
Photodermatitis (bullous)
(1989): Rivers JK+, *Med J Aust* 151, 167
Photosensitivity (<1%)
(1999): Litt JZ, Beachwood, OH, personal case (observation)
(1994): Berger TG+, *Arch Dermatol* 130, 609 (in HIV-infected)
(1991): Allen R+, *J Rheumatol* 18, 893
(1991): Lutzow-Holm C, *Tidsskr Nor Laegeforen* (Norwegian) 111, 2739
(1990): Suarez SM+, *Arthritis Rheum* 33, 903
(1990): Todd PA+, *Drugs* 40, 91
(1989): Kaidbey KH+, *Arch Dermatol* 125, 783
(1987): Sterling JC+, *Br J Rheumatol* 26, 210
(1986): Shelley WB+, *Cutis* 38, 169
(1986): Mayou S+, *Br J Dermatol* 114, 519
(1986): Judd LE+, *Arch Dermatol* 122, 451
(1986): Szczeklik A, *Drugs* 32 (Suppl 4), 148
(1985): Farr PM+, *Lancet* 1, 1166
(1983): Diffey BL+, *Br J Rheumatol* 22, 239
Phototoxic reaction
(1989): Kaidbey KH+, *Arch Dermatol* 125, 783
Pityriasis rosea
(1993): Yosipovitch G+, *Harefuah* (Hebrew) 124, 198; 247
Pruritus (3–9%)
(1990): Todd PA+, *Drugs* 40, 91 (1–5%)
(1985): Bigby M+, *J Am Acad Dermatol* 12, 866 (14%)
(1982): Bailin PL+, *Clin Rheum Dis* 8, 493 (passim)
(1978): Castles JJ+, *Arch Intern Med* 138, 362
(1975): Bowers DE+, *Ann Intern Med* 83, 470 (17%)
Pseudo-reactions (sic)
(1991): VanArsdel PP, *JAMA* 266, 3343
Purpura (<3%)
(1985): Bigby M+, *J Am Acad Dermatol* 12, 866
(1982): Bailin PL+, *Clin Rheum Dis* 8, 493 (passim)
(1979): Brogden RN+, *Drugs* 18, 241
(1975): Brogden RN+, *Drugs* 9, 326
Pustular eruption
(1989): Grattan CEH, *Dermatologica* 179, 57
(1986): Page SR+, *BMJ* 293, 510
Pyogenic granuloma
(1994): Shelley WB+, *Cutis* 53, 36 (observation)
Rash (sic) (3–9%)
(1995): Knulst AC+, *Br J Dermatol* 133, 647
Stevens–Johnson syndrome (<1%)
Toxic epidermal necrolysis (<1%)
(1993): Correia O+, *Dermatology* 186, 32
Urticaria
(1985): Bigby M+, *J Am Acad Dermatol* 12, 866 (1–5%)
(1984): Stern RS+, *JAMA* 252, 1433
(1979): Brogden RN+, *Drugs* 18, 241
(1975): Brogden RN+, *Drugs* 9, 326
Vasculitis
(1996): Lossos IS+, *Harefuah* (Hebrew) 130, 600
(1992): Jahangiri M+, *Postgrad Med J* 68, 766
(1992): Veraguth AJ+, *Schweiz Med Wochenschr* (German) 122, 923
(1990): Todd PA+, *Drugs* 40, 91 (1–5%) (necrotizing venulitis)
(1989): Singhal PC+, *Ann Allergy* 63, 107
(1985): Bigby M+, *J Am Acad Dermatol* 12, 866
(1980): Mordes JP, *Arch Intern Med* 140, 985
(1979): Brogden RN+, *Drugs* 18, 241
(1979): Grennan DM+, *N Z Med J* 89, 48
Vesiculobullous eruption
(1984): Stern RS+, *JAMA* 252, 1433

Hair

Hair – alopecia (<1%)
(1990): Todd PA+, *Drugs* 40, 91 (<1%)
(1989): Barter AC, *BMJ* 298, 325
(1989): Barth JH, *BMJ* 298, 675

Other

Anaphylactoid reaction (<1%)
Aphthous stomatitis
Myalgia (<1%)
Oral ulceration
Porphyria cutanea tarda
(1992): Shelley WB+, *Advanced Dermatologic Diagnosis*, WB Saunders, 414 (passim)
Pseudoporphyria
(1999): Al-Khenaizan S+, *J Cutan Med Surg* 3, 162
(1995): Creemers MC+, *Scand J Rheumatol* 24, 185
(1995): Girschick HJ+, *Scand J Rheumatol* 24, 108
(1994): Lang BA+, *J Pediatr* 124, 639
(1992): Petersen CS+, *Ugeskr Laeger* (Danish) 154, 1713
(1992): Cox NH+, *Br J Dermatol* 126, 86
(1991): Allen R+, *J Rheumatol* 18, 893
(1990): Suarez SM+, *Arthritis Rheum* 33, 903
(1990): Todd PA+, *Drugs* 40, 91
(1990): Sternberg A, *Acta Derm Venereol* 70, 354
(1990): Levy ML+, *J Pediatr* 117, 660
(1989): Kaidbey KH+, *Arch Dermatol* 125, 783
(1988): Diffey BL+, *Clin Exp Dermatol* 13, 207
(1987): Nicholls D, *N Z Med J* 100, 427
(1987): Taylor BJ+, *N Z Med J* 100, 322
(1987): Burns DA, *Clin Exp Dermatol* 12, 296
(1987): Sterling JC+, *Br J Rheumatol* 26, 210
(1987): Shelley ED+, *Cutis* 40, 314
(1986): Judd LE+, *Arch Dermatol* 122, 451
(1986): Mayou S+, *Br J Dermatol* 114, 519
(1985): Farr PM+, *Lancet* 1, 1166
(1985): Howard AM+, *Lancet* 1, 819
Salivary gland enlargement
(1995): Knulst AC+, *Br J Dermatol* 133, 647
Stomatitis (<3%)
Xerostomia

NARATRIPTAN

Trade name: Amerge (GlaxoWellcome)
Indications: Acute migraine attacks
Category: Antimigraine; serotonin agonist
Half-life: 6 hours
Clinically important, potentially serious interactions with: ergotamines, fluoxetine, fluvoxamine, methysergide, oral contraceptives, paroxetine, sertraline

Reactions

Skin
Acne (<1%)
Allergic reactions (sic) (<1%)
Atypical sensations (sic) (<1)%
Dermatitis (sic) (<1%)
Diaphoresis (<1%)
Edema (<1%)
Erythema (<1%)
Exanthems (<1%)
Folliculitis (<1%)
Photosensitivity (<1%)
Purpura (<1%)
Rash (sic) (<1%)
Urticaria (<1%)
Xerosis (<1%)

Hair
Hair – alopecia (<1%)

Other
Dysgeusia (<1%)
Hyperesthesia (<1%)
Hypesthesia (<1%)
Paresthesias (2%)
Photophobia (<1%)
Sialopenia (<1%)

NEBIVOLOL

Trade name: Nebilet (Menarini)
Indications: Hypertension
Category: Beta adrenergic blocking agent
Half-life: 8 hours
Clinically important, potentially serious interactions with: no data

Reactions

Skin
None

Other
Myalgia
Paresthesias
(1999): McNeely W+, *Drugs* 57, 633

NEFAZODONE

Trade name: Serzone (Bristol-Myers Squibb)
Indications: Depression
Category: Phenylpiperazine antidepressant
Half-life: 2–4 hours
Clinically important, potentially serious interactions with: alprazolam, astemizole, benzodiazepines, cisapride, CNS depressants, digoxin, fluoxetine, haloperidol, lovastatin, MAO inhibitors, phenytoin, pimozide, propranolol, simvastatin, terfenadine, trazodone, triazolam

Reactions

Skin
Acne (<1%)
Allergic reactions (sic) (<1%)
Burning (sic)
(2000): Lerner V+, *J Clin Psychiatry* 61, 216
Cellulitis (<1%)
Ecchymoses (<1%)
Eczema (sic) (<1%)
Exanthems (<1%)
Facial edema (<1%)
Flu-like syndrome (sic) (1–10%)
Flushing (4%)
Infection (sic) (8%)
Peripheral edema (3%)
Photosensitivity (<1%)
Pruritus (2%)
Rash (sic) (2%)
Urticaria (<1%)
Vesiculobullous eruption (<1%)
Xerosis (<1%)

Hair
Hair – alopecia (<1%)
(1998): Rademaker M, Hamilton, New Zealand (from Internet) (observation)
(1997): Gupta S+, *J Fam Pract* 44, 20

Other
Ageusia (<1%)
Dysgeusia (2%)
Foetor ex ore (halitosis) (<1%)
Gingivitis (<1%)
Glossitis (<1%)
Gynecomastia (<1%)
Hyperesthesia (<1%)
Mastodynia (1%)
Myalgia
Oral candidiasis (<1%)
Oral ulceration (<1%)
Paresthesias (4%)
(1999): Litt JZ, Beachwood, OH, personal case (observation)
Priapism (<1%)
Sialorrhea (<1%)
Stomatitis (<1%)
Vaginitis (2%)
Xerostomia (25%)

NELFINAVIR

Trade name: Viracept (Agouron)
Indications: HIV infection
Category: Antiretroviral; protease inhibitor*
Half-life: 3.5–5 hours
Clinically important, potentially serious interactions with: alcohol, alprazolam, amiodarone, astemizole, barbiturates, benzodiazepines, carbamazepine, cisapride, clorazepate, delavirdine, diazepam, estazolam, flurazepam, indinavir, nevirapine, oral contraceptives, phenobarbital, phenytoin, quinidine, rifabutin, rifampin, ritonavir, terfenadine, triazolam, zolpidem

Reactions

Skin

Allergic reactions (sic) (<1%)
Dermatitis (sic) (<1%)
Diaphoresis (<1%)
Pruritus (<1%)
Rash (sic) (1–10%)
(2000): Fortuny C+, *AIDS* 14, 335
Urticaria (<1%)

Other

Myalgia (<1%)
Oral ulceration (<1%)
Paresthesias (<1%)

***Note:** Protease inhibitors cause dyslipidemia which includes elevated triglycerides and cholesterol and redistribution of body fat centrally to produce the so-called "protease paunch," breast enlargement, facial atrophy, and "buffalo hump."

NEOMYCIN

Trade name: Neosporin (Warner-Lambert)
Other common trade names: *Gemicina; Myciguent; Neomicina; Neomycine Diamant; Neosulf; Nivemycin, etc.*
Indications: Various infections caused by susceptible organisms
Category: Aminoglycoside antibiotic
Half-life: 3 hours
Clinically important, potentially serious interactions with: aldesleukin, aminoglycosides, anticoagulants, bumetanide, digoxin, dimenhydrinate, ethacrynic acid, fenoprofen, furosemide, indomethacin, ketoprofen, methotrexate, naproxen, NSAIDs, piroxicam, succinylcholine, torsemide, vancomycin

Reactions

Skin

Allergic reactions (sic)
Angioedema
(1959): Pirilä V+, *Acta Derm Venereol* (Stockh) 39, 1470
Bullous eruption
Contact dermatitis
(1999): Lestringant GG+, *Int J Dermatol* 38, 181 (5.1%)
(1999): Giordano-Labadie F+, *Contact Dermatitis* 40, 192 (2.6%) (in atopics)
(1998): Kimura M+, *Contact Dermatitis* 39, 148
(1998): Katsarou-Katsari A+, *J Eur Acad Dermatol Venereol* 11, 9
(1997): Dasaraju P+, *Clin Infect Dis* 25, 33
(1996): Sheretz EF, *Arch Dermatol* 132, 461
(1994): Fisher AA, *Cutis* 54, 300
(1993): Lipozencic J+, *Arh Hig Rada Toksikol* (Serbo-Croatian-Roman) 44, 173
(1991): Barros MA+, *Contact Dermatitis* 25, 156
(1991): Mariani R+, *Contact Dermatitis* 24, 227
(1990): Grandinetti PJ+, *J Am Acad Dermatol* 23, 646
(1990): Smith IM+, *Clin Otolaryngol* 15, 155
(1989): Guin JD+, *Cutis* 43, 564
(1989): Massone L+, *Contact Dermatitis* 21, 344
(1988): Shupp DL+, *Cutis* 42, 528
(1987): Abdul-Gaffoor PM, *Indian J Dermatol* 32, 102
(1986): Baldinger J+, *Ann Ophthalmol* 18, 95
(1986): Rebandel P+, *Contact Dermatitis* 15, 92
(1986): Bajaj AK+, *Int J Dermatol* 25, 103
(1985): Fraki JE+, *Acta Otolaryngol Stockh* 100, 414
(1985): Frenzel U+, *Phlebologie* (French) 38, 389
(1985): Szarmach H+, *Przegl Dermatol* (Polish) 72, 521 (disseminated)
(1985): Fisher AA, *Cutis* 35, 315
(1984): Menne T+, *Hautarzt* (German) 35, 319
(1983): Macdonald RH+, *Clin Exp Dermatol* 8, 249
(1982): Fisher AA, *Ann Allergy* 49, 97
(1981): Fisher AA+, *Cutis* 28, 491
(1981): LeRoy R+, *Derm Beruf Umwelt* (German) 29, 168
(1981): Gordon W, *S Afr Med J* 59, 212
(1980): Epstein E, *Contact Dermatitis* 6, 219
(1979): Prystowsky SD+, *Arch Dermatol* 115, 959
(1979): Leyden JJ+, *JAMA* 242, 1276
(1979): Prystowsky SD+, *Arch Dermatol* 115, 713
(1978): Durocher LP, *Can Med Assoc J* (French) 118, 162
(1978): Forstrom L+, *Contact Dermatitis* 4, 312
(1977): Shouji A, *Nippon Rinsho* (Japanese) 35, 210
(1977): Sinka L+, *Bratisl Lek Listy* (Slovak) 67, 59
(1976): Fisher AA+, *Cutis* 18, 637
(1976): Carruthers JA+, *Contact Dermatitis* 2, 269
(1974): Peterkin GA, *J Laryngol Otol* 88, 15
(1974): Bandmann HJ+, *Internist Berl* (German) 15, 47
(1974): Malten KE+, *Phlebologie* (French) 27, 417
(1973): Ebner H, *Wien Klin Wochenschr* (German) 85, 203
(1973): *BMJ* 1, 250
(1973): Naess K, *Tidsskr Nor Laegeforen* (Norwegian) 93, 2498
(1972): Hattori S, *Nippon Ika Daigaku Zasshi* (Japanese) 39, 23
(1972): Hadida ME+, *J Med Lyon* (French) 53, 1093
(1971): Foussereau J+, *Bull Soc Fr Dermatol Syphiligr* (French) 78, 457
(1971): Bielicky T+, *Z Haut Geschlechtskr* (German) 46, 771
(1971): Epstein, E, *Arch Dermatol* 103, 562
(1970): Bandmann HJ, *Munch Med Wochenschr* (German) 112, 1125
(1970): Chilvers AS+, *Lancet* 1, 402
(1970): Bowczyc J+, *Przegl Dermatol* (Polish) 57, 763
(1969): Matner T, *Hautarzt* (German) 20, 446
(1969): Novak M+, *Cesk Dermatol* (Czech) 44, 177
(1968): Hjorth N+, *Br J Dermatol* 80, 163
(1968): Bartova J, *Cesk Dermatol* (Czech) 43, 271
(1968): Hiemisch I+, *Z Haut Geschlechtskr* (German) 43, 49
(1967): Pirila V+, *Acta Derm Venereol* (Stockh) 47, 419
(1967): Schwank R, *Cesk Dermatol* 42, 341
(1967): *Med Lett Drugs Ther* 9, 71
(1966): Pirila V+, *Acta Derm Venereol* (Stockh) 46, 489
(1966): Jensen OC+, *JAMA* 195, 131
(1965): Kirton V+, *Lancet* 1, 138
Dermatitis (sic) (1–10%)
(1990): Bouffioux B+, *Nouv Dermatol* (French) 9, 25
(1959): Pirilä V+, *Acta Derm Venereol* (Stockh) 39, 1470
Eczematous eruption (sic)
(1969): Ekelund A+, *Acta Derm Venereol* (Stockh) 49, 422
Erythema multiforme
(1986): Fisher AA, *Cutis* 37, 158
Exanthems
(1990): Bouffioux B+, *Nouv Dermatol* (French) 9, 25
Fixed eruption
(1985): Gomez B+, *Allergol Immunopathol Madr* (Spanish) 13, 87
Pruritus
Rash (sic) (1–10%)
Toxic epidermal necrolysis
(1969): Muresan D+, *Viata Med* (Romanian) 16, 731
(1959): Catto JVF, *BMJ* 2, 544
Ulceration
Urticaria (1–10%)
(1959): Pirilä V+, *Acta Derm Venereol* (Stockh) 39, 1470

Hair

Hair – alopecia

Other

Anaphylactoid reaction
(1986): Goh CL, *Australian J Dermatol* 27, 125

NEVIRAPINE

Trade name: Viramune (Roxane)
Indications: HIV infections
Category: Antiretroviral non-nucleoside reverse transcriptase inhibitor (NNRTI)
Half-life: 45 hours
Clinically important, potentially serious interactions with: cimetidine, estrogens, indinavir, ketoconazole, macrolides, nelfinavir, rifabutin, rifampin, ritonavir, saquinavir

Reactions

Skin

Dress syndrome*
(2000): Sissoko D+, *Presse Med* (French) 29, 1041
Exanthems
Pruritus
Rash (sic) (39.6%)
(1999): Anton P+, *AIDS* 13, 524
(1998): Ho TT+, *AIDS* 12, 2082
(1998): Bourezane Y+, *Clin Infect Dis* 27, 1321
(1998): Barner A+, *Lancet* 351, 1133
(1996): Luzuriaga K+, *J Infect Dis* 174, 713
(1995): Havlir D+, *J Infect Dis* 171, 537 (48%)
Stevens–Johnson syndrome (<1%)
(2000): Garcia Fernandez D+, *Rev Clin Esp* (Spanish) 200, 179
(1999): Wetterwald E+, *Br J Dermatol* 140, 980 (SJS/TEN overlap syndrome)
(1998): McClain SA, SUNY Stony Brook NY (from Internet) (observation)
(1998): Warren KJ+, *Lancet* 351–567
Toxic epidermal necrolysis
(1999): Wetterwald E+, *Br J Dermatol* 140, 980 (SJS/TEN overlap syndrome)
(1999): Descamps V+, *Lancet* 353, 1855
(1999): Phan TG+, *Australas J Dermatol* 40, 153

Other

Gingivitis (1–3%)
Hypersensitivity
(2000): Podzamczer D+, *AIDS* 14, 331
Lipodystrophy
(2000): Lewis RH+, *J Acquir Immune Defic Syndrom* 23, 355
(1999): Aldeen T+, *AIDS* 13, 865
Myalgia (1–10%)
Paresthesias (2%)
Ulcerative stomatitis (4%)

***Note:** The dress syndrome consists of "drug rash with eosinophilia and systemic symptoms".

NIACIN

Synonym: nicotinic acid
Trade names: Niaspan (Kos); Niacor (Upsher-Smith); Nicobid; Nicolar (Aventis); Nicotinex; Slo-Niacin (Upsher-Smith)
Other common trade names: *Apo-Nicotinamide; Nia-Bid; Niac; Niacels; Nicobion; Nicovital; Nicotinex; Pepeom Amide, Vitamin B_3*
Indications: Hyperlipidemia
Category: Antihyperlipidemic
Half-life: 45 minutes
Clinically important, potentially serious interactions with: adrenergic blocking agents, carbamazepine, lovastatin

Reactions

Skin

Acanthosis nigricans
(1994): Stals H+, *Dermatology* 189, 203
(1994): McKenney JM+, *JAMA* 271, 672
(1993): Stone OJ, *Med Hypotheses* 40, 154
(1992): Coates P+, *Br J Dermatol* 126, 412
(1990): Brown G+, *N Engl J Med* 323, 1289 (8.3%)
(1990): Audicana M+, *Contact Dermatitis* 22, 60
(1989): Larmi E, *Int J Dermatol* 28, 609
(1989): Ylipieti S+, *Contact Dermatitis* 21, 105
(1981): Elgart ML, *J Am Acad Dermatol* 5, 709
(1974): Pedro S, *N Engl J Med* 29, 422
(1971): Curth HO, *Birth Defects* 7, 31
(1967): Branehog I+, *Lakartidningen* (Swedish) 64, 1449
(1964): Tromovitch TA+, *Arch Dermatol* 89, 222
Contact dermatitis
(1995): Bilbao I+, *Contact Dermatitis* 33, 435
Erythema
(1995): Fisher AA, *Cutis* 55, 132
Exanthems
(1997): Blumenthal, HL, Beachwood, OH, personal case (observation)
(1997): Litt JZ, Beachwood, OH, two personal cases (observation)
(1990): Brown G+, *N Engl J Med* 323, 1289 (2.8%)
Fixed eruption (<1%)
(1992): de la Hoz-Caballer B+, *Med Clin (Barc)* (Spanish) 98, 357
Flushing (1–10%)
(1998): Knopp RH, *Am J Cardiol* 82, 24U
(1998): Guyton JR+, *Am J Cardiol* 82, 737 (4.8%)
(1998): Capuzzi DM+, *Am J Cardiol* 82, 74U
(1998): Morgan JM+, *Am J Cardiol* 82, 29U
(1997): Jungnickel PW+, *J Gen Intern Med* 12, 591
(1996): Glen AI+, *Prostaglandins Leukot Essent Fatty Acids* 55, 9
(1996): Crouse JR, *Coron Artery* 7, 321
(1994): Fivenson DP+, *Arch Dermatol* 130, 753
(1994): McKenney JM+, *JAMA* 271, 672
(1994): Sudan BJ, *Ann Pharmacother* 28, 1113
(1993): Fisher AA, *Cutis* 51, 225
(1992): Whelan AM+, *J Fam Pract* 34, 165 (passim)
(1992): Breathnach SM+, *Adverse Drug Reactions and the Skin*, Blackwell, Oxford, 265 (passim)
(1989): Warady B+, *Perit Dial Int* 9, 81
(1988): Figge HL+, *Pharmacotherapy* 8, 287
(1985): Mooney E, *Int J Dermatol* 24, 549
(1977): Estep DL+, *Clin Toxicol* 11, 325
(1973): Levy RI+, *Drugs* 6, 12
(1973): *Med Lett* 15, 102
Hyperpigmentation
(1992): Breathnach SM+, *Adverse Drug Reactions and the Skin*, Blackwell, Oxford, 265 (passim)
Ichthyosis
(1961): Berge KG+, *Am J Med* 31, 24
Keratoses, pigmented
(1974): Wittenborn JR+, *Adv Biochem Psychopharmacol* 9, 295
Pruritus (1–5%)
(1997): Jungnickel PW+, *J Gen Intern Med* 12, 591
(1997): Blumenthal, HL, Beachwood, OH, personal case (observation)
(1994): Fivenson DP+, *Arch Dermatol* 130, 753
(1994): McKenney JM+, *JAMA* 271, 672
(1992): Whelan AM+, *J Fam Pract* 34, 165 (passim)
(1992): Breathnach SM+, *Adverse Drug Reactions and the Skin*, Blackwell, Oxford, 265 (passim)
(1977): Estep DL+, *Clin Toxicol* 11, 325
(1973): Levy RI+, *Drugs* 6, 12
(1973): *Med Lett* 15, 102
Rash (sic) (<1%)
(1994): McKenney JM+, *JAMA* 271, 672
(1992): Breathnach SM+, *Adverse Drug Reactions and the Skin*, Blackwell, Oxford, 265 (passim)
(1988): Figge HL+, *Pharmacotherapy* 8, 287
Scaling (sic)
(1992): Breathnach SM+, *Adverse Drug Reactions and the Skin*, Blackwell, Oxford, 265 (passim)
Urticaria
(1995): Fisher AA, *Cutis* 55, 132
Xerosis

Other

Anaphylactoid reaction
Burning mouth syndrome
(1988): Haustein UF, *Contact Dermatitis* 19, 225
Gingival pain
(1998): Leighton RF+, *Chest* 114, 1472

Myopathy
(1994): Gharavi AG+, *Am J Cardiol* 74, 841
(1989): Goldstein MR, *Am J Med* 87, 248
(1989): Litin SC+, *Am J Med* 86, 481
Paresthesias (1–10%)
(1997): Jungnickel PW+, *J Gen Intern Med* 12, 591
(1992): Whelan AM+, *J Fam Pract* 34, 165 (passim)
Tooth pain (sic)
(1998): Leighton RF+, *Chest* 114, 1472
Xerostomia

NIACINAMIDE

Synonym: nicotinamide; vitamin B_3
Trade name: Niacinamide
Indications: Prophylaxis and treatment of pellagra
Category: Water-soluble nutritional supplement
Half-life: 45 minutes
Clinically important, potentially serious interactions with: adrenergic blocking agents, carbamazepine, lovastatin, oral hypoglycemics, probenecid, sulfinpyrazone

Reactions

Skin
Acanthosis nigricans
(1984): Papa CM, *Arch Dermatol* 120, 281
Pruritus (1–5%)
(1981): Zackheim HS+, *J Am Acad Dermatol* 4, 736
(1980): Bures FA, *J Am Acad Dermatol* 3, 530
Rash (sic)

Other
Paresthesias (1–10%)

NICARDIPINE

Trade name: Cardene (Wyeth-Ayerst)
Other common trade names: *Antagonil; Dagan; Loxen; Nicardal; Nicodel; Ranvil; Ridene; Rydene*
Indications: Angina, hypertension
Category: Calcium channel blocker; antianginal and antihypertensive; antimigraine
Half-life: 2–4 hours
Clinically important, potentially serious interactions with: amprenavir, azole antifungals, beta-blockers, calcium, carbamazepine, cimetidine, cyclosporine, digoxin, fentanyl, nelfinavir, procainamide, quinidine, rifampin, ritonavir, theophylline, **grapefruit juice**

Reactions

Skin
Allergic reactions (sic)
Cutaneous side effects (sic)
(1993): Kitamura K+, *J Dermatol* 20, 279 (psoriasiform)
Edema (1%)
Erythromelalgia
(1989): Levesque H+, *BMJ* 298, 1252
(1989): Drenth JH, *BMJ* 298, 1582
Exanthems
Flushing (5.6%)
(1998): Knowles S+, *J Am Acad Dermatol* 38, 201 (passim)
(1990): Webster J+, *Br J Clin Pharmacol* 29, 587P
Peripheral edema (7.1%)
(1998): Knowles S+, *J Am Acad Dermatol* 38, 201 (passim)
(1990): Webster J+, *Br J Clin Pharmacol* 29, 587P (leg edema)
Rash (sic) (1.2%)
(1998): Knowles S+, *J Am Acad Dermatol* 38, 201 (passim)
(1985): Deedwania PC+, *Clin Pharmacol Ther* 37, 190
(1985): Gelman JS+, *Am J Cardiol* 56, 232
Urticaria
(1983): Fisher JR+, *Ann Intern Med* 98, 671
(1983): Brodmerkel GJ, *Ann Intern Med* 99, 415
(1982): Grunwald Z, *Drug Intell Clin Pharm* 16, 492

Other
Gingival hyperplasia (<1%)
Myalgia (1%)
(1998): Knowles S+, *J Am Acad Dermatol* 38, 201 (passim)
Paresthesias (1%)
Parotitis
Xerostomia (1.4%)

NICOTINE*

Trade names: Habitrol Patch (Novartis); Nicoderm Patch (SmithKline Beecham); Nicorette Gum (SmithKline Beecham); Nicotrol Nasal Spray and Patch (McNeil); Polacrilex (SmithKline Beecham); Prostep Patch; Zyban (GlaxoWellcome)
Other common trade names: *Exodus, Nicabate, Nicolan; Nicorette Plus; Nicotinell-TTS; Nicotrans; Nikofrenon; Stubit*
Indications: Aid to smoking cessation
Category: Smoking deterrent
Half-life: varies with the delivery system*
Clinically important, potentially serious interactions with: acetaminophen, adenosine, beta-blockers, bupropion, caffeine, cimetidine, imipramine, insulin, oxazepam, pentazocine, propranolol, propoxyphene, theophylline, warfarin

Reactions

Skin
Contact dermatitis
(1993): Farm G, *Contact Dermatitis* 29, 214
Diaphoresis (1–3%)
Edema
Flushing
Erythema (>10%)
Pruritus (>10%)
Urticaria
Rash (sic)
Vasculitis
(1996): Van der Klauw MM+, *Br J Dermatol* 134, 361

Other
Application-site burning
Application-site erythema
Application-site pruritus
Dysgeusia
Hypersensitivity (<1%)
Myalgia (1–10%)
Paresthesias
Sialorrhea (>10%)
Stomatitis (>10%)
Tremor
Xerostomia (1–3%)

***Note:** Smoking cessation therapy has various delivery systems. These include: transdermal patches, chewing gum, nasal spray, inhaler, and oral forms.

NIFEDIPINE

Trade names: Adalat (Bayer); Procardia (Pfizer)
Other common trade names: *Adalate; Apo-Nifed; Aprical; Calcilat; Coracten; Corogal; Corotrend; Nifecor; Nu-Nifed; Pidilat*
Indications: Angina; hypertension
Category: Calcium channel blocker; antianginal and antihypertensive; antimigraine
Half-life: 2–5 hours
Clinically important, potentially serious interactions with: alcohol, amprenavir, azole antifungals, barbiturates, beta-blockers, calcium, carbamazepine, cimetidine, cisapride, cyclosporine, digoxin, diltiazem, fentanyl, nelfinavir, phenobarbital, prazosin, quinidine, rifampin, ritonavir, theophylline, vincristine, **grapefruit juice**

Reactions

Skin

Acute generalized exanthematous pustulosis (AGEP)
(1995): Moreau A+, *Int J Dermatol* 34, 263 (passim)
(1991): Roujeau J-C+, *Arch Dermatol* 127, 1333
Angioedema (<1%)
(1998): Knowles S+, *J Am Acad Dermatol* 38, 201 (passim)
(1989): Stern R+, *Arch Intern Med* 149, 829
Ankle edema
(1994): Mohammed KN, *Ann Pharmacother* 28, 967
(1991): Salmasi AM+, *Int J Cardiol* 30, 303
(1989): Williams SA+, *Eur J Clin Pharmacol* 37, 333
(1978): Bridgman JF, *BMJ* 276, 578
Bullous eruption
(1989): Stern R+, *Arch Intern Med* 149, 829
(1987): Alcalay J+, *Dermatologica* 175, 191
Chills (2%)
Cutaneous side effects (sic)
(1993): Kitamura K+, *J Dermatol* 20, 279 (psoriasiform)
Dermatitis (sic) (<2%)
Diaphoresis (<2%)
(1989): Stern R+, *Arch Intern Med* 149, 829
(1983): Lewis JG, *Drugs* 25, 196
Edema
(1983): Lewis JG, *Drugs* 25, 196
(1978): Bridgman JF, *BMJ* 276, 578 (erythematous, of legs)
Erysipelas
(1988): Leibovici V+, *Cutis* 41, 367
(1983): Lewis JG, *Drugs* 25, 196
Erythema
(1998): Knowles S+, *J Am Acad Dermatol* 38, 201 (passim)
(1992): Gonzalez-Castro U+, *Med Clin (Barc)* (Spanish) 98, 759
Erythema multiforme
(1998): Knowles S+, *J Am Acad Dermatol* 38, 201 (passim)
(1997): Springuel P, *Can Med Assoc J* 156, 90
(1989): Stern R+, *Arch Intern Med* 149, 829
(1986): Myrhed M+, *Acta Pharmacol Toxicol* 58, 133
Erythema nodosum
(1998): Knowles S+, *J Am Acad Dermatol* 38, 201 (passim)
(1989): Stern R+, *Arch Intern Med* 149, 829
Erythromelalgia (<0.5%)
(1989): Stern R+, *Arch Intern Med* 149, 829
(1987): Alcalay J+, *Dermatologica* 175, 191
(1983): Brodmerkel GJ, *Ann Intern Med* 99, 415
(1983): Fisher JR+, *Ann Intern Med* 98, 671
Exanthems
(1998): Knowles S+, *J Am Acad Dermatol* 38, 201 (passim)
(1995): Litt JZ, Beachwood, OH, personal case (observation)
(1992): Parish LC+, *Cutis* 49, 113 (morbilliform)
(1989): Stern R+, *Arch Intern Med* 149, 829
(1987): Alcalay J+, *Dermatologica* 175, 191
(1985): Findlay GH, *S Afr Med J* 68, 176
(1983): Lewis JG, *Drugs* 25, 196 (1%)
(1982): Grunwald Z, *Drug Intell Clin Pharm* 16, 492
(1980): Antman E+, *N Engl J Med* 302, 1269 (1%)
Exfoliative dermatitis (<1%)
(1994): Mohammed KN, *Ann Pharmacother* 28, 967
(1993): Collins P, *Br J Dermatol* 129, 630 (passim)
(1989): Stern R+, *Arch Intern Med* 149, 829
(1989): Reynolds HJ+, *Br J Dermatol* 121, 401
(1984): Scoble JE+, *Clin Nephrol* 21, 302
Facial edema (1%)
Fixed eruption
(1993): Litt JZ, Beachwood, OH, personal case (observation)
(1987): Alcalay J+, *Dermatologica* 175, 191
(1986): Alcalay J+, *BMJ* 292, 450
Flushing (3–25%)
(1992): Shelley WB+, *Advanced Dermatologic Diagnosis*, WB Saunders, 582 (passim)
(1985): Aberg H+, *Drugs* 29 (Suppl 2), 117 (22%)
(1983): Lewis JG, *Drugs* 25, 196 (5–15%)
(1980): Antman E+, *N Engl J Med* 302, 1269 (11%)
Lichenoid eruption
(1989): Reynolds HJ+, *Br J Dermatol* 121, 401
(1988): Leibovici V+, *Cutis* 41, 367
(1984): Scoble JE+, *Clin Nephrol* 21, 302
Lupus erythematosus
(1998): Callen JP, Academy '98 Meeting
Painful edema of extremities
(1985): Findlay GH, *S Afr Med J* 68, 176
(1982): Grunwald Z, *Drug Intell Clin Pharm* 16, 492
Pemphigoid nodularis
(2000): Ameen M+, *Br J Dermatol* 142, 575
Pemphigus foliaceus
(1993): Kim S-C+, *Acta Derm Venereol* (Stockh) 73, 210
Periorbital edema (1%)
(1985): Tordjman K+, *Am J Cardiol* 55, 1445
Peripheral edema (10–30%)
(1996): Tailor SA+, *Arch Dermatol* 132, 350 (with itraconazole)
Photosensitivity
(1996): Seggev JS+, *J Allergy Clin Immunol* 97, 852
(1991): Zenarola P+, *Dermatologica* 182, 196
(1990): Guarrera M+, *Photodermatology* 7, 25
(1988): Zlotogorski A, *Dermatologica* 177, 249
(1986): Thomas SE+, *BMJ* 292, 992
Prurigo nodularis
(1992): Shelley WB+, *Cutis* 50, 179 (observation)
Pruritus (<2%)
(1998): Knowles S+, *J Am Acad Dermatol* 38, 201 (passim)
(1993): Collins P, *Br J Dermatol* 129, 630 (passim)
(1989): Stern R+, *Arch Intern Med* 149, 829
Purpura (<2%)
(1990): Regazzini R+, *Chron Derm* (Italian) 21, 225
(1989): Oren R+, *Drug Intell Clin Pharm* 23, 88
(1985): Findlay GH, *S Afr Med J* 68, 176
Rash (sic) (<3%)
(1998): Knowles S+, *J Am Acad Dermatol* 38, 201 (passim)
(1989): Stern R+, *Arch Intern Med* 149, 829
Stevens–Johnson syndrome
(1998): Knowles S+, *J Am Acad Dermatol* 38, 201 (passim)
(1993): Collins P, *Br J Dermatol* 129, 630 (passim)
(1989): Stern R+, *Arch Intern Med* 149, 829
Telangiectases
(1994): Shelley WB+, *Cutis* 53, 40 (observation)
(1993): Collins P, *Br J Dermatol* 129, 630 (photodistribution)
(1992): Tsele E+, *Lancet* 339, 365
Toxic epidermal necrolysis
(1998): Knowles S+, *J Am Acad Dermatol* 38, 201 (passim)
(1993): Collins P, *Br J Dermatol* 129, 630 (passim)
Urticaria (<1%)
(1998): Knowles S+, *J Am Acad Dermatol* 38, 201 (passim)
(1991): Zenarola P+, *Dermatologica* 182, 196
(1989): Stern R+, *Arch Intern Med* 149, 829
(1988): Toner M+, *Chest* 93, 1320
(1986): Myrhed M+, *Acta Pharmacol Toxicol* 58, 133
(1978): Bridgman JF, *BMJ* 276, 578
Vasculitis
(1989): Oren R+, *Drug Intell Clin Pharm* 23, 88
(1987): Alcalay J+, *Dermatologica* 175, 191
(1985): Brenner S+, *Harefuah* (Hebrew) 108, 139

Hair

Hair – alopecia (1%)
(1998): Knowles S+, *J Am Acad Dermatol* 38, 201 (passim)
(1993): Collins P, *Br J Dermatol* 129, 630 (passim)

(1989): Stern R+, *Arch Intern Med* 149, 829
(1989): Reynolds HJ+, *Br J Dermatol* 121, 401
Hair – discoloration
(1989): Stern R+, *Arch Intern Med* 149, 829

Nails

Nails – dystrophy
(1989): Stern R+, *Arch Intern Med* 149, 829

Other

Dysgeusia (<1%)
Dysosmia
Erythromyalgia
(1989): Stern R+, *Arch Intern Med* 149, 829
Gingival hyperplasia (>10%)
(2000): James JA+, *J Clin Periodontol* 27, 109 (with cyclosporine)
(1999): Ellis JS+, *J Periodontol* 70, 63 (6.3%)
(1998): Desai P+, *J Can Dent Assoc* 64, 263
(1998): Nakou M+, *J Periodontol* 69, 664
(1998): Nohl F+, *Ther Umsch* (German) 55, 573
(1998): Bokor-Bratic M+, *Med Pregl* (Serbo-Croatian [Roman]) 51, 445
(1997): Jackson C+, *N Y State Dent J* 63, 46
(1997): Westbrook P+, *J Periodontol* 68, 645
(1997): Slezak R, *J West Soc Periodontal Periodontal Abstr* 45, 105
(1997): Thomason JM+, *Clin Oral Investig* 1, 35
(1996): Ciantar M, *Dent Update* 23, 374
(1996): Deen-Duggins L+, *Quintessence Int* 27, 163 (4 cases)
(1996): Saito K+, *J Periodontol Res* 31, 545
(1996): Darbar UR+, *J Clin Periodontol* 23, 941
(1996): Abitbol TE+, *N Y State Dent J* 63, 34
(1995): Harel-Raviv M+, *Oral Surg Oral Med Oral Pathol Oral Radiol Endoc* 79, 715
(1995): Nery EB+, *J Periodontol* 66, 572
(1995): Wynn RL, *Gen Dent* 43, 218
(1995): Ramsdale DR+, *Br Heart J* 73, 115
(1995): Silverstein LH+ *J Oral Implantol* 21, 116
(1994): Shelley WB+, *Cutis* 53, 282 (passim)
(1994): Henderson JS+ *Miss Dent Assoc J* 50, 12
(1993): Steele RM+, *Arch Intern Med* 120, 663
(1993): Morisaki I+, *J Periodontal Res* 28, 396
(1993): King GN+, *J Clin Periodontol* 20, 286
(1992): Hancock RH+, *J Clin Periodontol* 19, 12
(1991): Nishikawa SJ+, *J Periodontol* 62, 30
(1991): Wynn RL, *Gen Dent* 39, 240
(1989): Veraldi S+, *Clin Exp Dermatol* 14, 93
(1988): Boisnic S+, *Ann Dermatol Venereol* (French) 115, 373
(1988): Zlotogorski A, *Dermatologica* 177, 249
(1986): Jones CM, *Br Dent J* 160, 416
(1986): Bencini PL+, *G Ital Dermatol Venereol* (Italian) 121, 29
(1985): Bencini PL+, *Acta Derm Venereol* (Stockh) 65, 362
(1985): Lucas RM+, *J Periodontol* 56, 211
(1984): Ramon Y+, *Int J Cardiol* 5, 195
(1984): Lederman D+, *Oral Surg Oral Med Oral Pathol* 57, 620
Gynecomastia (<1%)
(1995): Marcos-Olea JL+, *Aten Primaria* (Spanish) 16, 115
(1988): Zlotogorski A, *Dermatologica* 177, 249
(1986): Clyne CAC, *BMJ* 292, 380
Myalgia (<1%)
Paresthesias (<3%)
(1982): Macdonald JB, *BMJ* 285, 1744
Parotitis
Shakiness (sic) (2%)
Tremor (2–8%)
Xerostomia (<3%)

NIMODIPINE

Trade name: Nimotop (Bayer)
Other common trade names: *Admon; Periplum; Vasotop*
Indications: Subarachnoid hemorrhage
Category: Calcium channel blocker
Half-life: 3 hours
Clinically important, potentially serious interactions with: amprenavir, barbiturates, beta-blockers, carbamazepine, cimetidine, cyclosporine, digoxin, fentanyl, nelfinavir, omeprazole, prazosin, propranolol, quinidine, ritonavir, theophylline, **grapefruit juice**

Reactions

Skin

Acne (<1%)
Acute generalized exanthematous pustulosis (AGEP)
(1999): Zabawski E+, Dallas TX (from Internet) (observation)
Diaphoresis (<1%)
Edema (2%)
Exanthems (2.4%)
(1989): Langley MS+, *Drugs* 37, 669
Flushing (2.1%)
Peripheral edema
Pruritus (<1%)
Purpura
Rash (sic) (3%)

Hair

Hair – alopecia
(1995): Daghfous R+, *Therapie* (French) 50, 590

NISOLDIPINE

Trade name: Sular (AstraZeneca)
Other common trade names: *Baymycard; Syscor*
Indications: Hypertension
Category: Calcium channel blocker; antihypertensive
Half-life: 7–12 hours
Clinically important, potentially serious interactions with: beta-blockers, carbamazepine, cimetidine, cyclosporine, digoxin, fentanyl, omeprazole, quinidine, theophylline, **grapefruit juice**

Reactions

Skin

Acne (<1%)
Angioedema
Cellulitis (<1%)
Chills (<1%)
Cutaneous side effects (sic)
(1993): Kitamura K+, *J Dermatol* 20, 279
Diaphoresis (<1%)
Ecchymoses (<1%)
Exanthems (<1%)
(1988): Friedel HA+, *Drugs* 36, 682 (0.7%)
Exfoliative dermatitis (<1%)
Facial edema (<1%)
Flu-like syndrome (sic) (<1%)
Flushing
(1988): Friedel HA+, *Drugs* 36, 682 (13.21%)
Herpes simplex (<1%)
Herpes zoster (<1%)
Peripheral edema (22%)
Petechiae (<1%)
Photosensitivity
Pigmentation (<1%)
Pruritus (<1%)
Pustular eruption (<1%)

Rash (sic) (2%)
Ulceration (<1%)
Urticaria (<1%)
Xerosis (<1%)

Hair

Hair – alopecia (<1%)

Other

Dysgeusia (<1%)
Gingival hyperplasia (<1%)
Glossitis (<1%)
Gynecomastia (<1%)
Hypersensitivity
Hypesthesia (<1%)
Oral ulceration (<1%)
Paresthesias (<1%)
Tremor (<1%)
Vaginitis (<1%)
Xerostomia (<1%)

NITROFURANTOIN

Trade names: Furadantin (Dura); Macrobid (Procter & Gamble); Macrodantin (Procter & Gamble)
Other common trade names: *Furadantina; Furadoine; Furalan; Furan; Furobactina; Infurin; Nephronex; Novo-Furan; Urofuran*
Indications: Various urinary tract infections caused by susceptible organisms
Category: Urinary tract antibiotic
Half-life: 20–60 minutes
Clinically important, potentially serious interactions with: probenecid, sulfinpyrazone

Reactions

Skin

Acute febrile neutrophilic dermatosis (Sweet's syndrome)
(1999): Retief CR+, *Cutis* 63, 177
Angioedema
(1982): Penn RG+, *BMJ* 284, 1440
(1981): Chisholm JC+, *J Nat Med Assoc* 73, 59 (passim)
(1977): Delaney RA+, *Am J Pharm* 149, 26 (passim)
(1971): Koch-Weser J+, *Ann Intern Med* 128, 399 (0.1%)
Bullous eruption
Chills
Contact dermatitis
(1978): Novak M, *Cesk Dermatol* (Czech) 53, 128
(1974): Bleumink E+, *Hautarzt* (German) 25, 403
(1970): Laubstein H+, *Dermatol Monatsschr* (German) 156, 1
Eczematous eruption (sic)
(1977): Delaney RA+, *Am J Pharm* 149, 26 (passim)
(1976): Mitchell J+, *Modern Med* 44, 63
Erythema multiforme
(1990): Chan HL+, *Arch Dermatol* 126, 43
(1986): Chapman JA, *Ann Allergy* 56, 16
(1971): Koch-Weser J+, *Ann Intern Med* 128, 399 (0.1%)
Erythema nodosum
(1981): Chisholm JC+, *J Nat Med Assoc* 73, 59
Exanthems (1–5%)
(1984): Paver R+, *Current Ther* 25, 55
(1983): Swinyer LJ, *Dermatol Clin* 1, 417
(1980): Calderwood SB+, *Surgical Clin N Amer* 60, 65
(1980): Holmberg L+, *Am J Med* 69, 733 (28%)
(1976): Stubb S, *Acta Derm Venereol* (Stockh) 56 (Suppl 76), 16
(1974): Eggers B+, *Z Hautkr* (German) 49, 704
(1972): Kauppinen K, *Acta Derm Venereol* (Stockh) 52 (Suppl), 68
(1971): Bailey RR+, *Lancet* 2, 1112 (1%)
(1971): Koch-Weser J+, *Ann Intern Med* 128, 399 (1%)
Exfoliative dermatitis
(1984): Paver R+, *Current Ther* 25, 55
(1983): Swinyer LJ, *Dermatol Clin* 1, 417
(1972): Kauppinen K, *Acta Derm Venereol* (Stockh) 52 (Suppl), 68
Fixed eruption
(1985): Kauppinen K+, *Br J Dermatol* 112, 575
Flushing
Lupus erythematosus
(1986): Chapman JA, *Annals Allergy* 56, 16
(1985): Stratton MA, *Clin Pharm* 4, 657
(1981): Fleck RM, *Pennsylvania Med* 84, 36
(1975): Selroos O+, *Acta Med Scand* 197, 125
(1974): Back O+, *Lancet* 1, 930
Photosensitivity
(1987): Australian Drug Evaluation Committee, 61 (Oct 15)
Pruritus (<1%)
(1987): Australian Drug Evaluation Committee, 61 (Oct 15)
(1981): Chisholm JC+, *J Nat Med Assoc* 73, 59 (passim)
Purpura
(1984): Paver R+, *Current Ther* 25, 55
(1983): Swinyer LJ, *Dermatol Clin* 1, 417
Rash (sic) (<1%)
(1982): Penn RG+, *BMJ* 284, 1440
(1977): Takala J+, *Acta Med Scand* 202, 75
Reticular hyperplasia
(1966): Korting GW+, *Dermatol Wochenschr* (German) 152, 257
Stevens–Johnson syndrome
(1971): Koch-Weser J+, *Ann Intern Med* 128, 399
Toxic epidermal necrolysis
(1993): Stables GI+, *Br J Dermatol* 128, 357
(1984): Kauppinen K+, *Acta Derm Venereol* (Stockh) 64, 320
(1983): Swinyer LJ, *Dermatol Clin* 1, 417
(1967): Duperrat B+, *Bull Soc Fr Dermatol Syphiligr* (French) 74, 423 (fatal)
(1963): Oswald FH, *Ned Tijdschr Geneesk* (Danish) 107, 999
Urticaria
(1999): Litt JZ, Beachwood, OH, personal case (observation)
(1996): Blumenthal HL, Beachwood, OH, personal case (observation)
(1983): Swinyer LJ, *Dermatol Clin* 1, 417
(1983): Griffin JP, *Practitioner* 227, 1283
(1982): Schneider RE, *Clin Ther* 4, 390
(1978): Watson B+, *Br J Dermatol* 99, 183
(1977): McLundie S, *Ann Allergy* 38, 71
(1972): Kauppinen K, *Acta Derm Venereol* (Stockh) 52 (Suppl), 68
(1971): Koch-Weser J+, *Ann Intern Med* 128, 399 (0.4%)
(1969): Aaronson CM, *JAMA* 210, 557

Hair

Hair – alopecia
(1983): Swinyer LJ, *Dermatol Clin* 1, 417
(1983): No Author, *Lakartidningen* (Swedish) 80, 4040
(1977): Delaney RA+, *Am J Pharm* 149, 26 (passim)
(1971): Coster C+, *Lakartidningen* (Swedish) 68, 3366
(1959): Johnson SH+, *J Urology* (Baltimore) 82, 162

Nails

Nails – onycholysis
(1982): Penn RG+, *BMJ* 284, 1440

Other

Anaphylactoid reaction
(1987): Australian Drug Evaluation Committee, 61 (Oct 15)
(1982): Penn RG+, *BMJ* 284, 1440
(1980): Calderwood SB+, *Surg Clin N Amer* 60, 65
Galactorrhea
(1986): Auwaerter A+, *Krankenhausarzt* (German) 59, 766
Hypersensitivity
(1976): Fine SR, *Cutis* 17, 1171
Mastodynia
(1986): Auwaerter A+, *Krankenhausarzt* (German) 59, 766
Myalgia
Panniculitis, nodular nonsuppurative
(1987): Sanford RG+, *Arthritis Rheum* 30, 1076
Paresthesias (1–10%)
Tooth discoloration
Xerostomia
(1977): Takala J+, *Acta Med Scand* 202, 75

NITROGLYCERIN

Synonyms: glyceryl trinitrate; nitroglycerol; NTG

Trade names:

Buccal tablets: Nitrogard
Lingual aerosol: Nitrolingual
Oral capsules: Nitro-Bid; Nitrocap; Nitrocine; Nitroglyn; Nitrospan
Oral tablets: Klavikordal; Niong; Nitronet; Nitrong
Parenteral: Nitro-Bid; Nitroject; Nitrol; Nitrostat; Tridil
Sublingual tablets: Nitrostat
Topical ointment: Nitro-Bid; Nitrol; Nitrong; Nitrostat
Topical transdermal systems: Deponit; Minitran; Nitrocine; Nitrodisc; Nitrodur; Transderm-Nitro. (Various pharmaceutical companies.)

Other common trade names: *Cardinit; Corditrine; Lenitral; Nitradisc; Nitroglin; Suscard; Sustac*

Indications: Acute angina

Category: Antianginal; vasodilator; antihypertensive

Half-life: 1–4 minutes

Clinically important, potentially serious interactions with: alcohol, alteplase, beta-blockers, calcium channel blockers, ergot, heparin, sildenafil

Reactions

Skin

Allergic reactions (sic) (<1%)
Angioedema
(1998): Rademaker M+, *New Zealand Adverse Drug Reactions Committee*, April, 1998 (from Internet)
Contact dermatitis (to topical systems) (<1%)
(1999): Machet L+, *Dermatology* 198, 106
(1994): de la Fuente-Prieto R+, *Ann Allergy* 72, 344
(1992): Torres V+, *Contact Dermatitis* 26, 53
(1991): Kanerva L+, *Contact Dermatitis* 24, 356
(1991): Laine R+, *Duodecim* (Finnish) 107, 41
(1990): Vaillant L+, *Contact Dermatitis* 23, 142
(1989): Di Landro A+, *Contact Dermatitis* 21, 115
(1989): Carmichael AJ+, *Contact Dermatitis* 21, 113
(1989): Holdiness MR, *Contact Dermatitis* 20, 3
(1988): Niedner R, *Hautarzt* (German) 39, 761
(1988): Apted J, *Med J Aust* 148, 482
(1987): Harari Z+, *Dermatologica* 174, 249
(1987): Gupta AK+, *Arch Dermatol* 123, 295
(1987): Topaz O+, *Ann Allergy* 59, 365
(1986): Weickel R+, *Hautarzt* (German) 37, 511
(1986): Schrader BJ+, *Pharmacotherapy* 6, 83
(1985): Fischer RG+, *South Med J* 78, 1523
(1984): Fisher AA, *Cutis* 34, 526
(1984): Rosenfeld AS+, *Am Heart J* 108, 1061
(1984): Letendre PW+, *Drug Intell Clin Pharm* 18, 69
(1983): Camarasa JG+, *Contact Dermatitis* 9, 320
(1979): Hendricks AA+, *Arch Dermatol* 115, 853
Cyanosis
Diaphoresis (<1%)
Eczematous eruption (sic)
(1989): Carmichael AJ+, *Contact Dermatitis* 21, 113
(1987): Topaz O+, *Ann Allergy* 59, 365
Edema
Erythema (to transdermal delivery system)
(1990): Hogan JD+, *J Am Acad Dermatol* 22, 811
Erythroderma
(1972): Ryan FP, *Br J Dermatol* 87, 498
Exanthems
Exfoliative dermatitis (1–10%)
(1972): Ryan FP, *Br J Dermatol* 87, 498
Flushing (>10%)
(1992): Shelley WB+, *Advanced Dermatologic Diagnosis*, WB Saunders, 582 (passim)
Pallor
Peripheral edema (<1%)
Purpura
(1989): Nishioka K+, *J Dermatol* 16, 220 (pigmented)
(1955): Shmushkovich J+, *Br J Dermatol* 67, 299
Rash (sic) (1–10%)
Rosacea (exacerbation)
(1980): Wilkin JK, *Arch Dermatol* 116, 598
Urticaria

Other

Anaphylactoid reaction (from perianal application)
(1999): Pietroletti R+, *Am J Gastroenterol* 94, 292
Oral burning and tingling (from sublingual)
Xerostomia (<1%)

NIZATIDINE

Trade name: Axid (Lilly)

Other common trade names: *Apo-Nizatidine; Calmaxid; Gastrax; Nizax; Nizaxid; Panaxid; Tazac; Zanizal*

Indications: Duodenal ulcer, gastroesophageal reflux disease (GERD)

Category: Histamine H_2-receptor antagonist and anti-ulcer

Half-life: 1–2 hours

Clinically important, potentially serious interactions with: antacids, aspirin, cephalosporins, ketoconazole, nifedipine, nisoldipine, quinolones

Reactions

Skin

Acne (<1%)
Allergic reactions (sic) (<1%)
Contact dermatitis
Diaphoresis (1%)
(1988): Price AH+, *Drugs* 36, 521 (1%)
(1987): Cloud ML, *Scand J Gastroenterol* 22, 39
Edema
Exanthems
Exfoliative dermatitis
Pruritus (1.7%)
(1988): Price AH+, *Drugs* 36, 521
(1987): Cloud ML, *Scand J Gastroenterol* 22, 39
Rash (sic) (1.9%)
(1987): Cloud ML, *Scand J Gastroenterol* 22, 39
Urticaria (<1%)
(1988): Price AH+, *Drugs* 36, 521 (0.5%)
Vasculitis
Xerosis (<1%)

Other

Gynecomastia
(1987): Cloud ML, *Scand J Gastroenterol* 22, 39
Myalgia (1.7%)
Paresthesias (<1%)
Pseudolymphoma
(1995): Magro CM+, *J Am Acad Dermatol* 32, 419
Serum sickness
Xerostomia (1.4%)

NORFLOXACIN

Trade names: Chibroxin (Merck); Noroxin (Merck; Roberts)
Other common trade names: *Barazan; Chibroxine; Chibroxol; Lexinor; Noroxine; Oranor; Utinor; Zoroxin*
Indications: Various urinary tract infections caused by susceptible organisms, conjunctivitis
Category: Broad-spectrum quinolone antibiotic
Half-life: 2.3–4 hours
Clinically important, potentially serious interactions with: antacids, caffeine, cimetidine, cyclosporine, didanosine, digoxin, iron, metoprolol, omeprazole, probenecid, propranolol, sucralfate, theophylline, warfarin, zinc

Reactions

Skin

Angioedema
Bullous eruption
(1993): Ramsey B+, *Br J Dermatol* 129, 500
Contact dermatitis
(1998): Silvestre JF+, *Contact Dermatitis* 39, 83
Diaphoresis (<1%)
Edema
Erythema (sic) (<1%)
Erythema multiforme
Exanthems
(1988): Wolfson JS+, *Ann Intern Med* 108, 238
(1985): Holmes B+, *Drugs* 30, 482 (0.2%)
Exfoliative dermatitis
Fixed eruption
(1997): Fenandez-Rivas M, *Allergy* 52, 477
Photosensitivity
(1963): Oswald FH, *Ned Tijdschr Geneesk* (Dutch) 107, 999
Phototoxic reaction
(2000): Traynor NJ+, *Toxicol Vitr* 14, 275
(1998): Martinez LJ+ *Photochem Photobiol* 67, 399
(1994): Fujita H+, *Photodermatol Photoimmunol Photomed* 10, 202
(1993): Ferguson J+, *Br J Dermatol* 128, 285
Pruritus (<1%)
(1985): Holmes B+, *Drugs* 30, 482 (0.2%)
Pustular eruption
(1992): Allegue F+, *Med Clin (Barc)* (Spanish) 99, 274
Rash (sic) (<1%)
Stevens–Johnson syndrome
(1992): Kubo-Shimasaki A+, *Rinsho Ketsueki* (Japanese) 33, 823
Stinging (from ophthalmic solution)
Subcorneal pustular dermatosis (Sneddon–Wilkinson)
(1988): Shelley ED+, *Cutis* 42, 24
Toxic epidermal necrolysis
(1993): Correia O+, *Dermatology* 186, 32
Toxic pustuloderma
(1993): Tsuda S+, *Acta Derm Venereol* (Stockh) 73, 382 (passim)
Urticaria
Vasculitis

Nails

Nails – photo-onycholysis
(1987): Baran R+, *J Am Acad Dermatol* 17, 1012
(1986): Baran R+, *Dermatologica* 173, 185

Other

Anaphylactoid reaction
Dysgeusia (<1%) (bitter taste)
Myalgia
Paresthesias
Stomatitis
Tendon rupture (<1%)
Vaginal candidiasis
Xerostomia (<1%)

NORTRIPTYLINE

Trade names: Aventyl (Lilly); Pamelor (Novartis)
Other common trade names: *Allegron; Apo-Nortriptyline; Aventyl; Noritren; Norpress; Nortrilen; Paxtibi; Vividyl*
Indications: Depression
Category: Tricyclic antidepressant and antipanic
Half-life: 28–31 hours
Clinically important, potentially serious interactions with: alcohol, anticoagulants, carbamazepine, chlorpropamide, cimetidine, clonidine, CNS depressants, diltiazem, epinephrine, fluoxetine, guanethidine, insulin, isoproterenol, lithium, MAO inhibitors, methylphenidate, phenothiazines, tolazamide, warfarin

Reactions

Skin

Acne
Allergic reactions (sic) (<1%)
Diaphoresis (1–10%)
Edema
Erythema
Exanthems
Flushing
Parkinsonism (1–10%)
Petechiae
Photosensitivity (<1%)
(1972): Macaione AS, *Bull Geisinger Med Cent* 24, 122
(1972): Richards DL+, *Adverse Drug Reactions*, Livingstone
Phototoxic reaction
Pruritus
Purpura
Rash (sic)
Urticaria
Vasculitis
Xerosis

Hair

Hair – alopecia (<1%)

Other

Acute intermittent porphyria
(1986): Krummel SJ+, *Drug Intell Clin Pharm* 20, 487
Black tongue
(1990): Vitiello B+, *Clin Pharm* 9, 421
Dysgeusia (>10%)
Galactorrhea (<1%)
Gynecomastia (<1%)
Paresthesias
Stomatitis
Tongue edema
Tremor
Vaginitis
Xerostomia (>10%)

NYSTATIN

Trade names: Mycostatin (Bristol-Myers Squibb); Nystop (Paddock)
Other common trade names: *Biofanal; Candio-Hermal; Mestatin; Moronal; Nistaquim; Nyaderm; Nystacid; Nystan; Nystex; Oranyst; Pedi-Dri*
Indications: Candidiasis
Category: Antifungal (anti-candidal) antibiotic
Half-life: no data
Clinically important, potentially serious interactions with: methotrexate

Reactions

Skin

Acrodermatitis perstans (exacerbation)
(1971): Petrozzi JW+, *Arch Dermatol* 103, 442
Acute generalized exanthematous pustulosis (AGEP)
(1999): Przybilla B+, *Hautarzt* (German) 50, 136
(1998): Rosenberger A+, *Hautarzt (German)* 49, 492
(1997): Kuchler A+, *Br J Dermatol* 137, 808 (3 cases)
Contact dermatitis (<1%)
(1994): Fisher AA, *Cutis* 54, 300
(1993): Hills RJ+, *Contact Dermatitis* 28, 48
(1990): de Groot AC+, *Dermatologic Clinics* 8, 153
(1987): Lechner T+, *Mykosen* (German) 30, 143
(1985): Lang E+, *Contact Dermatitis* 12, 182
(1971): Foussereau J+, *Bull Soc Fr Dermatol Syphiligr* (French) 78, 457
(1971): Chalmers D, *Arch Dermatol* 104, 437
(1971): Coskey RJ, *Arch Dermatol* 103, 228
(1971): Wasilewski C, *Arch Dermatol* 104, 437
(1970): Wasilewski C, *Arch Dermatol* 102, 216
Dermatitis (sic)
(1991): Quirce S+, *Contact Dermatitis* 25, 197 (generalized)
Eczematous eruption (sic)
(1987): Lechner T+, *Mykosen* (German) 30, 143
(1971): Coskey RJ, *Arch Dermatol* 103, 228
Erythema multiforme
(1991): Garty BZ, *Arch Dermatol* 127, 741
Erythroderma
(1980): Pareek SS, *Br J Dermatol* 103, 679
Exanthems
(1991): Quirce S+, *Contact Dermatitis* 25, 197
Fixed eruption
(1980): Pareek SS, *Br J Dermatol* 103, 679
(1969): Kandil E, *Dermatologica* 139, 37
Pruritus
(1987): Lechner T+, *Mykosen* (German) 30, 143
Rash (sic)
Stevens–Johnson syndrome (<1%)
(1991): Garty BZ, *Arch Dermatol* 127, 741
Urticaria

Other

Hypersensitivity (<1%)
Tongue edema
(1991): Quirce S+, *Contact Dermatitis* 25, 197

OCTREOTIDE

Trade name: Sandostatin (Novartis)
Other common trade names: *Sandostatina; Sandostatine*
Indications: Diarrhea
Category: Antidiarrheal; antihypotensive; growth hormone suppressant; antihypoglycemic; secretory inhibitor
Half-life: 1.5 hours
Clinically important, potentially serious interactions with: cyclosporine

Reactions

Skin

Allergic reactions (sic)
Cellulitis (1–4%)
Diaphoresis
Edema (1–10%)
Exanthems
(1990): Saltz L+, *Proc Am Soc Clin Oncol* 9, 97
Flushing (1–4%)
(2000): Caplin ME+, *Nucl Med Commun* 21, 97
Petechiae (1–4%)
Pruritus (1–4%)
Purpura (1–4%)
Rash (sic) (<1%)
Raynaud's phenomenon (1–4%)
Urticaria (1–4%)

Hair

Hair – alopecia (<1%)
(1995): Nakauchi Y+, *Endocr J* 42, 385
(1991): Jonsson A+, *Ann Intern Med* 115, 913

Other

Anaphylactoid reaction
Galactorrhea (1–4%)
Gynecomastia (1–4%)
Hyperesthesia (<1%)
Injection-site erythema (1%)
Injection-site local reaction
Injection-site pain (7.5%)
Thrombophlebitis (1–4%)
Vaginitis (1–4%)
Xerostomia

OFLOXACIN

Trade names: Floxin (Ortho-McNeil); Ocuflox (Allergan)
Other common trade names: *Bactocin; Exocine; Flobasin; Floxan; Floxil; Floxstat; Oflocet; Oflocin; Tabrin; Taravid*
Indications: Various infections caused by susceptible organisms
Category: Broad-spectrum fluoroquinolone antibiotic
Half-life: 4–8 hours
Clinically important, potentially serious interactions with: anticoagulants, caffeine, cimetidine, cyclosporine, didanosine, iron, metoprolol, NSAIDs, omeprazole, probenecid, procainamide, propranolol, sucralfate, theophylline, warfarin

Reactions

Skin

Angioedema
(1987): Monk JP, *Drugs* 33, 346
(1987): Jüngst G+, *Drugs* 34 (Suppl 1), 144
Bullous eruption
Candidiasis (sic)
(1987): Jüngst G+, *Drugs* 34 (Suppl 1), 144
Chills (<1%)
Cutaneous side effects (sic) (0.4%)
(1988): Fostini R+, *Drug Exp Clin Res* 14, 393
(1987): Monk JP, *Drugs* 33, 346
Dermatitis (sic)
(2000): Litt JZ, Beachwood, OH, personal case (observation)
(1987): Monk JP, *Drugs* 33, 346
Diaphoresis
Ecchymoses
Edema (<1%)
Erythema multiforme
Erythema nodosum
Exanthems
(1994): Shelley WB+, *Cutis* 55, 22 (observation)
(1994): Shelley WB+, *Cutis* 54, 146 (observation)
(1993): Litt JZ, Beachwood, OH, personal case (observation)
(1987): Monk JP, *Drugs* 33, 346
(1987): Jüngst G+, *Drugs* 34 (Suppl 1), 144
(1986): Baran R+, *Dermatologica* 173, 185
Exfoliative dermatitis
Fixed eruption
(1996): Kawada A+, *Contact Dermatitis* 34, 427
(1994): Kawada A+, *Contact Dermatitis* 31, 182
Petechiae
Photosensitivity (<1%)
(1994): Fujita H+, *Photodermatol Photoimmunol Photomed* 10, 202
(1993): Scheife RT+, *Int J Dermatol* 32, 413
(1990): Przybilla G+, *Dermatologica* 181, 98
(1988): Halkin H, *Rev Infect Dis* 10 (Suppl 1), 258
(1987): Jensen T+, *J Antimicrob Chemother* 20, 585
(1987): Jüngst G+, *Drugs* 34 (Suppl 1), 144
(1986): Baran R+, *Dermatologica* 173, 185
Phototoxic reaction
(2000): Traynor NJ+, *Toxicol Vitr* 14, 275
(1998): Martinez LJ+ *Photochem Photobiol* 67, 399
Pigmentation
Pruritus (1–3%)
(2000): Litt JZ, Beachwood, OH, personal case (observation)
(1987): Jüngst G+, *Drugs* 34 (Suppl 1), 144
(1987): Monk JP, *Drugs* 33, 346
Pruritus vulvae (1–3%)
Purpura
Rash (sic) (1–10%)
(1988): Kromann-Andersen B+, *J Antimicrob Chemother* 22 (Suppl C), 143
Stevens–Johnson syndrome
Toxic epidermal necrolysis
Toxic pustuloderma
(1993): Tsuda S+, *Acta Derm Venereol* (Stockh) 73, 382
Urticaria (<1%)
(1987): Jüngst G+, *Drugs* 34 (Suppl 1), 144
(1987): Monk JP, *Drugs* 33, 346
Vasculitis (<1%)
(1996): Pipek R+, *Am J Med Sci* 311, 82
(1989): Huminer D+, *BMJ* 299, 303
(1989): Pace JL+, *BMJ* 299, 658
(1987): Jüngst G+, *Drugs* 34 (Suppl 1), 144

Nails

Nails – photo-onycholysis
(1987): Baran R+, *J Am Acad Dermatol* 17, 1012
(1986): Baran R+, *Dermatologica* 173, 185

Other

Anaphylactoid reaction
(1987): Monk JP, *Drugs* 33, 346
(1987): Jüngst G+, *Drugs* 34 (Suppl 1), 144
Dysgeusia (1–3%)
(1995): Dark DS+, *Infections in Medicine* October, 551
Injection-site pain (1–10%)
Myalgia (<1%)
Oral mucosal eruption
(1987): Jüngst G+, *Drugs* 34 (Suppl 1), 144
(1987): Monk JP, *Drugs* 33, 346
Paresthesias (<1%)
Parosmia
Serum sickness

Tendon rupture (<1%)
Tourette's syndrome
Vaginitis (1–10%)
Xerostomia (1–3%)

OLANZAPINE

Synonym: LY170053
Trade name: Zyprexa (Lilly)
Indications: Psychotic disorders
Category: Benzodiazepine antipsychotic
Half-life: 21–54 hours
Clinically important, potentially serious interactions with: alcohol, antihypertensives, carbamazepine, ciprofloxacin, fluvoxamine, levodopa, omeprazole, rifampin, **cigarette smoking**

Reactions

Skin
Candidiasis (<1%)
Contact dermatitis (<1%)
Diaphoresis (>1%)
Ecchymoses (>1%)
Eczema (sic) (<1%)
Edema
Exanthems (<1%)
Facial edema (<1%)
Parkinsonism (1–10%)
Peripheral edema (2%)
Photosensitivity (<1%)
Pigmentation (<1%)
Pruritus (>1%)
Pustular eruption
(1999): Adams BB+, *J Am Acad Dermatol* 41, 851
Rash (>1%)
(1999): Green B, *Curr Med Res Opin* 15, 79 (2%)
Seborrhea (<1%)
Ulceration (<1%)
Urticaria (<1%)
Vesiculobullous eruption (2%)
Xerosis (<1%)

Hair
Hair – alopecia (<1%)
(2000): Mercke Y+, *Ann Clin Psychiatry* 12, 35
Hair – hirsutism (<1%)

Other
Aphthous stomatitis (<1%)
Dysgeusia (<1%)
Gingivitis (<1%)
Glossitis (<1%)
Hypesthesia (<1%)
Myalgia (>1%)
Oral candidiasis (<1%)
Oral ulceration (<1%)
Priapism (<1%)
(2000): Compton MT+, *Am J Psychiatry* 157, 659
(1999): Green B, *Curr Med Res Opin* 15, 79 (0.1%)
(1999): Gordon M+, *J Clin Psychopharmacol* 19, 192
(1998): Deirmenjian JM+, *J Clin Psychopharmacol* 18, 351
(1998): Heckers S+, *Psychosomatics* 39, 288
Sialorrhea (<1%)
(1998): Perkins DO+, *Am J Psychiatry* 155, 993
Stomatitis (<1%)
Tongue discoloration (<1%)
Tongue edema (<1%)
(1997): Litt JZ, Beachwood, OH, personal case, (observation)
Tremor (1–10%)
Twitching (2%)
Vaginitis (>1%)
Xerostomia (13%)
(1999): Green B, *Curr Med Res Opin* 15, 79 (7%)
(1998): Bever KA+, *Am J Health Syst Pharm* 55, 1003

OLOPATADINE

Trade name: Patanol (Alcon)
Indications: Pruritus due to allergic conjunctivitis
Category: Ophthalmic H_1 antagonist
Half-life: 3 hours
Clinically important, potentially serious interactions with: none

Reactions

SKIN
Eyelid burning (<5%)
Eyelid edema (<5%)
Eyelid stinging (<5%)
Pruritus

OTHER
Dysgeusia

OLSALAZINE

Trade name: Dipentum (Pharmacia & Upjohn)
Indications: Ulcerative colitis
Category: Inflammatory bowel disease suppressant
Half-life: 0.9 hours
Clinically important, potentially serious interactions with: none

Reactions

Skin
Acne
(1990): Zinberg J+, *Am J Gastroenterol* 85, 562
Exanthems (0.4%)
(1994): Shelley WB+, *Cutis* 53, 240 (observation)
(1991): Wadworth AN+, *Drugs* 41, 647
Lupus erythematosus
(1997): Gunnarsson I+, *Scand J Rheumatol* 26, 65
Pallor
Pruritus (1.1%)
Rash (sic) (2.3%)
(1990): *Drug Ther Bull* 28, 57
Urticaria (4.3%)
(1987): Meyers S+, *Gastroenterology* 93, 1255

Other
Stomatitis (1%)

OMEPRAZOLE

Trade name: Prilosec (AstraZeneca)
Other common trade names: *Antra; Audazol; Gastroloc; Inhibitron; Logastric; Losec; Mopral; Omed; Ozoken; Parizac; Ulsen*
Indications: Duodenal ulcer, gastroesophageal reflux disease (GERD)
Category: Gastric acid secretion inhibitor; proton pump inhibitor; anti-ulcer
Half-life: 0.5–1 hour
Clinically important, potentially serious interactions with: ampicillin, benzodiazepines, clorazepate, cyclosporine, diazepam, digoxin, iron, itraconazole, ketoconazole, methotrexate, phenytoin, quinolones, warfarin

Reactions

Skin

Allergic edema (sic)
(1989): Danish Omeprazole Study Group, *BMJ* 298, 645
Angioedema (<1%)
(1994): Bowlby HA+, *Pharmacotherapy* 14, 119
(1992): Haeney MR, *BMJ* 305, 870
Bullous eruption
(1995): Stenier C+, *Br J Dermatol* 133, 343
Bullous pemphigoid
(1991): Chosidow O+, *Ann Dermatol Venereol* (French) 118, 45
(1990): Joly P+, *Gastroenterol Clin Biol* (French) 14, 682
Burning (sic)
(1984): Blanchi A+, *Gastroenterol Clin Biol* (French) 8, 943
Diaphoresis (<1%)
(1989): Delchier JC+, *Gut* 30, 1173
Eczema (sic)
(1985): Classen M+, *Dtsch Med Wochenschr* (German) 110, 628 (scalp)
Edema (1–10%)
(2000): Natsch S+, *Ann Pharmacother* 34, 474
Erythema (sic)
(1984): Blanchi A+, *Gastroenterol Clin Biol* (French) 8, 943
Erythema multiforme (<1%)
Erythema nodosum
(1996): Ricci RM+, *Cutis* 57, 434
Erythroderma
(1999): Cockayne SE+, *Br J Dermatol* 141, 173
Exanthems
(1991): Langman MSJ, *BMJ* 303, 481
Exfoliative dermatitis
(1998): Rebuck JA+, *Pharmacotherapy* 18, 877
(1995): Epelde-Gonzalo FD+, *Ann Pharmacother* 29, 82
Fixed eruption
(1999): Kepekci Y+, *Int J Clin Pharmacol Ther* 37, 307 (hands)
Furunculosis
(1998): West BC+, *Clin Infect Dis* 26, 1234
Lichenoid eruption
(2000): Bong JL+, *BMJ* 320, 283
Lichen planus
(1997): Litt JZ, Beachwood, OH, personal case (observation)
(1986): Pounder RE+, *Scand J Gastroenterol* 21, 108
(1984): Sharma BK+, *Gut* 25, 957
Lichen spinulosus
(1989): Lee ML+, *Med J Aust* 150, 410
Lupus erythematosus
(1994): Sivakumar K+, *Lancet* 344, 619
Pemphigoid (exacerbation)
(1992): Cox NH, *Lancet* 340, 857
(1991): Chosidow D+, *Ann Dermatol Venereol* (French) 118, 45
Periorbital edema
(2000): Natsch S+, *Ann Pharmacother* 34, 474
Peripheral edema (<1%)
Pityriasis rosea
(1996): Buckley C, *Br J Dermatol* 135, 660
Pruritus (1–10%)
(2000): Natsch S+, *Ann Pharmacother* 34, 474
(1994): Bowlby HA+, *Pharmacotherapy* 14, 119
(1989): Danish Omeprazole Study Group, *BMJ* 298, 645
(1989): Lee ML+, *Med J Aust* 150, 410
(1987): Bertaccini G+, *Clin Ter* (Italian) 121, 201
(1987): Klinkenberg-Knol EC+, *Lancet* 1, 349
(1986): Bardhan KD+, *J Clin Gastroenterol* 8, 408
(1986): Rinetti M+, *Drugs Exp Clin Res* 12, 701
Psoriasis
(1984): Blanchi A+, *Gastroenterol Clin Biol* (French) 8, 943
Purpura
Rash (sic) (1.5%)
(1989): Delchier JC+, *Gut* 30, 1173
(1989): Lauritsen K+, *Aliment Pharmacol Ther* 3, 59
(1988): Hirschowitz BI+, *Gastroenterol* 94, A188
(1986): Bardhan KD+, *J Clin Gastroenterol* 8, 408
Stevens–Johnson syndrome (<1%)
Toxic epidermal necrolysis (<1%)
(1992): Cox NH, *Lancet* 340, 857
Urticaria (1–10%)
(1994): Bowlby HA+, *Pharmacotherapy* 14, 119
(1994): Schneider S+, *Gastroenterol Clin Biol* (French) 18, 534
(1993): Litt JZ, Beachwood, OH, personal case (observation)
(1992): Haeney MR, *BMJ* 305, 870
Xerosis (<1%)
(1988): Marks IN+, *S Afr Med J* (Suppl), 54

Hair

Hair – alopecia (<1%)
(1999): Litt JZ, Beachwood, OH, 2 personal cases (observations)
(1997): Borum ML+, *Am J Gastroenterol* 92, 1576
(1994): Bowlby HA+, *Pharmacotherapy* 14, 119 (passim)
Hair – discoloration

Other

Anaphylactoid reaction
(2000): Natsch S+, *Ann Pharmacother* 34, 474
(1999): Galindo PA+, *Ann Allergy Asthma Immunol* 82, 52
Dysesthesia (<1%)
Dysgeusia (1–10%)
(1996): Markitziu A+, *Scand J Gastroenterol* 31, 624
Gynecomastia
(2000): Hugues FC+, *Ann Med Interne (Paris)* (French) 151, 10 (passim)
(1998): N Z Medicines Adverse Reactions Committee, (from Internet) (observation) (3 cases)
(1995): Durand JM+, *Ann Med Interne* (Paris) (French) 146, 195
(1995): Carvajal A+, *Am J Gastroenterol* 90, 1028
(1994): Garcia-Rodriguez LA+, *BMJ* 308, 503
(1994): Pedrosa M+, *Med Clin (Barc)* (Spanish) 102, 435
(1994): Lindquist M+, *BMJ* 305, 451
(1991): Santucci L+, *N Engl J Med* 324, 635
(1991): Convens C+, *Lancet* 338, 1153
Myalgia (1–10%)
Oral candidiasis
(1995): Anderson PC, *Arch Dermatol* 131, 966
(1993): Mosimann F, *Transplantation* 56, 492
(1992): Larner AJ+, *Gut* 33, 860
Paresthesias (<1%)
(1986): Rinetti M+, *Drugs Exp Clin Res* 12, 701
(1984): Blanchi A+, *Gastroenterol Clin Biol* (French) 8, 943
Tremor (<1%)
Xerostomia (1–10%)
(1985): Classen M+, *Dtsch Med Wochenschr* (German) 110, 628

ONDANSETRON

Trade name: Zofran (GlaxoWellcome)
Other common trade names: *Emeset; Oncoden; Zofron*
Indications: Nausea and vomiting
Category: Antiemetic; serotonin antagonist
Half-life: 4 hours
Clinically important, potentially serious interactions with: barbiturates, carbamazepine, rifampin, phenytoin, phenylbutazone

Reactions

Skin

Angioedema
Chills (5–10%)
Exanthems
Fixed eruption
(1995): Iglesias ME+, *Dermatology* 191, 270
Flushing
(1994): Ahn MJ+, *Am J Clin Oncol* 17, 150
Pruritus (5%)
Rash (sic) (<1%)
Urticaria

Hair

Hair – alopecia

Other

Anaphylactoid reaction
(1998): Ross AK+, *Anesth Analg* 87, 779
(1991): Milne RJ+, *Drugs* 41, 574
Hypersensitivity (<1%)
(1996): Kataja V+, *Lancet* 347, 584
Injection-site burning
Injection-site erythema
Injection-site pain
Injection-site reaction (4%)
Paresthesias (2%)
Porphyria
(1992): DeWet M+, *S Afr Med J* 82, 480
Sialopenia (1–5%)
Xerostomia (1–10%)
(1994): Ahn MJ+, *Am J Clin Oncol* 17, 150
(1991): Milne RJ+, *Drugs* 41, 574

ORAL CONTRACEPTIVES

Trade names: Brevicon; Demulen; Desogen; Enovid; Estrostep; Jenest; Levlen; Loestrin; Lo/Ovral; Modicon; Nordette; Norinyl; Norlestrin; Ortho-Cept; Ortho-Novum; Ortho-Cyclen; Ortho Tri-Cyclen; Ovcon; Ovral; Tri-Levlen; Tri-Norinyl; Triphasil, etc. (Various pharmaceutical companies.)
Indications: Prevention of pregnancy
clinically important, potentially serious interactions with: anticonvulsants, caffeine, danazol, griseofulvin, metoprolol, penicillin, rifampin, tetracyclines, theophylline, tricyclic antidepressants, troleandomycin, tuberculostatics. Also **St John's wort**

Reactions

Skin

Acanthosis nigricans
(1975): Curth HO, *Arch Dermatol* 111, 1069
Acne
(1987): Kovacs G+, *Australasian J Dermatol* 28, 86
(1984): van der Meeren HL+, *Ned Tijdschr Geneeskd* (Dutch) 128, 1333
(1981): Scholz C+, *Zentralbl Gynakol* (German) 103, 1158
(1979): Harrison PV+, *BMJ* 2, 495
(1979): Marghescu S, *Ther Ggw* (German) 118, 1230
(1978): Amann W, *ZFA Stuttgart* (German) 54, 1809
(1974): Woodward RK, *Arch Dermatol* 110, 812
(1972): Gibbs WP, *Arch Dermatol* 109, 912
(1972): Olson RL+, *Arch Dermatol* 105, 928
(1972): Kligman AM, *Arch Dermatol* 105, 298
(1971): Peterson WC, *Minn Med* 54, 836
(1971): Jelinek JE, *Am Fam Physician* 4, 68
(1971): Prenen M+, *Arch Belg Dermatol Syphiligr* (French) 27, 253
(1971): Dugois P+, *Ann Dermatol Syphiligr Paris* (French) 98, 479
(1970): Jelinek JE, *Arch Dermatol* 101, 181
(1969): Racouchot J+, *Bull Soc Fr Dermatol Syphiligr* (French) 76, 132
(1969): Chanial G+, *Bull Soc Fr Dermatol Syphiligr* (French) 76, 125
Acute febrile neutrophilic dermatosis (Sweet's syndrome)
(1991): Tefany FJ+, *Aust J Dermatol* 32, 55
Angioedema
(2000): Bouillet L+, *Presse Med* (French) 29, 640
(1990): Borradori L+, *Dermatologica* 181, 78
(1967): Wolf RJ, *JAMA* 201, 982
Autoimmune progesterone dermatitis
(1981): Stone J+, *Int J Dermatol* 20, 50
Bullous eruption
(1981): Honeyman JF+, *Arch Dermatol* 117, 264
Candidiasis
(1983): Lebherz TB+, *Clin Ther* 5, 409
(1979): Marghescu S, *Ther Ggw* (German) 118, 1230
(1976): Aron-Brunetiere R, *Contracept Fertil Sex Paris* (French) 4, 175
(1971): Jelinek JE, *Am Fam Physician* 4, 68
(1970): Jelinek JE, *Arch Dermatol* 101, 181
(1969): Langer H, *Munch Med Wochenschr* (German) 111, 1748
(1968): Walsh H+, *Amer J Obstet Gynec* 101, 991
(1966): Porter PS+, *Arch Dermatol* 93, 402
(1966): Catterall RD, *Lancet* 2, 830
Chloasma
(1987): Kovacs G+, *Australasian J Dermatol* 28, 86
(1977): Smith AG+, *J Invest Dermatol* 68, 169
(1972): Ippen H+, *Hautarzt* (German) 23, 21
(1972): Ippen H+, *Hautarzt* (German) 23, 235
(1972): Ippen H, *Arch Dermatol Forsch* (German) 244, 500
(1971): Amblard P+, *Bull Soc Fr Dermatol Syphiligr* (French) 78, 561
(1969): Racouchot J+, *Bull Soc Fr Dermatol Syphiligr* (French) 76, 132
(1968): Carruthers R, *Practitioner* 200, 564
(1967): Merklen FP+, *Bull Soc Fr Dermatol Syphiligr* (French) 74, 801
(1967): Basset H, *Bull Soc Fr Dermatol Syphiligr* (French) 74, 166
(1967): Carruthers R, *BMJ* 3, 307
(1967): Quamina DB, *BMJ* 2, 638
(1966): Carruthers R, *Med J Aust* 2, 17
Cold urticaria
(1983): Burns MR+, *Ann Intern Med* 98, 1025
Dermatitis herpetiformis
(1972): Haim S+, *Dermatologica* 145, 199
Eczema (sic)
(1988): Edman B, *Acta Derm Venereol* 68, 402 (palmar)
Edema
Erythema
(1973): Delius L, *Dtsch Med Wochenschr* (German) 98, 1512 (flush-like)
Erythema multiforme
(1973): Naess K, *Tidsskr Nor Laegeforen* (Norwegian) 93, 2498
(1970): Savel H+, *Arch Dermatol* 101, 187
Erythema nodosum
(1981): Touboul JL+, *Nouv Presse Med* (French) 10, 712
(1980): Beaucaire G+, *Sem Hôp* (French) 56, 1426
(1980): Salvatore MA+, *Arch Dermatol* 116, 557
(1977): Bombardieri S+, *BMJ* 1, 1509
(1977): Taaffe A+, *BMJ* 2, 1353
(1976): Posternak F, *Rev Med Suisse Romande* (French) 96, 375
(1976): Bernstein MZ+, *J Am Podiatry Assoc* 66, 417
(1974): Darlington LG, *Br J Dermatol* 90, 209
(1974): Berant N, *Harefuah* (Hebrew) 87, 19.
(1973): Elias PM, *Arch Dermatol* 108, 716
(1973): Stumbo WG, *J Ky Med Assoc* 71, 433
(1973): Kariher DH, *Obstet Gynecol* 42, 323
(1972): Kirby J+, *Obstet Gynecol* 40, 409
(1971): Jelinek JE, *Am Fam Physician* 4, 68
(1970): Jelinek JE, *Arch Dermatol* 101, 181
(1970): Savel H+, *Arch Dermatol* 101, 187
(1968): Baden HP+, *Arch Dermatol* 98, 634
(1967): Matz MH, *N Engl J Med* 276, 351
Exanthems
(1981): Scholz C+, *Zentralbl Gynakol* (German) 103, 1158

Fixed eruption
(1977): Coskey R, *Arch Dermatol* 113, 333
Fox–Fordyce disease
(1971): Jelinek JE, *Am Fam Physician* 4, 68
Herpes genitalis (sic)
(1981): Scholz C+, *Zentralbl Gynakol* (German) 103, 1158
Herpes gestationis
(1989): Kemper T+, *Akt Dermatol* (German) 15, 121
(1975): Kocsis M+, *Acta Derm Venereol* (Stockh) 55, 25
(1968): Morgan JK, *Br J Dermatol* 80, 456
Lichenoid eruption
(1977): Coskey R, *Arch Dermatol* 113, 333
Livedo racemosa (Sneddon's syndrome)
(1991): Berchtold B+, *Hautarzt* (German) 45, 328
Lupus erythematosus
(1994): Hess EV+, *Curr Opin Rheumatology* 6, 474
(1994): Strom BL+, *Am J Epidemiol* 140, 632
(1993): Arden NK+, *Lupus* 2, 381
(1991): Furukawa F+, *J Dermatology* (Tokio) 18, 56
(1990): Zanetti R+, *Int J Epidemiol* 19, 522
(1990): Franceschi S+, *Tumori* (Italian) 76, 439
(1989): Beaumont V+, *Clin Physiol Biochem* 7, 263
(1989): Iskander MK+, *J Rheumatol* 16, 850
(1988): Mathur AK+, *J Rheumatology* 15, 1042
(1986): Asherson RA+, *Arthritis Rheum* 29, 1535
(1982): Jungers P+, *Nouv Presse Med* (French) 11, 3765
(1982): Jungers P+, *Arthritis Rheum* 25, 618
(1980): Garovich M+, *Arthritis Rheum* 23, 1396
(1975): Bielecka H, *Reumatologia* (Polish) 13, 223
(1974): Zurcher K+, *Dermatologica* 149, 321
(1973): Elias PM, *Arch Dermatol* 108, 716
(1972): Cordonnier V+, *J Sci Med Lille* (French) 90, 431
(1972): Tuffanelli DL, *Arch Dermatol* 106, 553
(1972): Dorfmann H+, *Nouv Presse Med* (French) 1, 2907
(1971): Laugier P+, *Bull Soc Fr Dermatol Syphiligr* (French) 78, 632
(1971): Cornet A+, *Ann Med Interne Paris* (French) 122, 1151
(1971): Chapel TA+, *Am J Obstet Gynecol* 110, 366
(1969): Rothfield NF, *Mayo Clin Proc* 44, 691
(1968): Schleicher EM, *Lancet* 1, 821
(1968): Dubois EL+, *Lancet* 2, 679
(1968): Pimstone BL, *Lancet* 1, 1153
Melanoma
(1992): Le MG+, *Cancer Causes Control* 3, 199
(1985): Quencez E+, *Ann Dermatol Venereol* (French) 112, 341
(1985): Gallagher RP+, *Br J Cancer* 52, 901
(1985): Bork K, *Hautarzt* (German) 36, 542
(1985): Green A+, *Med J Aust* 142, 446
Melasma
(1985): Lutfi RJ+, *J Clin Endocrinol Metab* 62, 28
(1981): Witkiewicz IM+, *Ned Tijdschr Geneeskd* (Dutch) 125, 609
(1970): Jelinek JE, *Arch Dermatol* 101, 181
(1968): *Northwest Med* 67, 251
(1967): Resnick SS, *Trans N Engl Obstet Gynecol Soc* 21, 107
(1967): Carruthers R, *BMJ* 3, 307
(1967): Resnick S, *JAMA* 199, 601
(1966): Resnick SS, *JAMA* 197, 25
Mucha–Habermann disease
(1973): Hollander A+, *Arch Dermatol* 107, 465
Perioral dermatitis
(1977): Kalkoff KW+, *Hautarzt* (German) 28, 74
(1975): Hornstein OP, *Internist Berl* (German) 16, 27
(1974): Buck A+, *Dtsch Med Wochenschr* (German) 99, 366
(1974): Reinken L+, *Int J Vitam Nutr Res* (German) 44, 75
(1972): Toyosi JO, *Hautarzt* (German) 23, 79
(1971): Kleine-Natrop HE, *Hautarzt* (German) 22, 508
(1969): Steigleder GK+, *Hautarzt* (German) 20, 288
(1989): Ehlers G, *Hautarzt* (German) 20, 287
Photosensitivity
(1994): Litt JZ, Beachwood, OH, personal case (observation)
(1979): Marghescu S, *Ther Ggw* (German) 118, 1230
(1977): Roberts DT+, *Br J Dermatol* 96, 549
(1973): Levantine A+, *Br J Dermatol* 89, 105
(1975): Horkay I+, *Arch Dermatol Res* 253, 53
(1971): Elgart ML+, *Med Ann Dist Columbia* 40, 501
(1971): Jelinek JE, *Am Fam Physician* 4, 68
(1970): Jelinek JE, *Arch Dermatol* 101, 181
(1970): Mathison IW+, *Obstet Gynecol Surv* 25, 389
(1968): Oosterhuis WW, *Ned Tijdschr Geneeskd* (Dutch) 112, 2154
(1968): Erickson LR+, *JAMA* 203, 980
Pigmentation
(1981): Granstein RD+, *J Am Acad Dermatol* 5, 1
(1981): Scholz C+, *Zentralbl Gynakol* (German) 103, 1158
(1980): Hertz RS+, *J Am Dent Assoc* 100, 713
(1979): Marghescu S, *Ther Ggw* (German) 118, 1230
(1978): Harlap S, *Lancet* 2, 39
(1976): Aron-Brunetiere R, *Contracept Fertil Sex Paris* (French) 4, 175
(1972): Ippen H, *Arch Dermatol Forsch* (German) 244, 500
(1972): Leonhardi G, *Arch Dermatol Forsch* (German) 244, 495
(1971): Bazex A, *Rev Fr Gynecol Obset* (French) 66, 575
(1971): Jelinek JE, *Am Fam Physician* 4, 68
(1971): Dugois P+, *Ann Dermatol Syphiligr Paris* (French) 98, 479
(1971): Kleine-Natrop HE, *Dermatol Monatsschr* (German) 157, 549
(1970): Jelinek JE, *Arch Dermatol* 101, 181
(1969): Chanial G+, *Bull Soc Fr Dermatol Syphiligr* (French) 76, 125
(1968): Gotz H+, *Munch Med Wochenschr* (German) 110, 1913
(1968): Sotaniemi E+, *BMJ* 2, 120
(1967): No Author, *S Afr Med J* 41, 709
(1965): No Author, *BMJ* 5471, 1180
Polymorphous light eruption
(1989): Boonstra H+, *Photodermatol* 6, 55
(1988): Neumann R, *Photodermatol* 5, 40
Pruritus (<1%)
(1976): Medline A+, *Am J Gastroenterol* 65, 156
(1975): Gagnaire JC+, *Nouv Presse Med* (French) 4, 1105
(1971): Dugois P+, *Rev Fr Gynecol Obstet* (French) 66, 589
(1970): Dahl MG, *Trans St Johns Hosp Dermatol Soc* 56, 11
(1969): Baker H, *Br J Dermatol* 81, 946 (passim)
Psoriasis
(1981): Scholz C+, *Zentralbl Gynakol* (German) 103, 1158
Purpura
(1983): McShane PM+, *Am J Obstet Gynecol* 145, 762
(1971): Jelinek JE, *Am Fam Physician* 4, 68
(1970): Jelinek JE, *Arch Dermatol* 101, 181
Seborrhea
(1981): Scholz C+, *Zentralbl Gynakol* (German) 103, 1158 (seborrheic dermatitis)
(1979): Marghescu S, *Ther Ggw* (German) 118, 1230
(1969): Chanial G+, *Bull Soc Fr Dermatol Syphiligr* (French) 76, 125
Spider angiomas
(1970): Jelinek JE, *Arch Dermatol* 101, 181
(1970): Goldman L, *Lancet* 2, 108
Stevens–Johnson syndrome
(1972): O'Callaghan J+, *Med J Aust* 1, 695
Telangiectases
(1983): Wilkin JK+, *J Am Acad Dermatol* 8, 468
(1971): Jelinek JE, *Am Fam Physician* 4, 68
(1970): Jelinek JE, *Arch Dermatol* 101, 181
(1970): Goldman L, *Lancet* 2, 108
(1968): Gotz H+, *Munch Med Wochenschr* (German) 110, 1913
(1964): Kopera H+, *Int J Fertil* 9, 69
Urticaria
(1981): Scholz C+, *Zentralbl Gynakol* (German) 103, 1158
(1970): Meyer-de-Schmid JJ+, *Bull Soc Fr Dermatol Syphiligr* (French) 77, 158
Varicosities

Hair

Hair – alopecia
(1989): Burke KE, *Postgrad Med* 85, 52
(1987): Kovacs G+, *Australasian J Dermatol* 28, 86
(1982): Hauser GA+, *Int J Tissue React* 4, 159
(1981): Scholz C+, *Zentralbl Gynakol* (German) 103, 1158
(1979): Marghescu S, *Ther Ggw* (German) 118, 1230
(1979): Price VH, *Int J Dermatol* 18, 95
(1978): Zaun H, *Dtsch Med Wochenschr* (German) 103, 240
(1978): Bergfeld W, *Cutis* 22, 190
(1974): Haim S, *Harefuah* (Hebrew) 86, 155
(1973): Levantine A+, *Br J Dermatol* 89, 549
(1973): No Author, *BMJ* 2, 499
(1973): Zaun H, *Z Geburtshilfe Perinatol* (German) 177, 67
(1971): Dawber RP+, *BMJ* 4, 234
(1971): Prenen M+, *Arch Belg Dermatol Syphiligr* (French) 27, 253
(1970): Zaun H, *Dtsch Med Wochenschr* (German) 95, 1433
(1969): Chanial G+, *Bull Soc Fr Dermatol Syphiligr* (French) 76, 125
(1968): *BMJ* 1, 593
(1967): Cormia FE, *JAMA* 201, 635

Hair – alopecia areata
(1971): Jelinek JE, *Am Fam Physician* 4, 68
(1966): Orentreich N+, *BMJ* 5485, 483
(1965): *BMJ* 5470, 1124
(1965): Vallings R, *BMJ* 2, 1005
Hair – hirsutism
(1994): Burdova M+, *Ceska Gynekol* (Czech) 59, 62
(1987): Kovacs G+, *Australasian J Dermatol* 28, 86
(1981): Scholz C+, *Zentralbl Gynakol* (German) 103, 1158
(1979): Marghescu S, *Ther Ggw* (German) 118, 1230
(1973): Zaun H, *Hautarzt* (German) 24, 1
(1973): Zaun H, *Z Geburtshilfe Perinatol* (German) 177, 67
(1971): Jelinek JE, *Am Fam Physician* 4, 68
(1971): Prenen M+, *Arch Belg Dermatol Syphiligr* (French) 27, 253
(1971): Dugois P+, *Ann Dermatol Syphiligr Paris* (French) 98, 479
(1969): Chanial G+, *Bull Soc Fr Dermatol Syphiligr* (French) 76, 125
(1968): Gotz H+, *Munch Med Wochenschr* (German) 110, 1913
(1966): Carruthers R, *Med J Aust* 2, 17

Nails

Nails – onycholysis
(1976): Byrne JPH+, *Postgrad Med J* 52, 536

Other

Acute intermittent porphyria
(1979): Brinkmann OH+, *ZFA Stuttgart* (German) 55, 1227
(1978): Gerlis LS, *J Int Med Res* 6, 255
(1977): Tasic D+, *Med Pregl* (Serbo-Croatian-Cyrillic) 30, 577
(1975): Schley G+, *Verh Dtsch Ges Inn Med* (German) 81, 1061
(1971): Contro L+, *Minerva Med* (Italian) 62, 2238
Galactorrhea
(1969): Friedman S+, *JAMA* 210, 1888
Gingival hyperplasia
(1967): Lindhe J+, *J Periodont Res* 2, 1
(1962): Sumner CF+, *J Periodont* 33, 344
Oral mucosal pigmentation
(1980): Hertz RS+, *J Am Dent Assoc* 100, 713 (gingival)
Porphyria cutanea prematura
(1977): Doss M, *Dtsch Med Wochenschr* (German) 102, 875
(1977): Leonhardi G+, *Dtsch Med Wochenschr* (German) 102, 160
Porphyria cutanea tarda
(1992): McKenna KE+, *Br J Dermatol* 127, 401
(1983): Doss M, *Dtsch Med Wochenschr* (German) 108, 1857
(1983): Zaumseil RP+, *Zentralbl Gynakol* (German) 105, 527
(1982): Zaumseil RP+, *Z Gesamte In Med* (German) 37, 703
(1981): Fiedler H+, *Dermatol Monatsschr* (German) 167, 481
(1979): Willerson D+, *Ann Ophthalmol* 11, 409
(1979): Grossman ME+, *Am J Med* 67, 277
(1977): Roberts DT+, *Br J Dermatol* 96, 549
(1976): Byrne JPH+, *Postgrad Med J* 52, 536
(1976): Curtis P, *Br J Clin Pract* 30, 47
(1976): Aron-Brunetiere R, *Contracept Fertil Sex Paris* (French) 4, 175
(1975): Austad WI+, *N Z Med J* 81, 8
(1974): Le Reun M+, *Concours Med* (French) 96, 2697
(1974): Vosmik F+, *Cesk Dermatol* (Czech) 49, 298
(1974): Nuss A+, *Z Haut* (German) 49, 273
(1974): Behm AR+, *Can Med Assoc J* 110, 1052
(1973): Ruszczak Z+, *Wiad Lek* (Polish) 26, 2177
(1973): Gutzwiller P, *Dermatologia* (German) 146, 342
(1973): Palma-Carlos AG+, *Nouv Presse Med* (French) 1, 1996
(1973): Constantinidis A+, *Minerva Ginecol* (Italian) 25, 192
(1973): Gajdos A+, *Nouv Presse Med* (French) 2, 1131
(1972): No Author, *BMJ* 3, 603
(1971): Goldswain PR+, *S Afr Med J* 25, 111
(1971): Jelinek JE, *Am Fam Physician* 4, 68
(1970): Roenigk HH+, *Arch Dermatol* 102, 260
(1969): Degos R+, *Ann Dermatol Syphiligr Paris* (French) 96, 5
(1967): Huber FB, *Schweiz Med Wochenschr* (German) 97, 1498
Porphyria variegata
(1975): Fowler CJ+, *BMJ* 1, 663
(1972): McKenzie AW+, *Br J Dermatol* 86, 453
Thrombophlebitis
(1967): Merklen FP+, *Bull Soc Fr Dermatol Syphiligr* (French) 74, 801

ORLISTAT

Trade name: Xenical (Roche)
Indications: Obesity; weight reduction
Category: Lipase inhibitor
Half-life: 1–2 hours
Clinically important, potentially serious interactions with: antidiabetic agents, phytonadione

Reactions

Skin

Dermatitis
Pedal edema
Rash (sic) (4.3%)
Xerosis

Other

Gingivitis (4.1%)
Myalgia (4.2%)
Tendinitis
Tooth disorder (sic) (4.3%)
Vaginitis (3.8%)

ORPHENADRINE

Trade names: Banflex (Forest); Norflex (3M)
Other common trade names: *Biorfen; Biorphen; Distalene; Disipal; Flexojet; Flexon; Myolin; Norgesic; Opheryl; Orfenace; Prolongatum*
Indications: Painful musculoskeletal conditions
Category: Skeletal muscle relaxant
Half-life: 14 hours
Clinically important, potentially serious interactions with: alcohol, CNS depressants, haloperidol, phenothiazines, propoxyphene

Reactions

Skin

Exanthems
Flushing (1–10%)
Pigment disorder (sic)
(1978): Rebhun J, *Ann Allergy* 40, 44
Pruritus
Rash (sic) (1–10%)
Urticaria

Other

Anaphylactoid reaction
Embolia cutis medicamentosa (Nicolau syndrome)
(1976): Brachtel R, *Med Klin* (German) 71, 504
Hypersensitivity
Paresthesias
Xerostomia

OSELTAMIVIR

Trade name: Tamiflu (Roche)
Indications: Influenza infection
Category: Antiviral (neuraminidase inhibitor)
Half-life: 6–10 hours
Clinically important, potentially serious interactions with: probenecid

Reactions

None

OXACILLIN

Trade name: Oxacillin
Other common trade names: *Bactocill; Bristopen; Prostaphlin; Stapenor*
Indications: Various infections caused by susceptible organisms
Category: Penicillinase-resistant penicillin antibiotic
Half-life: 23–60 minutes
Clinically important, potentially serious interactions with: anticoagulants, cyclosporine, disulfiram, methotrexate, oral contraceptives, probenecid, tetracycline

Reactions

Skin

Angioedema
Bullous eruption
  (1974): Hadida E+, *Bull Soc Fr Dermatol Syphiligr* (French) 81, 87
Ecchymoses
Erythema multiforme
Erythema nodosum
Exanthems
  (1978): Bruevich TS+, *Vestn Dermatol Venerol* (Russian) March, 74
  (1974): Spitzy KH, *Acta Med Austriaca* (German) 2, 46
Exfoliative dermatitis
Hematomas
Jarisch–Herxheimer reaction
Necrosis
  (1980): Tilden SJ+, *Am J Dis Child* 134, 1046
Pruritus
  (1998): Siegfried EC+, *J Am Acad Dermatol* 39, 797 (passim)
Rash (sic) (<1%)
Stevens–Johnson syndrome
  (1982): Sukovatykh TN+, *Pediatriia* (Russian) May, 76
Toxic epidermal necrolysis
Urticaria
  (1998): Siegfried EC+, *J Am Acad Dermatol* 39, 797 (passim)
Vasculitis

Other

Anaphylactoid reaction (0.04%)
  (1998): Siegfried EC+, *J Am Acad Dermatol* 39, 797 (passim)
Black tongue
Dysgeusia
Glossitis
Glossodynia
Hypersensitivity
Injection-site pain
Oral candidiasis
Phlebitis
Serum sickness (<1%)
Stomatitis
Stomatodynia
Thrombophlebitis
Tongue furry
Vaginitis
Xerostomia

OXAPROZIN

Trade name: Daypro (Searle)
Other common trade names: *Deflam; Duraprox*
Indications: Arthritis
Category: Nonsteroidal anti-inflammatory (NSAID)
Half-life: 42–50 hours
Clinically important, potentially serious interactions with: anticoagulants, aspirin, beta-blockers, cyclosporine, diuretics, heparin, lithium, loop diuretics, methotrexate, probenecid, salicylates, warfarin

Reactions

Skin

Angioedema (<1%)
Diaphoresis (<1%)
Ecchymoses (<1%)
Edema (<1%)
Erythema
Erythema multiforme (<1%)
  (1986): Todd PA+, *Drugs* 32, 291
Exanthems
  (1995): Litt JZ, Beachwood, OH, personal case (observation)
  (1994): Shelley WB+, *Cutis* 54, 72 (eczematous eruption) (observation)
  (1994): Litt JZ, Beachwood, OH, personal case (observation)
  (1983): Hubsher JA+, *Clin Pharmacol Ther* 33, 267
Exfoliative dermatitis (<1%)
Fixed eruption
  (1999): Blumenthal HL, Beachwood, OH, personal case (observation)
Linear IgA dermatosis
  (1999): Abate KL+, *Arch Dermatol* 135, 81–86 (off-center fold)
Photosensitivity (<1%)
Phototoxic reaction
  (1995): Shelley WB+, *Cutis* 55, 143 (observation)
  (1986): Todd PA+, *Drugs* 32, 291
Pruritus (1–10%)
  (1994): Shelley WB+, *Cutis* 53, 284 (observation)
Purpura
Rash (sic) (>10%)
  (1983): Kahn SB+, *J Clin Pharmacol* 23, 139
  (1978): Jamar R+, *Curr Med Res Op* 5, 433
Stevens–Johnson syndrome (<1%)
  (1998): Bell MJ+, *J Rheumatol* 25, 2027
Toxic epidermal necrolysis
  (1999): Carucci JA+, *Int J Dermatol* 38, 233
  (1998): Paul CD+, *J Burn Care Rehabil* 19, 321 (fatal)
Urticaria (<1%)
  (1997): Hicks A, Houston, TX (from Internet) (observation) [Note: Person is not a physician]
Vasculitis
  (1999): Reed BR, Denver, CO (from Internet) (observation)

Hair

Hair – alopecia

Other

Anaphylactoid reaction (<1%)
Dysgeusia
Pseudoporphyria
  (1999): Al-Khenaizan S+, *J Cutan Med Surg* 3, 162
  (1996): Ingrish G+, *Arch Dermatol* 132, 1519
  (1996): Jaffe PG, Columbia, SC (from Internet) (observation)
Serum sickness (<1%)
Stomatitis (<1%)

OXAZEPAM

Trade name: Oxazepam
Other common trade names: *Adumbran; Apo-Oxazepam; Azutranquil; Durazepam; Murelax; Novoxapam; Oxpam; Praxiten; Serax; Serepax; Zapex*
Indications: Anxiety, depression
Category: Benzodiazepine antianxiety and sedative-hypnotic; anticonvulsant
Half-life: 3–6 hours
Clinically important, potentially serious interactions with: alcohol, barbiturates, clarithromycin, CNS depressants, digoxin, diltiazem, levodopa, MAO inhibitors, narcotics, oral contraceptives, phenothiazines, phenytoin, theophylline, verapamil

Reactions

Skin
Dermatitis (sic) (1–10%)
Diaphoresis (>10%)
Edema
Erythema multiforme
(1986): McAlpine C, *BMJ* 293, 510
Exanthems
Fixed eruption
(1996): Krischer J, *Arch Dermatol* 132, 718
Pruritus
Purpura
Rash (sic) (>10%)
Urticaria

Other
Paresthesias
Sialopenia (>10%)
Sialorrhea (1–10%)
Tongue, coated
Tremor
Xerostomia (>10%)

OXCARBAZEPINE

Synonym: GP 47680
Trade name: Trileptal (Novartis)
Indications: Partial epileptic seizures
Category: Anticonvulsant
Half-life: 1–2.5 hours
Clinically important, potentially serious interactions with: carbamazepine, citalopram, diazepam, fosphenytoin, oral contraceptives, phenobarbital, phenytoin, propranolol, tolbutamide, topiramate, tricyclic antidepressants, valproic acid

Reactions

Skin
Acne
Angioedema
Allergy (sic) (2%)
(1994): Dam M, *Epilepsia* 35, S23
(1993): Beran RG, *Epilepsia* 34, 163
Contact dermatitis
Diaphoresis (3%)
Eczema
Edema (2%)
Erythema multiforme
Exanthems
(1999): Ruble R+, *CNS Drugs* 12, 215
Facial rash (sic)
Folliculitis
Genital pruritus
Hot flashes (2%)
Infection (sic) (2%)
Lupus erythematosus
Photosensitivity
Purpura (2%)
Rash (sic) (4%)
(1993): Friis ML+, *Acta Neurol Scand* 84, 224 (6%)
Sensitivity (sic)
(1991): Watts D+, *J Neurol Neurosurg Psychiatry 1991*, 54, 376
Stevens–Johnson syndrome
Toxic epidermal necrolysis
Vitiligo

Hair
Hair – alopecia

Other
Dysgeusia (5%)
Gingival hyperplasia
Hypersensitivity
Hypesthesia (3%)
Priapism
Stomatitis
Toothache (2%)
Tremor (4–6%)
Ulcerative stomatitis
Vaginitis (2%)
Xerostomia (3%)

OXYBUTYNIN

Trade name: Ditropan (Alza)
Other trade names: *Albert Oxybutynin; Cystrin; Dridase; Novitropan; Oxyban; Tropax*
Indications: Neurogenic bladder; urinary incontinence
Category: Urinary antispasmodic
Half-life: 1–2.3 hours
Clinically important, potentially serious interactions with: alcohol, antihistamines, CNS depressants, phenothiazines, tricyclic antidepressants

Reactions

Skin
Allergic reactions (sic) (<1%)
(1993): Jonville AP+, *Arch Fr Pediatr* (French) 50, 27
(1992): Jonville AP+, *Therapie* (French) 47, 389
Anhidrosis
Erythema multiforme
(1992): Jonville AP+, *Therapie* (French) 47, 389
Flushing
Hot flashes (1–10%)
Hypohidrosis (>10%)
Rash (sic) (1–10%)
Urticaria
Xerosis
(1998): Arango Toro O+, *Actas Urol Esp* (Spanish) 22, 124 (6%)

Other
Sialopenia
(1998): Arango Toro O+, *Actas Urol Esp* (Spanish) 22, 124 (42%)
(1995): Loesche WJ+, *J Am Geriatr Soc* 43, 401
Xerostomia (>10%)
(2000): Versi E+, *Obstet Gynecol* 95, 718
(1995): Loesche WJ+, *J Am Geriatr Soc* 43, 401

OXYCODONE

Trade names: Endocodone, OxyContin (Purdue), OxyIR (Purdue), Percolone (Endo), Percoset (Endo), Percodan (Endo), Roxicodone (Roxane), Tylox (McNeil)
Other common trade name: *Supeudol*
Indications: Pain
Category: Narcotic analgesic
Half-life: 4.6 hours
Clinically important, potentially serious interactions with: alcohol, CNS depressants, dextroamphetamine, MAO inhibitors, phenothiazines, sedatives, tricyclic antidepressants

Oxycodone is often combined with acetaminophen (Percoset, Roxicet, Tylox) or aspirin (Percodan, Roxiprin)

Reactions

Skin

Diaphoresis
Pruritus
(1999): Hale ME+, *Clin J Pain* 15, 179
(1999): Salzman RT+, *J Pain Symptom Manage* 18, 271
Rash (sic) (<1%)
Urticaria (<1%)

Other

Injection-site pain (1–10%)
Xerostomia (1–10%)

OXYTETRACYCLINE

Trade name: Terramycin (Pfizer)
Other common trade names: *Aknin; Cotet; Macocyn; Oxacycle; Oxitraklin; Oxy; Rorap; Terramycine; Uri-Tet*
Indications: Various infections caused by susceptible organisms
Category: Tetracycline antibiotic; antiprotozoal
Half-life: 6–10 hours
Clinically important, potentially serious interactions with: antacids, anticoagulants, carbamazepine, digoxin, iron, oral contraceptives, penicillin, phenytoin, warfarin. Also **herbals: barberry, goldenseal, Oregon grape**

Reactions

Skin

Angioedema
Contact dermatitis
(1976): Moller H, *Contact Dermatitis* 2, 289
(1974): Bojs G+, *Berufsdermatosen* (German) 22, 202
(1969): Walczynski Z+, *Wiad Lek* (Polish) 22, 929
Exanthems
Exfoliative dermatitis (<1%)
Fixed eruption
(1985): Gomez B+, *Allergol Immunopathol Madr* (Spanish) 13, 87
(1981): Shukla SR, *Dermatologica* 163, 160
(1975): Giminez-Garcia RM+, *N Engl J Med* 292, 819
(1970): Delaney TJ, *Br J Dermatol* 83, 357
(1952): Dougherty JW, *Arch Dermatol* 65, 485
Lupus erythematosus
Photosensitivity (1–10%)
(1987): Santucci B+, *G Ital Dermatol Venereol* (Italian) 122, IL-LII
(1982): Hawk JL, *Clin Exp Dermatol* 7, 341
(1977): Ramsay CA, *Clin Exp Dermatol* 2, 255
(1963): Tromovitch TA+, *Ann Intern Med* 58, 529 (1–5%)
Pigmentation
Pruritus (<1%)
Purpura
(1975): Kounis NG, *JAMA* 231, 734
Pustular eruption
(1971): Stevanovic DN, *Br J Dermatol* 85, 134
Sensitivity (sic)
(1997): Rudzki E+, *Contact Dermatitis* 37, 136
Urticaria
Vasculitis

Nails

Nails – pigmentation (<1%)

Other

Anaphylactoid reaction (<1%)
Black tongue
(1954): No Author, *Lancet* 2, 179
Hypersensitivity (<1%)
Oral mucosal lesions
(1971): Merdi T+, *Czas Stomatol* (Polish) 24, 1309
Paresthesias (<1%)
Porphyria cutanea tarda
(1982): Hawk JL, *Clin Exp Dermatol* 7, 341
Pseudotumor cerebri (<1%)
Thrombophlebitis (<1%)
Tooth discoloration (>10%) (in children)

PACLITAXEL

Trade name: Taxol (Bristol-Myers Squibb)
Other common trade name: *Paxene*
Indications: Metastatic carcinoma of the ovary
Category: Antineoplastic
Half-life: 5–17 hours
Clinically important, potentially serious interactions with: cisplatin, ketoconazole

Reactions

Skin

Acral erythema
(1996): de Argila D+, *Dermatology* 192, 377
(1995): Zimmerman GC+, *Arch Dermatol* 131, 202
Angioedema
(1990): Weiss RB+, *J Clin Oncol* 8, 1263
Cutaneous manifestations (sic)
(1995): Link CJ+, *Invest New Drugs* 13, 261
Edema (21%)
Erythema
(1995): Berghmans T+, *Support Care Cancer* 3, 203
(1995): Zimmerman GC+, *Arch Dermatol* 131, 202
Erythrodysesthesia
(1994): Zimmerman GC+, *J Natl Cancer Inst* 86, 557
(1993): Vukelja SJ+, *J Natl Cancer Inst* 85, 1423
Exanthems (<1%)
(1990): Weiss RB+, *J Clin Oncol* 8, 1263
Fixed eruption
(2000): Baykal C+, *Eur J Gynaecol Oncol* 21, 190
(1996): Young PC+, *J Am Acad Dermatol* 34, 313 (bullous)
Flushing (28%)
(1990): Weiss RB+, *J Clin Oncol* 8, 1263
Infections (sic) (>10%)
Pruritus (<1%)
(1995): Freilich RJ+, *J Natl Cancer Inst* 87, 933
(1990): Weiss RB+, *J Clin Oncol* 8, 1263
Purpura
Pustular eruption
(1997): Weinberg JM+, *Int J Dermatol* 36, 559
Radiation-recall (<1%)
(1996): McCarty MJ+, *Med Pediatr Oncol* 27, 185
(1995): Schweitzer VG+, *Cancer* 76, 1069
(1995): Phillips KA+, *J Clin Oncol* 13, 305
(1994): Shenkier T+, *J Clin Oncol* 12, 439
(1993): Raghavan VT+, *Lancet* 341, 1354
Rash (sic) (12%)
Urticaria
(1990): Weiss RB+, *J Clin Oncol* 8, 1263

Hair

Hair – alopecia (87%)
(1995): Lemenager M+, *Lancet* 346, 371
(1990): McGuire WP+, *Ann Intern Med* 111, 273 (total) (100%) (between days 14 and 21; reversible)

Nails

Nails – disorders (sic)
(1998): Luftner D+, *Ann Oncol* 9, 1139
Nails – onycholysis
(2000): Hussain S+, *Cancer* 88, 2367 (5 cases)
(1999): Flory SM+, *Ann Pharmacother* 33, 584
Nails – pigmentation (2%)
(1998): Auvinet M+, *Rev Med Interne* (French) 19, 353

Other

Anaphylactoid reaction
(1999): Smith ME, *Oncol Nurs Forum* 26, 516
Hypersensitivity (41%)
(1998): Tsavaris NB+, *Cancer Chemother Pharmacol* 42, 509
(1998): Lokich J+, *Ann Oncol* 9, 573
(1995): Del Priore G+, *Gynecol Oncol* 56, 316
(1994): Uziely B+, *Ann Oncol* 5, 474
(1993): Peereboom DM+, *J Clin Oncol* 11, 885
Injection-site cellulitis (>10%)
Injection-site extravasation (>10%)
(1997): Herrington JD+, *Pharmacotherapy* 17, 163
(1995): Raymond E+, *Rev Med Interne* (French) 16, 141
(1995): Berghmans T+, *Support Care Cancer* 3, 203
Injection-site pain (>10%)
Injection-site reaction (13%)
Mucocutaneous toxicity (sic)
(1996): Payne JY+, *South Med J* 89, 542
Mucositis (>10%)
Myalgia (60%)
(1999): Markman M+, *Gynecol Oncol* 72, 100
(1998): Savarese D+, *J Clin Oncol* 16, 3918
Oral mucosal lesions
(1990): McGuire WP+, *Ann Intern Med* 111, 273 (3–8%)
Paresthesias (>10%)
Phantom limb pain
(2000): Khattab J+, *Mayo Clin Proc* 75, 740
Recall at site of prior extravasation
(1996): du Bois A+, *Gynecol Oncol* 60, 94
(1994): Meehan JL+, *J Natl Cancer Inst* 86, 1250
Stomatitis (39%)

PAMIDRONATE

Trade name: Aredia (Novartis)
Indications: Hypercalcemia, Paget's disease
Category: Antidote (hypercalcemia)
Half-life: 1.6 hours
Clinically important, potentially serious interactions with: vitamin D

Reactions

Skin

Angioedema (<1%)
Candidiasis
Edema (1%)
Exanthems
(1984): Mantalen CA+, *BMJ* 288, 828 (1.2%)
Rash (sic) (<1%)

Other

Dysgeusia (<1%)
Hypersensitivity (<1%)
Infusion-site reaction (4%)
Myalgia (1%)
Stomatitis (1%)

PANTOPRAZOLE

Trade name: Protonix (WyethAyerst)
Indications: Esophagitis associated with gastroesophageal reflux disease (GERD)
Category: Proton pump (gastric acid secretion) inhibitor
Half-life: 1 hour
Clinically important, potentially serious interactions with: ampicillin, azole antifungals

Reactions

Skin

Abscess (<1%)
Acne (<1%)
Allergic reactions (<1%)
Angioedema (<1%)
Aphthous stomatitis (<1%)
Balanitis (<1%)
Contact dermatitis (<1%)

Diaphoresis (<1%)
(2000): Natsch S+, *Ann Pharmacother* 34, 474
Ecchymoses (<1%)
Eczema (<1%)
Edema (<1%)
Erythema multiforme (<1%)
Exanthems (<1%)
Facial edema (<1%)
Flu-like syndrome (sic) (1–10%)
Fungal infection (<1%)
Herpes simplex (<1%)
Herpes zoster (<1%)
Infection (sic) (1–10%)
Lichenoid eruption (<1%)
(2000): Bong JL+, *BMJ* 320, 283
Peripheral edema
(1994): Brunner G, *Aliment Pharmacol Ther* 8, 59
Pruritus (<1%)
(2000): Natsch S+, *Ann Pharmacother* 34, 474
Rash (sic) (<1%)
(1992): Muller P+, *Z Gastroenterol* 30, 771
Stevens–Johnson syndrome (<1%)
Toxic epidermal necrolysis (<1%)
Ulceration (<1%)
Urticaria (<1%)
(2000): Natsch S+, *Ann Pharmacother* 34, 474
Xerosis (<1%)

Hair

Hair – alopecia (<1%)

Other

Anaphylactoid reaction (<1%)
(2000): Natsch S+, *Ann Pharmacother* 34, 474
Dysgeusia (<1%)
Foetor ex ore (halitosis) (<1%)
Gingivitis (<1%)
Glossitis (<1%)
Hypesthesia (<1%)
Mastodynia (<1%)
Myalgia (<1%)
Oral candidiasis (<1%)
Paresthesias (<1%)
Sialorrhea (<1%)
Stomatitis (<1%)
Thrombophlebitis (<1%)
Tongue edema
(2000): Natsch S+, *Ann Pharmacother* 34, 474
Tongue pigmentation (<1%)
Tremor (<1%)
Vaginitis (<1%)
Xerostomia (<1%)

PANTOTHENIC ACID

Trade name: Dexol
Other common trade name: *Vitamin B_5*
Indications: Vitamin B complex malabsorption
Category: Water-soluble vitamin
Half-life: no data
Clinically important, potentially serious interactions with: none

Reactions

Skin

Exanthems
Pruritus
Urticaria

PAPAVERINE

Trade names: Genabid; Pavabid (Aventis); Pavatine
Other common trade names: *Angioverin; Genabid; Optenyl; Pameion; Papaverine 60; Papaverini; Pavagen; Pavased; Pavatine*
Indications: Peripheral and cerebral ischemia
Category: Peripheral vasodilator
Half-life: 0.5–2 hours
Clinically important, potentially serious interactions with: CNS depressants, levodopa, morphine

Reactions

Skin

Diaphoresis (<1%)
Exanthems
Fixed eruption
(1994): Kirby KA+, *Urology* 43, 886
Flushing (<1%)
Pruritus (<1%)
Pyogenic granuloma
(1990): Summers JL, *J Urol* 143, 1227
Rash (sic)
Toxic epidermal necrolysis
(1989): Simochkina ZA+, *Vrach Delo* (Russian) October, 91
Urticaria

Other

Injection-site thrombophlebitis (<1%)
Priapism
(1991): Schwarzer JU+, *J Urol* 146, 845
Xerostomia (<1%)

PARA-AMINOSALICYLIC ACID (PAS)

(See AMINOSALICYLATE SODIUM)

PARAMETHADIONE

Trade name: Paradione (Abbott)
Indications: Absence (petit-mal) seizures
Category: Anticonvulsant
Half-life: 12–24 hours
Clinically important, potentially serious interactions with: phenytoin, valproic acid

Reactions

Skin

Acne
Erythema multiforme
(1972): Levantine A+, *Br J Dermatol* 87, 646
(1961): Leblanc JL+, *Can Med Assoc J* 85, 200
Exanthems
Exfoliative dermatitis
(1946): Lennox WG, *Am J Psychiatry* 103, 159
Lupus erythematosus
Pruritus

Hair

Hair – alopecia

Other

Bleeding gums
Oral mucosal eruption
(1946): Lennox WG, *Am J Psychiatry* 103, 159
Paresthesias

PAROXETINE

Trade name: Paxil (SmithKline Beecham)
Other common trade name: *Aropax 20*
Indications: Depression
Category: Selective serotonin reuptake inhibitor (SSRI); antidepressant
Half-life: 21 hours
Clinically important, potentially serious interactions with: alcohol, anticoagulants, barbiturates, cimetidine, dextromethorphan, digoxin, fluoxetine, haloperidol, loop diuretics, MAO inhibitors, phenothiazines, phenytoin, selegiline, sertraline, tramadol, trazodone, tricyclic antidepressants, warfarin

Reactions

Skin

Acne (<1%)
Allergic reactions (sic) (<1%)
Angioedema (<1%)
(1996): Mithani H+, *J Clin Psychiatry* 57, 486
Candidiasis
Contact dermatitis (<1%)
Cutaneous reaction (sic)
(1998): Beauquier B+, *Encephale* (French) 24, 62
Diaphoresis (11.2%)
(1998): Stein MB+, *JAMA* 280, 708
(1997): Litt JZ, Beachwood, OH, personal case (observation)
(1992): Boyer WF+, *J Clin Psychiatry* 53, 61
(1991): Dechant KL+, *Drugs* 41, 225
(1990): Sindrup SH+, *Pain* 42, 135
(1985): Laursen AL+, *Acta Psychiatr Scand* 71, 249
Ecchymoses (<1%)
(1998): Cooper TA+, *Am J Med* 104, 197
Eczema (sic)
Edema (<1%)
Erythema nodosum (<1%)
Exanthems (<1%)
Facial edema (<1%)
Furunculosis (<1%)
Lymphedema
Melanoma (<1%)
Peripheral edema (<1%)
Photosensitivity (<1%)
Pigmentation (<1%)
Pruritus (<1%)
(1991): Dechant KL+, *Drugs* 41, 225
Purpura (<1%)
Rash (sic) (1.7%)
Toxic epidermal necrolysis
(2000): Nelson RA+, Nashville TN (Poster exhibit #16 from Academy 2000)
Urticaria (<1%)
Xerosis (<1%)

Hair

Hair – alopecia (<1%)
(2000): Umansky L+, *Harefuah* (Hebrew) 138, 547 ("massive")

Other

Ageusia (<1%)
(1997): Litt JZ, Beachwood, OH, personal case (observation)
Anosmia
(1997): Litt JZ, Beachwood, OH, personal case (observation)
Aphthous stomatitis (<1%)
Bruxism (<1%)
(1996): Romanelli F+, *Ann Pharmacother* 30, 1246
Dysgeusia (2.4%)
(1998): Litt JZ, Beachwood, OH, personal case (observation)
Galactorrhea
Gingivitis (<1%)
Glossitis (<1%)
Myalgia (1.7%)
Myopathy (1–10%)
Oral ulceration
Paresthesias (3.8%)
Priapism
(1996): Bertholon F+, *Ann Med Psychol Paris* (French) 154, 145
Sialorrhea (<1%)
Stomatitis (<1%)
Tongue edema (<1%)
(1996): Mithani H+, *J Clin Psychiatry* 57, 486
Tremor (1–10%)
Vaginal candidiasis (<1%)
Vaginitis
Xerostomia (18.1%)
(1998): Stein MB+, *JAMA* 280, 708
(1992): Boyer WF+, *J Clin Psychiatry* 53, 61
(1992): Shrivastava RK+, *J Clin Psychiatry* 53, 48
(1992): Fabre LF, *J Clin Psychiatry* 53, 40
(1992): Smith WT+, *J Clin Psychiatry* 53, 36
(1992): Claghorn JL, *J Clin Psychiatry* 53, 33
(1991): Dunbar GC+, *Br J Psychiatry* 159, 394
(1991): Dechant KL+, *Drugs* 1, 225
(1990): Sindrup SH+, *Pain* 42, 135
(1990): Cohn JB+, *Psychopharmacol Bull* 26, 185

PEMOLINE

Trade name: Cylert (Abbott)
Other common trade names: *Betanamin; Tradon*
Indications: Attention deficit disorder; narcolepsy
Category: Central nervous system stimulant; anorexient
Half-life: 9–14 hours
Clinically important, potentially serious interactions with: anticonvulsants, CNS depressants, CNS stimulants, sympathomimetics

Reactions

Skin

Exanthems (<1%)
(1992): Zürcher K and Krebs A, *Cutaneous Drug Reactions*, Karger, 280
Parkinsonism
Rash (sic) (>10%)

Other

Tourette's syndrome

PENBUTOLOL

Trade name: Levatol (Schwarz)
Other common trade names: *Betapresin; Betapressin*
Indications: Hypertension
Category: Beta-adrenergic blocker; antihypertensive
Half-life: 5 hours
Clinically important, potentially serious interactions with: clonidine, epinephrine, ergot, insulin, lidocaine, NSAIDs, naproxen, salicylates, theophylline, verapamil

Note: Cutaneous side-effects of beta-receptor blockaders are clinically polymorphous. They apparently appear after several months of continuous therapy. Atypical psoriasiform, lichen planus-like, and eczematous chronic rashes are mainly observed. (1983): Hödl St, *Z Hautkr* (German) 1:58, 17.

Reactions

Skin

Allergic reactions (sic)
(1985): Marone C+, *Curr Med Res Opin* 9, 417 (1–5%)
Ankle edema
Diaphoresis (1.6%)
Exanthems
(1985): Marone C+, *Curr Med Res Opin* 9, 417 (1–5%)

Flushing
(1985): Marone C+, *Curr Med Res Opin* 9, 417 (1–5%)
Peripheral edema
Pruritus
Psoriasis
Purpura
Rash (sic)

Hair

Hair – alopecia

Nails

Nails – bluish

Other

Dysgeusia
Paresthesias
Peyronie's disease

PENICILLAMINE

Trade names: Cuprimine (Merck); Depen (Wallace)
Other common trade names: *Artamin; Distamine; D-Penamine; Kelatin; Pendramine*
Indications: Wilson's disease, rheumatoid arthritis
Category: Antidote; chelating agent and antirheumatic
Half-life: 1.7–3.2 hours
Clinically important, potentially serious interactions with: antacids, antimalarials, chloroquine, digoxin, gold, immunosuppressants, iron, oxyphenbutazone, phenylbutazone, probenecid

Note: For excellent reviews of many of the cutaneous manifestations caused by penicillamine see (1983): Levy RS+, *J Am Acad Dermatol* 8, 548 and (1981): Sternlieb I+, *J Rheumatol* 8 (Suppl 7), 149

Reactions

Skin

Anetoderma
(1977): Davis W, *Arch Dermatol* 113, 976
Atrophy
(1982): Bailin PL+, *Clin Rheum Dis* 8, 493 (passim)
Bullous eruption
(1996): Bialy-Golan A+, *J Am Acad Dermatol* 35, 732 (passim)
(1982): Fulton RA+, *Br J Dermatol* 107 (Suppl 22), 95
(1977): Stewart WM+, *Ann Dermatol Venereol* (French) 104, 542
Bullous pemphigoid
(1998): Weller R+, *Ann Pharmacother* 32, 1368
(1996): Weller R+, *Clin Exp Dermatol* 21, 121
(1989): Rasmussen HB+, *J Cutan Pathol* 16, 154
(1987): Brown MD+, *Arch Dermatol* 123, 1119
(1986): Gall Y+, *Ann Dermatol Venereol* (French) 113, 55
Contact dermatitis
(1993): De Moor A+, *Contact Dermatitis* 29, 155 (eyedrops)
(1990): Coenraads PJ+, *Contact Dermatitis* 23, 371
Cutis laxa
(1994): Amichai B+, *Isr J Med Sci* 30, 667
(1983): Levy RS+, *J Am Acad Dermatol* 8, 548
(1983): Harpey JP+, *Lancet* 2, 858
(1982): Bailin PL+, *Clin Rheum Dis* 8, 493 (passim)
(1979): Linares A+, *Lancet* 2, 43
(1979): Walshe JM, *Lancet* 2, 144
(1977): Solomon L+, *N Engl J Med* 296, 54
Dermatomyositis
(1992): Kolsi R+, *Rev Rhum Mal Osteoartic* (French) 59, 341
(1991): Wilson CL+, *Int J Dermatol* 30, 148
(1987): Carroll CG+, *J Rheumatol* 14, 995
(1983): Levy RS+, *J Am Acad Dermatol* 8, 548
(1983): Doyle DR+, *Ann Intern Med* 98, 327
(1983): Lund HI+, *Scand J Rheumatol* 12, 350
(1982): Bailin PL+, *Clin Rheum Dis* 8, 493 (passim)
(1981): Major GA, *J R Soc Med* 74, 393
(1980): Wojnarowska F, *J R Soc Med* 73, 884
(1979): Simpson NB+, *Acta Derm Venereol* (Stockh) 59, 543
(1978): Petersen J+, *Scand J Rheumatol* 7, 113
(1977): Fernandes L+, *Ann Rheum Dis* 36, 94
Dermopathy
(1987): Dootson G+, *Clin Exp Dermatol* 12, 66
Discoid lupus erythematosus
(1978): Appelboom T+, *Scand J Rheumatol* 7, 64
Ecchymoses
Edema (1–10%)
(1999): Hsu HL+, *Taiwan Erh Ko I Hsueh Tsa Chih* 40, 448 (lip)
Ehlers–Danlos syndrome
(1982): Yung CW+, *J Am Acad Dermatol* 6, 317 (passim)
(1982): Bailin PL+, *Clin Rheum Dis* 8, 493 (passim)
Elastosis perforans serpiginosa
(2000): Hill VA+, *Br J Dermatol* 142, 560
(1994): Ratnavel RC+, *Dermatology* 189, 81
(1994): Wilhelm KP+, *Hautarzt* (German) 45, 45
(1994): Amichai B+, *Isr J Med Sci* 30, 667
(1989): Sahn EE+, *J Am Acad Dermatol* 20, 279
(1988): van Joost T+, *Ned Tijdschr Geneeskd* (Dutch) 132, 501
(1986): Price RG+, *Am J Dermatopathol* 8, 314
(1985): Meyrick-Thomas RHM+, *Clin Exp Dermatol* 10, 386
(1984): Venencie PY+, *Ann Med Interne (Paris)* (French) 135, 642
(1983): Levy RS+, *J Am Acad Dermatol* 8, 548
(1983): Rosenblum GA, *J Am Acad Dermatol* 8, 718
(1982): Bailin PL+, *Clin Rheum Dis* 8, 493 (passim)
(1982): Gloor M+, *Hautarzt* (German) 33, 291
(1982): Essigman WK, *Ann Rheum Dis* 41, 617
(1982): Raymond JL+, *J Cutan Pathol* 9, 352
(1981): Bardach H+, *Wien Klin Wochenschr* (German) 93, 117
(1979): Bardach H, *Hautarzt* (German) 30, 449
(1977): Abel M, *Arch Dermatol* 113, 1303
(1977): Kirsch N+, *Arch Dermatol* 113, 630
(1973): Pass F+, *Arch Dermatol* 108, 713
Epidermal inclusion cysts
(1967): Katz R, *Arch Dermatol* 95, 196
Epidermolysis bullosa
(1982): Yung CW+, *J Am Acad Dermatol* 6, 317 (passim)
(1982): Bailin PL+, *Clin Rheum Dis* 8, 493 (passim)
(1967): Beer WE+, *Br J Dermatol* 79, 123
Erythema multiforme (1–5%)
Erythema nodosum (<1%)
(1983): Grauer JL+, *Presse Med* (French) 12, 1997
Exanthems
(1999): Hsu HL+, *Taiwan Erh Ko I Hsueh Tsa Chih* 40, 448
(1983): Levy RS+, *J Am Acad Dermatol* 8, 548
(1982): Bailin PL+, *Clin Rheum Dis* 8, 493 (passim)
(1982): Egeland T+, *J Oral Pathol* 11, 183
(1981): Walshe JM, *J Rheumatol 8* (Suppl 7), 155
(1980): Stein HB+, *Ann Intern Med* 92, 24
(1979): Hill HFH, *Scand J Rheumatol* 28, 94
Exfoliative dermatitis
Facial edema
(1996): Bialy-Golan A+, *J Am Acad Dermatol* 35, 732 (passim)
Flushing
(1996): Bialy-Golan A+, *J Am Acad Dermatol* 35, 732 (passim)
Fragility (sic)
(1981): Shaw M+, *Clin Exp Dermatol* 6, 429
Graft-versus-host reaction
(1998): Jappe U+, *Hautarzt* (German) 49, 126 (passim)
Guillain–Barré syndrome
(1984): Knezevic W+, *Aust N Z J Med* 14, 50
Lathyrism
(1992): Godar JM+, *Arch Dermatol* 128, 977
Lichenoid eruption
(1983): Powell FC+, *J Am Acad Dermatol* 9, 540
(1983): Levy RS+, *J Am Acad Dermatol* 8, 548
(1982): Bailin PL+, *Clin Rheum Dis* 8, 493 (passim)
(1982): Powell FC+, *Br J Dermatol* 107, 616
(1981): Van Hecke E+, *Arch Dermatol* 117, 676
(1981): Seehafer JR+, *Arch Dermatol* 117, 140
(1975): Van de Staak WJBM+, *Dermatologica* 150, 372
Lichen planus
(1994): Thompson DF+, *Pharmacotherapy* 14, 561
(1986): Weismann K+, *Ugeskr Laeger* (Danish) 148, 456
(1981): Powell FC+, *Lancet* 2, 525
(1979): Krebs A, *Hautarzt* (German) 30, 281

Lupus erythematosus
(1996): Bialy-Golan A+, *J Am Acad Dermatol* 35, 732 (passim)
(1995): Barthel HR+, *Dtsch Med Wochenschr* (German) 120, 1253
(1994): Fritzler MJ, *Lupus* 3. 455
(1994): Yung RL+, *Rheum Dis Clin North Am* 20, 61
(1994): Borg AA, *Clin Rheumatol* 13, 522
(1993): Donnelly S+, *Br J Rheumatol* 32, 251
(1992): Skaer TL, *Clin Ther* 14, 496
(1992): Rubin RL+, *J Clin Invest* 90, 165
(1991): Weinstein A, *Arthritis Rheum* 34, 1343
(1991): Chin GL+, *J Rheumatol* 18, 947
(1990): Tsankov NK+, *Int J Dermatol* 29, 571
(1990): Suda M+, *Nippon Jinzo Gakkai Shi* (Japanese) 32, 1235
(1990): Enzenauer RJ+, *Arthritis Rheum* 33, 1582
(1987): Lopez-Guerra N+, *Med Clin (Barc)* (Spanish) 88, 552
(1985): Stratton MA, *Clin Pharm* 4, 657
(1985): Lovisetto P+, *Recenti Prog Med* (Italian) 76, 110
(1985): Kalina P+, *Bratisl Lek Listy* (Slovak) 84, 336
(1984): Clerc C+, *Ann Dermatol Venereol* (French) 135, 420
(1983): Levy RS+, *J Am Acad Dermatol* 8, 548
(1982): Bailin PL+, *Clin Rheum Dis* 8, 493 (passim)
(1982): Yung CW+, *J Am Acad Dermatol* 6, 317 (passim)
(1982): Chalmers A+, *Ann Intern Med* 97, 659
(1982): Egeland T+, *J Oral Pathol* 11, 183
(1981): Thorvaldsen J, *Dermatologia* 162, 277
(1981): Hughes GR+, *Arthritis Rheum* 24, 1070
(1981): Walshe JM, *J Rheumatol* Suppl 7, 155
(1979): Burns DA+, *Clin Exp Dermatol* 4, 389
(1978): Harkcom TM+, *Ann Intern Med* 89, 1012
(1978): Appelboom T+, *Scand J Rheumatol* 7, 64
(1975): Lee SL+, *Semin Arthritis Rheum* 5, 83
(1974): Harpey JP, *Ann Allergy* 33, 256
(1974): Crouzet J+, *Ann Med Interne Paris* (French) 125, 71
(1972): Oliver T+, *JAMA* 220, 588
(1971): Harpey JP+, *Lancet* 1, 292 (letter)
(1971): Harpey JP+, *Ann Med Interne Paris* (French) 122, 261
(1971): Boudin G+, *Ann Med Interne Paris* (French) 122, 269
(1971): Caille B+, *Ann Med Interne Paris* (French) 122, 255

Morphea
(1989): Liddle BJ, *Ann Rheum Dis* 48, 963
(1981): Bernstein RM+, *Ann Rheum Dis* 40, 42

Papular lesions at site of trauma
(1985): Thomas RHM+, *Clin Exp Dermatol* 10, 386

Pemphigoid
(1989): Marti-Huguet T+, *Arch Ophthalmol* 107, 1115
(1986): Peyri J+, *J Am Acad Dermatol* 14, 681 (cicatricial)
(1985): Lever LR+, *Br J Dermatol* 113, 88
(1985): Shuttleworth D+, *Br J Dermatol* 113, 89
(1985): Shuttleworth D+, *Clin Exp Dermatol* 10, 392 (cicatricial)
(1985): Velthuis PJ+, *Br J Dermatol* 112, 615

Pemphigus
(2000): Shapiro M+, *J Am Acad Dermatol* 42, 297
(1999): Jan V+, *Ann Dermatol Venereol* (French) 126, 153
(1997): Brenner S+, *J Am Acad Dermatol* 36, 919
(1997): Haimowitz JE+, Philadelphia, American Academy of Dermatology Meeting (SF), Gross and Microscopic
(1995): Ciompi ML+, *Rheumatol Int* 15, 95
(1993): Jones E+, *J Am Acad Dermatol* 28, 655
(1993): Brenner S+, *Clin Dermatol* 11, 501
(1992): Bauer-Vinassac D+, *Scand J Rheumatol* 21, 17
(1991): Korman NJ+, *J Invest Dermatol* 96, 273
(1990): Wouters EA+, *Acta Clin Belg* (French) 45, 15
(1990): Black AK+, *Br J Dermatol* 123, 277 (observation)
(1989): Civatte J, *Dermatol Monatsschr* (German) 175, 1
(1988): Buckley C+, *Ir J Med Sci* 157, 267
(1988): Blanken R+, *Acta Derm Venereol* (Stockh) 68, 456
(1987): Kind P+, *Hautarzt* (German) 38, 548
(1987): Walton S+, *Clin Exp Dermatol* 12, 275
(1987): Enjolras O+, *Ann Dermatol Venereol* (French) 114, 25
(1986): Peyri J+, *J Am Acad Dermatol* 14, 681
(1986): Civatte J, *Bull Soc Fr Dermatol Syphiligr* (French) 170, 1057
(1986): Tholen S, *Z Hautkr* (German) 61, 719
(1986): Dijkstra JW, *J Am Acad Dermatol* 14, 687
(1986): Steen VD+, *Ann Intern Med* 104, 699
(1985): Piette-Brion B+, *Dermatologica* (French) 170, 297
(1985): Ho VC+, *J Rheumatol* 12, 583
(1985): Velthuis PJ+, *Br J Dermatol* 112, 615
(1984): Hashimoto K+, *Arch Dermatol* 120, 762
(1984): Venencie PY+, *Ann Med Interne (Paris)* (French) 135, 642
(1983): Levy RS+, *J Am Acad Dermatol* 8, 548
(1983): Kaplan RP+, *Clin Dermatol* 1, 42
(1983): Tinozzi CC, *G Ital Dermatol Venereol* (Italian) 118, 45
(1983): Doutre MS+ *Rev Rhum Mal Osteoartic* (French) 50, 167
(1982): Ruocco V+, *Arch Dermatol Res* 274, 123
(1982): Benito-Urbino S+, *Rev Clin Esp* (Spanish) 166, 249
(1982): Barety M+, *Therapie* (French) 37, 471
(1982): Fye KH+, *J Rheumatol* 9, 331
(1982): Ruocco V+, *Dermatologica* 164, 236
(1982): Zone J+, *JAMA* 247, 2705
(1982): Yung CW+, *J Am Acad Dermatol* 6, 317 (pemphigus syndrome)
(1981): Trunnell TN+, *Cutis* 27, 402 (pemphigus-like)
(1981): Troy JL+, *J Am Acad Dermatol* 4, 547
(1981): Santa-Cruz DJ+, *Am J Dermatopathol* 3, 85
(1981): Livden JK+, *Scand J Rheumatol* 10, 95
(1980): Trau H+, *Arch Dermatol* 116, 721
(1980): Chouyet B+, *Dermatologica* (French) 160, 297
(1979): Delcambre B+, *Lille Med* (French) 24, 283
(1979): Hill HF, *Scand J Rheumatol Suppl* 28, 94
(1978): Christoph R+, *Med Welt* (German) 29, 1761
(1977): Marsden RA+, *Proc R Soc Med* 70, 103
(1977): Stewart WM+, *Ann Dermatol Venereol* (French) 104, 542
(1976): Colliard H+, *Rev Stomatol Chir Maxillofac* (French) 77, 741
(1976): Davies MG+, *Arch Dermatol* 112, 1308
(1976): From E+, *Dermatologica* 152, 358
(1976): Cairns RJ, *Proc R Soc Med* 69, 384
(1976): Tan SG+, *Br J Dermatol* 95, 99 (pemphigus-like)
(1975): Benveniste M+, *Nouv Presse Med* (French) 4, 3125
(1975): Hewitt J+, *BMJ* 3, 371
(1975): Asboe-Hansen G, *Acta Derm Venereol* 55, 461
(1971): Hewitt J+, *Ann Med Interne Paris* (French) 122, 1003
(1969): Degos R+, *Bull Soc Fr Dermatol Syphiligr* (French) 76, 751

Pemphigus erythematodes (Senear–Usher)
(1990): Willemsen MJ+, *Int J Dermatol* 29, 193
(1985): Amerian ML+, *Int J Dermatol* 24, 16
(1985): Gibson LE+, *J Am Acad Dermatol* 12, 883
(1984): Amerian ML+, *J Am Acad Dermatol* 10, 215
(1982): Yung CW+, *J Am Acad Dermatol* 6, 317
(1980): Keilhauer A+, *Z Hautkr* (German) 55, 948
(1979): Thorvaldsen J, *Dermatologica* 159, 167
(1978): Fellner MJ+, *Int J Dermatol* 17, 308
(1977): Scherak O+, *BMJ* 1, 838

Pemphigus foliaceus
(1999): Toth GG+, *Br J Dermatol* 141, 583
(1998): Brenner S+, *J Am Acad Dermatol* 39, 137
(1997): McGovern TW+, *Arch Dermatol* 133, 499
(1997): Peñas PF+, *J Am Acad Dermatol* 37, 121
(1995): Brenner S+, American Academy of Dermatology Meeting, New Orleans (observation)
(1993): Zillikens D+, *Hautarzt* (German) 44, 167
(1986): Kohn SR, *Arch Dermatol* 122, 17 (fatal)
(1985): Bahmer FA+, *Arch Dermatol* 121, 665
(1984): Knezevic W+, *Aust N Z J Med* 14, 50
(1983): Brenner S+, *Harefuah* (Hebrew) 104, 94
(1982): Kohn SR, *Dermatologic Capsule and Comment* 4, 11
(1981): Matkaluk RM+, *Arch Dermatol* 117, 156
(1977): Kristensen JK+, *Acta Derm Venereol* (Stockh) 57, 69
(1976): Marsden RA+, *BMJ* 2, 1423

Pemphigus herpetiformis
(1988): Weltfriend S+, *Hautarzt* (German) 39, 587
(1980): Morioka S+, *J Dermatol* 7, 425
(1977): Marsden RA+, *Br J Dermatol* 97, 451

Peripheral edema (1–10%)

Pruritus (44–50%)
(1982): Yung CW+, *J Am Acad Dermatol* 6, 317 (passim)
(1982): Bailin PL+, *Clin Rheum Dis* 8, 493 (passim)

Pseudoxanthoma elasticum
(1998): Coatesworth AP+, *J Clin Pathol* 51, 169 (pseudo-pseudoxanthoma elasticum [sic])
(1992): Bolognia JL+ *Dermatology* (Basel) 184, 12
(1992): Narron GH+, *Ann Plast Surg* 29, 367
(1991): Buckley C+, *Clin Exp Dermatol* 16, 310
(1990): Dalziel KL+, *Br J Dermatol* 123, 305
(1988): Burge S+, *Clin Exp Dermatol* 13, 255 (pseudo-pseudoxanthoma elasticum [sic])
(1987): Dootson G+, *Clin Exp Dermatol* 12, 66
(1986): Light N+, *Br J Dermatol* 114, 381

(1985): Bentley-Phillips B, *J R Soc Med* 78, 787
(1985): Meyrick-Thomas RH+, *Clin Exp Dermatol* 10, 386

Psoriasis
(1987): Forgie JC+, *BMJ* 294, 1101
(1986): Daunt SON+, *Br J Rheumatol* 25, 74
(1983): Levy RS+, *J Am Acad Dermatol* 8, 548
(1981): Sternlieb I+, *J Rheumatol* 8, 149

Purpura
(1983): Trice JM+, *Arch Intern Med* 143, 1487
(1982): Speth PA+, *J Rheumatol* 9, 812
(1982): Bailin PL+, *Clin Rheum Dis* 8, 493 (passim)
(1964): Sternlieb I+, *JAMA* 189, 748

Rash (sic) (44–50%)
(2000): Shannon MW+, *Ann Pharmacother* 34, 15
(1991): Barash J+, *Clin Exp Rheumatol* 9, 541
(1982): Smith PJ+, *Br Med J (Clin Res Ed)* 285, 595
(1982): Kean WF+, *J Am Geriatr Soc* 30, 94

Scleroderma
(1991): Bourgeois P+, *Baillieres Clin Rheumatol* 5, 13
(1987): Miyagawa S+, *Br J Dermatol* 116, 95
(1981): Bernstein RM+, *Ann Rheum Dis* 40, 42

Sjøgren's syndrome
(1996): Bialy-Golan A+, *J Am Acad Dermatol* 35, 732 (passim)

Stevens–Johnson syndrome
(1996): Kammler H-J, Jena, Germany (from Internet) (observation)

Toxic epidermal necrolysis (<1%)
(1984): Chan HL, *J Am Acad Dermatol* 10, 973
(1981): Ward K+, *Ir J Med Sci* 150, 252

Urticaria (44–50%)
(1983): Levy RS+, *J Am Acad Dermatol* 8, 548
(1979): Hill HFH, *Scand J Rheumatol* 28, 94

Vasculitis
(1998): Merkel PA, *Curr Opin Rheumatol* 10, 45
(1986): Gall Y+, *Ann Dermatol Venereol* (French) 113, 55
(1983): Curran JJ+, *J Rheumatol* 10, 344
(1983): Banfi G+, *Nephron* 33, 56
(1982): Bailin PL+, *Clin Rheum Dis* 8, 493 (passim)
(1974): Hill HFH, *Curr Med Res Opin* 2, 573

Vesicular eruption
(1992): Godar JM+, *Arch Dermatol* 128, 977

Wrinkling (sic)
(1983): Levy RS+, *J Am Acad Dermatol* 8, 548

Xerosis
(1982): Yung CW+, *J Am Acad Dermatol* 6, 317 (passim)

Hair

Hair – alopecia
(1983): Levy RS+, *J Am Acad Dermatol* 8, 548
(1981): Sternlieb I+, *J Rheumatol* 8 (Suppl 7), 149

Hair – hirsutism
(1990): Rose BI+, *J Reprod Med* 35, 43
(1983): Levy RS+, *J Am Acad Dermatol* 8, 548

Nails

Nails – dystrophy
(1987): Brown MD+, *Arch Dermatol* 123, 1119 (passim)

Nails – elkonyxis (punched-out appearance of the nail at lunulae)
(1989): Bjellerup M, *Acta Derm Venereol* (Stockh) 69, 339

Nails – leukonychia
(1967): Thivolet J+, *Bull Soc Fr Dermatol* (French) 75, 61

Nails – longitudinal ridges
(1967): Thivolet J+, *Bull Soc Fr Dermatol* (French) 75, 61

Nails – onychoschizia
(1989): Bjellerup M, *Acta Derm Venereol* (Stockh) 69, 339

Nails – yellow nail syndrome
(1991): Ichikawa Y+, *Tokai J Exp Clin Med* 16, 203
(1989): Bjellerup M, *Acta Derm Venereol* (Stockh) 69, 339
(1983): Ilchyshyn A+, *Acta Derm Venereol* (Stockh) 63, 534
(1979): Lubach D+, *Hautarzt* (German) 30, 547

Other

Ageusia (12%)
(1982): Yung CW+, *J Am Acad Dermatol* 6, 317 (passim)

Aphthous stomatitis
(1983): Levy RS+, *J Am Acad Dermatol* 8, 548

Benign mucous membrane pemphigoid
(1985): Shuttleworth D+, *Clin Exp Dermatol* 10, 392
(1977): Pegum JS+, *BMJ* 1, 1473

Bromhidrosis
(1996): Bialy-Golan A+, *J Am Acad Dermatol* 35, 732 (passim)

Dermatopathy with lymphangiectases
(1989): Goldstein JB+, *Arch Dermatol* 125, 92

Dysgeusia (metallic taste)
(1996): Bialy-Golan A+, *J Am Acad Dermatol* 35, 732 (passim)
(1983): Levy RS+, *J Am Acad Dermatol* 8, 548
(1982): Kean WF+, *J Am Geriatr Soc* 30, 94
(1980): Stein HB+, *Ann Intern Med* 92, 24

Gingivitis

Glossitis
(1967): Thivolet J+, *Bull Soc Fr Dermatol* (French) 75, 61

Gynecomastia
(1994): Desautels JE, *Can Assoc Radiol J* 45, 143 (gigantism)
(1985): Kahl LE+, *J Rheumatol* 12, 990
(1982): Reid DM+, *BMJ* 285, 1083

Hypersensitivity
(1999): Hsu HL+, *Taiwan Erh Ko I Hsueh Tsa Chih* 40, 448
(1994): Chan CY+, *Am J Gastroenterol* 89, 442

Hypogeusia (25–33%)
(1968): Keiser HR+, *JAMA* 203, 381
(1967): Henkin RI+, *Lancet* 2, 1268

Mucocutaneous reactions
(1982): Halla JT+, *Am J Med* 72, 423

Mucosal lesions (pemphigus-like)
(1981): Eisenberg E+, *Oral Surg Oral Med Oral Pathol* 51, 409
(1978): Hay KD+, *Oral Surg Oral Med Oral Pathol* 45, 385

Mucosal ulceration
(1981): Eisenberg E+, *Oral Surg* 51, 409

Oral lichenoid eruption
(1984): Blasberg B+, *J Rheumatol* 11, 348

Oral ulceration
(1996): Bialy-Golan A+, *J Am Acad Dermatol* 35, 732 (passim)
(1982): Egeland T+, *J Oral Pathol* 11, 183
(1980): Stein HB+, *Ann Intern Med* 92, 24
(1964): Sternlieb I+, *JAMA* 189, 748

Polymyositis
(1996): Bialy-Golan A+, *J Am Acad Dermatol* 35, 732 (passim)
(1991): Santos JC+, *Clin Exp Dermatol* 16, 76
(1978): Petersen J+, *Scand J Rheumatol* 7, 113

Serum sickness
(1996): Bialy-Golan A+, *J Am Acad Dermatol* 35, 732 (passim)

Stomatitis
(1996): Bialy-Golan A+, *J Am Acad Dermatol* 35, 732 (passim)
(1982): Yung CW+, *J Am Acad Dermatol* 6, 317 (passim)
(1981): Sternlieb I+, *J Rheumatol* 8 (Suppl 7), 149 (passim)
(1980): Stein HB+, *Ann Intern Med* 92, 24
(1968): Thivolet J+, *Bull Soc Fr Dermatol Syphiligr* (French) 75. 61

PENICILLINS

Generic names:

Amoxicillin
Trade names: Amoxil; Augmentin; Larotid; Polymox; Trimox; Wymox
Ampicillin
Trade names: Omnipen; Olycillin; Principen; Unasyn
Azlocillin
Trade names: Azlin
Bacampicillin
Trade name: Spectrobid
Carbenicillin
Trade name: Geopen
Cloxacillin
Trade names: Cloxapen; Tegopen
Cyclacillin
Trade name: none
Dicloxacillin
Trade names: Dycil; Dynapen; Pathocil
Methicillin
Trade name: Staphcillin
Mexlocillin
Trade name: Mezlin
Nafcillin
Trade names: Unipen
Oxacillin
Trade names: Bactocill; Prostaphlin
Penicillin G
Trade names: Bicillin; Crysticillin; Megacillin; Wycillin
Penicillin V
Trade names: Beepen; Betapen; Ledercillin; Pen Vee K; V-Cillin; etc.
Piperacillin
Trade names: Pipracil
Ticarcillin
Trade name: Ticar

(Various pharmaceutical companies.)

Indications: Various infections caused by susceptible organisms
Category: Antibiotic
Half-life: varies
Clinically important, potentially serious interactions with: aminoglycosides, anticoagulants, atenolol, beta-blockers, cyclosporine, doxycycline, erythromycin, methotrexate, minocycline, oral contraceptives, probenecid, tetracyclines

Note: "Patients with a history of penicillin allergy are about ten times more likely than the general population to experience a potentially fatal reaction to subsequent therapy with most other haptenating drugs." The degradation products of penicillin can bind with tissue or serum proteins to form an immunogenic complex that can elicit an immune response.

Reactions

Skin

Acral numbness
(1997): Takahashi H, *J Dermatol* 24, 50
Acute generalized exanthematous pustulosis (AGEP)
(1995): Gebhardt M+, *Contact Dermatitis* 33, 204
(1995): Moreau A+, *Int J Dermatol* 34, 263 (passim)
(1994): Manders SM+, *Cutis* 54, 194
(1991): Roujeau J-C+, *Arch Dermatol* 127, 1333
Allergy (sic)
(1984): Jolivet M+, *Union Med Can* (French) 113, 842
(1984): Cameron W+, *Ann Allergy* 53, 455
Angioedema
(1988): Van Arsdel PP Jr, *JAMA* 260, 2572
(1978): Girard JP, *Contact Dermatitis* 4, 309
(1968): Rosenblum AH, *J Allergy* 42, 309
Baboon syndrome
(1999): Panhans-Gross A+, *Contact Dermatitis* 41, 352
Bullous pemphigoid
(1992): Shelley WB+, *Advanced Dermatologic Diagnosis*, WB Saunders, 414 (passim)
(1988): Alcalay J+, *J Am Acad Dermatol* 18, 345
Contact dermatitis
(1990): Pecegueiro M, *Contact Dermatitis* 23, 190
(1991): Rudzki E+, *Contact Dermatitis* 25, 192
Contact urticaria
(1985): Rudzki E+, *Contact Dermatitis* 13, 192
(1983): Fisher AA, *Cutis* 32, 314
(1978): Girard JP, *Contact Dermatitis* 4, 309
Cutis laxa
(1971): Reed WB+, *Arch Dermatol* 103, 661
Dermatitis
(1984): Beckerman A+, *Int J Dermatol* 23, 149
Diaphoresis
Eczematous eruption (sic)
Erythema annulare centrifugum
(1978): Gupta HL+, *J Indian Med Assoc* 65, 307
(1964): Shelley WB, *Arch Dermatol* 90, 54
Erythema multiforme
(2000): Ibia EO+, *Arch Dermatol* 136, 849
(1990): Staretz LR+, *JADA* 121, 436
(1990): Garcia JJ+, *Clin Exp Allergy* 20 (Suppl 1), 121
(1985): Huff JC, *Dermatologic Clinics* 3(1), 141
(1983): Ansel J+, *Arch Dermatol* 119, 1006
Erythema nodosum
Exanthems
(2000): Ibia EO+, *Arch Dermatol* 136, 849
(2000): Schnyder B+, *Hautarzt* (German) 51, 46
(1995): Romano A+, *Allergy* 50, 113
(1986): de Haan P+, *Allergy* 41, 75
(1976): Lackner F+, *Int J Clin Pharmacol Biopharm* (German) 13, 90
(1976): Richter G, *Dermatol Monatsschr* (German) 162, 533
(1974): Spitzy KH, *Acta Med Austriaca* (German) 2, 46
(1970): Baer RL+, *Br J Dermatol* 83, 37
(1970): Fellner MN+, *J Invest Dermatol* 55, 390
Exfoliative dermatitis
(1986): Wengrower D+, *Respiration* 50, 301
Fixed eruption
(1993): Inadomi T+, *Eur J Dermatol* 3, 674
(1980): Haustein UF, *Dermatol Monatsschr* (German) 166, 680
(1979): Pasricha JS, *Br J Dermatol* 100, 183
(1975): Coskey RJ+, *Arch Dermatol* 111, 791
(1970): Dennison WL+, *Arch Dermatol* 101, 594
(1951): Canizares O, *Arch Dermatol* 63, 800
Jarisch–Herxheimer reaction (<1%)
(1977): Pareek SS, *Br J Vener Dis* 53, 389
Linear IgA bullous dermatosis
(1998): Wakelin SH+, *Br J Dermatol* 138, 310
(1994): Kuechle MK+, *J Am Acad Dermatol* 30, 187
(1993): Combemale P+, *Ann Dermatol Venereol* (French) 120, 847
Lupus erythematosus
Pemphigoid
(1988): Alcalay J+, *J Am Acad Dermatol* 18, 345
Pemphigus
(1997): Brenner S+, *J Am Acad Dermatol* 36, 919
(1991): Escallier F+, *Ann Dermatol Venereol* (French) 118, 381
(1988): Duhra P+, *Br J Dermatol* 118, 307
(1987): Seidenbaum M+, *Drug Intell Clin Pharm* 21, 1012
(1987): Brenner S+, *J Am Acad Dermatol* 17, 514
(1984): Ruocco V+, *Arch Dermatol Res* 274, 123
(1980): Ruocco V+, *Dermatologica* 159, 266
(1980): Fellner MJ, *Int J Dermatol* 9, 392
(1979): Ruocco V+, *Dermatologica* 159, 266
Pityriasis rosea
Pruritus
(1995): Litt JZ, Beachwood, OH, personal case (observation)
(1970): Baer RL+, *Br J Dermatol* 83, 37
Purpura
Pustular psoriasis
(1987): Katz M+, *J Am Acad Dermatol* 17, 918
(1976): Lindgren S+, *Acta Derm Venereol* (Stockh) 56, 139
(1971): Ryan TJ+, *Br J Dermatol* 85, 407
(1969): Hadida E+, *Bull Soc Fr Dermatol Syphiligr* (French) 76, 1095
(1969): Privat Y+, *Bull Soc Fr Dermatol Syphiligr* (French) 76, 505

Rash (sic) (<1%)
Stevens–Johnson syndrome
(1997): Shoji T+, *J Am Acad Dermatol* 37, 337
(1996): Kammler H-J, Jena, Germany (from Internet) (observation)
(1993): Leenutaphong V+, *Int J Dermatol* 32, 428
(1983): Sullivan M, *Dent Health London* 22, 10
(1983): Herold M+, *Ethiop Med J* 21, 227
(1971): Nava-Negrete A, *Alergia* (Spanish) 19, 29
Toxic epidermal necrolysis
(1993): Leenutaphong V+, *Int J Dermatol* 32, 428
(1983): Tagami H+, *Arch Dermatol* 119, 910
(1983): Herold M+, *Ethiop Med J* 21, 227
(1982): Herold M+, *Z Gesamte Inn Med* (German) 37, 706
(1979): Frontera-Izquierdo P+, *An Esp Pediatr* 12, 703
(1977): Ghosh JS, *Arch Dermatol* 113, 1162
(1972): Carli-Basset C+, *Sem Hôp* (French) 48, 497
(1969): Pustovaia AI+, *Vestn Dermatol Venerol* (Russian) 43, 73
(1966): Ulcova I+, *Cesk Pediatr* (Czech) 21, 923
Toxic erythema
(1995): Rademaker M, *N Z Med J* 108, 165 (with vancomycin)
Urticaria
(2000): Ibia EO+, *Arch Dermatol* 136, 849
(1988): Sorensen HT+, *Ugeskr Laeger* (Danish) 150, 2913
(1982): Boonk WJ+, *Br J Dermatol* 106, 183
(1971): Van Hecke E, *Ann Dermatol Syphiligr* (Paris) (French) 98, 147
(1970): Baer RL+, *Br J Dermatol* 83, 37
(1968): Rosenblum AH, *J Allergy* 42, 309
Vasculitis
Vesicular eruptions

Hair

Hair – alopecia
(1977): Pareek SS, *Br J Vener Dis* 53, 389

Other

Anaphylactoid reaction
(2000): Xi-Moy S+, *Anesthesiology* 93, 280
(1999): Dunn AB+, *J Reprod Med* 44, 381
(1993): van der Klauw MM+, *Br J Clin Pharmacol* 35, 400
(1977): Matveikov GP+, *Antibiotiki* (Russian) 22, 813
(1976): Kraus SJ+, *Cutis* 17, 765
(1972): Kelle L+, *Z Arztl Fortbild* (Jena) (German) 66, 538
(1969): Idsoe O+, *Schweiz Med Wochenschr* (German) 99, 1221 (151 deaths)
(1968): Rosenblum AH, *J Allergy* 42, 309
(1968): Bowszyc J, *Przegl Dermatol* (Polish) 55, 307
(1967): Fellner MJ+, *Arch Dermatol* 96, 687
(1953): Feinberg S+, *JAMA* 152, 114
Black tongue
Dysgeusia
Embolia cutis medicamentosa (Nicolau syndrome)
(1998): Saputo V+, *Pediatr Med Chir* (Italian) 20, 105
(1966): Deutsch J, *Dtsch Gesundheitw* (German) 21, 2433
Glossitis
Hypersensitivity (<1%)
(1998): Romano A, *Clin Exp Allergy* 28 (Suppl 4) 29
(1995): Bircher AJ, *Curr Probl Dermatol* 22, 31
(1988): Weiss ME+, *Clin Allergy* 18, 515
(1977): Reznikova ZT+, *Pediatriia* (Russian) April, 25
(1969): Leonhardi G+, *Hautarzt* (German) 20, 21
Injection-site aseptic necrosis
Injection-site reactions (1–10%)
(1990): Shen K, *Lancet* 336, 689
Injection-site urticaria
Oral candidiasis (>10%)
Oral ulceration
(1990): Staretz LR+, *JADA* 121, 436
Serum sickness
(2000): Ibia EO+, *Arch Dermatol* 136, 849
(1990): Heckbert SR+, *Am J Epidemiol* 132, 336
(1980): Brandslund I+, *Haemostasis* 9, 193
(1967): Fellner MJ+, *Arch Dermatol* 96, 687
(1967): Fellner MJ+, *J Invest Dermatol* 48, 384
Stomatitis
Thrombophlebitis (<1%)
Tongue, furry
Xerostomia

PENTAGASTRIN

Trade name: Peptavlon (Wyeth-Ayerst)
Other common trade name: *Gastrodiagnost*
Category: Diagnostic aid (gastric function)
Half-life: 10 minutes
Clinically important, potentially serious interactions with: no data

Reactions

Skin

Angioedema
(1985): Arnved J+, *Lancet* 2, 1068
(1975): Wastell C+, *BMJ* 1, 334
Diaphoresis
Exanthems
(1975): Wastell C+, *BMJ* 1, 334
Flushing
(1975): Wastell C+, *BMJ* 1, 334
Pruritus
(1975): Wastell C+, *BMJ* 1, 334
Purpura
(1985): Arnved J+, *Lancet* 2, 1068
Rash (sic)
Urticaria

Other

Hypersensitivity
Injection-site pain
Paresthesias

PENTAMIDINE

Trade names: NebuPent (Fujisawa); Pentacarinat; Pentam-300 (Fujisawa)
Other common trade name: *Pentacarinat*
Indications: *Pneumocystis carinii* infection; trypanosomiasis
Category: Antiprotozoal antibiotic; also indicated in the treatment of pneumocystis carinii pneumonia
Half-life: 9.1–13.2 hours (IM); 6.5 hours (IV)
Clinically important, potentially serious interactions with: didanosine, foscarnet

Note: The rate of adverse side-effects is increased in patients with AIDS.

Reactions

Skin

Bullous eruption
(1970): Wang JJ+, *J Pediatr* 77, 311
Cutaneous side effects (sic)
(1989): Berger TG+, *Ann Intern Med* 110, 1035
Edema
Erythema
Exanthems
(1992): Breathnach SM+, *Adverse Drug Reactions and the Skin*, Blackwell, Oxford, 179 (passim)
(1990): Soo Hoo GW+, *Ann Intern Med* 113, 195 (1–5%)
(1990): Monk JP+, *Drugs* 39, 741
(1990): Leoung GS+, *N Engl J Med* 323, 769 (0.25%)
(1989): Berger TG+, *Ann Intern Med* 110, 1035
(1988): Sattler FR+, *Ann Intern Med* 109, 280 (15%)
(1988): Leen CLS+, *Lancet* 2, 1250
(1987): Goa KL+, *Drugs* 33, 242 (1.5%)
(1984): Kovacs JA+, *Ann Intern Med* 100, 663 (6%)
(1984): Gordon FM+, *Ann Intern Med* 100, 495 (3%)
Jarisch–Herxheimer reaction (<1%)
(1987): Goa KL+, *Drugs* 33, 242
Pruritus
(1989): Berger TG+, *Ann Intern Med* 110, 1035
(1988): Leen CLS+, *Lancet* 2, 1250

Purpura
Rash (sic) (31–47%)
(1993): Dohn M+, *Int Conf AIDS* 9, 372
(1988): Leen CL+, *Lancet* 2, 1250
(1984): Gordin FM+, *Ann Intern Med* 100, 495
(1974): Walzer PD+, *Ann Intern Med* 80, 83 (1.5%)
Stevens–Johnson syndrome (0.2%)
Toxic epidermal necrolysis
(1988): Leen CLS+, *Lancet* 2, 1250 (passim)
(1987): Goa KL+, *Drugs* 33, 242
(1985): Heng MCY, *Br J Dermatol* 113, 597
Ulceration
(1985): Gottlieb JR+, *Plast Reconstr Surg* 76, 630
Urticaria
(1993): Belsito DV, *Contact Dermatitis* 29, 158 (contact)
(1992): Breathnach SM+, *Adverse Drug Reactions and the Skin*, Blackwell, Oxford, 179 (passim)
(1988): Leen CLS+, *Lancet* 2, 1250
Vasculitis
Xerosis

Other

Ageusia
Anosmia
Dysgeusia) (1.7%) (metallic taste)
Gingivitis
Injection-site calcification
(1987): Goa KL+, *Drugs* 33, 242
Injection-site cutaneous reaction (sic) (>10%)
(1992): Jones RS+, *Clin Infect Dis* 15, 561
Injection-site irritation
(1996): Herrero-Ambrosio A+, *Am J Health Syst Pharm* 53, 2881
(1996): Andersen JM, *Am J Health Syst Pharm* 53, 185
Injection-site ulceration
(1991): Bolognia JL, *Dermatologica* 183, 221
Myalgia (<5%)
Phlebitis
Xerostomia

PENTAZOCINE

Trade name: Talwin (Sanofi)
Other common trade names: *Fortral; Fortwin; Liticon; Ospronim; Pentafen; Sosegon; Susevin; Talacen*
Indications: Pain
Category: Narcotic; analgesic; sedative
Half-life: 2–3 hours
Clinically important, potentially serious interactions with: alcohol, anxiolytics, barbiturates, cimetidine, CNS depressants, diazepam, hypnotics, phenothiazines, tranquilizers, tripelennamine

Reactions

Skin

Cellulitis
(1992): Breathnach SM+, *Adverse Drug Reactions and the Skin*, Blackwell, Oxford, 212 (passim)
Dermatitis (sic)
Diaphoresis
Exanthems
(1987): Pedragosa R+, *Arch Dermatol* 123, 297
Facial edema
Flushing
(1973): Brogden RN+, *Drugs* 5, 6
Generalized eruption (sic)
(1992): Breathnach SM+, *Adverse Drug Reactions and the Skin*, Blackwell, Oxford, 212 (passim)
Hyperpigmentation (surrounding ulcers)
(1990): Furner BB, *J Am Acad Dermatol* 694 (passim)
Pruritus (<1%)
Rash (sic) (1–10%)
Scleroderma
(2000): D'Cruz D, *Toxicol Lett* 112 and 421
(1991): Bourgeois P+, *Baillieres Clin Rheumatol* 5, 13
Sclerosis
(1980): Palestine RF+, *J Am Acad Dermatol* 2, 47
(1974): Beckner TF, *JAMA* 227, 1383
(1973): Brogden RN+, *Drugs* 5, 6 (widespread)
Toxic epidermal necrolysis (<1%)
(1987): Pedragosa R+, *Arch Dermatol* 123, 297 (passim)
(1973): Hunter AAJ+, *Br J Dermatol* 88, 287
Tricotropism (sic)
(1987): Pedragosa R+, *Arch Dermatol* 123, 297 (passim)
Ulceration
(1992): Breathnach SM+, *Adverse Drug Reactions and the Skin*, Blackwell, Oxford, 212 (passim)
(1990): Furner BB, *J Am Acad Dermatol* 694
(1980): Palestine RF+, *J Am Acad Dermatol* 2, 47
(1979): Padilla RS+, *Arch Dermatol* 115, 975 (punched-out ulcers)
(1974): Winfield JB+, *South Med J* 67, 292
(1973): Winfield JB+, *JAMA* 226, 189
Urticaria

Other

Acute intermittent porphyria
Dysgeusia
Embolia cutis medicamentosa (Nicolau syndrome)
(1983): Bockers M+, *Med Welt* (German) 34, 1450
Fibrous myopathy
(1976): Johnson KR+, *Arthritis Rheum* 19, 923
(1975): Oh SJ+, *JAMA* 231, 271
Injection-site calcification
(1991): Magee KL+, *Arch Dermatol* 127, 1591
(1986): Hertzman A+, *J Rheumatol* 13, 210
Injection-site fibrosis
(1979): Padilla RS+, *Arch Dermatol* 115, 975
Injection-site granulomas and induration
(1982): Menon PA, *J Assoc Military Dermatol* 2, 65
(1972): Agache P+, *Bull Soc Fr Dermatol Syphiligr* (French) 79, 37
(1971): Schlicher JE+, *Arch Dermatol* 104, 90
Injection-site induration and ulcers
(1996): Bellman B+, *Arch Dermatol* 132, 1365
(1996): Gillum P, Oklahoma City, OK (from Internet) (observation)
(1984): Choucair AK+, *Neurology* 34, 524
(1983): Adams EM+, *Arch Intern Med* 143, 2203
(1977): Schiff BL+, *JAMA* 238, 1542
(1977): Cosman A+, *Plast Reconstr Surg* 59, 255
(1974): Seymour R+, *Am Surg* 40, 671
(1973): Hönigsmann H+, *Hautarzt* (German) 24, 128
(1971): Parks DL+, *Arch Dermatol* 104, 231
Injection-site pain
Injection-site pigmentation
(1980): Palestine RF+, *J Am Acad Dermatol* 2, 47
Lipogranulomas
(1973): Hönigsmann H, *Dermatol Monatsschr* (German) 159, 146
Myofibrosis
(1999): Jain A+, *J Dermatol* 26, 368
Panniculitis (chronic)
(1992): Breathnach SM+, *Adverse Drug Reactions and the Skin*, Blackwell, Oxford, 212 (passim)
Paresthesias
Phlebitis
(1992): Breathnach SM+, *Adverse Drug Reactions and the Skin*, Blackwell, Oxford, 212 (passim)
Soft tissue calcification
(1990): Furner BB, *J Am Acad Dermatol* 694 (passim)
Xerostomia (1–10%)

PENTOBARBITAL

Trade name: Nembutal (Abbott)
Other common trade names: *Medinox Mono; Mintal; Nova Rectal; Pentobarbitone; Prodromol; Sombutol*
Indications: Insomnia, sedation
Category: Hypnotic and sedative barbiturate; anticonvulsant
Half-life: 15–50 hours
Clinically important, potentially serious interactions with: acetaminophen, alcohol, anticoagulants, barbiturates, benzodiazepines, chloramphenicol, CNS depressants, calcium channel blockers, cimetidine, diltiazem, MAO inhibitors, metoprolol, nifedipine, theophylline, valproic acid

Reactions

Skin

Acne
Angioedema (< 1%)
Bullous eruption
(1970): Groeschel D+, *N Engl J Med* 283, 409
Erythema multiforme
(1975): Böttiger LE, *Acta Med Scand* 198, 229
Exanthems
(1943): Davison TC, *Curr Res Anesth Analg* 22, 52
Exfoliative dermatitis (< 1%)
(1944): Potter JK+, *Ann Intern Med* 21, 1041
Fixed eruption
(1970): Savin JA, *Br J Dermatol* 83, 546
Herpes simplex (activation)
Lupus erythematosus
(1967): Williams DI, *Proc R Soc Med* 60, 299
(1951): Grant Peterkin GA, *Edinb Med J* 58, 41
Necrosis
(1972): Almeyda J+, *Br J Dermatol* 86, 313
Photoreactions
(1939): Stryker GV, *J Mo Med Assn* 36, 484
Photosensitivity
Pruritus
Purpura
(1946): Grant Peterkin GA, *BMJ* 2, 52
Rash (sic) (< 1%)
Stevens–Johnson syndrome (< 1%)
Toxic epidermal necrolysis
(1973): Stüttgen G, *Br J Dermatol* 88, 291
Urticaria
Vasculitis

Other

Hypersensitivity
Injection-site pain (1–10%)
Injection-site reactions (< 1%)
Oral ulceration
Porphyria
(1968): Lang PA+, *Tex Rep Biol Med* 26, 525
Porphyria variegata
Thrombophlebitis (< 1%)

PENTOSAN

Synonym: PPS
Trade name: Elmiron (Alza)
Indications: Bladder pain, interstitial cystitis
Category: Urinary analgesic
Half-life: 4.8 hours
Clinically important, potentially serious interactions with: anticoagulants, NSAIDs, platelet inhibitors

Reactions

Skin

Allergic reactions (< 1%)
Ecchymoses
Photosensitivity (< 1%)
Pruritus (< 1%)
Purpura (< 1%)
Rash (sic) (1–10%)
Urticaria (< 1%)

Hair

Hair – alopecia (1–10%)

Other

Gingival bleeding (< 1%)
Oral ulceration (< 1%)

PENTOSTATIN

Trade name: Nipent (SuperGen)
Indications: Hairy-cell leukemia
Category: Antineoplastic; antimetabolite
Half-life: 5–15 hours
Clinically important, potentially serious interactions with: allopurinol, fludarabine, vidarabine

Reactions

Skin

Acne (<3%)
Allergic reactions (sic) (>10%)
Bullous eruption (3–10%)
Contact dermatitis (<3%)
Dermatitis (sic) (< 1%)
Diaphoresis (3–10%)
Ecchymoses (3–10%)
Eczema (sic) (3–10%)
Erythema
Erythroderma
(1999): Ghura HS+, *BMJ* 319, 549
Exanthems (3–10%)
(1997): Greiner D+, *J Am Acad Dermatol* 36, 950
(1989): O'Dwyer PJ+, *Cancer Chemother Pharmacol* 23, 173
Exfoliative dermatitis (<3%)
Facial edema (<3%)
Flushing (<3%)
Herpes simplex (3–10%)
Herpes zoster (3–10%)
Peripheral edema (3–10%)
Petechiae (3–10%)
Photosensitivity (<3%)
Pigmentation (3–10%)
Pruritus (3–10%)
Psoriasis (<3%)
Purpura (<3%)
(1999): Leach JW+, *Am J Hematol* 61, 268
Rash (sic) (26%)
Reactivation of pruritus and erythema of preexisting keratoses (sic)
(1989): Kerker BJ+, *Semin Dermatol* 8, 173

(1985): Camisa C+, *J Am Acad Dermatol* 12, 1108
Seborrhea (3–10%)
Skin disorder (sic) (17%)
Urticaria (<1%)
Xerosis (3–10%)

Hair
Hair – alopecia (<3%)

Other
Anaphylactoid reaction (<3%)
Candidiasis (<3%)
Dysgeusia (<3%)
Gingivitis (<3%)
Gynecomastia (<3%)
Injection-site hemorrhage (<3%)
Injection-site inflammation (<3%)
Leukoplakia (<3%)
Myalgia (>10%)
Paresthesias (3–10%)
Stomatitis (1–10%)
Thrombophlebitis (3–10%)
Vaginitis (<3%)

PENTOXIFYLLINE

Trade names: Pentoxil (Upsher-Smith); Trental (Aventis)
Other common trade names: *Apo-Pentoxifylline; Artal; Azupentat; Elorgan; Hemovas; Pentoxi; Pexal; Torental*
Indications: Peripheral vascular disease; intermittent claudication
Category: Blood viscosity-reducing agent
Half-life: 0.4–0.8 hours
Clinically important, potentially serious interactions with: antihypertensives, cimetidine, ciprofloxacin, theophylline, warfarin

Reactions

Skin
Allergic reactions (sic)
(1986): Bigby M+, *JAMA* 256, 3358
Angioedema (<1%)
(1994): Samlaska CP+, *J Am Acad Dermatol* 30, 603 (passim)
Diaphoresis
Edema (<1%)
Exanthems
Flushing
(1987): Ward A+, *Drugs* 34, 50 (2%)
(1976): *Drug Ther Bull* 14, 59
Pruritus (<1%)
(1994): Samlaska CP+, *J Am Acad Dermatol* 30, 603 (passim)
Purpura
Rash (sic) (<1%)
Urticaria

Nails
Nails – brittle (<1%)

Other
Dysgeusia (<1%)
Dysphagia
(1997): Puritz E, Smithtown, NY (from Internet) (observation)
(1997): Fetterman M, Miami, FL (from Internet) (observation)
Paresthesias
(1994): Samlaska CP+, *J Am Acad Dermatol* 30, 603 (passim)
Serum sickness
(1986): Panwalker AP+, *Drug Intell Clin Pharm* 20, 953
Sialorrhea (<1%)
Tremor
Xerostomia (<1%)
(1994): Samlaska CP+, *J Am Acad Dermatol* 30, 603 (passim)

PERGOLIDE

Trade name: Permax (Athena)
Other common trade names: *Celance; Parkotil; Pergolide*
Indications: Parkinsonism
Category: Antiparkinsonian; dopamine receptor agonist; ergot alkaloid
Half-life: 27 hours
Clinically important, potentially serious interactions with: dopamine antagonists, haloperidol, loxapine, methyldopa, metoclopramide, phenothiazines, thiothixene

Reactions

Skin
Acne
Chills (1–10%)
Diaphoresis (2.1%)
Discoloration (sic)
Edema (1.6%)
Erythromelalgia
(1989): Horn TD+, *Arch Dermatol* 125, 1512
(1984): Monk BE+, *Br J Dermatol* 111, 97 (on shins)
Exanthems
Facial edema (1.1%)
(1993): Garcia-Escrig M+, *Medicina Clinica* (Spanish) 101, 275
Flu-like syndrome (sic) (1–10%)
Peripheral edema (1–10%)
Pruritus
Rash (sic) (3.2%)
Seborrhea
Ulceration
Urticaria
Vasculitis
(1989): Horn TD+, *Arch Dermatol* 125, 1512
Xerosis

Hair
Hair – alopecia
Hair – hirsutism

Other
Dysgeusia (1.6%)
Gingivitis (<1%)
Mastodynia
Myalgia (<1%)
Paresthesias (1.6%)
Priapism
Tremor (1–10%)
Xerostomia (1–10%)

PERINDOPRIL

Trade name: Aceon (Solvay)
Other common trade names: *Acertil; Coversum; Coversyl; Prexum*
Indications: Hypertension
Category: Angiotensin-converting enzyme (ACE) inhibitor; antihypertensive
Half-life: 1.5–3 hours
Clinically important, potentially serious interactions with: amiloride, antihypertensives, diuretics, insulin, lithium, mercaptopurine, NSAIDs, spironolactone, triamterene

Reactions

Skin
Angioedema (<1%)
(1998): Lapostolle F+, *Am J Cardiol* 81, 523 (lingual)
Chills (<1%)
Cutaneous reactions (1.3%)
(1993): Desche P+, *Am J Cardiol* 71, 61E

Diaphoresis (0.3–1%)
Ecchymoses (0.3–1%)
Edema (3.9%)
Erythema (0.3–1%)
Exanthems
Facial edema (<1%)
Herpes simplex (0.3–1%)
Palmar-plantar pustulosis
(1995): Eriksen JG+, *Ugeskr Laeger* (Danish) 157, 3335
Pruritus (1–10%)
Psoriasis (<1%)
Purpura (<0.1%)
Rash (sic) (1–10%)
(1991): Dratwa M+, *J Cardiovasc Pharmacol* 18, S40
Xerosis (0.3–1%)

Other

Anaphylactoid reaction (<1%)
(1998): Speirs C+, *Br J Clin Pharmacol* 46, 63
Dysgeusia (<1%)
Myalgia (<1%)
Paresthesias (2.3%)
Vaginitis (0.3–1%)
Xerostomia (0.3–1%)

PERPHENAZINE

Trade names: Etrafon (Schering); Triavil (Lotus); Trilafon (Schering)
Other common trade names: *Apo-Perphenzine; Decentan; Fentazin; Leptopsique; Peratsin; Perphenan; Trilifan Retard; Triomin*
Indications: Psychotic disorders, nausea and vomiting
Category: Phenothiazine antipsychotic and antiemetic
Half-life: 9 hours
Clinically important, potentially serious interactions with: alcohol, anticholinergics, anticonvulsants, bromocriptine, chloroquine, CNS depressants, guanethidine, levodopa, MAO inhibitors, piperazine, propranolol, trazodone, **cigarette smoking**

Etrafon and Triavil are combinations of perphenazine and amitriptyline

Reactions

Skin

Angioedema
Contact dermatitis
Diaphoresis
Eczema (sic)
Erythema
Exanthems
(1976): Arndt KA+, *JAMA* 235, 918
(1959): Wright W, *JAMA* 171, 1642
Exfoliative dermatitis
Lupus erythematosus
(1988): Steen VD+, *Arthritis Rheum* 31, 923
(1986): Gupta MA+, *J Am Acad Dermatol* 14, 638
(1978): Gold MS+, *J Nerv Ment Dis* 166, 442
(1971): Fabius AJM+, *Acta Rheum Scand* 17, 137
Parkinsonism
Peripheral edema
Photosensitivity
Pigmentation (blue-gray) (<1%)
Pruritus
Purpura
Rash (sic) (1–10%)
Seborrhea
Urticaria
(1959): Wright W, *JAMA* 171, 1642
Xerosis

Other

Anaphylactoid reaction
Galactorrhea (black) (<1%)
(1985): Basler RSW+, *Arch Dermatol* 121, 418
Gynecomastia
Mastodynia (1–10%)
Priapism (<1%)
Pseudolymphoma
(1995): Magro CM+, *J Am Acad Dermatol* 32, 419
Sialorrhea
Xerostomia

PHENAZOPYRIDINE

Trade names: Baridium; Geridium; Prodium; Pyridiate; Pyridium (Parke-Davis)
Other common trade names: *Azodine; Eridium; Phenazo; Pyronium; Sedural; Urodine; Urogesic; Urohman; Uropyridin*
Indications: Urinary urgency, dysuria
Category: Urinary analgesic
Half-life: no data
Clinically important, potentially serious interactions with: none

Reactions

Skin

Allergic reactions (sic)
(1986): Bigby M+, *JAMA* 256, 3358 (0.88%)
Edema
Exanthems
(1976): Arndt KA+, *JAMA* 235, 918 (0.6%)
Pigmentation (<1%)
(1974): Eybel CE+, *JAMA* 228, 1027 (blue-gray; orange-yellow)
(1970): Alano FA+, *Ann Intern Med* 72, 89
Pruritus
Rash (sic) (<1%)

Nails

Nails – lemon-yellow
(1997): Amit G+, *Ann Intern Med* 127, 1137

Other

Anaphylactoid reaction

PHENDIMETRAZINE

Trade names: Bontril (Carnrick); Prelu-2 (Roxane)
Other common trade name: *Obesan-X*
Indications: Obesity
Category: Appetite suppressant
Half-life: 5–12.5 hours
Clinically important, potentially serious interactions with: diltiazem, doxycycline, MAO inhibitors, nifedipine, quinidine, tetracycline, tricyclic antidepressants

Reactions

Skin

Diaphoresis
Flushing
Urticaria

Other

Dysgeusia
Xerostomia

PHENELZINE

Trade name: Nardil (Parke-Davis)
Other common trade name: *Nardelzine*
Indications: Depression
Category: Monoamine oxidase (MAO) inhibitor; antidepressant and antipanic
Half-life: no data
Clinically important, potentially serious interactions with: barbiturates, buspirone, caffeine, carbamazepine, CNS depressants, dextroamphetamine, disulfiram, fluoxetine, guanethidine, levodopa, lithium, maprotiline, meperidine, phenothiazines, psychotropics, sertraline, sulfonylureas, sumatriptan, sympathomimetics, trazodone, venlafaxine. Also **tyramine-containing foods***

Reactions

Skin

Angioedema
(1962): Busfield BL+, *J Nerv Ment Dis* 134, 339
Ankle edema
(1977): Dunleavy DLF, *BMJ* 1, 1353
(1970): Kelly D+, *Br J Psychiatry* 116, 387
Diaphoresis
(1985): Levy AB+, *Can J Psychiatry* 30, 434
Edema
Exanthems
Lupus erythematosus
(1978): Swartz C, *JAMA* 239, 2693
Parkinsonism
Peripheral edema (1–10%)
Photosensitivity
(1988): Case JD+, *Photodermatology* 5, 101
(1962): Busfield BL+, *J Nerv Ment Dis* 134, 339 (13%)
Pruritus (13%)
(1962): Busfield BL+, *J Nerv Ment Dis* 134, 339
Rash (sic)
Telangiectases
Urticaria

Other

Black tongue
Glossitis
(1992): Zürcher K+, *Cutaneous Drug Reactions*, Karger, Basel (passim)
Priapism
Tremor
Twitching
Xerostomia (1–10%)
(1962): Busfield BL+, *J Nerv Ment Dis* 134, 339 (20%)

***Note:** Tyramine-containing foods include the following: aged cheeses, avocados, banana skins, bologna and other processed luncheon meats, chicken livers, chocolate, figs, canned pickled herring, meat extracts, pepperoni, raisins, raspberries, soy sauce, vermouth, sherry and red wines.

PHENINDAMINE

Trade name: Nolahist (Carnrick)
Indications: Allergic rhinitis, urticaria, angioedema
Category: H_1-receptor antihistamine and appetite stimulant
Half-life: no data
Clinically important, potentially serious interactions with: alcohol, CNS depressants

Reactions

Skin

Angioedema
Dermatitis (sic)
Diaphoresis
Erythema
Flushing
Lupus erythematosus
Photosensitivity
Purpura
Rash (sic)
Urticaria

Other

Xerostomia

PHENOBARBITAL

Synonyms: phenobarbitone; phenylethylmalonylurea
Trade names: Barbita; Luminal (Sanofi); Solfoton (ECR)
Other common trade names: *Alepsal; Barbilixir; Barbital; Gardenal; Luminal; Luminaletten; Phenaemal; Phenobarbitone*
Indications: Insomnia, seizures
Category: Sedative-hypnotic and anticonvulsant barbiturate
Half-life: 2–6 days
Clinically important, potentially serious interactions with: acetaminophen, alcohol, anticoagulants, benzodiazepines, beta-blockers, CNS depressants, chloramphenicol, diltiazem, doxycycline, estrogens, MAO inhibitors, methylphenidate, metoprolol, metronidazole, phenytoin, propoxyphene, quinidine, theophylline, tricyclic antidepressants, valproic acid, verapamil, warfarin

Reactions

Skin

Acne
(1992): Hesse S+, *Ann Dermatol Venereol* (French) 119, 655
Acute generalized exanthematous pustulosis (AGEP)
(1996): Wolkenstein P+, *Contact Dermatitis* 35, 234
Allergic reactions (sic)
(1987): Pigatto PD, *Contact Dermatitis* 16, 279
(1979): Montowska L+, *Pol Tyg Lek* (Polish) 34, 2029
Angioedema (<1%)
Bullous eruption
(1990): Dunn C+, *Cutis* 45, 43 (in coma)
(1970): Groeschel D+, *N Engl J Med* 283, 409
(1965): Beveridge GW+, *BMJ* 1, 835
(1940): Moss RE+, *Arch Dermatol* 46, 386
(1925): Birch CA, *Brit J Child Dis* 22, 280
Depigmentation
(1992): Mion N+, *Ann Dermatol Venereol* (French) 119, 927
Edema
Erythema multiforme
(1994): Shelley WB+, *Cutis* 53, 162 (observation)
(1994): Stewart MG+, *Otolaryngol Head Neck Surg* 111, 236
(1990): Salomon D+, *Br J Dermatol* 123, 797
(1988): Shear NH+, *J Clin Invest* 82, 1826
(1986): Palomeque A+, *An Esp Pediatr* (Spanish) 34, 328
(1975): Böttiger LE, *Acta Med Scand* 198, 229
(1940): Moss RE+, *Arch Dermatol* 46, 386
Erythroderma
(1993): Sakai C+, *Intern Med* 32, 182
Exanthems
(1997): Hyson C+, *Can J Neurol Sci* 24, 245
(1988): Shear NH+, *J Clin Invest* 82, 1826
(1986): Savich RD+, *Ill Med J* 169, 232
(1984): Fernandez de Corres L+, *Contact Dermatitis* 11, 319
(1979): Rudzki E, *Przegl Dermatol* (Polish) 66, 415
(1952): Sneddon IB+, *BMJ* 1, 1276
(1943): Davison TC, *Curr Res Anesth Analg* 22, 52
(1940): Moss RE+, *Arch Dermatol* 46, 386
(1925): Birch CA, *Brit J Child Dis* 22, 280
Exfoliative dermatitis (<1%)
(1993): Sakai C+, *Intern Med* 32, 182
(1986): Savich RD+, *Ill Med J* 169, 232
(1976): Weisburst M+, *South Med J* 69, 126
(1950): Welton DG, *JAMA* 143, 232
(1944): Potter JK+, *Ann Intern Med* 21, 1041

(1940): Moss RE+, *Arch Dermatol* 46, 386
Fixed eruption
(1989): Shiohara T+, *Arch Dermatol* 125, 1371
(1987): Savchak VI, *Vestn Dermatol Venerol* (Russian) 6, 62
(1979): Pasricha JS, *Br J Dermatol* 100, 183
(1974): Kuokkanen K, *Int J Dermatol* 13, 4 (genitalia and mucous membranes)
(1970): Savin JA, *Br J Dermatol* 83, 546
(1967): Schulz KH+, *Z Haut Geschlechtskr* (German) 42, 561
Graft-versus-host reaction
(1998): Jappe U+, *Hautarzt* (German) 49, 126 (passim)
Herpes simplex (activation)
Lupus erythematosus
(1967): Williams DI, *Proc R Soc Med* 60, 299
(1951): Grant Peterkin GA, *Edinb Med J* 58, 41
Necrosis
(1972): Almeyda J+, *Br J Dermatol* 86, 313
Pellagra
(1982): Stadler R+, *Hautarzt* (German) 33, 276
Pemphigus
(1986): Dourmishev AL+, *Dermatologica* 173, 256
Photoreactions
(1939): Stryker GV, *J Mo Med Assn* 36, 484
Photosensitivity
Pruritus
(1994): Sigl B, *Hautarzt* (German) 45, 409
Purpura
(1952): Sneddon IB+, *BMJ* 1, 1276
(1946): Grant Peterkin GA, *BMJ* 2, 52
Pustules (generalized)
(1991): Kleier RS+, *Arch Dermatol* 127, 1361
Rash (sic) (<1%)
Stevens–Johnson syndrome (<1%)
(1999): Rzany B+, *Lancet* 353, 2190
(1999): Duncan KO, *J Am Acad Dermatol* 40, 493 (at sites of radiation therapy)
(1995): Wolkenstein P+, *Arch Dermatol* 131, 544
(1995): Labandiera-Garcia J, *An Med Interna* (Spanish) 12, 569
(1994): Koukoulis A+, *An Med Interna* (Spanish) 11, 311
(1993): Leenutaphong V+, *Int J Dermatol* 32, 428
(1992): Lleonart R+, *Med Clin (Barc)* (Spanish) 99, 474
(1985): de Rego JA+, *Hillside J Clin Psychiatry* 7, 141
(1985): Avery JK, *J Tenn Med Assoc* 78, 764
(1982): Brahams D, *Lancet* 2, 1474
(1982): Oles KS+, *Clin Pharm* 1, 565
(1971): Adeloye A+, *Ghana Med J* 10, 56
Toxic epidermal necrolysis
(2000): Devidal R+, *Therapie* 55, 225 (2 cases)
(1999): Rzany B+, *Lancet* 353, 2190
(1996): Blum L+, *J Am Acad Dermatol* 34, 1088
(1995): Wolkenstein P+, *Arch Dermatol* 131, 544
(1994): Shelley WB+, *Cutis* 53, 162 (observation)
(1994): Errani A+, *Br J Dermatol* 131, 586
(1993): Leenutaphong V+, *Int J Dermatol* 32, 428
(1993): Correia O+, *Dermatology* 186, 32
(1989): Dominguez-Perez F+, *Rev Esp Anestesiol Reanim* (Spanish) 36, 350
(1988): Shear NH+, *J Clin Invest* 82, 1826
(1987): Teillac D+, *Arch Fr Pediatr* (French) 44, 583
(1985): de Rego JA+, *Hillside J Clin Psychiatry* 7, 141
(1984): Chan HL, *J Am Acad Dermatol* 10, 973
(1975): Giallorenzi AF+, *Oral Surg Oral Med Oral Pathol* 40, 611
(1975): Deviller G+, *Union Med Can* (French) 104, 399
(1973): Stüttgen G, *Br J Dermatol* 88, 291
(1966): Campos EC de+, *An Bras Dermatol* (Portuguese) 41, 165
(1966): Haraszti A+, *Orv Hetil* (Hungarian) 107, 2133 (fatal)
(1966): Kaczorowska-Hanke H+, *Przegl Dermatol* (Polish) 53, 197
Toxicodermia (sic)
(1998): Arima M+, *Jpn Circ J* 62, 132
Urticaria
(1940): Moss RE+, *Arch Dermatol* 46, 386
Vasculitis

Hair

Hair – depigmentation
(1992): Mion N+, *Ann Dermatol Venereol* (French) 119, 927

Nails

Nails – hypoplasia
(1991): Thakker JC+, *Indian Pediatr* 28, 73
(1990): Holder M+, *Monatsschr Kinderheilkr* (German) 138, 34

Other

Hypersensitivity (<1%)*
(1999): Moss DM+, *J Emerg Med* 17, 503
(1998): Chapman MS+, *Br J Dermatol* 138, 710
(1998): Schlienger RG+, *Epilepsia* 39, S3 (passim)
(1997): Morkunas AR+, *Crit Care Clin* 13, 727
(1992): Nagata T+, *Jpn J Clin Oncol* 22, 421
(1984): Fonseca JC+, *Med Cutan Ibero Lat Am* (Spanish) 12, 187
Hypoplasia of phalanges
(1991): Thakker JC+, *Indian Pediatr* 28, 73
(1990): Holder M+, *Monatsschr Kinderheilkr* (German) 138, 34
Injection-site bullous eruption
(1987): Haroun M+, *Cutis* 39, 233
Injection-site pain (>10%)
Injection-site thrombophlebitis (>10%)
Oral ulceration
Porphyria cutanea tarda
(1966): Ziprkowski L+, *Isr J Med Sci* 2, 338
Porphyria variegata
Xerostomia
(1952): Sneddon IB+, *BMJ* 1, 1276

***Note:** The antiepileptic drug hypersensitivity syndrome is a severe, occasionally fatal, disorder characterized by any or all of the following: pruritic exanthem, toxic epidermal necrolysis, Stevens–Johnson syndrome, exfoliative dermatitis, fever, hepatic abnormalities, eosinophilia, and renal failure.

PHENOLPHTHALEIN

Trade names: Agoral; Alophen; Caroid; Correctol; Doxidan; Espotabs; Evac-U-Gen; Ex-Lax; Feen-A-Mint; Medilax; Modane; Phenolax; Prulet, Trilax, etc. (Various pharmaceutical companies.)
Other common trade names: *Bom-Bon; Bonomint; Darmol; Easylax; Purganol; Ruguletts*
Indications: Constipation
Category: Laxative
Half-life: no data
Clinically important, potentially serious interactions with: no data

Reactions

Skin

Angioedema
(1972): Grillat JP+, *Rev Fr Allergie* (French) 12, 351
Bullous eruption
(1974): Magill M+, *Med J Aust* 1, 771
Diaphoresis
Erythema annulare (sic)
(1972): Grillat JP+, *Rev Fr Allergie* (French) 12, 351
Erythema multiforme
(1992): Breathnach SM+, *Adverse Drug Reactions and the Skin*, Blackwell, Oxford 344
(1972): Shelley WB+, *Br J Dermatol* 86, 118
Exanthems
(1972): Grilliat JP+, *Rev Fr Allergol* (French) 12, 351
(1969): Török H, *Dermatol Int* 8, 57
Exfoliative dermatitis
(1973): Nicolis GD+, *Arch Dermatol* 108, 788
Fixed eruption
(1997): Blumenthal HL, Beachwood, OH, 2 personal cases (observations)
(1993): Zanolli MD+, *Pediatrics* 91, 1199
(1991): Smoller BR+, *J Cutan Pathol* 18, 13
(1990): Gaffoor PMA+, *Cutis* 45, 242
(1987): Stroud MB+, *Arch Dermatol* 123, 1227
(1986): Kanwar AJ+, *Dermatologica* 172, 315
(1985): Kauppinen K+, *Br J Dermatol* 112, 575
(1984): Chan HL, *Int J Dermatol* 23, 607
(1978): Sehgal VN+, *Int J Dermatol* 17, 78

(1972): Shelley WB+, *Br J Dermatol* 86, 118 (bullous)
(1972): Wyatt E+, *Arch Dermatol* 106, 671
(1972): Louis P, *Z Haut Geschlechtskr* (German) 47, 387
(1972): Hunziker N, *Rev Med Suisse Romande* (French) 92, 237
(1970): Savin JA, *Br J Dermatol* 83, 546
(1969): Török H, *Dermatol Int* 8, 57
(1967): Schulz KH+, *Z Haut Geschlechtskr* (German) 42, 561
(1964): Browne SG, *BMJ* 2, 1041

Lupus erythematosus
(1992): Breathnach SM+, *Adverse Drug Reactions and the Skin*, Blackwell, Oxford 344

Perianal irritation

Pigmentation
(1973): Levantine A+, *Br J Dermatol* 89, 105

Pruritus
(1972): Grillat JP+, *Rev Fr Allergie* (French) 12, 351

Stevens–Johnson syndrome
(1972): Monnat A, *Schweiz Med Wochenschr* (French) 102, 1876

Toxic epidermal necrolysis
(1997): Artymowicz RJ+, *Ann Pharmacother* 31, 1157
(1986): Kar PK+, *J Indian Med Assoc* 84, 189
(1973): Björnberg A, *Acta Dermatol Venereol* (Stockh) 53, 149
(1973): Khamadullin LG, *Vestn Dermatol Venerol* (Russian) 47, 67
(1972): Monnat A, *Schweiz Med Wochenschr* (French) 102, 1876
(1967): Lowney ED+, *Arch Dermatol* 95, 359
(1966): Témime P+, *Bull Soc Fr Dermatol Syphiligr* (French) 73, 305
(1961): Browne SG+, *BMJ* 1, 550
(1957): Lang R+, *S Afr Med J* 31, 713

Urticaria
(1972): Grillat JP+, *Rev Fr Allergie* (French) 12, 351

Nails

Nails – discoloration of lunulae
(1984): Daniel CR+, *J Am Acad Dermatol* 10, 250

Other

Oral mucosal fixed eruption
Oral mucosal pigmentation
Oral mucosal ulceration

PHENOXYBENZAMINE

Trade name: Dibenzyline (SmithKline Beecham)
Other trade names: *Dibenyline; Dibenzyran*
Indications: Pheochromocytoma
Category: Alpha-adrenergic blocking agent; antihypertensive
Half-life: 24 hours
Clinically important, potentially serious interactions with: beta-blockers

Reactions

Skin

Contact dermatitis
(1975): MitchellJC+, *Contact Dermatitis* 1, 363

Reactions (sic)
(1973): Alexander SL+, *Lancet* 1, 317

Other

Priapism
(1974): Funderburk SJ+, *N Engl J Med* 290, 630

Xerostomia (1–10%)

PHENSUXIMIDE

Trade name: Milontin (Parke-Davis)
Indications: Petit mal seizures
Category: Anticonvulsant
Half-life: 5–12 hours
Clinically important, potentially serious interactions with: phenytoin, valproic acid

Reactions

Skin

Erythema multiforme (<1%)
Lupus erythematosus
Periorbital edema
Pruritus
Purpura
(1980): Miescher PA+, *Clin Haematol* 9, 505
Rash (sic)
Stevens–Johnson syndrome

Hair

Hair – alopecia
Hair – hirsutism

Other

Acute intermittent porphyria
Gingival hyperplasia
Oral ulceration

PHENTERMINE

Trade names: Adipex-P (Gate); Fastin (SmithKline Beecham); Ionamin (Medeva)
Other common trade names: *Behapront; Diminex; Minobese-Forte; Panbesy; Panbesyl; Redusa; Umine; Zantryl*
Indications: Obesity
Category: Appetite suppressant (anorexiant)
Half-life: 19–24 hours
Clinically important, potentially serious interactions with: barbiturates, CNS stimulants, MAO inhibitors, sympathomimetics, tricyclic antidepressants

Reactions

Skin

Diaphoresis (<1%)
Peripheral edema
Peripheral vasculopathy (sic)
(1999): Jefferson HJ+, *Nephrol Dial Transplant* 14, 1761
Purpura
Rash (sic)
Raynaud's phenomenon
(1990): Aeschlimann A+, *Scand J Rheumatol* 19, 87
Urticaria

Hair

Hair – alopecia (<1%)

Other

Dysgeusia
Myalgia (<1%)
Tremor
Xerostomia

PHENTOLAMINE

Trade name: Regitine (Novartis)
Other common trade names: *Regitin; Rogitene; Rogitine*
Indications: Hypertensive episodes in pheochromocytoma
Category: Alpha adrenergic blocking agent; antihypertensive; diagnostic aid for pheochromocytoma
Half-life: 19 minutes
Clinically important, potentially serious interactions with: ethanol, ephedrine, epinephrine

Reactions

Skin
Flushing (1–10%)

Other
Priapism

PHENYLEPHRINE

Trade names: AK-Dilate; L-Phrine; Isopto Frin; Neo-Synephrine; Prefrin; Sinarest; Vicks Sinest, etc. (Various pharmaceutical companies.)
Other trade names: *Dionephrine; Novahistine; Prefrin Liquifilm*
Indications: Nasal congestion, glaucoma, hypotension
Category: Alpha-adrenergic agonist; mydriatic ophthalmic agent
Half-life: 2.5 hours
Clinically important, potentially serious interactions with: beta-blockers, cocaine, furazolidone, guanethidine, MAO inhibitors, maprotiline, sympathomimetics, tricyclic antidepressants

Reactions

Skin
Contact dermatitis
(1999): Resano A+, *J Invest Allergol Clin Immunol* 9, 55 (blepharoconjunctivitis)
(1998): Rafael M+, *Contact Dermatitis* 39, 143 (blepharoconjunctivitis)
(1998): Wigger-Alberti W+, *Allergy* 53, 217 (blepharoconjunctivitis)
(1998): Thomas P+, *Contact Dermatitis* 38, 41 (blepharoconjunctivitis)
(1997): Marcos ML+, *Contact Dermatitis* 37, 189
(1997): Ockenfels HM+, *Dermatology* 195, 119 (periorbital)
(1997): Moreno-Ancillo M+, *Ann Allergy Asthma Immunol* 78, 569 (periorbital)
(1997): Mancuso G+, *Contact Dermatitis* 36, 110
(1995): Thomas P+, *Contact Dermatitis* 32, 249
(1993): Wilkinson SM+, *Contact Dermatitis* 29, 100
(1991): Anibarro B+, *Contact Dermatitis* 25, 323 (blepharoconjunctivitis)
(1991): Okamoto H+, *Cutis* 47, 357
(1991): Bardazzi F+, *Contact Dermatitis* 24, 56
(1990): Zucchi A+, *G Ital Dermatol Venereol* (Italian) 125, 155
(1986): Ducombs G+, *Contact Dermatitis* 15, 107
(1984): Camarasa JG, *Contact Dermatitis* 10, 182
(1983): Rarber KA, *Contact Dermatitis* 9, 274 (periorbital)
(1983): Hanna C+, *Am J Ophthalmol* 95, 703
(1979): De Vita L+, *Minerva Pediatr* (Italian) 31, 535
(1979): Mathias CG+, *Arch Ophthalmol* 97, 286
Pallor
Periorbital edema
(1998): Blum A+, *Hautarzt* (German) 49, 651
Stinging (from nasal or ophthalmic preparations) (1–10%)

Other
Hypersensitivity
(1991): Quirce Gancedo S+, *Med Clin (Barc)* (Spanish) 96, 317
Injection-site reaction
Paresthesias
Tremor

PHENYTOIN

Synonyms: diphenylhydantoin; DPH; phenytoin sodium
Trade name: Dilantin (Parke-Davis)
Other common trade names: *Di-Hydran; Diphenylan; Epanutin; Fenytoin; Phenhydan; Pyoredol; Zentropil*
Indications: Grand mal seizures
Category: Hydantoin anticonvulsant; antiarrhythmic
Half-life: 7–42 hours (dose dependent)
Clinically important, potentially serious interactions with: acetaminophen, amiodarone, chloramphenicol, cimetidine, corticosteroids, cyclosporine, diazoxide, dicumarol, disopyramide, disulfiram, doxycycline, ethosuximide, fluconazole, isoniazid, itraconazole, loop diuretics, meperidine, mexiletine, oral contraceptives, phenylbutazone, primidone, quinidine, rifampin, saquinavir, sulfonamides, theophylline, valproic acid, warfarin

Note: About 19% of patients receiving phenytoin develop skin reactions (1983): Rapp RP+, *Neurosurg* 13, 272. They typically develop 10 to 14 days following the start of treatment.

An excellent overview of cutaneous reactions to phenytoin can be found in (1988): Silverman AK+, *J Am Acad Dermatol* 18, 721.

Reactions

Skin
Acne
(1993): Shah M+, *Eur J Dermatol* 3, 576
(1990): Grunwald MH+, *Int J Dermatol* 29, 559
(1983): Greenwood R+, *Br Med J Clin Res Ed* 287, 1669
(1980): Stankler L+, *Br J Dermatol* 103, 453 (neonatal)
(1977): Frentz G, *Ugeskr Laeger* (Danish) 139, 338
(1972): Jenkins RB+, *N Engl J Med* 287, 148
(1964): Fegeler F, *Arch Klin Exp Derm* (German) 219, 335
Acute generalized exanthematous pustulosis (AGEP)
(1995): Moreau A+, *Int J Dermatol* 34, 263 (passim)
Angioedema
(1992): Schlaifer D+, *Eur J Hematol* 48, 274
(1967): Coleman WP, *Med Clin North Am* 51, 1073
Bullous eruption
(1988): Baird BJ+, *Int J Dermatol* 27, 170
Dermatomyositis
(1998): Dimachkie MM+, *J Child Neurol* 13, 577
Eosinophilic fasciitis
(1980): Buchanan RR+, *J Rheumatol* 7, 733
Epidermolysis bullosa
(1982): Bergfeld WF+, *J Am Acad Dermatol* 7, 275
Erythema multiforme
(1999): Micali G+, *Pharmacotherapy* 19, 223 (with cranial irradiation)
(1999): Marinella MA, *Ann Pharmacother* 33, 748
(1995): Rodriguez-Castellanos M+, *Arch Dermatol* 131, 620
(1990): Giroud M+, *Therapie* (French) 45, 23
(1988): Delattre JY+, *Neurology* 38, 194
(1988): Shear NH+, *J Clin Invest* 82, 1826
(1986): Green ST, *Clin Neuropharmacol* 9, 561
(1985): Tucker MS+, *J Am Osteopath Assoc* 85, 511
(1972): Almeyda J+, *Br J Dermatol* 87, 646
(1967): Coleman WP, *Med Clin North Am* 51, 1073
Erythroderma
(1996): Chopra S+, *Br J Dermatol* 134, 1109
(1991): Yamashina T+, *Nippon Shokakibyo Gakkai Zasshi* (Japanese) 88, 1269
(1983): Lillie MA+, *Arch Dermatol* 119, 415
(1966): Fischbeck R+, *Dtsch Gesundheitsw* (German) 21, 1273
Exanthems
(2000): Cohen AD+, *Isr Med Assoc J* 1, 95
(1997): Hyson C+, *Can J Neurol Sci* 24, 245
(1996): Leong KP+, *Asian Pac J Allergy Immunol* 14, 65 (71.4%)
(1992): Tone T+, *J Dermatol* 19, 27
(1991): Pelekanos J+, *Epilepsia* 32, 554
(1988): Shear NH+, *J Clin Invest* 82, 1826
(1984): Chadwick D+, *J Neurol Neurosurg Psychiatry* 47, 642 (6%)
(1983): Rapp RP+, *Neurosurgery* 13, 272
(1978): Wilson JT+, *BMJ* 1, 1583

(1975): Weedon AP, *Aust NZ J Med* 5, 561
(1970): Robinson HM+, *Arch Dermatol* 101, 462
(1969): Levene G+, *Br J Dermatol* 81, 712
(1967): Coleman WP, *Med Clin North Am* 51, 1073

Exfoliative dermatitis
(1997): Westhoven GS+, *Arch Dermatol* 133, 494
(1996): Leong KP+, *Asian Pac J Allergy Immunol* 14, 65 (2.4%)
(1996): Sigurdsson V+, *J Am Acad Dermatol* 35, 53
(1989): Danno K+, *J Dermatol* (Tokio) 16, 392
(1985): Matson JR+, *Hum Pathol* 16, 94
(1983): Rapp RP+, *Neurosurgery* 13, 272
(1972): Almeyda J+, *Br J Dermatol* 87, 646
(1963): Beerman H+, *Arch Dermatol* 87, 783
(1958): Chaiken BH+, *N Engl J Med* 242, 897
(1956): Gropper AL, *N Engl J Med* 254, 522
(1948): Van Wyck JJ+, *Arch Intern Med* 81, 605
(1942): Ritchie EB+, *Arch Dermatol* 46, 856

Fixed eruption
(1997): Chan HL+, *J Am Acad Dermatol* 36, 259
(1988): Baird BJ+, *Int J Dermatol* 27, 170 (bullous)
(1963): Goldstein N+, *Arch Dermatol* 87, 612

Heel pad thickening
(1975): Kattan KR, *AJR* 124, 52

Lichenoid eruption
(1992): Tone T+, *J Dermatol* 19, 27

Lichen planus
(1991): MacLeod SP+, *Br Dent J* 171, 237

Linear IgA bullous dermatosis
(1998): Acostamadiedo JM+, *J Am Acad Dermatol* 38, 352
(1994): Kuechle MK+, *J Am Acad Dermatol* 30, 187

Lupus erythematosus
(1993): Drory VE+, *Clin Neuropharmacol* 16, 19 (passim)
(1988): Jiang M, *Chung Kuo I Hsueh Ko Hsueh Yuan Hsueh Pao* (Chinese) 10, 379
(1985): Lovisetto P+, *Recenti Prog Med* (Italian) 76, 84
(1984): Wollina U, *Z Gesamte Int Med* (German) 39, 69
(1982): Gleichman H, *Arthritis Rheum* 25, 1387
(1977): Rybicka K+, *Pol Tyg Lek* (Polish) 32, 1269
(1976): Singsen BH+, *Pediatrics* 57, 529
(1974): Harpey JP, *Ann Allergy* 33, 256
(1970): Okuda M+, *Naika* (Japanese) 26, 989
(1967): Siegel M+, *Arthritis Rheum* 10, 407
(1966): Lee SL+, *Arch Intern Med* 117, 620
(1963): Jacobs JC, *Pediatrics* 32, 257
(1963): Goldstein N+, *Arch Dermatol* 87, 612
(1962): Benton JW+, *JAMA* 180, 115

Mycosis fungoides
(1991): Rijlaarsdam U+, *J Am Acad Dermatol* 24, 216
(1990): Souteyrand P+, *Curr Probl Dermatol* 19, 176
(1985): Wolf R+, *Arch Dermatol* 121, 1181
(1982): Rosenthal CH+, *Cancer* 49, 2305

Pellagra

Pemphigus
(1988): Seghal VN+, *Int J Dermatol* 27, 258

Pigmentation
(1964): Kuske H+, *Dermatologica* 129, 121

Pruritus
(1997): Litt JZ, Beachwood, OH, personal case (observation)
(1985): Rubinstein N+, *Int J Dermatol* 24, 54
(1967): Coleman WP, *Med Clin North Am* 51, 1073
(1963): Beerman H+, *Arch Dermatol* 87, 783

Pseudoacanthosis nigricans
(1972): Petko E+, *Arch Dermatol* 106, 918

Purple glove syndrome (sic)
(2000): Schmutz J+, *Ann Dermatol Venereol* (French) 127, 548
(1998): Cadenbach A+, *Dtsch Med Wochenschr* (German) 123, 318
(1994): Helfaer MA+, *J Neurosurg Anesthesiol* 6, 48

Purpura
(1975): Targan SR+, *Ann Intern Med* 83, 227 (fulminans)
(1967): Coleman WP, *Med Clin North Am* 51, 1073
(1963): Beerman H+, *Arch Dermatol* 87, 783
(1962): Weintraub RM+, *JAMA* 180, 528

Pustular eruption
(1993): O'Brien TJ+, *Australas J Dermatol* 34, 128
(1991): Kleier RS, *Arch Dermatol* 127, 1361
(1978): Stanley J+, *Arch Dermatol* 114, 1350

Rash (sic) (1–10%)
(1999): Mamon HJ+, *Epilepsia* 40, 341 (with cranial radiation)
(1987): Maguire JH+, *Br J Clin Pharmacol* 24, 554

Reticular hyperplasia
(1975): Wasik F+, *Hautarzt* (German) 26, 273
(1966): Korting GW+, *Dermatol Wochenschr* (German) 152, 257

Scleroderma
(1974): Kashiwazaki S+, *Ryumachi* (Japanese) 14, 220

Sezary syndrome
(1994): Doyle MF+, *Acta Hematol* 92, 204

Sjøgren's syndrome
(1996): Chakravarty K+, *Br J Rheumatol* 35, 1033

Stevens–Johnson syndrome
(2000): Madnani NA, Bombay, India (from Internet) (observation)
(1999): Rzany B+, *Lancet* 353, 2190
(1999): Ruble R+, *CNS Drugs* 12, 215
(1999): Khafaga YM+, *Acta Oncol* 38, 111 (with cranial irradiation)
(1996): Leong KP+, *Asian Pac J Allergy Immunol* 14, 65 (14.3%)
(1996): Cockey G+, *Am J Clin Oncol* 19, 32 (with irradiation of brain)
(1995): Wolkenstein P+, *Arch Dermatol* 131, 544
(1995): Cockey GH+, *Am J Clin Oncol* 19, 32
(1995): Borg M+, *Australas Radiol* 39, 42 (with irradiation of brain)
(1994): Marti J+, *An Med Interna* (Spanish) 11, 621
(1993): Leenutaphong V+, *Int J Dermatol* 32, 428
(1993): Schlienger RG+, *Schweiz Rundsch Med Prax* (German) 82, 888
(1993): Janinis J+, *Eur J Cancer* 29A, 478 (with cranial irradiation)
(1992): Tone T+, *J Dermatol* 19, 27
(1989): Kelly DF+, *Neurosurgery* 25, 976
(1988): Delattre JY+, *Neurology* 38, 194 (with cranial irradiation)
(1988): Shear NH+, *J Clin Invest* 82, 1826
(1985): Burge SM+, *J Am Acad Dermatol* 13, 665
(1985): de Rego JA+, *Hillside J Clin Psychiatry* 7, 141
(1985): Maiche A+, *Lancet* 2, 45 (with radiation therapy)
(1982): Oles KS+, *Clin Pharm* 1, 565
(1978): Assaad D+, *Can Med Assoc* 118, 154
(1976): Marg E, *Psychiatr Neurol Med Psychol Leipz* (German) 28, 436
(1971): Greenberg LM+, *Ann Ophthalmol* 3, 137
(1970): Rudner EJ, *Arch Dermatol* 102, 561

Toxic dermatitis (sic)
(1978): Huijgens PC+, *Acta Haematol* 59, 31

Toxic epidermal necrolysis
(2000): Cohen AD+, *Isr Med Assoc J* 1, 95 (2 patients)
(2000): Moussala M+, *J Fr Ophtalmol* (French) 23, 229
(1999): Ruble R+, *CNS Drugs* 12, 215
(1999): Rzany B+, *Lancet* 353, 2190
(1999): Cohen AD+, *Isr Med Assoc J* 1, 95 (2 cases)
(1997): Jester BA+, American Academy of Dermatology Meeting (SF), Poster #163
(1997): Sapadin A+, American Academy of Dermatology Meeting (SF), Poster #111 (with radiation)
(1996): Leong KP+, *Asian Pac J Allergy Immunol* 14, 65 (2.4%)
(1996): Frangogiannis NG+, *South Med J* 89, 1001
(1996): Creamer JD+, *Clin Exp Dermatol* 21, 116
(1995): Pion IA+, *N Engl J Med* 333, 1609
(1993): Leenutaphong V+, *Int J Dermatol* 32, 428
(1993): Janinis J+, *Eur J Cancer* 29A, 478
(1992): Tone T+, *J Dermatol* 19, 27
(1991): Rowe JE+, *Int J Dermatol* 30, 747
(1989): Kelly DF+, *Neurosurgery* 25, 976
(1989): Renfro L+, *Int J Dermatol* 28, 441
(1988): Dreyfuss DA+, *Ann Plast Surg* 20, 146
(1987): Birchall N+, *J Am Acad Dermatol* 16, 368
(1985): Sherertz EF+, *J Am Acad Dermatol* 12, 178
(1985): Muhar U, *Pediatr Dermatology* 3, 54
(1985): Burge SM+, *J Am Acad Dermatol* 13, 665
(1984): Smith DA+, *J Am Acad Dermatol* 10, 106 (followed by universal depigmentation)
(1984): Chan HL, *J Am Acad Dermatol* 10, 973
(1983): Schmidt D+, *Epilepsia* 24, 440 (fatal)
(1982): Peterson KA+, *Md State Med J* 31, 53
(1981): Spechler SJ+, *Ann Intern Med* 95, 455
(1979): Gately LE+, *Ann Intern Med* 91, 59
(1979): Lyell A, *Br J Dermatol* 100, 69
(1978): Assaad D+, *Can Med Assoc* 118, 154
(1975): Schopf E+, *Z Hautkr* (German) 50, 865
(1975): Giallorenzi AF+, *Oral Surg Oral Med Oral Pathol* 40, 611
(1968): Rodriguez-Adrados J+, *Rev Clin Esp* (Spanish) 110, 267
(1967): Coleman WP, *Med Clin North Am* 51, 1073

(1967): Vandvik IH, *Tidsskr Nor Laegeforen* (Norwegian) 87, 1068
Urticaria
(1995): Rodriguez-Castellanos M+, *Arch Dermatol* 131, 620
(1967): Coleman WP, *Med Clin North Am* 51, 1073
(1951): Jones DP, *BMJ* 1, 64
Vasculitis
(1999): Holt P, *N Z Med J* 112, 100
(1996): Parry RG+, *Nephrol Dial Transplant* 11, 357
(1996): Leong KP+, *Asian Pac J Allergy Immunol* 14, 65 (2.4%)
(1993): Drory VE+, *Clin Neuropharmacol* 16, 19 (passim)
(1983): Yermakov VM+, *Hum Pathol* 14, 182
(1967): Hass P, *Wiener Klin Wochenschr* (German) 75, 56
Warts
(1998): Kayal JD+, *Cutis* 61, 101

Hair

Hair – alopecia
(1984): Smith DA+, *J Am Acad Dermatol* 10, 106
(1973): Levantine A+, *Br J Dermatol* 89, 549
Hair – hirsutism
(1989): Vivard P+, *Ann Dermatol Venereol* (French) 116, 562
(1989): Backman K+, *Scand J Dent Res* 97, 222
(1972): Levantine A+, *Br J Dermatol* 87, 646
(1972): Leng JJ+, *Pediatr Clin North Am* 19, 681
(1970): Herberg KP, *South Med J* 70, 19
Hair – hypertrichosis
(1989): Rousseau C+, *Dermatologica* 179, 221

Nails

Nails – disorders
(1981): Krebs A, *Schweiz Rundsch Med Prax* (German) 70, 1951
Nails – hypoplasia
(1991): D'Souza SW+, *Arch Dis Child* 66, 320
(1981): Johnson RB+, *J Am Acad Dermatol* 5, 191
(1978): Prakash P+, *Indian Pediatr* 15, 866
Nails – malformation
(1975): Hanson JW+, *J Pediatrics* 87, 285
Nails – onychopathy
(1988): Verdeguer JM+, *Pediatr Dermatol* 5, 56
Nails – pigmentation
(1981): Johnson RB+, *J Am Acad Dermatol* 5, 191

Other

Acromegaloid features
(1972): Lefebvre EB+, *N Engl J Med* 286, 1301
Acute intermittent porphyria
(1989): Herrick AL+, *Br J Clin Pharmacol* 27, 491
Ageusia
(1998): Zeller JA+, *Lancet* 351, 1101
(1998): Henkin RI, *Lancet* 352, 68
Coarse facies (sic)
(1973): Falconer MA+, *Lancet* 2, 1112
(1972): Lefebvre EB+, *Med Intell* 286, 1301
Digital malformations
(1981): Johnson RB+, *J Am Acad Dermatol* 5, 191
(1978): Prakash P+, *Indian Pediatr* 15, 866
(1974): Barr M+, *J Pediatr* 84, 254 (hypoplasia)
Fetal hydantoin syndrome*
(1998): Ozkinay F+, *Turk J Pediatr* 40, 273 (2 siblings)
(1994): Buehler BA+, *Neurol Clin*, 12, 741
(1989): Nanda A+, *Pediatr Dermatol* 6, 130
(1989): Nanda A+, *Pediatr Dermatol* 6, 66
(1988): Verdeguer JM+, *Pediatr Dermatol* 5, 56
(1983): Tomsick RS, *Cutis* 32, 535
(1981): Nagy R, *Arch Dermatol* 117, 593
Gingival hyperplasia (>10%)
(1999): Wood WH, San Jose, CA (from Internet) (observation)
(1999): Kamali F+, *J Periodontal Res* 34, 145
(1998): Mattson JS+, *J Am Dent Assoc* 129, 78
(1998): Desai P+, *J Can Dent Assoc* 64, 263
(1998): Meraw SJ+, *Mayo Clin Proc* 73, 1196
(1998): Garzino-Demo P+, *Minerva Somatol* (Italian) 47, 387
(1997): Newland JR, *J Gt House Dent Soc* 69, 3
(1997): Silverstein LH+, *Gen Dent* 45, 371
(1997): Iacopino AM+, *J Periodontol* 68, 73
(1997): Mattioli A, *Minerva Stomatol* (Italian) 46, 525
(1996): Saito K+, *J Periodontol Res* 31, 545
(1996): Hayakawa I+, *Quintessence Int* 27, 235
(1995): Moghadam BKH+, *Cutis* 56, 46 (passim)
(1993): Lipton JM+, *J Indiana Dent Assoc* 72, 18
(1991): Hassell TM+, *Crit Rev Oral Biol Med* 2, 103
(1990): Hall WB, *Compendium* (Suppl) 14, 502
(1989): Dooley G+, *J N Z Soc Periodontol* 68, 19
(1989): Backman K+, *Scand J Dent Res* 97, 222
(1987): Stinnett E+, *J Am Dent Assoc* 114, 814
(1987): Norris JF+, *Int J Dermatol* 26, 602
(1976): Hassell TM+, *Proc Nat Acad Sci* 73, 2909
(1975): Angelopoulos AP, *J Can Dent Assoc* 2, 102
Gynecomastia
(1998): Ikeda A+, *J Neurol Neurosurg Psychiatry* 65, 803
Hypersensitivity syndrome**
(2000): Moore SJ+, *J Med Genet* 37, 489
(2000): Cohen AD+, *Isr Med Assoc J* 1, 95
(2000): Colombo-Arnet E, *Schweiz Rundsch Med Prax* (German) 89, 675
(1999): Quinones MD+, *Allergy* 54, 83 (fatal)
(1999): Hamer HM+, *Seizure* 8, 190
(1999): Moss DM+, *J Emerg Med* 17, 503
(1998): Galindo Bonilla PA+, *J Investig Allergol Clin Immunol* 8, 186
(1997): Tennis P+, *Neurology* 49, 542
(1997): Morkunas AR+, *Crit Care Clin* 13, 727
(1996): Conger LA+, *Cutis* 57, 223
(1996): Chopra S+, *Br J Dermatol* 134, 1109
(1994): Potter T+, *Arch Dermatol* 130, 856
(1993): Handfield-Jones SE+, *Br J Dermatol* 129, 175
(1983): Rapp RP+, *Neurosurgery* 13, 272
(1984): Fonseca JC+, *Med Cutan Ibero Lat Am* (Portuguese) 12, 187
(1978): Stanley J+, *Arch Dermatol* 114, 1350
(1975): Weedon AP, *Aust N Z J Med* 5, 561
(1973): Cohen BL+, *Clin Pediatr Phila* 12, 622
(1973): Sisca TS, *Am J Hosp Pharm* 30, 446
Injection-site necrosis
(1995): Hunt SJ, *Am J Dermatopathol* 17, 399
(1993): Hayes AG+, *J Am Acad Dermatol* 28, 360
Injection-site pain
Lymphadenopathy
(1971): Oates R+, *Med J Australia* 2/58, 371
Lymphoma (<1%)
(1985): Wolf R+, *Arch Dermatol* 121, 1181
(1978): Wilden JN+, *J Clin Pathol* 31, 761
(1975): Bichel J, *Acta Med Scand* 198, 327
(1975): Li FP+, *Cancer* 36, 1359
(1970): Anthony JJ, *Arch Neurol* 22, 450
Lymphoproliferative disease
(1992): Schlaifer D+, *Eur J Hematol* 48, 274
Mucocutaneous eruption
(1992): Tone T+, *J Dermatol* 19, 27
(1979): Pollack MA+, *Ann Neurol* 5, 262
Mucocutaneous lymph node syndrome
(1979): Anderson VM+, *Cutis* 23, 493
Myopathy
(1986): Engel JN+, *Am J Med* 81, 928
(1983): Harney J+, *Neurology* 33, 790
Oral ulceration
Paresthesias (<1%)
(1995): Rodriguez-Castellanos M+, *Arch Dermatol* 131, 620
Periarteritis nodosa
(1967): Haas P, *Wiener Klin Wochenschr* (German) 75, 56
(1948): Van Wyk JJ+, *Arch Intern Med* 81, 605
Peyronie's disease
Polyfibromatosis
(1979): Pierard GE+, *Br J Dermatol* 100, 335
Polymyositis
(1983): Harney J+, *Neurology* 33, 790
Porphyria
(1980): Fuchs T+, *Int J Biochem* 12, 955
Porphyria cutanea tarda
(1996): Ruggian JC+, *J Am Soc Nephrol* 7, 397
Pseudolymphoma (<1%)
(1997): Gigli GL+, *Int J Neurosci* 87, 181
(1995): Wolkenstein P+, *Arch Dermatol* 131, 544
(1993): Sigal M+, *Ann Dermatol Venereol* (French) 120, 175
(1992): Harris DW+, *Br J Dermatol* 127, 403
(1992): D'Incan M+, *Arch Dermatol* 128, 1371
(1992): Braddock SW+, *J Am Acad Dermatol* 27, 337
(1988): Cooke LE+, *Clin Pharm* 7, 153

(1988): Silverman AK+, *J Am Acad Dermatol* 18, 721
(1985): Brodell RT, *Dermatol Clin* 3, 719
(1983): Rapp RP+, *Neurosurgery* 13, 272
(1982): Rosenthal CJ+, *Cancer* 49, 2305
(1981): Adams JD, *Australas J Dermatol* 22, 28
(1980): Vellucci A+, *Clin Ter* (Italian) 94, 229
(1977): Halevy S+, *Dermatologica* 155, 321
(1977): Charlesworth EN, *Arch Dermatol* 113, 477
(1971): Oates RK+, *Med J Aust* 2, 371
(1968): Gams RA+, *Ann Intern Med* 69, 557
(1968): Schreiber MM+, *Arch Dermatol* 97, 297

Serum sickness
(1981): Menitove JE+, *Am J Hematol* 10, 277
(1975): Zidar BL+, *Am J Med* 58, 704

Thrombophlebitis (<1%)

***Note:** The fetal hydantoin syndrome (FHS) – children whose mothers receive phenytoin during pregnancy are born with FHS. The main features of this syndrome are mental and growth retardation, unusual facies, digital and nail hypoplasia, and coarse scalp hair. Occasionally neonatal acne will be present.

****Note:** The phenytoin hypersensitivity reaction (also known as the anticonvulsant hypersensitivity syndrome) is described in detail in (1978): Stanley J+, *Arch Dermatol* 114, 1350. The salient features of this reaction, which characteristically occur within the first 2 to 4 weeks of phenytoin therapy, are fever, generalized tender lymphadenopathy, hepatitis, leukocytosis, and a widespread, pruritic, irregular eruption consisting of ill-defined patches of macular erythema. Periorbital edema is common. The mucous membranes are frequently involved with erythema of the oral mucosa and pharynx. Papules, vesicles and pustules occasionally develop.

PHYTONADIONE

Synonyms: phylloquinone; phytomenadione; vitamin K_1
Trade names: AquaMEPHYTON (Merck); Konakion; Mephyton (Merck); Phytomenadione; Vitamin K1 (Abbott)
Other common trade names: *Kaywan; Vitak*
Indications: Coagulation disorders
Category: Fat-soluble nutritional supplement and antihemorrhagic
Half-life: 2–4 hours
Clinically important, potentially serious interactions with: anticoagulants

Reactions

Skin

Allergic reactions (sic)
(1999): Wong DA+, *Australas J Dermatol* 40, 147
(1990): Pigatto PD+, *Contact Dermatitis* 22, 307

Contact dermatitis
(1999): Drayton G, Los Angeles, CA (from Internet) (observation)
(1995): Bruynzeel I+, *Contact Dermatitis* 32, 78
(1995): Guy C+, *Therapie* (French) 50, 483
(1988): Dinis A+, *Contact Dermatitis* 18, 170
(1982): Camarasa JG+, *Contact Dermatitis* 8, 268
(1980): Romaguera C+, *Contact Dermatitis* 6, 355
(1979): Romaguera C+, *Actas Dermosifilogr* (Spanish) 70, 215

Diaphoresis (<1%)

Eczematous plaques
(1992): Lee MM+, *Arch Dermatol* 128, 257
(1988): Sanders MN+, *J Am Acad Dermatol* 19, 699

Erythema (annular)
(1986): Kay MH+, *Cutis* 37, 445

Exanthems
(1987): Finkelstein H+, *J Am Acad Dermatol* 16, 540

Flushing

Rash (sic)

Scleroderma
(1995): Morell A+, *Int J Dermatol* 34, 201
(1994): Guidetti MS+, *Contact Dermatitis* 31, 45
(1992): Fitzpatrick JE, *Dermatol Clin* 10, 19
(1989): Pujol RM+, *Cutis* 43, 365
(1988): Brunskill NJ+, *Clin Exp Dermatol* 13, 276
(1987): Finkelstein H+, *J Am Acad Dermatol* 16, 540
(1985): Janin-Mercier A+, *Arch Dermatol* 121, 1421
(1982): Rommel A+, *Ann Pediatr Paris* (French) 29, 64
(1981): Jean-Pastor MJ+, *Therapie* (French) 36, 369
(1975): Texier L+, *Bull Soc Fr Derm Syphiligr* (French) 82, 448
(1972): Texier L+, *Ann Dermatol Syphiligr Paris* (French) 99, 363
(1972): Texier L+, *Bord Med* (French) 5, 700

Urticaria
(1993): Ford G, *J Paediatr Child Health* 29, 241
(1988): Sanders MN+, *J Am Acad Dermatol* 19, 699
(1987): Mosser C+, *Ann Dermatol Venereol* (French) 114, 243
(1964): Piguet B+, *Bull Mem Soc Med Hop Paris* (French) 118, 1337

Vasculitis
(1964): Piguet B+, *Bull Mem Soc Med Hop Paris* (French) 118, 1337

Other

Anaphylactoid reaction (<1%)

Dysgeusia (<1%)

Hypersensitivity (<1%)

Injection-site eczematous eruption
(1996): Moreau-Cabarrot A+, *Ann Dermatol Venereol* (French) 123, 177
(1995): Keltz M+, American Academy of Dermatology Meeting, New Orleans (observation)
(1994): Giudetti MS+, *Contact Dermatitis* 31, 45
(1989): Allue-Bellosta L+, *Rev Clin Esp* (Spanish) 185, 217
(1988): Tsuboi R+, *J Am Acad Dermatol* 18, 386
(1988): Joyce JP+, *Arch Dermatol* 124, 27
(1987): Finkelstein H+, *J Am Acad Dermatol* 16, 540
(1978): Robison JW+, *Arch Dermatol* 114, 1790
(1978): Bullen AW+, *Br J Dermatol* 98, 561
(1970): Honda M+, *Hifuka no Rinsho* (Japanese) 12, 295
(1970): Anekoji K, *Chiryo* (Japanese) 52, 1577

Injection-site erythema
(1995): Keltz M+, American Academy of Dermatology Meeting, New Orleans (observation)
(1993): Lemlich G+, *J Am Acad Dermatol* 28, 345
(1992): Breathnach SM+, *Adverse Drug Reactions and the Skin*, Blackwell, Oxford, 265 (passim)

Injection-site indurated plaques (Texier's syndrome) (<1%)
(1999): Chung JY+, *Cutis* 63, 33 (2 cases)
(1996): Bourrat E+, *Ann Dermatol Venereol* (French) 123, 634 (6 cases)
(1996): Pank BK+, *Australas J Dermatol* 37, 44
(1995): Keltz M+, American Academy of Dermatology Meeting, New Orleans (observation)
(1994): Shelley WB+, *Cutis* 52, 203 (passim)
(1993): Lemlich G+, *J Am Acad Dermatol* 28, 345
(1993): Long CC+, *BMJ* 307, 336
(1992): Tuppal R+, *J Am Acad Dermatol* 27, 105
(1989): Pujol RM+, *Cutis* 43, 365
(1988): Joyce JP+, *Arch Dermatol* 124, 27
(1988): Brunskill NJ+, *Clin Exp Dermatol* 13, 276
(1988): Tsuboi R+, *J Am Acad Dermatol* 18, 386
(1977): Heydenreich G, *Br J Dermatol* 97, 697
(1976): Barnes HM+, *Br J Dermatol* 95, 653
(1972): Misson R+, *Bull Soc Fr Dermatol Syphiligr* (French) 79, 581
(1972): Bazex A+, *Bull Soc Fr Dermatol Syphiligr* (French) 79, 578

PILOCARPINE

Trade names: Adsorbocarbine; Akarpine; I-Pilopine; Isopto Carpine; Ocu-Carpine; Pilopine HS; Pilostat; Salagen; Storzine, etc. (Various pharmaceutical companies.)
Other trade names: *Diocarpine; Isopto Pilocarpine; Liocarpina; Miocarpine; Pilogel; Pilo Grin; Pilopt; Sno Pilo; Spersacarpine; Vistacarpin*
Indications: Glaucoma; miosis induction; xerostomia
Category: Cholinergic parasympathomimetic agent
Half-life: no data
Clinically important, potentially serious interactions with: anticholinergics, beta-blockers

Reactions

Skin

Burning (1–10%)

(1996): Rattenbury JM+, *Ann Clin Biochem* 33, 456
Chills
Contact dermatitis
(1993): Cusano F+, *Contact Dermatitis* 29, 99
(1991): Ortiz FJ+, *Contact Dermatitis* 25, 203
(1991): Helton J+, *Contact Dermatitis* 25, 133
Diaphoresis (<1%)
Edema (4%)
Flushing
Photocontact dermatitis
(1991): Helton J+, *Contact Dermatitis* 25, 133
Pruritus
Rash (sic)
Stinging (1–10%)
Urticaria
(1997): LeGrys VA+, *Pediatr Pulmonol* 24, 296

Other

Dysgeusia (2%)
Hypersensitivity (1–10%)
Myalgia (1%)
Ocular cicatricial pemphigoid
(2000): Plotkin A+, *Arch Dermatol* 136, 113
Sialorrhea (<1%)

PIMOZIDE

Trade name: Orap (Gate)
Other common trade names: *Frenal; Neurap; Pimodac*
Indications: Tourette's syndrome, schizophrenia
Category: Antipsychotic and antidyskinetic (Tourette's syndrome); neuroleptic agent
Half-life: 50 hours
Clinically important, potentially serious interactions with: alfentanil, amphetamines, azithromycin, azole antifungals, clarithromycin, CNS depressants, dirithromycin, erythromycin, fluoxetine, guanabenz, macrolide antibiotics, MAO inhibitors, methylphenidate, protease inhibitors

Reactions

Skin

Diaphoresis
Exanthems
Facial edema (1–10%)
Hyperpigmentation
(1991): Opler LA+, *J Clin Psychiatry* 52, 221
Periorbital edema
Photosensitivity
(1991): Opler LA+, *J Clin Psychiatry* 52, 221
Pruritus
Rash (sic) (8.3%)
Urticaria

Other

Dysgeusia
Galactorrhea
Gynecomastia (>10%)
Myalgia (2.7%)
Sialorrhea (13.8%)
(1987): Shapiro AK+, *Pediatrics* 79, 1032
Tremor
Xerostomia (>10%)
(1991): Opler LA+, *J Clin Psychiatry* 52, 221
(1990): Sandor P+, *J Clin Psychopharmacol* 10, 197
(1987): Shapiro AK+, *Pediatrics* 79, 1032

PINDOLOL

Trade name: Visken (Novartis)
Other common trade names: *Alti-Pindolol; Apo-Pindol; Barbloc; Durapindol; Gen-Pindolol; Nonspi; Pinbetol; Pinden; Syn-Pindol; Vypen*
Indications: Hypertension
Category: Beta-adrenergic blocker; antihypertensive
Half-life: 3–4 hours
Clinically important, potentially serious interactions with: calcium channel blockers, clonidine, epinephrine, ergot, flecainide, insulin, nifedipine, NSAIDs, oral contraceptives, salicylates, sulfonylureas, theophylline, verapamil

Note: Cutaneous side-effects of beta-receptor blockaders are clinically polymorphous. They apparently appear after several months of continuous therapy. Atypical psoriasiform, lichen planus-like, and eczematous chronic rashes are mainly observed. (1983): Hödl St, *Z Hautkr* (German) 1:58, 17.

Reactions

Skin

Diaphoresis (2%)
Eczematous eruption (sic)
Edema (6%)
Erythema multiforme
Exanthems
Exfoliative dermatitis
Hyperkeratosis (palms and soles)
Lichenoid eruption
(1978): Savage RL+, *BMJ* 1, 987
(1976): Palatsi R, *Ann Clin Res* 8, 239
Lupus erythematosus
(1979): Bensaid J+, *BMJ* 1, 1603
Peripheral edema
Pityriasis rubra pilaris
(1978): Finlay AY+, *BMJ* 1, 987
Pruritus (1–5%)
(1976): Palatsi R, *Ann Clin Res* 8, 239
Psoriasis
(1986): Czernielewski J+, *Lancet* 1, 808
(1986): Abel EA+, *J Am Acad Dermatol* 15, 1007
(1984): Arntzen N+, *Acta Derm Venereol* (Stockh) 64, 346
(1976): Palatsi R, *Ann Clin Res* 8, 239
(1976): Bonerandi JJ+, *Ann Dermatol Syphiligr* (Paris) (French) 103, 604
Purpura
Rash (sic) (1–10%)
Raynaud's phenomenon
(1984): Eliasson K+, *Acta Med Scand* 215, 333
(1976): Marshall AJ+, *BMJ* 1, 1498
Toxic epidermal necrolysis
Urticaria
Xerosis

Hair

Hair – alopecia

Nails

Nails – dystrophy
Nails – onycholysis

Other

Dysgeusia
Myalgia
Myopathy
(1980): Uusitupa M+, *BMJ* 1, 183
Oculo-mucocutaneous syndrome
(1982): Cocco G+, *Curr Ther Res* 31, 362
Oral lichenoid eruption
Paresthesias (3%)
Peyronie's disease
(1979): Pryor JP+, *Lancet* 1, 331

PIOGLITAZONE

Trade name: Actos (Takeda)
Indications: Type 2 diabetes
Category: Thiazolidinedione antidiabetic
Half-life: 3–7 hours
Clinically important, potentially serious interactions with: itraconazole, ketoconazole, oral contraceptives. Also **food**

Reactions

Skin
Edema (4.8%)
Other
Myalgia (5.4%)
Tooth disorder (sic) (2.3%)

PIPERACILLIN

Trade names: Pipracil (Lederle); Zosyn (Lederle)
Other common trade names: *Avocin; Ivacin; Picillin; Pipcil; Piperilline; Pipril; Piprilin; Pitamycin*
Indications: Various infections caused by susceptible organisms
Category: Beta-lactamase-sensitive penicillin antibiotic
Half-life: 0.6–1.2 hours
Clinically important, potentially serious interactions with: aminoglycosides, anticoagulants, chloramphenicol, erythromycin, heparin, methotrexate, neuromuscular blockers, probenecid, tetracyclines

Zosyn is piperacillin and tazobactam

Reactions

Skin
Allergic reactions (sic) (2–4%)
(1994): Pleasants RA+, *Chest* 106, 1124 (in patients with cystic fibrosis)
(1984): Holmes B+, *Drugs* 28, 375
Angioedema
Bullous eruption
Candidiasis
Ecchymoses
Edema
Erythema nodosum
Exanthems
(1993): Warrington RJ+, *J Allergy Clin Immunol* 92, 626
(1985): Mead GM+, *Lancet* 2, 499 (56%)
(1985): No Author, *Lancet* 2, 723
(1984): Holmes B+, *Drugs* 28, 375
Exfoliative dermatitis
Jarisch–Herxheimer reaction (<1%)
Pruritus
Purpura
Rash (sic) (1%)
Stevens–Johnson syndrome
(1995): Cheriyan S+, *Allergy Proc* 16, 85
Toxic epidermal necrolysis
Urticaria
(1995): Moscato G+, *Eur Respir J* 8, 467
(1984): Holmes B+, *Drugs* 28, 375
Vasculitis
Vesicular eruptions

Other
Anaphylactoid reaction (<1%)
Glossodynia
Hypersensitivity (<1%)
(1998): Cabanes R+, *Allergy* 53, 819
Injection-site pain (2%)
(1984): Holmes B+, *Drugs* 28, 375
Injection-site phlebitis (2%)
(1984): Holmes B+, *Drugs* 28, 375
Oral candidiasis
Serum sickness
Stomatodynia
Thrombophlebitis (<1%)
Vaginitis

PIRBUTEROL

Trade name: Maxair (3M)
Other trade names: *Exirel; Spirolair; Zeisin Autohaler*
Indications: Asthma, bronchospasm
Category: Bronchodilator; $beta_2$-adrenergic agonist
Half-life: 2–3 hours
Clinically important, potentially serious interactions with: MAO inhibitors, tricyclic antidepressants

Reactions

Skin
Edema
Pruritus
Purpura (<1%)
Rash (sic)

Hair
Hair – alopecia

Other
Dysgeusia (1–10%)
Glossitis
Paresthesias (<1%)
Trembling (>10%)
Xerostomia

PIROXICAM

Trade name: Feldene (Pfizer)
Other common trade names: *Antiflog; Apo-Piroxicam; Baxo; Doblexan; Felden; Larapam; Nu-Pirox; Rogal; Sotilen; Zunden*
Indications: Arthritis
Category: Nonsteroidal anti-inflammatory (NSAID); analgesic
Half-life: 50 hours
Clinically important, potentially serious interactions with: anticoagulants, aspirin, beta-blockers, diuretics, lithium, methotrexate, NSAIDs, probenecid, salicylates, warfarin

Reactions

Skin
Angioedema (<1%)
(1987): Gerber D, *Drug Intell Clin Pharm* 21, 707 (passim)
Bullous dermatosis
(1985): Guillaume JC+, *Ann Dermatol Venereol* (French) 112, 807
Contact dermatitis
(1995): Valsecchi R+, *Contact Dermatitis* 32, 63
(1993): Valsecchi R+, *Contact Dermatitis* 29, 167
(1993): Ophaswongse S+, *Contact Dermatitis* 29, 57
(1992): Green C+, *Contact Dermatitis* 27, 261 (to the gel)
(1990): Serrano G+, *J Am Acad Dermatol* 23, 479
Cutaneous side effects (sic) (46.9%)
(1987): Gerber D, *Drug Intell Clin Pharm* 21, 707 (passim)
Diaphoresis (<1%)
(1987): Gerber D, *Drug Intell Clin Pharm* 21, 707 (passim)
Dyshidrosis
(1985): Braunstein BL, *Cutis* 35, 485
Ecchymoses (<1%)
Edema (>1%)
Erythema (<1%)
Erythema annulare centrifugum
(1985): Hogan DJ+, *J Am Acad Dermatol* 13, 840

Erythema multiforme (<1%)
(1987): Gerber D, *Drug Intell Clin Pharm* 21, 707 (passim)
(1986): Stern RS, *J Am Acad Dermatol* 14, 276
(1986): Penso D, *J Am Acad Dermatol* 14, 275
(1985): Guillaume JC+, *Ann Dermatol Venereol* (French) 112, 807
(1985): Bigby M+, *J Am Acad Dermatol* 12, 866
(1985): O'Brien WM+, *J Rheumatol* 12, 13
(1984): Brogden RN+, *Drugs* 28, 292
(1984): Duro JC+, *J Rheumatol* 11, 554
(1984): Stern RS+, *JAMA* 252, 1433
(1982): Bertail MA, *Ann Dermatol Venereol* (French) 109, 261
(1982): Faure M, *Ann Dermatol Venereol* (French) 109, 255
Erythroderma
(1993): Sangla I+, *Rev Neurol Paris* (French) 149, 217
(1985): Guillaume JC+, *Ann Dermatol Venereol* (French) 112, 807
Exanthems (>5%)
(1994): Litt JZ, Beachwood, OH, personal case (observation)
(1987): Gerber D, *Drug Intell Clin Pharm* 21, 707 (passim)
(1985): Bigby M+, *J Am Acad Dermatol* 12, 866 (2.4%)
(1985): Guillaume JC+, *Ann Dermatol Venereol* (French) 112, 807
(1984): Brogden RN+, *Drugs* 28, 292 (0.8%)
(1984): Stern RS+, *JAMA* 252, 1433
(1982): Faure M+, *Ann Dermatol Venereol* (French) 109, 255
(1979): Dessain P+, *J Int Med Res* 7, 335
Exfoliative dermatitis (<1%)
(1987): Gerber D, *Drug Intell Clin Pharm* 21, 707 (passim)
Fixed eruption
(1998): Leal G, Fortaleza, Brazil (from Internet) (observation) 2 cases
(1995): Ordoqui E+, *Allergy* 50, 741
(1994): Ordoqui E+, *J Allergy Clin Immunology* 93, 242
(1993): Gastaminza G+, *Contact Dermatitis* 28, 43
(1993): No Author, *Dermatology* 186, 164
(1990): Stubb S+, *J Am Acad Dermatol* 22, 1111
(1990): de la Hoz B+, *Int J Dermatol* 29, 672
(1989): Shiohara T+, *Arch Dermatol* 125, 1371
(1989): Valsecchi R+, *J Am Acad Dermatol* 21, 1300
Hot flashes (<1%)
Lichenoid eruption
(1993): Veraldi S+, *Eur J Dermatol* 3, 156
(1992): Vaillant L+, *Ann Dermatol Venereol* (French) 119, 936
(1985): Guillaume JC+, *Ann Dermatol Venereol* (French) 112, 807
(1984): Stern RS+, *JAMA* 252, 1433
Linear IgA bullous dermatosis
(1998): Camilleri M+, *J Eur Acad Dermatol Venereol* 10, 70
Lupus erythematosus
(1991): Roura M+, *Dermatologica* 182, 56
Pemphigus
(1985): Guillaume JC+, *Ann Dermatol Venereol* (French) 112, 807
(1983): Martin RL, *N Engl J Med* 309, 795
Pemphigus foliaceus
(1984): Brogden RN+, *Drugs* 28, 292
Peripheral edema
Petechiae (<1%)
Photoreactions (<1%)
(1995): Gebhardt M+, *Z Rheumatol* (German) 54, 405
(1994): Sassolas B+, *Clin Exp Dermatol* 19, 189
(1989): Sunohara A, *Photodermatol* 6, 188
Photocontact dermatitis
(1992): Torinuki W, *Tohoku J Exp Med* 167, 267
Photosensitivity
(1998): Valentine M, Everett, WA (from Internet) (observation)
(1998): Varela P+, *Acta Med Port* (Portugese) 11, 997
(1998): Varela P+, *Contact Dermatitis* 38, 229
(1998): Varela P+, *Contact Dermatitis* 11, 997
(1996): Stingeni L+, *Contact Dermatitis* 34, 60
(1995): Gebhardt M+, *Z Rheumatol* (German) 54, 405
(1995): Mammen L+, *Am Fam Physician* 52, 575
(1993): Youn JI+, *Clin Exp Dermatol* 18, 52
(1993): Hariya T+, *J Dermatol Sci* 5, 165
(1992): Goncalo M+, *Contact Dermatitis* 27, 287
(1992): Serrano G+, *J Am Acad Dermatol* 26, 545
(1992): Izekawa Z+, *J Invest Dermatol* 98, 918
(1991): Roura M+, *Dermatologica* 182, 56
(1991): de Castro JL+, *Contact Dermatitis* 24, 187
(1990): Black AK+, *Br J Dermatol* 123, 277 (observation)
(1990): Serrano G+, *J Am Acad Dermatol* 23, 479
(1989): Kaidbey KH+, *Arch Dermatol* 125, 783
(1989): Cirne de Castro JL+, *J Am Acad Dermatol* 20, 706
(1989): De la Cuadra J+, *Contact Dermatitis* 21, 349
(1987): Gerber D, *Drug Intell Clin Pharm* 21, 707 (passim)
(1987): Morison WL+, *J Am Acad Dermatol* 17, 698
(1987): Figueiredo A+, *Contact Dermatitis* 17, 73
(1987): Magana-Garcia M+, *Rev Invest Clin* (Spanish) 39, 177
(1987): Halasz CL, *Cutis* 39, 37
(1986): Kochevar IE+, *Arch Dermatol* 122, 1283
(1986): McKerrow KJ+, *J Am Acad Dermatol* 15, 1237
(1985): Guillaume JC+, *Ann Dermatol Venereol* (French) 112, 807
(1985): Bigby M+, *J Am Acad Dermatol* 12, 866
(1985): Weigand DA, *J Am Acad Dermatol* 12, 373
(1985): Braunstein BL, *Cutis* 35, 485
(1985): Serrano G+, *J Am Acad Dermatol* 11, 113
(1984): Brogden RN+, *Drugs* 28, 292
(1984): Stern RS+, *JAMA* 252, 1433
(1983): Diffey BL+, *Br J Rheumatol* 22, 239
(1983): Fjellner B, *Acta Derm Venereol* (Stockh) 63, 557
(1982): Faure M+, *Ann Dermatol Venereol* (French) 109, 255
Pruritus (1–10%)
(1987): Gerber D, *Drug Intell Clin Pharm* 21, 707 (passim)
(1984): Brogden RN+, *Drugs* 28, 292
(1984): Stern RS+, *JAMA* 252, 1433
(1979): Dessain P+, *J Int Med Res* 7, 335
Purpura (<1%)
(1987): Gerber D, *Drug Intell Clin Pharm* 21, 707 (passim)
(1984): Brogden RN+, *Drugs* 28, 292
Rash (sic) (>10%)
Stevens–Johnson syndrome (<1%)
(1995): Katoh N+, *J Dermatol* 22, 677
(1985): Guillaume JC+, *Ann Dermatol Venereol* (French) 112, 807
Toxic dermatitis (sic)
(1991): Chosidow O+, *Ann Dermatol Venereol* (French) 118, 903
Toxic epidermal necrolysis (<1%)
(1996): Blum L+, *J Am Acad Dermatol* 34, 1088
(1993): Correia O+, *Dermatology* 186, 32
(1990): Black AK+, *Br J Dermatol* 123, 277 (observation)
(1987): Guillaume JC+, *Arch Dermatol* 123, 1166
(1987): Gerber D, *Drug Intell Clin Pharm* 21, 707 (passim)
(1986): Penso D+, *J Am Acad Dermatol* 14, 275 (letter)
(1986): Szczeklik A, *Drugs* 32 (Suppl 4), 148
(1985): Guillaume JC+, *Ann Dermatol Venereol* (French) 112, 807
(1985): Coscojuela C+, *Med Cutan Ibero Lat Am* (Spanish) 13, 291
(1982): Faure M+, *Ann Dermatol Venereol* (French) 109, 255
Urticaria (<1%)
(1987): Gerber D, *Drug Intell Clin Pharm* 21, 707 (passim)
(1985): Serrano G+, *J Am Acad Dermatol* 11, 113
(1984): Stern RS+, *JAMA* 252, 1433
(1982): Torras H+, *Med Cutan Ibero Lat Am* (Spanish) 10, 351
Vasculitis (<1%)
(1985): Guillaume JC+, *Ann Dermatol Venereol* (French) 112, 807
(1985): Bigby M+, *J Am Acad Dermatol* 12, 866
(1984): Stern RS+, *JAMA* 252, 1433
Vesicular eruption (<1%)
(1986): Stern RS, *J Am Acad Dermatol* 14, 276 (letter)
(1984): Stern RS+, *JAMA* 252, 1433

Hair

Hair – alopecia
(1987): Gerber D, *Drug Intell Clin Pharm* 21, 707
(1985): Bigby M+, *J Am Acad Dermatol* 12, 866
(1984): Stern RS+, *JAMA* 252, 1433

Nails

Nails – onycholysis

Other

Anaphylactoid reaction (<1%)
Aphthous stomatitis
(1991): Siegel MA+, *J Am Dent Assoc* 122, 75
Buccal ulceration
(1987): Gerber D, *Drug Intell Clin Pharm* 21, 707 (passim)
Paresthesias
(1987): Gerber D, *Drug Intell Clin Pharm* 21, 707
Serum sickness (<1%)
Stomatitis (>1%)
Xerostomia (<1%)

PLICAMYCIN

Synonym: mithramycin
Trade name: Mithracin (Bayer)
Other common trade name: *Mithraline*
Indications: Paget's disease, malignant testicular tumors
Category: Antineoplastic; antihypercalcemic; antihypercalciuric; bone resorption inhibitor
Half-life: 1 hour
Clinically important, potentially serious interactions with: calcitonin, etidronate, glucagon

Reactions

Skin

Bleeding tendency (5–12%)
Ecchymoses
(1970): Kennedy BJ, *Am J Med* 49, 494
Exanthems
Flushing (1–10%)
(1983): Bronner AK+, *J Am Acad Dermatol* 9, 645
(1982): Dunagin WG, *Semin Oncol* 9, 14
(1970): Kennedy BJ, *Am J Med* 49, 494 (35%)
Petechiae 1-(1–10%)
Purpura
(1970): Kennedy BJ, *Am J Med* 49, 494 (10%)
Seborrheic keratoses (inflammation of)
(1987): Johnson TM+, *J Am Acad Dermatol* 17, 192
Toxic epidermal necrolysis
(1978): Purpora D+, *N Engl J Med* 299, 1412

Other

Dysgeusia (metallic taste)
Injection-site cellulitis (1–10%)
Injection-site erythema (1–10%)
Injection-site pain (1–10%)
Oral mucosal lesions
(1989): Kerker BJ+, *Semin Dermatol* 8, 173 (1–5%)
(1970): Kennedy BJ, *Am J Med* 49, 494 (15%)
Stomatitis (>10%)

POLYTHIAZIDE

Trade names: Minizide (Pfizer); Renese (Pfizer)
Other common trade names: *Drenusil; Nephril*
Indications: Hypertension, edema
Category: Thiazide* diuretic; antihypertensive
Half-life: no data
Clinically important, potentially serious interactions with: antidiabetics, digoxin, lithium, methotrexate

Minizide is prazosin and polythiazide

Reactions

Skin

Exanthems
Photosensitivity (<1%)
Purpura
Rash (sic) (<1%)
Urticaria
Vasculitis

Other

Paresthesias

***Note:** Polythiazide is a sulfonamide and can be absorbed systemically. Sulfonamides can produce severe, possibly fatal, reactions such as toxic epidermal necrolysis and Stevens–Johnson syndrome.

POTASSIUM IODIDE

Synonyms: KI; Lugol's solution; strong iodine solution
Trade names: Pima (Fleming); Kie (Laser); SSKI (Upsher Smith); Thyroid-Block
Other common trade names: *Jodatum; Jodid; Kalium*
Indications: Hyperthyroidism
Category: Antihyperthyroid; thyroid inhibitor; antifungal; expectorant
Half-life: no data
Clinically important, potentially serious interactions with: lithium, methimazole, propylthiouracil

Reactions

Skin

Acne (1–10%)
Angioedema (1–10%)
(1979): Curd JG+, *Ann Intern Med* 91, 853
Bullous pemphigoid
(1994): Piletta P+, *Br J Dermatol* 131, 145
Dermatitis herpetiformis
(1989): Zone JJ+, *Immunol Ser* 46, 565
Diaphoresis
Exanthems
(1981): Farkas J, *Dermatol Monatsschr* (German) 167, 579
Iododerma
(1996): Alpay K+, *Pediatr Dermatol* 13, 51
(1990): Soria C+, *J Am Acad Dermatol* 22, 418 (vegetating)
(1989): Romanenko VN+, *Vestn Dermatol Venerol* (Russian) 12, 60
(1986): Raznatovskii IM+, *Vestn Dermatol Venerol* (Russian) 10, 71
(1987): O'Brien TJ, *Australas J Dermatol* 28, 119
(1985): Stone OJ, *Int J Dermatol* 24, 565
(1985): Wilkin JK+, *Cutis* 36, 335
(1981): Huang TY+, *Ann Allergy* 46, 264
(1978): Labohm EB, *Ned Tijdschr Geneeskd* (Dutch) 122, 1291 (vegetating)
(1978): Jezova J, *Cesk Dermatol* (Czech) 53, 240
(1974): Dienhart KJ, *N Engl J Med* 290, 521 (suppurative ulcerating)
(1973): Khan F+, *N Engl J Med* 289, 1018 (suppurative ulcerating)
(1971): Werbitt W, *J Am Osteopath Assoc* 70, 460
Lupus erythematosus
(1979): Curd JG+, *Ann Intern Med* 91, 853
Purpura
Pustular psoriasis
(1967): Shelley WB, *JAMA* 201, 1009
Rash (sic)
Systemic eczematous contact dermatitis
Urticaria (1–10%)
(1979): Curd JG+, *Ann Intern Med* 91, 853
Vasculitis
(1987): Eeckhout E+, *Acta Derm Venereol* (Stockh) 67, 362
(1981): Zone JJ, *Arch Dermatol* 117, 758
(1979): Curd JG+, *Ann Intern Med* 91, 853

Other

Dysgeusia (1–10%) (metallic taste)
Gingival pain
Paresthesias
Serum sickness
Sialorrhea
Stomatodynia

PRAMIPEXOLE

Trade name: Mirapex (Pharmacia & Upjohn)
Indications: Parkinsonism
Category: Antiparkinsonian
Half-life: ~8 hours
Clinically important, potentially serious interactions with: cimetidine, diltiazem, haloperidol, levodopa, metoclopramide, phenothiazines, quinidine, quinine, ranitidine, thiothixene, triamterene, verapamil

Reactions

Skin

Allergic reactions (sic) (>1%)
Diaphoresis (>1%)
Edema (5%)
Peripheral edema (5%)
(2000): Tan EK+, *Arch Neurol* 57, 729
Pruritus (>1%)
Rash (sic) (>1%)
Skin disorders (sic) (2%)

Other

Dysgeusia (>1%)
Hyperesthesia (3%)
Myalgia (>1%)
Paresthesias (>1%)
Sialorrhea (>1%)
Tooth disease (>1%)
Twitching (sic) (2%)
Xerostomia (7%)
(1998): Dooley M+, *Drugs Aging* 12, 495

PRAVASTATIN

Trade name: Pravachol (Bristol-Myers Squibb)
Other common trade names: *Elisor; Lipostat; Pravasin; Pravasine; Selectin; Selektine; Selipran*
Indications: Hypercholesterolemia
Category: Antihyperlipidemic; HMG-CoA reductase inhibitor
Half-life: ~2–3 hours
Clinically important, potentially serious interactions with: anticoagulants, cholestyramine, clofibrate, colestipol, cyclosporine, erythromycin, fenofibrate, gemfibrozil, niacin

Reactions

Skin

Allergic reactions (sic)
(1994): de Boer EM+, *Contact Dermatitis* 30, 238
Angioedema
Dermatomyositis
(1992): Schalke BB+, *N Engl J Med* 327, 649
Eczematous eruption (generalized)
(1993): Krasovec M+, *Dermatology* 186, 248
Erythema multiforme
Exanthems
Flu-like syndrome (sic)
Flushing
(1990): Wiklund O+, *J Intern Med* 228, 241
Lichenoid eruption
(1998): Keough GC+, *Cutis* 61, 98
(1997): Anthony JL, Montgomery, AL (from Internet) (observation)
Lupus erythematosus
Photosensitivity
Pruritus
(1992): Yoshimura N+, *Transplantation* 53, 94
(1991): Malini PL+, *Clin Ther* 13, 500
Purpura
Rash (sic) (1–10%)
(1992): Jungnickel PW+, *Clin Pharm* 11, 677
(1992): Betteridge DJ+, *BMJ* 304, 1335
(1991): McTavish D+, *Drugs* 42, 65
(1991): Raasch RH, *Drug Intell Clin Pharm* 25, 388
(1991): *Med Lett Drugs Ther* 33, 18
(1991): Crepaldi G+, *Arch Intern Med* 151, 146
(1990): Hunninghake DB+, *Atherosclerosis* 85, 81 (3.4%)
Stevens–Johnson syndrome
Toxic epidermal necrolysis
Urticaria
Vasculitis

Hair

Hair – alopecia
(1999): Oakley A, Hamilton, New Zealand (from Internet) (observation)
Hair – broken-off patches of scalp hair (greenish) (sic)
(1998): Fixler R, Cincinnati, OH, personal communication (observation)

Other

Anaphylactoid reaction
Dysgeusia (<1%)
Gynecomastia
(1999): Aerts J+, *Presse Med* (French) 28, 787
Hypersensitivity
Myalgia (2.7%)
Myopathy
(1992): Schalke BB+, *N Engl J Med* 327, 649
Paresthesias
Porphyria cutanea tarda
(1994): Perrot JL+, *Ann Dermatol Venereol* (French) 121, 817
Stomatitis

PRAZEPAM

Trade name: Centrax (Parke-Davis)
Other common trade names: *Centrac; Demetrin; Lysanxia; Prazene; Sedapran; Trepidan*
Indications: Anxiety, depression
Category: Benzodiazepine sedative-hypnotic, anxiolytic and antidepressant; anticonvulsant
Half-life: 30–100 hours
Clinically important, potentially serious interactions with: anticonvulsants, CNS depressants, cimetidine, clarithromycin, digoxin, disulfiram, verapamil

Reactions

Skin

Ankle edema
Dermatitis (sic) (1–10%)
Diaphoresis (>10%)
Exanthems
Facial edema
Pruritus
Purpura
Rash (sic) (>10%)
Urticaria

Hair

Hair – alopecia
Hair – hirsutism

Other

Gingivitis
Paresthesias
Sialopenia (>10%)
Sialorrhea (1–10%)
Xerostomia (>10%)

PRAZIQUANTEL

Trade name: Biltricide (Bayer)
Other common trade names: *Cisticid; Distocide; Flukacide; Kalcide; Prazite; Tecprazin; Teniken*
Indications: Helmintic infections
Category: Anthelmintic
Half-life: 0.8–1.5 hours
Clinically important, potentially serious interactions with: aminoquinolines, carbamazepine, phenytoin

Reactions

Skin

Diaphoresis (1–10%)
Edema
(1995): Stelma FF+, *Am J Trop Med Hyg* 53, 167
Pruritus (<1%)
Rash (sic) (<1%)
Urticaria (<1%)
(1996): Jaoko WG+, *East Afr Med J* 73, 499
(1995): Stelma FF+, *Am J Trop Med Hyg* 53, 167

PRAZOSIN

Trade names: Minipress (Pfizer); Minizide (Pfizer)
Other common trade names: *Alti-Prazosin; Apo-Prazo; Duramipress; Eurex; Hypovase; Nu-Prazo; Peripress; Pratisol; Pressin*
Indications: Hypertension
Category: Alpha-adrenergic blocker; antihypertensive
Half-life: 2–4 hours
Clinically important, potentially serious interactions with: beta-blockers, diltiazem, diuretics, nifedipine, NSAIDs, verapamil

Minizide is prazosin and polythiazide

Reactions

Skin

Angioedema
(1983): Ruzicka T+, *Lancet* 1, 473
Diaphoresis (<1%)
(1977): Lahon HFJ+, *Excerpta Med Int Congr* 431, 26
(1975): Pitts NE, *Postgraduate Medicine, Prazosin Clinical Symposium Proceedings* 20
Edema (1–4%)
(1975): Pitts NE, *Postgraduate Medicine, Prazosin Clinical Symposium Proceedings* 20
Exanthems (1–5%)
(1977): Lahon HFJ+, *Excerpta Med Int Congr* 431, 26 (0.7%)
Lichenoid eruption
Lichen planus (<1%)
Lupus erythematosus
(1979): Marshall AJ+, *BMJ* 1, 165
(1979): Wilson JD+, *Clin Pharmacol Ther* 26, 209
Pruritus (<1%)
(1975): Pitts NE, *Postgraduate Medicine, Prazosin Clinical Symposium Proceedings* 20
Rash (sic) (1–4%)
(1983): Stanaszek WF+, *Drugs* 25, 339
(1975): Pitts NE, *Postgraduate Medicine, Prazosin Clinical Symposium Proceedings* 20
Urticaria
(1983): Ruzicka T+, *Lancet* 1, 473

Hair

Hair – alopecia (<1%)

Other

Anaphylactoid reaction
(1983): Ruzicka T+, *Lancet* 1, 473
Myopathy
(1977): Tomlinson IW+, *BMJ* 1, 1319
Paresthesias (<1%)
Priapism (<1%)
(1980): Burke JR+, *Med J Aust* 1, 382
(1975): Pitts NE, *Postgraduate Medicine, Prazosin Clinical Symposium Proceedings* 20
Xerostomia (1–4%)
(1983): Stanaszek WF+, *Drugs* 25, 339
(1977): Lahon HFJ+, *Excerpta Med Int Congr* 431, 26 (5.6%)
(1975): Pitts NE, *Postgraduate Medicine, Prazosin Clinical Symposium Proceedings* 20

PRIMAQUINE

Synonym: prymaccone
Trade name: Primaquine (Sanofi)
Other common trade names: *Neo-Quipenyl; Palum*
Indications: Malaria
Category: Antiprotozoal; antimalarial
Half-life: 4–10 hours
Clinically important, potentially serious interactions with: quinacrine

Reactions

Skin

Angioedema
(1970): Stevenson DD+, *JAMA* 212, 624
Exanthems
(1976): Arndt KA+, *JAMA* 235, 918 (5%)
Pallor
Pruritus (<1%)
Psoriasis
(1963): Kirschenbaum MB, *JAMA* 185, 1044
Urticaria
(1970): Stevenson DD+, *JAMA* 212, 624

PRIMIDONE

Trade name: Mysoline (Elan)
Other common trade names: *Midone; Mylepsin; PMS Primidone; Prysoline; Sertan*
Indications: Seizures
Category: Anticonvulsant; barbiturate
Half-life: 10–12 hours
Clinically important, potentially serious interactions with: acetaminophen, anticoagulants, beta-blockers, carbamazepine, estrogens, felodipine, hydantoins, MAO inhibitors, methylphenidate, metronidazole, quinidine, theophyllines, valproic acid

Reactions

Skin

Acne
Allergic reactions (sic)
(1984): Steffan MA+, *Contact Dermatitis* 10, 184
Erythema multiforme (<1%)
(1979): Pollack MA+, *Ann Neurol* 5, 262
(1975): Böttiger LE+, *Acta Med Scand* 198, 229
Exanthems (1–5%)
(1980): Marghescu S+, *Fortschr Med* (German) 98, 723
Exfoliative dermatitis
Lupus erythematosus (<1%)
(1993): Drory VE+, *Clin Neuropharmacol* 16, 19 (passim)
(1977): Schubothe H+, *Verh Dtsch Ges Inn Med* (German) 83, 727
(1972): Levantine A+, *Br J Dermatol* 87, 646 (passim)
(1966): Ahuja GK+, *JAMA* 198, 201
Rash (sic) (<1%)

Toxic epidermal necrolysis
(1985): Muhar U+, *Pediatr Dermatol* 3, 54
(1979): Pollack MA+, *Ann Neurol* 5, 262
(1973): Stüttgen G, *Br J Dermatol* 88, 291
(1970): Hermann WA, *Dermatologica* 141, 366
Urticaria
(1984): Steffan MA+, *Contact Dermatitis* 10, 184

Other

Hypersensitivity*
(1998): Schlienger RG+, *Epilepsia* 39, S3 (passim)
Acute intermittent porphyria
Gingival hyperplasia
Mucocutaneous syndrome
(1975): Böttiger LE+, *Acta Med Scand* 198, 229

***Note:** The antiepileptic drug hypersensitivity syndrome is a severe, occasionally fatal, disorder characterized by any or all of the following: pruritic exanthem, toxic epidermal necrolysis, Stevens–Johnson syndrome, exfoliative dermatitis, fever, hepatic abnormalities, eosinophilia, and renal failure.

PROBENECID

Trade names: Benemid (Merck); Col-Benemid (Merck); Probalan
Other common trade names: *Bencid; Benecid; Benuryl; Panuric; Procid; Solpurin; Urocid*
Indications: Gouty arthritis
Category: Uricosuric
Half-life: 6–12 hours (dose-dependent)
Clinically important, potentially serious interactions with: acyclovir, benzodiazepines, beta-lactams, cephalosporins, dapsone, heparin, ketorolac, methotrexate, NSAIDs, penicillamine, sulfonylureas, thiopental, zidovudine

Reactions

Skin

Allergic reactions (sic)
Dermatitis (sic)
Erythema multiforme
(1985): Ting HC+, *Int J Dermatol* 24, 587
Exanthems:
Flushing (1–10%)
Pruritus (1–10%)
Rash (sic) (1–10%)
Urticaria (1–5%)

Hair

Hair – alopecia

Other

Anaphylactoid reaction (<1%)
Gingivitis (1–10%)
Hypersensitivity
(1998): Myers KW+, *Ann Allergy Asthma Immunol* 80, 416 (in AIDS)

PROCAINAMIDE

Trade names: Procan (Parke-Davis); Procanbid (Monarch); Pronestyl (Bristol-Myers Squibb); Rhythmin
Other common trade names: *Amisalen; Biocoryl; Procan SR; Promine; Ritmocamid*
Indications: Ventricular arrhythmias
Category: Antiarrhythmic class I-A
Half-life: 2.5–4.5 hours
Clinically important, potentially serious interactions with: amiodarone, astemizole, beta-blockers, cimetidine, cisapride, disopyramide, erythromycin, gatifloxacin, haloperidol, imipramine, lidocaine, moxifloxacin, ofloxacin, pimozide, quinidine, ranitidine, sotalol, sparfloxacin, terfenadine, thioridazine, trimethoprim

Reactions

Skin

Angioedema (<1%)
(1985): Ponte CD+, *Drug Intell Clin Pharm* 19, 139
Chills (<1%)
Dermatitis (sic)
(1985): Gorsulowsky DC+, *J Am Acad Dermatol* 12, 245 (6%)
Eczematous eruption (sic)
Exanthems (1–5%)
(1999): Numata T+, *Sangyo Ika Daigaku Zasshi* (Japanese) 21, 235
(1985): Gorsulowsky DC+, *J Am Acad Dermatol* 12, 245 (8%)
(1984): Christensen DJ+, *Ann Intern Med* 100, 918
(1973): Kosowski BD+, *Circulation* 47, 1204 (5%)
(1972): Blomgren SE+, *Am J Med* 52, 338
Flushing (<1%)
Lichen planus
(1988): Sherertz EF, *Cutis* 42, 51
Lupus erythematosus (>10%)
(1998): Kameda H+, *Br J Rheumatol* 37, 1236
(1998): Ohtani Y+, *Nihon Kokyuki Gakkai Zasshi* (Japanese) 36, 535
(1997): Yung R+, *Arthritis Rheum* 40, 1436
(1996): Miyasaka N, *Intern Med* 35, 527
(1995): Panine VV+, American Academy of Dermatology Meeting, New Orleans (observation)
(1995): Finger DR+, *J Rheumatol* 22, 574
(1995): Rubin RL+, *J Immunol* 154, 2483
(1995): Muramatsu M+, *Nippon Naika Gakkai Zasshi* (Japanese) 84, 1736
(1994): Cohen MG, *J Rheumatol* 21, 578
(1993): McDonald E+, *Hosp Pract Off ED* 28, 95
(1992): Rubin RL+, *J Clin Invest* 90, 165
(1992): Klimas NG+, *Am J Med Sci* 303, 99
(1992): Skaer TL, *Clin Ther* 14, 496
(1992): Rubin RL, *Clin Biochem* 25, 223
(1992): Stevens MB, *Hosp Pract Off Ed* 27, 27
(1990): Pauls JD+, *Mol Immunol* 27, 701
(1989): Adams LE+, *J Lab Clin Med* 113, 482
(1989): Asherson RA+, *Ann Rheum Dis* 48, 232
(1989): Turgeon PW+, *Ophthalmology* 96, 68
(1989): Nichols CJ+, *Ophthalmology* 96, 1535
(1989): Mohindra SK+, *Crit Care Med* 17, 961
(1989): Vivino FB+, *Arthritis Rheum* 32, 560
(1988): Uetrecht JP, *Chem Res Toxicol* 1, 133
(1988): Agudelo CA+, *J Rheumatol* 15, 1431
(1988): Forrester J+, *J Rheumatol* 15, 1384
(1988): No Author, *J Tenn Med Assoc* 81, 579
(1988): Hess E, *N Engl J Med* 318, 1460
(1988): Totoritis MC+, *N Engl J Med* 318, 1431
(1988): Sheretz EF, *Cutis* 42, 51
(1987): Craft JE+, *Arthritis Rheum* 30, 689
(1987): Shoenfeld Y+, *J Clin Immunol* 7, 410
(1986): Reidenberg MM+, *Angiology* 37, 968
(1986): Weisbart RH+, *Ann Intern Med* 104, 310
(1986): Harle JR+, *Ann Med Interne Paris* (French) 137, 599
(1986): Jackson C+, *Clin Exp Rheumatol* 4, 290
(1986): Vitas B+, *Lijec Vjesn* (Serbo-Croatian-Roman) 108, 137
(1986): Rubin RL+, *Am J Med* 80, 999
(1985): Stratton Ma, *Clin Pharm* 4, 657
(1985): Lovisetto P+, *Recenti Prog Med* (Italian) 76, 110
(1985): Cush JJ+, *Am J Med Sci* 290, 36

(1985): Kale SA, *Postgrad Med* 77, 231
(1985): Epstein A+, *Arthritis Rheum* 28, 158
(1985): Totoritis MC+, *Postgrad Med* 78, 149
(1985): Rubin RL+, *Clin Immunol Immunopathol* 36, 49
(1985): Gorsulowsky DC+, *J Am Acad Dermatol* 12, 245 (>5%)
(1985): Amadio P+, *Ann Intern Med* 102, 419
(1984): Tan EM+, *Allergy Clin Immunol* 74, 631
(1984): Wollina U, *Z Gesamte Inn Med* (German) 39, 69
(1984): Browning CA+, *Am J Cardiol* 53, 376
(1984): Goldberg SK+, *Am J Med* 76, 146
(1982): Tannen RH+, *Immunol Commun* 11, 33
(1982): Harmon CE+, *Clin Rheum Dis* 8, 121
(1982): Gupta AK+, *Indian J Dermatol* 27, 112
(1982): Chokron R+, *Nouv Presse Med* (French) 11, 2568
(1982): Hess EV, *Arthritis Rheum* 25, 857
(1981): Uetrecht JP+, *Arthritis Rheum* 24, 994
(1981): Reidenberg MM, *Arthritis Rheum* 24, 1004
(1981): Gonzalez ER, *JAMA* 246, 1634
(1981): Tan EM+, *Arthritis Rheum* 24, 1064
(1981): Schoen RT+, *Am J Med* 71, 5
(1981): Sheikh TK+, *Am J Clin Pathol* 75, 755
(1981): Hess EV, *Arthritis Rheum* 24, vi
(1981): Edwards RL+, *Arch Intern Med* 141, 1688
(1980): Ahmad S, *Circulation* 61, 865
(1980): Chubick A, *Adv Intern Med* 26, 467
(1980): Dixon JA+, *J Rheumatol* 7, 544
(1980): Weinstein A, *Prog Clin Immunol* 4, 1
(1980): Seligmann H+, *Harefuah* (Hebrew) 99, 166
(1979): Foucar E+, *J Clin Lab Immunol* 2, 79
(1979): Sonnhag C+, *Acta Med Scand* 206, 245
(1979): Bernstein RE, *Lancet* 2, 1076
(1979): Bluestein HG+, *Lancet* 2, 816
(1979): Stec GP+, *Ann Intern Med* 90, 799
(1979): Stein HB+, *J Rheumatol* 6, 543
(1979): Hoff BH, *Chest* 75, 107
(1979): McLain DA+, *Arthritis Rheum* 22, 305
(1978): Kaplan AI+, *Chest* 73, 875
(1978): Jones WN+, *Ariz Med* 35, 16
(1978): Woosley RL+, *N Engl J Med* 298, 1157
(1978): Wierzchowiecki M+, *Pol Arch Med Wewn* (Polish) 59, 197
(1978): Zeide MS+, *Clin Orthop* 134, 290
(1978): Nick J+, *Ann Med Interne Paris* (French) 129, 259
(1978): Robinson HM, *Z Hautkr* (German) 53, 349
(1977): Carel RS+, *Chest* 72, 670
(1977): Warner WA, *Ariz Med* 34, 172
(1977): Kahn MF+, *Sem Hôp* (French) 53, 2201
(1977): Schubothe H+, *Verh Dtsch Ges Inn Med* (German) 83, 727
(1977): Weiss RB, *W V Med J* 73, 101
(1977): Sahenk Z+, *Ann Neurol* 1, 378
(1977): Homma M, *Nippon Rinsho* (Japanese) 35, 1330
(1977): Bell WR+, *Arch Intern Med* 137, 1471
(1977): Schubothe H+, *Immun Infekt* 5, (German) 142
(1977): Healey LA, *Med Times* 105, 87
(1976): No Author, *Johns Hopkins Med J* 138, 289
(1976): Whittle TS+, *Arch Pathol Lab Med* 100, 469
(1976): Cohmen G, *Med Klin* (German) 71, 789
(1976): Demay-Wechsler P, *Rev Stomatol Chir Maxillofac* (French) 77, 727
(1976): Levo Y+, *Ann Rheum Dis* 35, 181
(1976): Utsinger PD+, *Ann Intern Med* 84, 293
(1975): Lee SL+, *Semin Arthritis Rheum* 5, 83
(1975): Dubois EL, *J Rheumatol* 2, 204
(1975): Novack MA+, *JAMA* 232, 1269
(1975): Falko JM+, *Ann Intern Med* 83, 832
(1975): Sunder SK+, *Am J Cardiol* 36, 960
(1975): Ghose MK, *Am J Med* 58, 581
(1975): Henningsen NC+, *Acta Med Scand* 198, 475 (>5%)
(1974): McEwen J, *Lancet* 2, 1570
(1974): Harpey JP, *Ann Allergy* 33, 256
(1974): No Author, *Va Med Mon* 101, 299
(1974): Winfield JB+, *Arthritis Rheum* 17, 97
(1974): Bareis RJ, *S D J Med* 27, 19
(1974): Frislid K+, *Tidsskr Nor Laegeforen* (Norwegian) 94, 1926
(1974): Winfield JB+, *Arthritis Rheum* 17, 325
(1974): No Author, *Med Lett Drugs Ther* 16, 34
(1974): Artinian B+, *Can Med Assoc J* 110, 314
(1973): Manigand G+, *Sem Hop* (French) 49, 3207
(1973): Auerbach RC+, *Radiology* 109, 287
(1973): Sokol SA, *J Maine Med Assoc* 64, 54
(1973): Swarbrick ET+, *Rheumatol Phys Med* 12, 94
(1973): Blomgren SE+, *Semin Hematol* 10, 345
(1973): Rosenberg DS+, *South Med J* 66, 1294
(1973): Durand JP+, *Can Med* (French) 14, 9
(1973): Kosowski BD+, *Circulation* 47, 1204 (>5%)
(1972): Hope RR+, *Med J Aust* 2, 298 (>5%)
(1972): Blomgren SE+, *Am J Med* 52, 338
(1972): Dorfmann H+, *Nouv Presse Med* (French) 1, 2967
(1972): Rasmussen K, *Tidsskr Nor Laegeforen* (Norwegian) 92, 709
(1972): Dorfmann H+, *Nouv Presse Med* (French) 1, 2967
(1972): Anastassiades TP+, *Can Med Assoc J* 107, 312
(1972): Donlan CJ+, *Chest* 61, 685
(1972): Swarbrick ET+, *Br Heart J* 34, 284
(1971): Maxon HR+, *Mil Med* 136, 617
(1971): Dabrowska B+, *Kardiol Pol* (Polish) 14, 316
(1971): Wehr KL+, *N C Med J* 32, 56
(1971): Sawaya J, *J Med Liban* (French) 24, 59
(1970): Whittingham S+, *Australas Ann Med* 19, 358
(1970): Hopkins BE, *Med J Aust* 2, 734
(1970): Sheldon PJ+, *Ann Rheum Dis* 29, 236
(1970): Waagstein F, *Nord Med* (Swedish) 83, 468
(1970): Baker H+, *Br J Dermatol* 82, 320
(1970): Heymans G+, *Acta Cardiol* (French) 25, 404
(1970): Merwe JP van de, *Ned Tijdschr Geneeskd* (Dutch) 114, 105
(1969): Gunther R+, *Dtsch Med Wochenschr* (German) 94, 2338
(1969): Atkins CJ+, *Proc R Soc Med* 62, 197
(1969): Alarcon-Segovia D, *Mayo Clin Proc* 44, 664
(1969): Russel AS+, *Ann Rheum Dis* 28, 328
(1969): Fellner MJ+, *Arch Belg Dermatol Syphiligr* (French) 25, 417
(1969): No Author, *JAMA* 208, 525
(1969): Byrd RB+, *Dis Chest* 55, 170
(1969): Dubois EL, *Medicine* (Baltimore) 48, 217
(1968): Lappat EJ+, *Am J Med* 45, 846
(1968): Cohen AI+, *Ariz Med* 25, 565
(1968): Puech P+, *Arch Mal Coeur Vaiss* (French) 61, 1550
(1968): Mehta BR, *Hawaii Med J* 28, 120
(1968): Rutherford BD, *N Z Med J* 68, 235
(1968): Petersen BN+, *Ugeskr Laeger* (Danish) 130, 2131
(1968): Hunt WH, *Tex Med* 64, 54
(1967): Compton-Smith RN+, *Br J Clin Pract* 21, 248
(1967): McDevitt DG+, *BMJ* 3, 780
(1967): Sanford HS+, *Dis Chest* 51, 172
(1967): Fakhro AM+, *Am J Cardiol* 20, 367 (>5%)
(1966): Alarcon-Segovia D, *Rev Invest Clin* (Spanish) 18, 445
(1966): London BL+, *Am Heart J* 72, 806
(1966): Oster ZH, *Isr J Med Sci* 2, 354
(1966): Prockop LD, *Arch Neuron* 14, 326
(1965): Paine R, *JAMA* 194, 23
(1965): Carabia AG+, *J Tenn Med Assoc* 58, 287
(1962): Ladd AT, *N Engl J Med* 267, 1357

Pruritus (<1%)

Purpura
(1984): Christensen DJ+, *Ann Intern Med* 100, 918
(1976): Bluming AZ+, *JAMA* 236, 2521
(1966): Stoffer RP, *J Kans Med Soc* 67, 20

Rash (sic) (<1%)

Sjøgren's syndrome
(1968): Taylor JA, *Lancet* 1, 978

Urticaria (1–5%)
(1988): Knox JP+, *Cutis* 42, 469

Vasculitis
(1988): Knox JP+, *Cutis* 42, 469
(1984): Ekenstam E+, *Arch Dermatol* 120, 484
(1968): Dolan DL, *Mo Med* 65, 365
(1967): Rosin JM, *Am J Med* 42, 625

Other

Dysgeusia (3–4%) (bitter taste)
(2000): Zervakis J+, *Physiol Behav* 68, 405

Myalgia (<1%)

Myopathy (<1%)
(1986): Lewis CA+, *BMJ* 292, 593
(1968): Taylor JA, *Lancet* 1, 978

Oral mucosal eruption
(1985): Gorsulowsky DC+, *J Am Acad Dermatol* 12, 245 (2%)

Tremor (<1%)

PROCARBAZINE

Trade name: Matulane (Sigma-Tau)
Other common trade name: *Natulan*
Indications: Hodgkin's disease, lymphomas
Category: Antineoplastic
Half-life: 60 minutes
Clinically important, potentially serious interactions with: alcohol, amphetamines, barbiturates, digoxin, epinephrine, MAO inhibitors, methotrexate, narcotics, tricyclic antidepressants, **tyramine-containing foods***

Reactions

Skin

Allergic reactions (sic) (<1%)
Angioedema
(1976): Glovsky MM+, *J Allergy Clin Immunol* 57, 134
Dermatitis (sic) (<1%)
Diaphoresis
Edema
Exanthems
(1980): Andersen E+, *Scand J Haematol* 24, 149 (9%)
(1972): Jones SE+, *Cancer* 29, 498
(1966): Witte S+, *Schweiz Med Wochenschr* (German) 96, 93 (2%)
(1965): Todd IDH, *BMJ* 1, 628
(1965): Brunner KW+, *Ann Intern Med* 63, 69 (4%)
Exfoliative dermatitis
(1976): Glovsky MM+, *J Allergy Clin Immunol* 57, 134
Fixed eruption
(1988): Giguere JK+, *Med Pediatr Oncol* 16, 378
Flu-like syndrome (sic) (<1%)
Flushing
(1966): Witte S+, *Schweiz Med Wochenschr* (German) 96, 93
(1965): Todd IDH, *BMJ* 1, 628
Herpes zoster
Petechiae
Photosensitivity
Pigmentation (1–10%)
Pruritus (<1%)
(1965): Brunner KW+, *Ann Intern Med* 63, 69
Purpura
Rash (sic)
Toxic epidermal necrolysis
(1980): Andersen E+, *Scand J Haematol* 24, 149
(1969): Guerrin J+, *Rev Med Dijon* (French) 4, 523
Urticaria
(1980): Andersen E+, *Scand J Haematol* 24, 149 (9%)
(1976): Glovsky MM+, *J Allergy Clin Immunol* 57, 134
(1972): Jones SE+, *Cancer* 29, 498

Hair

Hair – alopecia (1–10%)
(1970): Stolinsky DC+, *Cancer* 26, 984
(1965): Todd IDH, *BMJ* 1, 628

Other

Disulfiram-like reaction**(<1%)
Gynecomastia
Hypersensitivity (2%)
(1972): Jones SE+, *Cancer* 29, 498
Oral mucosal lesions
(1983): Bronner AK+, *J Am Acad Dermatol* 9, 645 (1–5%)
(1970): Stolinsky DC+, *Cancer* 26, 984
Myalgia (<1%)
Paresthesias (>10%)
Stomatitis (>10%)
Xerostomia

*Tyramine-containing foods include the following: aged cheeses, avocados, banana skins, bologna and other processed luncheon meats, chicken livers, chocolate, figs, canned pickled herring, meat extracts, pepperoni, raisins, raspberries, soy sauce, vermouth, sherry and red wines.

**Disulfiram-like reactions include headache, respiratory difficulties, nausea, vomiting, sweating, thirst, hypotension, and flushing.

PROCHLORPERAZINE

Trade name: Compazine (SmithKline Beecham)
Other common trade names: *Edisylate; Novamin; Novomit; Pasotomin; Prorazin; Stella; Stemetil; Tementil; Vertigon*
Indications: Psychotic disorders
Category: Phenothiazine antipsychotic and antiemetic
Half-life: 23 hours
Clinically important, potentially serious interactions with: alcohol, anticholinergics, anticonvulsants, barbiturates, chloroquine, cisapride, CNS depressants, epinephrine, guanethidine, levodopa, lithium, piperazine, propranolol, trazodone, tricyclic antidepressants, **cigarette smoking**

Reactions

Skin

Diaphoresis
Eczema (sic)
Erythema
Exanthems
(1959): Wright W, *JAMA* 171, 1642
Exfoliative dermatitis
Fixed eruption (<1%)
(1984): Reilly GD+, *Acta Derm Venereol* (Stockh) 64, 270
Hypohidrosis (>10%)
Lupus erythematosus
Parkinsonism
Peripheral edema
Photosensitivity (1–10%)
(1997): O'Reilly FM+, American Academy of Dermatology Meeting, Poster #14
(1988): Rasmussen HB+, *Ugeskr Laeger* (Danish) 150, 930
(1964): Hartman DL+, *Skin* 3, 198
Phototoxic reaction
Pigmentation (<1%) (blue-gray)
Pruritus (1–10%)
Purpura
(1965): Horowitz HI+, *Semin Hematol* 2, 287
Rash (sic) (1–10%)
Seborrhea
Toxic epidermal necrolysis
(1986): Mérot Y+, *Arch Dermatol* 122, 455
(1975): Benini G+, *Minerva Anestesiol* (Italian) 41, 314
Urticaria
Xerosis

Other

Anaphylactoid reaction (1–10%)
Blue tongue (sic)
(1989): Alroe C+, *Med J Aust* 150, 724
Galactorrhea (<1%)
Gynecomastia (1–10%)
Lip ulceration
(1984): Reilly GD+, *Acta Derm Venereol* (Stockh) 64, 270
Mastodynia
Priapism (<1%)
Sialorrhea
Tremor
Xerostomia (>10%)

PROCYCLIDINE

Trade name: Kemadrin (GlaxoWellcome)
Other common trade names: *Apricolin; Kemadren; Onservan; Procyclid*
Indications: Parkinsonism
Category: Anticholinergic, antidyskinetic, antiparkinsonian
Duration of action: 4 hours
Clinically important, potentially serious interactions with: amantadine, anticholinergics, atenolol, digoxin, donepezil, haloperidol, meperidine, phenothiazines, quinidine, rimantadine, tacrine, tricyclic antidepressants

Reactions

Skin
Hypohidrosis (>10%)
Photosensitivity (1–10%)
Rash (sic) (<1%)
Urticaria
Xerosis (>10%)

Other
Xerostomia (>10%)

PROGESTINS

Generic names:
Hydroxyprogesterone
Trade names: Delta-Lutin; Duralutin; Hylutin; Pro-Depo; Prodrox
Medroxyprogesterone
Trade names: Amen; Curretab; Cycrin; Provera
Megestrol
Trade name: Megace
Norethindrone
Trade names: Aygestin; Micronor; Norlutin; Norlutate; Nor-QD
Norgestrol
Trade name: Ovrette
Progesterone
Trade names: Gesterol 50; Progestaject
(Various pharmaceutical companies.)
Categories: Progestin; antineoplastic; contraceptive (systemic)

Reactions

Skin
Acne
(1995): Freeman EW+, *JAMA* 274, 51
Acute generalized exanthematous pustulosis (AGEP)
(1998): Kuno Y+, *Acta Derm Venereol* 78, 383
Angioedema
Ankle edema
Autoimmune dermatitis
(1991): Freychet F+, *Ann Dermatol Venereol* (French) 118, 551
(1990): Teelucksingh S+, *J Intern Med* 227, 143
(1985): Katayama I+, *Br J Dermatol* 112, 487
(1984): Anderson RH, *Cutis* 33, 490
(1978): Linse R+, *Dermatol Monatsschr* (German) 164, 656
(1974): Hipkin LJ, *BMJ* 3, 575
(1971): Farah FS+, *J Allergy Clin Immunol* 48, 257 (urticarial)
(1967): Tromovitch TA+, *Calif Med* 106, 211 (urticarial)
Dermatitis (sic)
(1974): Hipkin LJ, *BMJ* 3, 575
(1964): Shelley WB+, *JAMA* 190, 35
Diaphoresis
(1990): Willemse PHB+, *Eur J Cancer* 26, 337 (31%)
Edema
Erythema multiforme
(1985): Wojnarowska F+, *J R Soc Med* 78, 407
Erythema nodosum
Exanthems
Flushing
(1990): Willemse PHB+, *Eur J Cancer* 26, 337 (12%)
Hemorrhagic eruption (sic)
Melasma
Pruritus
Rash (sic)
Telangiectases
(1970): Aram H+, *Acta Derm Venereol* 50, 302
Urticaria
(1995): Shelley WB+, *Cutis* 55, 282 (observation)
(1994): Shelley WB+, *Cutis* 55, 21 (observation)
(1994): Yee KC+, *Br J Dermatol* 130, 121

Hair
Hair – alopecia
Hair – hirsutism

Other
Anaphylactoid reaction
Galactorrhea
Gynecomastia (painful)

PROMAZINE

Trade name: Sparine (Wyeth-Ayerst)
Other common trade names: *Liranol; Prazine; Protactyl; Savamine; Talofen*
Indications: Psychotic disorders, schizophrenia
Category: Phenothiazine antipsychotic; antiemetic
Half-life: 24 hours
Clinically important, potentially serious interactions with: alcohol, carbamazepine, chloroquine, CNS depressants, levodopa, lithium, piperazine, sympathomimetics, trazodone, tricyclic antidepressants, **cigarette smoking**

Reactions

Skin
Dermatitis (sic)
Edema
Exanthems
(1974): Rothstein E, *N Engl J Med* 290, 521
Hypohidrosis (>10%)
Parkinsonism
Photoreactions
Photosensitivity (1–10%)
(1964): Hartman DL+, *Skin* 3, 198
Phototoxic reaction
(1985): Chignell CF+, *Environ Health Perspect* 64, 103
(1985): Motten AG+, *Photochem Photobiol* 42, 9
Pigmentation (<1%) (slate-gray)
Purpura
Rash (sic) (1–10%)
Urticaria
Xerosis

Other
Galactorrhea (<1%)
Gynecomastia
Mastodynia (1–10%)
Priapism (<1%)
Xerostomia

PROMETHAZINE

Trade names: Anergan (Forest); Phenazine; Phenergan (Wyeth-Ayerst)
Other common trade names: *Atosil; Bonnox; Closin; Goodnight; Histantil; Pentazine; Prometh-50; Prothiazine; Pyrethia*
Indications: Allergic rhinitis, urticaria
Category: Phenothiazine H_1-receptor antihistamine and antiemetic; antivertigo and sedative-hypnotic
Half-life: 10–14 hours
Clinically important, potentially serious interactions with: alcohol, anticholinergics, antihypertensives, barbiturates, bromocriptine, chloroquine, cisapride, CNS depressants, epinephrine, lithium, MAO inhibitors, propranolol, trazodone, **cigarette smoking**

Reactions

Skin

Allergic reactions (sic) (<1%)
Angioedema (<1%)
Bullous eruption (<1%)
Chills
Contact dermatitis
(1997): Varela P, Porto, Portugal (from Internet) (observation)
(1970): Pirila V, *Allerg Asthma Leipz* (German) 16, 15 (endogenic)
(1968): Periss Z, *Lijec Vjesn* (Serbo-Croatian Cyrillic) 90. 15
(1955): Sidi I+, *J Invest Dermatol* 24, 345
Dermatitis
Diaphoresis
Eczematous eruption (sic)
(1955): Sidi E+, *J Invest Dermatol* 24, 345
Erythema multiforme
(1986): Fisher AA, *Cutis* 37, 158
(1986): Dikland WJ+, *Pediatr Dermatol* 3, 135
Exanthems
(1967): Lockey SD, *Med Sci* 18, 43
Fixed eruption
(1984): Chan HL, *Int J Dermatol* 23, 607
Flushing
Jaundice
Lupus erythematosus
(1971): Fabius AJM+, *Acta Rheumatol Scand* 17, 137
(1965): Grupper C+, *Bull Soc Fr Dermatol Syphiligr* (French) 72, 714
Parkinsonism
Photoreactions
Photosensitivity (<1%)
(1997): Varela P, Porto, Portugal (from Internet) (observation)
(1991): Bergner T+, *J Allergy Clin Immunol* 87, 278
(1988): Menz J+, *J Am Acad Dermatol* 18, 1044
(1982): Rosen K+, *Acta Derm Venereol* 62, 246
(1982): Torinuki W+, *Tohoku J Exp Med* 138, 223
(1974): Tay C, *Asian J Med* 10, 223
(1970): Leong YO, *Acta Rheumatol Scand* 17, 137
(1969): Kalivas J, *JAMA* 209, 1706
(1967): Lockey SD, *Med Sci* 18, 43
(1964): Hartman DL+, *Skin* 3, 198
(1961): Stevanovic DV, *Br J Dermatol* 73, 233
(1960): Newell RGD, *BMJ* 2, 359
(1957): Epstein S+, *J Invest Dermatol* 29, 319
Pigmentation
Purpura
(1967): Lockey SD, *Med Sci* 18, 43
(1965): Horowitz HI+, *Semin Hematol* 2, 287
Rash (sic) (<1%)
(1991): Blanc VF+, *Can J Anaesth* 38, 54
Stevens–Johnson syndrome
(1972): Monnat A, *Schweiz Med Wochenschr* (German) 102, 1876
Systemic eczematous contact dermatitis
Toxic epidermal necrolysis (<1%)
(1972): Monnat A, *Schweiz Med Wochenschr* (German) 102, 1876
(1959): Messaritakis J, *Ann Paediatr* (German) 207, 236
Urticaria
(1994): Myers P+, *Arch Ophthalmol* 112, 734
(1988): Mills PJ, *Anaesthesia* 43, 66 (with temazepam)
(1967): Lockey SD, *Med Sci* 18, 43

Other

Anaphylactoid reaction (with temazepam)
(1988): Mills PJ, *Anaesthesia* 43, 66
Embolia cutis medicamentosa (Nicolau syndrome)
(1995): Faucher L+, *Pediatr Dermatol* 12, 187
Galactorrhea
Gynecomastia
Hypersensitivity
(1996): Palop V+, *Aten Primaria* (Spanish) 18, 47
Injection-site reaction
Mastodynia
Myalgia (<1%)
Oral ulceration
(1967): Mackie BS, *Br J Dermatol* 79, 106
Paresthesias (<1%)
Priapism
Xerostomia (1–10%)
(1991): Blanc VF+, *Can J Anaesth* 38, 54

PROPAFENONE

Trade name: Rythmol (Knoll)
Other common trade names: *Arythmol; Norfenon; Normorytmin; Rythmex; Rytmonorm*
Indications: Ventricular arrhythmias
Category: Antiarrhythmic class I C
Half-life: 10–32 hours
Clinically important, potentially serious interactions with: anticoagulants, amprenavir, beta-blockers, cimetidine, cyclosporine, digoxin, metoprolol, propranolol, quinidine, ritonavir, theophylline, tricyclic antidepressants, warfarin

Reactions

Skin

Acne (1%)
Diaphoresis (1%)
Edema (<1%)
Exanthems
(1975): Harron DWG+, *Drugs* 34, 617
Flushing (<1%)
Lupus erythematosus (<1%)
(1986): Guindo J+, *Ann Intern Med* 104, 589
(1975): Harron DWG+, *Drugs* 34, 617
Pruritus (<1%)
Purpura (<1%)
Rash (sic) (1–3%)
Urticaria

Hair

Hair – alopecia (<1%)

Other

Dysgeusia (3–23%)
(2000): Zervakis J+, *Physiol Behav* 68, 405
Oral mucosal lesions
(1975): Harron DWG+, *Drugs* 34, 617 (>5%)
Paresthesias (<1%)
Parosmia (<1%)
Tremor (<1%)
Xerostomia (2%)

PROPANTHELINE

Trade name: Propantheline
Other common trade names: *Bropantil; Corrigast; Ercoril; Ercotina; Norproban; Propantel*
Indications: Peptic ulcer
Category: Gastrointestinal anticholinergic; antispasmodic
Half-life: 1.6 hours
Clinically important, potentially serious interactions with: adenosine, amiodarone, amoxapine, analgesics, anticholinergics, beta-blockers, bretylium, CNS depressants, corticosteroids, disopyramide, haloperidol, phenothiazines, tricyclic antidepressants

Reactions

Skin

Allergic reactions (sic)
Contact dermatitis
(1996): Jansen T+, *Dtsch Med Wochenschr* (German) 121, 41
(1983): Przybilla B+, *Hautarzt* (German) 34, 459 (from antiperspirant)
(1982): Gall H+, *Derm Beruf Umwelt* (German) 30, 55 (from antiperspirant)
(1976): Agren-Jonsson S+, *Contact Dermatitis* 2, 79 (from antiperspirant)
(1975): Osmundsen PE, *Contact Dermatitis* 1, 251
(1975): Hannuksela M, *Contact Dermatitis* 1, 244
Diaphoresis (>10%)
Exanthems
Hypohidrosis
Rash (sic) (<1%)
Urticaria
Xerosis (>10%)

Other

Ageusia
Anaphylactoid reaction
Dysgeusia
Sialopenia
Xerostomia (>10%)

PROPOFOL

Trade name: Diprivan (AstraZeneca)
Indications: Induction and maintenance of anesthesia
Category: General anesthetic; sedative
Half-life: initial: 40 minutes; terminal: 3 days
Clinically important, potentially serious interactions with: alcohol, atracurium, barbiturates, benzodiazepines, CNS depressants, phenothiazines, theophylline, tricyclic antidepressants

Reactions

Skin

Allergic reactions (sic)
(1988): Jamieson V+, *Anaesthesia* 43, 70
Edema (<1%)
Exanthems
(1987): Boittiaux P+, *Ann Fr Anesth Reanim* (French) 6, 324 (6.6%)
(1987): Coursange F+, *Ann Fr Anesth Reanim* (French) 6, 258 (6.6%)
Fixed eruption (1%)
Flushing (>1%)
Pruritus (>1%)
(1987): Coursange F+, *Ann Fr Anesth Reanim* (French) 6, 258
Rash (sic) (5%)
Raynaud's phenomenon
(1999): Gilston A, *Anaesthesia* 54, 307
Urticaria
(1988): Aitken HA, *Anaesthesia* 43, 170
(1987): Coursange F+, *Ann Fr Anesth Reanim* (French) 6, 258

Hair

Hair – color change (sic)
(1994): Motsch J+, *Eur J Anaesthesiol* 11, 499 (passim)
(1992): Bublin JG+, *J Clin Pharm Ther* 17, 297

Other

Anaphylactoid reaction (1–10%)
(2000): Ducart AR+, *J Cardiothorac Vasc Anesth* 14, 200
Dysgeusia (<1%)
Injection-site erythema (<1%)
Injection-site pain (>10%)
(2000): Picard P+, *Anesth Analg* 90, 963
(2000): Pickford A+, *Pediatr Anaesth* 10, 129
(2000): Levecque JP+, *Can J Anaesth* (French) 47, 291
(1998): Nathanson MH+, *Anaesthesia* 53, 608
(1998): Tan CH+, *Anaesthesia* 53, 468
(1998): Ozturk E+, *Anesthesiology* 89, 1041
(1988): Langley MS+, *Drugs*
Injection-site pruritus (<1%)
Myalgia (>1%)
Phlebitis
Sialorrhea (>1%)
Twitching (1–10%)
Xerostomia (<1%)

PROPOXYPHENE

Trade names: Darvocet-N (Lilly); Darvon (Lilly); Darvon Compound (Lilly)
Other common trade names: *Algafan; Antalvic; Develin; Dolotard; Doloxene; Liberan; Parvon*
Indications: Pain
Category: Narcotic analgesic
Half-life: 8–24 hours
Clinically important, potentially serious interactions with: alcohol, alprazolam, carbamazepine, CNS depressants, MAO inhibitors, phenobarbital, ritonavir, tricyclic antidepressants, warfarin, **cigarette smoking**

Darvocet is propoxyphene and acetaminophen; Darvon Compound is propoxyphene and aspirin

Reactions

Skin

Diaphoresis
Exanthems
(1976): Arndt KA+, *JAMA* 235, 918
Facial edema
Flushing
Pruritus
Rash (sic) (<1%)
Urticaria (<1%)

Other

Ano-recto-vaginal ulcerations
(1984): Laplanche G+, *Ann Dermatol Venereol* (French) 111, 347 (from suppositories)
Injection-site nodules
(1987): Pedragosa R+, *Arch Dermatol* 123, 297
Injection-site pain (1–10%)
Trembling
Xerostomia (1–10%)

PROPRANOLOL

Trade names: Inderal (Wyeth-Ayerst); Inderide (Wyeth-Ayerst)
Other common trade names: *Acifol; Apsolol; Betabloc; Cinlol; Detensol; Inderex; Inderalici; Novo-Pranol; Prosin; Sinal; Tesnol*
Indications: Hypertension; angina pectoris
Category: Beta-adrenergic blocker; antianginal; antihypertensive; antiarrhythmic class II
Half-life: 2–6 hours
Clinically important, potentially serious interactions with: antidiabetics, barbiturates, calcium channel blockers, cimetidine, clonidine, diltiazem, epinephrine, ergot, flecainide, fluoxetine, haloperidol, hydralazine, insulin, nifedipine, NSAIDs, oral contraceptives, phenothiazines, prazosin, quinidine, rifampin, salicylates, terazosin, theophylline, verapamil, **cigarette smoking**

Inderide is propranolol and hydrochlorothiazide

Note: Cutaneous side-effects of beta-receptor blockaders are clinically polymorphous. They apparently appear after several months of continuous therapy. Atypical psoriasiform, lichen planus-like, and eczematous chronic rashes are mainly observed. (1983): Hödl St, *Z Hautkr* (German) 58, 17.

Reactions

Skin

Acne
(1973): Almeyda J+, *Br J Dermatol* 88, 313
Angioedema
(1983): Hannaway PJ+, *N Engl J Med* 308, 1536
Bullous eruption
(1979): Faure M+, *Ann Dermatol Venereol* (French) 106, 161
Contact dermatitis
(1994): Valsecchi R+, *Contact Dermatitis* 30, 177 (occupational)
(1990): Rebandel P+, *Contact Dermatitis* 23, 199
Diaphoresis
Eczematous eruption (sic)
(1981): van Joost T+, *Arch Dermatol* 117, 600
(1979): Faure M+, *Ann Dermatol Venereol* (French) 106, 161
Edema
Erythema multiforme
(1969): Pimstone B+, *S Afr Med J* 43, 1203
Exanthems
(1976): Jensen HA+, *Acta Med Scand* 199, 363
(1974): Greenblatt DJ+, *Drugs* 7, 118. (0.8%)
(1973): Almeyda J+, *Br J Dermatol* 88, 313
(1966): Stephen SA+, *Am J Cardiol* 18, 463 (0.4%)
Exfoliative dermatitis
(1976): Jensen HA+, *Acta Med Scand* 199, 363
Flushing
(1973): Almeyda J+, *Br J Dermatol* 88, 313
(1966): Stephen SA+, *Am J Cardiol* 18, 463
Hyperkeratosis (palms and soles)
Lichenoid eruption
(1991): Massa MC+, *Cutis* 48, 41
(1980): Hawk JLM, *Clin Exp Dermatol* 5, 93
(1976): Cochran REI+, *Arch Dermatol* 112, 1173
Lupus erythematosus
(1982): Hughes GRV, *BJM* 284, 1358
(1976): Harrison T+, *Postgrad Med* 59, 241
Necrosis
Pemphigus
(1982): Ruocco V+, *Arch Dermatol Res* 274, 123
(1980): Godard W+, *Ann Dermatol Venereol* (French) 107, 1213
Peripheral edema
Peripheral skin necrosis (sic)
(1979): Gokal R+, *BMJ* 1, 721
(1979): Hoffbrand BI, *BMJ* 1, 1082
Photosensitivity
(1979): Faure M+, *Ann Dermatol Venereol* (French) 106, 161
Phototoxic reaction
(1992): Shelley WB+, *Cutis* 50, 182 (observation)
Pruritus
(1973): Almeyda J+, *Br J Dermatol* 88, 313
Psoriasis
(1993): Halevy S+, *J Am Acad Dermatol* 29, 504
(1992): Raychaudhuri SP+, *J Am Acad Dermatol* 27, 787
(1990): Halevy S+, *Arch Dermatol Res* 283, 472
(1988): Heng MCY+, *Int J Dermatol* 27, 619
(1987): Savola J+, *BMJ* 295, 637
(1987): Altomare GF+, *G Ital Dermatol Venereol* (Italian) 122, 531
(1986): Czernielewski J, *Lancet* 1, 808 (exacerbation)
(1986): Abel EA+, *J Am Acad Dermatol* 15, 1007
(1984): Arntzen K+, *Acta Derm Venereol* (Stockh) 64, 346
(1983): Kaur S+, *Indian Heart J* 35, 181
(1979): Halevy S+, *Cutis* 24, 95
(1979): Faure M+, *Ann Dermatol Venereol* (French) 106, 161
(1976): Enger E, *Tidsskr Nor Laegeforen* (Norwegian) 96, 1103
(1976): Wadskov S+, *Ugeskr Laeger* (Danish) 138, 784
(1976): Jensen HA+, *Acta Med Scand* 199, 363
(1975): Padfield PL+, *BMJ* 1, 626
Purpura
(1966): Harris A, *Am J Cardiol* 18, 431
Pustular psoriasis
(1988): Heng MCY+, *Int J Dermatol* 27, 619
(1985): Hu C-H+, *Arch Dermatol* 121, 1326
Rash (sic) (1–10%)
Raynaud's phenomenon
(1976): Marshall AJ+, *BMJ* 1, 1498 (59%)
Sclerosis
(1980): Graham JR, *Trans Am Clin Climatol Assoc* 92, 122
Stevens–Johnson syndrome
(1990): Zukervar P+, *J Toxicol Clin Exp* (French) 10, 169
(1989): Mukul+, *J Assoc Physicians India* 37, 797
Systemic erythematous eruption (sic)
(1975): Felix RH+, *BMJ* 1, 626
Toxic epidermal necrolysis
(1977): van Ketel WG+, *Ned Tijdschr Geneeskd* (Dutch) 121, 1475
Toxicoderma
(1981): Danilov LN, *Vestn Dermatol Venerol* (Russian) January 42
Urticaria
(1983): Hannaway PJ+, *N Engl J Med* 308, 1536
(1983): Oliver R, *Cent Afr J Med* 29, 91
(1975): Seides SF+, *Chest* 67, 496
Xerosis

Hair

Hair – alopecia
(1994): Friedman M, *J Fam Pract* 39, 114
(1983): Hödl St, *Z Hautkr* (German) 58, 17.
(1982): England JRF+, *Aust Fam Physician* 11, 225
(1979): Hilder RJ, *Cutis* 24, 63
(1977): Scribner MD, *Arch Dermatol* 113, 1303
(1973): Martin CM+, *Am Heart J* 86, 236

Nails

Nails – discoloration
(1976): Jensen HA+, *Acta Med Scand* 199, 363
Nails – onycholysis
(1983): Hödl St, *Z Hautkr* (German) 58, 17.
Nails – pitting (psoriasiform)
(1976): Jensen HA+, *Acta Med Scand* 199, 363
Nails – thickening
(1983): Hödl St, *Z Hautkr* (German) 58, 17.
(1979): Faure M+, *Ann Dermatol Venereol* (French) 106, 161

Other

Anaphylactoid reaction
(1983): Hannaway PJ+, *N Engl J Med* 308, 1536
Cheilostomatitis (sic)
(1977): Tangsrud SE+, *BMJ* 2, 1385
Dupuytren's contracture
(1966): Coupland WW, *Med J Aust* 2, 137
Dysgeusia
(2000): Zervakis J+, *Physiol Behav* 68, 405
Myalgia
Myopathy
(1980): Uuisitupa M+, *BMJ* 1, 183
Oral ulceration
(1980): Hawk JLM, *Clin Exp Dermatol* 5, 93
Paresthesias

Peyronie's disease
(1981): Neumann HAM+, *Dermatologica* 162, 330
(1979): Pryor JP+, *Lancet* 1, 824
(1977): Osborne DR, *Lancet* 1, 1111
(1977): Wallis AA+, *Lancet* 2, 980
(1977): Yudkin JS, *Lancet* 2, 1355 (passim)
(1966): Coupland WW, *Med J Aust* 2, 137
Serum sickness
(1983): Yen MC+, *Postgrad Med* 74, 291
Tongue pigmentation
(1975): Raleigh F, *Drug Intell Clin Pharm* 9, 455
Xerostomia

PROPYLTHIOURACIL

Trade name: Propylthiouracil (Lederle)
Other common trade names: *Propacil; Propycil; Propyl-Thyracil; Tiotil*
Indications: Hyperthyroidism
Category: Antithyroid
Half-life: 1–5 hours
Clinically important, potentially serious interactions with: amiodarone, anticoagulants, beta-blockers, digoxin, iodine, metoprolol, theophylline

Reactions

Skin

Acne
(1980): Vasily DB+, *JAMA* 243, 458
Angioedema
(1980): Vasily DB+, *JAMA* 243, 458
(1970): Amrhein JA+, *J Pediatr* 76, 54 (1%)
(1965): Shelley WB, *Arch Dermatol* 91, 165
Dermatitis (sic)
(1993): Elias AN+, *J Am Acad Dermatol* 29, 78
Edema (<1%)
Erythema nodosum
(1985): Keren G+, *Isr J Med Sci* 21, 62
Exanthems
(1987): Wing SS+, *Can Med Assoc J* 136, 121
(1982): Gammeltoft M+, *Acta Dermatol Venereol* (Stockh) 62, 171 (3–5%)
(1980): Vasily DB+, *JAMA* 243, 458
(1972): Wiberg JJ+, *Ann Intern Med* 77, 414
(1970): Amrhein JA+, *J Pediatr* 76, 54
Exfoliative dermatitis (<1%)
Lichenoid eruption
(1967): Coleman WP, *Med Clin North Am* 51, 1073
Lupus erythematosus (1–10%)
(1994): Sato-Matsumura KC+, *J Dermatol* 21, 501
(1992): Skaer TL, *Clin Ther* 14, 496
(1991): Alarcon-Segovia D+, *Baillieres Clin Rheumatol* 5, 1
(1989): Horton RC+, *Lancet* 2, 568
(1987): Wing SS+, *Can Med Assoc J* 136, 121 (20% ANA)
(1985): Bulvik S+, *Harefuah* (Hebrew) 109, 13
(1983): Berkman EM+, *Transfusion* 23, 135
(1981): Searles RP+, *J Rheumatol* 8, 498
(1981): Takuwa N+, *Endocrinol Jpn* 28, 663
(1973): Hung W+, *J Pediatr* 82, 852
(1970): Amrhein JA+, *J Pediatr* 76, 54
(1966): Faber V+, *Acta Med Scand* 179, 257
(1964): Best MM+, *J Ky Med Assoc* 62, 47
Photosensitivity
(1997): Ohtsuka M+, *Eur Resp J* 10, 1405
Pigmentation
Pruritus (<1%)
(1980): Vasily DB+, *JAMA* 243, 458
Purpura
(1987): Wing SS+, *Can Med Assoc J* 136, 121
(1962): Walzer RA, *Arch Dermatol* 86, 826
Pyoderma gangrenosum
(1999): Darben T+, *Australas J Dermatol* 40, 144
Rash (sic) (>10%)
Rosacea
(1980): Vasily DB+, *JAMA* 243, 458
Skin reaction (sic)
(1982): Pacini F+, *J Endocrinol Invest* 5, 403
Ulceration
(1987): Wing SS+, *Can Med Assoc J* 136, 121
Urticaria (<1%)
(1980): Vasily DB+, *JAMA* 243, 458
(1970): Amrhein JA+, *J Pediatr* 76, 54
Vasculitis (<1%)
(2000): Lopez-Marina V+, *Med Clin (Barc)* (Spanish) 114, 398
(1998): Harper L+, *Nephrol Dial Transplant* 13, 455
(1998): Merkel PA, *Curr Opin Rheumatol* 10, 45
(1998): Miller RM+, *Australas J Dermatol* 39, 96
(1997): Kitahara T+, *Clin Nephrol* 47, 336
(1997): Yarman S+, *Int J Clin Pharm Ther* 35, 282
(1993): Dolman KM+, *Lancet* 342, 651
(1992): Wolf D+, *Cutis* 49, 253
(1992): Stankus SJ+, *Chest* 102, 1595
(1987): Wing SS+, *Can Med Assoc J* 136, 121
(1987): Carrasco MD+, *Arch Intern Med* 147, 1677
(1986): Gleisner A+, *Rev Child Pediatr* (Spanish) 57, 64
(1985): Cox NH+, *Clin Exp Dermatol* 10, 292
(1982): Gammeltoft M+, *Acta Dermatol Venereol* (Stockh) 62, 171
(1982): Reidy TJ+, *South Med J* 75, 1297
(1980): Vasily DB+, *JAMA* 243, 458
(1979): Houston BD+, *Arthritis Rheum* 22, 925
(1978): Griswold WR+, *West J Med* 128, 543
(1973): Hung W+, *J Pediatr* 82, 852
(1965): Shelley WB, *Arch Dermatol* 91, 165
(1965): McCombs RP, *JAMA* 194, 1059
(1962): Walzer RA, *Arch Dermatol* 86, 826
Vesicular eruption (in newborn)
(1980): Vasily DB+, *JAMA* 243, 458
(1977): Caplan RH+, *Wis Med J* 76, S88

Hair

Hair – alopecia (<1%)
(1997): Ohtsuka M+, *Eur Resp J* 10, 1405
(1980): Vasily DB+, *JAMA* 243, 458
(1951): Clarke MLB, *JAMA* 147, 1711
Hair – depigmentation
(1980): Vasily DB+, *JAMA* 243, 458

Other

Ageusia (1–10%)
Dysgeusia (1–10%) (metallic taste)
(1993): Elias AN+, *J Am Acad Dermatol* 29, 78
Hypersensitivity
(1999): Chastain MA+, *J Am Acad Dermatol* 41, 757
(1991): Fong PC+, *Horm Res* 35, 132
(1963): Walzer RA+, *JAMA* 184, 743
Myalgia
Oral mucosal lesions
(1970): Amrhein JA+, *J Pediatr* 76, 54
Oral ulceration
(1979): Houston BD+, *Arthritis Rheum* 22, 925
(1970): Amrhein JA+, *J Pediatr* 76, 54
Paresthesias (<1%)

PROTAMINE

Trade name: Protamine Sulfate (Lilly)
Indications: Heparin overdose
Category: Heparin antagonist
Duration of action: 2 hours
Clinically important, potentially serious interactions with: heparin

Reactions

Skin

Angioedema
(1991): Roelofse JA+, *Anesth Prog* 38, 99
Exanthems
(1989): Weiss ME+, *N Engl J Med* 320, 886

Flushing (<1%)
Urticaria
(1989): Weiss ME+, *N Engl J Med* 320, 886

Other

Anaphylactoid reaction
(1991): Roelofse JA+, *Anesth Prog* 38, 99
(1988): Oswald-Mammosser M+, *Rev Fr Allergol* (French) 28, 173
Hypersensitivity (<1%)

PROTEASE INHIBITORS*

Generic names:
Amprenavir
Trade name: Agenerase
Indinavir
Trade name: Crixivan
Nelfinavir
Trade name: Viracept
Ritonavir
Trade name: Norvir
Saquinavir
Trade names: Invirase; Fortovase
Indications: HIV infection
Half-life: varies
Clinically important, potentially serious interactions with: cisapride, clarithromycin, disulfiram, itraconazole, ketoconazole, metronidazole, oral contraceptives, rifabutin, rifampin,

Reactions

Skin

Acute generalized exanthematous pustulosis
(1998): Aquilina C+, *Arch Intern Med* 158, 2160
Striae
(1999): Darvay A+, *J Am Acad Dermatol* 41, 467

Nails

Nails – ingrown
(2000): Miot HA, Sao Paulo, Brasil (from Internet) (observation)
Nails – paronychia
(2000): Panse I+, *Br J Dermatol* 142, 496

Other

Buffalo hump
(2000): Carr A+, *AIDS* 14, F25
(1998): Dieleman JP+, *Ned Tijdschr Geneeskd* (Dutch) 142, 2856 (3 patients)
(1998): Saint-Marc T+, *Lancet* 352, 319
(1998): De Luca A+, *Lancet* 352, 320
(1998): Lo JC+, *Lancet* 351, 867
(1998): Schindler JT+, *Ann Intern Med* 129, 164
(1998): Lo JC+, *Lancet* 351, 867 (8 patients)
Buffalo neck
(1999): Milpied-Homsi B+, *Ann Dermatol Venereol* (French) 126, 254
Bull neck (sic)
(1998): Meinrenken S, *Dtsch Med Wochenschr* (German) 123, A9
Fat distribution abnormality
(1999): Mann M+, *Aids Patient Care* 13, 287
(1998): Ho TT+, *Lancet* 351, 1736
(1998): Wurtz R, *Lancet* 351, 1735
(1998): Mishriki YY, *Postgrad Med* 104, 45 ("bulging belly")
Hypersensitivity
(1997): Bonfanti P+, *AIDS* 11, 1301
Lipoatrophy
(2000): Carr A+, *AIDS* 14, F25
(2000): Panse I+, *Br J Dermatol* 142, 496
Lipodystrophy
(2000): Hartmann M+, *Hautarzt* (German) 51, 159
(2000): Behrens GM+, *MMM Fortschr Med* (German) 142, 68
(2000): Panse I+, *Br J Dermatol* 142, 496
(2000): Lyon DE+, *J Assoc Nurses AIDS Care* 11, 36
(2000): Reus S+, *An Med Interna* (Spanish) 17, 123
(2000): Paparizos VA+, *AIDS* 14, 903
(1999): Yanovski JA+, *J Clin Endocrinol Metab* 84, 1925
(1999): Ponce-de-Leon S+, *Lancet* 353, 1244
(1998): Dieleman JP+, *Ned Tijdschr Geneeskd* (Dutch) 142, 2856 (3 patients)
(1998): Fischer T+, *Dtsch Med Wochenschr* (German) 123, 1512
(1998): Carr A+, *N Engl J Med* 339, 1296
(1998): Carr A+, *AIDS* 12, F51
(1998): *Drugs and Ther Perspect* 12, 11
(1998): Lipsky J, *Lancet* 351, 847
(1998): Miller KD+, *Lancet* 351, 871 (indinavir)

*Please see individual generic drugs for more references.

Note: Protease inhibitors cause dyslipidemia which includes elevated triglycerides and cholesterol and redistribution of body fat centrally to produce the so-called "protease paunch," breast enlargement, facial atrophy, and "buffalo hump."

PROTRIPTYLINE

Trade name: Vivactil (Merck)
Other common trade names: *Concordin; Triptil*
Indications: Depression
Category: Tricyclic antidepressant and antinarcolepsy adjunct
Half-life: 54–92 hours
Clinically important, potentially serious interactions with: alcohol, anticholinergics, CNS depressants, cimetidine, clonidine, dicumarol, epinephrine, fluoxetine, guanethidine, indinavir, lithium, MAO inhibitors, phenothiazines, quinidine, ritonavir, sympathomimetics, tricyclic antidepressants, warfarin

Reactions

Skin

Acne
Allergic reactions (sic) (<1%)
Angioedema
Dermatitis (sic) (3%)
(1967): Gilbert MM, *Int J Neuropsychiatry* 3, 36
Diaphoresis (1–10%)
Edema
Erythema
Exanthems
Flushing
Parkinsonism (1–10%)
Petechiae
Photosensitivity (<1%)
(1972): Bruinsma W, *Dermatologica* 145, 377
Phototoxic reaction
(1980): Kochevar IE, *Toxicol App Pharmacol* 54, 258
Pruritus (1–5%)
(1967): Gilbert MM, *Int J Neuropsychiatry* 3, 36
Purpura
Rash (sic)
Urticaria
Vasculitis
Xerosis

Hair

Hair – alopecia (<1%)

Other

Black tongue
Dysgeusia (>10%)
Galactorrhea (<1%)
Glossitis
Gynecomastia (<1%)
Oral mucosal eruption
Paresthesias
Stomatitis
Tremor
Xerostomia (>10%)

PSEUDOEPHEDRINE

Trade names: Actifed; Afrinol; Allerid; Cenafed; Decofed; Drixoral; Entex; Novafed; Seldane-D, Sudafed; Trinalin; etc. (Various pharmaceutical companies.)
Other common trade names: *Balminil; Eltor 120; Maxiphed; Robidrine*
Indications: Nasal congestion
Category: Nasal decongestant; sympathomimetic; adrenergic agonist
Half-life: 9–16 hours
Clinically important, potentially serious interactions with: antihypertensives, beta-blockers, bromocriptine, caffeine, furazolidone, guanethidine, MAO inhibitors, methyldopa, procarbazine, propranolol, sympathomimetics, tricyclic antidepressants

Reactions

Skin

Angioedema
(1997): Rademaker M, Hamilton, New Zealand, (3 personal cases) (observation)
(1993): Cavanah DK+, *Ann Intern Med* 119, 302
Baboon syndrome
(2000): Sanchez TS+, *Contact Dermatitis* 42, 312
Contact dermatitis
(1998): Downs AM+, *Contact Dermatitis* 39, 33
Dermatitis (sic)
(1998): Vega F+, *Allergy* 53, 218
Diaphoresis (1–10%)
Eczematous eruption (sic)
(1991): Tomb RR+, *Contact Dermatitis* 24, 86
Exanthems
(1995): Rochina A+, *J Invest Allergol Clin Immunol* 5, 235
(1994): Shelley WB+, *Cutis* 52, 203 (observation)
(1993): Cavanah DK+, *Ann Intern Med* 119, 302 (generalized)
(1978): Frankland AW, *Practitioner* 211, 828
Exfoliative dermatitis
(1993): Cavanah DK+, *Ann Intern Med* 119, 302
Fixed eruption
(1997): Garcia Ortiz JC+, *Allergy* 52, 229 (non-pigmenting)
(1998): Hindioglu U+, *J Am Acad Dermatol* 38, 499 (non-pigmenting solitary)
(1998): Litt JZ, Beachwood, OH, personal case (observation)
(1998): Anibarro B+, *Allergy* 53, 902
(1998): Vidal C+, *Ann Allergy Asthma Immunol* 80, 309 (non-pigmenting)
(1996): Alanko K+, *J Am Acad Dermatol* 35, 647
(1996): Quan MB+, *Int J Dermatol* 35, 367 (non-pigmenting)
(1994): Shelley WB+, *Cutis* 54, 240 (observation)
(1994): Krivda SJ+, *J Am Acad Dermatol* 31, 291 (non-pigmenting)
(1994): Shelley WB+, *Cutis* 53, 116 (observation)
(1994): Hauken M, *Ann Intern Med* 120, 442
(1988): Camisa C, *Cutis* 41, 339
(1987): Shelley WB+, *J Am Acad Dermatol* 17, 403 (non-pigmenting)
(1968): Brownstein MH, *Arch Dermatol* 97, 115
Pallor
Pseudo-scarlatina (sic)
(1988): Taylor BJ+, *Br J Dermatol* 118, 827
Systemic contact dermatitis
(1991): Tomb RR+, *Contact Dermatitis* 24, 86
Toxic erythema
(1999): Oakley A, (from Internet) (2 observations)
Toxic shock syndrome
(1994): Shelley WB+, *Cutis* 52, 203 (observation)
(1993): Cavanah DK+, *Ann Intern Med* 119, 302
Urticaria
(1997): Rademaker M, Hamilton, New Zealand, (3 personal cases))observation)
(1994): Shelley WB+, *Cutis* 54, 375 (observation)

Other

Trembling
Tremor
Xerostomia

PSORALENS

Trade names: 8-MOP (ICN); Oxsoralen (ICN); Trisoralen (ICN)
Indications: Vitiligo
Category: Repigmenting agents
Half-life: 2 hours
Clinically important, potentially serious interactions with: other photosensitizing agents

Reactions

Skin

Acne
(1978): Nielsen EB+, *Acta Derm Venereol* (Stockh) 58, 374
Basal cell carcinoma
(1999): Hannuksela-Svahn A+, *J Am Acad Dermatol* 40, 694
Blistering (sic)
(1993): Sheehan MP+, *Br J Dermatol* 129, 431 (PUVA)
(1991): No Author, *Ned Tijdschr Geneeskd* (Dutch) 135, 1764
Bowen's disease
(1979): Hofmann C+, *Br J Dermatol* 101, 685
Bullous pemphigoid (with UVA)
(1996): George PM, *Photodermatol Photoimmunol Photomed* 11, 185
(1996): Perl S+, *Dermatology* 193, 245
(1994): Fryer EJ+, *J Am Acad Dermatol* 30, 651 (passim)
(1989): Weber PJ+, *Arch Dermatol* 125, 690
(1985): Grunwald MH+, *J Am Acad Dermatol* 13, 224
(1982): Stüttgen G, *Int J Dermatol* 21, 198
(1979): Abel EA+, *Arch Dermatol* 115, 988
(1978): Robinson JK, *Br J Dermatol* 99, 709
(1977): Melski JW+, *J Invest Dermatol* 68, 328
(1976): Thomsen K+, *Br J Dermatol* 95, 568
Burning (1–10%)
(1996): Nettelblad H+, *Burns* 22, 633
(1982): Stüttgen G, *Int J Dermatol* 21, 198 (passim)
Cheilitis (1–10%)
Contact dermatitis
(1994): Korffmacher H+, *Contact Dermatitis* 30, 283
(1991): Takashima A+, *Br J Dermatol* 124, 37
(1990): Fleming D+, *Allergy Proc* 11, 125
(1990): Moller H, *Photodermatol Photoimmunol Photomed* 7, 43
(1979): Saihan EM, *BMJ* 2, 20
Eczematous eruption (sic)
(1994): Korffmacher H+, *Contact Dermatitis* 30, 283
(1979): Saihan EM, *BMJ* 2, 20
Edema (1–10%)
Erythema
(2000): Yeo UC+, *Br J Dermatol* 142, 733
Folliculitis
Freckles (1–10%)
(1993): Sheehan MP+, *Br J Dermatol* 129, 431 (PUVA)
(1984): Kietzmann E+, *Dermatologica* 168, 306
(1983): Kietzmann H+, *Ann Dermatol Venereol* (French) 110, 63
(1983): Kanerva L+, *Dermatologica* 166, 281
(1978): Bleehen SS, *Br J Dermatol* 99, 20
Granuloma annulare
(1979): Dorval JC+, *Ann Dermatol Venereol* (French) 106, 79
Herpes simplex
(1993): Sheehan MP+, *Br J Dermatol* 129, 431 (PUVA)
(1982): Stüttgen G, *Int J Dermatol* 21, 198
Herpes zoster
(1982): Stüttgen G, *Int J Dermatol* 21, 198
(1977): Roenigk HH+, *Arch Dermatol* 113, 1667
Hypopigmentation (1–10%)
Keratoacanthoma
(1979): Hofmann C+, *Br J Dermatol* 101, 685
Lichen planus
(1980): Dupre A+, *Ann Dermatol Venereol* (French) 107, 557
Lupus erythematosus
(1991): Lehmann P, *J Am Acad Dermatol* 24, 515 (discoid)
(1985): Bruze M+, *Acta Derm Venereol* (Stockh) 65, 31
(1979): Eyanson S+, *Arch Dermatol* 115, 54 (systemic)
(1979): Domke HF+, *Arch Dermatol* 115, 642
(1978): Millns J+, *Arch Dermatol* 114, 1177

Melanoma
(1999): Lindelof B, *Drug Saf* 20, 289
(1994): Reseghetti A+, *Dermatology* 189, 75
(1980): Forrest JB+, *J Surg Oncol* 13, 337
Miliaria
Pemphigoid
(1980): Lutowiecka-Wranicz A+, *Przegl Dermatol* (Polish) 67, 641
Pemphigus vulgaris
(1994): Fryer EJ+, *J Am Acad Dermatol* 30, 651
Photoreactions
(1978): Plewig G+, *Arch Dermatol Res* 261, 201
Photocontact dermatitis
(1998): Clark SM+, *Contact Dermatitis* 38, 289
(1991): Takashima A+, *Br J Dermatol* 124, 37
(1990): Moller H, *Photodermatol Photoimmunol Photomed* 7, 43
(1982): Kavli G+, *Acta Derm Venereol* 62, 435
(1982): Weiss W+, *Dermatol Monatsschr* (German) 168, 116
(1981): Bleehen SS, *Br J Dermatol* 105, 23
Photosensitivity
(1986): Morliere P, *Biochimie* (French) 68, 849
(1986): Jeanmougin M, *Biochimie* (French) 68, 891
(1986): Lerman S, *Ophthalmology* 93, 304
(1982): Haudenschild-Falb E+, *Ther Umsch* (German) 39, 178
(1980): Dupre A+, *Ann Dermatol Venereol* (French) 107, 557
(1980): Heidbreder G, *Z Hautkr* (German) 55, 84
Phototoxic reaction
(1997): Morison WL+, *J Am Acad Dermatol* 36, 183
(1997): Morison WL, *Arch Dermatol* 133, 1609
(1997): Neumann NJ+, *Acta Derm Venereol* 77, 385
(1990): Ljunggren B, *Arch Dermatol* 126, 1334
(1989): Morison WL, *Arch Dermatol* 125, 433 (topical)
(1986): Toback AC+, *Dermatol Clin* 4, 223
(1986): Lowe NJ, *Br J Dermatol* 115, 86
(1983): Kavli G+, *Contact Dermatitis* 9, 257
(1980): Barth J+, *Z Arztl Fortbild Jena* (German) 74, 789
(1980): Kornhauser A, *Ann N Y Acad Sci* 346, 398
(1980): Wolska H+, *Przegl Dermatol* (Polish) 67, 439
Phytophotodermatitis
(1998): Adams SP, *Can Fam Physician* 44, 503
(1994): Finkelstein E+, *Int J Dermatol* 33, 116
(1993): Leopold JC+, *Am J Dis Child* 147, 311
(1985): Lembo G+, *Photodermatol* 2, 119
(1984): Goitre M, *G Ital Dermatol Venereol* (Italian) 119, 435
(1983): Heskel NS+, *Contact Dermatitis* 9, 278
Pigmentation
(1994): Burrows NP+, *Clin Exp Dermatol* 19, 380
(1993): Poskitt BL+, *J R Soc Med* 86, 665
(1990): Trattner A+, *Int J Dermatol* 29, 310
(1989): Weiss E+, *Int J Dermatol* 28, 188
(1987): Bruce DR+, *J Am Acad Dermatol* 16, 1087
(1986): MacDonald KJS+, *Br J Dermatol* 114, 395
(1985): Rodighiero G, *Farmaco Prat* 40, 173
(1983): Farber EM+, *Arch Dermatol* 119, 426
(1981): No Author, *Br Med J Clin Red Ed* 283, 335
Porokeratosis (actinic)
(1988): Beiteke U+, *Photodermatology* 5, 274
(1985): Hazen PG+, *J Am Acad Dermatol* 12, 1077
(1980): Reymond JL, *Acta Derm Venereol* (Stockh) 60, 539
Prurigo
(1982): Stüttgen G, *Int J Dermatol* 21, 198 (passim)
Pruritus (>10%)
(1990): Roelandts R+, *Photodermatol Photoimmunol Photomed* 7, 141
(1982): Stüttgen G, *Int J Dermatol* 21, 198 (passim)
(1979): Jordan WP, *Arch Dermatol* 115, 636
Psoriasis
Rash (sic) (1–10%)
Rosacea
(1989): McFadden JP+, *Br J Dermatol* 121, 413
Scleroderma
(1976): Duperrat B+, *Bull Soc Franc Dermatol Syphiligr* (French) 83, 79
Seborrheic dermatitis
(1983): Tegner E, *Acta Derm Venereol* (Stockh) Suppl 107, 5
Skin pain
(1993): Burrows NP+, *Br J Dermatol* 129, 504
(1987): Norris PG+, *Clin Exp Dermatol* 12, 403
(1983): Tegner E, *Acta Derm Venereol* (Stockh) Suppl 107, 5
Squamous cell carcinoma
(1986): Kahn JR+, *Clin Exp Dermatol* 11, 398
Tumors (for the most part malignant)
(1995): Weinstock MA+, *Arch Dermatol* 131, 701
(1994): Altman JS+, *J Am Acad Dermatol* 31, 505
(1994): Lewis FM+, *Lancet* 344, 1157
(1994): Lever LR+, *Clin Exp Dermatol* 19, 443 (malignant)
(1993): Lindelof B+, *Br J Dermatol* 129, 39
(1990): Young AR, *J Photochem Photobiol* B 6, 237
(1989): Stern RS+, *Carcinog Compr Surv* 11, 85
(1989): Hannuksela M+, *J Am Acad Dermatol* 21, 813
(1988): Gupta AK+, *J Am Acad Dermatol* 19, 67
(1987): Henseler T+, *J Am Acad Dermatol* 16, 108
(1983): Shafrir A, *Harefuah* (Hebrew) 104, 364
(1983): Farber EM+, *Arch Dermatol* 119, 426
(1981): No Author, *Br Med J Clin Red Ed* 283, 335
(1980): Halprin KM, *J Am Acad Dermatol* 2, 432
(1980): Brown FS+, *J Am Acad Dermatol* 2, 393
(1980): Halprin KM, *J Am Acad Dermatol* 2, 334
(1978): Bridges BA, *Clin Exp Dermatol* 3, 349
Urticaria
(1994): Bech-Thomsen N+, *J Am Acad Dermatol* 31, 1063
Vasculitis
(1981): Barriere H+, *Presse Med* (French) 10, 37
Vitiligo
(1983): Tegner E, *Acta Derm Venereol* (Stockh) 107 (Suppl), 5
(1976): Duperrat B+, *Bull Soc Franc Dermatol Syphiligr* (French) 83, 79
Warts
(1982): Stüttgen G, *Int J Dermatol* 21, 198

Hair

Hair – hypertrichosis
(1992): Shelley WB+, *Advanced Dermatologic Diagnosis*, WB Saunders, 725 (passim)
(1983): Rampen FHJ, *Br J Dermatol* 109, 657
(1967): Singh G+, *Br J Dermatol* 79, 501
(1959): Elliot JA, *J Invest Dermatol* 32, 311

Nails

Nails – photo-onycholysis
(1979): Warin AP, *Arch Dermatol* 115, 235
(1978): Ortonne JP+, *Ann Dermatol Venereol* (French) 105, 887
Nails – pigmentation
(1990): Trattner A+, *Int J Dermatol* 29, 310
(1989): Weiss E+, *Int J Dermatol* 28, 188
(1986): MacDonald KJS+, *Br J Dermatol* 114, 395
(1982): Naik RPC+, *Int J Dermatol* 21, 275

Other

Lymphoproliferative disease
(1989): Aschinoff R+, *J Am Acad Dermatol* 21, 1134

PYRAZINAMIDE

Trade names: Pyrazinamide (Lederle); Rifater (Aventis)
Other common trade names: *Braccopril; Dipimide; Isopas; Lynamide; Pirilene; Pyrazide; Rozide; Tebrazid; Zinastat*
Indications: Tuberculosis
Category: Antibacterial; antitubercular
Half-life: 9–10 hours
Clinically important, potentially serious interactions with: allopurinol, colchicine, cyclosporine, probenecid, rifampin, sulfinpyrazone

Reactions

Skin

Acne (<1%)
Erythema multiforme
(1996): Perdu D+, *Allergy* 51, 340
Exanthems
(1990): Goday J+, *Contact Dermatitis* 22, 181
Fixed eruption
(1990): Goday J+, *Contact Dermatitis* 22, 181
Flushing

Pellagra
(1983): Jorgensen J, *Int J Dermatol* 22, 44
Photodermatitis (<1%)
(1999): Choonhakarn C+, *J Am Acad Dermatol* 40, 645 (lichenoid)
Pruritus (<1%)
Purpura
Rash (sic) (<1%)
(2000): Gordin F+, *JAMA* 283, 1445
(1998): Olivier C+, *Arch Pediatr* (French) 5, 289
(1998): Radal M+, *Rev Mal Respir* (French) 15, 305 (3 cases)
Urticaria

Other

Acute intermittent porphyria
(1976): Treece GL+, *Am Rev Respir Dis* 113, 233
Hypersensitivity
Myalgia (1–10%)
Oral mucosal lesions
Porphyria cutanea tarda (<1%)

PYRIDOXINE

Synonym: vitamin B_6
Trade names: Hexabetalin (Lilly); Nestrex
Other common trade names: *B(6)-Vicotrat;Beesix; Benadon; Godabion B6; Hexa-Betalin; Nestrex*
Indications: Pyridoxine deficiency
Category: Water-soluble nutritional supplement and antidote
Half-life: 15–20 days
Clinically important, potentially serious interactions with: cycloserine, hydralazine, isoniazid, levodopa, oral contraceptives, penicillamine, phenobarbital, phenytoin

Reactions

Skin

Acne
(1991): Sherertz EF, *Cutis* 48, 119
(1976): Braun-Falco O+, *MMW Münch Med Wochenschr* (German) 118, 155
(1964): Fegeler F, *Arch Klin Exp Dermatoi* (German) 219, 335
Allergic reactions (sic) (<1%)
Bullous eruption
(1984): Ruzicka T+, *Hautarzt* (German) 35, 197
Contact dermatitis
(1990): Camarasa JG+, *Contact Dermatitis* 23, 115
(1985): Yoshikawa K+, *Contact Dermatitis* 12, 55
(1983): Fujita M+, *Contact Dermatitis* 9, 61
Fixed eruption
(1972): Kuokkanen K, *Acta Allergol* 27, 407
Photoreactions
(1996): Tanaka M+, *J Dermatol* 23, 708
Photosensitivity
(1998): Murata Y+, *J Am Acad Dermatol* 39, 314 (2 cases)
Purpura
Toxic epidermal necrolysis
(1980): Andriushchenko OM+, *Klin Med Mosk* (Russian) 58, 101
Vasculitis
(1984): Ruzicka T+, *Hautarzt* (German) 35, 197
Vesicular eruption
(1986): Friedman MA+, *J Am Acad Dermatol* 14, 915

Hair

Hair – pigmentation
(1972): Shelley WB+, *Arch Dermatol* 106, 228

Other

Hypersensitivity
(1969): Zheltakov MM+, *Vestn Dermatol Venerol* (Russian) 43, 62
Injection-site burning
Injection-site stinging
Paresthesias (<1%)
Porphyria cutanea tarda
(1992): Shelley WB+, *Advanced Dermatologic Diagnosis*, WB Saunders, 414 (passim)
Pseudoporphyria
(1984): Baer RL+, *J Am Acad Dermatol* 10, 527

PYRILAMINE

Trade name: Triaminic (Novartis)
Indications: Allergic rhinitis
Category: H_1-receptor antihistamine
Half-life: no data
Clinically important, potentially serious interactions with: no data

Reactions

Skin

Angioedema
Dermatitis (sic)
Diaphoresis
Flushing
Lupus erythematosus
Photosensitivity
Purpura
Rash (sic)
Urticaria

Other

Anaphylactoid reaction
Gynecomastia
Paresthesias
Stomatitis
Xerostomia

PYRIMETHAMINE

Trade names: Daraprim (GlaxoWellcome); Fansidar (Roche)
Other common trade names: *Erbaprelina; Malocide; Pirimecidan*
Indications: Malaria
Category: Antimalarial
Half-life: 80–95 hours
Clinically important, potentially serious interactions with: co-trimoxazole, folic acid, methotrexate, sulfonamides

Fansidar is pyrimethamine and sulfadoxine

Reactions

Skin

Acute generalized exanthematous pustulosis (AGEP)
(1995): Moreau A+, *Int J Dermatol* 34, 263 (passim)
Angioedema
(1992): Breathnach SM+, *Adverse Drug Reactions and the Skin*, Blackwell, Oxford, 176 (passim)
Bullous eruption
(1992): Breathnach SM+, *Adverse Drug Reactions and the Skin*, Blackwell, Oxford, 176 (passim)
(1989): Caumes E+, *Presse Med* (French) 18, 1708
Dermatitis (sic) (<1%)
Erythema multiforme (<1%)
(1993): Sturchler D+, *Drug Saf* 8, 160
(1991): Porteous DM+, *Arch Dermatol* 127, 740 (IN HIV+ patients)
(1987): Hellgren U+, *Br Med J Clin Res Ed* 295, 365
(1986): Miller KD+, *Am J Trop Med Hyg* 35, 451
Exanthems
(1989): Ortel B+, *Dermatologica* 178, 39 (papular)
(1987): Groth H+, *Schweiz Rundsch Med Prax* (German) 76, 570
Exfoliative dermatitis
(1987): Elsas T+, *Tidsskr Nor Laegeforen* (Norwegian) 107, 1231
(1986): Langtry JA+, *Br Med J Clin Res Ed* 292, 1107

Fixed eruption
(1988): Tham SN+, *Singapore Med J* 29, 300
Lichenoid eruption
(1989): Zain RB, *Southeast Asian J Trop Med Public Health* 20, 253 (oral)
(1980): Cutler TP, *Clin Exp Dermatol* 5, 253
Lymphoma
(1997): Costello JM+, *N Z Med J* 86, 430
Photosensitivity (>10%)
(1992): Breathnach SM+, *Adverse Drug Reactions and the Skin*, Blackwell, Oxford, 176 (passim)
(1989): Ortel B+, *Dermatologica* 178, 39
(1974): Craven SA, *BMJ* 2, 556
Pigmentation (<1%)
(1991): Poizot-Martin I+, *Presse Med* (French) 20, 632
(1990): Poizot-Martin I+, *Int Conf AIDS* 6, 357
(1977): Costello JM+, *N Z Med J* 86, 430
(1965): TenPas A+, *Am J Med Sciences* 249, 448
Pruritus
(1987): Groth H+, *Schweiz Rundsch Med Prax* (German) 76, 570
Purpura
(1965): TenPas A+, *Am J Med Sciences* 249, 448
Pustular eruption
(1973): Macmillan AL, *Dermatologica* 146, 285 (generalized)
Rash (sic) (<1%)
Stevens–Johnson syndrome (1–10%)
(1995): Caumes E+, *Clin Infect Dis* 21, 656
(1993): Schlienger RG+, *Schweiz Rundsch Med Prax* (German) 82, 888
(1993): Sturchler D+, *Drug Saf* 8, 160
(1992): Breathnach SM+, *Adverse Drug Reactions and the Skin*, Blackwell, Oxford, 176 (passim)
(1991): Porteous DM+, *Arch Dermatol* 127, 740 (in HIV+ patients)
(1990): Thiel HJ+, *Klin Monatsbl Augenheilkd* (German) 197, 142
(1989): Phillips-Howard PA+, *Lancet* 2, 803
(1989): Ortel B+, *Dermatologica* 178, 39
(1988): Mimoun G+, *Bull Soc Ophtalmol Fr* (French) 88, 961
(1987): Lenox-Smith I, *J Infect* 14, 90 (fatal)
(1987): Hellgren U+, *Br Med J Clin Res Ed* 295, 365
(1987): Lyn PC+, *Med J Aust* 146, 335
(1986): Gascon-Brustenga J+, *Med Clin (Barc)* (Spanish) 87, 821
(1986): Bamber MG+, *J Infect* 13, 31 (fatal)
(1986): Miller KD+, *Am J Trop Med Hyg* 35, 451
(1985): Clareus BW+, *Lakartidningen* (Swedish) 82, 4211
(1985): Adams SJ+, *Postgrad Med J* 61, 263
(1983): Ligthelm RJ+, *Ned Tijdschr Geneeskd* (Dutch) 127, 1735
(1982): Hornstein OP+, *N Engl J Med* 307, 1529
Toxic dermatitis (sic)
(1995): Piketty C+, *Presse Med* (French) 24, 1710
Toxic epidermal necrolysis (<1%)
(1998): Schmidt-Westhausen A+, *Oral Dis* 4, 90
(1998): Moussala M+, *J Fr Ophtalmol* (French) 21, 72
(1995): Caumes E+, *Clin Infect Dis* 21, 656
(1993): Sturchler D+, *Drug Saf* 8, 160
(1992): Breathnach SM+, *Adverse Drug Reactions and the Skin*, Blackwell, Oxford, 176 (passim)
(1991): Kimura S+, *Jpn J Med* 30, 553
(1990): Ward DJ+, *Burns* 16, 97
(1988): Phillips-Howard PA+, *Br Med J Clin Res Ed* 296, 1605
(1988): Raviglione MC+, *Arch Intern Med* 148, 2683 (fatal)
(1988): *MMWR Morb Mortal Wkly Rep* 37, 571
(1987): Hellgren U+, *Br Med J Clin Res Ed* 295, 365
(1986): Miller KD+, *Am J Trop Med Hyg* 35, 451
Urticaria
Vasculitis

Hair

Hair – alopecia

Other

Anaphylactoid reaction (<1%)
Dysgeusia
Glossitis (<1%) (atrophic)
Hypersensitivity (>10%)
Lymphoproliferative disease
(1977): Costello JM+, *N Z Med J* 86, 430
Xerostomia (<1%)

QUAZEPAM

Trade name: Doral (Wallace)
Other common trade names: *Oniria; Pamerex; Quazium; Quiedorm; Selepam; Temodal*
Indications: Insomnia
Category: Benzodiazepine sedative-hypnotic; antidepressant
Half-life: 25–41 hours
Clinically important, potentially serious interactions with: alcohol, anesthetics, barbiturates, cimetidine, ciprofloxacin, clarithromycin, clozapine, CNS depressants, digoxin, diltiazem, disulfiram, erythromycin, fluconazole, fluoxetine, fluvoxamine, isoniazid, itraconazole, ketoconazole, labetalol, levodopa, loxapine, MAO inhibitors, metoprolol, metronidazole, miconazole, narcotics, nefazodone, omeprazole, phenothiazines, phenytoin, rifabutin, rifampin, theophylline, tricyclic antidepressants, valproic acid, verapamil, **grapefruit juice**

Reactions

Skin

Dermatitis (sic) (1–10%)
Diaphoresis (>10%)
Pruritus
(1991): Roth T+, *J Clin Psychiatry* 52 Suppl 38–41
Purpura
Rash (sic) (>10%)
(1991): Roth T+, *J Clin Psychiatry* 52 Suppl 38–41
Urticaria

Hair

Hair – alopecia
Hair – hirsutism

Other

Dysgeusia
Oral ulceration
Paresthesias
Sialopenia (>10%)
Sialorrhea (1–10%)
Xerostomia (1–5%)
(1991): Roth T+, *J Clin Psychiatry* 52 Suppl 38–41

QUETIAPINE

Trade name: Seroquel (AstraZeneca)
Indications: Psychotic disorders; schizophrenia
Category: Antipsychotic
Half-life: ~6 hours
Clinically important, potentially serious interactions with: alcohol, barbiturates, carbamazepine, cimetidine, CNS depressants, levodopa, lorazepam, phenothiazines, phenytoin, rifampin, thioridazine

Reactions

Skin

Angioedema
(1999): Drayton G, Los Angeles, CA (from Internet) (observation) (patient is also allergic to sulfa)
Candidiasis (<1%)
Diaphoresis (1–10%)
Edema
Facial edema (<1%)
Photosensitivity (<1%)
Rash (sic) (4%)
Xerosis (<1%)

Other

Bruxism (<1%)
Gingivitis (<1%)
Glossitis (<1%)
Myalgia (<1%)
Oral ulceration (<1%)
Paresthesias (1%)
Priapism
Sialorrhea (<1%)
Stomatitis (<1%)
Tongue edema (<1%)
Thrombophlebitis (<1%)
Xerostomia (7%)

QUINACRINE

Trade name: Atabrine (Sanofi)
Other common trade name: *Atabil*
Indications: Various infections caused by susceptible helminths
Category: Anthelmintic; antimalarial
Half-life: 4–10 hours
Clinically important, potentially serious interactions with: primaquine

Reactions

Skin

Contact dermatitis
Erythema dyschromicum perstans
(1970): Tolman MM, *Arch Dermatol* 102, 113
Erythematous plaques
(1981): Bauer F, *J Am Acad Dermatol* 4, 239
Exanthems
(1981): Bauer F, *J Am Acad Dermatol* 4, 239 (eczematous) (80%)
(1963): Nagy E+, *Dermatologica* (German) 126, 13 (1.4%)
(1955): Alexander HL, *Reactions with Drug Therapy*, Philadelphia, WB Saunders
(1953): Zeller F, *Hautarzt* (German) 4, 384
Exfoliative dermatitis
(1981): Bauer F, *J Am Acad Dermatol* 4, 239 (8%)
(1967): Lockey SD, *Med Sci* 18, 43
(1955): Alexander HL, *Reactions with Drug Therapy*, Philadelphia, WB Saunders
Fixed eruption
(1967): Lockey SD, *Med Sci* 18, 43
(1964): Browne SG, *BMJ* 2, 1041
(1961): Welch AL+, *Arch Dermatol* 84, 1004
(1955): Alexander HL, *Reactions with Drug Therapy*, Philadelphia, WB Saunders
Hypomelanosis
(1967): Lockey SD, *Med Sci* 18, 43
Keratoderma
(1978): Bauer F, *Aust J Dermatol* 19, 9
Lichenoid eruption
(1981): Bauer F, *J Am Acad Dermatol* 4, 239 (12%)
(1979): Callaway JL, *J Am Acad Dermatol* 1, 456
(1978): Bauer F, *Aust J Dermatol* 19, 9
(1971): Almeyda J+, *Br J Dermatol* 85, 604
(1964): Baker H, *Br J Dermatol* 76, 186
(1963): Nagy E+, *Dermatologica* (German) 126, 13 (1.4%)
(1955): Alexander HL, *Reactions with Drug Therapy*, Philadelphia, WB Saunders
Ochronosis
(1976): Egorin MJ+, *JAMA* 236, 385
(1976): Tuffanelli DL, *JAMA* 236, 2491
Photosensitivity
(1997): Hindson C, Worcestershire UK, *The Schoch Letter* 47, 53
Pigmentation
(1982): Sokol RJ+, *Pediatrics* 69, 232 (yellow)
(1981): Koranda FC, *J Am Acad Dermatol* 4, 650
(1981): Zuehlke RL+, *Int J Dermatol* 20, 57
(1979): Leigh IM+, *Br J Dermatol* 101, 147
(1978): Bauer F, *Aust J Dermatol* 19, 9
(1969): *Med Lett* 11, 27 (yellowish)
Pruritus (<1%)
Squamous cell carcinoma
(1979): Callaway JL, *J Am Acad Dermatol* 1, 456

(1978): Bauer F, *Aust J Dermatol* 19, 9
Urticaria
(1969): *Med Lett* 11, 27 (1–5%)
(1955): Alexander HL, *Reactions with Drug Therapy*, Philadelphia, WB Saunders

Hair
Hair – alopecia
(1981): Bauer F, *J Am Acad Dermatol* 4, 239 (eczematous) (80%)
(1978): Bauer F, *Aust J Dermatol* 19, 9

Nails
Nails – changes (sic)
(1978): Bauer F, *Aust J Dermatol* 19, 9
Nails – pigmentation
(1969): *Med Lett* 11, 27

Other
Oral pigmentation
(1970): Brynolf I, *Sven Tandlak Tidskr* (Swedish) 63, 585

QUINAPRIL

Trade name: Accupril (Parke-Davis)
Other common trade names: *Accuprin; Accupro; Acuitel; Acupril; Asig; Korec; Quinazil*
Indications: Hypertension
Category: Angiotensin-converting enzyme (ACE) inhibitor; antihypertensive and vasodilator
Half-life: 1–2 hours
Clinically important, potentially serious interactions with: alcohol, allopurinol, bumetanide, digoxin, diuretics, indomethacin, lithium, phenothiazines, potassium-sparing diuretics, salicylates, tetracycline

Reactions

Skin
Angioedema (<1%)
(1997): Sigler C+, *Arch Dermatol* 113, 972
(1996): Boxer M, *J Allergy Clin Immunol* 98, 471
(1995): Maier C, *Anaesthesist* (German) 44, 875
(1994): Cosano L+, *Med Clin (Barc)* (Spanish) 102, 275
(1993): Mendez-Mora JL+, *Med Clin (Barc)* (Spanish) 101, 76
(1992): Materson BJ, *Am J Cardiol* 69, 46C
(1989): Sedman AJ+, *Angiology* 40 (4 Pt 2), 360
Ankle edema
(1992): Bahena JH+, *Clin Ther* 14, 527
Bullous eruption
(1998): Sienkiewicz G, Johnson City, NY (from Internet) (observation)
Diaphoresis (<1%)
(1991): Morant J+, *Arzneimittel-Kompendium der Schweiz* (German) Basel, Documed, 1990
(1989): Maclean D, *Angiology* 40 (4 Pt 2), 370
(1989): Frank GJ+, *Angiology* 40 (4 Pt 2), 405
Edema
(1989): Frank GJ+, *Angiology* 40 (4 Pt 2), 405
(1989): Frank GJ, *Cardiology* 76 (Suppl 2), 56
Exanthems
(1991): Morant J+, *Arzneimittel-Kompendium der Schweiz* (German) Basel, Documed, 1990
Exfoliative dermatitis (<1%)
Facial edema (sic)
(1989): Sedman AJ+, *Angiology* 40 (4 Pt 2), 360
Flushing (<1%)
Pemphigus (<1%)
Peripheral edema (<1%)
(1991): Wadworth AN+, *Drugs* 41, 378
Photosensitivity (<1%)
(1989): Maclean D, *Angiology* 40 (4 Pt 2), 370
Pruritus (<1%)
(1991): Cetnarowski-Cropp AB, *Drug Intell Clin Pharm* 25, 499
(1991): Morant J+, *Arzneimittel-Kompendium der Schweiz* (German) Basel, Documed, 1990
(1990): Swartz RD+, *J Clin Pharmacol* 30, 1136
(1990): Frishman WH, *Clin Cardiol* 13 (Suppl 7), VII19
(1989): Maclean D, *Angiology* 40 (4 Pt 2), 370
(1989): Frank GJ+, *Angiology* 40 (4 Pt 2), 405
(1989): Frank GJ, *Cardiology* 76 (Suppl 2), 56
Rash (sic) (1.2%)
(1992): Materson BJ, *Am J Cardiol* 69, 46C
(1989): Frank GJ+, *Angiology* 40 (4 Pt 2), 405
(1989): Frank GJ, *Cardiology* 76 (Suppl 2), 56
(1989): Maclean D, *Angiology* 40 (4 Pt 2), 370
(1989): Taylor SH, *Angiology* 40 (4 Pt 2), 382
Urticaria (<1%)
Vasculitis (<1%)

Hair
Hair – alopecia (<1%)

Other
Dysgeusia
(1991): Cetnarowski-Cropp AB, *Drug Intell Clin Pharm* 25, 499
(1989): Taylor SH, *Angiology* 40 (4 Pt 2), 382
Hypersensitivity
Myalgia (1.5%)
Paresthesias (<1%)
Xerostomia (<1%)

QUINESTROL

Trade name: Estrovis (Parke-Davis)
Indications: Atrophic vaginitis, menopausal symptoms
Category: Estrogen
Half-life: 120 hours
Clinically important, potentially serious interactions with: corticosteroids

Reactions

Skin
Angioedema
(1970): Aitken DA+, *BMJ* 2, 177
Chloasma (<1%)
Edema (<1%)
Erythema
Melasma (<1%)
Peripheral edema (>10%)
Photosensitivity
Rash (sic) (<1%)
Urticaria
(1970): Aitken DA+, *BMJ* 2, 177

Other
Acute intermittent porphyria
Gynecomastia (>10%)
Mastodynia (>10%)
Thrombophlebitis

QUINETHAZONE

Trade name: Hydromox (Lederle)
Other common trade name: *Aquamox*
Indications: Hypertension; edema
Category: Sulfonamide* diuretic and antihypertensive
Half-life: no data
Clinically important, potentially serious interactions with: antidiabetics, diazoxide, digoxin, furosemide, lithium, loop diuretics

Reactions

Skin
Bullous eruption (<1%)
(1966): Miller RC+, *Arch Dermatol* 93, 346

Exanthems
(1966): Miller RC+, *Arch Dermatol* 93, 346
Photoreactions
Photosensitivity (<1%)
(1969): Kalivas J, *JAMA* 209, 1706
(1966): Miller RC+, *Arch Dermatol* 93, 346
Pruritus
(1969): Kalivas J, *JAMA* 209, 1706
Purpura
Rash (sic) (<1%)
Urticaria
Vasculitis

Other

Hypersensitivity
Paresthesias
Xanthopsia
Xerostomia

***Note:** Quinethazone is a sulfonamide and can be absorbed systemically. Sulfonamides can produce severe, possibly fatal, reactions such as toxic epidermal necrolysis and Stevens–Johnson syndrome.

QUINIDINE

Trade names: Cardioquin (Purdue Frederick); Cin-Quin; Quinaglute (Berlex); Quinalan; Quinidex (Robins); Quinora
Other common trade names: *Cardine; Cardioquin; Gluquine; Kinidin; Quinate; Quinidex; Quini Durules*
Indications: Tachycardia; atrial fibrillation
Category: Antiarrhythmic class I-A
Half-life: 6–8 hours
Clinically important, potentially serious interactions with: amiloide, amiodarone, amprenavir, anticoagulants, astemizole, beta-blockers, cimetidine, cisapride, coumarin, digoxin, diltiazem, gatifloxacin, nelfinavir, nifedipine, pimozide, propafenone, propranolol, rifampin, ritonavir, sparfloxacin, terfenadine, verapamil, warfarin

Reactions

Skin

Acne
(1981): Burkhart CG, *Arch Dermatol* 117, 603
Acute generalized exanthematous pustulosis (AGEP)
(1995): Moreau A+, *Int J Dermatol* 34, 263 (passim)
(1991): Roujeau J-C+, *Arch Dermatol* 127, 1333
Allergic reactions (sic)
(1986): Bigby M+, *JAMA* 256, 3358 (1.34%)
Angioedema (<1%)
Bullous eruption
Contact dermatitis
(1985): Fowler JF, *Contact Dermatitis* 13, 280
(1981): Wahlberg JE+, *Contact Dermatitis* 7, 27 (occupational)
(1965): Fernstrom AI, *Acta Derm Venereol* 45, 129
Cutaneous side effects (sic)
(1977): Cohen IS+, *Prog Cardiovasc Dis* 20, 151 (1%)
Eczematous eruption (sic)
Erythema multiforme
(1989): Alanko K, *Acta Derm Venereol* (Stockh) 69, 223
Exanthems
(1990): Lou CP+, *Postgrad Med J* 66, 406
(1985): Bruce S+, *J Am Acad Dermatol* 12, 332
(1982): Holt RJ, *Drug Intell Clin Pharm* 16, 615
(1980): Harrison DC+, *Am Heart J* 100, 1046 (16.6%)
(1976): Geltner D+, *Gastroenterology* 70, 650 (0.8%)
(1976): Arndt KA+, *JAMA* 235, 918 (generalized) (1.2%)
Exfoliative dermatitis (<1%)
(1996): Sigurdsson V+, *J Am Acad Dermatol* 35, 53
(1987): Bellogini GC+, *Minerva Cardioangiol* (Italian) 35, 457
(1985): Bruce S+, *J Am Acad Dermatol* 12, 332
(1965): Gouffault J+, *Sem Hôp* (French) 41, 1350
(1951): Taylor DR+, *JAMA* 145, 641
Exudative dermatitis (sic)
(1942): Goldschlag F, *Med J Australia* 2, 501
Fixed eruption
(1960): Engelhardt AW, *Hautarzt* (German) 11, 49
Flushing (<1%)
(1991): Ross EV+, *J Assoc Military Dermatol* XVII (1), 16
(1985): Bruce S+, *J Am Acad Dermatol* 12, 332
Granuloma annulare
(1991): Ross EV+, *J Assoc Military Dermatol* XVII (1), 16
Lichenoid eruption
(1988): de Larrard G+, *Ann Dermatol Venereol* (French) 115, 1172
(1987): Jeanmougin M+, *Ann Dermatol Venereol* (French) 114, 1397 (photosensitive)
(1982): Berger TC+, *Cutis* 29, 595
(1981): Haim S+, *Harefuah* (Hebrew) 101, 310
(1976): Gammer S+, *Cutis* 17, 72
(1968): Pegum JS, *Br J Dermatol* 80, 343
Lichen planus
(1994): Thompson DF+, *Pharmacotherapy* 14, 561
(1985): Rebondy JP+, *Ann Dermatol Venereol* (French) 112, 989
(1985): Bruce S+, *J Am Acad Dermatol* 12, 332 (passim)
(1980): Maltz BL+, *Int J Dermatol* 19, 96
(1967): Anderson TE, *Br J Dermatol* 79, 500
(1967): Sarkany I, *Br J Dermatol* 79, 123
(1954): Wechsler HL, *Arch Dermatol* 69, 741
Livedo reticularis (<1%)
(1989): Manzi S+, *Arch Dermatol* 125, 417 (photosensitive)
(1985): Bruce S+, *J Am Acad Dermatol* 12, 332 (photosensitive)
(1977): Cohen IS+, *Prog Cardiovasc Dis* 20, 151
(1974): de Groot WP+, *Dermatologica* 148, 371 (photosensitive)
(1973): Marion DF+, *Arch Dermatol* 108, 100 (photosensitive)
Lupus erythematosus (<1%)
(1996): Rich MW, *Postgrad Med* 100, 299
(1995): Alloway JA+, *Semin Arthritis Rheum* 24, 315
(1994): Yung RL+, *Rheum Dis Clin North Am* 20, 61
(1992): Skaer TL, *Clin Ther* 14, 496
(1992): Rubin RL, *Clin Biochem* 25, 223
(1992): Rubin RL+, *J Clin Invest* 90, 165
(1991): Alarcon-Segovia D+, *Baillieres Clin Rheumatol* 5, 1
(1991): Tebas P+, *Rev Clin Esp* (Spanish) 189, 123
(1989): Cohen MG, *Geriatric Med Today* 8, 95
(1988): Cohen MG+, *Ann Intern Med* 108, 369
(1988): Schmid FR, *Ann Intern Med* 109, 247
(1988): Webb J+, *Med J Aust* 149, 53
(1987): Sukenik S+, *Isr J Med Sci* 23, 1232
(1986): Bar-El Y+, *Am Heart J* 111, 1209
(1985): Stratton MA, *Clin Pharm* 4, 657
(1985): Gastineau DA+, *Arch Intern Med* 145, 1926
(1985): McCormack GD+, *Semin Arthritis Rheum* 15, 73
(1985): Lavie CJ+, *Arch Intern Med* 145, 446
(1985): Rebondy JP+, *Ann Dermatol Venereol* (French) 112, 989
(1985): Krainin MJ+, *Arch Intern Med* 145, 1740
(1985): Amadio P+, *Ann Intern Med* 102, 419
(1984): West SG+, *Ann Intern Med* 100, 840
(1982): Chagnon A+, *Nouv Presse Med* (French) 11, 2020
(1981): Barrier J+, *Nouv Presse Med* (French) 10, 2991
(1978): Robinson HM, *Z Hautkr* (German) 53, 349
(1977): Tweed JM, *N Z Med J* 86, 40
(1977): Cohen IS+, *Prog Cardiovasc Dis* 20, 151
(1976): Yudis M+, *JAMA* 235, 2000
(1974): Donoho CR+, *Arthritis Rheum* 17, 322
(1973): Hanauer LB, *Ann Intern Med* 78, 308
(1973): Marion DF+, *Arch Dermatol* 108, 100
(1972): Anderson FP+, *Conn Med* 36, 84
(1970): Kendall MJ+, *Postgrad Med J* 46, 729
Palmoplantar keratosis
(1988): De Larrard G+, *Ann Dermatol Venereol* (French) 115, 1172
Photoreactions
(1991): Schürer NY+, *Hautarzt* (German) 42, 158
(1990): Fertin C+, *Nouv Dermatol* (French) 9, 446
(1986): Jeanmougin M+, *Ann Dermatol Venereol* (French) 113, 985
(1976): Gammer S+, *Cutis* 17, 72
Photosensitivity (<1%)
(1992): Schürer NY+, *Photodermatol Photoimmunol Photomed* 9, 78
(1989): Rosen C, *Semin Dermatol* 8, 149
(1988): De Larrard G+, *Ann Dermatol Venereol* (French) 115, 1172
(1987): Bonnetblanc JM+, *Ann Dermatol Venereol* (French) 114, 957 (lichenoid)

(1987): Ferguson J+, *Br J Dermatol* 117, 631
(1987): Wolf R+, *Dermatologica* 174, 285 (lichenoid and eczematous)
(1986): Ljunggren B+, *Photodermatol* 3, 26
(1985): Rebondy JP+, *Ann Dermatol Venereol* (French) 112, 989
(1985): Armstrong RB+, *Arch Dermatol* 121, 525
(1985): Bonnetblanc JM+, *Ann Dermatol Venereol* (French) 112, 671
(1984): Fisher DA, *Arch Dermatol* 120, 298
(1983): Marx JL+, *Arch Dermatol* 119, 39
(1983): Lang PS, *J Am Acad Dermatol* 9, 124
(1982): Berger TC+, *Cutis* 29, 595 (lichenoid)
(1976): Pariser RJ+, *Arch Dermatol* 112, 1610
(1976): Bogoch ER+, *Arch Dermatol* 112, 559
(1975): Pariser DM+, *Arch Dermatol* 111, 1440

Pigmentation (<1%)
(1996): Conroy EA+, *Cutis* 57, 425
(1996): Messina JL+, *J Geriatr Dermatol* 4, 198
(1995): Rippis G+, American Academy of Dermatology Meeting, New Orleans (observation)
(1986): Mahler R+, *Arch Dermatol* 122, 1062

Pruritus (<1%)
(1985): Bruce S+, *J Am Acad Dermatol* 12, 332 (passim)
(1982): Holt RJ, *Drug Intell Clin Pharm* 16, 615
(1976): Geltner D+, *Gastroenterology* 70, 650 (0.8%)

Psoriasis (<1%)
(1998): Smith KC, Niagara Falls, Canada (from Internet) (observation)
(1993): Brenner S+, *Arch Dermatol* 129, 1331
(1986): Abel EA+, *J Am Acad Dermatol* 15, 1007
(1983): Harwell WB, *J Am Acad Dermatol* 9, 278
(1977): Cohen IS+, *Prog Cardiovasc Dis* 20, 151 (with erythroderma)
(1973): Almeyda J+, *Br J Dermatol* 88, 313 (with erythroderma)

Purpura
(1993): Kaufman DW+, *Blood* 82, 2714
(1991): Salom IL, *JAMA* 266, 1220 (letter)
(1988): Reid DM+, *Ann Intern Med* 108, 206
(1981): Barrier J+, *Nouv Presse Med* (French) 10, 2991
(1981): Conri C+, *Nouv Presse Med* (French) 7, 3361
(1980): Miescher PA+, *Clin Haematol* 9, 505
(1976): Khaleeli AA, *BMJ* 2, 562
(1976): Geltner D+, *Gastroenterology* 70, 650 (1.4%)
(1962): Weintraub RM+, *JAMA* 180, 528
(1959): Bishop RC+, *Ann Intern Med* 50, 1227
(1958): Shaftel N+, *Angiology* 9, 34
(1956): Freedman AL+, *J Lab Clin Med* 48, 205
(1956): Bolton FG, *Blood* 11, 547

Pustular eruption
(1951): Taylor DR+, *JAMA* 145, 641

Rash (sic) (1–10%)

Subcorneal pustular dermatosis (Sneddon–Wilkinson)
(1983): Halevy S+, *Acta Derm Venereol* (Stockh) 63, 441

Toxic epidermal necrolysis
(2000): Adornato MC, *N Y State Dent J* 66, 38
(1974): Callaway JL+, *Arch Dermatol* 109, 909

Urticaria (<1%)
(1985): Bruce S+, *J Am Acad Dermatol* 12, 332

Vasculitis (<1%)
(1990): Zax RH+, *Arch Dermatol* 126, 69
(1989): Cohen MG, *Geriatric Med Today* 8, 99
(1988): Quin J+, *Med J Aust* 148, 145 (allergic granulomatous)
(1985): Shalit M+, *Arch Intern Med* 145, 2051

Hair

Hair – alopecia
(1988): de Larrard G+, *Ann Dermatol Venereol* (French) 115, 1172

Other

Dysgeusia (>10%) (bitter taste)

Hypersensitivity
(1966): Martt JM+, *Mo Med* 63, 908

Lymphoproliferative disease
(1987): Gay RG+, *Am J Med* 82, 143

Myalgia (<1%)

Oral mucosal eruption
(1988): De Larrard G+, *Ann Dermatol Venereol* (French) 115, 1172
(1958): Shaftel N+, *Angiology* 9, 34

Oral mucosal pigmentation
(1988): Birek C+, *Oral Surg Oral Med Oral Pathol* 66, 59

Oral ulceration

Polymyalgia
(1995): Alloway JA+, *Semin Arthritis Rheum* 24, 315

Porphyria
(1971): Sayag J+, *Bull Soc Franc Dermatol Syphiligr* (French) 78, 664

Pseudoporphyria
(1992): Petersen CS+, *Ugeskr Laeger* (Danish) 154, 1713

Sicca syndrome (<1%)
(1983): Naschitz JE+, *J Toxicol Clin Toxicol* 20, 367

Tremor (2%)

QUININE

Trade names: Formula-Q; Legatrin (Columbia), M-KYA; Q-Vel; Quiphile (Geneva)
Other common trade names: *Adaquin; Chinine; Genin; Quinate; Quinoctal; Quinsan; Quinsul*
Indications: Malaria; nocturnal leg cramps
Category: Antiprotozoal and antimyotonic
Half-life: 8–14 hours
Clinically important, potentially serious interactions with: amiodarone, anticoagulants, astemizole, beta-blockers, cimetidine, coumarin, digoxin, mefloquine, quinidine, terfenadine, verapamil

Reactions

Skin

Acne
(1981): Burkhart CC, *Arch Dermatol* 117, 603
(1967): Hitch JM, *JAMA* 200, 879

Angioedema (<1%)

Bullous eruption

Contact dermatitis
(1994): Tapadinhas C+, *Contact Dermatitis* 31, 127 (from hair lotion)
(1994): Isaksson M+, *Acta Derm Venereol* 74, 286
(1994): Dias M+, *Contact Dermatitis* 30, 121
(1978): Hardie RA+, *Contact Dermatitis* 4, 121 (occupational)
(1978): Calnan CD+, *Contact Dermatitis* 4, 58
(1961): Calnan CD+, *BMJ* 2, 1750

Diaphoresis

Eczematous eruption (sic)

Erythema

Erythema multiforme (<1%)
(1967): Coleman WP, *Med Clin North Am* 51, 1073

Exanthems (1–5%)
(1969): Török H, *Dermatol Int* 8, 57

Exfoliative dermatitis
(1975): Jarratt M+, *Arch Dermatol* 111, 132
(1974): Callaway JL+, *Arch Dermatol* 109, 909

Facial edema

Fixed eruption
(2000): Litt JZ, Beachwood, OH, personal case (observation)
(1993): Litt JZ, Beachwood, OH, personal case (from quinine water) (observation)
(1990): Gaffoor PMA+, *Cutis* 45, 242 (passim)
(1974): Kuokkanen K, *Int J Dermatol* 13, 4
(1970): Savin JA, *Br J Dermatol* 83, 546
(1967): Kogoj F, *Med Glas* (Serbo-Croatian-Roman) 21, 351
(1961): Welsh AL+, *Arch Dermatol* 84, 1004
(1960): Engelhardt AW, *Hautarzt* (German) 11, 49

Flushing (<1%)

Hyperpigmentation
(1999): Rosen T+, Houston, TX, personal case (observation)

Lichenoid eruption
(1995): Dawson TA, *BMJ* 310, 738
(1989): Tan SV+, *Clin Exp Dermatol* 14, 335
(1987): Ferguson J+, *Br J Dermatol* 117, 631

Lichen planus
(1994): Litt JZ, Beachwood, OH, personal case (observation)
(1986): Meyrick-Thomas RH+, *Clin Exp Dermatol* 11, 97 (in a photosensitive distribution)
(1986): Dawson TAJ, *Clin Exp Dermatol* 11, 670
(1979): Krebs A, *Hautarzt* (German) 30, 281

Livedo racemosa (photosensitive)
(1988): Diffey BL+, *Br J Dermatol* 118, 679

(1974): de Groot WP+, *Dermatologica* 148, 371
(1973): Marion DF, *Arch Dermatol* 108, 100

Lupus erythematosus
(1996): Rosa-Re D+, *Ann Rheum Dis* 55, 559

Ochronosis
(1986): Bruce S+, *J Am Acad Dermatol* 15, 357

Photoreactions

Photosensitivity
(1998): Rademaker M, Hamilton, New Zealand (from Internet) (observation)
(1995): Dawson TA, *BMJ* 310, 738
(1995): Delmas A+, *Presse Med* (French) 24, 1707
(1994): Wagner GH+, *Br J Dermatol* 131, 734 (from tonic water)
(1994): Isaksson M+, *Acta Derm Venereol* 74, 286
(1994): Okun MM+, *Clin Exp Dermatol* 19, 246 (mycosis-fungoides-like)
(1994): Litt JZ, Beachwood, OH, personal case (observation)
(1992): Ljunggren B+, *Contact Dermatitis* 26, 1
(1992): Fitzpatrick JE, *Dermatol Clin* 10, 19
(1990): Guzzo C+, *Photodermatol Photoimmunol Photomed* 7, 166
(1988): Diffey BL+, *Br J Dermatol* 118, 679
(1987): Ferguson J+, *Br J Dermatol* 117, 631
(1986): Ljunggren B+, *Arch Dermatol* 122, 909
(1986): Ljunggren B+, *Photodermatol* 3, 26
(1986): Dawson TAJ, *Clin Exp Dermatol* 11, 670 (lichenoid)
(1984): Jeanmougin M+, *Ann Dermatol Venereol* (French) 11, 565
(1978): Calnan CD+, *Contact Dermatitis* 4, 58
(1975): Johnson BE+, *Br J Dermatol* 93 (Suppl 11), 21
(1969): Kalivas J, *JAMA* 209, 1706

Pigmentation
(1994): Litt JZ, Beachwood, OH, personal case (observation)
(1986): Mahler R+, *Arch Dermatol* 122, 1062
(1986): Bruce S+, *J Am Acad Dermatol* 15, 357 (from injections)
(1964): Dummett CO, *J Oral Ther Pharmacol* 1, 106
(1963): Tuffanelli D+, *Arch Dermatol* 88, 419

Pruritus (<1%)

Psoriasis
(1998): Smith KC, Niagara Falls, Canada (from Internet) (observation)

Purpura
(1993): Kaufman DW+, *Blood* 82, 2714
(1985): Ambriz-Fernandez R+, *Rev Invest Clin* (Spanish) 37, 347
(1980): Miescher PA+, *Clin Haematol* 9, 505
(1969): Török H, *Dermatol Int* 8, 57
(1967): Helmly RB+, *Arch Intern Med* 120, 59
(1967): Belkin CA, *Ann Intern Med* 66, 583
(1965): Horowitz HI+, *Semin Hematol* 2, 287
(1962): Weintraub RM+, *JAMA* 180, 528
(1952): Lincoln RB+, *Am Pract* 3, 42
(1946): Schrager J+, *Am J Med Sci* 212, 54

Rash (sic) (<1%)
(1993): Siderov J, *J Am Geriatr Soc* 41, 498

Stevens–Johnson syndrome
(1986): Gascon-Brustenga J+, *Med Clin (Barc)* (Spanish) 87, 821
(1967): Coleman WP, *Med Clin North Am* 51, 1073

Toxic epidermal necrolysis (<1%)
(1975): Jarratt M+, *Arch Dermatol* 111, 132
(1974): Callaway JL+, *Arch Dermatol* 109, 909 (tonic water)

Urticaria
(1969): Török H, *Dermatol Int* 8, 57

Vasculitis
(1992): Price EJ+, *Br J Clin Pract* 46, 138
(1991): Harland CC+, *BMJ* 302, 295
(1990): Mathur S+, *BMJ* 300, 613
(1968): Rockl H+, *Munch Med Wochenschr* (German) 110, 2549
(1952): Lincoln RB+, *Am Pract* 3, 42

Vitiligo
(1998): Rademaker M, Hamilton, New Zealand (from Internet) (observation) (following photosensitivity)

Nails

Nails – photo-onycholysis
(1989): Tan SV+, *Clin Exp Dermatol* 14, 335

Other

Hypersensitivity (<1%)
(1998): Schattner A, *Am J Med* 104–488

Oral mucosal eruption
(1964): Dummett CO, *J Oral Ther Pharmacol* 1, 106

Oral ulceration

Porphyria
(1971): Sayag J+, *Bull Soc Franc Dermatol Syphiligr* (French) 78, 664

QUINUPRISTIN/DALFOPRISTIN

Synonym: pristinamycin; RP59500
Trade name: Synercid (Aventis)
Indications: Serious life-threatening bacterial infections
Category: Streptogramin antibiotic
Half-life: 1.3–1.5 hours
Clinically important, potentially serious interactions with: astemizole, cisapride, cyclosporine, midazolam, nifedipine, terfenadine

Reactions

Skin

Allergic reactions (sic) (<1%)
Candidiasis (<1%)
Diaphoresis (<1%)
Exanthems (<1%)
Peripheral edema (<1%)
Pruritus (1.5%)
Rash (sic) (2.5%)
Ulceration (<1%)
Urticaria (<1%)

Other

Anaphylactoid reaction (<1%)
Infusion-site edema (17.3%)
Infusion-site inflammation (42%)
Infusion-site pain (40%)
Infusion-site reactions (sic) (13.4%)
Myalgia (<1–5%)
Oral candidiasis (<1%)
Paresthesias (<1%)
Phlebitis (<1%)
Stomatitis (<1%)
Thrombophlebitis (2.4%)
Tremor (<1%)
Vaginitis (<1%)

RABEPRAZOLE

Synonym: pariprazole
Trade name: Aciphex (Janssen)
Indications: Gastroesophageal reflux disease (GERD)
Category: Proton pump (gastric acid secretion) inhibitor
Half-life: 1–2 hours
Clinically important, potentially serious interactions with: ampicillin, cyclosporine, diazepam, digoxin, itraconazole, ketoconazole

Reactions

Skin
- Allergic reactions (sic) (<1%)
- Chills (<1%)
- Diaphoresis (<1%)
- Ecchymoses (<1%)
- Edema
- Eruptions (sic) (<1%)
- Facial edema (<1%)
- Herpes zoster (<1%)
- Peripheral edema (<1%)
- Photosensitivity (<1%)
- Pigmentation (<1%)
- Pruritus (<1%)
- Psoriasis (<1%)
- Purpura
- Rash (sic) (<1%)
- Urticaria (<1%)
- Xerosis (<1%)

Hair
- Hair – alopecia (<1%)

Other
- Gingivitis (<1%)
- Glossitis (<1%)
- Gynecomastia (<1%)
- Myalgia (<1%)
- Oral ulceration
- Paresthesias (<1%)
- Stomatitis (<1%)
- Thrombophlebitis (<1%)
- Tremor (<1%)
- Twitching (<1%)
- Xerostomia (<1%)

RALOXIFENE

Synonym: Keoxifene
Trade name: Evista (Lilly)
Indications: Osteoporosis
Category: Selective estrogen receptor modulator
Half-life: 27.7 hours
Clinically important, potentially serious interactions with: ampicillin, anticoagulants, cholestyramine, clofibrate, diazepam, diazoxide, ibuprofen, indomethacin, naproxen, warfarin

Reactions

Skin
- Diaphoresis (3.1%)
- Edema
- Flu-like syndrome (sic) (~2%)
- Hot flashes (24.6%)
  - (1999): Scott JA+, *Am Fam Physician* 60, 1131
  - (1999): Ettinger B+, *JAMA* 282, 637 (10%)
  - (1998): Walsh BW+, *JAMA* 279, 1445 (22%)
- Infection (sic) (~2%)
- Peripheral edema (3.3%)
  - (1999): Ettinger B+, *JAMA* 282, 637 (5%)
  - (1999): Cummings SR+, *JAMA* 281, 2189
- Rash (sic) (5.5%)

Other
- Mastodynia (4.4%)
  - (1999): Cummings SR+, *JAMA* 281, 2189
  - (1998): Walsh BW+, *JAMA* 279, 1445 (4%)
- Myalgia (7.7%)
- Vaginitis (4.3%)

RAMIPRIL

Trade name: Altace (Monarch)
Other common trade names: *Delix; Hytren; Pramace; Quark; Ramace; Triatec; Tritace; Unipril*
Indications: Hypertension
Category: Angiotensin-converting enzyme (ACE) inhibitor; antihypertensive and vasodilator
Half-life: 3–17 hours
Clinically important, potentially serious interactions with: alcohol, allopurinol, digoxin, furosemide, indomethacin, insulin, lithium, NSAIDs, phenothiazines, potassium-sparing diuretics, salicylates

Reactions

Skin
- Acne
  - (1987): Predel HG+, *Am J Cardiol* 59, 143D
- Angioedema (0.3%)
  - (1995): Epeldo-Gonzalo F+, *Ann Pharmacother* 29, 431
  - (1990): Todd PA+, *Drugs* 39, 110
- Dermatitis (sic) (<1%)
- Diaphoresis (<1%)
  - (1988): Zabludowski J+, *Curr Med Res Opin* 11, 93
  - (1987): Walter U+, *Am J Cardiol* 59, 125D
- Dry feeling on face (sic)
  - (1987): Fukiyama K+, *Am J Cardiol* 59, 121D
- Edema (<1%)
  - (1990): Todd PA+, *Drugs* 39, 110
- Erythema (circumscribed) (sic)
  - (1987): Predel HG+, *Am J Cardiol* 59, 143D
- Erythema multiforme (<1%)
- Exanthems
  - (1990): Todd PA+, *Drugs* 39, 110
- Flushing
  - (1988): Zabludowski J+, *Curr Med Res Opin* 11, 93
  - (1987): Kaneko Y+, *Am J Cardiol* 59, 86D
- Lichen planus pemphigoides
  - (1997): Ogg GS+, *Br J Dermatol* 136, 412
- Pemphigus (<1%)
  - (1996): Vignes S+, *Br J Dermatol* 135, 657
- Photosensitivity (<1%)
  - (1994): Shelley WB+, *Cutis* 53, 39 (observation)
  - (1993): Shelley WB+, *Cutis* 52, 81 (observation)
- Pruritus (<1%)
  - (1990): Todd PA+, *Drugs* 39, 110
  - (1987): Predel HG+, *Am J Cardiol* 59, 143D
  - (1987): Walter U+, *Am J Cardiol* 59, 125D
- Purpura (<1%)
- Rash (sic) (<1%)
  - (1990): Janka HU+, *Arzneimittelforschung* (German) 40, 432
  - (1990): Todd PA+, *Drugs* 39, 110
  - (1987): Walter U+, *Am J Cardiol* 59, 125D
  - (1987): Ball SG+, *Am J Cardiol* 59, 23D
- Urticaria (<1%)
- Vasculitis (<1%)

Hair
- Hair – alopecia (1–10%)

Other

Ageusia (<1%)
Anaphylactoid reaction (<1%)
Dysgeusia (<1%)
(1990): Todd PA+, *Drugs* 39, 110
Hypersensitivity (<1%)
Paresthesias (<1%)
(1987): Walter U+, *Am J Cardiol* 59, 125D
Sialorrhea (<1%)
Tremor (<1%)
Xerostomia (<1%)

RANITIDINE

Trade name: Zantac (GlaxoWellcome; Warner Lambert)
Other common trade names: *Apo-Ranitidine; Axoban; Azantac; Nu-Ranit; Raniben; Raniplex; Ranisen; Sostril; Zantab; Zantac-C; Zantic*
Indications: Duodenal ulcer
Category: Histamine H_2-receptor antagonist; antiulcer drug
Half-life: 2.5 hours
Clinically important, potentially serious interactions with: cyclosporine, diazepam, fentanyl, gentamicin, glipizide, glyburide, ketoconazole, metoprolol, midazolam, nifedipine, pentoxifylline, phenytoin, quinidine, quinolones, warfarin

Note: Ranitidine is present in mother's milk in relatively large amounts. It is thought that gynecomastia develops as a result of ranitidine blocking the androgen receptors at the end organs.

Reactions

Skin

Acute generalized exanthematous pustulosis (AGEP)
(1996): Sawhney RA+, *Int J Dermatol* 35, 826
Angioedema (<1%)
Contact dermatitis
(1988): Romaguera C+, *Contact Dermatitis* 18, 177
(1987): Alomar A+, *Contact Dermatitis* 17, 54
(1984): Goh CL+, *Contact Dermatitis* 4, 252
(1983): Rycroft RJ, *Contact Dermatitis* 9, 456 (occupational)
Eczematous eruption (sic)
(1992): Juste S+, *Contact Dermatitis* 27, 339
(1988): Romaguera C+, *Contact Dermatitis* 18, 177
Erythema multiforme
Exanthems
(1993): Devuyst O+, *Acta Clin Belg* 48, 109
(1989): Grant SM+, *Drugs* 37, 801
(1988): Haboubi N+, *Br Med J Clin Res Ed* 296, 897
(1984): Khandheria BK, *JAMA* 253, 3252
Fixed eruption
(1990): Black AK+, *Br J Dermatol* 123, 277
Lichenoid eruption
(1996): Horiuchi Y+, *J Dermatol* 23, 510
Photosensitivity
(1995): Todd P+, *Clin Exp Dermatol* 20, 146
Pruritus (<1%)
(1985): Classen M+, *Dtsch Med Wochenschr* (German) 110, 628
Psoriasis
(1991): Andersen M, *Ugeskr Laeger* (Danish) 153, 132
Purpura
(1989): Gafter U+, *Gastroenterol* 84, 560
(1987): Gafter U+, *Ann Intern Med* 106, 477
Pustular eruption
Rash (sic) (1–10%)
(1988): Haboubi N+, *Br Med J Clin Res Ed* 296, 897
Stevens–Johnson syndrome
Toxic epidermal necrolysis
(2000): Velez A+, *J Am Acad Dermatol* 42, 305
(1995): Miralles ES+, *J Am Acad Dermatol* 32, 133
Urticaria
(1997): Sancho Calabuig A+, *Aten Primaria* 20, 396
(1989): Grant SM+, *Drugs* 37, 801
(1984): Khandheria BK, *JAMA* 253, 3252
(1983): Picardo M+, *Contact Dermatitis* 4, 327
Vasculitis
(1988): Haboubi N+, *BMJ* 296, 897
Xerosis

Hair

Hair – alopecia
(1995): Shelley WB+, *Cutis* 55, 148 (observation)

Other

Anaphylactoid reaction
(1993): Lazaro M+, *Allergy* 48, 385
(1993): Powell JA+, *Anaesth Intensive Care* 21, 702
Dysgeusia
(1985): Classen M+, *Dtsch Med Wochenschr* (German) 110, 628
Gynecomastia (>1%)
(1994): Garcia-Rodriguez LA+, *BMJ* 308, 503
(1984): Bianchi Porro G+, *It J Gastroenterol* (Italian) 16, 56
(1982): Tosi S+, *Lancet* 2, 160
Hypersensitivity
(1996): Gonzalo-Garijo MA+, *Allergy* 51, 659
Injection-site burning
Injection-site pain
Myalgia
Porphyria
(1988): Tripathi SK, *J Assoc Physicians India* 36, 680
(1988): Bhadoria DP+, *J Assoc Physicians India* 36, 295
(1988): Pratap D+, *J Assoc Physicians India* 36, 237
Pseudolymphoma
(1995): Magro CM+, *J Am Acad Dermatol* 32, 419

REPAGLINIDE

Trade name: Prandin (Novo Nordisk)
Indications: Non-insulin dependent diabetes type II
Category: Antidiabetic
Half-life: 1 hour
Clinically important, potentially serious interactions with: barbiturates, beta-blockers, carbamazepine, erythromycin, hydantoins, ketoconazole, MAO inhibitors, miconazole, NSAIDs, probenecid, rifampin, salicylates, sulfonamides, troglitazone, warfarin

Reactions

Skin

Allergy (sic) (2%)

Other

Anaphylactoid reaction (<1%)
Paresthesias (3%)
Tooth disorder (sic)

RESERPINE

Trade names: Resa; Ser-Ap-Es (Novartis); Serpalan; Serpasil (Ciba); Serpatabs
Other common trade names: *Anserpin; Inerpin; Novo-Reserpine; Reserfia; Sedaraupin; Serpasol; Tionsera*
Indications: Hypertension
Category: Nondiuretic antihypertensive; rauwolfia alkaloid
Half-life: 50–100 hours
Clinically important, potentially serious interactions with: levodopa, MAO inhibitors, sympathomimetics, tricyclic antidepressants

Ser-Ap-Es is reserpine, hydralazine and hydrochlorothiazide

Reactions

Skin

Ankle edema
Bullous eruption
(1994): Watanabe S+, *Reg Anesth* 19, 59 (following intravenous block)

Edema
Exanthems
Flushing
Lupus erythematosus (exacerbation)
(1963): Rivero I+, *Arthritis Rheum* 6, 293
Parkinsonism
Peripheral edema (1–10%)
Pruritus
Purpura
Rash (sic) (<1%)
Toxic epidermal necrolysis
(1979): Kats GL+, *Vrach Delo* (Russian) November, 97
Urticaria

Other

Gynecomastia
Sialorrhea
Xerostomia (>10%)

RETEPLASE

Synonyms: recombinant plasminogen activator; r-PA
Trade name: Retavase (Centocor)
Indications: Acute myocardial infarction
Category: Tissue plasminogen activator; thrombolytic agent
Half-life: 13–16 minutes
Clinically important, potentially serious interactions with: abciximab, anticoagulants, aspirin, dipyridamole, heparin, NSAIDs, ticlopidine, valproic acid, warfarin

Reactions

Skin

Allergic reactions (sic) (<1%)
Bleeding
Ecchymoses
Purpura

Other

Anaphylactoid reaction (<1%)
Injection-site bleeding (1–10%)

RIBAVIRIN

Synonyms: RTCA; tribavirin
Trade names: Rebetol; Rebetron (Schering); Virazole (ICN)
Other common trade names: *Viramid; Virazid*
Indications: Respiratory syncytial viral infections
Category: Antiviral (against respiratory syncytial virus [RSV])
Half-life: 24 hours
Clinically important, potentially serious interactions with: zidovudine

Rebetron is interferon and ribavirin

Reactions

Skin

Erythema multiforme
(1960): Heijer A+, *Acta Derm Venereol* (Stockh) 40, 35
Exanthems
(1990): Janai HK+, *Pediatr Infect Dis J* 9, 209 (0.5%)
Flu-like syndrome (sic) (10%)*
Grover's disease
(2000): Antunes I+, *Br J Dermatol* 142, 1257
Herpes simplex (activation)
Photosensitivity
(1999): Stryjek-Kaminska D+, *Am J Gastroenterol* 94, 1686
Pruritus (>10%)*
(1999): Stryjek-Kaminska D+, *Am J Gastroenterol* 94, 1686
Rash (sic) (<10%)*
Urticaria
(1999): Stryjek-Kaminska D+, *Am J Gastroenterol* 94, 1686

Hair

Hair – alopecia (>10%)*

Skin

Dysgeusia (1–10%)*
Myalgia (>10%)*

***Note:** Please note that the reaction patterns with the asterisk occurred while receiving combination therapy with interferon alpha 2-b.

RIBOFLAVIN

Synonyms: Lactoflavin; Vitamin B_2; Vitamin G
Trade name: Riobin
Indications: Riboflavin deficiency
Category: Water-soluble nutritional supplement
Half-life: 66–84 minutes
Clinically important, potentially serious interactions with: probenecid

Reactions

Skin

Acne
(1964): Fegeler F, *Arch Klin Exp Dermatol* (German) 219, 335
Allergic reactions (sic)
(1975): Soloshenko EN+, *Sov Med* (Russian) October, 141
Angioedema
(1972): Kuokkanen K, *Acta Allergol* 27, 407
Ichthyosis
(1985): Spirov G+, *Dermatol Venereol* (Sofia) 24, 50
Urticaria
(1972): Kuokkanen K, *Acta Allergol* 27, 407

RIFABUTIN

Trade name: Mycobutin (Pharmacia & Upjohn)
Indications: Prevention of disseminated mycobacterium avium infection
Category: Antitubercular antibiotic
Half-life: 45 hours
Clinically important, potentially serious interactions with: anticoagulants, benzodiazepines, beta-blockers, bisoprolol, chloramphenicol, clarithromycin, corticosteroids, cyclosporine, disopyramide, erythromycin, hydantoins, indinavir, itraconazole, ketoconazole, oral contraceptives, protease inhibitors, quinidine, ritonavir, sulfonylureas, tacrolimus, theophylline, zidovudine

Reactions

Skin

Lupus erythematosus
(1997): Berning SE+, *Lancet* 349, 1521
Pigmentation
(1995): Smith JF+, *Clin Infect Dis* 21, 1515
Rash (sic) (11%)
Urticaria

Other

Ageusia
(1993): Morris JT+, *Ann Intern Med* 119, 171
Discolored sputum (sic)
Dysgeusia (3%)
Myalgia (2%)
Paresthesias (<1%)

RIFAMPIN

Synonym: rifampicin
Trade names: Rifadin (Aventis); Rimactane (Geneva)
Other common trade names: *Abrifam; Corifam; Ramicin; Rifaldin; Rifamed; Rimpin; Rimycin; Rofact*
Indications: Tuberculosis
Category: Tuberculostatic and antileprotic antibiotic
Half-life: 3–5 hours
Clinically important, potentially serious interactions with: anticoagulants, amprenavir, barbiturates, benzodiazepines, beta-blockers, chloramphenicol, corticosteroids, cyclosporine, digoxin, diltiazem, enalapril, hydantoins, isoniazid, ketoconazole, methadone, non-nucleoside reverse transcriptase inhibitors, oral contraceptives, phenytoin, probenecid, quinidine, ritonavir, sertraline, tacrolimus, theophylline, verapamil

Reactions

Skin

Acne
(1990): Mimouni A+, *Drug Intell Clin Pharm* 24, 947
(1985): Holdiness MR, *Int J Dermatol* 24, 280
(1974): Nwokolo U, *BMJ* 3, 473 (1–5%) (only men)
Angioedema
(1989): Holdiness MR, *Med Toxicol Adv Drug Exp* 4, 444 (72%)
Bullous eruption (<1%)
Contact dermatitis
(1986): Milpied B+, *Contact Dermatitis* 14, 252
(1986): Holdiness MR. *Contact Dermatitis* 15, 282
Cutaneous side effects (sic)
(1985): Holdiness MR, *Int J Dermatol* 24, 280 (5%)
Diaphoresis (1–10%)
Erythema multiforme (<1%)
(1990): Mimouni A+, *Drug Intell Clin Pharm* 24, 947
(1988): Hira SK+, *J Am Acad Dermatol* 19, 451 (in AIDS patients)
(1979): Nigam P+, *Lepr India* 51, 249
(1977): Nyirenda R+, *BMJ* 2, 1189
Exanthems (1–5%)
(1998): Zimmerli W+, *JAMA* 279, 1537
(1989): Wurtz RM+, *Lancet* 1, 955 (in AIDS patients)
(1985): Holdiness MR, *Int J Dermatol* 24, 280
(1976): Mangi RJ, *N Engl J Med* 294, 113 (3%)
(1971): Esposito R+, *Lancet* 2, 491 (1–5%)
(1971): Poole G+, *BMJ* 3, 343 (1–5%)
Exfoliative dermatitis
(1987): Goldin HM+, *Ann Intern Med* 107, 789
Facial edema
Fixed eruption
(2000): Jaiswal AK+, *Lepr Rev* 71, 217
(1998): John SS, *Lepr Rev* 69, 397
(1993): Pavithran K, *Indian J Lepr* 65, 339
(1990): Mimouni A+, *Drug Intell Clin Pharm* 24, 947
(1985): Naik RPC+, *Indian J Lepr* 57, 648
Flushing
(1995): Hoss DM+, *Arch Dermatol* 131, 647
(1993): Tsankov NK+, *Int J Dermatol* 32, 401 (passim)
(1990): Mimouni A+, *Drug Intell Clin Pharm* 24, 947
(1985): Holdiness MR, *Int J Dermatol* 24, 280
(1982): Girling DJ, *Drugs* 23, 56 (5%)
(1976): Mangi RJ, *N Engl J Med* 294, 113 (7%)
(1972): Girling HM+, *BMJ* 1, 765
(1971): Girling DJ+, *BMJ* 4, 231
Linear IgA bullous dermatosis
(1994): Kuechle MK+, *J Am Acad Dermatol* 30, 187
Pemphigus
(1995): Hoss DM+, *Arch Dermatol* 131, 647
(1993): Tsankov NK+, *Int J Dermatol* 32, 401 (passim)
(1987): Honeybourne D+, *Br J Clin Pract* 41, 937
(1986): Miyagawa S+, *Br J Dermatol* 114, 729 (exacerbation)
(1984): Lee CW+, *Br J Dermatol* 111, 619 (foliaceus)
(1982): Ruocco V+, *Arch Dermatol Res* 274, 123
(1976): Gange RW+, *Br J Dermatol* 95, 445
Pruritus (<1%)
(1995): Hoss DM+, *Arch Dermatol* 131, 647
(1995): Walker-Renard P, *Ann Pharmacother* 29, 267
(1993): Tsankov NK+, *Int J Dermatol* 32, 401 (passim)
(1989): Holdiness MR, *Med Toxicol Adv Drug Exp* 4, 444 (62%)
(1987): Goldin HM+, *Ann Intern Med* 107, 789
(1972): Girling HM+, *BMJ* 1, 765
(1971): Girling DJ+, *BMJ* 4, 231
Purpura
(1980): Miescher PA+, *Clin Haematol* 9, 505
(1972): Girling HM+, *BMJ* 1, 765 (0.5–1%)
(1971): Esposito R+, *Lancet* 2, 491
(1971): Girling DJ+, *BMJ* 4, 231 (0.5–1%)
(1971): Poole G+, *BMJ* 3, 343
(1970): Blajckman MA+, *BMJ* 3, 24
Rash (sic) (1–5%)
(2000): Gordin F+, *JAMA* 283, 1445
(1995): Chaisson RE, *Infections in Medicine* 12, 48
Red man syndrome
(1995): Dayavathi+, *J Assoc Physicians India* 43, 724
(1992): Gupta M+, *Indian Pediatr* 29, 1315
(1989): Holdiness MR, *Med Toxicol Adv Drug Exp* 4, 444
(1988): Gross DJ+, *Cutis* 42, 175 (red/orange person syndrome)
(1986): Bolan G+, *Pediatrics* 77, 633
(1980): Meisel S+, *Ann Intern Med* 92, 262
(1975): Newton RW+, *Scott Med J* 20, 55
Stevens–Johnson syndrome
(1994): Marfatia YS, *Arch Dermatol* 130, 1074 (passim)
(1993): Tsankov NK+, *Int J Dermatol* 32, 401 (passim)
(1988): Hira SK+, *J Am Acad Dermatol* 19, 451 (in AIDS patients)
(1977): Nyirenda R+, *BMJ* 2, 1189
Toxic epidermal necrolysis
(1996): Blum L+, *J Am Acad Dermatol* 34, 1088
(1994): Marfatia YS, *Arch Dermatol* 130, 1074 (passim)
(1990): Prazuck T+, *Scand J Infect Dis* 22, 629
(1987): Guillaume JC+, *Arch Dermatol* 123, 1166
(1987): Okano M+, *J Am Acad Dermatol* 17, 303
Urticaria
(1997): Sharma VK+, *Lepr Rev* 68, 331
(1987): Gupta CM+, *Lepr Rev* 58, 308
(1985): Holdiness MR, *Int J Dermatol* 24, 280
(1972): Girling HM+, *BMJ* 1, 765
(1971): Girling DJ+, *BMJ* 4, 231
Vasculitis
(1995): Hoss DM+, *Arch Dermatol* 131, 647
(1990): Chan CH+, *Tubercle* 71, 297
(1989): Iredale JP+, *Chest* 96, 215

Other

Anaphylactoid reaction
(1999): Garcia F+, *Allergy* 54, 527 (to topical)
(1989): Wurtz RM+, *Lancet* 1, 955 (in AIDS patients)
Glossodynia
Injection-site erythema
(1988): Fan-Havard P+, *Clin Pharm* 7, 616
Mucosal bleeding (sic)
(1971): Poole G+, *BMJ* 3, 343
Myalgia
Myopathy
Oral mucosal eruption
(1971): Poole G+, *BMJ* 3, 343
Porphyria
(1985): Holdiness MR, *Int J Dermatol* 24, 280
(1982): Igual JP+, *Presse Med* (French) 11, 2846
Porphyria cutanea tarda
(1980): Millar JW, *Br J Dis Chest* 74, 405
Serum sickness
(1994): Parra FM+, *Ann Allergy* 73, 123
Stomatitis (<1%)

RIFAPENTINE

Trade name: Priften (Aventis)
Indications: Tuberculosis
Category: Antitubercular antibiotic
Half-life: 14–17 hours
Clinically important, potentially serious interactions with: anticoagulants, barbiturates, benzodiazepines, beta-blockers, chloramphenicol, corticosteroids, cyclosporine, digoxin, diltiazem, enalapril, hydantoins, isoniazid, ketoconazole, methadone, oral contraceptives, phenytoin, probenecid, protease inhibitors, quinidine, sildenafil, tacrolimus, theophylline, verapamil, zidovudine

Reactions

Skin

Acne (1–10%)
Peripheral edema (<1%)
Pigmentation (<1%)
Purpura (<1%)
Pruritus (1–10%)
Rash (sic) (1–10%)
Urticaria (<1%)

RILUZOLE

Synonym: RP54274
Trade name: Rilutek (Aventis)
Indications: Amyotrophic lateral sclerosis (ALS)
Category: Amyotrophic lateral sclerosis (ALS) agent
Half-life: no data
Clinically important, potentially serious interactions with: amitriptyline, caffeine, omeprazole, quinolones, rifampin, tacrine, theophylline, **cigarette smoking**

Reactions

Skin

Candidiasis
Cellulitis
Chills
Eczema (sic) (1.6%)
Edema
Exfoliative dermatitis
Facial edema
Granuloma (sic)
Peripheral edema (3%)
Petechiae
Photosensitivity
Pruritus
Purpura

Hair

Hair – alopecia (1%)

Other

Dysgeusia
Glossitis
Gum hemorrhage
Hypesthesia
Injection-site reaction
Mastodynia
Oral candidiasis (0.6%)
Paresthesias
Phlebitis (1%)
Stomatitis (1%)
Tongue discoloration
Tooth disorder (sic) (1%)
Vaginal candidiasis
Xerostomia (3.5%)

RIMANTADINE

Trade name: Flumadine (Forest)
Other common trade name: *Ruflual*
Indications: Various infections caused by the influenza virus
Category: Oral antiviral
Half-life: 25–30 hours
Clinically important, potentially serious interactions with: acetaminophen, aspirin, cimetidine

Reactions

Skin

Edema (pedal) (1–10%)
Rash (sic) (<1%)
(1989): Hayden FG+, *N Engl J Med* 321, 1696 (1%)

Other

Ageusia (<0.3%)
Dysgeusia
Hypesthesia
Parosmia (<0.3%)
Stomatitis
Xerostomia (1.6%)

RISEDRONATE

Trade name: Actonel (Procter & Gamble)
Indications: Paget's disease of bone; postmenopausal osteoporosis
Category: Biphosphonate bone-resorption inhibitor
Half-life: terminal: 220 hours
Clinically important, potentially serious interactions with: antacids, calcium supplements, NSAIDs

Reactions

Skin

Ecchymoses (4.3%)
Edema
Flu-like syndrome (sic) (9.8%)
Peripheral edema (8.2%)
Pruritus (3.0%)
Rash (sic) (11.5%)

Other

Glossitis (<1%)
Myalgia (6.6%)
Paresthesias (2.1%)
Tendon disorder (sic) (3.0%)
Tooth disorder (sic) (2.1%)

RISPERIDONE

Trade name: Risperdal (Janssen)
Indications: Psychotic disorders
Category: Antipsychotic
Half-life: 3–30 hours
Clinically important, potentially serious interactions with: alcohol, beta-blockers, bromocriptine, carbamazepine, clozapine, CNS depressants, levodopa, quinidine, warfarin

Reactions

Skin

Acne (<1%)
Allergic reactions (<1%)
(1998): Terao T+, *J Clin Psychiatry* 59, 82

Angioedema
(1995): Cooney C+, *BMJ* 311, 1204
Bullous eruption (<1%)
Bullous pemphigoid
(1996): Wijeratne C+, *Am J Psychiatry* 153, 735
Dermatitis (sic)
Diaphoresis (<1%)
Edema
(1996): Baldassano CF+, *J Clin Psychiatry* 57, 422 (generalized)
Exfoliative dermatitis (0.1–1%)
Flushing (<1%)
Furunculosis (<1%)
Hyperkeratosis (sic) (<1%)
Hypohidrosis (<1%)
Lichenoid eruption (<1%)
Parkinsonism
Photosensitivity (1–10%)
(1998): Almond DS+, *Postgrad Med J* 74, 252
Pigmentation (1%)
Pruritus (<1%)
Psoriasis (<1%)
Purpura (<1%)
Rash (sic) (5%)
Seborrhea
Ulceration (<1%)
Urticaria (<0.1%)
Warts (<1%)
Xerosis (2%)

Hair

Hair – alopecia (<1%)
(2000): Mercke Y+, *Ann Clin Psychiatry* 12, 35
Hair – hypertrichosis (<1%)

Other

Anaphylactoid reaction
Dysgeusia (<1%)
Galactorrhea (1–10%)
(1998): Popli A+, *Ann Clin Psychiatry* 10, 31
Gingivitis (<1%)
Gynecomastia (1–10%)
(1999): Benazzi F, *Pharmacopsychiatry* 32, 41
Hypesthesia (<1%)
Mastodynia (<1%)
Myalgia (<1%)
Paresthesias (<1%)
Priapism (1–10%)
Sialopenia (5%)
Sialorrhea (2%)
Stomatitis (<1%)
Thrombophlebitis (<1%)
Tongue edema (<1%)
Tongue pigmentation (<1%)
Xerostomia (1–10%)

RITODRINE

Trade names: Pre-Par; Yutopar (AstraZeneca)
Indications: Preterm labor
Category: Tocolytic (uterine relaxant); adrenergic agonist
Half-life: 1.3–12 hours
Clinically important, potentially serious interactions with: atropine, beta-blockers, corticosteroids, diazoxide, diuretics, meperidine

Reactions

Skin

Chills (3–10%)
Diaphoresis (1–3%)
(1978): Hauser GA, *Ther Umsch* (German) 35, 422 (3–14%)
Erythema (10–15%)
Erythema multiforme
(1988): Beitner O+, *Drug Intell Clin Pharm* 22, 724
Exanthems
Pustular eruption (in a pregnant woman with psoriasis)
(1998): D'Incan M+, *J Eur Acad Dermatol Venereol* 11, 91
Rash (sic) (1–3%)
Urticaria
Vasculitis
(1991): Bosnyak S+, *Am J Obstet Gyn* 165, 427

Other

Anaphylactoid reaction (1–3%)
Tremor (>10%)

RITONAVIR

Trade name: Norvir (Abbott)
Indications: HIV infection
Category: Antiretroviral; protease inhibitor*
Half-life: 3–5 hours
Clinically important, potentially serious interactions with: amiodarone, amprenavir, astemizole, benzodiazepines, bepridil, bupropion, carbamazepine, cisapride, clozapine, desipramine, flecainide, HMG-CoA reductase inhibitors, indinavir, ketoconazole, meperidine, phenytoin, pimozide, piroxicam, propafenone, propoxyphene, quinidine, rifabutin, rifampin, sildenafil, terfenadine, theophylline, warfarin, etc.

Reactions

Skin

Acne (<2%)
Allergic reactions (sic) (<2%)
Angioedema
Bullous eruption (<2%)
Cheilitis (<2%)
Contact dermatitis (<2%)
Diaphoresis (1–10%)
Ecchymoses (<2%)
Eczema (sic) (<2%)
Edema
Exanthems (<2%)
(1997): Bachmeyer C+, *Dermatology* 195, 301 (in 2 HIV patients)
Facial edema (<2%)
Folliculitis (<2%)
Peripheral edema (<2%)
Photosensitivity (<2%)
Pruritus (<2%)
Psoriasis (<2%)
Rash (sic) (1–10%)
Seborrhea (<2%)
Stevens–Johnson syndrome
Urticaria (<2%)
Xerosis (<2%)

Other

Ageusia (<2%)
Anaphylactoid reaction
Dysgeusia (10.3%)
Gingivitis (<2%)
Hyperesthesia (<2%)
Myalgia (1–10%)
Oral candidiasis (<2%)
Oral ulceration (<2%)
Paresthesias (2.6%)
Parosmia (<2%)
Xerostomia (<2%)

*Protease inhibitors cause dyslipidemia which includes elevated triglycerides and cholesterol and redistribution of body fat centrally to produce the so-called "protease paunch," breast enlargement, facial atrophy, and "buffalo hump."

RITUXIMAB

Trade name: Rituxan (IDEC; Genentech)
Indications: Non-Hodgkin's lymphoma
Category: Monoclonal antibody; antineoplastic
Half-life: 60 hours (after first infusion)
Clinically important, potentially serious interactions with: no data

Reactions

Skin
Angioedema (>10%)
Chills (10%)
Diaphoresis
Exanthems (10%)
Flushing (<5%)
Peripheral edema
Pruritus (10%)
Rash (sic) (10%)
Urticaria (10%)

Other
Myalgia (7%)
Injection-site reactions

RIVASTIGMINE

Trade name: Exelon (Novartis)
Indications: Alzheimer's disease and dementia
Category: Acetylcholinesterase inhibitor, cholinergic agent
Half-life: 1–2 hours
Clinically important, potentially serious interactions with: atropine, benztropine, bethanechol, calcium channel blockers, donepezil, NSAIDs, tacrine, trihexyphenidyl

Reactions

Skin
Allergy (sic) (~1%)
Bullous eruption (~1%)
Cellulitis (~1%)
Clammy skin (~1%)
Contact dermatitis (~1%)
Diaphoresis (10%)
Edema (~1%)
Exanthems (~1%)
Exfoliative dermatitis (~1%)
Facial edema (~1%)
Flushing (~1%)
Herpes simplex (~1%)
Hot flashes (~1%)
Infection (sic) (~2%)
Peripheral edema (~2%)
Periorbital edema (~1%)
Psoriasis (~1%)
Purpura (~1%)
Rash (sic) (~2%)
Ulceration (~1%)
Urticaria (~1%)

Hair
Hair – alopecia (~1%)

Other
Ageusia (~1%)
Dysgeusia (~1%)
Foetor ex ore (halitosis) (~1%)
Gingivitis (~1%)
Glossitis (~1%)
Hypesthesia (~1%)
Paresthesias (~1%)
Mastodynia (~1%)
Myalgia (20%)
Sialorrhea (~1%)
Thrombophlebitis (<2%)
Tremor (4%)
Ulcerative stomatitis (~1%)
Vaginitis (~1%)
Xerostomia (~1%)

RIZATRIPTAN

Synonym: MK462
Trade name: Maxalt (Merck)
Indications: Migraine
Category: Antimigraine; serotonin agonist
Half-life: 2–3 hours
Clinically important, potentially serious interactions with: ergot-containing drugs, MAO inhibitors, propranolol, SSRIs

Reactions

Skin
Chills (<1%)
Diaphoresis (<1%)
Facial edema (<1%)
Flushing (1–10%)
Hot flashes (1–10%)
Pruritus (<1%)

Other
Hypesthesia
Myalgia (<1%)
Paresthesias
Tongue edema
Xerostomia (<5%)

ROFECOXIB

Trade name: Vioxx (Merck)
Indications: Osteoarthritis, acute pain
Category: Nonsteroidal anti-inflammatory (Cox-2 inhibitor); analgesic
Half-life: 17 hours
Clinically important, potentially serious interactions with: ACE-inhibitors, aspirin, cimetidine, corticosteroids, diuretics, lithium, methotrexate, rifampin, thiazide diuretics, warfarin

Reactions

Skin
Abrasion (<2%)
Allergy (sic)(<2%)
Angioedema
(2000): Medicines Control Agency and Committee on Safety of Medicines Reports (5 cases)
Atopic dermatitis (<2%)
Basal cell carcinoma (<2%)
Bullous eruption (<2%)
Cellulitis (<2%)
Contact dermatitis (<2%)
Diaphoresis (<2%)
Edema (3.7%)
(2000): Medicines Control Agency and Committee on Safety of Medicines Reports (101 cases)
Erythema (<2%)
(2000): Wright WL, Castro Valley, CA, (from Internet) (observation) (after the second day)
Exanthems
(2000): Blumenthal HL, Beachwood, OH, personal case (observation)

Flu-like syndrome (sic) (2.9%)
Flushing (<2%)
Fungal infection (<2%)
Granuloma annulare
(2000): Rotman H, Houston, TX (personal communication) (observation)
Herpes simplex (<2%)
Herpes zoster (<2%)
Peripheral edema (6%)
Photosensitivity
(2000): Valentine M, Everett, WA (from Internet) (observation)
(1999): Gregg LJ, Tulsa, OK (from Internet) (observation)
Pruritus (<2%)
Rash (sic)(<2%)
Urticaria (<2%)
(2000): Wright WL, Castro Valley, CA, (from Internet) (2 observations) (after the second day)
Xerosis (<2%)

Hair

Hair – alopecia (<2%)

Nails

Nails – disorder (sic)(<2%)

Other

Aphthous stomatitis (<2%)
Hypesthesia (<2%)
Myalgia (<2%)
Oral ulceration (<2%)
Paresthesias (<2%)
Tendinitis (<2%)
Xerostomia (<2%)

ROPINIROLE

Trade name: Requip (SmithKline Beecham)
Indications: Parkinsonism
Category: Antiparkinsonian; dopamine agonist
Half-life: ~6 hours
Clinically important, potentially serious interactions with: cimetidine, ciprofloxacin, CNS depressants, diltiazem, enoxacin, erythromycin, fluvoxamine, metoclopramide, mexiletine, norfloxacin, omeprazole, phenothiazines, tacrine, thioxanthenes

Reactions

Skin

Balanoposthitis (<1%)
Basal cell carcinoma (>1%)
Cellulitis (<1%)
Dermatitis (sic) (<1%)
Diaphoresis (6%)
Eczema (sic) (<1%)
Edema (<1%)
Exanthems (<1%)
Flushing (3%)
Fungal dermatitis (sic) (<1%)
Furunculosis (<1%)
Herpes simplex (<1%)
Herpes zoster (<1%)
Hyperkeratosis (<1%)
Hypertrophy (sic) (<1%)
Peripheral edema (<1%)
Photosensitivity (<1%)
Pigmentation (<1%)
Pruritus (<1%)
Psoriasis (<1%)
Purpura (<1%)
Rash (sic) (>1%)
Ulceration (<1%)
Urticaria (<1%)
Viral infection

Hair

Hair – alopecia (<1%)

Other

Gingivitis (>1%)
Glossitis (<1%)
Gynecomastia (<1%)
Hypesthesia (4%)
Mastitis (<1%)
Paresthesias (5%)
Peyronie's disease (<1%)
Sialorrhea (>1%)
Stomatitis (<1%)
Thrombophlebitis (<1%)
Tongue edema (<1%)
Tremor (6%)
Ulcerative stomatitis (<1%)
Vaginal candidiasis (<1%)
Xerostomia (5%)

ROSIGLITAZONE

Trade name: Avandia (SmithKline Beecham)
Indications: Type 2 diabetes
Category: Thiazolidinedione antidiabetic
Half-life: 3.5 hours
Clinically important, potentially serious interactions with: no data

Reactions

Skin

Edema (4.8%)
Exanthem
(1999): Rehbein HM, Jacksonville, FL (from Internet) (observation)

SACCHARIN

Trade names: Saccharin; Sweet 'n Low
Indications: Sugar substitute
Category: Sulfonamide* sweetening agent
Half-life: no data
Clinically important, potentially serious interactions with: none

Reactions

Skin

Dermatitis (sic)
(1989): Birbeck J, *N Z Med J* 102, 24
(1972): Gordon H, *Cutis* 10, 77
(1972): Gordon H H *Am J Obstet Gynecol* 15, 1145
Exanthems
(1965): Boros E, *JAMA* 194, 571
(1965): Fujita H+, *Acta Derm* 60, 303
Fixed eruption
(1956): Stritzler C+, *Arch Dermatol* 74, 433
Notalgia paresthetica
(1986): Fishman HC, *J Am Acad Dermatol* 15, 1304
Photosensitivity
(1972): Gordon H, *Cutis* 10, 77
(1972): Taub SJ, *Eye Ear Nose Throat Mon* 51, 405
(1961): Kennedy B+, *J Louisiana Med Soc* 113, 365
Pruritus
(1989): Birbeck J, *N Z Med J* 102, 24
(1972): Gordon H, *Cutis* 10, 77
(1965): Boros E, *JAMA* 194, 571
Sensitivity (sic)
(1966): Kingsley HJ, *Cent Afr J Med* 12, 243
Urticaria
(1989): Birbeck J, *N Z Med J* 102, 24
(1974): Miller R+, *J Allergy Clin Immunol* 53, 240
(1972): Gordon H, *Cutis* 10, 77
(1956): Stritzler C+, *Arch Dermatol* 74, 433
(1955): Stritzler C+, *New York J Med* 55, 3479

Other

Dysgeusia
(1965): Boros E, *JAMA* 194, 571

***Note:** Saccharin is a sulfonamide and can be absorbed systemically. Sulfonamides can produce severe, possibly fatal, reactions such as toxic epidermal necrolysis and Stevens–Johnson syndrome.

SALMETEROL

Trade name: Serevent (GlaxoWellcome)
Other common trade names: *Salmeter; Serobid; Zantirel*
Indications: Asthma
Category: Sympathomimetic bronchodilator; adrenergic agonist
Half-life: 3–4 hours
Clinically important, potentially serious interactions with: beta-blockers, MAO inhibitors, tricyclic antidepressants

Reactions

Skin

Angioedema
Eczematoid eruption (sic)
(1997): Leal GB, Fortaleza, Brazil (from Internet) (observation)
Exanthems
Pruritus
Rash (sic) (1–3%)
(1994): D'Alonzo GE+, *JAMA* 271, 1412
(1991): Hatton MQ+, *Lancet* 337, 1169
Urticaria (1–3%)
(1991): Hatton MQF+, *Lancet* 337, 1169

Other

Hypersensitivity (<1%)
Myalgia (1–3%)
Paresthesias
Trembling
Tremor (1–10%)

SALSALATE

Synonyms: disalicylic acid; salicylsalicylic acid
Trade names: Disalcid (3M); Mono-Gesic (Schwarz); Salflex (Carnrick); Salsitab (Upsher Smith)
Other common trade names: *Argesic-SA; Artha-G; Atisuril; Disalgesic; Marthritic; Nobegyl; Salgesic; Salina; Umbradol*
Indications: Arthritis
Category: Nonsteroidal anti-inflammatory (NSAID); salicylate; analgesic
Half-life: 7–8 hours
Clinically important, potentially serious interactions with: ACE-inhibitors, alcohol, anticoagulants, beta-blockers, heparin, hypoglycemics, methotrexate, NSAIDs, valproic acid, vancomycin

Reactions

Skin

Angioedema
Dermatitis (sic)
Exanthems
Pruritus
Purpura
Rash (sic) (1–10%)
Urticaria
(1986): Chudwin DS+, *Ann Allergy* 57, 133

Other

Anaphylactoid reaction (1–10%)

SAQUINAVIR

Trade names: Fortovase (Roche); Invirase (Roche)
Indications: Advanced HIV infection
Category: Antiretroviral; protease inhibitor*
Half-life: 12 hours
Clinically important, potentially serious interactions with: calcium channel blockers, cisapride, clarithromycin, clindamycin, dapsone, ergot derivatives, ketoconazole, midazolam, quinidine, rifabutin, rifampin, ritonavir, triazolam, **grapefruit juice**

Reactions

Skin

Acne (<2%)
Bullous eruption
Candidiasis (<2%)
Cheilitis (<2%)
Dermatitis (<2%)
Diaphoresis (<2%)
Eczema (sic) (<2%)
Erythema (<2%)
Erythema multiforme
(1998): Garat H+, *Ann Dermatol Venereol* (French) 125, 42
Exanthems (<2%)
Folliculitis (<2%)
Fixed eruption
(2000): Smith KJ+, *Cutis* 66, 29 (2 cases)
Furunculosis
Guillain–Barré syndrome
Herpes simplex (<2%)
Herpes zoster (<2%)

Papulovesicular lesions
(2000): Smith KJ+, *Cutis* 66, 29 (2 cases)
Photosensitivity (<2%)
(1997): Winter AJ+, *Genitourin Med* 73, 323
Pigmentary changes (<2%)
(2000): Smith KJ+, *Cutis* 66, 29 (2 cases)
Pruritus
(2000): Smith KJ+, *Cutis* 66, 29 (2 cases)
Rash (sic) (1.3%)
Seborrheic dermatitis (<2%)
Stevens–Johnson syndrome
Ulceration (<2%)
Urticaria (<2%)
Warts (<2%)
Xerosis (<2%)

Hair

Hair – alopecia
Hair – changes (sic) (<2%)

Other

Dysesthesia (<2%)
Dysgeusia (<2%)
Gingivitis (<2%)
Glossitis (<2%)
Gynecomastia
(1999): Donovan B+, *Int J STD AIDS* 10, 49
Hyperesthesia (<2%)
Lingual lesions (sic)
(1998): Ruscin JM+, *Ann Pharmacother* 32, 1248
Oral ulceration (2.5%)
Paresthesias (2.6%)
Stomatitis (<2%)
Xerostomia (<2%)

***Note:** Protease inhibitors cause dyslipidemia which includes elevated triglycerides and cholesterol and redistribution of body fat centrally to produce the so-called "protease paunch," breast enlargement, facial atrophy, and "buffalo hump."

SARGRAMOSTIN

(See GRANULOCYTE COLONY-STIMULATING FACTOR [GCSF])

SCOPOLAMINE

Trade names: Isopto Hyoscine Ophthalmic*; Scopase; Transderm-Scop Patch (Novartis)
Other common trade names: *Scopace; Scopoderm-TTS; Transdermal-V*
Indications: Nausea and vomiting, excess salivation
Category: Anticholinergic, antispasmodic
Half-life: 8 hours
Clinically important, potentially serious interactions with: acetaminophen, amantadine, anticholinergics, digoxin, haloperidol, ketoconazole, levodopa, phenothiazines, riboflavin, tacrine, tricyclic antidepressants

Reactions

Skin

Contact dermatitis
(1989): Gordon CR+, *BMJ* 298, 1220
Dermatitis (transdermal patch and ophthalmic)
(1990): Hogan DJ+, *J Am Acad Dermatol* 22, 811
(1989): Holdiness MR, *Contact Dermatitis* 20, 3
(1988): van der Willigen AH+, *J Am Acad Dermatol* 18, 146
(1985): Clissold SP+, *Drugs* 29, 189
(1985): Trozak DJ, *J Am Acad Dermatol* 13, 247
(1984): Fisher AA, *Cutis* 34, 526
Edema (<1%) (ophthalmic)
Erythema
Erythema multiforme
(1986): Fisher AA, *Cutis* 37, 158; 262
(1979): Guill MA+, *Arch Dermatol* 115, 742
Exanthems
(1985): Clissold SP+, *Drugs* 29, 189 (transdermal patch)
Fixed eruption
(1981): Kanwar AJ+, *Dermatologica* 162, 378
Flushing
Hypohidrosis (>10%)
Photosensitivity (1–10%)
Rash (sic) (<1%)
Urticaria
Xerosis (>10%)

Other

Anaphylactoid reaction
(1995): Manhart AR+, *J Toxicol Clin Toxicol* 33, 189 (fatal)
(1994): Watanabe F+, *J Toxicol Clin Toxicol* 32, 593 (fatal)
Injection-site irritation (>10%)
Oral mucosal lesions
(1985): Clissold SP+, *Drugs* 29, 189 (transdermal patch) (>5%)
Xerostomia (>60%)
(1985): Clissold SP+, *Drugs* 29, 189 (transdermal patch) (66%)
(1981): Price NM+, *Clin Pharmacol Ther* 29, 414

***Note:** Systemic adverse effects have been reported following ophthalmic administration

SECOBARBITAL

Synonym: quinalbarbitone
Trade name: Seconal (Lilly)
Other common trade names: *Immenoctal; Novo-Secobarb; Secanal*
Indications: Insomnia
Category: Short-acting barbiturate; hypnotic-sedative
Half-life: 15–40 hours
Clinically important, potentially serious interactions with: acetaminophen, anticoagulants, beta-blockers, CNS depressants, chloramphenicol, chlorpropamide, MAO inhibitors, quinidine, theophylline, verapamil

Reactions

Skin

Angioedema (<1%)
Exanthems
Exfoliative dermatitis (<1%)
Purpura
Rash (sic) (<1%)
Stevens–Johnson syndrome (<1%)
Urticaria

Other

Hypersensitivity
Injection-site pain (>10%)
Serum sickness
Thrombophlebitis (<1%)

SECRETIN

Trade name: Secretin-Ferring (Ferring)
Indications: Diagnosis of gastrinoma (Zollinger–Ellison syndrome)
Category: Gastrointestinal peptide hormone
Half-life: no data
Clinically important, potentially serious interactions with: no data

Reactions

Skin

Allergic reactions (sic)
Urticaria
(1975): Baenkler HW+, *BMJ* 2, 747

Other

Injection-site reactions (sic)
(1975): Baenkler HW+, *BMJ* 2, 747

SELEGILINE

Synonyms: deprenyl; L-deprenyl
Trade name: Eldepryl (Somerset)
Other common trade names: *Apo-Selegiline; Carbex; Eldeprine; Jumex; Movergan; Novo-Selegiline; Plurimen*
Indications: Parkinsonism
Category: Monoamine oxidase (MAO) inhibitor; antiparkinsonian
Half-life: 9 minutes
Clinically important, potentially serious interactions with: dextroamphetamine, dextromethorphan, dopamine, ephedrine, fenfluramine, fluoxetine, levodopa, methylphenidate, meperidine, opioids, paroxetine, sertraline, sibutramine, sympathomimetics, tricyclic antidepressants, venlafaxine, **tyramine-containing foods***

Reactions

Skin

Diaphoresis
Peripheral edema
Photosensitivity
Rash (sic)

Hair

Hair – alopecia
Hair – hypertrichosis (facial)

Other

Bruxism (1–10%)
Dysgeusia
Paresthesias
Tremor
Xerostomia (>10%)
(1988): Golbe LI+, *Clin Neuropharmacol* 11, 45

***Note:** Tyramine-containing foods include the following: aged cheeses, avocados, banana skins, bologna and other processed luncheon meats, chicken livers, chocolate, figs, canned pickled herring, meat extracts, pepperoni, raisins, raspberries, soy sauce, vermouth, sherry and red wines.

SERTRALINE

Trade name: Zoloft (Pfizer)
Other common trade name: *Atruline*
Indications: Depression; panic disorders; obsessive compulsive disorders
Category: Selective serotonin reuptake inhibitor (SSRI); antidepressant
Half-life: 24–26 hours
Clinically important, potentially serious interactions with: beta-blockers, lithium*, MAO inhibitors*, rifampin, sumatriptan*, trazodone, tricyclic antidepressants*, warfarin, **St John's wort**

Reactions

Skin

Acne (<1%)
Allergic reactions (sic)
(1991): Guthrie SK, *Drug Intell Clin Pharm* 25, 952
Angioedema
(1994): Gales BJ+, *Am J Hosp Pharm* 51, 118
Balanoposthitis (<1%)
Bullous eruption (<1%)
Cutaneous reaction (sic)
(1998): Beauquier B+, *Encephale* (French) 24, 62
Dermatitis (sic) (<1%)
Diaphoresis (8.4%)
(2000): Henney JE, *JAMA* 283, 596
(1991): Guthrie SK, *Drug Intell Clin Pharm* 25, 952
(1990): Reimherr FW+, *J Clin Psychiatry* 51, 18
(1988): Doogan DP+, *J Clin Psychiatry* 49, 46
Discoloration (sic) (<1%)
Edema (<1%)
Erythema
Erythema multiforme (<1%)
(1994): Gales BJ+, *Am J Hosp Pharm* 51, 118
Exanthems (<1%)
(2000): Kittay SA, (from Internet) (observation)
(2000): Fernandes B+, *Contact Dermatitis* 42, 287
(1999): Blumenthal, HL, Beachwood, OH, personal case (observation)
(1998): Litt JZ, Beachwood, OH, personal case (observation)
Fixed eruption
(1997): Sawada KY, Wheat Ridge, CO (from Internet) (observation)
Flushing (2.2%)
Lupus erythematosus
(1998): Hill VA+, *J R Army Med Corps* 144, 109
Periorbital edema (<1%)
Peripheral edema (<1%)
Photosensitivity (<1%)
Pruritus (<1%)
(1999): Blumenthal, HL, Beachwood, OH, personal case (observation)
Purpura (<1%)
Rash (sic) (2.1%)
Stevens–Johnson syndrome
(1999): Jan V+, *Acta Derm Venereol* 79, 401
Urticaria (<1%)
Xerosis (<1%)

Hair

Hair – abnormal texture (sic) (<1%)
Hair – alopecia (<1%)
(1996): Bourgeois JA, *J Clin Psychopharmacol* 16, 91
Hair – hirsutism (<1%)

Other

Aphthous stomatitis (<1%)
Bromhidrosis (<1%)
Bruxism (<1%)
Dysgeusia
Galactorrhea
(1993): Bronzo MR+, *Am J Psychiatry* 150, 1269
Gingival hyperplasia (<1%)
Glossitis (<1%)
Gynecomastia (<1%)

Halitosis (<1%)
Hyperesthesia (<1%)
Hypesthesia (2%)
Paresthesias (2%)
Priapism
(1998): Rand EH, *J Clin Psychiatry* 59, 538
Sialorrhea (<1%)
Stomatitis (<1%)
Tongue edema (<1%)
Tongue ulceration (<1%)
Tremor (1–10%)
Vaginitis (atrophic)
Xerostomia (16.3%)
(2000): Brady K+, *JAMA* 283, 1837
(1992): Berman H+, *Hosp Community Psychiatry* 43, 671
(1991): Guthrie SK, *Drug Intell Clin Pharm* 25, 952
(1990): Reimherr FW+, *J Clin Psychiatry* 51, 18
(1988): Doogan DP+, *J Clin Psychiatry* 49, 46

*These medications, along with sertraline, may precipitate the serotonin syndrome consisting of restlessness, confusion, agitation, myoclonus, hyperreflexia, diarrhea, diaphoresis, shivering, tremor, fever, and mental changes.

SIBUTRAMINE

Trade name: Meridia (Knoll)
Indications: Obesity
Category: Obesity management; anorexiant
Half-life: 1.1 hours
Clinically important, potentially serious interactions with: alcohol, bupropion, ephedrine, ergot, erythromycin, fentanyl, fluoxetine, ketoconazole, lithium, MAO inhibitors, meperidine, paroxetine, pseudoephedrine, SSRIs, sumatriptan, tetracyclic antidepressants, tricyclic antidepressants, venlafaxine

Reactions

Skin

Acne (1.0%)
Allergic reactions (sic) (1.5%)
Diaphoresis (2.5%)
Ecchymoses (0.7%)
Edema (2%)
Flu-like syndrome (sic) (1–10%)
Herpes simplex (1.3%)
Peripheral edema (>1%)
Pruritus (>1%)
Rash (sic) (3.8%)

Other

Dysgeusia (2.2%)
Myalgia (1.9%)
Paresthesias (2.0%)
Tooth disorder (sic)
Vaginal candidiasis (1.2%)
Xerostomia (17.2%)

SILDENAFIL

Trade name: Viagra (Pfizer)
Indications: Erectile dysfunction
Category: Phosphodiesterase (type 5) enzyme inhibitor
Half-life: 4 hours
Clinically important, potentially serious interactions with: amprenavir, cimetidine, erythromycin, itraconazole, ketoconazole, mibefradil, protease inhibitors, ritonavir

Reactions

Skin

Allergic reactions (sic) (<2%)
Contact dermatitis (<2%)
Diaphoresis (<2%)
Edema (<2%)
Exfoliative dermatitis (<2%)
Flushing (10%)
Facial edema (<2%)
Fixed eruption (urticarial)
(1998): Reed BR, Denver, CO (from Internet) (observation)
Genital edema (<2%)
Herpes simplex (<2%)
Lichenoid eruption
(2000): Goldman BD, *Cutis* 66, 282
Peripheral edema (<2%)
Photosensitivity (<2%)
Pruritus (<2%)
Rash (sic) (2%)
Ulceration (<2%)
Urticaria (<2%)

Other

Dyschromatopsia (3%) (blue-green vision)
(1998): Craig D+, *Cleveland Clinic Foundation* 52, 963 (11%)
Gingivitis (<2%)
Glossitis (<2%)
Gynecomastia (<2%)
Hypesthesia (<2%)
Myalgia (<2%)
Paresthesias (<2%)
Photophobia (<2%)
Priapism
(2000): Sur RL+, *Urology* 55, 950
Stomatitis (<2%)
Xerostomia (<2%)

SIMVASTATIN

Trade name: Zocor (Merck)
Other common trade names: *Denan; Lipex; Liponorm; Lodales; Simovil; Sivastin; Zocord*
Indications: Hypercholesterolemia
Category: Antihyperlipidemic (cholesterol-lowering); HMG-CoA reductase inhibitor
Half-life: 1.9 hours
Clinically important, potentially serious interactions with: amprenavir, anticoagulants, clarithromycin, cyclosporine, danazol, digoxin, diltiazem, erythromycin, fluconazole, fluvoxamine, gemfibrozil, indinavir, itraconazole, ketoconazole, miconazole, nefazodone, niacin, ritonavir, saquinavir, verapamil, warfarin

Reactions

Skin

Actinic dermatitis (sic)
(1998): Granados MT+, *Contact Dermatitis* 38, 294
Angioedema

Ankle edema
(1991): Borland Y+, *Nephron* 57, 365
Cheilitis
(1998): Mehregan DR+, *Cutis* 62, 197
Dermatomyositis
(1994): Khattak FH+, *Br J Rheumatol* 32(2), 199
Diaphoresis
(1991): Scott RS+, *N Z Med J* 104, 493
Eczema (sic)
(1995): Proksch E, *Hautarzt* (German) 46, 76
(1991): Steyn K+, *S Afr Med J* 79, 639
Eczematous eruption (generalized)
(1993): Krasovec M+, *Dermatology* 186, 248
(1993): Feldmann R+, *Dermatology* 186, 272
Erythema multiforme
Erythematous scaly plaques
(1993): Feldmann R+, *Dermatology* 186, 272
Exanthems
(1991): McDowell IF+, *Br J Clin Pharmacol* 31, 340
Flushing
Lichenoid eruption
(1994): Roger D+, *Clin Exp Dermatol* 19, 88
Lichen planus
(1991): Steyn K+, *S Afr Med J* 79, 639
Lupus erythematosus
(1998): Khosia R+, *South Med J* 91, 873
(1998): Hanson J+, *Lancet* 352, 1070
(1992): Bannwarth B+, *Arch Intern Med* 152, 1093
Petechiae
(1997): Horiuchi Y+, *J Dermatol* 24, 549
Photosensitivity
(1995): Morimoto K+, *Contact Dermatitis* 33, 274
(1991): Brocard JJ+, *Schweiz Med Wochenschr* (German) 121, 977
Pruritus
(1993): Feldmann R+, *Dermatology* 186, 272
(1991): Steyn K+, *S Afr Med J* 79, 639
Purpura
(1998): Koduri PR, *Lancet* 352, 2020
(1991): Steyn K+, *S Afr Med J* 79, 639
Pustular eruption
Radiation recall
(1995): Abadir R+, *Clin Oncol R Coll Radiol* 7, 325
Rash (sic) (1–10%)
(1993): Feldmann R+, *Dermatology* 186, 272
(1990): Ziegler O+, *Cardiology* 77 (Suppl 4), 50
Rosacea
(1991): Brocard JJ+, *Schweiz Med Wochenschr* (German) 121, 977
Stevens–Johnson syndrome
Thrombocytopenic purpura
(1998): McCarthy LJ+, *Lancet* 352, 1284
Toxic epidermal necrolysis
Urticaria
Vasculitis

Hair

Hair – alopecia
(1999): Litt JZ, Beachwood, OH, personal case (observation)
(1998): Robb-Nicholson C, *Harv Womens Health Watch* 5, 8 (anecdote)
(1997): Shelley WB+, *Cutis* 60, 20 (observation)
(1995): Litt JZ, Beachwood, OH, personal case (observation)
(1994): Litt JZ, Beachwood, OH, personal case (observation)

Other

Anaphylactoid reaction
Dysgeusia (<1%)
(1991): Saito Y+, *Arterioscler Thromb* 11, 816
Gynecomastia
Hypersensitivity
Myalgia (1.6%)
Myopathy (1–10%)
(1994): al-Jubouri MA+, BMJ 308, 588
(1991): Deslypere JP+, *Ann Intern Med* 114, 342
(1990): Bilheimer DW, *Cardiology* 77 (Suppl 4), 58
Paresthesias
Porphyria cutanea tarda
(1994): Perrot JL+, *Ann Dermatol Venereol* (French) 121, 817

SIROLIMUS

Trade name: Rapamune (Wyeth-Ayerst)
Indications: Prophylaxis of organ rejection in renal transplants
Category: Immunosuppressant
Half-life: 62 hours
Clinically important, potentially serious interactions with: bromocriptine, cimetidine, cisapride, clarithromycin, clotrimazole, danazol, diltiazem, erythromycin, fluconazole, indinavir, itraconazole, ketoconazole, metoclopramide, nicardipine, ritonavir, verapamil, **grapefruit juice**

Reactions

Skin

Abscess (3–20%)
Acne (20–31%)
(2000): Vasquez EM, *Am J Health Syst Pharm* 57, 437
Cellulitis (3–20%)
Chills (3–20%)
Diaphoresis (3–20%)
Ecchymoses (3–20%)
Edema (16–24%)
Facial edema (3–20%)
Flu-like syndrome (sic)
Fungal dermatitis (3–20%)
Hypertrophy (3–20%)
Infection (sic) (3–20%)
Peripheral edema (54–64%)
Pruritus (3–20%)
Purpura
Rash (sic) (10–20%)
(2000): Vasquez EM, *Am J Health Syst Pharm* 57, 437
Scrotal edema (3–20%)
Ulceration (3–20%)

Hair

Hair – hirsutism (3–20%)

Other

Gingival hyperplasia
Gingivitis
Hypesthesia (3–20%)
Myalgia
Oral candidiasis (3–20%)
Oral ulceration (3–20%)
Paresthesias (3–20%)
Stomatitis (3–20%)
Thrombophlebitis (3–20%)
Tremor (21–31%)

SODIUM CROMOGLYCATE

(See CROMOLYN)

SOTALOL

Trade name: Betapace (Berlex)
Other common trade names: *Beta-Cardone; Betades; Cardol; Sotacor; Sotahexal; Sotalex; Sotacor*
Indications: Ventricular arrhythmias
Category: Beta-adrenergic blocker; antiarrhythmic class III
Half-life: 7–18 hours
Clinically important, potentially serious interactions with: amiodarone, antidiabetics, astemizole, calcium channel blockers, clonidine, disopyramide, flecainide, guanethidine, insulin, naproxen, nifedipine, NSAIDs, oral contraceptives, phenothiazines, procainamide, quinidine, sertraline, sulfonylureas, terfenadine, tricyclic antidepressants

Reactions

Skin

Cold extremities (sic)
Cutaneous thickening (sic)
Diaphoresis (<1%)
(1995): Schmutz JL+, *Dermatology* 190, 86
Edema (5%)
Exanthems
Lichenoid eruption
(1994): O'Brien TJ+, *Australas J Dermatol* 35, 93
Peripheral edema
Photosensitivity (<1%)
Pruritus (1–10%)
Psoriasis
(1988): Heng MCY+, *Int J Dermatol* 27, 619
(1986): Czernielewski J+, *Lancet* 1, 808
(1984): Arntzen N+, *Acta Derm Venereol* (Stockh) 64, 346
Rash (sic) (3%)
Raynaud's phenomenon (<1%)
Scleroderma
(1988): Ahmad N+, *Scott Med J* 33, 210
(1979): Michel JP+, *Lancet* 1, 54
(1979): Bonnetblanc JM+, *Ann Dermatol Venereol* (French) 106, 927
Skin irritation (sic)
Urticaria
Vasculitis
(1998): Rustmann WC+, *J Am Acad Dermatol* 38, 111

Hair

Hair – alopecia (<1%)

Other

Dysgeusia
Injection-site extravasation (<1%)
Myalgia (<1%)
Myopathy
(1979): Forfar JC+, *BMJ* 2, 1331
Paresthesias (3%)
Phlebitis (<1%)
Xerostomia (<1%)

SPARFLOXACIN

Trade name: Zagam (Bertek)
Other common trade names: *Spara; Sparlox; Torospar*
Indications: Community-acquired pneumonia
Category: Quinolone antibiotic
Half-life: 16–30 hours
Clinically important, potentially serious interactions with: bumetanide, caffeine, cimetidine, cisapride, cyclosporine, digoxin, erythromycin, iron salts, lithium, pentamidine, phenothiazines, probenecid, salicylates, tricyclic antidepressants, warfarin, zinc salts

Reactions

Skin

Acne (<1%)
Allergic reactions (sic) (<1%)
Angioedema (<1%)
Bullous eruption (<1%)
Cellulitis (<1%)
Contact dermatitis (<1%)
Diaphoresis (<1%)
Ecchymoses (<1%)
Edema (<1%)
Erythema nodosum
Exanthems (<1%)
Exfoliative dermatitis (<1%)
Facial edema (<1%)
Furunculosis (<1%)
Herpes simplex (<1%)
Lichenoid eruption
(1998): Hamanaka H+, *J Am Acad Dermatol* 38, 945
Peripheral edema (<1%)
Petechiae (<1%)
Photosensitivity (3.6%)
(2000): Schentag JJ, *Clin Ther* 22, 372
(1999): Hamanaka H, *J Dermatol Sci* 21, 27
(1999): Lipsky BA+, *Clin Ther* 21, 148
(1998): Hamanaka H+, *J Am Acad Dermatol* 38, 945
(1997): Burrow WH, Jackson MS (from Internet) (observation)
(1996): Tokura Y+, *Arch Dermatol Res* 288, 45
(1995): Hiramoto T+, *Rinsho Dermatol* (Japanese) 37, 1681
(1995): Hamanaka H+, *Jpn J Dermatol* 105, 601
Phototoxic reaction (7.9%)
(2000): Pierfitte C+, *Br J Clin Pharmacol* 49, 609
(1999): Blondeau JM, *Clin Ther* 21, 6
(1996): Tokura Y+, *Arch Dermatol Res* 288, 45
Pigmentation (<1%)
Pruritus (3.3%)
Purpura
Pustular eruption (<1%)
Rash (sic) (1.1%)
Stevens–Johnson syndrome
Toxic epidermal necrolysis
Urticaria (<1%)
Vasculitis
Xerosis (<1%)

Hair

Hair – alopecia (<1%)

Other

Anaphylactoid reaction (<1%)
Anosmia
Dysgeusia (1.4%)
(1999): Lipsky BA+, *Clin Ther* 21, 148
Gingivitis (<1%)
Hyperesthesia (<1%)
Hypersensitivity
Hypesthesia (<1%)
Mastodynia (<1%)
Myalgia (<1%)
Oral candidiasis (<1%)

Oral ulceration (<1%)
Paresthesias (<1%)
Serum sickness
Stomatitis (<1%)
Tendon rupture
Tongue disorder (<1%)
Vaginal candidiasis (2.8%)
Vaginitis (<1%)
Xerostomia (1.4%)

SPECTINOMYCIN

Trade name: Trobicin (Pharmacia & Upjohn)
Other common trade name: *Spectam*
Indications: Gonorrhea
Category: Antibiotic
Half-life: 1–3 hours
Clinically important, potentially serious interactions with: none

Reactions

Skin

Chills
Contact dermatitis
(1994): Dal-Monte A+, *Contact Dermatitis* 31, 204 (occupational)
(1991): Vilaplana J+, *Contact Dermatitis* 24, 225
Exanthems
Pruritus (<1%)
(1974): Bogden C+, *Schweiz Med Wochenschr* (German) 104, 46
Rash (sic) (<1%)
Urticaria (<1%)
(1971): *Med Lett* 13, 105

Other

Anaphylactoid reaction
(1977): Raab W, *Z Hautkr* (German) 9, 14
Hypersensitivity
(1977): Raab W, *Z Hautkr* (German) 9, 14
Injection-site induration
Injection-site pain (<1%)
Oral mucosal lesions

SPIRONOLACTONE

Trade names: Aldactazide (Searle); Aldactone (Searle)
Other common trade names: *Aldopur; Almatol; Diram; Merabis; Novo-Spiroton, Osiren; Spiroctan; Tensin*
Indications: Hyperaldosteronism; hirsutism; hypertension
Category: Potassium-sparing antihypertensive; diuretic
Half-life: 78–84 minutes
Clinically important, potentially serious interactions with: ACE-inhibitors, amiloride, benazepril, digoxin, diuretics, enalapril, fosinopril, heparin, indomethacin, lisinopril, mitotane, NSAIDs, potassium chloride, salicylates, triamterene. Also **foods and licorice candy**

Aldactazide is spironolactone and hydrochlorothiazide

Reactions

Skin

Chills
Chloasma
(1988): Hughes BR+, *Br J Dermatol* 118, 687
Contact dermatitis
(1996): Corazza M+, *Contact Dermatitis* 35, 365
(1994): Balato N+, *Contact Dermatitis* 31, 203
(1994): Aguirre A+, *Contact Dermatitis* 30, 312
(1994): Fernandez-Vozmediano JM+, *Contact Dermatitis* 30, 118
(1993): Vincenzi C+, *Contact Dermatitis* 29, 277 (from an anti-acne cream)
(1984): Klijn J, *Contact Dermatitis* 10, 105
Cutaneous side effects (sic)
(1973): Almeyda J+, *Br J Dermatol* 88, 313
Diaphoresis
Eczematous eruption (sic)
(1994): Balato N+, *Contact Dermatitis* 31, 203
(1994): Fernandez-Vozmediano JM+, *Contact Dermatitis* 30, 118
Erythema
Erythema annulare centrifugum
(1987): Carsuzaa F+, *Ann Dermatol Venereol* (French) 114, 375
Erythema multiforme
(1986): Greenberger PA+, *N Engl Reg Allergy Proc* 7, 343
Exanthems
(1994): Gupta AK+, *Dermatol* 189, 402
(1988): Hughes BR+, *Br J Dermatol* 118, 687 (9.3%)
(1986): Wathen CG+, *Lancet* 1, 919
(1979): Uddin MS+, *Cutis* 24, 198 (passim)
(1977): Ferguson RK+, *Clin Pharmacol Ther* 21, 62 (1–5%)
(1973): Greenblatt DJ+, *JAMA* 225, 40 (0.5%)
Facial edema
(1998): Lubbos HG+, *Arch Dermatol* 134, 1163
Flushing (<1%)
Graft-versus-host reaction
(1998): Jappe U+, *Hautarzt* (German) 49, 126 (passim)
Lichenoid eruption
(1998): Clark C+, *Clin Exp Dermatol* 23, 43
(1994): Schon MP+, *Acta Derm Venereol* 74, 476
Lichen planus
(1978): Downham TF, *JAMA* 240, 1138
Lupus erythematosus
(1987): Leroy D+, *Ann Dermatol Venereol* (French) 114, 1237
Melasma
(2000): Shaw JC, *J Am Acad Dermatol* 43, 498
(1979): Uddin MS+, *Cutis* 24, 198
Necrotizing angiitis
Pemphigoid
(1997): Grange F+, *Ann Dermatol Venereol* (French) 124, 700
Photosensitivity
Pigmentation
(1988): Hughes BR, *Dermatology Times* June, 10 (chloasma-like)
(1988): Hughes BR+, *Br J Dermatol* 118, 687 (chloasma-like)
(1983): Luderschmidt C, *Dtsch Med Wochenschr* (German) 108, 1922
(1975): Davies DL+, *Drugs* 9, 214
Pruritus
(1988): Hughes BR, *Dermatology Times* June, 10
(1986): Wathen CG+, *Lancet* 1, 919
Purpura
Rash (sic) (1–10%)
(1988): Hughes BR, *Dermatology Times* June, 10
(1973): Greenblatt DJ+, *JAMA* 225, 40
Raynaud's phenomenon
(1975): Davies DL+, *Drugs* 9, 214
Urticaria
(1988): Helfer EL+, *J Clin Endocrinol Metab* 66, 208
(1979): Uddin MS+, *Cutis* 24, 198 (passim)
Vasculitis
(1984): Phillips GWL+, *BMJ* 288, 368
Xerosis
(2000): Shaw JC, *J Am Acad Dermatol* 43, 498
(1988): Hughes BR+, *Br J Dermatol* 118, 687 (40%)
(1988): Hughes BR, *Dermatology Times* June, 10

Hair

Hair – alopecia
(1988): Helfer EL+, *J Clin Endocrinol Metab* 66, 208
(1975): Davies DL+, *Drugs* 9, 214
Hair – hirsutism

Other

Acute intermittent porphyria
Ageusia
Anaphylactoid reaction
Gynecomastia (<1%)
(2000): Hugues FC+, *Ann Med Interne (Paris)* (French) 151, 10 (passim)
(1994): *BMJ* 308, 503
(1994): Dove F, *Hosp Pract Off Ed* 29, 27

(1993): Thompson DF+, *Pharmacotherapy* 13, 37
(1988): Hughes BR+, *Br J Dermatol* 118, 687
(1977): Rose LI+, *Ann Intern Med* 87, 398
(1976): Loriaux DL, *Ann Intern Med* 85, 630
(1973): Greenblatt DJ+, *JAMA* 225, 40 (passim)
(1965): Clark E, *JAMA* 193, 163
(1963): Mann NM, *JAMA* 190, 160

Mastodynia
(2000): Shaw JC, *J Am Acad Dermatol* 43, 498

Oral lichen planus
(1990): Lamey PJ+, *Oral Surg Oral Med Oral Pathol* 70, 184

Paresthesias

Xerostomia

STANOZOLOL

Trade name: Winstrol (Sanofi)
Other common trade names: *Menabol; Stromba*
Indications: Hereditary angioedema
Category: Anabolic steroid; androgen
Half-life: no data
Clinically important, potentially serious interactions with: ACTH, adrenal steroids, anticoagulants, antidiabetics, insulin, sulfonylureas

Reactions

Skin

Acne (>10%)
(1995): Helfman T+, *J Am Acad Dermatol* 32, 254

Chills (1–10%)

Edema

Exanthems

Folliculitis
(1995): Helfman T+, *J Am Acad Dermatol* 32, 254

Hyperpigmentation (1–10%)

Rosacea
(1995): Helfman T+, *J Am Acad Dermatol* 32, 254

Seborrheic dermatitis
(1995): Helfman T+, *J Am Acad Dermatol* 32, 254

Urticaria

Hair

Hair – alopecia (in women)

Hair – hirsutism (in women)
(1995): Helfman T+, *J Am Acad Dermatol* 32, 254
(1987): Sheffer AL+, *J Allergy Clin Immunol* 80, 855

Other

Gynecomastia (>10%)
(1995): Helfman T+, *J Am Acad Dermatol* 32, 254

Priapism (>10%)

STAVUDINE

Synonym: d4T
Trade name: Zerit (Bristol-Myers Squibb)
Indications: Human immunodeficiency virus (HIV)
Category: Antiretroviral; nucleoside reverse transcriptase inhibitor (NRTI)
Half-life: 1.44 hours
Clinically important, potentially serious interactions with: didanosine, hydroxyurea, phenylpropanolamine, probenecid, zidovudine

Reactions

Skin

Allergic reactions (sic) (9%)

Buffalo hump

Chills (50%)

Diaphoresis (19%)

Neutrophilic eccrine hidradenitis
(1998): Krischer J+, *J Dermatol* 25, 199

Rash (sic) (~40%)

Other

Gynecomastia
(1998): Melbourne KM+. *Ann Pharmacother* 32, 1108

Lipodystrophy
(1999): Ruel M+, *Ann Med Interne (Paris)* (French) 150, 269

Myalgia (32%)
(2000): Miller KD+, *Ann Intern Med* 133, 192

Paresthesias

STREPTOKINASE

Trade names: Kabikinase (Pharmacia & Upjohn); Streptase (AstraZeneca)
Indications: Pulmonary embolism, acute myocardial infarction
Category: Thrombolytic
Half-life: 83 minutes
Clinically important, potentially serious interactions with: anticoagulants, dipyridamole, NSAIDs, sulfinpyrazone, valproic acid, warfarin

Reactions

Skin

Allergic reactions (sic) (4.4%)
(1998): Stephens MB+, *Postgrad Med* 103, 89
(1997): Cannas S+, *G Ital Cardiol* (Italian) 27, 278

Angiitis
(1988): Sorber WA+, *Cutis* 42, 57

Angioedema (>10%)
(1994): Cooper JP+, *Postgrad Med J* 70, 592

Cutaneous bleeding
(1990): Goa KL+, *Drugs* 39, 693 (3.6%)

Diaphoresis (1–10%)

Ecchymoses

Exanthems (1–5%)
(1990): Goa KL+, *Drugs* 39, 693
(1976): Kohner GM+, *BMJ* 1, 550

Flushing (<1%)

Periorbital edema (>10%)

Pruritus (1–10%)

Purpura

Rash (sic) (1–10%)

Urticaria (1–5%)
(1990): Goa KL+, *Drugs* 39, 693

Vasculitis
(1994): Penswick J+, *BMJ* 309, 378
(1991): Patel A+, *J Am Acad Dermatol* 24, 652
(1988): Ong AC+, *Int J Cardiology* 21, 71
(1988): Davidson JR+, *Clin Exp Rheumatol* 6, 381
(1986): Manoharan A+, *Aust N Z J Med* 16, 815
(1985): Thompson RF+, *Clin Pharm* 4, 383

Other

Anaphylactoid reaction (<1%)
(1993): Hohage H+, *Wien Klin Wochenschr* (German) 105, 176

Injection-site bleeding
(1990): Goa KL+, *Drugs* 39, 693 (3%)

Injection-site phlebitis

Serum sickness
(1995): Creamer JD+, *Clin Exp Dermatol* 20, 468
(1994): Proctor BD+, *N Engl J Med* 330, 576
(1991): Patel A+, *J Am Acad Dermatol* 24, 652
(1984): Alexopoulos D+, *Eur Heart J* 5, 1010
(1982): Totty WG+, *Am J Roentgenol* 138, 143

Stomatitis (following local application)

Tongue edema (with hemorrhagic swelling)

STREPTOMYCIN

Trade name: Streptomycin (Pfizer)
Indications: Tuberculosis
Category: Aminoglycoside antibiotic; tuberculostatic
Half-life: 2–5 hours
Clinically important, potentially serious interactions with: aminoglycosides, amphotericin B, bumetanide, ethacrynic acid, furosemide, loop diuretics, polypeptide antibiotics, torsemide

Reactions

Skin

Acute generalized exanthematous pustulosis (AGEP)
(1995): Moreau A+, *Int J Dermatol* 34, 263 (passim)
Allergic reactions (sic)
(1961): Chakravarty S+, *Acta Tuberc Pneumol Scand* 41, 144 (11%)
(1947): Steiner K+, *Arch Dermatol* 56, 511 (18%)
Angioedema (<1%)
(1959): Bereston ES, *J Invest Dermatol* 33, 427
Bullous eruption (<1%)
Cheilitis (2%)
(1949): Cohen AC+, *Arch Dermatol* 60, 373
Contact dermatitis
(1988): Holdiness MR, *Contact Dermatitis* 15, 282
(1983): Fisher AA, *Cutis* 32, 314
Eczematous eruption (sic)
(1958): Wilson HT, *BMJ* 1, 1378
Edema
Erythema multiforme (<1%)
(1988): Hira SK+, *J Am Acad Dermatol* 19, 451 (in AIDS patient)
(1985): Holdiness MR, *Int J Dermatol* 24, 280 (1–5%)
(1985): Ting HC+, *Int J Dermatol* 24, 587
(1947): Steiner K+, *Arch Dermatol* 56, 511
Erythema nodosum (<1%)
Exanthems (>5%)
(1968): Sarkany I, *Proc R Soc Med* 61, 891
(1966): Smith JW+, *Ann Intern Med* 65, 629
(1961): Gupta SK, *Indian J Dermatol* 6, 115
(1960): Heijer A+, *Acta Derm Venereol* (Stockh) 40, 35
(1955): Yow EM, *Ann Intern Med* 43, 323 (10%)
(1949): Bunn PA+, *Streptomycin*, Williams and Wilkins, Baltimore, 524
(1949): Cohen AC+ *Arch Dermatol* 60, 373 (11%)
(1948): Keefer CS+, *The Therapeutic Value of Streptomycin*, Edwards, Ann Arbor
(1947): Steiner K+, *Arch Dermatol* 56, 511
Exfoliative dermatitis
(1992): Matsuzawa Y+, *Kekkaku* (Japanese) 67, 413
(1986): Sehgal VN+, *Dermatologica* 173, 278
(1985): Holdiness MR, *Int J Dermatol* 24, 280
(1973): Nicolis GD+, *Arch Dermatol* 108, 788
(1972): Kauppinen K, *Acta Derm Venereol* (Stockh) 52, 68
(1969): Agrawal R, *BMJ* 4, 540
(1965): McQueen A, *N Z Med J* 64, 663
(1961): Gupta SK, *Indian J Dermatol* 6, 115
(1959): Bereston ES, *J Invest Dermatol* 33, 427
(1949): Cohen AC+, *Arch Dermatol* 60, 373
(1949): Bunn PA+, *Streptomycin*, Williams and Wilkins, Baltimore, 524
(1948): Coombs FC+, *N Y State J Med* 48, 2024
Fixed eruption (<1%)
Follicular pustular eruption (sic)
(1981): Kushimoto H+, *Arch Dermatol* 117, 444
Lichenoid eruption
(1958): Renkin A, *Arch Belg Dermatol Syph* (French) 14, 185
Lupus erythematosus
(1993): Toyoshima M+, *Kekkaku* (Japanese) 68, 319
(1986): Layer P+, *Dtsch Med Wochenschr* (German) 111, 1603
(1980): Agarwal MB+, *J Postgrad Med* 26, 263
(1959): Popkhristov P+, *Surv Med* (Sofia) 10, 81
Photosensitivity
(1971): Girard JP, *Helv Med Acta* 36, 3
Pruritus (<1%)
(1972): Levantine A+, *Br J Dermatol* 86, 651
Purpura
(1969): Peterkin GAG+, *Practitioner* 202, 117
(1965): Horowitz HI+, *Semin Hematol* 2, 287
(1955): Yow EM, *Ann Intern Med* 43, 323 (10%)
(1949): Bunn PA+, *Streptomycin*, Williams and Wilkins, Baltimore, 524
Pustular eruption
(1981): Kushimoto H+, *Arch Dermatol* 117, 444
Rash (sic) (<1%)
Stevens–Johnson syndrome
(1988): Hira SK+, *J Am Acad Dermatol* 19, 451 (in AIDS patient)
(1985): Holdiness MR, *Int J Dermatol* 24, 280
(1982): Sarkar SK+, *Tubercle* 63, 137
Systemic eczematous contact dermatitis
Toxic epidermal necrolysis
(1994): *Drug Facts and Comparisons*, 1926
(1988): Fesenko IP+, *Vrach Delo* (Russian) April, 93
(1980): Jain VK+, *Indian J Chest Dis Allied Sci* 22, 73
(1979): Odinokova VA+, *Arkh Patol* (Russian) 41, 37
(1979): Frontera-Izquierdo P+, *An Esp Pediatr* (Spanish) 12, 703
(1974): Ruiz-Maldonado R+, *Bol Med Hosp Infant Mex* (Spanish) 31, 1201
(1973): Sehgal VN+, *Indian J Chest Dis* 15, 57
(1967): Lowney ED+, *Arch Dermatol* 95, 359
Toxic erythema (sic)
(1981): Kushimoto H+, *Arch Dermatol* 117, 444
Urticaria
(1961): Gupta SK, *Indian J Dermatol* 6, 115
(1960): Heijer A+, *Acta Derm Venereol* (Stockh) 40, 35
(1949): Bunn PA+, *Streptomycin*, Williams and Wilkins, Baltimore, 524
(1949): Cohen AC+, *Arch Dermatol* 60, 373 (11%)
Vasculitis
(1971): Girard JP, *Helv Med Acta* 36, 3
(1949): Bunn PA+, *Streptomycin*, Williams and Wilkins, Baltimore, 524

Hair

Hair – hypertrichosis
(1992): Shelley WB+, *Advanced Dermatologic Diagnosis*, WB Saunders, 725 (passim)

Other

Anaphylactoid reaction
(1969): Levene GM+, *Trans St Johns Hosp Dermatol Soc* 55, 184
Black tongue
(1954): No Author, *Lancet* 2, 179
Embolia cutis medicamentosa (Nicolau syndrome)
(1972): Labouche F+, *Bull Soc Fr Dermatol Syphiligr* (French) 79, 559
Glossitis (2%)
(1949): Cohen AC+, *Arch Dermatol* 60, 373
Injection-site granuloma
Injection-site reaction (sic)
Oral mucosal eruption
(1972): Levantine A+, *Br J Dermatol* 86, 651
(1964): Dummett CO, *J Oral Ther Pharmacol* 1, 106
Oral ulceration
Paresthesias (<1%)
Stomatitis
(1964): Dummett CO, *J Oral Ther Pharmacol* 1, 106
(1948): Beham H+, *JAMA* 138, 495
Tremor (<1%)

STREPTOZOCIN

Trade name: Zanosar (Pharmacia & Upjohn)
Indications: Carcinoma of the pancreas, carcinoid tumor, Hodgkin's disease
Category: Antineoplastic
Half-life: 35 minutes
Clinically important, potentially serious interactions with: doxorubicin, immunosuppressives

Reactions

Skin

Edema
Exanthems
(1978): Levine N+, *Cancer Treat Rev* 5, 67

Pruritus
(1978): Levine N+, *Cancer Treat Rev* 5, 67
Purpura
Toxic epidermal necrolysis
(1975): Hadida E+, *Bull Soc Fr Dermatol Syphiligr* (French) 81, 76

Other

Injection-site erythema
Injection-site necrosis
(1987): Dufresne RG, *Cutis* 39, 197
Injection-site pain (1–10%)

SUCCINYLCHOLINE

Synonym: suxamethonium
Trade name: Anectine (GlaxoWellcome)
Indications: Skeletal muscle relaxation during general anesthesia
Category: Skeletal muscle relaxant; cholinergic
Half-life: no data
Clinically important, potentially serious interactions with: aminoglycosides, anticholinesterase drugs, beta-blockers, chloroquine, cimetidine, cyclophosphamide, digoxin, ketamine, lidocaine, lithium, MAO inhibitors, metoclopramide, oral contraceptives, quinidine, quinine, tacrine, thiotepa, vancomycin

Reactions

Skin

Contact dermatitis
(1996): Delgado J+, *Contact Dermatitis* 35, 120
Erythema (<1%)
(1975): Fisher MMcD, *Anaesth Intensive Care* 3, 180
Exanthems
Flushing
Pruritus (<1%)
Rash (sic) (<1%)
Urticaria

Other

Anaphylactoid reaction
(1999): Porter JM+, *Ir J Med Sci* 168, 99
(1999): Villas Martinez F+, *J Investig Allergol Clin Immunol* 9, 126
(1998): Tresch K+, *Ann Fr Anesth Reanim* (French) 17, 1181
(1981): Moneret-Vautrin DA+, *Clin Allergy* 11, 175 (13 cases)
(1975): Mandappa JM+, *Br J Anaesth* 47, 523 (2 cases)
Hypersensitivity
(1983): Yamaya R+, *Masui* (Japanese) 32, 1464
Myalgia (<1%)
(1996): van den Berg AA+, *Anaesth Intensive Care* 24, 116
Myopathy
(1990): Shoji S, *Nippon Rinsho* (Japanese) 48, 1517
Sialorrhea (1–10%)

SUCRALFATE

Trade name: Carafate (Aventis)
Other common trade names: *Antepsin; Sucrabest; Sulcrate; Ulcar; Ulcogant; Ulcyte; Urbal*
Indications: Duodenal ulcer
Category: Antiulcer; gastric mucosa protectant
Half-life: no data
Clinically important, potentially serious interactions with: antacids, cimetidine, ciprofloxacin, digoxin, ketoconazole, penicillamine, phenytoin, quinidine, quinolones, ranitidine, tetracycline, theophylline

Reactions

Skin

Angioedema
Exanthems
(1984): Brogden RN+, *Drugs* 17, 233
Facial edema
Pruritus (<0.5%)
Rash (sic) (<0.5%)
Urticaria

Other

Xerostomia (<1%)

SUFENTANIL

Trade name: Sufenta (Taylor)
Indications: Epidural and general anesthesia
Category: Narcotic analgesic
Half-life: 152 minutes
Clinically important, potentially serious interactions with: beta-blockers, CNS depressants

Reactions

Skin

Chills
Cold clammy skin (<1%)
Erythema
Pruritus (25%)
Rash (sic) (<1%)
Urticaria (<1%)

Other

Dysesthesia (<1%)

SULFADIAZINE

Trade name: Microsulfon
Other trade name: *Coptin*
Indications: Various infections caused by susceptible organisms
Category: Sulfonamide* antibiotic
Half-life: 17 hours
Clinically important, potentially serious interactions with: anticoagulants, cyclosporine, hypoglycemics, methotrexate, phenytoin, sulfonylureas, warfarin

Reactions

Skin

Allergy (sic)
(1991): de la Hoz Caballer B+, *J Allergy Clin Immunol* 88, 137
Argyria
(1992): Payne CM+, *Lancet* 340, 126 (from silver sulfadiazine)
(1992): Fraser-Moodie A, *Burns* 18, 74 (from silver sulfadiazine)
Chills
Erythema multiforme
(1983): Lockhart SP+, *Burns Incl Therm Inj* 10, 9
Exanthems
(1984): Finland M+, *JAMA* 251, 1467
Exfoliative dermatitis
Fixed eruption
(1991): Thankappen TP+, *Int J Dermatol* 30, 867 (12.4%)
Lupus erythematosus
Periorbital edema
Photosensitivity (>10%)
Pigmentation
(1985): Dupuis LL+, *J Am Acad Dermatol* 12, 1112
Pruritus (>10%)
Purpura
Rash (sic) (>10%)
Stevens–Johnson syndrome (1–10%)
(1999): Carrion-Carrion C+, *Ann Pharmacother* 33, 379 (fatal) (in AIDS patient)
(1965): Sharma R+, *J Assoc Physicians India* 13, 727

Toxic epidermal necrolysis (1–10%)
(1993): Correia O+, *Dermatology* 186, 32
Urticaria

Other

Anaphylactoid reaction
Hypersensitivity
(1987): Volckaert A+, *Acta Clin Belg* 42, 381
(1985): Jia XM, *Chung Hua Cheng Hsing Shao Shang Wai Ko Tsa Chih* (Chinese) 1, 232
Serum sickness (<1%)
Stomatitis

***Note:** Sulfadiazine is a sulfonamide and can be absorbed systemically. Sulfonamides can produce severe, possibly fatal, reactions such as toxic epidermal necrolysis and Stevens–Johnson syndrome.

SULFADOXINE

Trade name: Fansidar (Roche)
Other common trade names: *Cryodoxin; Malocide; Methipox*
Indications: Malaria
Category: Sulfonamide* antimalarial; folic acid antagonist
Half-life: 5–8 days
Clinically important, potentially serious interactions with: co-trimoxazole, methotrexate, other sulfonamides

Fansidar is sulfadoxine and pyrimethamine (this combination is almost always prescribed)

Reactions

Skin

Bullous eruption
(1985): Hernborg A, *Lancet* 1, 1072
Erythema multiforme (<1%)
(1993): Sturchler D+, *Drug Saf* 8, 160
(1989): Ortel B+, *Dermatologica* 178, 39
(1986): Miller KD+, *Am J Trop Med Hyg* 35, 451
Exanthems
(1987): Groth H+, *Schweiz Rundsch Med Prax* (German) 76, 570
Exfoliative dermatitis
(1987): Zitelli BJ+, *Ann Intern Med* 106, 393
(1987): Elsas T+, *Tidsskr Nor Laegeforen* (Norwegian) 107, 1231
(1986): Langtry JA+, *Br Med J Clin Res Ed* 292, 1107
Lupus erythematosus
Necrosis (<1%)
Periorbital edema
Photosensitivity (>10%)
(1989): Ortel B+, *Dermatologica* 178, 39
(1985): Hernborg A, *Lancet* 1, 1072 (passim)
Pruritus
(1987): Groth H+, *Schweiz Rundsch Med Prax* (German) 76, 570
Purpura
(1985): Hernborg A, *Lancet* 1, 1072 (passim)
Pustular eruption
Rash (sic) (<1%)
Stevens–Johnson syndrome (1–10%)
(1993): Sturchler D+, *Drug Saf* 8, 160
(1990): Thiel HJ+, *Klin Monatsbl Augenheilkd* (German) 197, 142
(1989): Phillips-Howard PA+, *Lancet* 2, 803
(1989): Ortel B+, *Dermatologica* 178, 39
(1987): Hellgren U+, *Br Med J Clin Res Ed* 295, 365
(1987): Lenox-Smith I, *J Infect* 14, 90 (fatal)
(1986): Jeffrey RF, *Postgrad Med J* 62, 893
(1986): Gascon-Brustenga J+, *Med Clin (Barc)* (Spanish) 87, 821
(1986): Bamber MG+, *J Infect* 13, 31 (fatal)
(1986): Steffen R+, *Lancet* 1, 610
(1986): Miller KD+, *Am J Trop Med Hyg* 35, 451
(1985): Hernborg A, *Lancet* 2, 1072
(1985): Navin TR+, *Lancet* 1, 1332
(1985): Clareus BW+, *Lakartidningen* (Swedish) 82, 4211
(1985): Adams SJ+, *Postgrad Med J* 61, 263
(1983): Ligthelm RJ+, *Ned Tijdschr Geneeskd* (Dutch) 127, 1735
(1982): Hornstein OP+, *N Engl J Med* 307, 1529
(1982): Olsen VV+, *Lancet* 2, 994
(1982): Aberer W+, *Hautarzt* (German) 33, 484
Toxic epidermal necrolysis
(2000): Moussala M+, *J Fr Ophtalmol* (French) 23, 229
(1998): Moussala M+, *J Fr Ophtalmol* (French) 21, 72
(1998): Schmidt-Westhausen A+, *Oral Dis* 4, 90
(1993): Correia O+, *Dermatology* 186, 32
(1993): Sturchler D+, *Drug Saf* 8, 160
(1991): Kimura S+, *Jpn J Med* 30, 553
(1990): Ward DJ+, *Burns* 16, 97
(1989): Caumes E+, *Presse Med* (French) 18, 1708 (fatal)
(1988): No Author, *MMWR Morb Mortal Wkly Rep* 37, 571 (fatal)
(1988): Raviglione MC+, *Arch Intern Med* 148, 2863 (fatal)
(1988): No Author, *JAMA* 260, 2193 (fatal)
(1986): Miller KD+, *Am J Trop Med Hyg* 35, 451
(1984): Chan HL, *J Am Acad Dermatol* 10, 973
(1983): Ghinelli F+, *Acta Biomed Ateneo Parmense* (Italian) 54, 363
Urticaria

Other

Ageusia
Anaphylactoid reaction
Glossitis (>10%)
Hypersensitivity (>10%)
Oral lichenoid eruption
(1989): Zain RB, *Southeast Asian J Trop Med Public Health* 20, 253
Oral ulceration
(1985): Hernborg A, *Lancet* 1, 1072
Stomatitis
(1985): Hernborg A, *Lancet* 1, 1072 (passim)
Tremors (>10%)
Urogenital ulceration
(1985): Hernborg A, *Lancet* 1, 1072

***Note:** Sulfadoxine is a sulfonamide and can be absorbed systemically. Sulfonamides can produce severe, possibly fatal, reactions such as toxic epidermal necrolysis and Stevens–Johnson syndrome.

SULFAMETHOXAZOLE

Trade names: Bactrim (Roche); Septra (Monarch)
Other common trade names: *Sinomin; Urobak*
Indications: Various infections caused by susceptible organisms
Category: Antibacterial and antiprotozoal sulfonamide*
Half-life: 7–12 hours
Clinically important, potentially serious interactions with: anticoagulants, cyclosporine, hydantoins; hypoglycemics, MAO inhibitors, methotrexate

Note: Sulfamethoxazole is commonly used in conjunction with trimethoprim (see co-trimoxazole)

Reactions

Skin

Acute febrile neutrophilic dermatosis (Sweet's syndrome)
(1996): Walker DC+, *J Am Acad Dermatol* 34, 918
(1989): Cobb MW, *J Am Acad Dermatol* 21, 339 (passim)
(1986): Su WPD+, *Cutis* 37, 167
Acute generalized exanthematous pustulosis (AGEP)
(1995): Moreau A+, *Int J Dermatol* 34, 263 (passim)
Angioedema
(1988): Fihn SD+, *Ann Intern Med* 108, 350 (1–5%)
Bullous eruption
(1989): Caumes E+, *Presse Med* (French) 18, 1708
Cutaneous side effects (sic)
(1994): Roudier C+, *Arch Dermatol* 130, 1383 (48% in AIDS patients)
(1971): Koch-Weser J+, *Arch Intern Med* 128, 399 (2.1%)
Dermatitis (sic)
(1989): Atahan IL+, *Br J Radiol* 62, 1107 (at previously irradiated area)
(1984): Shelley WB+, *J Am Acad Dermatol* 11, 53 (at site of previous sunburn)
(1987): Vukelja SJ+, *Cancer Treat Rep* 71, 668 (at previously irradiated area)

(1971): Cotterill JA+, *Br J Dermatol* 84, 366

Erythema multiforme

(1997): Rieder MJ+, *Pediatr Infect Dis J* 16, 1028 (70% in children with HIV)
(1991): Tilden ME+, *Arch Ophthalmol* 109, 67
(1990): Chan HL+, *Arch Dermatol* 126, 43
(1989): Alanko K+, *Acta Derm Venereol* (Stockh) 69, 223
(1988): Hira SK+, *J Am Acad Dermatol* 19, 451
(1988): Platt R+, *J Infect Dis* 158, 474
(1987): Schöpf E, *Infection* 15 (Suppl 5P), S254
(1987): Penmetcha M, *BMJ* 295, 556
(1985): Heer M+, *Gastroenterology* 88, 1954
(1982): Brettle RP+, *J Infect* 4, 149
(1979): Beck MH+, *Clin Exp Dermatol* 4, 201
(1978): Assaad D+, *Can Med Assoc J* 118, 154
(1978): Azinge NO+, *J Allergy Clin Immunol* 62, 125
(1975): Bernstein LS, *Can Med Assoc J* 112 (Suppl), 96
(1971): Koch-Weser J+, *Arch Intern Med* 128, 399 (0.15%)

Erythema nodosum

(1974): Delaney TJ+, *Br J Dermatol* 90, 205
(1971): Koch-Weser J+, *Arch Intern Med* 128, 399

Erythroderma

(1979): Kennedy C+, *BMJ* 1, 1356

Exanthems

(1998): Hattori N+, *J Dermatol* 25, 269
(1997): Caumes E+, *Arch Dermatol* 133, 465
(1995): Wolkenstein P+, *Arch Dermatol* 131, 544
(1995): Hertl M+, *Br J Dermatol* 132, 215
(1994): Litt JZ, Beachwood, OH, personal case (observation)
(1993): Litt JZ, Beachwood, OH, personal case (observation)
(1993): Malnick SDH+, *Ann Pharmacotherapy* 27, 1139
(1993): Agarwal BR+, *Indian Pediatr* 30, 1026
(1990): Medina I+, *N Engl J Med* 323, 776 (47% in AIDS patients)
(1988): Sattler FR+, *Ann Intern Med* 109, 280 (44% in AIDS patients)
(1988): Weinke T+, *Dtsch Med Wochenschr* (German) 113, 1129 (25% in AIDS patients)
(1988): Fihn SD+, *Ann Intern Med* 108, 350 (1–5%)
(1988): DeRaeve L+, *Br J Dermatol* 119, 521 (in AIDS patient)
(1987): Goa KL+, *Drugs* 33, 242 (65% in AIDS patients)
(1987): Schöpf E, *Infection* 15 (Suppl 5P), S254
(1986): Sonntag MR+, *Schweiz Med Wochenschr* (German) 116, 142
(1985): DeHovitz JA+, *Ann Intern Med* 103, 479
(1985): Maayan S+, *Arch Intern Med* 145, 1607
(1984): Kovacs JA+, *Ann Intern Med* 100, 663 (29% in AIDS patients)
(1984): Gordon FM+, *Ann Intern Med* 100, 495 (51% in AIDS patients)
(1983): Mitsuyasu R+, *N Engl J Med* 308, 1535 (69% in AIDS patients.)
(1982): Goetz MB+, *JAMA* 247, 3118
(1980): Fennell RS+, *Clin Pediatr* 19, 124
(1979): Abengowe CU, *Curr Med Res Opin* 5, 749 (3.2%)
(1977): Taylor B+, *BMJ* 2, 552 (12%)
(1976): Gower PE+, *BMJ* 1, 684 (>5%)
(1976): Arndt KA+, *JAMA* 235, 918 (5.9%)
(1975): Sallam MA+, *Curr Med Res Opin* 3, 229 (3.4%)
(1975): Bernstein LS, *Can Med Assoc J* 112 (Suppl), 96 (1.9%)
(1975): Gleckman RA, *JAMA* 233, 427 (0.84%)
(1972): Halpern GM, *BMJ* 1, 691
(1971): Koch-Weser J+, *Arch Intern Med* 128, 399 (1%)

Exfoliative dermatitis

(1990): Ponte CD+, *Drug Intell Clin Pharm* 24, 140 (feet)
(1975): Bernstein LS, *Can Med Assoc J* 112 (Suppl), 96
(1971): Koch-Weser J+, *Arch Intern Med* 128, 399

Fixed eruption

(1997): Gruber F+, *Clin Exp Dermatol* 22, 144
(1996): Sharma VK+, *J Dermatol* 23, 530
(1995): Wolkenstein P+, *Arch Dermatol* 131, 544
(1993): Oleaga JM+, *Contact Dermatitis* 29, 155
(1993): Ramam M+, *Indian Pediatr* 30, 110 (in an infant)
(1992): Lim JT+, *Ann Acad Med Singapore* 21, 408
(1991): Smoller BR+, *J Cutan Pathol* 18, 13
(1991): Jain VK+, *Ann Dent* 50, 9 (oral mucous membrane)
(1990): Gaffoor PMA+, *Cutis* 45, 242 (genitalia)
(1989): Gupta R, *Indian J Dermatol* 55, 181 (in an infant)
(1989): Varsano I+, *Dermatologica* 178, 232
(1989): Bharija SC+, *Australas J Dermatol* 30, 43
(1989): Basomba A+, *J Allergy Clin Immunol* 84, 409
(1988): Baird BJ+, *Int J Dermatol* 27, 170 (bullous and generalized)
(1988): Bharija SC+, *Dermatologica* 176, 108 (in an infant)
(1987): Amir J+, *Drug Intell Clin Pharm* 21, 41
(1987): Hughes BR+, *Br J Dermatol* 116, 241
(1987): Van Voorhees A+, *Am J Dermatopathol* 9, 528
(1986): Kanwar AJ+, *Dermatologica* 172, 230
(1985): Gomez B+, *Allergol Immunopathol Madr* (Spanish) 13, 87
(1984): Pandhi RK+, *Sex Transm Dis* 11, 164
(1982): Gibson JR, *BMJ* 284, 1529
(1980): Talbot MD, *Practitioner* 224, 823
(1978): Verbov J, *Arch Dermatol* 114, 963
(1972): Aoyama H+, *Jpn J Dermatol B* 82, 16

Flushing

(1984): Jick SS+, *Lancet* 2, 631

Lichenoid eruption

(1994): Berger TG+, *Arch Dermatol* 130, 609

Linear IgA bullous dermatosis

(1994): Kuechle MK+, *J Am Acad Dermatol* 30, 187

Lupus erythematosus

(1985): Stratton MA, *Clin Pharm* 4, 657
(1975): Grennan DM+, *BMJ* 4, 385

Mucocutaneous syndrome

(1982): Brettle RP+, *J Infect* 4, 149

Photosensitivity (>10%)

(1994): Shelley WB+, *Cutis* 53, 162 (observation)
(1994): Berger TG+, *Arch Dermatol* 130, 609 (in HIV-infected) (4 cases)
(1987): Schöpf E, *Infection* 15 (Suppl 5P), S254
(1986): Chandler MJ, *J Infect Dis* 153, 1001

Pruritus (>10%)

(1997): Caumes E+, *Arch Dermatol* 133, 465
(1997): Thaler D, Monona, WI (from Internet) (observation)
(1996): Litt JZ, Beachwood, OH, personal case (observation)
(1990): Medina I+, *N Engl J Med* 323, 776 (1–5%)
(1987): Colebunders R+, *Ann Intern Med* 107, 599 (4% in AIDS patients)
(1986): Sher MR, *J Allergy Clin Immunol* 77, 133
(1984): Kramer BS+, *Cancer* 53, 329
(1975): Gleckman RA, *JAMA* 233, 427 (0.84%)
(1971): Koch-Weser J+, *Arch Intern Med* 128, 399 (0.15%)

Pruritus vulvae

(1981): *Modern Medicine* 49, 111

Psoriasis

(1979): Kennedy C+, *BMJ* 1, 1356

Purpura

(1993): Kaufman DW+, *Blood* 82, 2714
(1989): Saxena SK, *J Assoc Physicians India* 37, 479
(1971): Koch-Weser J+, *Arch Intern Med* 128, 399

Pustular eruption

(1994): Spencer JM+, *Br J Dermatol* 130, 514
(1990): Guy C+, *Nouv Dermatol* (French) 9, 540
(1989): Grattan CEH, *Dermatologica* 179, 57 (passim)
(1986): Macdonald KJS+, *BMJ* 293, 1279
(1978): Braun-Falco O+, *Hautarzt* (German) 29, 371
(1977): Knudsen L+, *Ugeskr Laeger* (Danish) 139, 1007

Radiation recall

(1990): Leslie MD+, *Br J Radiol* 63, 661
(1987): Vukelja SJ+, *Cancer Treat Rep* 71, 668 (at previously irradiated area)
(1984): Shelley WB+, *J Am Acad Dermatol* 11, 53 (at site of previous sunburn)

Rash (sic) (>10%)

(1995): Williams JW+, *JAMA* 273, 1015
(1993): Malnick SD+, *Ann Pharmacother* 27, 1139

Stevens–Johnson syndrome (1–10%)

(1997): Douglas R+, *Clin Infect Dis* 25, 1480
(1997): Rieder MJ+, *Pediatr Infect Dis J* 16, 1028 (10% in children with HIV)
(1996): Caumes E, *Rev Mal Respir* (French) 13, 101
(1996): McCarty J, Fort Worth, TX (from Internet) (observation)
(1995): Kuper K+, *Ophthalmologe* (German) 92, 823
(1995): Sharma VK+, *Pediatr Dermatol* 12, 178
(1995): Wolkenstein P+, *Arch Dermatol* 131, 544
(1994): Shelley WB+, *Cutis* 53, 159 (observation)
(1993): Litt JZ, Beachwood, OH, personal case (observation)
(1990): Chan HL+, *Arch Dermatol* 126, 43
(1988): Platt R+, *J Infect Dis* 158, 474
(1985): Heer M+, *Gastroenterology* 88, 1954
(1982): Brettle RP+, *J Infect* 4, 149
(1979): Beck MH+, *Clin Exp Dermatol* 4, 201
(1978): Azinge NO+, *J Allergy Clin Immunol* 62, 125
(1978): Kikuchi S+, *Lancet* 2, 580

(1978): Thorpe JA+, *Lancet* 1, 276 (fatal)
(1975): Bernstein LS, *Can Med Assoc J* 112 (Suppl), 96
(1970): Shaw DJ+, *Johns Hopkins Med J* 126, 130

Toxic epidermal necrolysis (1–10%)
(2000): Moussala M+, *J Fr Ophtalmol* (French) 23, 229
(1996): Caumes E, *Rev Mal Respir* 13, 101
(1996): Rehbein H, Jacksonville, FL (from Internet) (observation)
(1995): Sharma VK+, *Pediatr Dermatol* 12, 178
(1995): Wolkenstein P+, *Arch Dermatol* 131, 544 (7 cases)
(1993): Correia O+, *Dermatology* 186, 32
(1990): Kobza Black A+, *Br J Dermatol* 123, 277
(1990): Ward DJ+, *Burns* 16, 97
(1990): Chan HL+, *Arch Dermatol* 126, 43
(1990): Roujeau JC+, *Arch Dermatol* 126, 37
(1989): Carmichael AJ+, *Lancet* 2, 808
(1989): Whittington RM, *Lancet* 2, 574
(1988): De Raeve L+, *Br J Dermatol* 119, 521 (passim)
(1987): Guillaume JC+, *Arch Dermatol* 123, 1166
(1987): Schöpf E, *Infection* 15 (Suppl 5P), S254
(1986): Miller KD+, *Am J Trop Med Hyg* 33, 451
(1986): Roman O+, *Rev Pediatr Obstet Ginecol Pediatr* (Romanian) 35, 261
(1986): Revuz J, *J Dermatol Paris* 153
(1984): Westly ED+, *Arch Dermatol* 120, 721
(1984): Fong PH+, *Singapore Med J* 25, 184
(1983): Petersen P+, *Ugeskr Laeger* (Danish) 145, 3345
(1982): Ortiz JE+, *Ann Plast Surg* 9, 249
(1978): Assaad D+, *Can Med Assoc J* 118, 154
(1978): Petricevic I+, *Lijec Vjesn* (Serbo-Croatian-Roman) 100, 596
(1975): Bernstein LS, *Can Med Assoc J* 112 (Suppl), 96
(1973): Beyvin AJ+, *Anesth Analg Paris* (French) 30, 767
(1972): Chanial G+, *J Med Lyon* (French) 53, 859
(1971): Chanial G+, *Bull Soc Fr Dermatol Syphiligr* (French) 78, 565

Urticaria
(1994): Blumenthal HL, Beachwood, OH, personal case (observation)
(1993): Litt JZ, Beachwood, OH, personal case (observation)
(1991): Greenberger PA, *JAMA* 265, 458
(1987): Schöpf E, *Infection* 15 (Suppl 5P), S254
(1985): Maayan S+, *Arch Intern Med* 145, 1607
(1985): Goolamali SK, *Postgrad Med J* 61, 925
(1984): Kramer BS+, *Cancer* 53, 329
(1981): Abi-Mansur P+, *Am J Gastroenterol* 76, 356
(1971): Koch-Weser J+, *Arch Intern Med* 128, 399

Vasculitis (<1%)
(1989): Verne-Pignatelli J+, *Postgrad Med J* 65, 51
(1987): Schöpf E, *Infection* 15 (Suppl 5P), S254
(1978): Coquin Y+, *Nouv Presse Med* (French) 7, 3145
(1978): Braun-Falco O+, *Hautarzt* (German) 29, 371
(1976): Wåhlin A+, *Lancet* 2, 1415
(1971): Koch-Weser J+, *Arch Intern Med* 128, 399

Vulvovaginitis
(1985): Wong ES+, *Ann Intern Med* 102, 302

Other

Anaphylactoid reaction
(1988): Arnold PA+, *Drug Intell Clin Pharm* 22, 43
(1985): Gossius G+, *Scand J Infect Dis* 16, 373

Aphthous stomatitis
(1981): *J Antimicrob Chemother* 7, 179

Black tongue
(1993): Blumenthal HL, Beachwood, OH, personal case (observation)

Dysgeusia
(1988): Fischl MA+, *JAMA* 259, 1185

Glossitis

Hypersensitivity
(1998): Chen D, Chicagi, IL (from Internet) (observation)
(1997): Hicks ME+, *Ann Pharmacother* 31, 1259
(1993): Mehta J+, *J Assoc Physicians India* 41, 235
(1993): Marinac JS+, *Clin Infect Dis* 16, 178
(1993): Martin GJ+, *Clin Infect Dis* 16, 175
(1993): Mathelier-Fusade P+, *Presse Med* (French) 22, 1363

Oral mucosal eruption
(1991): Tilden ME+, *Arch Ophthalmol* 109, 67
(1988): Fihn SD+, *Ann Intern Med* 108, 350 (1–5%)

Oral ulceration
(1987): Hughes WT+, *N Engl J Med* 316, 1627
(1981): Orenstein WA+, *Am J Med Sci* 282, 27

Pseudolymphoma
(1978): Laugier P+, *Z Hautkr* (German) 53, 353

Serum sickness (<1%)
(1988): Platt R+, *J Infect Dis* 158, 474

Stomatitis

Tongue ulceration
(1981): *J Antimicrob Chemother* 7, 179

***Note:** Sulfamethoxazole is a sulfonamide and can be absorbed systemically. Sulfonamides can produce severe, possibly fatal, reactions such as toxic epidermal necrolysis and Stevens–Johnson syndrome.

SULFASALAZINE

Synonym: salicylazosulfapyridine
Trade name: Azulfidine (Pharmacia & Upjohn)
Other common trade names: *Colo-Pleon; Salazopyrin; Salisulf; Saridine; SAS-500; Sulfazine; Ulcol*
Indications: Ulcerative colitis; rheumatoid arthritis
Category: Inflammatory bowel disease; sulfonamide*
Half-life: 5–10 hours
Clinically important, potentially serious interactions with: anticoagulants, anticonvulsants, digoxin, folic acid, oral hypoglycemics, methotrexate, sulfonylureas, warfarin

Reactions

Skin

Acute generalized exanthematous pustulosis (AGEP)
(1999): Kawaguchi M+, *J Dermatol* 26, 359
(1998): Mitchell D, Thomasville, GA (from Internet) (observation)
(1993): Wainwright NJ+, *Drug Saf* 9, 437
(1993): Marce S+, *Presse Med* (French) 22, 271

Angioedema
(1990): Petterson T+, *Br J Rheumatol* 29, 239
(1990): Donovan S+, *Br J Rheumatol* 29, 201

Bullous eruption

Bullous pemphigoid
(1970): Bean SF+, *Arch Dermatol* 102, 205

Cheilitis
(1986): Farr M+, *Drugs* 32 (Suppl 1), 49

Cutaneous side effects (sic)
(1986): Amos RS+, *BMJ* 293, 420 (5.5%)

Dermatitis (sic)
(1989): Challier P+, *Presse Med* (French) 18, 778

Diaphoresis
(1986): Farr M+, *Drugs* 32 (Suppl 1), 49

Eczematous eruption (sic)
(1947): Sulzberger MB+, *J Allergy* 18, 92

Erythema multiforme
(1987): Penmetcha M, *BMJ* 295, 556
(1986): Garcia e Silva L, *Acta Med Port* (Portuguese) 7, 71
(1985): Hernborg A, *Lancet* 2, 1072
(1985): Huff JC, *Dermatol Clin* 3, 141
(1985): Heer M+, *Gastroenterology* 88, 1954
(1982): Hornstein OP+, *N Engl J Med* 307, 1529
(1979): Beck MH+, *Clin Exp Dermatol* 4, 201
(1966): Cameron HA+, *BMJ* 2, 1174

Erythema nodosum
(1986): Areias E+, *Ann Dermatol Venereol* (French) 113, 197
(1971): Koch-Weser J+, *Arch Intern Med* 128, 399

Erythroderma
(1984): Sala F+, *Cronica Dermatol* (Italian) 15, 209

Exanthems
(1995): Wolkenstein P+, *Arch Dermatol* 131, 544
(1994): Akahoshi K+, *J Gastroenterol* 29 772
(1992): Bodokh I+, *Presse Med* (French) 21, 630
(1991): Hertzberger-ten-Cate R+, *Clin Exp Rheumatol* 9, 85
(1990): Gupta AK+, *Arch Dermatol* 126, 487 (23%)
(1990): Petterson T+, *Br J Rheumatol* 29, 239
(1990): Donovan S+, *Br J Rheumatol* 29, 201 (4.1%)
(1989): Gremse DA+, *J Pediatr Gastroenterol Nutr* 9, 261
(1989): Alanko K+, *Acta Derm Venereol* (Stockh) 69, 223
(1988): Williams HJ+, *Arthritis Rheum* 31, 702 (7%)
(1986): Farr M+, *Drugs* 32 (Suppl 1), 49
(1986): Poland GA+, *Am J Med* 81, 707

(1985): Maayan S+, *Arch Intern Med* 145, 1607
(1984): Purdy BH+, *Ann Intern Med* 100, 512
(1984): Iwatsuki K+, *Arch Dermatol* 120, 964
(1984): Peppercorn MA, *Ann Intern Med* 101, 377
(1982): Goetz MB+, *JAMA* 247, 3118
(1980): Fennell RS+, *Clin Pediatr* 19, 124
(1976): Arndt KA+, *JAMA* 235, 918 (2%)
(1973): Das KM+, *N Engl J Med* 289, 491 (2%)
(1972): Halpern GM, *BMJ* 1, 691
(1968): Baron JH+, *Lancet* 1, 1094
(1962): Truelove SC+, *BMJ* 2, 1708 (3%)

Exfoliative dermatitis
(1990): Donovan S+, *Br J Rheumatol* 29, 201
(1984): Sala F+, *Cronica Dermatol* (Italian) 15, 209
(1978): Mihas AA+, *JAMA* 239, 2590
(1975): Bernstein LS, *Can Med Assoc J* 112, 96S
(1971): Koch-Weser J+, *Arch Intern Med* 128, 399

Fixed eruption
(1996): Kawada A+, *Contact Dermatitis* 34, 155
(1988): Bharija SC+, *Dermatologica* 176, 108
(1987): Hughes BR+, *Br J Dermatol* 116, 241
(1987): Kanwar AJ+, *Dermatologica* 174, 104
(1986): Kanwar AJ+, *Dermatologica* 172, 230
(1982): Gibson JR, *BMJ* 284, 1529
(1980): Talbot MD, *Practitioner* 224, 823

Flushing
(2000): Jung JH+, *Clin Exp Rheumatol* 18, 245
(1984): Jick SS+, *Lancet* 2, 631

Lichen planus
(1995): Kaplan S+, *J Rheumatol* 22, 191
(1991): Alstead EM+, *J Clin Gastroenterol* 13, 335

Lupus erythematosus
(1997): Gunnarsson I+, *Br J Rheumatol* 36, 1089
(1996): Khattak FH+, *Br J Rheumatol* 35, 104
(1995): Veale DJ+, *Br J Rheumatol* 34, 383
(1994): Fritzler MJ, *Lupus* 3, 455
(1994): Bray VJ+, *J Rheumatol* 21, 2157
(1994): Borg AA+, *Clin Rheumatol* 13, 522
(1994): Mongey AB+, *Br J Rheumatol* 33, 789
(1994): Walker EM+, *Br J Rheumatol* 33, 175
(1994): Caulier M+, *J Rheumatol* 21, 750
(1993): Wildhagen K+, *Clin Rheumatol* 12, 265
(1993): Siam AR+, *J Rheumatol* 20, 207
(1992): Skaer TL, *Clin Ther* 14, 496
(1991): Alarcon-Segovia D+, *Baillieres Clin Rheumatol* 5, 1
(1989): Sugimoto M+, *Nippon Naika Gakkai Zasshi* (Japanese) 78, 583
(1989): Deboever G+, *Am J Gastroenterol* 84, 85
(1988): Clementz GL+, *Am J Med* 84, 535
(1987): Hobbs RN+, *Ann Rheum Dis* 46, 408
(1985): Stratton MA, *Clin Pharm* 4, 657
(1985): Lovisetto P+, *Recenti Prog Med* (Italian) 76, 110
(1983): Vanheule BA+, *Eur J Pediatr* 140, 66
(1982): Carr-Locke DL, *Am J Gastroenterol* 77, 614
(1980): Crisp AJ+, *J R Soc Med* 73, 60
(1980): Rouleau L+, *Union Med Can* (French) 109, 1326
(1979): Weiller PJ+, *Ann Med Interne Paris* (French) 130, 665
(1978): Jaup BH, *Dtsch Med Wochenschr* (German) 103, 1211
(1977): Griffiths ID+, *BMJ* 2, 1188
(1969): Alarcon-Segovia D, *Mayo Clin Proc* 44, 664
(1966): Cohen P+, *JAMA* 197, 817

Necrosis
(1988): Krakamp B+, *Med Klin* (German) 83, 611

Periorbital edema

Photosensitivity (>10%)
(1999): Bouyssou-Gauthier ML, *Dermatology* 198, 388
(1994): Shelley WB+, *Cutis* 53, 240 (observation)
(1986): Chandler MJ, *J Infect Dis* 153, 1001
(1986): Amos RS+, *BMJ* 293, 420 (1–5%)

Pigmentation
(1992): Gabazza EC+, *Am J Gastroenterol* 87, 1654 (orange-yellow)
(1970): Morse MO+, *Arch Dermatol* 102, 112
(1968): Yell J+, *BMJ* 4, 452

Pruritus (>10%)
(1993): Gran JT+, *Scand J Rheumatol* 22, 229
(1990): Donovan S+, *Br J Rheumatol* 29, 201
(1990): Peppercorn MA, *Ann Intern Med* 112, 50 (1–5%)
(1987): Colebunders R+, *Ann Intern Med* 107, 599
(1986): Farr M+, *Drugs* 32 (Suppl 1), 49
(1986): Sher MR, *J Allergy Clin Immunol* 77, 133
(1984): Kramer BS+, *Cancer* 53, 329

Pruritus vulvae
(1981): *Modern Medicine* 49, 111

Psoriasis
(1991): Bliddal H+, *Clin Rheumatol* 10, 178

Purpura
(1989): Gremse DA+, *J Pediatr Gastroenterol Nutr* 9, 261

Pustular eruption
(1994): Gallais V+, *Ann Dermatol Venereol* (French) 121, 11
(1976): Lindgren S+, *Acta Derm Venereol* (Stockh) 56, 139

Rash (sic) (>10%)
(2000): Jung JH+, *Clin Exp Rheumatol* 18, 245
(1999): Besnard M+, *Arch Pediatr* 6, 643
(1994): McCarthy C+, *Ir J Med Sci* 163, 238
(1993): Koski JM, *Clin Exp Dermatol* 11, 169
(1992): Brooks H+, *Clin Rheumatol* 11, 566
(1989): Gyssens IC+, *Ned Tijdschr Geneeskd* (Dutch) 133, 1608
(1989): Scott DL+, *J Rheumatol* Suppl 16, 17
(1986): Bax DE+, *Ann Rheum Dis* 45, 139
(1984): Purdy BH+, *Ann Intern Med* 100, 512
(1984): Farr M+, *Clin Rheumatol* 3, 473
(1978): Mihas AA+, *JAMA* 239, 2590

Raynaud's phenomenon
(1984): Peppercorn MA, *Ann Intern Med* 101, 377
(1980): Reid J+, *Postgraduate Med J* 56, 106

Skin reactions (sic)
(1993): Gran JT+, *Scand J Rheumatol* 22, 229

Stevens–Johnson syndrome (<1%)
(1966): Cameron HA+, *BMJ* 2, 1174

Toxic epidermal necrolysis (1–10%)
(1995): Jullien D+, *Arthritis Rheum* 38, 573
(1987): Guillaume JC+, *Arch Dermatol* 123, 1166
(1985): Heng MCY, *Br J Dermatol* 113, 597
(1985): Curley RK+, *Br Med J Clin Res Ed* 290, 471 (fatal)
(1984): Peppercorn MA, *Ann Intern Med* 101, 377
(1981): Hensen E, *Tijdschr Ziekenverpl* (Dutch) 34, 563
(1981): Hensen EJ+, *Lancet* 2, 151
(1980): Maddocks JL+, *J R Soc Med* 73, 587
(1976): Varkonyi V+, *Orv Hetil* (Hungarian) 117, 971
(1975): Bernstein LS, *Can Med Assoc J* 112, 96S

Urticaria (<3%)
(2000): Jung JH+, *Clin Exp Rheumatol* 18, 245
(1989): Alanko K+, *Acta Derm Venereol* (Stockh) 69, 223
(1986): Farr M+, *Drugs* 32 (Suppl 1), 49
(1986): Amos RS+, *BMJ* 293, 420 (1–5%)
(1985): Maayan S+, *Arch Intern Med* 145, 1607
(1984): Purdy BH+, *Ann Intern Med* 100, 512
(1984): Peppercorn MA, *Ann Intern Med* 101, 377
(1984): Kramer BS+, *Cancer* 53, 329
(1981): Abi-Mansur P+, *Am J Gastroenterol* 76, 356
(1971): Koch-Weser J+, *Arch Intern Med* 128, 399

Vasculitis
(1971): Koch-Weser J+, *Arch Intern Med* 128, 399
(1965): McCombs RP, *JAMA* 194, 1059

Vulvovaginitis
(1985): Wong ES+, *Ann Intern Med* 102, 302

Xerosis
(1990): Donovan S+, *Br J Rheumatol* 29, 201

Hair

Hair – alopecia
(1988): Fich A+, *J Clin Gastroenterol* 10, 466
(1987): Codeluppi P+, *Dig Dis Sci* 32, 221
(1986): Farr M+, *Drugs* 32 (Suppl 1), 49
(1986): Breen EG+, *BMJ* 292, 802
(1983): Taffet SL+, *Dig Dis Sci* 28, 833
(1981): Attar A+, *Gastroenterology* 80, 1102

Other

Anaphylactoid reaction
(1990): Donovan S+, *Br J Rheumatol* 29, 201
(1988): Arnold PA+, *Drug Intell Clin Pharm* 22, 43
(1985): Gossius G+, *Scand J Infect Dis* 16, 373

Aphthous stomatitis
(1981): *J Antimicrob Chemother* 7, 179

Dysgeusia
(1991): Marcus RW, *J Rheumatol* 18, 634

Glossitis
Hypersensitivity (1–5%)
(1998): Tohyama M+, *Arch Dermatol* 134, 1113
(1997): Otero S+, *Gastroenterol Hepatol* (Spanish) 20, 446
(1995): Tolia V, *Am J Gastroenterol* 87, 1029
(1992): Leroux JL+, *Clin Exp Rheumatol* 10, 427
(1987): Ackerman Z+, *Postgrad Med J* 63, 55
(1984): Korelitz BI+, *J Clin Gastroenterol* 6, 27
(1978): Sotolongo RP+, *Gastroenterology* 75, 95
(1978): Mihas AA+, *JAMA* 289, 2590
Hypogeusia
Lymphoproliferative disease
(1989): Lafeuillade A+, *Presse Med* (French) 18, 1709
Mononucleosis
(1984): Iwatsuki K+, *Arch Dermatol* 120, 964
Mucocutaneous side effects (sic)
(1990): Donovan S+, *Br J Rheumatol* 29, 201 (6.3%)
(1986): Farr M+, *Drugs* 32 (Suppl 1), 49 (5.5%)
Myalgia
Myopathy
(1994): Norden DK+, *Am J Gastroenterology* 89, 801
Oral mucosal eruption
(1990): Petterson T+, *Br J Rheumatol* 29, 239
(1986): Amos RS+, *BMJ* 293, 420 (0.3%)
(1984): Iwatsuki K+, *Arch Dermatol* 120, 964
(1966): Cameron HA+, *BMJ* 2, 1174
Oral ulceration
(1987): Hughes WT+, *N Engl J Med* 316, 1627
(1986): Farr M+, *Drugs* 32 (Suppl 1), 49
(1981): Orenstein WA+, *Am J Med Sci* 282, 27
Pseudolymphoma
(1994): Gallais V+, *Ann Dermatol Venereol* (French) 121, 11
(1975): Delage C+, *Union Med Can* (French) 104, 579
Serum sickness (<1%)
(1992): Brooks H+, *Clin Rheumatol* 11, 566
(1990): Petterson T+, *Br J Rheumatol* 29, 239
(1975): Delage C+, *Union Med Can* (French) 104, 579
Stomatitis
(1993): Gran JT+, *Scand J Rheumatol* 22, 229
Tongue ulceration
(1981): *J Antimicrob Chemother* 7, 179
Xerostomia
(1990): Donovan S+, *Br J Rheumatol* 29, 201

***Note:** Sulfasalazine is a sulfonamide and can be absorbed systemically. Sulfonamides can produce severe, possibly fatal, reactions such as toxic epidermal necrolysis and Stevens–Johnson syndrome.

SULFINPYRAZONE

Trade name: Anturane (Novartis)
Other common trade names: *Antazone; Antiran; Anturan; Anturano; Enturen; Falizal; Novopyrazone*
Indications: Gouty arthritis
Category: Antigout; antihyperuricemic sulfonamide*
Half-life: 2–7 hours
Clinically important, potentially serious interactions with: acetaminophen, anticoagulants, beta-blockers, hypoglycemics, salicylates, sulfonylureas, verapamil

Reactions

Skin
Dermatitis (sic) (1–10%)
Edema
Exanthems (<3%)
Flushing (<1%)
Purpura
Rash (sic) (1–10%)

***Note:** Sulfinpyrazone is a sulfonamide and can be absorbed systemically. Sulfonamides can produce severe, possibly fatal, reactions such as toxic epidermal necrolysis and Stevens–Johnson syndrome.

SULFISOXAZOLE

Trade name: Pediazole (Ross)
Other common trade names: *Isoxazine; Novo-Soxazole; Oxazole; Sulfazin; Sulfazole; Sulizole; Thiazin; Urazole*
Indications: Various infections caused by susceptible organisms
Category: Urinary tract antibacterial and antiprotozoal sulfonamide*
Half-life: 3–7 hours
Clinically important, potentially serious interactions with: cyclosporine, hydantoins, oral anticoagulants, oral hypoglycemics, MAO inhibitors, methotrexate, sulfonylureas, warfarin

Reactions

Skin
Allergic reactions (sic)
(1971): Koch-Weser J+, *Arch Intern Med* 128, 399 (2.8%)
Angioedema (<1%)
(1971): Koch-Weser J+, *Arch Intern Med* 128, 399 (0.15%)
Bullous eruption (<1%)
(1966): Falk AB+, *Arch Dermatol* 94, 249
Cutaneous side effects (sic)
(1971): Koch-Weser J+, *Arch Intern Med* 128, 399 (2.1%)
Eczematous eruption (sic)
(1947): Sulzberger MB+, *J Allergy* 18, 92
Erythema multiforme (<1%)
(1987): Penmetcha M, *BMJ* 295, 556
(1985): Hernborg A, *Lancet* 2, 1072
(1985): Heer M+, *Gastroenterology* 88, 1954
(1979): Beck MH+, *Clin Exp Dermatol* 4, 201
(1975): Bernstein LS, *Can Med Assoc J* 112, 96S
(1971): Koch-Weser J+, *Arch Intern Med* 128, 399 (0.15%)
(1970): Shaw DJ+, *Johns Hopkins Med J* 126, 130
Erythema nodosum
(1971): Koch-Weser J+, *Arch Intern Med* 128, 399
Exanthems (1–5%)
(1985): Maayan S+, *Arch Intern Med* 145, 1607
(1982): Goetz MB+, *JAMA* 247, 3118
(1980): Fennell RS+, *Clin Pediatr* 19, 124
(1976): Arndt KA+, *JAMA* 235, 918 (1.7%)
(1972): Halpern GM, *BMJ* 1, 691
(1972): Kauppinen K, *Acta Derm Venereol* (Stockh) 52 (Suppl), 68
(1971): Koch-Weser J+, *Arch Intern Med* 128, 399 (1%)
(1967): Lehr D, *Ann N Y Acad Sci* 69, 417 (2%)
(1956): Davis JB, *JAMA* 161, 228
Exfoliative dermatitis
(1975): Bernstein LS, *Can Med Assoc J* 112, 96S
(1971): Koch-Weser J+, *Arch Intern Med* 128, 399
Fixed eruption (<1%)
(1988): Bharija SC+, *Dermatologica* 176, 108
(1987): Hughes BR+, *Br J Dermatol* 116, 241
(1986): Kanwar AJ+, *Dermatologica* 172, 230
(1982): Gibson JR, *BMJ* 284, 1529
(1980): Talbot MD, *Practitioner* 224, 823
(1968): Sarkany I, *Proc R Soc Med* 61, 891
Flushing
(1984): Jick SS+, *Lancet* 2, 631
Linear IgA bullous dermatosis
(1981): Safai B+, *J Am Acad Dermatol* 4, 435
Lupus erythematosus
(1975): Grossman J+, *Am J Dis Child* 129, 123
(1966): Cohen P+, *JAMA* 197, 817
Periorbital edema
Photoreactions
Photosensitivity (>10%)
(1986): Chandler MJ, *J Infect Dis* 153, 1001
(1981): Flach AJ+, *Arch Ophthalmol* 100, 1206 (from topical application)
(1981): Flach AJ+, *Arch Ophthalmol* 99, 609 (from topical application)
(1972): Kauppinen K, *Acta Derm Venereol* (Stockh) 52 (Suppl), 68
Phototoxic reaction
(1982): Flach AJ+, *Arch Ophthalmol* 100, 1286 (from topical application)
Pruritus (>10%)
(1987): Colebunders R+, *Ann Intern Med* 107, 599
(1986): Sher MR, *J Allergy Clin Immunol* 77, 133

(1984): Kramer BS+, *Cancer* 53, 329
(1971): Koch-Weser J+, *Arch Intern Med* 128, 399 (0.15%)
Pruritus vulvae
(1981): *Modern Medicine* 49, 111
Purpura
(1980): Miescher PA+, *Clin Haematol* 9, 505
(1977): Cimo PL+, *Am J Hematol* 2, 65
(1956): Green TW+, *JAMA* 161, 1563
(1951): Gale GL, *Can Med Assoc J* 64, 252
Pustular eruption
Rash (sic) (>10%)
Stevens–Johnson syndrome (1–10%)
(1983): Fischer PR+, *Am J Dis Child* 137, 914
(1970): Shaw DJ+, *Johns Hopkins Med J* 126, 130
(1956): Davis JB, *JAMA* 161, 228
Toxic epidermal necrolysis (1–10%)
(1995): Raymond F+, *Arch Pediatr* (French) 2, 494
(1990): Jacqz-Aigrain E+, *Lancet* 336, 1010
(1989): Alanko K+, *Acta Derm Venereol* (Stockh) 69, 223
(1975): Bernstein LS, *Can Med Assoc J* 112, 96S
(1972): Kauppinen K, *Acta Derm Venereol* (Stockh) 52 (Suppl), 68
Urticaria
(1985): Maayan S+, *Arch Intern Med* 145, 1607
(1984): Kramer BS+, *Cancer* 53, 329
(1981): Abi-Mansur P+, *Am J Gastroenterol* 76, 356
(1971): Koch-Weser J+, *Arch Intern Med* 128, 399 (0.04%)
Vasculitis (<1%)
(1971): Koch-Weser J+, *Arch Intern Med* 128, 399
(1967): Lee DK+, *JAMA* 200, 720
(1965): McCombs RP, *JAMA* 194, 1059
Vulvovaginitis
(1985): Wong ES+, *Ann Intern Med* 102, 302

Hair

Hair – alopecia
(1975): Grossman J+, *Am J Dis Child* 129, 123

Other

Anaphylactoid reaction
(1988): Arnold PA+, *Drug Intell Clin Pharm* 22, 43
(1985): Gossius G+, *Scand J Infect Dis* 16, 373
Aphthous stomatitis
(1981): *J Antimicrob Chemother* 7, 179
Dysgeusia
(1988): Fischl MA+, *JAMA* 259, 1185
Glossitis
Hypersensitivity
Myalgia
Oral psoriasis (sic)
(1974): Yaffee HS, *Int J Dermatol* 13, 185
Oral ulceration
(1987): Hughes WT+, *N Engl J Med* 316, 1627
(1981): Orenstein WA+, *Am J Med Sci* 282, 27
Serum sickness (<1%)
(1969): Mukherjee DN, *J Indian Med Assoc* 52, 225
Stomatitis
Temporal arteritis
(1967): Lee DK+, *JAMA* 200, 720
Tongue ulceration
(1981): *J Antimicrob Chemother* 7, 179

***Note:** Sulfisoxazole is a sulfonamide and can be absorbed systemically. Sulfonamides can produce severe, possibly fatal, reactions such as toxic epidermal necrolysis and Stevens–Johnson syndrome.

SULINDAC

Trade name: Clinoril (Merck)
Other common trade names: *Aflodac; Algocetil; APO-Sulin; Arthrocine; Mobilin; Novo-Sundac; Sulene; Sulic; Suloril*
Indications: Arthritis
Category: Nonsteroidal anti-inflammatory (NSAID); analgesic
Half-life: 7.8–16.4 hours
Clinically important, potentially serious interactions with: aminoglycosides, anticoagulants, cyclosporine, digoxin, diuretics, lithium, loop diuretics, methotrexate, NSAIDs, probenecid

Reactions

Skin

Angioedema (<1%)
Dermatitis (sic)
(1991): Renaut JJ, *Allerg Immunol Paris* (French) 23, 365
Diaphoresis
Ecchymoses (<1%)
Edema
Erythema
(1991): Renaut JJ, *Allerg Immunol Paris* (French) 23, 365
Erythema multiforme (<1%)
(1987): Jeanmougin M+, *Ann Dermatol Venereol* (French) 114, 1400
(1985): O'Brien WM+, *J Rheumatol* 12, 13
(1985): Bigby M+, *J Am Acad Dermatol* 12, 866
(1984): Stern RS+, *JAMA* 252, 1433
(1982): Park GD+, *Arch Intern Med* 142, 1292
(1981): Husain Z+, *J Rheumatol* 8, 176
(1981): Maguire FW, *Del Med J* 53, 193
(1980): Russell IJ, *Ann Intern Med* 92, 716
Exanthems (1–5%)
(1993): Litt JZ, Beachwood, OH, personal case (observation)
(1991): Hyson CP+, *Arch Intern Med* 151, 387
(1987): Jeanmougin M+, *Ann Dermatol Venereol* (French) 114, 1400
(1985): Bigby M+, *J Am Acad Dermatol* 12, 866
(1984): Stern RS+, *JAMA* 252, 1433
(1982): Park GD+, *Arch Intern Med* 142, 1292
(1981): Dhand A+, *Gastroenterology* 80, 585
(1980): Russell IJ, *Ann Intern Med* 92, 716
(1979): Anderson R, *N Engl J Med* 300, 735
(1977): Calabro JJ+, *Clin Pharmacol Ther* 22, 358 (3%)
Exfoliative dermatitis (<1%)
Exfoliative erythroderma
(1984): Stern RS+, *JAMA* 252, 1433
Facial erythema
(1979): Anderson R, *N Engl J Med* 300, 735
Fixed eruption (<1%)
(1987): Jeanmougin M+, *Ann Dermatol Venereol* (French) 114, 1400
(1986): Bruce DR+, *Cutis* 38, 323
(1985): Bigby M+, *J Am Acad Dermatol* 12, 866
(1984): Aram H, *Int J Dermatol* 23, 421
(1984): Stern RS+, *JAMA* 252, 1433
Hot flashes (<1%)
Jaundice
(1979): Wolfe PB, *Ann Intern Med* 91, 656
Lichen planus
(1983): Hamburger J+, *BMJ* 287, 1258
Pernio
(1981): Reinertsen JL, *Arthritis Rheum* 24, 1215
Photosensitivity (<1%)
(1987): Jeanmougin M+, *Ann Dermatol Venereol* (French) 114, 1400
(1984): Stern RS+, *JAMA* 252, 1433
Phototoxic reaction
Pruritus (1–10%)
(1987): Jeanmougin M+, *Ann Dermatol Venereol* (French) 114, 1400
(1985): Bigby M+, *J Am Acad Dermatol* 12, 866
(1984): Stern RS+, *JAMA* 252, 1433
(1982): Park GD+, *Arch Intern Med* 142, 1292
(1980): Russell IJ, *Ann Intern Med* 92, 716
Purpura (<1%)
(1987): Jeanmougin M+, *Ann Dermatol Venereol* (French) 114, 1400
(1984): Stern RS+, *JAMA* 252, 1433

Rash (sic) (>10%)
Raynaud's phenomenon
(1981): Reinertsen JL, *Arthritis Rheum* 24, 1215 (passim)
Skin pain (sic)
(1984): Stern RS+, *JAMA* 252, 1433
Stevens–Johnson syndrome (<1%)
(1993): Awaya N+, *Ryumachi* (Japanese) 33, 432
(1983): Klein SM+, *J Rheumatol* 10, 512
(1981): Maguire FW, *Del Med J* 53, 193
(1981): Husain Z+, *J Rheumatol* 8, 176
(1980): Levitt L+, *JAMA* 243, 1262
Toxic epidermal necrolysis (<1%)
(1990): Hovde O, *Tidsskr Nor Laegeforen* (Norwegian) 110, 2537
(1988): Small RE+, *Clin Pharm* 7, 766
(1987): Jeanmougin M+, *Ann Dermatol Venereol* (French) 114, 1400
(1987): Ikeda N+, *Z Rechtsmed* (German) 98, 141
(1986): Rodt SA+, *Tidsskr Nor Laegeforen* (Norwegian) 106, 2982
(1985): Chevrant-Breton JC, *Therapie* (French) 40, 67
(1985): Heng MCY, *Br J Dermatol* 113, 597
(1985): Bigby M+, *J Am Acad Dermatol* 12, 866
(1984): Stern RS+, *JAMA* 252, 1433
(1983): Klein SM+, *J Rheumatol* 10, 512
(1982): Park GD+, *Arch Intern Med* 142, 1292
(1980): Russell IJ, *Ann Intern Med* 92, 716
(1980): Levitt L+, *JAMA* 243, 1262
Urticaria (<1%)
(1987): Jeanmougin M+, *Ann Dermatol Venereol* (French) 114, 1400
(1985): Bigby M+, *J Am Acad Dermatol* 12, 866
(1984): Stern RS+, *JAMA* 252, 1433
(1981): Burrish G+, *Ann Emerg Med* 10, 154
Vasculitis (<1%)

Hair

Hair – alopecia (<1%)

Other

Ageusia (<1%)
Anaphylactoid reaction (<1%)
(1991): Hyson CP+, *Arch Intern Med* 151, 387
(1985): O'Brien WM+, *J Rheumatol* 12, 13
(1981): Burrish G+, *Ann Emerg Med* 10, 154
(1980): Smith F+, *JAMA* 244, 269
Aphthous stomatitis
Dysesthesia
(1980): Russell IJ, *Ann Intern Med* 92, 716
Dysgeusia (<1%)
Glossitis (<1%)
Gynecomastia
(1983): Kapoor A, *JAMA* 250, 2284
Hypersensitivity (<1%) (potentially fatal)
Oral lichenoid eruption
(1983): Hamburger J+, *BMJ* 287, 1258
Oral mucosal eruption
(1985): Bigby M+, *J Am Acad Dermatol* 12, 866
(1977): Calabro JJ+, *Clin Pharmacol Ther* 22, 358 (3%)
Oral mucosal erythema
(1979): Anderson RJ, *N Engl J Med* 300, 735
Oral ulceration
Paresthesias (<1%)
Serum sickness
(1984): Stern RS+, *JAMA* 252, 1433
Stomatitis (<1%)
(1991): Renaut JJ, *Allerg Immunol Paris* (French) 23, 365
(1978): Brogden R+, *Drugs* 16, 97
Xerostomia
(1980): Smith F+, *JAMA* 244, 269
(1978): Huskinson L+, *Ann Rheum Dis* 37, 89

SUMATRIPTAN

Trade name: Imitrex (GlaxoWellcome)
Other common trade name: *Imigrane*
Indications: Migraine attacks
Category: Antimigraine; serotonin agonist
Half-life: 2.5 hours
Clinically important, potentially serious interactions with: ergot-containing drugs, MAO inhibitors, SSRIs

Reactions

Skin

Angioedema
(1995): Dachs R+, *Am J Med* 99, 684
Burning (sic) (1–10%)
Diaphoresis (1.6%)
Erythema (<1%)
Exanthems
Flushing (6.6%)
Hot flashes (>10%)
Hot sensations
(1991): Multiple authors, *N Engl J Med* 325, 316
Photosensitivity (<1%)
Pruritus (<1%)
Rash (sic) (<1%)
Raynaud's phenomenon (<1%)
Sensitivity (sic)
(1994): Black P+, *N Z Med J* 107, 20
Urticaria
(1996): Pradalier A+, *Cephalalgia* 16, 280

Other

Anaphylactoid reaction
Dysesthesia (<1%)
Dysgeusia (<1%)
Glossodynia
Hyperesthesia (<1%)
Injection-site reactions (sic) (58%)
(1991): Multiple authors, *N Engl J Med* 325, 316 (10–20%)
Myalgia (1.8%)
Parageusia (<1%)
Paresthesias (13.5%)
Parosmia (<1%)
Xerostomia

TACRINE

Synonym: THA
Trade name: Cognex (Parke-Davis)
Indications: Dementia of Alzheimer's disease
Category: Anticholinesterase; cholinergic
Half-life: 1.5–4 hours
Clinically important, potentially serious interactions with: benztropine, beta-blockers, cholinesterase inhibitors, cimetidine, levodopa, NSAIDs, succinylcholine, theophylline, **cigarette smoking**

Reactions

Skin

Acne (<1%)
Basal cell carcinoma
Bullous eruption
Cellulitis
Cyst (sic)
Dermatitis (sic) (<1%)
Desquamation (sic)
Diaphoresis
Eczema (sic)
Edema (<1%)
Exanthems (7%)
Facial edema (<1%)
Flushing (3%)
Furunculosis (<1%)
Herpes simplex (<1%)
Herpes zoster (<1%)
Melanoma (<1%)
Necrosis (<1%)
Parkinsonism
(1999): Cabeza-Alvarez CI+, *Neurologia* (Spanish) 14, 96
Peripheral edema (<1%)
Petechiae
Pruritus (7%)
Psoriasis (<1%)
Purpura (2%)
Rash (sic) (7%)
Seborrhea
Squamous cell carcinoma
Ulceration (<1%)
Urticaria (7%)
Xerosis (<1%)

Hair

Hair – alopecia (<1%)

Other

Dysgeusia (<1%)
Gingivitis (<1%)
Glossitis (<1%)
Myalgia (9%)
Paresthesias (<1%)
Sialorrhea (<1%)
Stomatitis (<1%)
Tremor (1–10%)
Xerostomia (<1%)

TACROLIMUS

Synonym: FK506
Trade name: Prograf (Fujisawa); Protopic (Fujisawa)
Indications: Prophylaxis of organ rejection; atopic dermatitis (topical)
Category: Immunosuppressant; topical for atopic dermatitis
Half-life: ~8.7 hours
Clinically important, potentially serious interactions with: amphotericin B, bromocriptine, cimetidine, clarithromycin, clotrimazole, cyclosporine, danazol, diltiazem, erythromycin, fluconazole, itraconazole, ketoconazole, methylprednisolone, metoclopramide, nicardipine, phenobarbital, phenytoin, rifampin, vaccines, verapamil, **grapefruit juice**

Reactions

Skin

Burning
(2000): Reitamo S+, *Arch Dermatol* 136, 999 (46.8%)
Connective tissue nevi (sic)
(1999): Reed BR, Denver CO, (from Internet) (observation) (confirmed by biopsies)
Diaphoresis (>3%)
Ecchymoses (>3%)
Edema (>10%)
Erythema
(2000): Reitamo S+, *Arch Dermatol* 136, 999 (12.3%)
Exanthems
(2000): Reitamo S+, *Arch Dermatol* 136, 999 (4.1%)
Flushing
(2000): Reitamo S+, *Arch Dermatol* 136, 999
(1997): Sandborn WJ, *Am J Gastroenterol* 92, 876
Folliculitis
(2000): Reitamo S+, *Arch Dermatol* 136, 999 (10.8%)
Herpes simplex
(2000): Reitamo S+, *Arch Dermatol* 136, 999 (13%)
Infection (sic) (>10%)
Peripheral edema (26%)
Photosensitivity (>3%)
Pruritus (36%)
(2000): Reitamo S+, *Arch Dermatol* 136, 999 (25.3%)
(2000): Emre S+, *Transpl Int* 13, 73
Purpura
(1996): Nash RA+, *Blood* 88, 3634
Pustular eruption
(2000): Reitamo S+, *Arch Dermatol* 136, 999 (6.3%)
Rash (sic) (24%)

Hair

Hair – alopecia (>3%)
(1999): Ushigome H+, *Transplant Proc* 31, 2885 (2 cases)
(1998): Shapiro R+, *Transplantation* 65, 1284
(1997): Talbot D+, *Transplantation* 64, 1631
Hair – growth (sic)
(1994): Yamamoto S+, *J Dermatol Sci* 7, S47
Hair – hirsutism

Other

Anaphylactoid reaction (<1%)
Application-site burning
(1997): Ruzicka T+, *N Engl J Med* 337, 816
Dysphagia (>3%)
Gingival hyperplasia
(1998): Basile C+, *Nephrol Dial Transplant* 13, 2980
Hyperesthesia
Myalgia (>3%)
Oral candidiasis (>3%)
Paresthesias (40%)
(1997): Sandborn WJ, *Am J Gastroenterol* 92, 876
(1996): *Arch Dermatol* 132, 419
Tremor (>10%)

TAMOXIFEN

Trade name: Nolvadex (AstraZeneca)
Other common trade names: *Apo-Tamox; Bilim; Istubol; Kessar; Mamofen; Novofen; Tamaxin; Tamofen; Tamoxan; Taxus; Valodex*
Indications: Advanced breast cancer
Category: Antiestrogen; antineoplastic estrogen receptor
Half-life: 7 days
Clinically important, potentially serious interactions with: allopurinol, aminoglutethimide, anticoagulants, cyclosporine, warfarin

Reactions

Skin

Dermatomyositis
(1982): Harris AL+, *BMJ* 284, 1674
Diaphoresis
(1986): Buchanan RB+, *J Clin Oncology* 4, 1326
(1980): Pritchard KI+, *Cancer Treat Rep* 64, 787
Edema (3.8%)
(1986): Buchanan RB+, *J Clin Oncology* 4, 1326
(1978): Heel RC+, *Drugs* 16, 1 (2–6%)
Exanthems
(1999): Descamps V+, *Ann Dermatol Venereol* (French) 126, 716
(1980): Pritchard KI+, *Cancer Treat Rep* 64, 787
(1978): Heel RC+, *Drugs* 16, 1 (3.6%)
Flushing (>10%)
(1999): Drayton G, Los Angeles, CA (from Internet) (observation)
(1992): Shelley WB+, *Advanced Dermatologic Diagnosis*, WB Saunders, 583 (passim)
(1989): Buckley MMT+, *Drugs* 37, 451 (10–20%)
(1986): Buchanan RB+, *J Clin Oncology* 4, 1326
(1981): Ingle JN+, *N Engl J Med* 304, 16 (29%)
(1980): Pritchard KI+, *Cancer Treat Rep* 64, 787
(1978): Heel RC+, *Drugs* 16, 1 (14%)
(1977): Kiang DT+, *Ann Intern Med* 87, 687 (21%)
(1973): Ward HWC, *BMJ* 1, 13 (12%)
Hot flashes
Peripheral edema
Pruritus
(1980): Pritchard KI+, *Cancer Treat Rep* 64, 787
Pruritus vulvae
(1980): Pritchard KI+, *Cancer Treat Rep* 64, 787
(1978): Heel RC+, *Drugs* 16, 1 (2–3%)
Purpura
(1978): Heel RC+, *Drugs* 16, 1
Radiation recall
(1999): Bostrom A+, *Acta Oncol* 38, 955
(1992): Parry BR, *Lancet* 340, 49
Rash (sic) (1–10%)
Urticaria
Vaginal pruritus
Vasculitis
(1994): Rzany B+, *J Am Acad Dermatol* 30, 509
(1990): Drago F+, *Ann Intern Med* 112, 965
Xerosis
(1978): Heel RC+, *Drugs* 16, 1 (7%)

Hair

Hair – alopecia
(1993): Litt JZ, Beachwood, OH, personal case (observation)
(1980): Pritchard KI+, *Cancer Treat Rep* 64, 787
(1978): Heel RC+, *Drugs* 16, 1 (2%)
Hair – color change (sic)
(1995): Hampson JP+, *Br J Dermatol* 132, 483
Hair – hirsutism
(1980): Pritchard KI+, *Cancer Treat Rep* 64, 787
Hair – hypertrichosis

Other

Dysgeusia
Galactorrhea (1–10%)
Myopathy
(1982): Harris AL+, *BMJ* 284, 1674
Thrombophlebitis
(1996): Zimmet S, *The Schoch Letter* 46, 22 (#86) (observation)
Xerostomia
(1978): Heel RC+, *Drugs* 16, 1 (7%)

TAMSULOSIN

Trade name: Flomax (Boehringer Ingelheim)
Indications: Benign prostatic hypertrophy
Category: Alpha-adrenergic blocking agent
Half-life: 9–13 hours
Clinically important, potentially serious interactions with:, cimetidine, doxazosin, prazosin, terazosin, warfarin

Reactions

Skin

Angioedema
Eczematous eruption (sic)
(2000): Frederickson KS, Novalo, CA (from Internet) (observation)
Erythema multiforme
(1999): Reed BR, Denver, CO (from Internet) (observation)
Pruritus
Rash (sic)

Other

Tooth disorder (sic)

TELMISARTAN

Trade name: Micardis (Boehringer Ingelheim)
Indications: Hypertension
Category: Angiotensin II receptor antagonist antihypertensive
Half-life: 24 hours
Clinically important, potentially serious interactions with: digoxin, lithium

Reactions

Skin

Allergic reactions (sic) (<1%)
Angioedema (>0.3%)
Dermatitis (sic) (>0.3%)
Diaphoresis (>0.3%)
Eczema (sic) (>0.3%)
Flu-like syndrome (sic) (1%)
Flushing (>0.3%)
Fungal infection (sic) (>0.3%)
Leg edema (>0.3%)
Peripheral edema (1%)
Pruritus (>0.3%)
Rash (sic) (>0.3%)

Other

Hypesthesia (>0.3%)
Myalgia (1%)
Paresthesias (>0.3%)
Xerostomia (>0.3%)

TEMAZEPAM

Trade name: Temazepam
Other common trade names: *Apo-Temazepam; Cerepax; Euhypnos; Lenal; Levanxene; Normison; Nu-Temazepam; Planum*
Indications: Insomnia, anxiety
Category: Benzodiazepine sedative and hypnotic
Half-life: 8–15 hours
Clinically important, potentially serious interactions with: alcohol, CNS depressants, cimetidine, clarithromycin, digoxin, diltiazem, levodopa, theophylline, verapamil

Reactions

Skin

Bullous eruption
(1999): Verghese J+, *Acad Emerg Med* 6, 1071
Dermatitis (sic) (1–10%)
Diaphoresis (>10%)
Exanthems
Fixed eruption
(1988): Archer CB+, *Clin Exp Dermatol* 13, 336
Lichenoid eruption
(1986): Norris P+, *BMJ* 293, 510
Pruritus
Purpura
Rash (sic) (>10%)
Skin disorders (sic)
(1984): Stricker BH, *Ned Tijdschr Geneeskd* (Dutch) 128, 870
Urticaria

Other

Anaphylactoid reaction
(1988): Mills PJ, *Anaesthesia* 43, 66
Dysgeusia
Paresthesias
Sialopenia (>10%)
Sialorrhea (1–10%)
Tremor (<1%)
Xerostomia (1.7%)

TEMOZOLOMIDE

Trade name: Temodar (Schering)
Indications: Anaplastic astrocytoma
Category: Antineoplastic
Half-life: 1.8 hours
Clinically important, potentially serious interactions with: anticoagulants, immunosuppressives, NSAIDs, platelets inhibitors, salicylates, thrombolytic agents, vaccines

Reactions

Skin

Infections (sic)
Peripheral edema (11%)
Pruritus (8%)
Rash (sic) (8%)
Viral infection (sic) (11%)

Other

Mastodynia (6%)
Myalgia (5%)
Paresthesias (9%)

TERAZOSIN

Trade name: Hytrin (Abbott)
Other common trade names: *Heitrin; Hitrin; Hytrine; Hytrinex; Itrin; Vicard*
Indications: Hypertension, benign prostatic hypertrophy
Category: $Alpha_1$-adrenergic blocking agent; antihypertensive
Half-life: 12 hours
Clinically important, potentially serious interactions with: beta-blockers, diuretics, NSAIDs, verapamil

Reactions

Skin

Diaphoresis (>1%)
Edema (1–10%)
Exanthems
(1998): Hernandez-Cano N+, *Lancet* 352, 202 (generalized)
(1998): Rosen R, (from Internet) (observation) (following PUVA)
Facial edema (>1%)
Flu-like syndrome (sic) (<1%)
Lichenoid eruption
(1993): Shelley WB+, *Cutis* 52, 88 (observation)
Peripheral edema (5.5%)
Phototoxic reaction
(1993): Shelley WB+, *Cutis* 52, 259 (observation)
Pruritus (>1%)
(1998): Hernandez-Cano N+, *Lancet* 352, 202
Rash (sic) (>1%)

Other

Anaphylactoid reaction
Myalgia (>1%)
Paresthesias (2.9%)
Priapism (<1%)
(1998): Vaidyanathan S+, *Spinal Cord* 36, 805
Xerostomia (1–10%)

TERBINAFINE

Trade name: Lamisil (Novartis)
Indications: Fungal infections of the skin and nails
Category: Antifungal
Half-life: 22–26 hours
Clinically important, potentially serious interactions with: alcohol, caffeine, cimetidine, cyclosporine, rifampin, terfenadine, warfarin

Reactions

Skin

Acute generalized exanthematous pustulosis (AGEP)
(2000): Hall AP+, *Australas J Dermatol* 41, 42
(1998): Condon CA+, *Br J Dermatol* 138, 709
(1997): Kempinaire A+, *J Am Acad Dermatol* 37, 653
(1996): Dupin N+, *Arch Dermatol* 132, 1253 (2 cases)
Allergic reactions (sic) (1–10%)
(1989): Savin R, *Clin Exp Dermatol* 14, 116
Angioedema
(1997): Hall M+, *Arch Dermatol* 133, 1213
Contact dermatitis (1–10%)
Cutaneous side effects (sic) (2.7%)
(1990): Villars V+, *J Dermatol Treat* 1, 33
Desquamation (sic)
(1995): Wachs F+, *Arch Dermatol* 131, 960 (passim)
Eczema (sic)
(1997): Hall M+, *Arch Dermatol* 133, 1213 (0.2%)
(1990): Villars V+, *J Dermatol Treat* 1, 33
Erythema multiforme
(1998): Gupta AK+, *Br J Dermatol* 138, 529 (5 patients)
(1997): Hall M+, *Arch Dermatol* 133, 1213
(1995): Todd P+, *Clin Exp Dermatol* 20, 247

(1995): Tramaloni S+, *Therapie* (French) 50, 594
(1994): Carstens J+, *Acta Derm Venereol* (Stockh) 74, 391
(1994): McGregor JM+, *Br J Dermatol* 131, 587
(1994): Rzany B+, *J Am Acad Dermatol* 30, 509

Erythroderma
(1998): Gupta AK+, *Br J Dermatol* 138, 529
(1996): Mitchell D, Charleston, SC (from Internet) (observation)
(1990): Villars V+, *J Dermatol Treat* 1, 33

Exanthems
(1999): Valentine MC, Everett, WA (from Internet) (observation)
(1997): Sidhu JS, Malaysia (from Internet) (observation)
(1995): Wachs F+, *Arch Dermatol* 131, 960 (passim)
(1995): Hofmann H+, *Arch Dermatol* 131, 919
(1990): Villars V+, *J Dermatol Treat* 1, 33

Fixed eruption
(1995): Munn SE+, *Br J Dermatol* 133, 815

Lupus erythematosus
(2000): Reed BR, Denver, CO (personal communication) (from a meeting presented by Callen JP, Louisville, KY) (4 cases)
(1999): *Ann Dermatol Venereol* (French) 126, 463 (Announced as the first published case!)
(1999): Poster Exhibit #239, AAD Meeting, March 1999 (Reported by ED and WB Shelley) (3 patients)
(1998): Murphy M+, *Br J Dermatol* 138, 708
(1998): Holmes S+, *Br J Dermatol* 139, 1133
(1998): Brooke R+, *Br J Dermatol* 139, 1132

Peripheral edema
(1997): Hall M+, *Arch Dermatol* 133, 1213

Photosensitivity
(1998): Litt JZ, Beachwood, OH, personal case (observation)
(1997): Sidhu JS, Malaysia (from Internet) (observation)

Pityriasis rosea
(1998): Gupta AK+, *Br J Dermatol* 138, 529

Pruritus (2.8%)
(1998): Litt JZ, Beachwood, OH, personal case (observation)
(1997): Hall M+, *Arch Dermatol* 133, 1213 (0.3%)
(1995): Wachs F+, *Arch Dermatol* 131, 960 (passim)
(1990): Villars V+, *J Dermatol Treat* 1, 33

Psoriasis
(1998): Gupta AK+, *Br J Dermatol* 138, 529 (2 patients)
(1997): Gupta AK+, *J Am Acad Dermatol* 36, 858
(1995): Wachs F+, *Arch Dermatol* 131, 960 (erythema annulare centrifugum-like [SIC])

Pustular eruption
(1999): Bennett ML+, *Int J Dermatol* 38, 596

Pustular psoriasis
(2000): Le Guyadec T+, *Ann Dermatol Venereol* (French) 127, 279
(1998): Papa CA+, *J Am Acad Dermatol* 39, 115
(1998): Wilson NJ+, *Br J Dermatol* 139, 168
(1995): Gupta AK+, unpublished findings

Rash (sic) (5.6%)
(1995): Haroon TS+, *Br J Dermatol* 135, 86

Stevens–Johnson syndrome
(1999): Rosen R, (from Internet) (observation)
(1994): Rzany B+, *J Am Acad Dermatol* 30, 509

Toxic epidermal necrolysis
(1996): White SI+, *Br J Dermatol* 134, 188
(1994): Carstens J+, *Acta Derm Venereol* (Stockh) 74, 391
(1993): Beutler M+, *BMJ* 307, 26

Toxicoderma
(1997): Hall M+, *Arch Dermatol* 133, 1213

Urticaria (1.1%)
(1998): Gupta AK+, *Br J Dermatol* 138, 529
(1997): Hall M+, *Arch Dermatol* 133, 1213 (0.3%)
(1998): Rademaker M+, *New Zealand Adverse Drug Reactions Committee,* April, 1998 (from Internet)
(1997): :Billon S, *The Schoch Letter* 47, 32 (observation)
(1995): Wachs F+, *Arch Dermatol* 131, 960 (passim)
(1990): Savin RC, *J Am Acad Dermatol* 23, 807
(1990): Villars V+, *J Dermatol Treat* 1, 33

Hair

Hair – alopecia (1–10%)

Hair – alopecia areata
(1990): Del Palacio Hernanz A+, *Clin Exp Dermatol* 15, 210

Nails

Nails – onychocryptosis
(2000): Weaver TD+, *Cutis* 66, 211
(1995): Arenas R+, *Int J Dermatol* 34, 138

Other

Ageusia
(2000): Schmutz JL+, *Ann Dermatol Venereol* (French) 127, 341 (persistent)
(1999): Villota Hoyos R+, *Aten Primaria* (Spanish) 23, 102
(1999): Private Patient Query from the Internet
(1998): Bong JL+, *Br J Dermatol* 139, 747
(1997): Hall M+, *Arch Dermatol* 133, 1213 (0.3%)
(1995): Haroon TS+, *Br J Dermatol* 135, 86
(1995): Martinez-Yelamos S+, *Med Clin (Barc)* (Spanish) 105, 276
(1994): Cribier B+, *Ann Dermatol Venereol* (French) 121, 15
(1993): Stricker BHC, *Ned Tijdschr Geneeskd* 137, 617
(1992): Stricker BHC, *Ned Tijdschr Geneeskd* 136, 2438
(1992): Ottervanger JP+, *Lancet* 340, 728
(1992): Juhlin L, *Lancet* 339, 1483
(1992): Back D, *Lancet* 340, 252

Anaphylactoid reaction

Anosmia
(1993): Beutler M+, *BMJ* 307, 26

Aphthous stomatitis
(1998): Litt JZ, Beachwood, OH, personal case (observation)

Dyschromatopsia (green vision)
(1996): Gupta AK+, *Arch Dermatol* 132, 845

Dysgeusia (2.8%) (metallic taste)
(2000): Duxbury AJ+, *Br Dent J* 188, 295 ("persistent")
(1999): Marmelzat J, Los Angeles, CA (from Internet) (observation) (lasted for 6 months)
(1997): Hall M+, *Arch Dermatol* 133, 1213 (0.4%)
(1997): Danby FW, Kingston, Ontario (from Internet) (observation)
(1997): Marmelzat J, Los Angeles, CA (from Internet) (observation)
(1997): Sidhu JS, Malaysia (from Internet) (observation)
(1993): Beutler M+, *BMJ* 307, 26
(1992): Ottervanger JP+, *Lancet* 340, 728

Gingivitis
(1998): Gupta AK+, *J Am Acad Dermatol* 38, 765

Hypersensitivity*
(1998): Schlienger RG+, *Epilepsia* 39, S3 (passim)
(1998): Gupta AK+, *Australas J Dermatol* 39, 171
(1997): Gupta AK+, *J Am Acad Dermatol* 36, 1018
(1996): Marmelzat J, Los Angeles, CA (from Internet) (observation)
(1996): Uhleman J, St. Charles, MO (from Internet) (observation)
(1996): Gupta AK+, London, Ontario (observation)

Hypogeusia
(1992): Ottervanger JP+, *Lancet* 340, 728

Hyposmia
(1999): Villota Hoyos R+, *Aten Primaria* (Spanish) 23, 102

Parosmia
(1997): Hall M+, *Arch Dermatol* 133, 1213 (0.02%)

Parotid gland swelling
(1998): Torrens JK+, *BMJ* 316, 440

Serum sickness
(1995): Kruczynski K+, *Can J Clin Pharmacol* 2, 1

Stomatitis
(1998): Gupta AK+, *J Am Acad Dermatol* 38, 765

Tongue pigmentation
(1992): Ottervanger JP+, *Lancet* 340, 728

***Note:** The antiepileptic drug hypersensitivity syndrome is a severe, occasionally fatal, disorder characterized by any or all of the following: pruritic exanthem, toxic epidermal necrolysis, Stevens–Johnson syndrome, exfoliative dermatitis, fever, hepatic abnormalities, eosinophilia, and renal failure.

TERBUTALINE

Trade names: Brethaire (Novartis); Brethine (Novartis); Bricanyl (Aventis)
Other common trade names: *Ataline; Brothine; Bucaril; Butaline; Convon; Respirol; Vacanyl*
Indications: Bronchospasm
Category: $Beta_2$-adrenergic bronchodilator; sympathomimetic; tocolytic
Half-life: 11–16 hours
Clinically important, potentially serious interactions with: beta-blockers, digoxin, MAO inhibitors, sympathomimetics, tricyclic antidepressants

Reactions

Skin

Contact dermatitis (irritant)
(1988): Eedy DJ+, *Postgrad Med J* 64, 306
Diaphoresis (1–10%)
Exanthems
(1996): Drugge R, Stamford, CT (from Internet) (observation)
Flushing
Pruritus
(1996): Drugge R, Stamford, CT (from Internet) (observation)
Urticaria
Vasculitis
(1988): Enat R+, *Ann Allergy* 61, 275

Other

Dysgeusia (1–10%)
Oral ulceration
(1987): High S, *BMJ* 294, 375
Xerostomia (1–10%)

TERCONAZOLE

Synonym: triaconazole
Trade name: Terazol (Ortho-McNeil)
Other trade names: *Fungistat; Gyno-Terazol; Tercospor*
Indications: Vulvovaginal candidiasis
Category: Antifungal
Half-life: no data
Clinically important, potentially serious interactions with: none

Reactions

Skin

Chills
Pruritus (2.3%)
Toxic epidermal necrolysis
(1998): Searles GE+, *J Cutan Med Surg* 3, 85 (from vaginal suppository)

Other

Vulvovaginal burning (1–10%)

TERFENADINE*

Trade name: Seldane (Aventis)
Other common trade names: *Alergist; Allerplus; Cyater; Ferdin; Teldane; Teldanex; Triludan*
Category: H_1-receptor antihistamine
Half-life: 16–22 hours
Clinically important, potentially serious interactions with: amiodarone, astemizole, azithromycin, bepridil, carbamazepine, cimetidine, clarithromycin, disopyramide, erythromycin, fluconazole, fluoxetine, fluvoxamine, hydrochlorothiazide, itraconazole, ketoconazole, metronidazole, miconazole, nefazodone, nifedipine, omeprazole, procainamide, pseudoephedrine, quinidine, ritonavir, saquinavir, sotalol, troleandomycin, verapamil, **grapefruit juice**

Reactions

Skin

Angioedema (<1%)
(1986): Stricker BHC+, *BMJ* 293, 536
Atopic dermatitis (exacerbation)
(1986): Goodfield MJD+, *BMJ* 293, 1103
Cutaneous side effects (sic)
(1995): McClintock AD+, *N Z Med J* 108, 208
Diaphoresis
Exanthems
(1986): Stricker BHC+, *BMJ* 293, 536
Fixed eruption
(1994): Gani F+, *Ann Allergy* 72, 76
Flushing
Lupus erythematosus
Peeling skin (sic)
(1986): Stricker BHC+, *BMJ* 293, 536
Photosensitivity (<1%)
(1994): Shelley WB+, *Cutis* 53, 121 (observation)
(1994): Berger TG+, *Arch Dermatol* 130, 609 (in HIV-infected) (2 cases)
(1986): Fenton D+, *BMJ* 293, 823
(1986): Stricker BHC+, *BMJ* 293, 536
Pruritus
Psoriasis (exacerbation)
(1990): Navaratnam AE+, *Clin Exp Dermatol* 15, 78
(1988): Harrison PV+, *Clin Exp Dermatol* 13, 275
Purpura
Rash (sic) (<1%)
Urticaria
(1986): Stricker BHC+, *BMJ* 293, 536

Hair

Hair – alopecia
(1993): Shelley WB+, *Cutis* 52, 81 (observation)
(1992): Frazier CA, *N C Med J* 53, 390
(1985): Jones SK+, *BMJ* 291, 940

Other

Anaphylactoid reaction
Galactorrhea
Gynecomastia
Myalgia (<1%)
Oral mucosal eruption
(1990): McTavish D+, *Drugs* 39, 552
Paresthesias (<1%)
Pseudolymphoma
(1995): Magro CM+, *J Am Acad Dermatol* 32, 419
Stomatitis
Xerostomia (1–10%)
(1990): McTavish D+, *Drugs* 39, 552

***Note:** Terfenadine has been withdrawn in the USA.

TESTOSTERONE

Trade names: Androderm (Watson); AndroGel; Andro-L.A; Andronaq; Delatest; Delatestryl (BTG); depAndro; Duratest; Histerone; Testoderm (Alza), etc.
Other common trade names: *Malogen; Testandro; Testex; Testopel*
Indications: Androgen replacement; hypogonadism, postpartum breast pain
Category: Androgen
Half-life: 10–100 minutes
Clinically important, potentially serious interactions with: anticoagulants, cyclosporine, tricyclic antidepressants

Reactions

Skin

Acne (>10%)
(1998): Kwon PS+, *Arch Dermatol* 134, 376
(1995): Tabata N+, *J Am Acad Dermatol* 33, 676 (infantile)
(1992): Fyrand O+, *Acta Derm Venereol* 72, 148
(1990): Fuchs E+, *J Am Acad Dermatol* 23, 125
(1989): Hartmann AA+, *Monatsschr Kinderheilkd* (German) 137, 466
(1989): Fyrand O+, *Tidsskr Nor Laegeforen* (Norwegian) 109, 239
(1989): von Muhlendahl KE+, *Dtsch Med Wochenschr* (German) 114, 712
(1989): Heydenreich G, *Arch Dermatol* 125, 571 (fulminans)
(1989): Scott MJ+, *Cutis* 44, 30
(1988): Traupe H+, *Arch Dermatol* 124, 414 (fulminans)
(1987): Kiraly CL+, *Am J Dermatopathol* 9, 515
(1984): Lamb DR, *Am J Sports Med* 12, 31
(1965): Rook A, *Br J Dermatol* 77, 115
(1965): Kennedy BJ, *J Am Geriatr Soc* 13, 230
Contact dermatitis (4%)
(1998): Buckley DA+, *Contact Dermatitis* 39, 91 (from patch)
(1989): Holdiness MR, *Contact Dermatitis* 20, 3 (from patch)
Edema (1–10%)
Exanthems
Flushing (1–10%)
(1965): Kennedy BJ, *J Am Geriatr Soc* 13, 230
Folliculitis
(1998): Kwon PS+, *Arch Dermatol* 134, 376
Furunculosis
(1989): Scott MJ+, *Cutis* 44, 30
Lichenoid eruption
(1989): Aihara M+, *J Dermatol* (Tokio) 16, 330
Lupus erythematosus
(1978): Robinson HM, *Z Haut* (German) 53, 349
Peripheral edema
Pruritus
Psoriasis
(1990): O'Driscoll JB+, *Clin Exp Dermatol* 15, 68
Rash (sic) (2%)
Seborrhea (sic) (<1%)
Seborrheic dermatitis
(1989): Scott MJ+, *Cutis* 44, 30
Striae
(1989): Scott MJ+, *Cutis* 44, 30
Urticaria

Hair

Hair – alopecia (<1%)
(1989): Scott MJ+, *Cutis* 44, 30
(1965): Kennedy BJ, *J Am Geriatr Soc* 13, 230
Hair – hirsutism (1–10%)
(1994): Castillo-Ceballos A+, *Med Clin (Barc)* (Spanish) 102, 78
(1991): Bates GW+, *Clin Obstet Gynecol* 34, 848
(1991): No Author, *Obstet Gynecol* 78, 474
(1991): Parker LU+, *Cleve Clin J Med* 58, 43
(1991): Urman B+, *Obstet Gynecol* 77, 595
(1989): Scott MJ+, *Cutis* 44, 30
(1974): Baron J, *Zentralbl Gynakol* (German) 96, 129
(1971): Fusi S+, *Folia Endocrinol* (Italian) 24, 412
(1965): Kennedy BJ, *J Am Geriatr Soc* 13, 230

Other

Anaphylactoid reaction (<1%)
Application-site bullae (12%)
Application-site burning (3%)
Application-site erythema (7%)
Application-site induration (3%)
Application-site pruritus (37%)
Application-site vesicles (6%)
Gynecomastia (<1%)
Hypersensitivity (<1%)
Injection-site pain
Mastodynia (>10%)
Paresthesias (<1%)
Priapism (>10%)
Stomatitis

TETRACYCLINE

Trade names: Achromycin V (Lederle); Ala-Tet (Del-Ray); Panmycin (Pharmacia & Upjohn); Robitet (Robins); Sumycin (Bristol-Myers Squibb), etc.
Other common trade names: *Apo-Tetra; Economycin; Florocycline; Steclin; Teflin; Tetramig; Teline; Topicycline (Topical) Zorbenal-G*
Indications: Various infections caused by susceptible organisms
Category: Antibiotic
Half-life: 6–11 hours
Clinically important, potentially serious interactions with: amoxicillin, ampicillin, antacids, carbamazepine, cholestyramine, didanosine, etretinate, iron, isotretinoin, oral contraceptives, sucralfate, vitamin A, warfarin, zinc. Also **food: dairy products; herbals: barberry, goldenseal, Oregon grape**

Reactions

Skin

Acne
(1971): Bean SF, *Br J Dermatol* 85, 585
(1969): Weary PE+, *Arch Dermatol* 100, 179
Angioedema
(1997): Shapiro LE+, *Arch Dermatol* 133, 1224
(1978): Jolly HW+, *Arch Dermatol* 114, 1485
Bullous eruption
(1971): Benazeraf C+, *Bull Soc Fr Dermatol Syphiligr* (French) 78, 19
Candidiasis
(1970): Lehner T+, *Br J Dermatol* 83, 161 (oral)
(1965): Clendenning WE, *Arch Dermatol* 91, 628
Cheilitis
(1978): Jolly HW+, *Arch Dermatol* 114, 1485
Dermatitis (sic)
(1970): Chilvers AS+, *Lancet* 1, 402 (leg)
Diaphoresis
Eczematous eruption (sic)
Erythema multiforme
(1988): Lewis-Jones MS+, *Clin Exp Dermatol* 13, 245
(1987): Curley RK+, *Clin Exp Dermatol* 12, 124
(1987): Shoji A+, *Arch Dermatol* 123, 18
(1987): Leroy D+, *Photodermatol* 4, 52 (photodistributed)
(1983): Albengres E+, *Therapie* (French) 38, 577
(1968): Bianchine JR+, *Am Med J* 44, 390
(1965): Clendenning WE, *Arch Dermatol* 91, 628
Exanthems
(1993): Chaffins ML+, *J Am Acad Dermatol* 28, 988
(1979): Patriarca G+, *Boll Ist Sieroter Milan* (Italian) 57, 805 (fixed)
(1978): Jolly HW+, *Arch Dermatol* 114, 1485
Exfoliative dermatitis (<1%)
(1978): Jolly HW I, *Arch Dermatol* 114, 1485
(1972): Kauppinen K, *Acta Derm Venereol* (Stockh) 52 (Suppl) 68
Fixed eruption
(1998): Leal G, Fortaleza, Brazil (from Internet) (observation) (pulsating)
(1994): Bielan B, *Dermatol Nurs* 6, 198
(1991): Thankappen TP+, *Int J Dermatol* 30, 867 (15.9%)
(1990): Gaffoor PMA+, *Cutis* 45, 242
(1988): Chan HL+, *Ann Acad Med Singapore* 17, 514
(1986): Sehgal VH+, *Genitourin Med* 62, 56 (genital)

(1985): Pandhi RK+, *Australas J Dermatol* 26, 88
(1985): Kauppinen K+, *Br J Dermatol* 112, 575
(1985): Chan HL+, *J Am Acad Dermatol* 13, 302
(1985): Dodds PR+, *J Urol* 133, 1044 (balanitis)
(1984): Kanwar AJ+, *J Dermatol* 11, 383
(1984): Pandhi RK+, *Sex Transm Dis* 11, 164 (male genitalia)
(1984): Chan HL, *Int J Dermatol* 23, 607
(1982): Kanwar AJ+, *Dermatologica* 164, 115
(1981): Fiumara NJ+, *Sex Transm Dis* 8, 258
(1981): Fiumara NJ+, *Sex Transm Dis* 8, 23 (penile)
(1981): Bhargava NC+, *Int J Dermatol* 20, 435
(1979): Pasricha JS, *Br J Dermatol* 101, 361
(1979): Patriarca G+, *Boll Ist Sieroter Milan* (Italian) 57, 805
(1979): Pasricha JS, *Br J Dermatol* 100, 183
(1978): Parish LC+, *Acta Derm Venereol* (Stockh) 58, 545 (pulsating)
(1978): Jolly HW+, *Arch Dermatol* 114, 1485
(1976): Farkas J, *Dermatol Monatsschr* (German) 162, 250
(1976): Epstein JH+, *Arch Dermatol* 112, 661 (porphyria-like)
(1974): Sehgal VN, *Dermatologica* 148, 120
(1974): Brown ST, *JAMA* 227, 801 (balanitis)
(1973): Armati RP, *Australas J Dermatol* 14, 75
(1971): Csonka GW+, *Br J Ven Dis* 47, 42 (balanitis)
(1970): Tarnowski WM, *Acta Derm Venereol* (Stockh) 50, 117
(1970): Savin JA, *Br J Dermatol* 83, 546
(1970): Delaney TJ, *Br J Dermatol* 83, 357
(1970): Duricic S, *Med Arh* (Serbo-Croatian-Roman) 24, 143
(1970): Brodin MB, *Arch Dermatol* 101, 621
(1970): Tarnowski WM, *Arch Dermatol* 102, 234
(1969): Minkin W+, *Arch Dermatol* 100, 749
(1969): Kandil E, *Dermatologica* 139, 37
(1963): Reiner E+, *Arch Dermatol* 88, 465
(1962): Post CF+, *Arch Dermatol* 86, 678
(1961): Welsh AL+, *Arch Dermatol* 84, 1004
(1952): Dougherty JW, *Arch Dermatol* 65, 485
(1950): Peck SM+, *JAMA* 142, 1137

Granulomas
(1979): Hagedorn M+, *Dermatologica* 158, 93 (multiple and pyogenic)

Lichenoid eruption
(1974): Tay C, *Asian J Med* 10, 223
(1974): Maibach HI+, *Arch Dermatol* 109, 97
(1971): Almeyda J+, *Br J Dermatol* 85, 604

Lupus erythematosus
(1999): Sturkenboom MCJM+, *Arch Int Med* 159, 493
(1985): Stratton MA, *Clin Pharm* 4, 657
(1964): Sulkowski SR+, *JAMA* 189, 152
(1959): Domz CA+, *Ann Intern Med* 50, 1217

Lymphoepithelioma
(1973): Sadoff L+, *Lancet* 1, 675

Photosensitivity (1–10%)
(1997): Shapiro LE+, *Arch Dermatol* 133, 1224
(1993): Wainwright NJ+, *Drug Saf* 9, 437
(1989): Rosen C, *Semin Dermatol* 8, 149
(1977): Epstein E, *Arch Dermatol* 113, 236
(1975): Breit R, *MMW Munch Med Wochenschr* (German) 117, 23
(1969): Moller H, *Lakartidningen* (Swedish) 66, 1446
(1969): Levene G+, *Br J Dermatol* 81, 712
(1967): Tarsitani F+, *Policlinico Prat* (Italian) 74, 329
(1967): Ippen H, *Z Haut Geschlechtskr* (German) 42, 47
(1966): Cullen SI+, *Arch Dermatol* 93, 77
(1965): Clendenning WE, *Arch Dermatol* 91, 628

Phototoxic reaction
(1980): Stern RS+, *Arch Dermatol* 116, 1269
(1975): Breit R, *MMW Munch Med Wochenschr* (German) 117, 23

Pigmentation
(1983): White SW+, *Arch Dermatol* 119, 1
(1981): Brothers DM+, *Ophthalmology* 88, 1212 (conjunctival)
(1981): Granstein RD+, *J Am Acad Dermatol* 5, 1 (blue-black)

Pruritus (<1%)
(1995): Nowakowski J+, *J Am Acad Dermatol* 32, 223

Pruritus ani

Psoriasis (exacerbation)
(1990): Bergner T+, *J Am Acad Dermatol* 23, 770
(1988): Tsankov N+, *J Am Acad Dermatol* 19, 629

Purpura
(1965): Horowitz HI+, *Semin Hematol* 2, 287

Pustular eruption
(1973): Thomsen K+, *Br J Dermatol* 89, 293 (palms and soles)

Rash (sic)
(1997): Shapiro LE+, *Arch Dermatol* 133, 1224

Stevens–Johnson syndrome
(1997): Shoji T+, *J Am Acad Dermatol* 37, 337
(1993): Leenutaphong V+, *Int J Dermatol* 32, 428
(1985): Burge SM+, *J Am Acad Dermatol* 13, 665
(1968): Bianchine JR+, *Am Med J* 44, 390

Sunburn (exaggerated)
(1965): Clendenning WE, *Arch Dermatol* 91, 628

Toxic epidermal necrolysis
(1993): Leenutaphong V+, *Int J Dermatol* 32, 428
(1989): Davies MG+, *BMJ* 298, 1523
(1988): Gimova EK+, *Sov Med* (Russian) 6, 119
(1987): Curley RK+, *Clin Exp Dermatol* 12, 124
(1985): Tatnall FM+, *Br J Dermatol* 113, 629
(1985): Burge SM+, *J Am Acad Dermatol* 13, 665
(1984): Chan HL, *J Am Acad Dermatol* 10, 973
(1979): Izmailov GA+, *Khirurgiia Mosk* (Russian) September 102
(1974): Maibach HI+, *Arch Dermatol* 109, 97
(1970): Ocheret'ko MP, *Pediatriia* (Russian) 49, 86
(1967): Lowney ED+, *Arch Dermatol* 95, 359
(1966): Messaritakis J, *Ann Paediatr* 207, 236
(1959): Evans C, *BMJ* 2, 827

Urticaria
(1997): Shapiro LE+, *Arch Dermatol* 133, 1224
(1978): Jolly HW+, *Arch Dermatol* 114, 1485
(1977): McLundie S, *Ann Allergy* 38, 71

Vasculitis
(1960): Calnan CD+, *Trans A Rep St John's Hosp Derm Soc* (London) 44, 69

Warts (flat)
(1975): Gould WM, *Arch Dermatol* 111, 930

Nails

Nails – discoloration (<1%)
(1980): Hendricks AA, *Arch Dermatol* 116, 438 (yellow lunulae)

Nails – onycholysis
(1979): Kanwar AJ+, *Cutis* 23, 657
(1976): Sanders CV+, *South Med J* 69, 1090
(1974): Merrill RH, *South Med J* 67, 677
(1972): Kestel JL, *Arch Dermatol* 106, 766
(1965): Clendenning WE, *Arch Dermatol* 91, 628

Nails – photo-onycholysis
(1987): Baran R+, *J Am Acad Dermatol* 17, 1012
(1983): Ibsen HH+, *Acta Derm Venereol* 63, 555
(1978): Lasser AE+, *Pediatrics* 61, 98
(1978): Hatch DJ+, *J Am Podiatry Assoc* 68, 172
(1977): Rothstein MS, *Arch Dermatol* 113, 520
(1973): Verma KC+, *Indian J Dermatol* 18, 23
(1971): Frank SB+, *Arch Dermatol* 103, 520

Other

Anaphylactoid reaction (<1%)
(1965): Clendenning WE, *Arch Dermatol* 91, 628

Black tongue
(1954): Annotations, *Lancet* 2, 179

Fixed intraoral eruption
(1982): Murray VK+, *J Periodontology* 53, 267

Gingivitis

Glossitis
(1978): Jolly HW+, *Arch Dermatol* 114, 1485

Hypersensitivity (<1%)
(1997): Shapiro LE+, *Arch Dermatol* 133, 1224
(1972): No Author, *Tidsskr Nor Laegeforen* (Norwegian) 92, 1478

Mucocutaneous febrile syndrome
(1972): *Tidsskr Nor Laegeforen* (Norwegian) 92, 175

Mucous membrane pigmentation

Oral ulceration

Paresthesias (<1%)
(1996): Sorkin M, *The Schoch Letter* 45 (5), 18 (observation)
(1994): Blanchard L, *The Schoch Letter* 44, (6) (observation)

Porphyria cutanea tarda
(1992): Shelley WB+, *Advanced Dermatologic Diagnosis*, WB Saunders, 414 (passim)

Pseudoporphyria
(1976): Epstein JH+, *Arch Dermatol* 112, 661

Pseudotumor cerebri
(1999): Quinn AG+, *J Aapos* 3, 53
(1998): Noll K, La Crosse, WI (from Internet) (observation)
(1995): Lee AG, *Cutis* 55, 165
(1986): Pierog SH+, *J Adolesc Health Care* 7, 139
(1981): Steigleder GK, *Z Haut* 56, 839
(1978): Stuart BH+, *J Pediatr* 92, 679
Serum sickness
(1997): Shapiro LE+, *Arch Dermatol* 133, 1224
Thrombophlebitis (<1%)
Tongue pigmentation
Tooth discoloration (commonly in under 8-year-olds) (>10%)
(1998): Livingston HM+, *Ann Pharmacother* 32, 607
(1994): Hofmann H, *Hautarzt* (German) 45, 803
(1979): Jackson R, *Cutis* 23, 613
(1974): Moffitt JM+, *J Am Dent Ass* 88, 547
(1971): Grossman ER+, *Pediatrics* 47, 567
(1970): Conchie JM+, *Can Med Ass J* 103, 351
(1968): *Med Lett* 10, 76
(1964): Stewart DJ, *Br J Dermatol* 76, 374
(1962): Wallman IS+, *Lancet* 1, 827 (>5%)
Vaginitis
(1977): Hall JH+, *Cutis* 20, 97
(1972): Gilgor RS, *N C Med J* 33, 331
(1972): Litt IF, *Pediatrics* 49, 637

THALIDOMIDE

Trade names: Contergan, Distaval, Kevadon, Thalidomid (Celgene)
Indications: Graft-versus-host reactions, recalcitrant aphthous stomatitis
Category: Immunosuppressant; treatment for graft-versus-host disease and nodose leprosy
Half-life: 8.7 hours
Clinically important, potentially serious interactions with: no data

Reactions

Skin

Bullous eruption
(1975): Sheskin J, *Hautarzt* (German) 26, 1 (5%)
Burning
(1989): Gutierrez-Rodriguez O+, *J Rheumatol* 16, 158
Dermatitis (sic)
(1971): Waters MFR, *Lepr Rev* 42, 26
Diaphoresis
(1978): Smithells RW, *Lancet* 1, 1042
Edema
(1997): Duran McKinster C, *Skin and Allergy News* August, 37
(1996): Tseng S+, *J Am Acad Dermatol* 35, 969 (passim)
(1989): Grinspan D+, *J Am Acad Dermatol* 20, 1060
(1984): Gutierrez-Rodriguez O, *Arthritis Rheum* 27, 1118
Erythema
(1989): Gutierrez-Rodriguez O+, *J Rheumatol* 16, 158
Erythema nodosum
(1988): Viraben R+, *Dermatologica* 176, 107
Erythroderma
(1996): Tseng S+, *J Am Acad Dermatol* 35, 969 (passim)
(1994): Bielsa I+, *Dermatology* (Basel) 189, 178
Exanthems
(1999): Burrow WH, Jackson, MS, (from Internet) (observation)
(1991): Williams I+, *Lancet* 337, 436 (37% in AIDS patients)
Exfoliative dermatitis
(1996): Tseng S+, *J Am Acad Dermatol* 35, 969 (passim)
(1988): Salafia A+, *Int J Lepr Other Mycobact Dis* 56, 625
Facial erythema
(1989): Gutierrez-Rodriguez O+, *J Rheumatol* 16, 158
(1975): Sheskin J, *Hautarzt* (German) 26, 1 (1–5%)
Pedal edema
(2000): Bahl S+, *Skin and Aging*, May, 41
Pruritus
(1996): Tseng S+, *J Am Acad Dermatol* 35, 969 (passim)
(1989): Gutierrez-Rodriguez O+, *J Rheumatol* 16, 158
Purpura
(1996): Tseng S+, *J Am Acad Dermatol* 35, 969 (passim)
Pustuloderma
(1999): Rua-Figuero I+, *Lupus* 8, 248
Rash (sic)
(1997): Jacobson JM+, *New Engl J Med* 336, 1487 (>50%)
(1997): Haslett P+, *Infect Med* 14, 393
(1993): Holm AL+, *Arch Dermatol* 129, 1548 (passim)
(1986): Hamza MH, *Clin Rheumatol* 5, 365
Red palms
(1996): Tseng S+, *J Am Acad Dermatol* 35, 969 (passim)
Shakes (sic)
(1999): Duong DJ, *Arch Dermatol* 135, 1079
Toxic epidermal necrolysis
(1999): Horowitz SB+, *Pharmacotherapy* 19, 1177
Toxic pustuloderma
(1997): Darvay A+, *Clin Exp Dermatol* 22, 297
Urticaria
(1975): Sheskin J, *Hautarzt* (German) 26, 1 (3%)
Vasculitis
(1996): Tseng S+, *J Am Acad Dermatol* 35, 969 (passim)
Xerosis
(2000): Bahl S+, *Skin and Aging*, May, 41
(1989): Gutierrez-Rodriguez O+, *J Rheumatol* 16, 158

Hair

Hair – alopecia
(1989): Gutierrez-Rodriguez O+, *J Rheumatol* 16, 158

Nails

Nails – brittle
(1996): Tseng S+, *J Am Acad Dermatol* 35, 969 (passim)

Other

Dysesthesia
(1989): Grinspan D+, *J Am Acad Dermatol* 20, 1060
Galactorrhea
(1996): Tseng S+, *J Am Acad Dermatol* 35, 969 (passim)
Hypesthesia
(2000): Bahl S+, *Skin and Aging*, May, 41
Paresthesias
(2000): Bahl S+, *Skin and Aging*, May, 41
(2000): Ordi-Ros J+, *J Rheumatol* 27, 1429
(1999): Duong DJ, *Arch Dermatol* 135, 1079
(1998): Lee JB+, *J Am Acad Dermatol* 39, 835
Xerostomia
(2000): Bahl S+, *Skin and Aging*, May, 41
(1996): Tseng S+, *J Am Acad Dermatol* 35, 969 (passim)
(1989): Gutierrez-Rodriguez O+, *J Rheumatol* 16, 158
(1989): Grinspan D+, *J Am Acad Dermatol* 20, 1060

THEOPHYLLINE

(See AMINOPHYLLINE)

THIABENDAZOLE

Synonym: tiabendazole
Trade name: Mintezol (Merck)
Other common trade name: *Triasox*
Indications: Various infections caused by susceptible helminths
Category: Anthelmintic
Half-life: 1.2 hours
Clinically important, potentially serious interactions with: theophylline

Reactions

Skin

Angioedema
Contact dermatitis
(1994): Mancuso G, *Contact Dermatitis* 31, 207

(1993): Izu R+, *Contact Dermatitis* 28, 243 (photoaggravated)
(1968): De Irureta-Goyena A, *Arch Dermatol* 97, 348

Erythema multiforme (<1%)
(1988): Kardaun SH+, *Br J Dermatol* 118, 545
(1988): Humphreys F+, *Br J Dermatol* 118, 855

Exanthems (>5%)
(1982): Sanchez del Rio J+, *Actas Dermosifiliogr* (Spanish) 73, 125
(1977): Casado-Jiminez M+, *Actas Dermosifiliogr* (Spanish) 68, 675
(1976): Marron-Gasca J+, *Actas Dermosifiliogr* (Spanish) 67, 701
(1965): Bowen J+, *Arch Dermatol* 91, 425

Fixed eruption (<1%)
(1976): Marron-Gasca J+, *Actas Dermosifiliogr* (Spanish) 67, 701

Flushing

Jarisch–Herxheimer reaction

Perianal rash

Pruritus (<1%)
(1965): Bowen J+, *Arch Dermatol* 91, 425

Psoriasis (exacerbation)

Rash (sic) (1–10%)

Sjøgren's syndrome
(1995): Bion E+, *J Hepatol* 23, 672
(1979): Fink AI+, *Ophthalmology* 86, 1892

Stevens–Johnson syndrome (1–10%)

Toxic epidermal necrolysis (<1%)
(1993): Correia O+, *Dermatology* 186, 32
(1976): Robinson HM+, *Arch Dermatol* 112, 1757

Urticaria (1–5%)
(1970): Tanowitz HB+, *J Trop Med Hyg* 73, 141

Other

Anaphylactoid reaction

Dry mucous membranes (sic)

Hypersensitivity (<1%)

Paresthesias

Xanthopsia (<1%)

Xerostomia
(1979): Fink AI+, *Ophthalmology* 86, 1892

THIAMINE

Synonym: vitamin B_1
Trade names: Betalin; Thiamilate
Other common trade names: *Actamin; Beneuril; Betabion; Betamin; Betaxin; Bewon; Biamine; Thiamilate; Tiamina; Vitantial*
Indications: Thiamine deficiency
Category: Water-soluble vitamin; nutritional supplement
Half-life: no data
Clinically important, potentially serious interactions with: none

Reactions

Skin

Allergic reactions (sic)
(1969): Zheltakov MM+, *Vestn Dermatol Venerol* (Russian) 43, 62

Angioedema (<1%)

Contact dermatitis
(1989): Ingemann-Larsen A+, *Contact Dermatitis* 20, 387
(1958): Hjorth N, *J Invest Dermatol* 30, 261

Diaphoresis

Eczematous eruption (sic)
(1958): Hjorth N, *J Invest Dermatol* 30, 261

Exanthems
(1980): Kolz R+, *Hautarzt* (German) 31, 657

Pruritus (<1%)

Purpura
(1989): Nishioka K+, *J Dermatol* 16, 220
(1980): Nishioka K+, *Clin Exp Dermatol* 5, 213

Rash (sic) (<1%)

Systemic eczematous contact dermatitis

Urticaria

Vasculitis
(1989): Nishioka K+, *J Dermatol* 16, 220

Other

Anaphylactoid reaction
(1998): Morinville V+, *Schweiz Med Wochenschr* 128, 1743
(1997): Fernandez M+, *Allergy* 52, 958

Foetor ex ore (halitosis)

Injection-site reactions

Paresthesias (<1%)

THIOGUANINE

Synonyms: TG; 6-TG; 6-thioguanine; tioguanine
Trade name: Thioguanine (GlaxoWellcome)
Other common trade name: *Lanvis*
Indications: Leukemias
Category: Antineoplastic; antimetabolite
Half-life: 11 hours
Clinically important, potentially serious interactions with: busulfan

Reactions

Skin

Cutaneous malignancies
(1997): Zackheim HS+, *J Am Acad Dermatol* 30, 452 (nonmelanoma)

Exanthems
(1988): Zimm S+, *J Clin Oncol* 6, 696

Painful red hands
(1988): Shall L+, *Br J Dermatol* 119, 249

Petechiae

Photosensitivity (<1%)
(1988): Zimm S+, *J Clin Oncol* 6, 696

Pruritus
(1999): Silvis NG+, *Arch Dermatol* 135, 433

Psoriasis
(1999): Silvis NG+, *Arch Dermatol* 135, 433

Purpura

Rash (sic) (1–10%)

Hair

Hair – alopecia
(1999): Murphy FP+, *Arch Dermatol* 135, 1495
(1988): Zimm S+, *J Clin Oncol* 6, 696

Other

Oral mucosal lesions

Stomatitis (1–10%)

Xerostomia
(1999): Silvis NG+, *Arch Dermatol* 135, 433

THIOPENTAL

Trade name: Thiopental (Baxter)
Other common trade names: *Anesthal; Hypnostan; Intraval; Nesdonal; Sodipental; Trapanal*
Indications: Induction of anesthesia
Category: Barbiturate anesthetic; anticonvulsant; sedative
Half-life: 3–12 hours
Clinically important, potentially serious interactions with: antidepressants, benzodiazepines, chloramphenicol, CNS depressants, codeine, fentanyl, ketamine, MAO inhibitors, meperidine, methadone, narcotic analgesics, pentazocine, phenothiazines, probenecid, sulfisoxazole

Reactions

Skin

Angioedema
(1975): Brown TP, *Anaesth Intensive Care* 3, 257
(1972): Almeyda J+, *Br J Dermatol* 86, 313
(1971): Fox GS+, *Anesthesiology* 35, 655

(1957): Hayward JR+, *J Oral Surg* 15, 61
Bullous eruption
(1987): Saiag P+, *Ann Dermatol Venereol* (French) 114, 1440
(1977): Evans JM+, *BMJ* 2, 735
Erythema (<1%)
Erythema multiforme
(1947): Hunter AR, *Lancet* 1, 47
(1946): Peterkin GAG, *BMJ* 2, 52
Exanthems
(1987): Boittiaux P+, *Ann Fr Anesth Reanim* (French) 6, 324 (3.3%)
(1971): Fox GS+, *Anesthesiology* 35, 655
(1946): Peterkin GAG, *BMJ* 2, 52
Exfoliative dermatitis
Fixed eruption
(1995): Bremang JA+, *Can J Anaesth* 42, 628
(1990): Desmeules H, *Anesth Analg* 70, 216 (non-pigmenting)
(1987): Saiag P+, *Ann Dermatol Venereol* (French) 114, 1440
Hypopigmentation
(1979): Coote N+, *Anaesthesia* 34, 336
Pruritus (<1%)
Purpura
(1972): Almeyda J+, *Br J Dermatol* 86, 313
(1946): Peterkin GAG, *BMJ* 2, 52
Rash (sic)
Stevens–Johnson syndrome
(1946): Peterkin GAG, *BMJ* 2, 52
Toxic epidermal necrolysis
(1987): Saiag P+, *Ann Dermatol Venereol* (French) 114, 1440
Urticaria
(1972): Almeyda J+, *Br J Dermatol* 86, 313
(1972): Barjenbruch KP+, *Anesth Analg* 51, 113
(1957): Hayward JR+, *J Oral Surg* 15, 61
(1946): Peterkin GAG, *BMJ* 2, 52

Other

Anaphylactoid reaction (<1%)
(1993): Seymour DG, *JAMA* 270, 2503 (letter)
(1992): Breathnach SM+, *Adverse Drug Reactions and the Skin*, Blackwell, Oxford, 193 (passim)
(1988): Cheema AL+, *J Allergy Clin Immunol* 81, 220
(1975): Brown TP, *Anaesth Intensive Care* 3, 257
(1973): Kelly AJ+, *Anaesth Intensive Care* 1, 332
(1972): Barjenbruch KP+, *Anesth Analg* 51, 113
(1971): Davis J, *Br J Anaesth* 43, 1191
(1971): Sargent NW, *Br J Anaesth* 43, 591
Injection-site necrosis
Injection-site pain (>10%)
Injection-site phlebitis
(1981): Clark RSJ, *Drugs* 22,26 (6%)
Porphyria
(1993): Harrison GG+, *Anaesthesia* 48, 1008–1010
(1976): Panica D+, *Folia Med Plovdiv* 18, 161
(1975): Mees DE+, *South Med J* 68, 29
(1966): Eales L, *Anesthesiology* 27, 703
Shivering
(1987): Boittiaux P+, *Ann Fr Anesth Reanim* (French) 6, 324 (27%)
Thrombophlebitis (<1%)
Twitching (<1%)

THIORIDAZINE

Trade name: Mellaril (Novartis)
Other common trade names: *Aldazine; Apo-Thioridazine; Calmaril; Dazine; Melleril; Ridazin; Thinin; Thioril*
Indications: Psychotic disorders
Category: Phenothiazine antipsychotic
Half-life: 21–25 hours
Clinically important, potentially serious interactions with: alcohol, beta-blockers, CNS depressants, epinephrine, levodopa, lithium, pindolol, propranolol, sulfadoxine, trazodone, tricyclic antidepressants, **cigarette smoking**

Reactions

Skin

Acanthosis nigricans
(1979): Arnold HL+, *J Am Acad Dermatol* 1, 93
Angioedema (<1%)
(1964): Welsh AL, *Med Clin North Am* 48, 459
Dermatitis (sic)
(1968): Wolpert A+, *Clin Pharmacol Ther* 9, 456
Erythema multiforme
(1985): Rees TD, *J Periodontol* 56, 480
Exanthems
(1974): Rothstein E, *N Engl J Med* 290, 521
Exfoliative dermatitis
Hypohidrosis (>10%)
Lupus erythematosus
(1971): Fabius AJM+, *Acta Rheumatol Scand* 17, 137
Parkinsonism (>10%)
Peripheral edema
Photoreactions
(1987): Röhrborn W+, *Contact Dermatitis* 17, 241
(1976): Suhonen R, *Contact Dermatitis* 2, 179
Photosensitivity (1–10%)
Phototoxic reaction
(1967): Satanove A+, *JAMA* 200, 209
(1960): Barsa JA+, *Am J Psychiatry* 116, 1028
Pigmentation (<1%) (blue-gray)
(1970): Ayd FJ, *Int Drug Ther Newsletter* 5, 24
(1969): Berger H, *Arch Dermatol* 100, 487
Purpura
Rash (sic) (1–10%)
(1981): Georgotas A+, *Psychopharmacology* 73, 292
(1969): Doyle JA+, *Curr Ther Res* 11, 429
(1960): May RH+, *J Nerv Mental Dis* 130, 230
Seborrhea
Toxic epidermal necrolysis
(1987): Harnar TJ+, *J Burn Care Rehabil* 8, 554
Urticaria
Xerosis

Hair

Hair – alopecia
Hair – hypertrichosis
(1979): Phillips P+, *JAMA* 241, 920

Other

Anaphylactoid reaction
Galactorrhea (<1%)
Gynecomastia
Hypersensitivity
Lymphoproliferative disease
(1992): Aguilar JL+, *Arch Dermatol* 128, 121
Mastodynia (1–10%)
Oral mucosal eruption
(1985): Rees TD, *J Periodontol* 56, 480
Paresthesias
Parotitis
(1974): Rothstein E, *N Engl J Med* 290, 521
Porphyria
(1985): Kamal S+, *Union Med Can* (French) 114, 330

Priapism (<1%)
Pseudolymphoma
(1988): Kardaun SH+, *Br J Dermatol* 118, 545
Tremor
Xerostomia
(1981): Georgotas A+, *Psychopharmacology* 73, 292

THIOTEPA

Synonym: TSPA
Trade name: Thioplex (Immunex)
Indications: Breast, ovarian and bladder carcinomas
Category: Antineoplastic
Half-life: 109 minutes
Clinically important, potentially serious interactions with: neuromuscular blocking agents, succinylcholine

Reactions

Skin

Allergic reactions (sic) (1–10%)
Angioedema
(1992): Breathnach SM+, *Adverse Drug Reactions and the Skin*, Blackwell, Oxford, 292 (passim)
(1987): Lee M+, *J Urol* 138, 143
(1985): Levine N+, *Cancer Treat Rev* 5, 67
(1981): Weiss RB+, *Ann Intern Med* 94, 66
(1969): Veenema RJ+, *J Urol* 101, 711
Bruising
Ecchymoses
Eccrine squamous syringometaplasia
(1997): Valks R+, *Arch Dermatol* 133, 873
Leucoderma
(1979): Harben DJ+, *Arch Dermatol* 115, 973 (passim)
(1976): Rosai J+, *Hum Pathol* 7, 83
(1969): Berkow JW+, *Arch Ophthalmol* 82, 415 (periorbital)
(1966): Reed RJ+, *Arch Dermatol* 94, 396
Pigmentation (1–10%)
(1992): Breathnach SM+, *Adverse Drug Reactions and the Skin*, Blackwell, Oxford, 292 (passim)
(1989): Horn TD+, *Arch Dermatol* 125, 524
(1974): Hornblass A+, *Ann Ophthalmol* 6, 1155
(1969): Howitt D+, *Am J Ophthalmol* 68, 473
Pruritus (1–10%)
(1992): Breathnach SM+, *Adverse Drug Reactions and the Skin*, Blackwell, Oxford, 292 (passim)
(1987): Lee M+, *J Urol* 138, 143
(1985): Levine N+, *Cancer Treat Rev* 5, 67
(1981): Weiss RB+, *Ann Intern Med* 94, 66
(1969): Veenema RJ+, *J Urol* 101, 711
Rash (sic) (1–10%)
Urticaria
(1992): Breathnach SM+, *Adverse Drug Reactions and the Skin*, Blackwell, Oxford, 292 (passim)
(1987): Lee M+, *J Urol* 138, 143
(1985): Levine N+, *Cancer Treat Rev* 5, 67
(1981): Weiss RB+, *Ann Intern Med* 94, 66
(1977): Greenspan E+, *JAMA* 237, 2288 (3.8%)
(1969): Veenema RJ+, *J Urol* 101, 711

Hair

Hair – alopecia (1–10%)
(1966): Clavert W, *BMJ* 2, 831

Other

Anaphylactoid reaction (<1%)
Injection-site pain (>10%)
Stomatitis (<1%)

THIOTHIXENE

Synonym: tiotixene
Trade name: Navane (Pfizer)
Other common trade name: *Orbinamon*
Indications: Psychotic disorders
Category: Antipsychotic
Half-life: >24 hours
Clinically important, potentially serious interactions with: alcohol, anticholinergics, benztropine, bromocriptine, chloroquine, CNS depressants, guanethidine, levodopa, lithium, propranolol, quinidine, trazodone, tricyclic antidepressants, **cigarette smoking**

Reactions

Skin

Diaphoresis
(1968): Wolpert A+, *Clin Pharmacol Ther* 9, 456 (14%)
Exanthems
(1994): Shelley WB+, *Cutis* 54, 71 (observation)
(1968): Wolpert A+, *Clin Pharmacol Ther* 9, 456 (14%)
Hypohidrosis (>10%)
Parkinsonism (>10%)
Palmar erythema
(1982): Matsuoka LY, *J Am Acad Dermatol* 7, 405
Peripheral edema
Photosensitivity (1–10%)
(1970): *Med Lett* 12, 104
(1966): Gallant DM+, *Am J Psychiatry* 123, 345
Pigmentation (blue-gray) (<1%)
Pruritus
Rash (sic) (1–10%)
Raynaud's phenomenon
(1991): McCance-Katz EF, *J Clin Psychiatry* 52, 89
Seborrheic dermatitis
(1984): Binder RL+, *J Clin Psychiatry* 45, 125
(1983): Binder RL+, *Arch Dermatol* 119, 473
Sensitivity (sic)
(1982): Matsuoka LY, *J Am Acad Dermatol* 7, 405
Telangiectases
(1982): Matsuoka LY, *J Am Acad Dermatol* 7, 405
Urticaria

Hair

Hair – alopecia

Other

Anaphylactoid reaction
Black tongue
(2000): Heymann WR, *Cutis* 66, 25
Dysgeusia
(2000): Heymann WR, *Cutis* 66, 25
Galactorrhea (<1%)
Gynecomastia
Mastodynia (1–10%)
Paresthesias
Priapism (<1%)
Sialorrhea
Xerostomia
(2000): Heymann WR, *Cutis* 66, 25
(1987): Sarai K+, *Pharmacopsychiatry* 20, 38

TIAGABINE

Trade name: Gabitril (Abbott)
Indications: Partial seizures
Category: Anticonvulsant
Half-life: 7–9 hours
Clinically important, potentially serious interactions with: carbamazepine, phenobarbital, phenytoin, primidone, valproic acid

Reactions

Skin

Acne (>1%)
Allergic reactions (sic) (<1%)
Carcinoma (sic) (<1%)
Contact dermatitis (<1%)
Diaphoresis (<1%)
Ecchymoses (>1%)
Eczema (sic) (<1%)
Edema (<1%)
Exanthems (<1%)
Exfoliative dermatitis (<1%)
Facial edema (<1%)
Furunculosis (<1%)
Herpes simplex (<1%)
Herpes zoster (<1%)
Neoplasms (benign) (<1%)
Nodules (<1%)
Peripheral edema (<1%)
Petechiae (<1%)
Photosensitivity (<1%)
Pigmentation (<1%)
Pruritus (2%)
Psoriasis (<1%)
Rash (sic) (5%)
Stevens–Johnson syndrome
Ulcerations (<1%)
Urticaria (<1%)
Vesiculobullous eruption (<1%)
Xerosis (<1%)

Hair

Hair – alopecia (<1%)
Hair – hirsutism (<1%)

Other

Ageusia (<1%)
Dysgeusia (<1%)
Gingival hyperplasia (<1%)
Gingivitis (<1%)
Glossitis (<1%)
Gynecomastia (<1%)
Halitosis (<1%)
Mastodynia (<1%)
Myalgia (>1%)
Oral ulceration (2%)
Paresthesias (4%)
Parosmia (<1%)
Sialorrhea (<1%)
Stomatitis (<1%)
Thrombophlebitis (<1%)
Tremor (>1%)
Ulcerative stomatitis (<1%)
Vaginitis (<1%)
Xerostomia (>1%)

TICARCILLIN

Trade name: Ticar (SmithKline Beecham)
Indications: Various infections caused by susceptible organisms
Category: Penicillinase-sensitive penicillin antibiotic
Half-life: 1.0–1.2 hours
Clinically important, potentially serious interactions with: aminoglycosides, anticoagulants, chloramphenicol, cyclosporine, erythromycin, heparin, methotrexate, neuromuscular blockers, oral contraceptives, probenecid, tetracyclines

Reactions

Skin

Allergic reactions (sic)
(1994): Pleasants RA+, *Chest* 106, 1124 (in patients with cystic fibrosis)
Angioedema
Bullous eruption
Ecchymoses
Erythema multiforme
Erythema nodosum
Exanthems
(1980): Brogden RN+, *Drugs* 20, 325 (1%)
Exfoliative dermatitis
Hematomas
Jarisch–Herxheimer reaction (<1%)
Pruritus
Purpura
Rash (sic) (<1%)
Stevens–Johnson syndrome
Toxic epidermal necrolysis
Urticaria
Vasculitis

Other

Anaphylactoid reaction (<1%)
Black tongue
Dysgeusia
Glossitis
Glossodynia
Hypersensitivity (<1%)
Injection-site pain
(1980): Brogden RN+, *Drugs* 20, 325
Injection-site phlebitis
(1980): Brogden RN+, *Drugs* 20, 325
Oral candidiasis
Serum sickness
Stomatitis
Stomatodynia
Thrombophlebitis (<1%)
Vaginitis
Xerostomia

TICLOPIDINE

Trade name: Ticlid (Roche)
Other common trade names: *Anagregal; Panaldine; Ticlidil; Ticlodix; Ticlodone; Tiklid; Tiklyd*
Indications: To reduce risk of thrombotic stroke
Category: Antithrombotic; platelet aggregation inhibitor
Half-life: 24 hours
Clinically important, potentially serious interactions with: antacids, anticoagulants, antipyrine, aspirin, carbamazepine, cimetidine, cyclosporine, NSAIDs, phenytoin, theophylline

Reactions

Skin

Acute generalized exanthematous pustulosis
(2000): Cannavò SP+, *Br J Dermatol* 142, 577

Angioedema (<1%)
(1999): Chassany O+, *Presse Med* (French) 28, 18
Cutaneous bleeding (sic)
(1990): McTavish D+, *Drugs* 40, 238 (1–5%)
(1984): Stiegler H+, *Dtsch Med Wochenschr* (German) 109, 1240 (4.4%)
Cutaneous side effects (sic)
(1984): Stiegler H+, *Dtsch Med Wochenschr* (German) 109, 1240 (8%)
Dermatitis (sic)
(1998): Ceylan C+, *Am J Hematol* 59, 260
Diaphoresis
(1984): Stiegler H+, *Dtsch Med Wochenschr* (German) 109, 1240 (1.7%)
Ecchymoses (<1%)
Erythema
(1990): McTavish D+, *Drugs* 40, 238
Erythema multiforme (<1%)
(1999): Yosipovitch G+, *J Am Acad Dermatol* 41, 473
Erythema nodosum (<1%)
Erythromelalgia
(1999): Yosipovitch G+, *J Am Acad Dermatol* 41, 473
Exanthems (<1%)
(2000): Prost C+, *Presse Med* (French) 29, 303
(1999): Yosipovitch G+, *J Am Acad Dermatol* 41, 473
(1997): Litt JZ, Beachwood, OH, personal case (observation)
(1990): McTavish D+, *Drugs* 40, 238 (7%)
(1989): Hass WK+, *N Engl J Med* 321, 501 (11.9%)
(1987): Saltiel E+, *Drugs* 34, 222 (1–5%)
Exfoliative dermatitis (<1%)
Facial erythema
(1999): Yosipovitch G+, *J Am Acad Dermatol* 41, 473
Fixed eruption
(1999): Yosipovitch G+, *J Am Acad Dermatol* 41, 473
Hematomas
(1984): Stiegler H+, *Dtsch Med Wochenschr* (German) 109, 1240 (2.7%)
Lupus erythematosus (positive ANA) (<1%)
Petechiae
(1984): Stiegler H+, *Dtsch Med Wochenschr* (German) 109, 1240 (1.7%)
Phenytoin toxicity (sic)
(1998): Klaasen SL, *Ann Pharmacother* 32, 1295
Pruritus (1.3%)
(1999): Yosipovitch G+, *J Am Acad Dermatol* 41, 473
(1990): McTavish D+, *Drugs* 40, 238
(1987): Saltiel E+, *Drugs* 34, 222
Purpura (2.2%)
(2000): Chemnitz JM+, *med Klin* (German) 95, 96
(2000): Tsai HM+, *Ann Intern Med* 132, 794
Rash (sic) (5.1%)
(1999): Quinn MJ+, *Circulation* 100, 1667
(1999): Whetsel TR+, *Pharmacotherapy* 19, 228
Stevens–Johnson syndrome (<1%)
Thrombocytopenic purpura (2.2%)
(2000): Tsai H-M+, *Ann Intern Med* 132, 794
(1999): Elangovan L, *Arch Int Med* 159, 1624
(1999): Bennett CL+, *Ann Intern Med* 159, 2524
(1999): Steinhubl SR+, *JAMA* 281, 806
(1999): Chen DK+, *Arch Intern Med* 159, 311
(1999): Mauro M+, *Blood* 94, 1–646a
(1998): Bennett CL+, *Lancet* 352, 1036
(1998): Bennett CL+, *Ann Intern Med* 128, 541
(1998): Muszkat M+, *Pharmacotherapy* 18, 1352
(1998): Mukamal KJ+, *Ann Intern Med* 129, 837
(1998): Jamar S+, *Acta Cardiol* 53, 285
(1997): Kupfer Y+, *N Engl J Med* 337, 1245
(1996): Wysowski DK+, *JAMA* 276, 952
(1991): Page Y+, *Lancet* 337, 774
(1990): McTavish D+, *Drugs* 40, 238 (1–5%)
(1990): Takishita S+, *N Engl J Med* 323, 1487
(1989): Hass WK+, *N Engl J Med* 321, 501 (4%)
(1984): Stiegler H+, *Dtsch Med Wochenschr* (German) 109, 1240 (1–5%)
(1982): de Fraiture WH+, *Ned Tijdschr Geneeskd* (Dutch) 126, 1051
Toxic erythroderma (sic)
(1999): Hsi DH+, *N Engl J Med* 340, 1212
Urticaria (<1%)
(1999): Yosipovitch G+, *J Am Acad Dermatol* 41, 473
(1990): McTavish D+, *Drugs* 40, 238
(1989): Hass WK+, *N Engl J Med* 321, 501 (2%)
(1987): Saltiel E+, *Drugs* 34, 222 (1–5%)
Vasculitis (<1%)

Other
Serum sickness

TIMOLOL

Trade names: Blocadren (Merck); CoSopt (Merck); Timolide (Merck); Timoptic (ophthalmic) (Merck)
Other common trade names: *Apo-Timol; Aquanil; Blocadren; Dispatim; Nu-Timolol; Tenopt; Tiloptic; Timacor; Timoptic; Timoptol*
Indications: Hypertension
Category: Beta-adrenergic blocker; antihypertensive
Half-life: 2–2.7 hours
Clinically important, potentially serious interactions with: calcium channel blockers, ciprofloxacin, clonidine, epinephrine, ergot, flecainide, insulin, nifedipine, NSAIDs, oral contraceptives, prazosin, propafenone, salicylates, theophylline, verapamil

Note: Cutaneous side-effects of beta-receptor blockaders are clinically polymorphous. They apparently appear after several months of continuous therapy. Atypical psoriasiform, lichen planus-like, and eczematous chronic rashes are mainly observed. (1983): Hödl St, *Z Hautkr* (German) 1:58, 17.

CoSopt is timolol and dorzolamide*; Timolide is timolol and hydrochlorothiazide*

Reactions

Skin
Angioedema
Burning (from ophthalmic)
Contact dermatitis (eyedrops)
(2000): Quiralte J+, *Contact Dermatitis* 42, 245
(1995): Koch P, *Contact Dermatitis* 33, 140
(1993): Corazza M+, *Contact Dermatitis* 28, 188)
(1993): O'Donnell BF+, *Contact Dermatitis* 28, 121)
(1991): Cameli N+, *Contact Dermatitis* 25, 129
(1991): Kubota K+, *Br J Clin Pharmacol* 31, 471
(1988): Kanzaki T+, *Contact Dermatitis* 19, 388
(1986): Romaguera C,+ *Contact Dermatitis* 14, 248
(1986): Fernandez-Vozmediano JM+, *Contact Dermatitis* 14, 252
Dermatitis (sic)
(1998): Lewis B, Colorado Springs, CO (from Internet) (observation) (glans penis)
Diaphoresis
Eczematous eruption (sic)
(1991): Cameli N+, *Contact Dermatitis* 25, 129
(1979): van Joost T, *Br J Dermatol* 101, 171
Edema (0.6%)
Erythema multiforme
Erythroderma
(1997): Shelley WB+, *J Am Acad Dermatol* 37, 799
(1993): Shelley WB+, *Cutis* 51, 330 (observation)
Exanthems
Exfoliative dermatitis
Hyperkeratosis (palms and soles)
Lichenoid eruption
(1978): Savage RL+, *BMJ* 1, 987
Lupus erythematosus
(1994): Cohen MG, *J Rheumatol* 21, 578
(1992): Zamber RW+, *J Rheumatol* 19, 977
Pemphigoid
(1987): Fiore PM+, *Arch Ophthalmol* 105, 1660
Photosensitivity
Pigmentation
Pityriasis rubra pilaris
(1978): Finlay AY+, *BMJ* 1, 987
Pruritus (1–5%)
(1996): Lazarov A+, *Cutis* 58, 363 (from eye drops)
Psoriasis
(1992): Germain ML+, *Therapie* (French) 47, 447
(1989): Puig L+, *Am J Ophthalmol* 108, 455

(1987): Savola J+, *BMJ* 295, 637 (also aggravation of psoriasis)
(1986): Czernielewski J+, *Lancet* 1, 808
(1984): Arntzen N+, *Acta Derm Venereol* (Stockh) 64, 346

Purpura
Rash (sic) (1–10%)
Raynaud's phenomenon
(1984): Eliasson K+, *Acta Med Scand* 215, 333
(1976): Marshall AJ+, *BMJ* 1, 1498
Stinging (from ophthalmic)
Toxic epidermal necrolysis
Urticaria
Xerosis

Hair

Hair – alopecia (also from Timoptic eye drops) (1–10%)
(1990): Fraunfelder FT+, *JAMA* 263, 1493

Nails

Nails – dystrophy
Nails – onycholysis
Nails – pigmentation
(1981): Feiler-Ofry V, *Ophthalmologica* (Basel) 182, 153

Other

Anaphylactoid reaction
Digital necrosis
(1989): Dompmartin A+, *Ann Dermatol Venereol* (French) 115, 593
Dysgeusia
Myalgia
Ocular pemphigoid
(1992): Shelley WB+, *Advanced Dermatologic Diagnosis*, WB Saunders, 554 (passim)
Oculo-mucocutaneous syndrome
(1982): Cocco G+, *Curr Ther Res* 31, 362
Oral lichenoid eruption
Paresthesias (<1%)
Peyronie's disease
(1979): Pryor JP+, *Lancet* 1, 331

***Note:** Dorzolamide and hydrocholorothiazide are sulfonamides and can be absorbed systemically. Sulfonamides can produce severe, possibly fatal, reactions such as toxic epidermal necrolysis and Stevens–Johnson syndrome.

TIOPRONIN

Trade name: Thiola (Mission)
Other common trade names: *Acadione; Captimer*
Indications: Cystinuria
Category: Antiurolithic
Half-life: no data
Clinically important, potentially serious interactions with: none

Reactions

Skin

Angioedema
(1988): Sigaud M+, *Rev Rhum Mal Osteoartic* (French) 55, 467 (14.5%)
Bullous pemphigoid
(1988): Nakajima H+, *Nippon Hifuka Gakkai Zasshi* (Japanese) 98, 803
Contact dermatitis
(1995): Romano A+, *Contact Dermatitis* 33, 269
Cutaneous side effects (sic)
(1988): Sigaud M+, *Rev Rhum Mal Osteoartic* (French) 55, 467 (27.5%)
Ecchymoses
Edema
Elastosis perforans serpiginosa
Erythema
(1990): Sany J+, *Rev Rhum Mal Osteoartic* (French) 57, 105
Erythema multiforme
(1988): Nakajima H+, *Nippon Hifuka Gakkai Zasshi* (Japanese) 98, 803
Exanthems
(1988): Sigaud M+, *Rev Rhum Mal Osteoartic* (French) 55, 467 (14.5%)
(1984): Shichiri M+, *Arch Intern Med* 144, 89
Lichenoid eruption
(1994): Pierard E+, *J Am Acad Dermatol* 31, 665
(1990): Kurumaji Y+, *J Dermatol* (Tokio) 17, 176
(1988): Kawabe Y+, *J Dermatol* (Tokio) 15, 434 (bullous)
Lupus erythematosus
(1986): Katayama I+, *J Dermatol* (Tokio) 13, 151
Pemphigus
(1994): Verdier-Sevrain S+, *Br J Dermatol* 130, 238
(1990): Sany J+, *Rev Rhum Mal Osteoartic* (French) 57, 105
(1990): Meuhier L+, *Ann Dermatol Venereol* (French) 117, 959
(1988): Sigaud M+, *Rev Rhum Mal Osteoartic* (French) 55, 467 (5.8%)
(1987): Enjolras O+, *Ann Dermatol Venereol* (French) 114, 25
Pemphigus erythematosus
(1982): Alinovi A+, *Acta Derm Venereol* (Stockh) 62, 452
Pemphigus foliaceus
(1983): Lucky PA+, *J Am Acad Dermatol* 8, 667
Photosensitivity
(1988): Sigaud M+, *Rev Rhum Mal Osteoartic* (French) 55, 467 (1.5%)
Pityriasis rosea
(1990): Sany J+, *Rev Rhum Mal Osteoartic* (French) 57, 105
(1988): Sigaud M+, *Rev Rhum Mal Osteoartic* (French) 55, 467 (5.8%)
Pruritus
Rash (sic)
Toxic epidermal necrolysis
Urticaria
Wrinkling (sic)

Hair

Hair – alopecia
(1990): Sany J+, *Rev Rhum Mal Osteoartic* (French) 57, 105
Hair – hypertrichosis
(1993): Arnaud M+, *Joint Bone Spine Dis* 60, 548

Other

Hypogeusia
Mucocutaneous side effects (sic)
(1990): Sany J+, *Rev Rhum Mal Osteoartic* (French) 57, 105 (32.8%)
Myopathy
(1988): Menkes CJ+, *Presse Med* (French) 17, 1156
Oral mucosal lesions
(1988): Sigaud M+, *Rev Rhum Mal Osteoartic* (French) 55, 467 (4.4%)
(1984): Shichiri M+, *Arch Intern Med* 144, 89
Oral ulceration
Parageusia
Parosmia
Polymyositis
(1999): Cacoub B+, *Presse Med* (French) 28, 911
Stomatitis
(1990): Sany J+, *Rev Rhum Mal Osteoartic* (French) 57, 105
(1988): Sigaud M+, *Rev Rhum Mal Osteoartic* (French) 55, 467
Xerostomia

TIROFIBAN

Trade name: Aggrastat (Merck)
Indications: Acute coronary syndrome
Category: Antiplatelet
Half-life: 2 hours
Clinically important, potentially serious interactions with: anticoagulants, aspirin, cephalosporins, heparin, NSAIDs, warfarin

Reactions

Skin

Bleeding (sic)
Diaphoresis (2%)
Edema (2%)
Rash (sic) (<1%)
Urticaria (<1%)

Other

Leg pain (3%)

TIZANIDINE

Trade name: Zanaflex (Athena)
Other common trade names: *Sirdalud; Ternalax; Ternelin*
Indications: Muscle spasticity, multiple sclerosis
Category: Alpha$_2$-adrenergic agonist
Half-life: 2.5 hours
Clinically important, potentially serious interactions with: alcohol, antihypertensives, baclofen, CNS depressants, diuretics, oral contraceptives, phenytoin

Reactions

Skin
Acne (<1%)
Allergic reactions (sic) (<1%)
Candidiasis (<1%)
Cellulitis (<1%)
Diaphoresis (>1%)
Ecchymoses (<1%)
Edema (<1%)
Exanthems (<1%)
Exfoliative dermatitis (<1%)
Herpes simplex (<1%)
Herpes zoster (<1%)
Petechiae (<1%)
Pruritus (1–10%)
Purpura (<1%)
Rash (sic) (1–10%)
Ulceration (>1%)
Urticaria (<1%)
Xerosis (<1%)

Hair
Hair – alopecia (<1%)

Other
Paresthesias (>1%)
Tremor (1–10%)
Vaginal candidiasis (<1%)
Xerostomia (49%)

TOBRAMYCIN

Trade names: Nebcin (Lilly); TOBI (Pathogenesis); TobraDex (Alcon)
Other common trade names: *AKTob Ophthalmic; Oftalmotrisol-T; Tobra*
Indications: Various serious infections caused by susceptible organisms, superficial ocular infections
Category: Aminoglycoside antibiotic
Half-life: 2–3 hours
Clinically important, potentially serious interactions with: aminoglycosides, amphotericin B, cephalosporins, furosemide, loop diuretics, neuromuscular blockers, penicillins, torsemide, vancomycin

TobraDex is tobramycin and dexamethasone

Reactions

Skin
Contact dermatitis (from ophthalmic preparations) (<1%)
(1998): Litt JZ, Beachwood, OH, personal case (observation)
(1995): Caraffini S+, *Contact Dermatitis* 32, 186
(1990): Menendez-Ramos F+, *Contact Dermatitis* 22, 305
Cutaneous side effects (sic)
(1976): Brogden RN+, *Drugs* 12, 166 (<1%)
Eczematous eruption (sic)
Erythema multiforme
(1983): Ansel J+, *Arch Dermatol* 119, 1006
Exanthems
(1991): Karp S+, *Cutis* 47, 331
(1976): Brogden RN+, *Drugs* 12, 166
Exfoliative dermatitis
(1991): Karp S+, *Cutis* 47, 331
Eyelid edema (from ophthalmic preparations) (<1%)
Pruritus (<1%)
(1976): Brogden RN+, *Drugs* 12, 166
Purpura
Rash (sic) (<1%)
Urticaria

Other
Hypersensitivity
(1995): Schretlen-Doherty JS+, *Ann Pharmacother* 29, 704
Injection-site pain
Paresthesias (<1%)
Sialorrhea
Tremor (<1%)

TOCAINIDE

Trade name: Tonocard (AstraZeneca)
Indications: Ventricular arrhythmias
Category: Antiarrhythmic class I B
Half-life: 11–14 hours
Clinically important, potentially serious interactions with: beta-blockers, caffeine, cimetidine, metoprolol, phenobarbital, phenytoin, rifampin, theophylline

Reactions

Skin
Clammy skin
Diaphoresis (<1%)
Erythema multiforme (<1%)
Exanthems
(1988): Dunn JM+, *Drug Intell Clin Pharm* 22, 142
Exfoliative dermatitis (<1%)
Lupus erythematosus (<1%)
(1994): Gelfand MS+, *South Med J* 87, 839
(1988): Oliphant LD+, *Chest* 94, 427
Pallor (<1%)
Pruritus (<1%)
Rash (sic) (0.5–8.4%)
Allergic reactions (sic)
(1987): Arrowsmith JB+, *Ann Intern Med* 107, 693
(1985): Coulter DM+, *N Z Med J* 98, 553
Stevens–Johnson syndrome (<1%)
Vasculitis (<1%)

Hair
Hair – alopecia (<1%)

Other
Dysgeusia (8.4%)
Gingival bleeding
(1988): Dunn JM+, *Drug Intell Clin Pharm* 22, 142
Hypersensitivity (<1%)
Myalgia (<1%)
Parosmia (<1%)
Paresthesias (3.5–9%)
Stomatitis (<1%)
Xerostomia (<1%)

TOLAZAMIDE

Trade name: Tolinase (Pharmacia & Upjohn)
Other common trade names: *Diabewas; Diadutos; Norglycin; Tolanase; Tolisan*
Indications: Non-insulin dependent diabetes type II
Category: First generation sulfonylurea* hypoglycemic
Half-life: 7 hours
Clinically important, potentially serious interactions with: alcohol, anticoagulants, beta-blockers, chloramphenicol, clofibrate, fluconazole, gemfibrozil, methyldopa, MAO inhibitors, phenylbutazones, probenecid, salicylates, sulfinpyrazone, sulfonamides, thiazides, tricyclic antidepressants

Reactions

Skin

Dermatitis (sic)
(1966): Beidleman P+, *J Fla Med Assoc* 53, 191
Diaphoresis
Eczematous eruption (sic)
(1985): Frosch PJ+, *Contact Dermatitis* 13, 272
Erythema (0.4%)
Exanthems (0.4%)
Lichenoid eruption
(1990): Franz CB+, *J Am Acad Dermatol* 22, 128
(1984): Barnett JH+, *Cutis* 34, 542
Lupus erythematosus
Photosensitivity (1–10%)
Pruritus (0.4%)
Purpura
Rash (sic) (1–10%)
Urticaria (1–10%)

Other

Acute intermittent porphyria
Dysgeusia
Paresthesias
Porphyria cutanea tarda
Tongue ulceration
(1984): Barnett JH+, *Cutis* 34, 542

***Note:** Tolazamide is a sulfonamide and can be absorbed systemically. Sulfonamides can produce severe, possibly fatal, reactions such as toxic epidermal necrolysis and Stevens–Johnson syndrome.

TOLAZOLINE

Trade name: Priscoline (Novartis)
Indications: Pulmonary hypertension in the newborn
Category: Alpha-adrenergic blocking agent; peripheral vasodilator antihypertensive (of the newborn)
Half-life: 3–10 hours (neonates)
Clinically important, potentially serious interactions with: disulfiram, dopamine, epinephrine

Reactions

Skin

Contact dermatitis
(1985): Frosch PJ+, *Contact Dermatitis* 13, 272
Edema
Exanthems
(1989); Cambazard F+, *Ann Dermatol Venereol* (French) 116, 499
Flushing
(1972): Coffman JD+, *Ann Intern Med* 76, 35 (66%)
Rash (sic)
Urticaria

Other

Injection-site burning (>10%)

TOLBUTAMIDE

Trade name: Orinase (Pharmacia & Upjohn)
Other common trade names: *Abemin; Aglycid; Diaben; Diatol; Dolipol; Mobenol; Novo-Butamid; Orabet; Rastinon*
Indications: Non-insulin dependent diabetes type II
Category: First generation sulfonylurea* hypoglycemic
Half-life: 4–25 hours
Clinically important, potentially serious interactions with: beta-blockers, chloramphenicol, clofibrate, dicumarol, fluconazole, gemfibrozil, MAO inhibitors, methyldopa, phenylbutazone, probenecid, salicylates, sulfinpyrazone, sulfonamides, tricyclic antidepressants

Reactions

Skin

Allergic reactions (sic)
(1965): Bernhard H, *Diabetes* 14, 59 (0.8%)
Bullous eruption (<1%)
Bullous pemphigoid
(1975): Glander HJ+, *Derm Monatsschr* (German) 161, 455
Contact dermatitis
(1982): Fisher AA, *Cutis* 29, 551 (systemic)
Cutaneous side effects (sic)
(1967): McKiddie MT+, *Scott Med J* 12, 6 (1.65%)
(1965): Ferguson BD, *Med Clin North Am* 49, 929 (0.35%)
(1959): O'Donovan CJ, *Curr Ther Res* 1, 69 (1.1%)
Erythema (1.1%)
Erythema multiforme (<1%)
Exanthems (1–5%)
(1972): Kuokkanen K, *Acta Allergol* 27, 407
(1971): Harris EL, *BMJ* 3, 29 (1–5%)
(1969): *Postgrad Med* 45, 211
Fixed eruption (<1%)
Flushing
(1981): Capretti L+, *BMJ* 283, 1361
(1966): Cohen P+, *JAMA* 197, 817
(1966): Muller SA, *Proc Staff Meet Mayo Clin* 41, 689
Lichenoid eruption
(1963): Hurlbut WB, *Arch Dermatol* 88, 105
Photoreactions
Photosensitivity (1–10%)
(1984): Kar PK+, *J Indian Med Assoc* 82, 289
(1978): Meneghini CL+, *Z Haut* (German) 53, 329
Poikiloderma
(1965): Esteves J+, *Hautarzt* (German) 16, 281
Pruritus (1.1%)
Purpura
(1965): Horowitz HI+, *Semin Hematol* 2, 287
(1959): Bradley RF, *Ann N Y Acad Sci* 82, 513
Rash (sic) (1–10%)
Toxic epidermal necrolysis (<1%)
Urticaria (1–10%)
(1960): Boshell BR, *N Engl J Med* 262, 80

Other

Acute intermittent porphyria
Disulfiram-type reaction
Dysgeusia
Hypersensitivity (<1%)
Injection-site thrombophlebitis (<1%)
Oral lichenoid eruption
Paresthesias
Porphyria
(1968): De Matteis F, *Semin Hematol* 5, 409
Porphyria cutanea tarda
(1960): Rook A+, *BMJ* 1, 860
Thrombophlebitis (<1%)

***Note:** Tolbutamide is a sulfonamide and can be absorbed systemically. Sulfonamides can produce severe, possibly fatal, reactions such as toxic epidermal necrolysis and Stevens–Johnson syndrome.

TOLCAPONE

Trade name: Tasmar (Roche)
Indications: Parkinsonism
Category: Antiparkinsonian adjunct
Half-life: 2–3 hours
Clinically important, potentially serious interactions with: MAO inhibitors

Reactions

Skin

Allergic reactions (sic) (<1%)
Burning (sic) (2%)
Cellulitis (<1%)
Diaphoresis (7%)
Eczema (sic) (<1%)
Edema (<1%)
Erythema multiforme (<1%)
Facial edema (<1%)
Fungal infection (sic) (<1%)
Furunculosis (<1%)
Herpes simplex (<1%)
Herpes zoster (<1%)
Pigmentation (<1%)
Pruritus (<1%)
Rash (sic) (<1%)
Seborrhea (<1%)
Tumor (sic) (1%)
Urticaria (<1%)

Hair

Hair – alopecia (1%)

Other

Hypesthesia (<1%)
Myalgia (<1%)
Oral ulceration (<1%)
Paresthesias (3%)
Parosmia (<1%)
Sialorrhea (<1%)
Tongue disorder (<1%)
Tooth disorder (<1%)
Twitching (<1%)
Vaginitis (<1%)
Xerostomia (5%)

TOLMETIN

Trade name: Tolectin (Ortho-McNeil)
Other common trade names: *Donison; Midocil; Novo-Tolmetin; Reutol; Safitex*
Indications: Arthritis
Category: Nonsteroidal anti-inflammatory (NSAID); analgesic
Half-life: 1–2 hours
Clinically important, potentially serious interactions with: aminoglycosides, anticoagulants, aspirin, cyclosporine, digoxin, diuretics, insulin, lithium, methotrexate, sulfonylureas

Reactions

Skin

Angioedema (<1%)
(1994): Shapiro N, *J Oral Maxillofac Surg* 52, 626
(1985): Ponte CD+, *Drug Intell Clin Pharm* 19, 479
Bullous eruption
Diaphoresis
Edema (3–9%)
Erythema multiforme (<1%)
Exanthems
(1985): Bigby M+, *J Am Acad Dermatol* 12, 866
(1984): Stern RS+, *JAMA* 252, 1433
(1981): Reimer GW, *S Afr Med J* 60, 843
(1977): Aylward M+, *Curr Res Med Opin* 4, 695 (9%)
Hot flashes (<1%)
Photodermatitis
(1993): Shelley WB+, *Cutis* 52, 201 (observation)
Pruritus (1–10%)
(1985): Bigby M+, *J Am Acad Dermatol* 12, 866
(1981): Reimer GW, *S Afr Med J* 60, 843
(1978): Restivo C+, *JAMA* 240, 246
Purpura
(1984): Stern RS+, *JAMA* 252, 1433
Rash (sic) (>10%)
Stevens–Johnson syndrome (<1%)
Toxic epidermal necrolysis (<1%)
(1992): Breathnach SM+, *Adverse Drug Reactions and the Skin*, Blackwell, Oxford, 191 (passim)
(1985): Bigby M+, *J Am Acad Dermatol* 12, 866
(1984): Stern RS+, *JAMA* 252, 1433
Urticaria (1–5%)
(1985): Bigby M+, *J Am Acad Dermatol* 12, 866
(1985): Ponte CD+, *Drug Intell Clin Pharm* 19, 479
(1984): Stern RS+, *JAMA* 252, 1433
(1980): Ahmad S, *N Engl J Med* 303, 1417
(1978): Restivo C+, *JAMA* 240, 246

Other

Anaphylactoid reaction
(1985): O'Brien WM, *J Rheumatol* 12, 13
(1985): Bretza JA+, *Western J Med* 143, 55
(1983): Paulus HE, *Arthritis Rheum* 26, 1397
(1982): Rossi AC+, *N Engl J Med* 307, 499
(1980): Ahmad S, *N Engl J Med* 303, 1417
(1980): McCall CY+, *JAMA* 243, 1263
(1978): Restivo C+, *JAMA* 240, 246
Aphthous stomatitis
Dysgeusia
Gingival ulceration
Glossitis (<1%)
Gynecomastia
Myalgia
Oral ulceration
Serum sickness (<1%)
Stomatitis (<1%)
Xerostomia

TOLTERODINE

Trade name: Detrol (Pharmacia & Upjohn)
Indications: Urinary incontinence
Category: Muscarinic antagonist for overactive bladder; anticholinergic
Half-life: 2–4 hours
Clinically important, potentially serious interactions with: azole antifungals, erythromycin, fluoxetine

Reactions

Skin

Erythema (1.9%)
Flu-like syndrome (sic) (4.4%)
Fungal infection (sic) (1.1%)
Pruritus (1.3%)
Rash (sic) (1.9%)
Upper respiratory infection (sic) (5.9%)
Xerosis (1.7%)

Other

Paresthesias (1.1%)
Xerostomia (40%)
(1999): Millard R+, *J Urol* 161, 1551
(1999): Ruscin JM+, *Ann Pharmacother* 33, 1073

(1999): Drutz HP+, *Int Urogynecol J Pelvic Floor Dysfunct* 10, 283
(1997): Jonas U+, *World J Urol* 15, 144 (9%)
(1997): Appell RA, *Urology* 50, 90

TOPIRAMATE

Trade name: Topamax (Ortho-McNeil)
Indications: Partial onset seizures
Category: Anticonvulsant
Half-life: 21 hours
Clinically important, potentially serious interactions with: acetazolamide, alcohol, carbamazepine, CNS depressants, digoxin, oral contraceptives, phenytoin, valproic acid

Reactions

Skin

Acne (>1%)
Basal cell carcinoma (<1%)
Dermatitis (sic) (<1%)
Diaphoresis (1.8%)
Eczema (sic) (<1%)
Edema (1.8%)
Exanthems (<1%)
Facial edema (<1%)
Flu-like syndrome (sic) (1–10%)
Flushing (<1%)
Folliculitis (<1%)
Hot flashes (1–10%)
Hypohidrosis (<1%)
Photosensitivity (<1%)
Pigmentation (<1%)
Pruritus (1.8%)
Purpura (<1%)
Rash (sic) (4.4%)
Seborrhea (<1%)
Urticaria (<1%)
Xerosis (<1%)

Hair

Hair – abnormal texture (<1%)
Hair – alopecia (>1%)

Nails

Nails – disorder (sic) (<1%)

Other

Ageusia (<1%)
Bromhidrosis (1.8%)
Dysgeusia (>1%)
Foetor ex ore (halitosis)
Gingival hyperplasia (<1%)
Gingivitis (1.8%)
Gynecomastia (8.3%)
Hyperesthesia (<1%)
Hypesthesia (2.7%)
Mastodynia (3–9%)
Myalgia (1.8%)
Paresthesias (15%)
(1999): Glauser TA, *Epilepsia* 40, S71
Parosmia (<1%)
Stomatitis (<1%)
Tongue edema (<1%)
Tremor (>10%)
Vaginitis
Xerostomia (2.7%)

TOPOTECAN

Synonyms: hycamptamine; SKF 104864; TOPO; TPT
Trade name: Hycamtin (SmithKline Beecham)
Indications: Metastatic ovarian carcinoma
Category: Antineoplastic antibiotic
Half-life: 3 hours
Clinically important, potentially serious interactions with: cisplatin, filgrastim, sargramostim

Reactions

Skin

Erythema (<1%)
Purpura (<1%)

Hair

Hair – alopecia (59%)
(1999): Ormrod D+, *Drugs* 58, 533

Other

Paresthesias (9%)
Stomatitis (24%)

TOREMIFENE

Trade name: Fareston (Schering)
Indications: Metastatic breast cancer
Category: Antineoplastic; antiestrogen
Half-life: ~5 days
Clinically important, potentially serious interactions with: erythromycin, ketoconazole, thiazides, warfarin

Reactions

Skin

Dermatitis (sic)
Diaphoresis (20%)
(1997): Wiseman LR+, *Drugs* 54, 141
(1990): Valavaara R+, *J Steroid Biochem* 36, 229
Edema (5%)
(1997): Wiseman LR+, *Drugs* 54, 141
Hot flashes (35%)
(1997): Wiseman LR+, *Drugs* 54, 141
Pigmentation
Pruritus

Other

Galactorrhea (1–10%)
Priapism (1–10%)
Thrombophlebitis (1%)
Vaginal discharge (13%)
(1997): Wiseman LR+, *Drugs* 54, 141

TORSEMIDE

Trade name: Demadex (Roche)
Other common trade name: *Unat*
Indications: Edema
Category: A sulfonylurea* loop diuretic; antihypertensive
Half-life: 2–4 hours
Clinically important, potentially serious interactions with: ACE-inhibitors, aminoglycosides, anticoagulants, beta-blockers, cisplatin, digoxin, lithium, NSAIDs, salicylates, sulfonylureas, thiazides

Reactions

Skin

Angioedema
Edema (1.1%)
Exanthems
Lichenoid eruption
(1997): Byrd DR+, *Mayo Clin Proc* 72, 930 (photosensitive)
Photosensitivity (1–10%)
Pruritus
Purpura
(1998): Sanfelix Genoves J+, *Aten Primaria* (Spanish) 21, 252
Rash (sic) (<1%)
Stevens–Johnson syndrome
(1997): Billon S, *The Schoch Letter* 47, 32 (observation)
Urticaria (1–10%)
Vasculitis
(1998): Sanfelix Genoves J+, *Aten Primaria* (Spanish) 21, 252
(1998): Palop-Larrea V+, *Lancet* 352, 1909

Other

Injection-site erythema (<1%)
Myalgia (1.6%)
Xerostomia

***Note:** Torsemide is a sulfonamide and can be absorbed systemically. Sulfonamides can produce severe, possibly fatal, reactions such as toxic epidermal necrolysis and Stevens–Johnson syndrome.

TRAMADOL

Trade name: Ultram (Ortho-McNeil)
Other common trade names: *Contramal; Tadol; Tradol; Tramal; Tramed; Tramol; Tridol; Zipan*
Indications: Pain
Category: Centrally-acting synthetic analgesic
Half-life: 6–7 hours
Clinically important, potentially serious interactions with: alcohol, carbamazepine, cimetidine, CNS depressants, MAO inhibitors, quinidine, ritonavir, tricyclic antidepressants

Reactions

Skin

Allergic reactions (sic) (<1%)
Angioedema
(1996): Kind B+, *Schweiz Med Wochenschr* (German) 85, 567
Diaphoresis (9%)
Exanthems
(1999): Ghislain PD+, *Ann Dermatol Venereol* (French) 126, 38
Pruritus (10%)
(1999): Ghislain PD+, *Ann Dermatol Venereol* (French) 126, 38
Rash (sic) (1–5%)
Toxic dermatitis (sic)
(1999): Ghislain PD+, *Ann Dermatol Venereol* (French) 126, 38
Urticaria (<1%)

Other

Anaphylactoid reaction
(1999): Moore PA, *J Am Dent Assoc* 130, 1075
Dysgeusia (<1%)
Paresthesias (<1%)
Stomatitis
Tremor (5–10%)
Xerostomia (10%)

TRANDOLAPRIL

Trade names: Mavik (Knoll); Tarka (Knoll)
Other common trade names: *Gopten; Odrik; Udrik*
Indications: Hypertension
Category: Angiotensin-converting enzyme (ACE) inhibitor, calcium channel blocker (with verapamil); antihypertensive
Half-life: 24 hours
Clinically important, potentially serious interactions with: alcohol, allopurinol, beta-blockers, bumetanide, carbamazepine, cyclosporine, digoxin, diuretics, fentanyl, lithium, mercaptopurine, quinidine, salicylates, theophylline

Tarka is trandolapril and verapamil

Reactions

Skin

Angioedema (0.15%)
(1996): *Med Lett Drugs Ther* 38, 104
Edema (>3%)
Flushing (>3%)
Pemphigus (<1%)
Pruritus (>3%)
Rash (sic) (>10%)

Other

Hypesthesia (>3%)
Myalgia (>3%)
Paresthesias (>3%)
Xerostomia (>3%)

TRANYLCYPROMINE

Trade name: Parnate (SmithKline Beecham)
Other common trade name: *Siciton*
Indications: Depression
Category: Monoamine oxidase (MAO) inhibitor; antidepressant and antimanic
Half-life: 2.5 hours
Clinically important, potentially serious interactions with: amphetamines, barbiturates, caffeine, CNS depressants, dextroamphetamine, disulfiram, fluoxetine, fluvoxamine, levodopa, meperidine, nefazodone, paroxetine, phenothiazines, reserpine, sertraline, sumatriptan, sympathomimetics, trazodone, tricyclic antidepressants, venlafaxine, **tyramine-containing foods***

Reactions

Skin

Diaphoresis
(1963): Adams PH+, *Lancet* 2, 692
Edema (<1%)
Exanthems
Flushing
(1963): Adams PH+, *Lancet* 2, 692
Peripheral edema
Photosensitivity (<1%)
Pruritus
Rash (sic) (<1%)
Urticaria

Other

Acute intermittent porphyria
(1963): Adams PH+, *Lancet* 2, 692
Black tongue
Paresthesias
Priapism
Tremor
Twitching
Xerostomia (<1%)

***Note:** Tyramine-containing foods include the following: aged cheeses, avocados, banana skins, bologna and other processed luncheon meats, chicken livers, chocolate, figs, canned pickled herring, meat extracts, pepperoni, raisins, raspberries, soy sauce, vermouth, sherry and red wines.

TRAZODONE

Trade name: Desyrel (Apothecon)
Other common trade names: *Alti-Trazodone; Bimaran; Deprax; Desirel; Molipaxin; Sideril; Taxagon; Trazalon*
Indications: Depression
Category: Heterocyclic antidepressant and antineuralgic
Half-life: 3–6 hours
Clinically important, potentially serious interactions with: alcohol, CNS depressants, digoxin, fluoxetine, fluvoxamine, MAO inhibitors, paroxetine, phenytoin, sertraline, tricyclic antidepressants, venlafaxine

Reactions

Skin

Diaphoresis (>1%)
Edema (1–10%)
Erythema multiforme
(1985): Ford HE+, *J Clin Psychiatry* 46, 294
Exanthems
(1988): Warnock JK+, *Am J Psychiatry* 145, 425
(1986): Rongioletti F+, *J Am Acad Dermatol* 14, 274
(1984): Cohen LE, *J Am Acad Dermatol* 11, 526
(1984): Cohen LE, *J Am Acad Dermatol* 10, 303
(1980): Al-Yassiri MM+, *Neuropharmacology* 19, 1191
(1979): Trapp GA+, *Psychopharmacol Bull* 15, 25
Exfoliative dermatitis
(1983): Chu AG+, *Ann Intern Med* 99, 128
Photosensitivity
(1994): Berger TG+, *Arch Dermatol* 130, 609 (in HIV-infected)
(1986): Rongioletti F+, *J Am Acad Dermatol* 14, 274
Pruritus (<1%)
Psoriasis (exacerbation)
(1992): Breathnach SM+, *Adverse Drug Reactions and the Skin*, Blackwell, Oxford, 197 (passim)
(1986): Barth JH+, *Br J Dermatol* 115, 629 (generalized and pustular)
Purpura
Rash (sic) (<1%)
(1985): Longstreth GF+, *J Am Acad Dermatol* 13, 149
Urticaria
(1988): Warnock JK+, *Am J Psychiatry* 145, 425
(1984): Cohen LE, *J Am Acad Dermatol* 10, 303
(1983): Fabre LF+, *J Clin Psychiatry* 44, 17
Vasculitis
(1984): Mann SC+, *J Am Acad Dermatol* 10, 669

Hair

Hair – alopecia
(2000): Mercke Y+, *Ann Clin Psychiatry* 12, 35
(1988): Warnock JK+, *Am J Psychiatry* 145, 425

Nails

Nails – leukonychia
(1985): Longstreth GF+, *J Am Acad Dermatol* 13, 149

Other

Dysgeusia (>10%)
Formication
(1987): Peabody CA, *J Clin Psychiatry* 48, 385
Hypersensitivity
Galactorrhea
Gynecomastia
Myalgia (1–10%)
Paresthesias (>1%)
Priapism (<1%)
(1998): Myrick H+, *Ann Clin Psychiatry* 10, 81
(1994): Thavundayil JX+, *Neuropsychobiology* 30, 4
(1993): Pescatori ES+, *J Urol* 149, 1557
Sialorrhea
Tremor (1–10%)
Xerostomia (>10%)
(1982): Rawls WN, *Drug Intell Clin Pharm* 16, 7

TRIAMTERENE

Trade names: Dyazide (SmithKline Beecham); Dyrenium (SmithKline Beecham); Maxzide (Bertek)
Other common trade names: *Amterene; Diarrol; Diuteren; Dytac; Reviten; Suloton; Trian*
Indications: Edema
Category: Potassium-sparing diuretic; antihypertensive
Half-life: 1–2 hours
Clinically important, potentially serious interactions with: ACE-inhibitors, amantadine, amiloride, diclofenac, ibuprofen, indomethacin, spironolactone

Dyazide is triamterene and hydrochlorothiazide*; Maxzide is triamterene and hydrochlorothiazide*

Reactions

Skin

Chills
Diaphoresis
(1979): Fan WJ+, *Pediatrics* 64, 698
Edema (1–10%)
Exanthems
Flushing (<1%)
Lupus erythematosus (in combination with hydrochlorothiazide)
(1991): Wollenberg A+, *Hautarzt* (German) 42, 709
(1988): Darken M+, *J Am Acad Dermatol* 18, 38
Perleche
Photosensitivity
(1989): Rosen C, *Semin Dermatol* 8, 149
(1987): Fernandez de Corres L+, *Contact Dermatitis* 17, 114
Pruritus
Purpura
Rash (sic) (1–10%)
Urticaria
Vasculitis

Other

Anaphylactoid reaction
Dysgeusia
(1999): Sorkin M, Denver, CO (from Internet) (observation)
Glossitis
Gynecomastia (<1%)
Paresthesias
Pseudoporphyria
(1990): Motley RJ, *BMJ* 300, 1468
Stomatodynia
(1999): Sorkin M, Denver, CO (from Internet) (observation)
Xerostomia
(1987): Fernandez de Corres L+, *Contact Dermatitis* 17, 114

***Note:** Hydrochlorothiazide is a sulfonamide and can be absorbed systemically. Sulfonamides can produce severe, possibly fatal, reactions such as toxic epidermal necrolysis and Stevens–Johnson syndrome.

TRIAZOLAM

Trade name: Halcion (Pharmacia & Upjohn)
Other common trade names: *Dumozolam; Novo-Triolam; Nuctane; Nu-Triazo; Somese; Somniton; Songar; Trialam*
Indications: Insomnia
Category: Benzodiazepine sedative-hypnotic
Half-life: 1.5–5.5 hours
Clinically important, potentially serious interactions with: alcohol, amprenavir, carbamazepine, CNS depressants, cimetidine, clarithromycin, diltiazem, erythromycin, nefazodone, nelfinavir, rifabutin, rifampin, ritonavir, verapamil, **grapefruit juice**

Reactions

Skin

Dermatitis (sic) (1–10%)
(1984): Greenblatt DJ+, *J Clin Psychiatry* 45, 192
Diaphoresis (>10%)
(1983): Kroboth PD+, *Drug Intell Clin Pharm* 17, 495
(1979): van der Kroef C, *Lancet* 2, 526
Exanthems
Photosensitivity
(1984): Hussar DA, *Am Drug* 190, 109
Pruritus
(1983): Poeldinger W+, *Neuropsychobiology* 9, 135
(1981): Cobden I+, *Postgrad Med J* 57, 730
Purpura
Rash (sic) (>10%)
(1985): Jerram TC, *Side Effects Drugs Annu* 9, 39
Urticaria

Hair

Hair – alopecia
Hair – hirsutism

Other

Dysesthesia (<1%)
Dysgeusia (<1%)
(1979): van der Kroef C, *Lancet* 2, 526
(1978): Fabre LF Jr+, *J Clin Psychiatry* 39, 679
Gingivitis
Glossitis (<1%)
Glossodynia (<1%)
Paresthesias (<1%)
(1979): van der Kroef C, *Lancet* 2, 526
Sialopenia (>10%)
(1995): Loesche WJ+, *J Am Geriatr Soc* 43, 401
Sialorrhea (1–10%)
Stomatitis (<1%)
Tremor (1–10%)
Xerostomia (>10%)
(1995): Loesche WJ+, *J Am Geriatr Soc* 43, 401
(1986): Hughes RRL+, *Br J Clin Pract* 40, 279
(1984): Greenblatt DJ+, *J Clin Psychiatry* 45, 192
(1983): Cohn JB, *J Clin Psychiatry* 44, 401

TRICHLORMETHIAZIDE

Trade names: Metahydrin (Aventis); Naqua (Schering)
Other common trade names: *Anatran; Aquacot; Carvacron; Diurese; Doqua; Esmarin; Flute; Iopran; Niazide; Trichlon; Trichlorex*
Indications: Edema, hypertension
Category: Thiazide* diuretic; antihypertensive
Half-life: no data
Clinically important, potentially serious interactions with: allopurinol, amphotericin B, antidiabetics, calcium, diazoxide, digoxin, furosemide, lithium, loop diuretics, methotrexate, methyldopa

Reactions

Skin

Exanthems
Lichenoid eruption (<1%)
Lupus erythematosus
(1978): Pereyo-Torellas N, *Arch Dermatol* 114, 1097
Photosensitivity (<1%)
Purpura
(1962): Loftus LR+, *JAMA* 180, 410
Rash (sic)
Urticaria
Vasculitis
(1962): Loftus LR+, *JAMA* 180, 410

Other

Anaphylactoid reaction
Paresthesias
Xerostomia

***Note:** Trichlormethiazide is a sulfonamide and can be absorbed systemically. Sulfonamides can produce severe, possibly fatal, reactions such as toxic epidermal necrolysis and Stevens–Johnson syndrome.

TRIENTINE

Trade name: Syprine (Merck)
Indications: Wilson's disease
Category: Chelating agent; antidote (copper toxicity)
Half-life: no data
Clinically important, potentially serious interactions with: iron

Reactions

Skin

Dermatitis (sic)
(1980): Rudzki E, *Contact Dermatitis* 6, 235
Desquamation
Lupus erythematosus (<1%)
Thickening (sic) (<1%)

Other

Aphthous stomatitis
Oral mucosal lesions

TRIFLUOPERAZINE

Trade name: Stelazine (SmithKline Beecham)
Other common trade names: *Calmazine; Domilium; Flupazine; Fluzine; Nerolet; Psyrazine; Sedizine; Tfp*
Indications: Psychoses, anxiety
Category: Phenothiazine tranquilizer; anxiolytic; antipsychotic
Half-life: 10–20 hours
Clinically important, potentially serious interactions with: alcohol, barbiturates, chloroquine, CNS depressants, levodopa, lithium, MAO inhibitors, piperazine, propranolol, trazodone, tricyclic antidepressants, **cigarette smoking**

Reactions

Skin

- Angioedema
  - (1974): Panikarskii VG, *Vrach Delo* (Russian) February, 118
- Contact dermatitis
- Diaphoresis
- Eczema (sic)
- Erythema
- Exanthems
- Exfoliative dermatitis
- Fixed eruption
  - (1987): Kanwar AJ+, *Br J Dermatol* 117, 798
- Hypohidrosis
- Lupus erythematosus
- Parkinsonism (>10%)
- Peripheral edema
- Photosensitivity (1–10%)
  - (1970): *Med Lett* 12, 104
- Pigmentation (blue-gray) (<1%)
  - (1994): Buckley C+, *Clin Exp Dermatol* 19, 149
- Pruritus
- Purpura
- Rash (sic) (1–10%)
- Seborrhea
- Urticaria
- Xerosis

Other

- Anaphylactoid reaction
- Galactorrhea (<1%)
- Gynecomastia
- Mastodynia (1–10%)
- Oral mucosal eruption
  - (1988): Ward DF+, *Postgrad Med* 84, 99
- Priapism (<1%)
- Tongue edema
  - (1988): Ward DF+, *Postgrad Med* 84, 99
- Tremor
- Xerostomia

TRIHEXYPHENIDYL

Trade name: Artane (Lederle)
Other common trade names: *Acamed; Aparkane; Bentex; Hexinal; Hipokinon; Parkines; Partane; Tridyl; Trihexy; Trihexyphen*
Indications: Parkinsonism
Category: Antidyskinetic; antiparkinsonian; anticholinergic
Half-life: 3–4 hours
Clinically important, potentially serious interactions with: amantadine, anticholinergics, digoxin, haloperidol, levodopa, phenothiazines, quinidine, rimantadine, tacrine, tricyclic antidepressants

Reactions

Skin

- Chills
- Diaphoresis
- Flushing
- Hypohidrosis (>10%)
- Photosensitivity (1–10%)
- Rash (sic) (<1%)
- Spider angiomas
  - (1953): Holt CL, *N Engl J Med* 249, 318
- Urticaria
- Xerosis (>10%)

Other

- Glossitis
- Glossodynia
- Paresthesias
- Xerostomia (30–50%)

TRIMEPRAZINE

Trade name: Temaril (Allergan)
Other common trade names: *Nedeltran; Panectyl; Theralene; Vallergan; Variargil*
Indications: Pruritus, urticaria
Category: Phenothiazine H_1-receptor antihistamine and sedative-hypnotic
Duration of action: 3–6 hours
Clinically important, potentially serious interactions with: alcohol, CNS depressants, MAO inhibitors, oral contraceptives, progesterone, reserpine

Reactions

Skin

- Angioedema (<1%)
  - (1959): Wright W, *JAMA* 171, 1642
- Dermatitis (sic)
- Diaphoresis
- Edema (<1%)
- Exanthems
  - (1959): Wright W, *JAMA* 171, 1642
- Lupus erythematosus
- Peripheral edema
- Photosensitivity (<1%)
- Pruritus
  - (1959): Wright W, *JAMA* 171, 1642
- Purpura
- Rash (sic) (<1%)
- Urticaria

Other

- Anaphylactoid reaction
- Gynecomastia
- Myalgia (<1%)
- Paresthesias (<1%)

Stomatitis
Xerostomia (1–10%)
(1992): Chambers FA+, *Anaesthesia* 47, 585

TRIMETHADIONE

Trade name: Tridione (Abbott)
Other common trade name: *Mino Aleviatin*
Category: Anticonvulsant
Half-life: no data
Clinically important, potentially serious interactions with: phenytoin, valproic acid

Reactions

Skin

Acne
Bullous eruption
Erythema multiforme
(1992): Breathnach SM+, *Adverse Drug Reactions and the Skin*, Blackwell, Oxford, 210 (passim)
(1972): Levantine A+, *Br J Dermatol* 87, 646
(1961): Rallison ML+, *Am J Dis Child* 101, 725
(1948): Kevin JC, *Lancet* 1, 267
Exanthems
(1972): Levantine A+, *Br J Dermatol* 87, 646
(1962): LeVan P+, *Arch Dermatol* 86, 254
(1948): Kevin JC, *Lancet* 1, 267
Exfoliative dermatitis
(1992): Breathnach SM+, *Adverse Drug Reactions and the Skin*, Blackwell, Oxford, 210 (passim)
(1948): Kevin JC, *Lancet* 1, 267
Fixed eruption
Lupus erythematosus
(1993): Drory VE+, *Clin Neuropharmacol* 16, 19
(1976): Singsen BH+, *Pediatrics* 57, 529
(1973): Beernink DH+, *J Pediatr* 82, 113
(1962): LeVan P+, *Arch Dermatol* 86, 254
(1961): Rallison ML+, *Am J Dis Child* 101, 725
Petechiae
Photosensitivity
(1962): LeVan P+, *Arch Dermatol* 86, 254
Pruritus
(1961): Weingartner L, *Monatsschr Kinderheilkd* (German) 109, 517
Purpura
(1956): Wintrobe MM+, *Arch Intern Med* 98, 559
Stevens–Johnson syndrome
(1961): Rallison ML+, *Am J Dis Child* 101, 725
Urticaria
(1992): Breathnach SM+, *Adverse Drug Reactions and the Skin*, Blackwell, Oxford, 210 (passim)
(1964): Beall GN, *Medicine* (Baltimore) 43, 131
(1948): Kevin JC, *Lancet* 1, 267
Vasculitis
(1993): Drory VE+, *Clin Neuropharmacol* 16, 19
(1986): Hannedouche T+, *Ann Med Interne Paris* (French) 137, 57

Hair

Hair – alopecia
(1960): Holowach J+, *N Engl J Med* 263, 1187

Other

Acute intermittent porphyria
Gingivitis
Paresthesias

TRIMETHOBENZAMIDE

Trade names: Arrestin; Benzacot; Bio-Gan; Navogan; Stemetic; Tebamide; T-Gene; Tegamide; Ticon; Tigan (Roberts); Triban; Tribenzagen; Trimazide. (Various pharmaceutical companies.)
Other common trade names: *Anaus; Elen; Ibikin*
Indications: Prevention and treatment of nausea and vomiting
Category: Antiemetic
Half-life: no data
Clinically important, potentially serious interactions with: oral anticoagulants

Reactions

Skin

Parkinsonism
Allergic reactions (sic) (<1%)

Other

Hypersensitivity (<1%)
Injection-site reactions

TRIMETHOPRIM*

Trade names: Bactrim (Roche): Septra (Monarch)
Other common trade names: *Abaprim; Alprim; Bactin; Idotrim; Ipral; Lidaprim; Methoprim; Monotrim; Primosept; Syraprim; Tiempe; Triprim; Unitrim; Wellcprim*
Indications: Various urinary tract infections caused by susceptible organisms
Category: Antibiotic
Half-life: 8–10 hours
Clinically important, potentially serious interactions with: amantadine, cyclosporine, dapsone, digoxin, methotrexate, phenytoin, procainamide, pyrimethamine, rifampin, triamterene, trimetrexate, valproic acid, warfarin

Reactions

Skin

Erythema multiforme
Erythema nodosum
(1983): *Ugeskr Laeger* (Danish) 145, 1070
Exanthems
Exfoliative dermatitis (<1%)
Photosensitivity
Pruritus (1–10%)
Rash (sic) (2.9–6.7%)
Stevens–Johnson syndrome
Toxic epidermal necrolysis

Other

Anaphylactoid reactions
Dysgeusia
Glossitis

***Note:** Although trimethoprim has been known to elicit occasional adverse reactions by itself, it is most commonly used in conjunction with sulfamethoxazole (co-trimoxazole). The trade names for this combination are: Bactrim; Cotrim; Septra. Please see co-trimoxazole for the specific reaction patterns and references.

TRIMETREXATE

Trade name: Neutrexin (US Bioscience)
Indications: *Pneumocystis carinii* pneumonia; antiprotozoal
Category: Antineoplastic, folate antagonist
Half-life: 15–17 hours
Clinically important, potentially serious interactions with: acetaminophen, cimetidine, erythromycin, fluconazole, ketoconazole, miconazole, rifabutin, rifampin, zidovudine

Reactions

Skin

Angioedema
(1990): Grem JL+, *Drugs* 8, 211
Exanthems
(1987): Leiby J+, *Invest New Drugs* 5, 136
Fixed eruption
Flu-like syndrome (sic) (1–10%)
Flushing
(1990): Grem JL+, *Drugs* 8, 211
Photosensitivity
Pruritus (5.5%)
(1990): Grem JL+, *Drugs* 8, 211
Rash (1–10%)

Other

Hypersensitivity (1–10%)
Oral mucosal lesions
(1987): Leiby J+, *Invest New Drugs* 5, 136
Stomatitis (1–10%)

TRIMIPRAMINE

Trade name: Surmontil (Wyeth-Ayerst)
Other common trade names: *Apo-Trimip; Rhotrimine; Stangyl; Sumontil*
Indications: Major depression
Category: Tricyclic antidepressant, antineuralgic and antiulcer
Half-life: 20–26 hours
Clinically important, potentially serious interactions with: alcohol, amphetamines, anticholinergics, CNS depressants, cimetidine, clonidine, epinephrine, guanethidine, MAO inhibitors, methylphenidate, phenothiazines, quinidine, SSRIs, warfarin, **grapefruit juice**

Reactions

Skin

Allergic reactions (sic) (<1%)
Diaphoresis (1–10%)
Exanthems
Parkinsonism (1–10%)
Petechiae
Photosensitivity (<1%)
Pruritus
Purpura
Rash (sic)
Urticaria

Hair

Hair – alopecia (<1%)

Other

Dysgeusia (>10%)
Galactorrhea (<1%)
Glossitis
Gynecomastia (<1%)
Paresthesias
Stomatitis
Tremor
Xerostomia (>10%)

TRIOXSALEN

Trade name: Trisoralen (ICN)
Other common trade names: *Neosoralen; Puvadin*
Indications: Vitiligo, hypopigmentation
Category: Repigmenting agent and antipsoriatic; psoralen
Half-life: ~2 hours
Clinically important, potentially serious interactions with: sulfonamides, tetracyclines

Reactions

Skin

Acne
(1978): Nielsen EB+, *Acta Derm Venereol* (Stockh) 58, 374
Bullous eruption (with UVA)
(1999): Chuan MT+, *J Formos Med Assoc* 98, 335
(1979): Abel EA+, *Arch Dermatol* 115, 988
(1977): Melski JW+, *J Invest Dermatol* 68, 328
(1976): Thomsen K+, *Br J Dermatol* 95, 568
Eczematous eruption (sic)
(1979): Saihan EM, *BMJ* 2, 20
Freckles
(1984): Kietzmann E+, *Dermatologica* 168, 306
(1983): Kanerva L+, *Dermatologica* 166, 281
Granuloma annulare
(1979): Dorval JC+, *Ann Dermatol Venereol* (French) 106, 79
Herpes simplex
(1982): Stüttgen G, *Int J Dermatol* 21, 198
Herpes zoster
(1982): Stüttgen G, *Int J Dermatol* 21, 198
(1977): Roenigk HH+, *Arch Dermatol* 113, 1667
Lupus erythematosus
(1985): Bruze M+, *Acta Derm Venereol* (Stockh) 65, 31
Melanoma
(1980): Forrest JB+, *J Surg Oncol* 13, 337
Pemphigoid
(1978): Robinson JK, *Br J Dermatol* 99, 709
Photoreactions
(1978): Plewig G+, *Arch Derm Res* 261, 201
(1977): Ljunggren B, *Contact Dermatitis* 3, 85
Photosensitivity
(1976): Jonelis FJ+, *Arch Dermatol* 112, 1036
Phototoxic reaction
(1992): George SA+, *Br J Dermatol* 127, 444
(1979): Fischer T+, *Acta Derm Venereol* (Stockh) 59, 171
Pigmentation
(1989): Weiss E+, *Int J Dermatol* 28, 188
(1987): Bruce DR+, *J Am Acad Dermatol* 16, 1087
(1986): MacDonald KJS+, *Br J Dermatol* 114, 395
Porokeratosis (actinic)
(1988): Beiteke U+, *Photodermatology* 5, 274
(1985): Hazen PG+, *J Am Acad Dermatol* 12, 1077
(1980): Reymond JL, *Acta Derm Venereol* (Stockh) 60, 539
Pruritus (>10%)
(1999): Chuan MT+, *J Formos Med Assoc* 98, 335
Scleroderma
(1976): Duperrat B+, *Bull Soc Franc Dermatol Syphiligr* (French) 83, 79
Seborrheic dermatitis
(1983): Tegner E, *Acta Derm Venereol* (Stockh) Suppl 107, 5
Skin pain (sic)
(1987): Norris PG+, *Clin Exp Dermatol* 12, 403
(1983): Tegner E, *Acta Derm Venereol* (Stockh) Suppl 107, 5
Tumors (sic)
(1995): Halder RM+, *Arch Dermatol* 131, 734
(1989): Hannuksela M+, *J Am Acad Dermatol* 21, 813
(1988): Gupta AK+, *J Am Acad Dermatol* 19, 67
(1987): Henseler T+, *J Am Acad Dermatol* 16, 108
(1986): Kahn JR+, *Clin Exp Dermatol* 11, 398
Vasculitis
(1981): Barriere H+, *Presse Med* (French) 10, 37
Vitiligo
(1983): Tegner E, *Acta Derm Venereol* (Stockh) Suppl 107, 5
(1976): Duperrat B+, *Bull Soc Franc Dermatol Syphiligr* (French) 83, 79

Xerosis
(1999): Chuan MT+, *J Formos Med Assoc* 98, 335

Hair

Hair – hypertrichosis
(1983): Rampen FHJ, *Br J Dermatol* 109, 657
(1967): Singh G+, *Br J Dermatol* 79, 501

Nails

Nails – photo-onycholysis
(1987): Baran R+, *J Am Acad Dermatol* 17, 1012
Nails – pigmentation
(1990): Trattner A+, *Int J Dermatol* 29, 310
(1989): Weiss E+, *Int J Dermatol* 28, 188
(1986): MacDonald KJS+, *Br J Dermatol* 114, 395
(1982): Naik RPC+, *Int J Dermatol* 21, 275

Other

Lymphoproliferative disease
(1989): Aschinoff R+, *J Am Acad Dermatol* 21, 1134

TRIPELENNAMINE

Trade name: PBZ (Novartis)
Other common trade names: *Azaron; Pyribenzamine; Triplen*
Indications: Allergic rhinitis, urticaria
Category: H_1-receptor blocker; antihistamine
Half-life: no data
Clinically important, potentially serious interactions with: alcohol, CNS depressants, MAO inhibitors

Reactions

Skin

Angioedema (<1%)
(1951): Guiducci A+, *Arch Dermatol* 63, 263
Diaphoresis
Edema (<1%)
Fixed eruption
(1961): Welsh AL+, *Arch Dermatol* 84, 1004
Flushing
Lichenoid eruption
(1947): Epstein E, *JAMA* 134, 782
Lupus erythematosus
Peripheral edema
Photosensitivity (<1%)
Pityriasis rosea
(1947): Epstein E, *JAMA* 134, 782
Purpura
(1956): Wintrobe MM+, *Arch Intern Med* 98, 559
(1951): Uvitsky IH, *J Allergy* 22, 544
Rash (sic) (<1%)
Systemic eczematous contact dermatitis
Urticaria
(1949): London ID, *J Invest Dermatol* 13, 317

Other

Anaphylactoid reaction
Myalgia (<1%)
Paresthesias (<1%)
Stomatitis
Tremor (<1%)
Xerostomia (1–10%)

TRIPROLIDINE

Trade names: Actagen; Actidil; Actifed; Allerphed; Cenafed; Genac; Myidil; Trifed; Triofed; Triposed. (Various pharmaceutical companies.)*
Other common trade name: *Actidilon*
Indications: Allergic rhinitis
Category: H_1-receptor antihistamine; sympathomimetic
Half-life: no data
Clinically important, potentially serious interactions with: alcohol, CNS depressants, MAO inhibitors, sympathomimetics

Reactions

Skin

Angioedema (<1%)
Diaphoresis (1–10%)
Edema (<1%)
Exanthems
Fixed eruption
(1968): Brownstein MH, *Arch Dermatol* 97, 115
Flushing
Lichenoid eruption
(1964): Alexander S, *BMJ* 2, 512
Photosensitivity (<1%)
Purpura
Rash (sic) (<1%)
Urticaria

Other

Myalgia (<1%)
Paresthesias (<1%)
Xerostomia (1–10%)

***Note:** Most of the trade name drugs contain pseudoephedrine as well

TROGLITAZONE*

Trade name: Rezulin (Parke-Davis)
Indications: Type 2 diabetes
Category: Oral antihyperglycemic (antidiabetic)
Half-life: 16–34 hours
Clinically important, potentially serious interactions with: cholestyramine, cyclosporine, HMG-CoA reductase inhibitors, oral contraceptives, tacrolimus, terfenadine

Reactions

Skin

Edema
(1999): Bando Y+, *J Int Med Res* 27, 53
Peripheral edema (5%)

Other

Rhabdomyolysis
(2000): Yokomaya M+, *Diabetes Care* 23, 421

***Note:** Troglitazone was withdrawn from the USA market on March 21, 2000

TROLEANDOMYCIN

Trade name: TAO (Pfizer)
Indications: Various infections caused by susceptible organisms
Category: Macrolide antibiotic
Half-life: no data
Clinically important, potentially serious interactions with: astemizole, carbamazepine, cisapride, cyclosporine, ergot alkaloids, oral contraceptives, pimozide, terfenadine, theophylline, triazolam

Reactions

Skin

Angioedema
(1971): *Med Lett* 13, 55
Erythema multiforme
Exanthems
(1961): Saslaw S, *Med Clin North Am* 45, 839
(1960): Welsh AL+, *Antibiotic Med Clin Ther* 7, 179
Pruritus
(1971): *Med Lett* 13, 55
Rash (sic) (1–10%)
Urticaria (1–10%)
(1971): *Med Lett* 13, 55

Other

Anaphylactoid reaction
Oral mucosal lesions
(1971): *Med Lett* 13, 55

TROVAFLOXACIN*

Trade name: Trovan (Pfizer)
Indications: Various infections caused by susceptible organisms
Category: 4th generation fluoroquinolone antibiotic
Half-life: 9.5 hours
Clinically important, potentially serious interactions with: antacids, iron, morphine, sucralfate, **dairy products**

Reactions

Skin

Acne
Allergic reactions (sic) (<1%)
Angioedema (<1%)
Balanoposthitis (<1%)
Candidiasis (<1%)
Cheilitis (<1%)
Dermatitis (sic) (<1%)
Diaphoresis (<1%)
Edema (<1%)
Erythema multiforme
Exanthems
(1999): Litt JZ, Beachwood, OH, personal case (observation)
Exfoliation (<1%)
Facial edema (<1%)
Flushing (<1%)
Lichen planus
(1999): Smith KC, Niagara Falls, NY (from Internet) (observation)
Periorbital edema (<1%)
Peripheral edema (<1%)
Photosensitivity (0.03%)
(2000): Ferguson J+, *J Antimicrob Chemother* 45, 503
Phototoxic reaction
(2000): Traynor NJ+, *Toxicol Vitr* 14, 275
Pruritus (2%)
(1999): Litt JZ, Beachwood, OH, personal case (observation)
(1998): Mayne JT+, *J Antimicrob Chemother* 39, 67
Pruritus ani (<1%)
Rash (sic) (2%)
Seborrhea (<1%)
Stevens–Johnson syndrome (<1%)
Toxic epidermal necrolysis
(1999): Matthews MR+, *Arch Intern Med* 159, 2225
Ulceration (<1%)
Urticaria (<1%)
Vasculitis

Other

Anaphylactoid reaction (<1%)
Dysgeusia (<1%)
Foetor ex ore (halitosis) (<1%)
Hypersensitivity
Injection-site edema (<1%)
Injection-site inflammation (<1%)
Injection-site pain (<1%)
Gingivitis (<1%)
Myalgia (<1%)
Paresthesias (<1%)
Serum sickness
Sialorrhea (<1%)
Stomatitis (<1%)
Tendon rupture
Thrombophlebitis (<1%)
Tongue disorder (<1%)
Tongue edema (<1%)
Vaginitis (<10%)
Xerostomia (<1%)

***Note:** Trovafloxacin has been withdrawn in the USA except for intravenous hospital use.

UROKINASE

Trade name: Abbokinase (Abbott)
Other common trade name: *Ukidan*
Indications: Acute myocardial infarction; coronary artery thrombosis; pulmonary embolism
Category: Thrombolytic enzyme
Half-life: 10–20 minutes
Clinically important, potentially serious interactions with: anticoagulants, antiplatelet drugs, aspirin, dextran, indomethacin

Reactions

Skin
Angioedema (>10%)
Bleeding (44%)
Bullous eruption (hemorrhagic)
(1995): Ejaz AA+, *Am J Nephrol* 15, 178
Chills
Diaphoresis (<1%)
Ecchymoses
Exanthems
Flushing
Periorbital edema (>10%)
Pruritus
Purpura
Rash (sic) (<1%)
Urticaria

Other
Anaphylactoid reaction (>10%)
Injection-site phlebitis

URSODIOL

Trade names: Actigall (Novartis); Urso (Axcan; Schwarz)
Other common trade names: *Arsacol; Cholit-Ursan; Destolit; Litanin; Urso; Ursochol; Ursolvan*
Indications: Cholelithiasis
Category: Gallstone dissolution agent
Half-life: 100 hours
Clinically important, potentially serious interactions with: cholestyramine, clofibrate, colestipol, estrogens

Reactions

Skin
Diaphoresis
Lichen planus
(1992): Ellul JP+, *Dig Dis Sci* 37, 628
Pruritus (<1%)
Rash (sic) (<1%)
Urticaria
Xerosis

Hair
Hair – alopecia

Other
Dysgeusia (<1%) (metallic taste)
Myalgia
Stomatitis

VALACYCLOVIR

Trade name: Valtrex (GlaxoSmithKline)
Indications: Herpes zoster
Category: Antiviral
Half-life: 3 hours
Clinically important, potentially serious interactions with: cimetidine, probenecid

Reactions

Skin

Facial edema
(2000): Colin J+, *Ophthalmology* 107, 1507 (3–5%)
Periorbital edema
(2000): Colin J+, *Ophthalmology* 107, 1507 (3–5%)
Purpura
(2000): Rivaud E+, *Arch Intern Med* 160, 1705

VALPROIC ACID

Synonym: divalproex
Trade names: Depakene (Abbott); Depakote (Abbott)
Indications: Seizures; migraine
Category: Anticonvulsant
Half-life: 6–16 hours
Clinically important, potentially serious interactions with: alcohol, aspirin, barbiturates, carbamazepine, cimetidine, clonazepam, clozapine, CNS depressants, diazepam, ethosuximide, felbamate, isoniazid, lamotrigine, phenobarbital, phenytoin, primidone, rifampin, salicylates, tolbutamide, warfarin, zidovudine

Reactions

Skin

Acne
Allergic reactions (sic) (<5%)
Contact dermatitis
(1994): Garcia-Bravo B+, *Contact Dermatitis* 30, 40
Ecchymoses (<5%)
Edema
Erythema multiforme (<1%)
(1990): Chan HL+, *Arch Dermatol* 126, 43
Exanthems (5%)
(1983): Bruni J+, *Arch Neurol* 40, 135
(1978): Lewis JR, *JAMA* 240, 2190
Facial edema (>5%)
Fixed eruption
(1997): Chan HL+, *J Am Acad Dermatol* 36, 259
Furunculosis (<5%)
Lupus erythematosus
(1996): Park-Matsumoto YC+, *J Neurol Sci* 143, 185
(1994): Fritzler MJ, *Lupus* 3, 455
(1993): Drory VE+, *Clin Neuropharmacol* 16, 19 (passim)
(1990): Bleck TP+, *Epilepsia* 31, 343
Morphea
(1980): Goihman-Yahr M+, *Arch Dermatol* 116, 621
Peripheral edema (<5%)
Petechiae (<5%)
Photosensitivity
Pruritus (>5%)
Psoriasis
Purpura
(1984): *Drugs Ther Bull* 22, 23
(1976): Winfield DA+, *BMJ* 2, 981
Rash (sic) (>5%)
(1978): Lewis JR, *JAMA* 240, 2190
Scleroderma
(1980): Goihman-Yahr M+, *Arch Dermatol* 116, 621
Seborrhea
Stevens-Johnson syndrome
(1999): Rzany B+, *Lancet* 353, 2190
(1998): Tsai SJ+, *J Clin Psychopharmacol* 18, 420
Toxic epidermal necrolysis
(1999): Rzany B+, *Lancet* 353, 2190
(1991): Porteous DM+, *Arch Dermatol* 127, 740
Urticaria
Vasculitis
(1991): Kamper AM+, *Lancet* 1, 497

Hair

Hair – alopecia (7%)
(1998): Fetterman M, Miami FL (from Internet) (observation)
(1996): Wallace SJ, *Drug Saf* 15, 378
(1996): McKinney PA+, *Ann Clin Psychiatry* 8, 183
(1995): Fatemi SH+, *Ann Pharmacother* 29, 1302
(1981): Herranz JL, *Dev Med Child Neurol* 23, 386
(1978): *Drug Ther Bull* 16, 77 (UP TO 10%)
(1978): Lewis JR, *JAMA* 240, 2190
(1977): Pinder RM+, *Drugs* 13, 81 (<0.5%)
(1976): Winfield DA+, *BMJ* 2, 981
(1975): Barnes SE+, *Dev Med Child Neurol* 17, 175
(1974): Jeavons PM+, *BMJ* 2, 584
Hair – curly
(1977): Jeavons PM+, *Lancet* 1, 359
Hair – depigmentation
(1981): Herranz JL+, *Dev Med Child Neurol* 23, 386
Hair – perming effect (sic)
(1988): Gupta AK, *Br J Clin Pract* 42, 75

Other

Acute intermittent porphyria
(1989): Herrick AL+, *Br J Clin Pharmacol* 27, 491
(1980): Garcia-Merino JA+, *Lancet* 2, 856
Aplasia cutis congenita
Dysgeusia (<5%)
Galactorrhea
(1983): Kollipara S+, *J Pediatr* 103, 501
Gingival hyperplasia
(1997): Anderson HH+, *ASDC J Dent Child* 64, 294
(1991): Behari M, *J Neurol Neurosurg Psychiatry* 54, 279
Glossitis (<5%)
Gynecomastia
(1983): Kollipara S+, *J Pediatr* 103, 501
Hypersensitivity
Hypesthesia
Myalgia (<5%)
Paresthesias (<5%)
Porphyria
(1991): Jalil P+, *Rev Med Chil* 119, 920
(1981): Doss M+, *Lancet* 2, 91
Sialorrhea
Stomatitis (<5%)
Vaginitis (<5%)
Xerostomia (<5%)

VALSARTAN

Trade name: Diovan (Novartis)
Indications: Hypertension
Category: Angiotensin II antagonist; antihypertensive
Half-life: 9 hours
Clinically important, potentially serious interactions with: cimetidine

Reactions

Skin

Allergic reactions (sic) (>2%)
Angioedema (>2%)
(1998): Frye CB+, *Pharmacotherapy* 18, 866

Edema (>1%)
(1996): Corea L+, *Clin Pharmacol Ther* 60, 341
Photosensitivity
(1998): Frye CB+, *Pharmacotherapy* 18, 866
Pruritus (>2%)
Rash (sic) (>2%)

Other

Dysgeusia (>10%)
Myalgia (>2%)
Paresthesias (>2%)
Xerostomia (>2%)

VANCOMYCIN

Trade name: Vancocin (Lilly)
Other common trade names: *Balcoran; Diatracin; Vanmicina*
Indications: Various infections caused by susceptible organisms
Category: Narrow-spectrum antibiotic
Half-life: 5–11 hours
Clinically important, potentially serious interactions with: aminoglycosides, anesthetics, bumetanide, carmustine, cholestyramine, cisplatin, colestipol, cyclosporine, ethacrynic acid, furosemide, streptozocin, succinylcholine

Reactions

Skin

Acute generalized exanthematous pustulosis (AGEP)
(1996): Sawhney RA+, *Int J Dermatol* 35, 826
(1995): Moreau A+, *Int J Dermatol* 34, 263 (passim)
(1991): Roujeau J-C+, *Arch Dermatol* 127, 1333
Allergic reactions (sic) (<5%)
(1997): Kahata S+, *Bone Marrow Transplant* 20, 1001
(1992): Breathnach SM+, *Adverse Drug Reactions and the Skin*, Blackwell, Oxford, 158 (passim)
Angioedema
(1989): Koestner B+, *Schweiz Med Wochenschr* (German) 119, 28
(1959): Rothenberg HJ, *JAMA* 171, 1102
Bullous eruption
(1996): Heald PW, *Skin and Allergy News* 27, 18
(1992): Carpenter S+, *J Am Acad Dermatol* 26, 45
(1990): Forrence EA+, *Drug Intell Clin Pharm* 24, 369
(1988): Baden LA+, *Arch Dermatol* 124, 1186
Chills (>10%)
Cutaneous reactions (sic)
(1997): Korman TM+, *J Antimicrob Chemother* 39, 371
Erythema multiforme
(1992): Laurencin CT, *Ann Pharmacotherapy* 26, 1520
(1988): Gutfeld MB+, *Drug Intell Clin Pharm* 22, 881
Exanthems
(1991): McCullough JM+, *Drug Intell Clin Pharm* 25, 1326
(1991): Valero R+, *J Cardiothorac Vasc Anesth* 5, 574
(1988): Neal D+, *BMJ* 296, 137
(1988): Schlemmer B+, *N Engl J Med* 318, 1127
(1987): Lacouture PG+, *J Pediatr* 111, 615 (35%)
(1987): Longon P+, *Presse Med* (French) 16, 682
(1986): Davis RL+, *Ann Intern Med* 104, 285
(1986): McElrath MJ+, *Lancet* 1, 47
(1986): Markman M+, *South Med J* 79, 382 (passim)
(1985): Schifter S+, *Lancet* 2, 499 (8%)
(1984): Rimailho A+, *Presse Med* (French) 13, 567
(1984): Odio C+, *Am J Dis Child* 138, 17
(1960): Kirby WMM+, *N Engl J Med* 262, 49 (1–5%)
Exfoliative dermatitis
(1990): Forrence EA+, *Drug Intell Clin Pharm* 24, 369
(1988): Gutfeld MB+, *Drug Intell Clin Pharm* 22, 881
(1988): Neal D+, *BMJ* 296, 137
Flushing (1–10%)
Linear IgA bullous dermatosis
(2000): Klein PA+, *J Am Acad Dermatol* 42, 316
(1999): Nousari HC+, *Medicine* 78, 1
(1998): Nousari HC+, *Ann Intern Med* 129, 507
(1998): Bernstein EF+, *Ann Intern Med* 129, 508
(1997): Norland A, Minneapolis, American Academy of Dermatology Meeting (SF), Gross and Microscopic
(1996): Primka E+, *J Cutan Pathol* 23, 58
(1996): Whitworth JM+, *J Am Acad Dermatol* 34, 890
(1996): Richards SS+, *Arch Dermatol* 131, 1447
(1996): Tranvan A+, *J Am Acad Dermatol* 35, 865
(1996): Bitman LM+, *Arch Dermatol* 132, 1289
(1995): Geissmann C+, *J Am Acad Dermatol* 32, 296
(1995): Richards S+, *Arch Dermatol* 131, 1447
(1994): Piketty C+, *Br J Dermatol* 130, 130
(1994): Kuechle MK+, *J Am Acad Dermatol* 30, 187
(1992): Carpenter S+, *J Am Acad Dermatol* 26, 45
(1988): Baden LA+, *Arch Dermatol* 124, 1186
Lupus erythematosus
(1993): Ena J+, *JAMA* 269, 598
(1986): Markman M+, *South Med J* 79, 382
Pruritus
(1991): Killian AD+, *Ann Intern Med* 115, 410
(1991): McCullough JM+, *Drug Intell Clin Pharm* 25, 1326
(1989): Koestner B+, *Schweiz Med Wochenschr* (German) 119, 28
(1986): Davis RL+, *Ann Intern Med* 104, 285
(1959): Rothenberg HJ, *JAMA* 171, 1102
Purpura
(1998): Michael S+, *Scand J Rheumatol* 27, 233
Rash (sic)
(1997): Reis AG+, *Rev Paul Med* 115, 1452
(1993): Ena J+, *JAMA* 269, 598
(1983): Farber BF+, *Antimicrob Agents Chemother* 23, 138
(1978): Hook EW+, *Am J Med* 65, 411
(1976): Arndt KA+, *JAMA* 235, 918 (10%)
Red man syndrome* (1–10%)
(1999): Khurana C+, *Postgrad Med J* 75, 41
(1998): Polk RE, *Ann Pharmacother* 32, 840
(1996): Szymusiak-Mutnick BA+, *Am J Health Syst Pharm* 53, 2098
(1995): Lilley LL+, *Am J Nurs* 95, 14
(1994): Bergeron L+, *Ann Pharmacother* 28, 581
(1993): Polk RE+, *Antimicrob Agents Chemother* 37, 2139
(1993): O'Sullivan TL+, *J Infect Dis* 168, 773
(1993): Ena J+, *JAMA* 269, 598
(1992): Rengo C+, *Recenti Prog Med* (Italian) 83, 726
(1992): Levy M+, *Harefuah* (Hebrew) 122, 36
(1991): Valero R+, *J Cardiothorac Vasc Anesth* 5, 574
(1991): Maccabruni A+, *Recenti Prog Med* (Italian) 82, 17
(1991): Wallace MR+, *J Infect Dis* 164, 1180
(1991): Killian AD+, *Ann Intern Med* 115, 410
(1990): Healey DP+, *Antimicrob Agents Chemother* 34, 550
(1990): Sahai J+, *Antimicrob Agents Chemother* 34, 765
(1990): No Author, *Lancet* 335, 1006
(1990): Bailie GR+, *Clin Pharm* 9, 671
(1990): Levy M+, *Pediatrics* 86, 572
(1989): Sahai J+, *J Infect Dis* 160, 876
(1989): Pearson DA, *J Am Dent Assoc* 118, 59
(1988): Rubin M+, *Ann Intern Med* 108, 30 (3%)
(1988): Polk RE+, *J Infect Dis* 157, 502
(1987): Duro JC+, *Med Clin (Barc)* (Spanish) 89, 218
(1986): Daly BM+, *Drug Intell Clin Pharm* 20, 986
(1986): Rolston KV+, *JAMA* 255, 2445
(1986): Wade TP+, *Arch Surg* 121, 859
(1986): Davis RL+, *Ann Intern Med* 104, 285
(1985): Cole DR+, *Lancet* 2, 280
(1985): Holliman R, *Lancet* 1, 1399
(1985): Garrelts JC+, *N Engl J Med* 312, 245
Red neck syndrome (sic)
(1985): Pau AK+, *N Engl J Med* 313, 756
(1985): Ackerman BH+, *Ann Intern Med* 102, 723
Stevens–Johnson syndrome (<1%)
(1996): Alexander II+, *Allergy Asthma Proc* 17, 75
(1995): Patterson R+, *Allergy Proc* 16, 115
(1992): Laurencin CT+, *Ann Pharmacother* 26, 1520
(1990): Forrence EA+, *Drug Intell Clin Pharm* 24, 369
Toxic epidermal necrolysis
(2000): Chan-Tack K, *Mo Med* 97, 131
(1992): Vidal C+, *Ann Allergy* 68, 345
(1990): Hannah BA+, *South Med J* 83, 720
(1985): Heng MCY, *Br J Dermatol* 113, 597
Urticaria
(1989): Koestner B+, *Schweiz Med Wochenschr* (German) 119, 28
(1988): Neal D+, *BMJ* 296, 137

(1987): Longon P+, *Presse Med* (French) 16, 682
(1986): Davis RL+, *Ann Intern Med* 104, 285
(1986): Markman M+, *South Med J* 79, 382 (passim)
(1960): Kirby WMM+, *N Engl J Med* 262, 49 (1–5%)
(1959): Rothenberg HJ, *JAMA* 171, 1102 (1–5%)
Vasculitis (<1%)
(1987): Rawlinson WD+, *Med J Australia* 147, 470
(1986): Markman M+, *South Med J* 79, 382

Other

Anaphylactoid reaction
(2000): Chopra N+, *Ann Allergy Asthma Immunol* 84, 633
(1992): Breathnach SM+, *Adverse Drug Reactions and the Skin*, Blackwell, Oxford, 158 (passim)
(1988): Rubin M+, *Ann Intern Med* 108, 30 (1 IN 63 patients)
(1987): Longon P+, *Presse Med* (French) 16, 682
(1986): Markman M+, *Southern Med J* 79, 382 (passim)
Dysgeusia (>10%)
Hypersensitivity
(1997): Marik PE+, *Pharmacotherapy* 17, 1341
Injection-site thrombophlebitis
Paresthesias
Phlebitis
(1983): Farber BF+, *Antimicrob Agents Chemother* 23, 138
(1978): Hook EW+, *Am J Med* 65, 411
Priapism
(1998): Czachor JS+, *N Engl J Med* 338, 1701

***Note:** The vancomycin-induced red man syndrome is characterized by pruritus, erythema and, in severe cases, angioedema, hypotension, and cardiovascular collapse.

VASOPRESSIN

Synonyms: ADH; antidiuretic hormone
Trade name: Pitressin (Parke-Davis)
Other common trade name: *Pressyn*
Indications: Diabetes insipidus
Category: Vasoconstrictor and antidiuretic pituitary hormone; vasopressor; antidiuretic
Half-life: 10–20 minutes
Clinically important, potentially serious interactions with: carbamazepine, chlorpropamide, phenformin, urea

Reactions

Skin

Allergic reactions (sic) (<1%)
Angioedema
Bullous eruption
(1997): Lin RY+, *Dermatology* 195, 271
(1991): Colemont LJ+, *J Clin Gastroenterol* 13, 91
(1986): Korenberg RJ+, *J Am Acad Dermatol* 15, 393
Diaphoresis (1–10%)
Ecchymoses
(1997): Lin RY+, *Dermatology* 195, 271
(1985): Thomas TK, *Am J Gastroenterol* 80, 704
Exanthems
Gangrene
(1997): Lin RY+, *Dermatology* 195, 271
Pallor (1–10%)
Purpura
(1996): Lemlich G+, *Cutis* 57, 330
(1985): Thomas TK, *Am J Gastroenterol* 80, 704
Rash (sic)
Urticaria (1–10%)

Hair

Hair – alopecia
(1994): Maceyko RD+, *J Am Acad Dermatol* 31, 111

Other

Anaphylactoid reaction
Infusion-site necrosis
(1997): Lin RY+, *Dermatology* 195, 271 (amber-like)
(1996): Lemlich G+, *Cutis* 57, 330
(1991): Colemont LJ+, *J Clin Gastroenterol* 13, 91
(1990): Stump DL+, *Drugs* 39, 38
(1986): Korenberg RJ+, *J Am Acad Dermatol* 15, 393
(1985): Thomas TK, *Am J Gastroenterol* 80, 704
Trembling
Tremor (1–10%)

VENLAFAXINE

Trade name: Effexor (Wyeth-Ayerst)
Indications: Depression
Category: Heterocyclic antidepressant; selective serotonin reuptake inhibitor (SSRI)
Half-life: 3–7 hours
Clinically important, potentially serious interactions with: antiarrhythmics, beta-blockers, cimetidine, fluoxetine, MAO inhibitors, phenothiazines, sertraline, trazodone, tricyclic antidepressants, warfarin

Reactions

Skin

Acne (<1%)
Allergic reactions (sic) (<1%)
Candidiasis
Contact dermatitis
Diaphoresis (12%)
(2000): Pierre JM+, *J Clin Psychopharmacol* 20, 269
(2000): Gelenberg AJ+, *JAMA* 283, 3082
Ecchymoses (<1%)
Eczema (sic) (<1%)
Edema (<1%)
Exanthems (<1%)
Exfoliative dermatitis (<1%)
Facial edema (<1%)
Furunculosis (<1%)
Herpes simplex (<1%)
Herpes zoster (<1%)
Lichenoid eruption (<1%)
Peripheral edema
Photosensitivity (<1%)
Pruritus (1–10%)
Psoriasis (<1%)
Pustular eruption (<1%)
Rash (sic) (3%)
Urticaria (<1%)
Vesiculobullous eruption (<1%)
Xerosis (<1%)

Hair

Hair – alopecia (<1%)
Hair – discoloration (<1%)
Hair – hirsutism (<1%)

Other

Ageusia (<1%)
Bromhidrosis (<1%)
Dysgeusia (2%)
Gingivitis (<1%)
Glossitis (<1%)
Gynecomastia (<1%)
Hyperesthesia (<1%)
Hypesthesia (>1%)
Mastodynia
(1996): Bhatia SC+, *J Clin Psychiatry* 57, 423
Myalgia (>1%)
Oral ulceration (<1%)
Paresthesias (3%)
Parosmia (<1%)
Sialorrhea (<1%)
Stomatitis (<1%)
Thrombophlebitis (<1%)

Tongue edema (<1%)
Tongue pigmentation (<1%)
Tremor (1–10%)
Vaginal candidiasis (<1%)
Vaginitis
Xerostomia (22%)
(2000): Gelenberg AJ+, *JAMA* 283, 3082

VERAPAMIL

Trade names: Calan (Searle); Covera-HS (Searle); Isoptin (Knoll); Tarka (Knoll); Verelan (Schwarz)
Other common trade names: *APO-Verap; Arpamyl LP; Azupamil; Berkatens; Chronovera; Cordilox; Geangin; Isoptine; Nu-Verap; Veraken*
Indications: Angina, hypertension
Category: Calcium channel blocker; antianginal, antihypertensive and antiarrhythmic
Half-life: 2–8 hours
Clinically important, potentially serious interactions with: aspirin, atorvastatin, barbiturates, beta-blockers, calcium salts, carbamazepine, cerivastatin, cimetidine, clonidine, cyclosporine, dantrolene, digoxin, disopyramide, erythromycin, fentanyl, flecainide, lithium, lovastatin, phenytoin, prazosin, quinidine, rifampin, simvastatin, tacrolimus, theophylline, **grapefruit juice**

Tarka is trandolapril and verapamil

Reactions

Skin

Acne
(1989): Stern R+, *Arch Intern Med* 149, 829
Acute febrile neutrophilic dermatosis (Sweet's syndrome)
(1998): Knowles S+, *J Am Acad Dermatol* 38, 201 (passim)
Angioedema
(1998): Knowles S+, *J Am Acad Dermatol* 38, 201 (passim)
(1989): Sadick NS+, *J Am Acad Dermatol* 21, 132
(1989): Stern R+, *Arch Intern Med* 149, 829
Ankle edema
Cutaneous side effects (sic)
(1993): Kitamura K+, *J Dermatol* 20, 279 (psoriasiform)
(1989): McTavish D+, *Drugs* 38, 19. (0.6%)
Dermatitis (sic)
Diaphoresis (<1%)
(1989): Stern R+, *Arch Intern Med* 149, 829
(1983): Lewis JG, *Drugs* 25, 196
Ecchymoses (<1%)
(1989): Sadick NS+, *J Am Acad Dermatol* 21, 132
Edema (1.9%)
Erythema multiforme (<1%)
(1991): Kürkçüoglu N+, *J Am Acad Dermatol* 24, 511
(1989): Lin AYF+, *Drug Intell Clin Pharm* 23, 987
(1989): Stern R+, *Arch Intern Med* 149, 829
(1987): Naito S+, *Skin Res* (Japanese) 29, 602
Erythema nodosum
(1998): Knowles S+, *J Am Acad Dermatol* 38, 201 (passim)
Exanthems
(1998): Knowles S+, *J Am Acad Dermatol* 38, 201 (passim)
(1989): McTavish D+, *Drugs* 38, 19
(1989): Stern R+, *Arch Intern Med* 149, 829
(1989): Sadick NS+, *J Am Acad Dermatol* 21, 132
(1983): Lewis JG, *Drugs* 25, 196 (3.2%)
(1982): Anon, *Lakartidningen* (Swedish) 79, 3822
(1980): Midtbo K+, *Curr Ther Res* 27, 830
Exfoliative dermatitis
(1998): Knowles S+, *J Am Acad Dermatol* 38, 201 (passim)
(1989): Stern R+, *Arch Intern Med* 149, 829
Flushing (0.6%)
(1992): Shelley WB+, *Advanced Dermatologic Diagnosis*, WB Saunders, 583 (passim)
(1989): McTavish D+, *Drugs* 38, 19 (1–5.4%)
(1983): Lewis JG, *Drugs* 25, 196 (4–7%)
(1980): Raftos J, *Med J Aust* 2, 78
Hyperkeratosis (palms) (<1%)
(1989): Sadick NS+, *J Am Acad Dermatol* 21, 132
(1983): Major P, *Tidsskr Nor Laegeforen* (Norwegian), 103, 2061
Lichenoid eruption
Lupus erythematosus
(1998): Callen JP, Academy '98 Meeting (4 patients)
Parkinsonism
Peripheral edema (1–10%)
Photosensitivity
(1994): Berger TG+, *Arch Dermatol* 130, 609 (in HIV-infected)
(1989): McTavish D+, *Drugs* 38, 19
(1983): Lewis JG, *Drugs* 25, 196
(1979): Anon, *Med J Aust* 2, 204
Prurigo (sic)
(1983): Lewis JG, *Drugs* 25, 196
Pruritus
(1998): Knowles S+, *J Am Acad Dermatol* 38, 201 (passim)
(1989): McTavish D+, *Drugs* 38, 19
(1989): Stern R+, *Arch Intern Med* 149, 829
(1988): Burgunder JM+, *Hepatogastroenterology* 35, 169
(1983): Lewis JG, *Drugs* 25, 196
(1982): Fischer Hansen J+, *Clin Exp Pharmacol Physiol* 6, 31
Purpura (<1%)
(1982): *Lakartidningen* (Swedish) 79, 3822
Rash (sic) (1.2%)
(1989): Stern R+, *Arch Intern Med* 149, 829
(1987): Johnson BF+, *Clin Pharmacol Ther* 42, 66
Stevens–Johnson syndrome (<1%)
(1998): Knowles S+, *J Am Acad Dermatol* 38, 201 (passim)
(1992): Gonski PN, *Med J Aust* 156, 672
(1989): Stern R+, *Arch Intern Med* 149, 829
(1989): Lin AYF+, *Drug Intell Clin Pharm* 23, 987
Urticaria (<1%)
(1998): Knowles S+, *J Am Acad Dermatol* 38, 201 (passim)
(1989): McTavish D+, *Drugs* 38, 19
(1989): Stern R+, *Arch Intern Med* 149, 829
(1989): Sadick NS+, *J Am Acad Dermatol* 21, 132
(1983): Lewis JG, *Drugs* 25, 196
Vasculitis (<1%)
(1989): Sadick NS+, *J Am Acad Dermatol* 21, 132
(1983): Lewis JG, *Drugs* 25, 196

Hair

Hair – alopecia (<1%)
(1994): Litt JZ, Beachwood, OH, personal case (observation)
(1991): Shelley WB+, *Cutis* 48, 364 (observation)
(1989): Stern R+, *Arch Intern Med* 149, 829
(1989): Sadick NS+, *J Am Acad Dermatol* 21, 132
(1981): Rosing DR+, *Am J Cardiol* 48, 545
(1980): Rosing DR+, *Chest* 78 (Suppl), 239
Hair – hypertrichosis
(1991): Sever PS, *Lancet* 338, 1215
Hair – pigmentation
(1991): Read GM, *Lancet* 338, 1520

Nails

Nails – dystrophy
(1989): Stern R+, *Arch Intern Med* 149, 829

Other

Erythermalgia
(1992): Drenth JP+, *Br J Dermatol* 127, 292
Galactorrhea (<1%)
Gingival hyperplasia (19%)
(1995): Moghadam BKH+, *Cutis* 56, 46 (passim)
(1993): Steele RM+, *Arch Intern Med* 120, 663
(1989): Pernu HE+, *J Oral Pathol Med* 18, 422
(1987): Giustiniani S+, *Int J Cardiol* 15, 247
Gynecomastia (<1%)
(2000): Hugues FC+, *Ann Med Interne (Paris)* (French) 151, 10 (passim)
(1994): *BMJ* 308, 503
(1994): Deniel-Rosanas J, *Med Clin (Barc)* (Spanish) 102, 399
(1988): Tanner LA+, *Arch Intern Med* 148, 379
Paresthesias (<1%)
Serum sickness
(1989): Pascual-Velasco F, *Med Clin (Barc)* (Spanish) 92, 719
Xerostomia (<1%)

VIDARABINE

Synonyms: adenine arabinoside; ara-A
Trade name: Vira-A Ophthalmic (Parke-Davis)
Other common trade names: *Adena a Ungena; Arasena*
Indications: Herpetic keratoconjunctivitis
Category: Ophthalmic antiviral
Half-life: 3.3 hours
Clinically important, potentially serious interactions with: corticosteroids

Reactions

Skin

Ocular burning
Ocular erythema
Ocular pruritus
Pruritus
Rash (sic)

VINBLASTINE

Trade name: Velban (Lilly)
Indications: Lymphomas, melanoma, carcinomas
Category: Antineoplastic
Half-life: initial phase: 3.7 minutes; terminal phase: 24.8 hours
Clinically important, potentially serious interactions with: interferon, mitomycin, phenytoin

Reactions

Skin

Acne
(1962): Falkson G+, *Br J Dermatol* 74, 229
Acral gangrene
(1998): Reiser M+, *Eur J Clin Microbiol Infect Dis* 17, 58
(1997): Hladunewich M+, *J Rheumatol* 24, 2371
Bullous eruption (<1%)
Cellulitis
(1983): Bronner AK+, *J Am Acad Dermatol* 9, 645
Dermatitis (sic) (1–10%)
Erythema
(1969): Lampkin BC, *Lancet* 1, 891
Erythema multiforme
(1991): Arias D+, *J Cutan Pathol* 18, 344
Exanthems
Hyperpigmentation
(1997): Smith KJ+, *J Am Acad Dermatol* 36, 329
(1994): Cecchi R+, *Dermatology* 188, 244
Photosensitivity (1–10%)
(1992): Breathnach SM+, *Adverse Drug Reactions and the Skin*, Blackwell, Oxford, 302 (passim)
(1975): Breza TS+, *Arch Dermatol* 111, 1168
Phototoxic reaction
Purpura
Radiation recall
(1992): Nemechek PM+, *Cancer* 70, 1605
Radiodermatitis (reactivation)
(1969): Lampkin BC, *Lancet* 1, 891
Rash (sic) (1–10%)
Raynaud's phenomenon (1–10%)
(1998): Reiser M+, *Eur J Clin Microbiol Infect Dis* 17, 58
(1997): Hladunewich M+, *J Rheumatol* 24, 2371
(1993): von Gunten CF+, *Cancer* 72, 2004
(1981): Harvey HA+, *Ann Intern Med* 94, 542
(1981): Vogelzang NJ+, *Ann Intern Med* 95, 288
(1978): Rothberg H, *Cancer Treat Rep* 62, 569
(1977): Teutsch C+, *Cancer Treat Rep* 61, 925
Urticaria

Hair

Hair – alopecia (>10%)
(1992): Breathnach SM+, *Adverse Drug Reactions and the Skin*, Blackwell, Oxford, 302 (passim)
Hair – changes (sic)
(1971): Kostanecki W+, *Z Haut Geschlechtskr* (German) 46, 704

Other

Dysgeusia (>10%) (metallic taste)
Injection-site necrosis
(1992): Misery L+, *Presse Med* (French) 21, 2153
(1991): Arias D+, *J Cutan Pathol* 18, 344
Injection-site pain
Myalgia (1–10%)
Oral mucosal lesions
(1978): Levine N+, *Cancer Treat Rev* 5, 67 (1–5%)
Paresthesias (1–10%)
Phlebitis
(1989): Kerker BJ+, *Semin Dermatol* 8, 173
Stomatitis (>10%)
Ulceration due to extravasation
Vesiculation of mouth (sic)

VINCRISTINE

Trade names: Oncovin (Lilly); Vincasar (Pharmacia & Upjohn)
Indications: Leukemias, lymphomas, neuroblastoma, Wilm's tumor
Category: Antineoplastic
Half-life: 24 hours
Clinically important, potentially serious interactions with: digoxin, itraconazole, mitomycin, nifedipine, paclitaxel, quinolones

Reactions

Skin

Angioedema
(1984): Gassel WD+, *Oncology* 41, 403
Dermatitis herpetiformis
(1986): Gottlieb D+, *Med J Aust* 145, 241 (flare)
Edema
Erythroderma
(1989): Matsumoto N+, *Gan To Kagaku Ryoho* (Japanese) 16, 2297
(1984): Gassel WD+, *Oncology* 41, 403
Exanthems
(1984): Gassel WD+, *Oncology* 41, 403
(1978): Levine N+, *Cancer Treat Rev* 5, 67
(1972): Zanoni G+, *Blut* (German) 25, 20
Palmar-plantar erythema
(1990): Pagliuca A+, *Postgrad Med J* 66, 242
Pruritus
(1978): Levine N+, *CancerTreat Rev* 5, 67
Rash (sic) (1–10%)
Raynaud's phenomenon
(1998): Reiser M+, *Eur J Clin Microbiol Infect Dis* 17, 58
Serpentine supravenous hyperpigmentation (sic)
(2000): Marcoux D+, *J Am Acad Dermatol* 43, 540 (with dactinomycin)
Sjøgren's syndrome
(1989): Monno S+, *Jpn J Med* 28, 399
Urticaria

Hair

Hair – alopecia (20–70%)
(1987): David J+, *Nurs Times* 83, 36
(1973): Levantine A+, *Br J Dermatol* 89, 549 (>5%)
(1971): Helson L+, *N Engl J Med* 284, 336
(1970): O'Brien R+, *N Engl J Med* 283, 1469
(1966): Simister JM, *BMJ* 2, 1138
(1964): Knock FE, *Med Clin North Am* 48, 501 (>5%)
(1963): Martin J+, *Lancet* 2, 1080 (47%)

Nails

Nails – Beau's lines (transverse nail bands)
(1994): Ben-Dayan D+, *Acta Haematol* 91, 89

Nails – leukonychia
(1990): Bader-Meunier B+, *Ann Pediatr Paris* (French) 37, 337 (transverse)
Nails – Mees' lines
(1983): James WD+, *Arch Dermatol* 119, 334
(1982): Jeanmougin M+, *Ann Dermatol Venereol* (French) 109, 169
Nails – onychodermal band
(1993): Kowal-Vern A+, *Cutis* 52, 43 (plus erythema of proximal nail fold)

Other

Anaphylactoid reaction
Dysgeusia (1–10%) (metallic taste)
Injection-site cellulitis (>10%)
(1983): BronnerAK+, *J Am Acad Dermatol* 9, 645
Injection-site necrosis (>10%)
Myalgia (1–10%)
Oral mucosal lesions (1–10%)
(1989): KerkerBJ+, *Semin Dermatol* 8, 173 (1–5%)
(1964): Knock FE, *Med Clin North Am* 48, 501
Oral ulceration (1–10%)
Paresthesias (1–10%)
Phlebitis (1–10%)
Stomatitis (<1%)

VINORELBINE

Trade name: Navelbine (GlaxoWellcome)
Indications: Nonsmall cell lung cancer
Category: Antineoplastic
Half-life: 28–44 hours
Clinically important, potentially serious interactions with: cisplatin, mitomycin

Reactions

Skin

Angioedema
Erythema
Flushing
Hand-foot syndrome
(1998): Hoff PM+, *Cancer* 82, 965
Pigmentation
(1994): Cecchi R+, *Dermatology* 188, 244
Pruritus
Rash (sic) (<5%)
Toxic epidermal necrolysis
(1992): Misery L+, *Presse Med* (French) 21, 2153

Hair

Hair – alopecia (12%)
(1994): Gasparini G+, *J Clin Oncol* 12, 2094
(1989): Marty M+, *Nouv Rev Fr Hematol* (French) 31, 77

Other

Anaphylactoid reaction
Dysgeusia (>10%) (metallic taste)
Hyperesthesia (1–10%)
Injection-site irritation (1–10%)
Injection-site necrosis (1–10%)
Injection-site pain (1.6%)
Injection-site phlebitis
(1998): Sauter C+, *Schweiz Med Wochenschr* (German) 128, 343
(1989): Marty M+, *Nouv Rev Fr Hematol* (French) 31, 77 (12%)
Myalgia (<5%)
Paresthesias (1–10%)
Phlebitis (7%)
Stomatitis (>10%)
(1989): Marty M+, *Nouv Rev Fr Hematol* (French) 31, 77 (12%)

VITAMIN A

Trade names: Aquasol A (AstraZeneca); Del-Vi-A (DelRay); Palmitate A
Other common trade names: *Acaren; Acon; Afaxin; Arovit; Avipur; Avitin; Axerol; Dolce; Vogan*
Indications: Vitamin A deficiency
Category: Nutritional fat-soluble vitamin supplement
Half-life: no data
Clinically important, potentially serious interactions with: acitretin, isotretinoin

Reactions

Skin

Cheilitis
Contact dermatitis
(1996): Bazzano C+, *Contact Dermatitis* 35, 261
(1995): Heidenheim M+, *Contact Dermatitis* 33, 439
(1994): Manzano A+, *Contact Dermatitis* 31, 324
(1994): Sanz de Galdeano C+, *Contact Dermatitis* 30, 50
(1984): Blondeel A, *Contact Dermatitis* 11, 191
Dermatitis (dry, scaly and keratotic – mainly palms and soles)
(1971): Muenter MD+, *Am J Med* 50, 129
(1958): Oliver TK, *Am J Dis Child* 95, 57
Eczematous eruption (pellagra-like)
(1982): Hamann K+, *Hautarzt* (German) 33, 559
Erythema
(1992): Breathnach SM+, *Adverse Drug Reactions and the Skin*, Blackwell, Oxford, 254 (passim)
Erythema multiforme (<1%)
(1971): Muenter MD+, *Am J Med* 50, 129
Exanthems
(1971): Muenter MD+, *Am J Med* 50, 129
Exfoliative dermatitis
Fissuring
(1992): Breathnach SM+, *Adverse Drug Reactions and the Skin*, Blackwell, Oxford, 254 (passim)
Generalized peeling (sic)
(1970): Nater P+, *Acta Derm Venereol* (Stockh) 50, 109
Hyperkeratosis
(1992): Breathnach SM+, *Adverse Drug Reactions and the Skin*, Blackwell, Oxford, 254 (passim)
Perleche
(1971): Muenter MD+, *Am J Med* 50, 129
Photosensitivity
Pigmentation (yellow-orange)
(1971): Muenter MD+, *Am J Med* 50, 129
Pruritus (<1%)
(1992): Breathnach SM+, *Adverse Drug Reactions and the Skin*, Blackwell, Oxford, 254 (passim)
(1971): Muenter MD+, *Am J Med* 50, 129
Shedding
Stevens–Johnson syndrome
(1971): Muenter MD+, *Am J Med* 50, 129
Xerosis (1–10%)
(1975): Stüttgen G, *Acta Derm Venereol* (Stockh) 55 (Suppl 74), 174

Hair

Hair – alopecia
(1992): Breathnach SM+, *Adverse Drug Reactions and the Skin*, Blackwell, Oxford, 254 (passim)
(1979): Schmunes E, *Arch Dermatol* 115, 882
(1975): Stüttgen G, *Acta Derm Venereol* (Stockh) 55 (Suppl 74), 174
(1973): Levantine A+, *Br J Dermatol* 89, 549
(1972): Mausle R+, *Fortschr Med* (German) 90, 687
(1971): Muenter MD+, *Am J Med* 50, 129
(1970): Ippen H, *Dtsch Med Wochenschr* (German) 95, 1411
(1967): di Benedetto RJ, *JAMA* 201, 700
(1965): Rook A, *Br J Dermatol* 77, 115
(1960): Morrice G+, *JAMA* 173, 1802

Other

Anaphylactoid reaction
Gingivitis

Hypersensitivity
(1995): Shelley WB+, *BMJ* 311, 232
Oral mucosal eruption
(1971): Muenter MD+, *Am J Med* 50, 129
(1964): Smith JH, *Oral Surg* 17 (Suppl 3), 305
Pseudotumor cerebri
Stomatodynia
Xerostomia
(1992): Breathnach SM+, *Adverse Drug Reactions and the Skin*, Blackwell, Oxford, 254 (passim)

VITAMIN B_1

(See THIAMINE)

VITAMIN B_2

See RIBOFLAVIN)

VITAMIN B_3

(See NIACINAMIDE)

VITAMIN B_5

(See PANTOTHENIC ACID)

VITAMIN B_6

(See PYRIDOXINE)

VITAMIN B_9

(See FOLIC ACID)

VITAMIN B_{12}

(See CYANOCOBALAMIN)

VITAMIN C

(See ASCORBIC ACID)

VITAMIN D

(See ERGOCALCIFEROL)

VITAMIN E

Synonym: alpha tocopherol
Trade names: Aquasol E; Eprolin; E-Vitamin Succinate; Pheryl-E; Vita Plus E; Vitec. (Various pharmaceutical companies.)
Other common trade names: *Bio E; Davitamon E; Detulin; E Perle; Ephynal; Optovit-E; Vita-E*
Indications: Vitamin E deficiency
Category: Fat-soluble vitamin
Half-life: no data
Clinically important, potentially serious interactions with: anticoagulants

Reactions

Skin

Contact dermatitis (<1%)
(1997): Parsad D+, *Contact Dermatitis* 37, 294 (xanthomatous)
(1994): Manzano D+, *Contact Dermatitis* 31, 324
(1994): Perrenoud D+, *Dermatology* 189, 225
(1992): Garcia-Bravo B+, *Contact Dermatitis* 26, 280 (generalized)
(1991): Fisher AA, *Cutis* 48, 272
(1991): de Groot AC+, *Contact Dermatitis* 25, 302
(1986): Goldman MP+, *J Am Acad Dermatol* 14, 133
(1976): Roed-Petersen J+, *Br J Dermatol* 94, 233
(1975): Schorr WF, *Am Fam Physician* 12, 90
(1975): Roed-Petersen J+, *Contact Dermatitis* 1, 391
(1973): Aeling JL+, *Arch Dermatol* 108, 579
Dermatitis (sic)
(1991): Hunter D+, *Cutis* 47, 193
Erythema multiforme
(1994): Spreux A+, *Therapie* (French) 49, 460
(1986): Fisher AA, *Cutis* 37, 158 and 262 (topical administration)
(1984): Saperstein H+, *Arch Dermatol* 120, 906
Exanthems
Lupus erythematosus
(1995): Whittam J+, *Am J Clin Nutr* 62, 1025
Urticaria

Hair

Hair – depigmentation (at injection sites)
(1972): Sehgal VN, *Dermatologica* 145, 56

Other

Gingival bleeding
(1998): Liede KE+, *Ann Med* 30, 542
Gynecomastia
(1994): Roberts HJ, *Hosp Pract Off Ed* 29, 12
Sclerosing lipogranuloma
(1983): Foucar E+, *J Am Acad Dermatol* 9, 103
Thrombophlebitis
(1979): Roberts HS, *Angiology* 30, 169
Yellow spots on dental enamel

VITAMIN K

(See PHYTONADIONE)

WARFARIN

Trade name: Coumadin (DuPont)
Other common trade names: *Aldocumar; Coumadine; Marevan; Waran; Warfilone*
Indications: Thromboembolic disease; pulmonary embolism
Category: Oral anticoagulant
Half-life: 1.5–2.5 days (highly variable)
Clinically important, potentially serious interactions with: scores of drugs; too extensive a list for review here

Note: Alternative remedies, including herbals, may potentially increase the risk of bleeding or potentiate the effects of warfarin therapy. Some of these include the following: angelica root, arnica flower, anise, asafetida, bogbean, borage seed oil, bromelain, capsicum, celery, chamomile, clove, dan shen, devil's claw, fenugreek, feverfew, garlic, ginger, ginkgo biloba, ginseng, horse chestnut, licorice root, lovage root, meadowsweet, onion, parsley, passionflower herb, poplar, quassia, red clover, rue, sweet clover, turmeric and willow bark. Also coenzyme Q_{10}, danshen, devil's claw, dong quai, ginseng, green tea, papain and vitamin E.

Reactions

Skin

Abscess
(1997): Clayton BD, *J Geriatr Dermatology* 5, 314
Acral purpura
(1986): Stone MS+, *J Am Acad Dermatol* 14, 796
Angioedema (<1%)
Bullous eruption
(1993): Elis A+, *J Intern Med* 234, 615 (hemorrhagic)
(1986): Stone MS+, *J Am Acad Dermatol* 14, 796 (passim)
Dermatitis (sic)
(1992): Breathnach SM+, *Adverse Drug Reactions and the Skin*, Blackwell, Oxford, 248 (passim)
(1991): Quintavalla R+, *Int Angiol* 10, 103
Ecchymoses
(1988): Cole MS+, *Surgery* 103, 271 (passim)
Exanthems
(1993): Antony SJ+, *South Med J* 86, 1413
(1989): Kruis-de Vries MH+, *Dermatologica* 178, 109
(1988): Cole MS+, *Surgery* 103, 271 (passim)
(1978): Kwong P+, *JAMA* 239, 1884
(1968): Schiff BL+, *Arch Dermatol* 98, 136
(1960): Adams CW+, *Circulation* 22, 947
Exfoliative dermatitis
Hemorrhagic skin infarcts
(1989): Geoghegan+, *BMJ* 298, 902
(1988): Cole MS, *Surgery* 103, 271
(1980): Schleicher SM+, *Arch Dermatol* 116, 444
Livedo reticularis
(1993): Park S+, *Arch Dermatol* 129, 775
Necrosis (>10%)
(2000): Chan YC+, *Br J Surgery* 87, 266
(1999): Stewart AJ+, *Postgrad Med J* 75, 233
(1999): Martin FL, *Am J Nursing* 99, 53
(1999): Gailine D+, *Am J Hematol* 60, 231
(1999): Yang Y+, *N Engl J Med* 340, 735
(1998): Sallah S+, *Haemostasis* 28, 25
(1998): Gelwix TJ+, *Am J Emerg Med* 16, 541
(1998): Essex DW+, *Am J Hematol* 57, 233
(1997): Wynn SS+, *Haemostasis* 27, 246
(1997): Sallah S+, *Thromb Haemost* 78, 785
(1997): English JC+, *J Am Acad Dermatol* 37, 1 (passim)
(1997): Hermes B+, *Acta Derm Venereol* 77, 35
(1996): Makris M+, *Thromb Haemost* 75, 523
(1996): Jillella AP+, *Am J Hematol* 52, 117
(1995): DeFranzo AJ+, *Ann Plast Surg* 34, 203
(1995): Sternberg ML+, *Ann Emerg Med* 26, 94
(1995): Hauben M, *N Engl J Med* 332, 959
(1994): Soisson AP+, *Mil Med* 159, 252
(1994): Lewandowski K+, *Thromb Haemost* 69, 311
(1993): Yates P+, *Clin Exp Dermatol* 18, 138
(1993): Bauer KA, *Arch Dermatol* 129, 766
(1993): Eby CS, *Hematol Oncol Clin North Am* 7, 1291
(1993): Colman RW+, *Am J Hematol* 43, 300
(1993): LaPrade RF+, *Orthopedics* 16, 703
(1993): Locht H+, *J Intern Med* 233, 287
(1993): Hiers CL, *J Ark Med Soc* 89, 443
(1993): Schramm W+, *Arch Dermatol* 129, 753
(1992): Sharafuddin MA+, *Arch Dermatol* 128, 105
(1992): Anderson DR+, *Haemostasis* 22, 124
(1992): McKnight JT+, *Arch Fam Med* 1, 105
(1992): Viegas GV, *J Am Podiatr Med Assoc* 82, 463
(1991): Berkompas DC, *Indiana Med* 84, 788
(1991): Ritchie AJ+, *Ulster Med J* 60, 248
(1991): Brooks LW+, *J Am Osteopath Assoc* 91, 601
(1991): Humphries JE+, *Am J Hematol* 37, 197
(1990): Comp PC+, *Semin Thromb Hemost* 16, 293
(1989): Grimaudo V+, *BMJ* 289, 233
(1989): Barkley C+, *J Urology* 141, 946
(1988): Kandrotas RJ+, *Pharmacotherapy* 8, 351
(1988): Conlan MG+, *Am J Hematol* 29, 226
(1988): Cole MS+, *Surgery* 103, 271
(1988): Dominic W+, *Burns Incl Therm Inj* 14, 139
(1988): Konrad P+, *Vasa*, 17, 208
(1987): Norris PG, *Clin Exp Dermatol* 12, 370
(1987): Haimovici H+, *J Vasc Surg* 5, 655
(1987): Gladson CL+, *Arch Dermatol* 123, 1701
(1986): Sjoberg A+, *Lakartidningen* (Swedish) 83, 4089
(1986): Rowbotham B+, *Aust N Z J Med* 16, 513
(1986): Everett RN+, *Postgrad Med* 79, 97
(1986): Zauber NP+, *Ann Intern Med* 104, 659
(1986): Brennan M+, *J Tenn Med Assoc* 79, 210
(1984): Franson TR+, *Arch Dermatol* 120, 927
(1984): McGehee WG+, *Ann Intern Med* 101, 59
(1984): Slutzki S+, *Int J Dermatol* 23, 117
(1984): Schwartz RA+, *Dermatologica* 168, 31 (linear localized)
(1983): Papa MA+, *Harefuah* (Hebrew) 104, 504
(1983): Caldwell EH+, *Plast Reconstr Surg* 72, 231
(1983): Leath MC, *Tex Med* 79, 62
(1982): Torngren S+, *Acta Chir Scand* 148, 471
(1982): Faraci PA, *Int J Dermatol* 21, 329
(1981): Horn JR+, *Am J Hosp Pharm* 38, 1763
(1980): Hislop IG+, *Aust N Z J Med* 10, 51
(1980): Schleicher SM+, *Arch Dermatol* 116, 444
(1979): Jones RR+, *Br J Dermatol* 101, 561
(1979): Boss JM+, *Br J Dermatol* 100, 617
(1978): Kirby JD+, *Br J Dermatol* 98, 707
(1978): Faraci PA+, *Surg Gynecol Obstet* 146, 695
(1976): Kirby JD+, *Br J Dermatol* 94, 97
(1976): Renick AM, *South Med J* 69, 775
(1975): Lacy JP+, *Ann Intern Med* 82, 381
(1971): Nalbandian RM+, *Obstet Gynecol* 38, 395
(1970): Martin CM+, *Calif Med* 113, 78
(1969): Korbitz BD+, *Am J Cardiol* 24, 420
(1969): Vaughan ED+, *JAMA* 210, 2282 (genitalia)
(1969): Lipp H+, *Med J Aust* 2, 351
(1954): Verhagen H, *Acta Med Scand* 148, 453
Pruritus (<1%)
(1978): Kwong P+, *JAMA* 239, 1884
Purplish erythema (feet and toes) (sic) (<1%)
(1998): Krahn MJ+, *Can J Cardiol* 14, 90 ("purple toes")
(1997): Sallah S+, *Thromb Haemost* 78, 785 ("purple toes")
(1994): Soisson AP+, *Mil Med* 159, 252
(1993): Park S+, *Arch Dermatol* 129, 775
(1982): Lebsack CS+, *Postgrad Med* 71, 81 ("purple toes")
(1981): Akle CA+, *J R Soc Med* 74, 219 (purple toe syndrome)
(1978): Kwong P+, *JAMA* 239, 1884
(1961): Feder W+, *Ann Intern Med* 55, 911
Purpura
(1988): Cole MS+, *Surgery* 103, 271 (passim)
(1978): Friedenberg WR+, *Arch Dermatol* 114, 578 (fulminans)
Rash (sic) (<1%)
Urticaria
(1988): Cole MS+, *Surgery* 103, 271 (passim)
(1986): Stone MS+, *J Am Acad Dermatol* 14, 796 (passim)
(1959): Sheps ES+, *Am J Cardiol* 3, 118
Vasculitis
(1998): Krahn MJ+, *Can J Cardiol* 14, 90
(1994): Tamir A+, *Acta Derm Venereol* 74, 138
(1982): Howitt AJ+, *Postgrad Med J* 58, 233
(1982): Tanay A+, *Dermatologica* 165, 178

Vesicular eruption
(1986): Stone MS+, *J Am Acad Dermatol* 14, 796 (passim)

Hair

Hair – alopecia (>10%)
(1995): Nagao T+, *Lancet* 346, 1004
(1989): Kruis-de Vries MH+, *Dermatologica* 178, 109 (passim)
(1988): Umlas J+, *Cutis* 42, 63
(1986): Stone MS+, *J Am Acad Dermatol* 14, 796 (passim)
(1969): Baker H+, *Br J Dermatol* 81, 236
(1957): Cornbleet T+, *Arch Dermatol* 75, 440

Other

Gangrene
(1978): Hardisty CA, *Postgrad Med J* 54, 123
(1976): Shnider M+, *Can J Surg* 19, 64
(1973): Chua FS+, *J Thorac Cardiovasc Surg* 65, 238
Hematomas
(1997): Clayton BD, *J Geriatr Dermatology* 5, 314
Hypersensitivity
(1968): Schiff BL+, *Arch Dermatol* 98, 136
Oral ulceration (<1%)
Priapism
(1997): Daryanani S+, *Clin Lab Haematol* 19, 213

YOHIMBINE

Trade names: Actibine (Consolidated Midland); Aphrodyne (Star); Yocon (Palisades); Yohimex (Kramer); Yomax
Indications: Impotence, orthostatic hypertension
Category: Impotence therapy agent; alpha$_2$-adrenergic blocking agent
Half-life: 36 minutes
Clinically important, potentially serious interactions with: clonidine

Reactions

Skin

Diaphoresis
Exfoliative dermatitis
(1993): Sandler B+, *Urology* 41, 343
Flushing
Lupus erythematosus
(1993): Sandler B+, *Urology* 41, 343

ZAFIRLUKAST

Trade name: Accolate (AstraZeneca)
Indications: Asthma
Category: Antiasthmatic; leukotriene receptor antagonist
Half-life: 10 hours
Clinically important, potentially serious interactions with: aspirin, erythromycin, terfenadine, theophylline, warfarin

Reactions

Skin

Allergic granulomatous angiitis (Churg–Strauss syndrome)
(1999): Green RL+, *Lancet* 353, 725 (2 cases)
(1999): Wechsler ME+, *Chest* 116, 266
(1999): Wechsler ME+, *Lancet* 353, 1970
(1998): Wechsler ME+, *JAMA* 279, 457
(1998): Holloway J+, *J Am Osteopath Assoc* 98, 275
(1998): Knoell DL+, *Chest* 114, 332
(1998): Churg J+, *JAMA* 279, 1949
(1998): Honsinger RW, *JAMA* 279, 1949
(1998): Katz RS+, *JAMA* 279, 1949
Lupus erythematosus
(1999): Finkel TH+, *J Allergy Clin Immunol* 103, 533

Other

Myalgia (1.6%)

ZALCITABINE

Synonyms: ddC; dideoxycytidine
Trade name: Hivid (Roche)
Indications: Advanced HIV disease
Category: Antiretroviral; nucleoside reverse transcriptase inhibitor (NRTI)
Half-life: 2.9 hours
Clinically important, potentially serious interactions with: aminoglycosides, amphotericin, didanosine, foscarnet, lamivudine, probenecid, stavudine

Reactions

Skin

Acne (<1%)
Angioedema
(1988): Yarchoan R+, *Lancet* 1, 76 (5%)
Ankle edema
(1989): Jeffries DJ, *J Antimicrob Chemother* 23, 29
Bullous eruption (<1%)
Cutaneous side effects (sic)
(1991): Yarchoan R+, *Blood* 78, 859
(1990): Broder S+, *Am J Med* 88, 31S
Dermatitis (sic) (<1%)
Diaphoresis (<1%)
Edema (<1%)
(1991): Pluda JM+, *Hematol Oncol Clin North Am* 5, 229
(1991): Yarchoan R+, *Blood* 78, 859
(1989): McNeely MC+, *J Am Acad Dermatol* 21, 1213 (70%) (dose-related)
Erythema multiforme
(1995): Wardropper AG+, *Int J STD AIDS* 6, 450
Erythroderma
(1989): McNeely MC+, *J Am Acad Dermatol* 21, 1213 (10%)
Exanthems (<1%)
(1991): Pluda JM+, *Hematol Oncol Clin North Am* 5, 229
(1991): Fischl MA, *Recent Advances in Antiretroviral Therapy*, New York, Triclinica Communications
(1991): Merigan TC, *Am J Med* 90, 8S
(1990): Pizzo PA+, *J Pediatr* 117, 799
(1989): McNeely MC+, *J Am Acad Dermatol* 21, 1213 (40%)
(1989): Merigan TC+, *Ann Intern Med* 110, 189 (66%)
(1989): Yarchoan R+, *N Engl J Med* 321, 726 (1–5%)
(1988): Yarchoan R+, *Lancet* 1, 76 (65%)
(1987): Richman DD+, *N Engl J Med* 317, 192 (1–5%)
Exfoliative dermatitis (<1%)
Flushing (<1%)
Folliculitis
Photosensitivity (<1%)
Pruritus (3–5%)
Rash (sic) (2–11%)
(1990): Bozzette SA+, *Am J Med* 88, 24S
(1989): Jeffries DJ, *J Antimicrob Chemother* 23, 29
Urticaria (3.4%)
(1992): Roche Laboratories Monograph
Xerosis (<1%)

Hair

Hair – alopecia

Nails

Nails – changes
(1989): Jeffries DJ, *J Antimicrob Chemother* 23, 29

Other

Ageusia (<1%)
Anaphylactoid reaction
(1992): Roche Laboratories Monograph
Aphthous stomatitis
(1991): Fischl MA, *Recent Advances in Antiretroviral Therapy.* New York, Triclinica Communications
(1991): Merigan TC, *Am J Med* 90, 8S
(1991): Pluda JM+, *Hematol Oncol Clin North Am* 5, 229
(1989): Jeffries DJ, *J Antimicrob Chemother* 23, 29
(1989): Yarchoan R+, *N Engl J Med* 321, 726
(1988): Yarchoan R+, *Lancet* 1, 76
Dysgeusia (<1%)
Gingivitis (<1%)
Glossitis (<1%)
Glossodynia (<1%)
Myalgia (1–6%)
Myopathy (<1%)
Oral mucosal lesions (3%)
(1991): Fischl MA, *Recent Advances in Antiretroviral Therapy.* New York, Triclinica Communications
(1989): Merigan TC+, *Ann Intern Med* 110, 189 (73%)
(1988): Yarchoan R+, *Lancet* 1, 76 (40%)
Oral ulceration (3–7%)
(1990): Bozzette SA+, *Am J Med* 88, 24S
(1990): Pizzo PA+, *J Pediatr* 117, 799 (painful)
(1989): McNeely MC+, *J Am Acad Dermatol* 21, 1213 (64%)
Paresthesias
Parosmia (<1%)
Penile edema (<1%)
Stomatitis (3%)
(1991): Yarchoan R+, *Blood* 78, 859
Tongue disorder (sic) (<1%)
Xerostomia (<1%)

ZALEPLON

Trade name: Sonata (Wyeth-Ayerst)
Indications: Insomnia
Category: Nonbenzodiazepine hypnotic and sedative
Half-life: 1 hour
Clinically important, potentially serious interactions with: alcohol, cimetidine, imipramine, rifampin, thioridazine

Reactions

Skin

Acne (<1%)
Cheilitis (<1%)
Chills (<1%)
Contact dermatitis (<1%)

Diaphoresis (<1%)
Ecchymoses (<1%)
Eczema (<1%)
Edema (<1%)
Exanthems (<1%)
Facial edema (<1%)
Peripheral edema (1–10%)
Photosensitivity (1–10%)
Pigmentation (<1%)
Pruritus (<1%)
Psoriasis (<1%)
Purpura (<1%)
Pustular eruption (<1%)
Rash (sic) (<1%)
Xerosis (<1%)
Vesiculobullous eruption (<1%)

Hair

Hair – alopecia (<1%)

Other

Ageusia (<1%)
Aphthous stomatitis (<1%)
Gingival hemorrhage (<1%)
Gingivitis (<1%)
Glossitis (<1%)
Hyperesthesia (<1%)
Hypesthesia (2%)
Mastodynia (<1%)
Myalgia (5%)
Oral ulceration (<1%)
Paresthesias (3%)
Parosmia (2%)
Sialorrhea (<1%)
Stomatitis (<1%)
Thrombophlebitis (<1%)
Tongue discoloration (<1%)
Tremor (1–10%)
Vaginitis (<1%)
Xerostomia (1–10%)

ZANAMIVIR

Trade name: Relenza (GlaxoWellcome)
Indications: Influenza A and B
Category: Inhibitor of viral neuranimidase (by oral inhalation)
Half-life: 2.5–5.1 hours
Clinically important, potentially serious interactions with: no data

Reactions

Skin

Infections (sic) (2%)
Urticaria (<1.5%)

Other

Myalgia (<1.5%)

ZIDOVUDINE

Synonyms: azidothymidine; AZT; compound S
Trade names: Combivir (GlaxoWellcome); Retrovir (GlaxoWellcome)
Other common trade names: *Novo-AZT; Retrovis*
Indications: HIV infection
Category: Antiretroviral; nucleoside reverse transcriptase inhibitor (NRTI)
Half-life: 1 hour
Clinically important, potentially serious interactions with: acetaminophen, acyclovir, amphotericin B, aspirin, cimetidine, dapsone, flucytosine, ganciclovir, indomethacin, lorazepam, pentamidine, probenecid, valproic acid, vinblastine, vincristine

Reactions

Skin

Acne (<5%)
(1988): McEvoy GK, *Am Hosp Formulary Service: Drug Info* 392
Blue vitiligo (sic)
(1994): Ivker R+, *J Am Acad Dermatol* 30, 829
Bullous eruption
(1989): Caumes E+, *Presse Med* (French) 18, 1708 (fatal in AIDS)
Diaphoresis (5–19%)
(1988): McEvoy GK, *Am Hosp Formulary Service: Drug Info* 392
Ecchymoses
(1992): Breathnach SM+, *Adverse Drug Reactions and the Skin*, Blackwell, Oxford, 172 (passim)
Erythema multiforme
(1989): Yarchoan R+, *N Engl J Med* 321, 726
(1989): Langtry HD+, *Drugs* 37, 408
Erythroderma
(1996): Duque S+, *J Allergy Clin Immunol* 98, 234
Exanthems
(1990): Petty BG+, *Lancet* 335, 1044 (1–5%) (in AIDS patients)
(1989): Gelman K+, *AIDS* 3, 555 (>5%)
(1989): Langtry HD+, *Drugs* 37, 408
(1987): Richman DD+, *N Engl J Med* 317, 192
Heightened cutaneous reactions to mosquito bites (sic)
(1988): Diven DG+, *Arch Intern Med* 148, 2296
Neutrophilic eccrine hidradenitis
(1990): Smith KJ+, *J Am Acad Dermatol* 23, 945
Pigmentation
(1993): Hermanns-Le T+, *Ann Pathol* (French) 13, 328
(1992): Hill DA+, *Hosp Pract Off Ed* 27, 29
(1992): Baudo F+, *Eur J Dermatol* 2, 448
(1991): Tal A+, *Cutis* 48, 153
(1991): Poizot-Martin I+, *Presse Med* (French) 20, 632
(1990): Greenberg RG+, *J Am Acad Dermatol* 22, 327
(1989): Bendick C+, *Arch Dermatol* 125, 1285 (palms and soles)
(1989): Merenich JA+, *Am J Med* 86, 469
(1989): Valencia ME+, *Med Clin (Barc)* (Spanish) 92, 357
Pruritus
(1989): Gelman K+, *AIDS* 3, 555 (>5%)
(1988): McEvoy GK, *Am Hosp Formulary Service: Drug Info* 392
Purpura
Rash (sic) (17%)
(1996): Henry K+, *Ann Intern Med* 124, 855
(1987): Richman DD+, *N Engl J Med* 317, 192
Stevens–Johnson syndrome
(1989): Langtry HD+, *Drugs* 37, 408
(1989): Yarchoan R+, *N Engl J Med* 321, 726
Toxic epidermal necrolysis
(1996): Murri R+, *Clin Infect Dis* 23, 640
Urticaria (<5%)
(1990): McKinley GF+, *Lancet* 336, 384
(1988): McEvoy GK, *Am Hosp Formulary Service: Drug Info* 392
Vasculitis
(1992): Torres RA+, *Arch Intern Med* 152, 850
(1990): Lee MH+, *Int Conf AIDS* 6, 360 (leukocytoclastic)

Hair

Hair – alopecia
(1996): Geletko SM+, *Pharmacotherapy* 16, 69

Hair – hypertrichosis (eyelashes)
(1991): Klutman NE+, *N Engl J Med* 324, 1896
(1991): Sahai J+, *AIDS* 5, 1395

Nails

Nails – blue lunulae
(1990): Don PC+, *Ann Intern Med* 112, 145 (30–67%)
Nails – paronychia
(1999): Russo F+, *J Am Acad Dermatol* 40, 322
Nails – pigmentation (1–10%)
(1992): Rahav G+, *Scand J Infect Dis* 24, 557
(1991): Sahai J+, *AIDS* 5, 1395
(1990): Ramos C+, *Rev Clin Esp* (Spanish) 187, 94
(1990): Poizot-Martin I+, *Int Conf AIDS* 6, 357
(1990): Greenberg RG+, *J Am Acad Dermatol* 22, 327
(1990): Don PC+, *Ann Intern Med* 112, 145 (42%)
(1989): Yarchoan R+, *N Engl J Med* 321, 726
(1989): Langtry HD+, *Drugs* 37, 408
(1989): Fisher CA+, *Cutis* 43, 552
(1989): Groark SP+, *J Am Acad Dermatol* 21, 1032
(1989): Anders KH+, *J Am Acad Dermatol* 21, 792
(1989): Bendick C+, *Arch Dermatol* 125, 1285
(1989): Merenich JA+, *Am J Med* 86, 469
(1989): Depaoli MA+, *G Ital Dermatol Venereol* (Italian) 124, 71
(1989): Dupon M+, *Scand J Infect Dis* 21, 237
(1988): Gonzalez-Lahoz JM+, *Rev Clin Esp* (Spanish) 183, 278 (bluish)
(1988): Vaiopoulos G+, *Ann Intern Med* 108, 777
(1988): Azon-Masoliver A+, *Arch Dermatol* 124, 1570
(1987): Furth PA+, *Ann Intern Med* 107, 350
Nails – pigmented bands
(1991): Tadini G+, *Arch Dermatol* 127, 267
(1990): Grau-Massanes M+, *J Am Acad Dermatol* 22, 687
(1990): Tosti A+, *Dermatologica* 180, 217 (longitudinal)
(1989): Valencia ME+, *Rev Clin Esp* (Spanish) 185, 167 (blue striae)
(1989): Bendick C+, *Z Hautkr* (German) 64, 91

Other

Bromhidrosis (<5%)
(1988): McEvoy GK, *Am Hosp Formulary Service: Drug Info* 392
Dysgeusia (5–19%)
(1988): McEvoy GK, *Am Hosp Formulary Service: Drug Info* 392
(1987): Richman DD+, *N Engl J Med* 317, 192
Edema of lip (<5%)
(1988): McEvoy GK, *Am Hosp Formulary Service: Drug Info* 392
Foetor ex ore (halitosis)
Gingival bleeding
Hypersensitivity
Myopathy (<1%)
(1993): Simpson DM+, *Neurology* 43, 971
(1989): Gertner E+, *Am J Medicine* 86, 814
(1988): Helbert M+, *Lancet* 2, 689
Oral lichenoid eruption
(1993): Ficarra G+, *Oral Surg Oral Med Oral Pathol* 76, 460
Oral mucosal eruption
(1989): Gelman K+, *AIDS* 3, 555 (>5%)
Oral mucosal pigmentation
(1991): Poizot-Martin I+, *Presse Med* (French) 20, 632
(1991): Tadini G+, *Arch Dermatol* 127, 267
(1990): Ficarra G+, *Oral Surg Oral Med Oral Pathol* 70, 748
(1990): Poizot-Martin I+, *Int Conf AIDS* 6, 357
(1990): Grau-Massanes M+, *J Am Acad Dermatol* 22, 687
(1990): Greenberg RG+, *J Am Acad Dermatol* 22, 327
(1989): Merenich JA+, *Am J Med* 86, 469
Oral ulceration (<5%)
(1988): McEvoy GK, *Am Hosp Formulary Service: Drug Info* 392
Paresthesias (<8%)
(1988): McEvoy GK, *Am Hosp Formulary Service: Drug Info* 392
Polymyositis
(1988): Bessen LJ+, *N Engl J Med* 318, 708 (4 patients)
Porphyria cutanea tarda
(1988): Ong EL+, *Postgrad Med J* 64, 956
Tongue edema (<5%)
(1988): McEvoy GK, *Am Hosp Formulary Service: Drug Info* 392
Tongue pigmentation
(1991): Tadini G+, *Arch Dermatol* 127, 267
(1991): Tal A+, *Cutis* 48, 153
(1990): Greenberg RG+, *J Am Acad Dermatol* 22, 327
(1990): Grau-Massanes M+, *J Am Acad Dermatol* 22, 687
Tongue ulceration
(1993): Schwander S+, *Med Klin* (German) 88, 60

ZILEUTON

Trade name: Zyflo (Abbott)
Indications: Asthma
Category: Antiasthmatic bronchodilator; leukotriene receptor inhibitor
Half-life: 2.5 hours
Clinically important, potentially serious interactions with: anticoagulants, astemizole, cisapride, nifedipine, propranolol, terfenadine, theophylline, xanthines, warfarin

Reactions

Skin

Erythema nodosum
(2000): Dellaripa PF+, *Mayo Clin Proc* 75, 643
Pruritus (>1%)

Other

Myalgia (3.2%)
Paresthesias (1%)
Vaginitis (>1%)

ZOLMITRIPTAN

Trade name: Zomig (AstraZeneca)
Indications: Migraine attacks
Category: Antimigraine; serotonin agonist
Half-life: 3 hours
Clinically important, potentially serious interactions with: cimetidine, ergot, estrogens, fluoxetine, fluvoxamine, MAO inhibitors, paroxetine, sertraline, SSRIs

Reactions

Skin

Allergy (sic) (<1%)
Diaphoresis (2%)
Ecchymoses (<1%)
Edema (<1%)
Facial edema (<1%)
Flushing
Hot flashes (>10%)
Photosensitivity (<1%)
Pruritus (<1%)
Rash (sic) (<1%)
Urticaria (<1%)

Other

Hyperesthesia (<1%)
Hypesthesia (2%)
Myalgia (2%)
Paresthesias (9%)
(1998): Multiple Authors, *Headache* 38, 173 (11%)
Parosmia (<1%)
Thrombophlebitis (<1%)
Tongue edema (<1%)
Twitching (<1%)
Xerostomia (3%)
(1997): Edmeads JG+, *Cephalalgia* 17, 41

ZOLPIDEM

Trade name: Ambien (Searle)
Other common trade names: *Niotal; Stilnoct; Stilnox*
Indications: Insomnia
Category: Nonbenzodiazepine sedative-hypnotic
Half-life: 2.6 hours
Clinically important, potentially serious interactions with: alcohol, CNS depressants, flumazenil, ritonavir, sertraline, food

Reactions

Skin

Acne (<1%)
Allergic reactions (sic) (4%)
Bullous eruption (<1%)
Dermatitis (sic) (<1%)
Diaphoresis (<1%)
Edema (<1%)
Facial edema (<1%)
Flushing (<1%)
Furunculosis (<1%)
Herpes simplex (<1%)
Herpes zoster (<1%)
Hot flashes (<1%)
Periorbital edema (<1%)
Photosensitivity (<1%)
Pruritus
(1994): Litt JZ, Beachwood, OH, personal case (observation)
Purpura (<1%)
Rash (sic) (2%)
Urticaria (<1%)

Other

Anaphylactoid reaction (<1%)
Dysgeusia (<1%)
Hypesthesia (<1%)
Injection-site inflammation (<1%)
Mastodynia (<1%)
Myalgia (7%)
Paresthesias (<1%)
Tremor (<1%)
Vaginitis (<1%)
Xerostomia (3%)

ZONISAMIDE

Trade name: Zonegran (Elan Pharma)
Indications: Epilepsy
Category: Anticonvulsant, sulfonamide*
Half-life: 63 hours
Clinically important, potentially serious interactions with: carbamazepine, phenobarbital, phenytoin, valproate

Reactions

Skin

Acne (<1%)
Allergic reactions (<1%)
Diaphoresis (<1%)
Ecchymoses (2%)
Eczema (<1%)
Edema (<1%)
Exanthems (<1%)
Facial edema (<1%)
Lupus erythematosus (<1%)
Peripheral edema (<1%)
Petechiae (<1%)
Pruritus (<1%)
Purpura (2%)
Pustular eruption (<1%)
Rash (sic) (3%)
Stevens–Johnson syndrome
(1985): Wilensky AJ+, *Epilepsia* 26, 212
Toxic epidermal necrolysis
Urticaria (<1%)
Vesiculobullous eruption (<1%)
Xerosis (<1%)

Hair

Hair – alopecia (<1%)
Hair – hirsutism (<1%)

Other

Dysgeusia (2%)
Gingival hyperplasia (<1%)
Gingivitis (<1%)
Glossitis (<1%)
Gynecomastia (<1%)
(1998): Ikeda A+, *J Neurol Neurosurg Psychiatry* 65, 803
Hyperesthesia (<1%)
Hyperpyrexia
(1997): Shimizu T+, *Brain Dev* 19, 366
Hypersensitivity
Myalgia (<1%)
Oligohydrosis
(1999): Isumi H+, *No To Hattatsu* (Japanese) 31, 468
(1997): Shimizu T+, *Brain Dev* 19, 366
(1996): Okumura A+, *No To Hattatsu* (Japanese) 28, 44
Oral ulceration (<1%)
Paresthesias (4%)
Parosmia (<1%)
Stomatitis (<1%)
Thrombophlebitis (<1%)
Tremor (<1%)
(1992): Taira T, *No To Shinkei* (Japanese) 44, 61
Ulcerative stomatitis (<1%)
Xerostomia (2%)

***Note:** Zonisamide is a sulfonamide and can be absorbed systemically. Sulfonamides can produce severe, possibly fatal, reactions such as toxic epidermal necrolysis and Stevens–Johnson syndrome.

HERBALS, BOTANICALS, TRACE ELEMENTS, SUPPLEMENTS AND MISCELLANEOUS

Botanicals have become more and more popular in the past few years. More than five billion dollars are being spent in the United States each year on these untested, purported remedies, and this number is growing. People have been using herbs to treat and prevent medical problems long before modern drugs arrived on the scene. Eighty percent of the world's population still uses herbs – leaves, roots, berries or extracts – as their primary source of medicine.

One in three Americans are now self-medicating with herbals routinely to promote good health or cure illness. One of the perils of this new craze is that three out of every four people taking these so-called medications never impart this information to their physicians.

Herbal medicines come in a variety of forms: flowers, fruit, leaves, stems, seeds, bark and roots of plants; these are available raw and whole, brewed into teas, dried and pulverized into powders, dissolved in liquid tinctures, or processed into pills, capsules or topical remedies.

Medicinal herbs are most commonly used for minor complaints such as aches and pains, digestive problems, premenstrual symptoms and menstrual cramps, upper respiratory infections, insomnia, and skin ailments.

There are few, if any, data supporting claimed benefits from the list below. These so-called nutraceuticals are not regulated as drugs, and rigid quality control standards are not required for them. Since they are not rigorously tested, they cannot be marketed for the cure, diagnosis or prevention of disease.

Although patients may believe that herbal products are inherently safe because they are "natural," there are, in fact, many interactions of herbals to prescription and over-the-counter medications as well as adverse reactions that can ensue.

Some of the common herbals and their interactions and adverse reactions on the skin and hair (almost all of which are anecdotal) follow. I have employed the common names of these products and I will follow with the formal and precise botanical name, where accessible.

ARNICA

Scientific names: *Arnica montana, Arnica fulgens, Arnica sororia*, etc.
Other common names: Arnica Flos, Arnica Flower, Leopard's Bane, Wolf's Bane, etc.
Family: Asteraceae; Compositae
Purported indications: Inflammation and immune system stimulation associated with bruises, aches and sprains; insect bites; superficial phlebitis. Diuretic (Historically used as an abortifacient.)
Other uses: Flavoring agent, candy, puddings; found in hair tonics, anti-dandruff shampoos, etc.
Clinically important, potentially serious interactions with: anticoagulants, antiplatelets

Adverse side-effects

Skin
Allergic reactions (sic)
Contact dermatitis
Dermal irritation (sic)
Sweet's syndrome

Other
Mucous membrane irritation (sic)

BLACK COHOSH

Scientific names: *Cimicifuga racemosa, Actaea racemosa, Actaea macrotys*
Other common names: Baneberry, Black Snakeroot, Bugbane, Cimifuga, Rattle Root, Rattle Snakeroot, Rattleweed, Squawroot, etc.
Family: Ranunculaceae
Purported indications: Hormone replacement therapy; dysmenorrhea; hot flashes
Other uses: Dyspepsia, rheumatism, fever, sore throat, cough, insect repellent. Fresh root applied topically for rattlesnake bites
Clinically important, potentially serious interactions with: tamoxifen

Adverse side-effects

Skin
Diaphoresis
Toxic reactions (sic)

Note: Black cohosh was also used as an ingredient in Lydia Pinkham's Vegetable Compound

BLOODROOT

Scientific name: *Sanguinaria canadensis*
Other common names: Blood Root, Coon Root, Indian Plant, Indian Red Paint, Red Puccoon, Red Root, Sanguinaria, Snakebite, Sweet Slumber, Tetterwort
Family: Papaveraceae
Purported indications: Orally, used as an emetic, cathartic, expectorant and antispasmodic. Topically, used as an irritant and debriding agent and, in dentistry, to remove plaque
Other uses: Bronchitis, asthma, croup, laryngitis, pharyngitis, scabies, eczema, athlete's foot, nasal polyps, rheumatism, arts, cancer, dental analgesia, fever, anemia and general tonic
Clinically important, potentially serious interactions with: no data

Adverse side-effects

Skin

Contact dermatitis
(1998): Brinker F, *Contraindications and Drug Interactions*, Eclectic Medical Publications
Irritation (sic)

CHAMOMILE

Scientific names: *Chamomilla recutita; Matricaria chamomilla; Matricaria recutita*
Other common names: German Chamomile; Camomille Allemande; Echte Kamille; Fleur de Camomile; Manzanilla; Pin Heads; Wild Chamomile, etc.
Family: Asteraceae; Compositae
Purported indications: Flatulence; travel sickness; nervous diarrhea; restlessness; menstrual cramps
Other uses: Hemorrhoids, mastitis, leg ulcers, inflammation of the respiratory tract. Used in flavoring, cosmetics, soaps and mouthwashes
Clinically important, potentially serious interactions with: anticoagulants, benzodiazepines, sedatives

Adverse side-effects

SKIN

Allergic reactions (to those allergic to ragweed, marigolds, daisies)
Contact dermatitis
Irritation

Other

Anaphylactoid reaction
(1989): Subiza J+, *J Allergy Clin Immunol* 84, 353
Hypersensitivity

CHONDROITIN

Scientific names: Chondroitin 4-sulfate; chondroitin 4- and 6-sulfate
Other common names: CDS; Chondroitin Sulfate A; Chondroitin Sulfate C, CSA, CSC, GAG
Family: N/A
Purported indications: Osteoarthritis (often in combination with glucosamine); ischemic heart disease; osteoporosis; hyperlipidemia
Other uses: Keratoconjunctivitis, an agent in cataract surgery
Clinically important, potentially serious interactions with: ardeparin, aspirin, dalteparin, dextran, dipyridamole, exoxaparin, heparin, NSAIDs, warfarin

Adverse side-effects

Skin

Allergic reactions (sic)
Eyelid edema
(2000): Leeb BF+, *J Rheumatology* 27, 205
Peripheral edema

HAIR

Hair – alopecia

DAN-SHEN

Scientific names: *Salvia miltiorrhiza* (red sage); *Gansu danshen*; Southern danshen
Other common names: Chinese Red Sage; Huang Ken; Red Rooted Sage; Red Sage; Salvia Root; Tzu Tan-Ken
Family: Labiatae/Lamiaceae
Purported indications: Circulation problems; ischemic stroke; angina pectoris; cardiovascular disease
Other uses: menstrual problems, chronic hepatitis, abdominal masses, insomnia, acne, psoriasis, eczema, bruising
Clinically important, potentially serious interactions with: anticoagulants, antiplatelets, warfarin, **herbs with anticoagulant/antiplatelet potential**

Adverse side-effects

Skin

Pruritus

ECHINACEA

Scientific names: *Echinacea angustifola; Echinacea pallida; Echinacea purpurea*
Other common names: American Cone Flower; Black Sampson; Black Susans; Comb Flower; Indian Head; Purple-Cone Flower; Snakeroot, etc.
Family: Asteraceae; Compositae
Purported indications: Colds and upper respiratory infections; antiseptic; antiviral; immune stimulant; peripheral vasodilator; urinary tract infections; yeast infections
Other uses: skin wounds, skin ulcers, psoriasis, herpes simplex, septicemia, tonsillitis, boils, abscesses, rheumatism, migraines, dyspepsia, pain, eczema, rattlesnake bites, syphilis, typhoid, malaria, diphtheria, bee stings and hemorrhoids
Clinically important, potentially serious interactions with: CYP450 3A4 isoenzymes, econazole

Adverse side-effects

SKIN

Allergic reactions (sic)
Angioedema
(2000): www.aaaai.org/media/pressreleases/2000/03/000307.html
Urticaria
(2000): www.aaaai.org/media/pressreleases/2000/03/000307.html

OTHER

Anaphylactoid reaction
(2000): www.aaaai.org/media/pressreleases/2000/03/000307.html
(1998): Mullins RJ, *Med J Aust* 168, 170
Hypersensitivity
(2000): www.aaaai.org/media/pressreleases/2000/03/000307.html (23 cases)
Paresthesias
Sialorrhea

Note: Individuals with atopy may be more likely to experience an allergic reaction when taking Echinacea

EPHEDRA

Scientific names: *Ephedra sinica; Ephedra intermedia; Ephedra equisetina; Ephedra distachya; Ephedra gerardiana*
Other common names: Desert Herb; Joint Fir; Ma Huang; Mahuang; Popotillo; Sea Grape; Teamster's Tea; Yellow Astringent; Yellow Horse, etc.
Family: Ephedraceae
Purported indications: Bronchospasm; asthma; bronchitis; allergic disorders; central nervous stimulant; cardiovascular stimulant; appetite suppressant
Other uses: Colds, flu, fever, chills, edema, headache, anhidrosis, diuretic, joint and bone pain
Clinically important, potentially serious interactions with: amitriptyline, caffeine, dexamethasone, digoxin, MAO inhibitors, oxytocin, reserpine, theophylline, **coffee, tea**

Adverse side-effects

Skin
Flushing

Other
Eosinophilia-myalgia syndrome
(1999): Zaacks SM+, *J Toxicol Clin Toxicol* 37, 485
Hypersensitivity
Myalgia
Myopathy
Tremor

FEVERFEW

Scientific names: *Tanacetum parthenium; Chrysanthemum parthenium; Pyrethrum parthenium*
Other common names: Atamisa; Bachelor's Button; Featerfoiul; Featherfew; Featherfoil; Santa Maria
Family: Asteraceae; Compositae
Purported indications: fever; headache; migraine; menstrual irregularites; arthritis; psoriasis; allergies; asthma; tinnitus; vertigo; nausea; vomiting
Other uses: Infertility, cancer, common cold, earache, liver disease, prevention of miscarriage, orthopedic disorders, swollen feet, diarrhea, dyspepsia. General stimulant and tonic
Clinically important, potentially serious interactions with: anticoagulants, antiplatelets, NSAIDs

Adverse side-effects

Skin
Angioedema (lips)
(1998): Awang DVC, *Int Med* 1, 11
(1985): Johnson ES+, *BMJ (Clin Res Ed)* 291, 569
Contact dermatitis
(1996): Lamminpaa A+, *Contact Dermatitis* 34, 330

Other
Ageusia
(1998): Awang DVC, *Int Med* 1, 11
(1985): Johnson ES+, *BMJ (Clin Res Ed)* 291, 569
Oral ulceration
(1998): Awang DVC, *Int Med* 1, 11
(1985): Johnson ES+, *BMJ (Clin Res Ed)* 291, 569

GARLIC

Scientific name: *Allium sativum*
Other common names: Ail; Ajo; Allium; Camphor of the Poor; Clove Garlic; Nectar of the Gods; Poor Man's Treacle; Rust Treacle; Stinking Rose
Family: Amaryllidaceae; Liliaceae
Purported indications: Hypertension; hypercholesterolemia; preventing atherosclerosis; earaches; menstrual disorders; cancer prevention; immune system stimulation
Other uses: Diabetes, allergies, 'flu, arthritis, traveler's diarrhea, bacterial and fungal infections, tinea corporis, tines pedis and onychomycosis. Vaginitis. Flavor component
Clinically important, potentially serious interactions with: anticoagulants, antiplatelets, aspirin, clopidogrel, enoxaparin, insulin, **ginger**

Adverse side-effects

Skin
Bullous eruption
(1993): Garty BZ, *Pediatrics* 91, 658
Contact dermatitis
(1987): Cronin E, *Contact Dermatitis* 17, 265

Other
Anaphylactoid reaction
Foetor ex ore (halitosis)
Stomatodynia

GINGER

Scientific names: *Zingiber officinale*
Other common names: African Ginger; Black Ginger; Cochin Ginger; Gingembre; Ginger Root; Jamaica Ginger; Race Ginger; Zingiberis rhizoma
Family: Zingiberaceae
Purported indications: Motion sickness; colic; dyspepsia; flatulence; rheumatoid arthritis; loss of appetite; post-surgical nausea and vomiting; discontinuing SSRI drug therapy
Other uses: Anorexia, upper respiratory infections, cough, bronchitis. thermal burns, flavoring agent, fragrance component in soaps and cosmetics
Clinically important, potentially serious interactions with: antacids, antiplatelet medications, proton pump inhibitors, sucralfate, **garlic**

Adverse side-effects

Skin
Dermatitis (sic)

GINKGO BILOBA

Scientific names: *Ginkgo biloba*
Other common names: Fossil Tree; Ginkgo; Ginkgo Folium; Ginkyo; Japanese Silver Apricot; Kew Tree; Maidenhair Tree; Salisburia
Family: Ginkgoaceae
Purported indications: Dementia; Alzheimer's disease; memory loss; headache; tinnitus; vertigo; dizziness; mood disturbances; hearing disorders; intermittent claudication; attention deficit-hyperactivity disorder
Other uses: Premenstrual syndrome, thrombosis, heart disease, hypercholesterolemia, dysentery, filariasis, diabetic retinopathy. Wound dressings, psychiatric conditions in the elderly
Clinically important, potentially serious interactions with: anticoagulants, antiplatelets, aspirin, dipyridamole, MAO inhibitors, thiazides, ticlopidine, trazodone, warfarin, vitamin E, **garlic, ginger, ginseng, licorice**, etc.

Adverse side-effects

Skin
Allergic reactions (sic)
Contact dermatitis
Erythema
Pruritus
Rash
Vasculitis
Vesicular eruption

Other
Phlebitis
Rectal burning (sic)
Stomatitis

Note: *Ginkgo biloba* is the oldest living tree species in the world. Ginkgo trees can live as long as 1000 years. Ginkgo is the most frequently prescribed herbal medicine in Germany

GINSENG

Scientific names: *Panax ginseng*
Other common names: Asian Ginseng; Asiatic Ginseng; Chinese Ginseng; Ginseng Radix; Ginseng Root; Japanese Ginseng; Jintsam; Korean Ginseng; Korean Red; Ninjin; Oriental Ginseng; Panax Ginseng; Red Ginseng; Ren She; Sang; Seng
Family: Araliaceae
Purported indications: General tonic; stimulating the immune system. improving physical stamina; athletic stamina; cognitive function; concentration and work efficiency; diuretic; antidepressant
Other uses: Premature ejaculation, anemia, diabetes, gastritis, neurasthenia, impotence, fever and hangover. Used in soaps, cosmetics and flavorings
Clinically important, potentially serious interactions with: anticoagulants, antidiabetics, antiplatelets, antipsychotics, caffeine, furosemide, insulin, warfarin

Adverse side-effects

SKIN
Allergic reactions (sic)
Edema
Pruritus
Stevens–Johnson syndrome
(1996): Dega H+, *Lancet* 313, 756

Other
Mastodynia
(1978): Palmer BV+, *BMJ* 1, 1284
Penile pain

Note: Ginseng has been used for medicinal purposes for more than 2000 years. Approximately 6,000,000 Americans use it regularly

GREEN TEA

Scientific names: *Camellia sinensis; Camellia thea; Camellia theifera; Thea sinensis; Thea bohea; Thea viridis*
Other common names: Chinese tea; tea
Family: Theaceae
Purported indications: Improving cognitive performance; stomach disorders; nausea; vomiting; diarrhea; headaches
Other uses: Crohn's disease, reduces risk of prostate and colon cancer, protects against heart disease, dental caries, kidney stones. Prevents skin cancer related to UV radiation. Topically, green tea bags are used as a wash to soothe sunburn, a compress for headaches, a poultice for bags under eyes, to stop bleeding of gum sockets. To stop increased sweating. Tea is consumed as a beverage
Clinically important, potentially serious interactions with: acetaminophen, adenosine, anticoagulants, antiplatelets, antipsychotics, aspirin, barbiturates, benzodiazepines, beta-adrenergic agonists, chlorpromazine, cimetidine, clozapine, disulfiram, ephedrine, ergotamine, lithium, MAO-inhibitors, mexiletine, oral contraceptives, phenytoin, phenylpropanolamine, quinolones, theophylline, verapamil, warfarin, **grapefruit juice**

Adverse side-effects

Skin
None

KAVA

Scientific names: *Piper methysticum*
Other common names: Ava; Awa; Intoxicating Pepper; Kava Kava; Kawa Kawa; Kew; Sakau; Tonga
Family: Piperaceae
Purported indications:: Anxiety disorders; stress; insomnia; restlessness
Other uses: Epilepsy, psychosis, depression, sedative, headaches, migraines, colds, tuberculosis, rheumatism, cystitis, vaginal prolapse, leprosy, otitis, abscesses, etc.
Clinically important, potentially serious interactions with: alcohol, alprazolam, barbiturates, CNS depressants, levodopa

Adverse side-effects

Skin
Allergic reactions (sic)
Dermopathy (pellagra-like syndrome)
(1998): Brown DJ+, *Quart Rev Natural Med* Dec, 329
Lymphocytic inflammation of the dermis (sic)
Parkinsonism
Photosensitivity
Pigmentation (yellow)
(1999): Pizzorno JE+, *Textbook of Natural Medicine*, Churchill Livingstone, Edinburgh
Pruritus
Rash (sic)
Scaly rash (sic)
Xerosis
(1999): Pizzorno JE+, *Textbook of Natural Medicine*, Churchill Livingstone, Edinburgh

HAIR
Hair – pigmentation
(1999): Pizzorno JE+, *Textbook of Natural Medicine*, Churchill Livingstone, Edinburgh

NAILS
Nails – pigmentation
(1999): Pizzorno JE+, *Textbook of Natural Medicine*, Churchill Livingstone, Edinburgh

OTHER
Mouth numbness (sic)

Note: Kava was discovered by Captain Cook, who named the plant "intoxicating pepper." In the South Pacific, kava is a popular social drink, similar to alcohol in Western societies

LAVENDER

Scientific names: *Lavandula angustifolia; Lavandula vera; Lavandula spica; Lavandula latifolia; Lavandula dentata; Lavandula pubescens*
Other common names: Alhucema; Common Lavender; English Lavender; French Lavender; Garden Lavender; Spanish Lavender; Spike Lavender; True Lavender
Family: Lamiaceae
Purported indications: Restlessness; insomnia; nervous stomach; loss of appetite
Other uses: Flatulence, colic spasms, giddiness, nervous headaches, migraines, toothaches, sprains, neuralgia, rheumatism, acne, pimples, sores, nausea and vomiting. Lavender products are used as flavor components, in pharmaceuticals, as fragrance ingredients in soaps and cosmetics, as an insect repellent
Clinically important, potentially serious interactions with: barbiturates, chloral hydrate, CNS depressants, HMG-CoA reductase inhibitors

Adverse side-effects

Skin
Contact dermatitis

LICORICE

Scientific names: *Glycyrrhiza glabra; Glycyrrhiza uralensis*
Other common names: Alcacuz; Alcazuz; Chinese Licorice; Gan Cao; Gan Zao; Glycyrrhiza; Licorice Root; Liquorice; Orozuz; Reglisse; Russian Licorice; Spanish Licorice; Subholz; Sweet Root
Family: Fabaceae; Leguminaceae
Purported indications: Inflammation of the upper respiratory tract mucous membranes; gastric and duodenal ulcers; bronchitis; colic; dry cough; arthritis; lupus; hepatitis B and C; cholestatic liver disorders
Other uses: Increase fertility in women, prostate cancer (in combination with seven other herbs – PC-Spes), sore throats, malaria, tuberculosis, sores, abscesses, food poisoning, diabetes insipidus, contact dermatitis. Also used as a flavoring agent in foods, beverages and tobacco
Clinically important, potentially serious interactions with: antihypertensives, CYP450 (3A4) enzymes, digoxin, ethacrynic acid, furosemide, insulin, **grapefruit juice**

Adverse side-effects

SKIN
Contact dermatitis
Edema

OTHER
Myopathy

MEADOWSWEET

Scientific names: *Filipendula ulmaria; Spiraea ulmaria*
Other common names: Bridewort; Dolloff; Dropwort; Filipendula; Lady of the Meadow; Meadow Queen; Meadowsweet; Meadow-Wart; Queen of the Meadow; Ulmaria
Family: Rosaceae
Purported indications: Colds; fevers
Other uses: Cough, bronchitis, dyspepsia, heartburn, peptic ulcer, gout, rheumatic disorders. Diuretic
Clinically important, potentially serious interactions with: alcohol, anticoagulants, heparin, methotrexate, salicylates, sulfonylureas, valproic acid

Adverse side-effects

Skin
Rash (sic)

Other
Hypersensitivity

MELATONIN

Scientific name: *N*-acetyl-5-methoxytryptamine
Other common name: MEL
Family: None
Purported indications: Jet lag; sleep disorders; "shift-work" disorder; Alzheimer's disease; tinnitus; depressive disorders; migraine and cluster headaches; hypertension; hyperpigmentation; preventing osteoporosis, cancer of the breast, brain, lung and prostate
Other uses: Anti-aging; immune system enhancer, antioxidant, epilepsy, contraceptive. Skin protectant against sunburn
Clinically important, potentially serious interactions with: CNS depressants, fluvoxamine, immunosuppressants, nifedipine

Adverse side-effects

SKIN
Fixed eruption
Photosensitivity

MILK THISTLE*

Scientific names: *Silibum marianum; Carduus marainum*
Other common names: Cardui mariae fructus; Holy Thistle; Lady's Thistle; Marian Thistle; Mary Thistle; St. Mary Thistle; Silibum; Silymarin
Family: Asteraceae; Compositae
Purported indications: Dyspepsia; liver protectant; chronic hepatitis; loss of appetite
Other uses: Liver and gallbladder complaints, diseases of the spleen, supportive treatment for mushroom poisoning. Historically the fruit and seed are roasted for use as a coffee substitute
Clinically important, potentially serious interactions with: acetaminophen, alcohol, aspirin

Adverse side-effects

Skin
Allergic reactions (sic)
Diaphoresis

*Fruit and seed as opposed to the "above ground parts"

PROPOLIS

Scientific name: Propolis
Other common names: Bee Glue; Bee Propolis; Hive Dross; Propolis Balsam; Propolis Resin; Propolis Wax; Russian Penicillin
Family: None
Purported indications: Tuberculosis; bacterial and fungal infections; protozoal infections; nasopharyngeal carcinoma; improving immune response; duodenal ulcer
Other uses: *Helicobacter pylori* infection, common cold, wound cleansing, mouth rinse, genital herpes. Used as an ingredient in cosmetics
Clinically important, potentially serious interactions with: none

Adverse side-effects

Skin
Allergic reactions (sic)
Contact dermatitis
Dermatitis (sic)

Other
Mucositis
(1990): Hay KD+, *Oral Surg Oral Med Oral Pathol* 70, 584
Oral ulceration
(1990): Hay KD+, *Oral Surg Oral Med Oral Pathol* 70, 584

SAW PALMETTO

Scientific names: *Serenoa repens; Serenoa serrulata; Sabal serrulata*
Other common names: American Dwarf Palm Tree; Cabbage Palm; Ju-Zhong; Palmier Nain; Sabal; Sabal Fructus; Saw Palmetto Berry
Family: Arecacaea/Palmaceae
Purported indications: Benign prostatic hyperplasia; diuretic; sedative; anti-inflammatory; antiseptic
Other uses: Prostate cancer (in combination with seven other herbs – PC-Specs), aphrodisiac, hair growth, colds, coughs, sore throat, asthma, chronic bronchitis, migraines, cancer
Clinically important, potentially serious interactions with: finasteride

Adverse side-effects

Skin
None

ST JOHN'S WORT

Scientific name: *Hypericum perforatum*
Other common names: Amber, Demon Chaser; Fuga Daemonum; Goatweed; Hardhay; Hypereikon; Hypericum; Johns Wort; Klamath Weed; Rosin Rose; SJW; Tipton Weed
Family: Hypericaceae
Purported indications: Depression; dysthymic disorder; fatigue; insomnia; loss of appetite; anxiety; obsessive-compulsive disorders; mood disturbances; migraine headaches; neuralgia; fibrositis; sciatica; palpitations; exhaustion; headache; muscle pain
Other uses: Cancer, vitiligo, HIV/AIDS, diuretic, bruises, abrasions, muscle pain, first degree burns, hemorrhoids, neuralgia
Clinically important, potentially serious interactions with: antidepressants, barbiturates, cyclosporine, digoxin, fenfluramine, indinavir, MAO inhibitors, nefazodone, NNRTIs, nortriptyline, oral contraceptives, paroxetine, photosensitizing drugs, protease inhibitors, reserpine, sertraline, theophylline, triptans, warfarin, **tyramine-containing foods***

Adverse side-effects

Skin
Irritation (sic)
Photosensitivity
(1999): Gulick RM+, *Ann Intern Med* 130, 510
(1997): Brockmoller J+, *Pharmacopsychiatry* 30, 94
(1997): Golsch S+, *Hautarzt* (German) 48, 249
(1997): Upton R+, Santa Cruz, CA, *American Herbal Pharmacopoeia* 1–32

Other
Hypersensitivity
Paresthesias
(1998): Ernst E+, *Eur J Clin Pharmacol* 54, 589
Serotonin syndrome
(2000): Brown TM, *Am J Emerg Med* 18, 231
Xerostomia

*Tyramine-containing foods include the following: aged cheeses, avocados, banana skins, bologna and other processed luncheon meats, chicken livers, chocolate, figs, canned pickled herring, meat extracts, pepperoni, raisins, raspberries, soy sauce, vermouth, sherry and red wines

Note: St John's wort is a natural source of flavoring in Europe. Although not indigenous to Australia, and long considered a weed, St John's wort is now grown there as a cash crop and produces 20% of the world's supply. The flowers of St John's wort can have the brightest appearance on June 24, the birthday of St. John the Baptist

TRYPTOPHAN

Scientific name: L-2-amino-3-(indole-3yl) propionic acid
Other common names: L-trypt; L-tryptophan
Family: None
Purported indications: Insomnia; depression; myofascial pain; presmenstrual syndrome
Other uses: Smoking cessation, bruxism
Clinically important, potentially serious interactions with: benxzodiazepines, MAO inhibitors, phenothiazines, SSRIs, trazodone, **herbs with sedative properties**

Adverse side-effects

Skin
None

Other
Eosinophilia myalgia syndrome
Parkinsonism

Note: Tryptophan is an essential amino acid. It is a precursor of serotonin and is also converted to nicotinic acid and nicotinamide

VALERIAN

Scientific names: *Valeriana officinalis; Valeriana jatamansii; Valeriana wallichii; Valeriana edulis; Valeriana sitchensis*
Other common names: Amantilla; All-Heal; Baldrian; Common Valerian; Garden Heliotrope; Valeriana; Valariane
Family: Valerianaceae
Purported indications: Sedative–hypnotic; anxiolytic; depression; tremors; epilepsy; attention deficit–hyperactivity disorder
Other uses: Rheumatic pain, nervous asthma, gastric spasms, colic, menstrual cramps, hot flashes. Bath additive for restlessness and sleep disorders. Used as flavoring in foods and beverages
Clinically important, potentially serious interactions with: alcohol, barbiturates, benzodiazepines

Adverse side-effects

Skin
None

WILLOW BARK

Scientific names: *Salix alba; Salix fragilis; Salix purpurea*, etc.
Other common names: Basket Willow; Bay Willow; Brittle Willow; Crack Willow; Daphne Willow; Laurel Willow; Purple Osier; Violet Willow; White Willow; Willowbark
Family: Salicaceae
Purported indications: Colds; infections; headaches; pain; muscle and joint aches; influenza; gouty arthritis; ankylosing spondylitis; rheumatoid arthritis
Other uses: Diseases accompanied by fever, rheumatic ailments
Clinically important, potentially serious interactions with: anticoagulants, antiplatelets, salicylates

Adverse side-effects

Skin
Rash (sic)

Drugs responsible for 100 common reaction patterns

Acanthosis nigricans
Azathioprine
Corticosteroids
Diethylstilbestrol
Estrogens
Gemfibrozil
Heroin
Lithium
Mechlorethamine
Methsuximide
Methyltestosterone
Niacin
Niacinamide
Oral contraceptives
Thioridazine

Acne
Acyclovir
Alosetron
Alprazolam
Amitriptyline
Amobarbital
Amoxapine
Atorvastatin
Azathioprine
Betaxolol
Bexarotene
Bisoprolol
Buspirone
Cabergoline
Carteolol
Cefamandole
Cefpodoxime
Ceftazidime
Cetirizine
Chloral hydrate
Cidofovir
Cimetidine
Ciprofloxacin
Clofazimine
Clomiphene
Clomipramine
Corticosteroids
Cyanocobalamin
Cyclosporine
Dactinomycin
Danazol
Dantrolene
Deferoxamine
Demeclocycline
Desipramine
Diazepam
Diltiazem
Disulfiram
Eflornithine
Erythromycin
Esmolol
Estazolam
Estrogens
Ethionamide
Famotidine
Felbamate
Fenoprofen
Fexofenadine
Fluconazole
Fluoxetine
Fluoxymesterone
Fluvoxamine
Folic acid
Foscarnet
Fosphenytoin
Gabapentin
Ganciclovir
Gold & gold compounds
Granulocyte colony-stimulating factor (GCSF)
Grepafloxacin
Haloperidol
Halothane
Heroin
Imipramine
Interferons, alfa-2
Isoniazid
Isotretinoin
Lamotrigine
Lansoprazole
Leflunomide
Leuprolide
Levothyroxine
Lithium
Maprotiline
Medroxyprogesterone
Mephenytoin
Mesalamine
Methotrexate
Methoxsalen
Methyltestosterone
Minoxidil
Mirtazapine
Mycophenolate
Nabumetone
Nafarelin
Naratriptan
Nefazodone
Nimodipine
Nisoldipine
Nizatidine
Nortriptyline
Olsalazine
Oral contraceptives
Oxcarbazepine
Pantoprazole
Paramethadione
Paroxetine
Pentobarbital
Pentostatin
Pergolide
Phenobarbital
Phenytoin
Potassium iodide
Primidone
Propafenone
Propranolol
Propylthiouracil
Protriptyline
Psoralens
Pyrazinamide
Pyridoxine
Quinidine
Quinine
Ramipril
Riboflavin
Rifampin
Rifapentine
Risperidone
Ritonavir
Saquinavir
Sertraline
Sibutramine
Sirolimus
Sparfloxacin
Stanozolol
Tacrine
Testosterone
Tetracycline
Tiagabine
Tizanidine
Topiramate
Trimethadione
Trioxsalen
Trovafloxacin
Venlafaxine
Verapamil
Vinblastine
Zalcitabine
Zaleplon
Zidovudine
Zolpidem
Zonisamide

Acral erythema
Bleomycin
Capecitabine
Cisplatin
Cyclophosphamide
Cytarabine
Didanosine
Fluorouracil
Hydroxyurea
Idarubicin
Lomustine
Mercaptopurine
Methotrexate
Mitotane

Acute febrile neutrophilic dermatosis
Clofazimine
Co-trimoxazole
Cytarabine
Furosemide
Gabapentin
Glucagon
Granulocyte colony-stimulating factor (GCSF)
Hydralazine
Minocycline
Nitrofurantoin
Oral contraceptives
Sulfamethoxazole
Verapamil

Acute generalized exanthematous pustulosis
Acetaminophen
Acetazolamide
Allopurinol
Amoxapine
Amoxicillin
Ampicillin
Aspirin
Bacampicillin
Carbamazepine
Cefaclor
Cefazolin
Cefuroxime
Cephalexin
Cephradine
Chloramphenicol
Chloroquine
Clindamycin
Clozapine
Co-trimoxazole
Codeine
Corticosteroids
Diltiazem
Doxycycline
Erythromycin
Furosemide
Hydroxychloroquine
Imipenem/cilastatin
Isoniazid
Itraconazole
Lansoprazole
Metronidazole
Minocycline
Nifedipine
Nimodipine
Nystatin
Penicillins
Phenobarbital
Phenytoin
Progestins
Protease inhibitors
Pyrimethamine
Quinidine
Ranitidine
Streptomycin
Sulfamethoxazole
Sulfasalazine

Terbinafine
Ticlopidine
Vancomycin

Ageusia

Acarbose
Acetazolamide
Amitriptyline
Aspirin
Atorvastatin
Azelastine
Benazepril
Betaxolol
Captopril
Cetirizine
Cisplatin
Clidinium
Clomipramine
Clopidogrel
Cocaine
Cyclobenzaprine
Diazoxide
Dicyclomine
Enalapril
Etidronate
Fluoxetine
Fluvoxamine
Fosinopril
Grepafloxacin
Indomethacin
Isotretinoin
Levodopa
Losartan
Methantheline
Methimazole
Mirtazapine
Nefazodone
Paroxetine
Penicillamine
Pentamidine
Phenytoin
Propantheline
Propylthiouracil
Ramipril
Rifabutin
Rimantadine
Ritonavir
Rivastigmine
Spironolactone
Sulfadoxine
Sulindac
Terbinafine
Tiagabine
Topiramate
Venlafaxine
Zalcitabine
Zaleplon

Alopecia – see Hair – alopecia

Alopecia areata see Hair – alopecia areata

Anaphylactoid reaction

Abacavir
Abciximab
Acetaminophen
Acetazolamide
Acyclovir
Alteplase
Amiloride
Aminocaproic acid
Aminoglutethimide
Amitriptyline
Amoxicillin
Amphotericin B
Ampicillin
Anistreplase
Aprotinin
Asparaginase
Aspartame
Aspirin
Astemizole
Atenolol
Azathioprine
Azithromycin
Aztreonam
Bacampicillin
Benactyzine
Bendroflumethiazide
Betaxolol
Bisoprolol
Bleomycin
Bromfenac
Bromocriptine
Butalbital
Calcitonin (human & salmon)
Captopril
Carbenicillin
Carboplatin
Carisoprodol
Carteolol
Carvedilol
Cefaclor
Cefadroxil
Cefamandole
Cefazolin
Cefdinir
Cefepime
Cefixime
Cefmetazole
Cefonicid
Cefotaxime
Cefotetan
Cefoxitin
Cefpodoxime
Ceftazidime
Ceftizoxime
Ceftriaxone
Cefuroxime
Cephalexin
Cephalothin
Cephapirin
Cephradine
Cerivastatin
Cetirizine
Chloramphenicol
Chlorhexidine
Chlorothiazide
Chlorpromazine
Chlorzoxazone
Cimetidine
Cinoxacin
Ciprofloxacin
Cisplatin
Clarithromycin
Clemastine
Clidinium
Clindamycin
Cloxacillin
Co-trimoxazole
Codeine
Colchicine
Corticosteroids
Cromolyn
Cyanocobalamin
Cyclobenzaprine
Cyclophosphamide
Cyclosporine
Cyproheptadine
Cytarabine
Dacarbazine
Dactinomycin
Dalteparin
Dantrolene
Daunorubicin
Deferoxamine
Demeclocycline
Denileukin
Dexchlorpheniramine
Dextromethorphan
Diazepam
Diclofenac
Dicloxacillin
Dicyclomine
Didanosine
Diflunisal
Dimenhydrinate
Diphenhydramine
Diphenoxylate
Dipyridamole
Dirithromycin
Dolasetron
Doxorubicin
Doxycycline
Edrophonium
Enalapril
Enoxaparin
Epirubicin
Epoetin alfa
Eptifibatide
Erythromycin
Ethambutol
Ethanolamine
Etoposide
Felbamate
Fenoprofen
Fentanyl
Fluconazole
Flucytosine
Fluorouracil
Fluoxetine
Fluoxymesterone
Fluphenazine
Flurbiprofen
Fluvastatin
Fluvoxamine
Folic acid
Fosfomycin
Fosinopril
Furosemide
Ganciclovir
Gatifloxacin
Gemcitabine
Gemfibrozil
Gentamicin
Gold & gold compounds
Goserelin
Granisetron
Granulocyte colony-stimulating factor (GCSF)
Griseofulvin
Heparin
Ibuprofen
Ifosfamide
Indapamide
Indomethacin
Insulin
Ipodate
Ipratropium
Isoetharine
Itraconazole
Ketoconazole
Ketoprofen
Ketorolac
Labetalol
Lamotrigine
Lansoprazole
Leflunomide
Leucovorin
Levamisole
Levofloxacin
Lidocaine
Lincomycin
Lisinopril
Loratadine
Losartan
Marihuana
Mechlorethamine
Medroxyprogesterone
Mefenamic acid
Meloxicam
Melphalan
Meprobamate
Mesoridazine
Metaxalone
Methantheline
Methicillin
Methocarbamol
Methohexital
Methotrexate
Methyclothiazide
Methyltestosterone
Metolazone
Mezlocillin
Miconazole
Midazolam
Minocycline
Misoprostol
Moexipril
Nabumetone
Nafcillin
Nalidixic acid
Naproxen
Neomycin
Niacin
Nitrofurantoin
Nitroglycerin

Norfloxacin
Octreotide
Ofloxacin
Omeprazole
Ondansetron
Orphenadrine
Oxacillin
Oxaprozin
Oxytetracycline
Penicillins
Pentostatin
Perindopril
Perphenazine
Phenazopyridine
Phytonadione
Piperacillin
Piroxicam
Pravastatin
Prazosin
Probenecid
Prochlorperazine
Progestins
Promethazine
Propantheline
Propofol
Propranolol
Protamine
Pyrilamine
Pyrimethamine
Quinupristin/dalfopristin
Ramipril
Ranitidine
Repaglinide
Reteplase
Rifampin
Risperidone
Ritodrine
Ritonavir
Salsalate
Scopolamine
Simvastatin
Sparfloxacin
Spectinomycin
Spironolactone
Streptokinase
Streptomycin
Succinylcholine
Sulfadiazine
Sulfadoxine
Sulfamethoxazole
Sulfasalazine
Sulfisoxazole
Sulindac
Sumatriptan
Tacrolimus
Temazepam
Terazosin
Terbinafine
Terfenadine
Testosterone
Tetracycline
Thiabendazole
Thiamine
Thiopental
Thioridazine
Thiotepa
Thiothixene
Ticarcillin
Timolol
Tolmetin
Tramadol
Triamterene
Trichlormethiazide
Trifluoperazine
Trimeprazine
Tripelennamine
Troleandomycin
Trovafloxacin
Urokinase
Vancomycin
Vasopressin
Vincristine
Vinorelbine
Vitamin A
Zalcitabine
Zolpidem

Angioedema

Acetaminophen
Albuterol
Aldesleukin
Allopurinol
Alteplase
Aminoglutethimide
Aminosalicylate sodium
Amitriptyline
Amobarbital
Amoxicillin
Amphotericin B
Ampicillin
Anistreplase
Aprobarbital
Aprotinin
Ascorbic acid
Asparaginase
Aspartame
Aspirin
Astemizole
Azatadine
Azathioprine
Azithromycin
Aztreonam
Bacampicillin
Benactyzine
Benazepril
Betaxolol
Bisoprolol
Bleomycin
Brompheniramine
Butabarbital
Candesartan
Captopril
Carbamazepine
Carbenicillin
Carisoprodol
Carteolol
Carvedilol
Cefaclor
Cefadroxil
Cefepime
Cefoxitin
Cefprozil
Ceftazidime
Ceftriaxone
Cefuroxime
Cephalexin
Cerivastatin
Cetirizine
Chloral hydrate
Chlorambucil
Chloramphenicol
Chlordiazepoxide
Chloroquine
Chlorpheniramine
Chlorpromazine
Chlorpropamide
Chlorzoxazone
Cimetidine
Cinoxacin
Ciprofloxacin
Cisplatin
Clemastine
Clonazepam
Clonidine
Cloxacillin
Co-trimoxazole
Cocaine
Codeine
Colchicine
Corticosteroids
Cromolyn
Cyanocobalamin
Cyclamate
Cyclobenzaprine
Cyclophosphamide
Cyclosporine
Cyproheptadine
Dacarbazine
Danazol
Daunorubicin
Deferoxamine
Delavirdine
Demeclocycline
Desipramine
Dexchlorpheniramine
Dexfenfluramine
Diazepam
Diclofenac
Dicloxacillin
Dicumarol
Diethylstilbestrol
Diflunisal
Digoxin
Diltiazem
Dimenhydrinate
Diphenhydramine
Diphenoxylate
Dipyridamole
Disopyramide
Docetaxel
Dofetilide
Doxorubicin
Doxycycline
Enalapril
Epoetin alfa
Eprosartan
Estrogens
Ethambutol
Etidronate
Etodolac
Famotidine
Fenoprofen
Fluconazole
Fluorouracil
Fluoxetine
Fluphenazine
Flurbiprofen
Fluvastatin
Fluvoxamine
Fosfomycin
Fosinopril
Gatifloxacin
Gemfibrozil
Glucagon
Glyburide
Gold & gold compounds
Griseofulvin
Halothane
Heparin
Heroin
Hydralazine
Hydroxychloroquine
Hydroxyzine
Ibuprofen
Imipenem/cilastatin
Imipramine
Indapamide
Indomethacin
Insulin
Isoniazid
Itraconazole
Ketoconazole
Ketoprofen
Ketorolac
Labetalol
Lamivudine
Lamotrigine
Levamisole
Levothyroxine
Lidocaine
Lincomycin
Lisinopril
Lithium
Loratadine
Losartan
Mebendazole
Mechlorethamine
Meclizine
Meclofenamate
Medroxyprogesterone
Mefenamic acid
Meloxicam
Melphalan
Meperidine
Mephenytoin
Mephobarbital
Meprobamate
Mesna
Mesoridazine
Methadone
Methicillin
Methohexital
Methylphenidate
Metoclopramide
Metoprolol

Metronidazole
Mezlocillin
Mibefradil
Miconazole
Midazolam
Minocycline
Mitomycin
Mitotane
Moexipril
Montelukast
Nabumetone
Nafcillin
Nalidixic acid
Naloxone
Naproxen
Neomycin
Nifedipine
Nisoldipine
Nitrofurantoin
Nitroglycerin
Norfloxacin
Ofloxacin
Omeprazole
Ondansetron
Oral contraceptives
Oxacillin
Oxaprozin
Oxcarbazepine
Oxytetracycline
Pamidronate
Pantoprazole
Paroxetine
Penicillins
Pentagastrin
Pentobarbital
Pentoxifylline
Perindopril
Perphenazine
Phenelzine
Phenindamine
Phenobarbital
Phenolphthalein
Phenytoin
Piperacillin
Piroxicam
Potassium iodide
Pravastatin
Prazosin
Primaquine
Procainamide
Procarbazine
Progestins
Promethazine
Propranolol
Propylthiouracil
Protamine
Protriptyline
Pseudoephedrine
Pyrilamine
Pyrimethamine
Quetiapine
Quinapril
Quinestrol
Quinidine
Quinine
Ramipril
Ranitidine
Riboflavin
Rifampin
Risperidone
Ritonavir
Rituximab
Rofecoxib
Salmeterol
Salsalate
Secobarbital
Sertraline
Simvastatin
Sparfloxacin
Streptokinase
Streptomycin
Sucralfate
Sulfamethoxazole
Sulfasalazine
Sulfisoxazole
Sulindac
Sumatriptan
Tamsulosin
Telmisartan
Terbinafine
Terfenadine
Tetracycline
Thiabendazole
Thiamine
Thiopental
Thioridazine
Thiotepa
Ticarcillin
Ticlopidine
Timolol
Tiopronin
Tolmetin
Torsemide
Tramadol
Trandolapril
Trifluoperazine
Trimeprazine
Trimetrexate
Tripelennamine
Triprolidine
Troleandomycin
Trovafloxacin
Urokinase
Vancomycin
Vasopressin
Verapamil
Vincristine
Vinorelbine
Warfarin
Zalcitabine

Anosmia

Acetazolamide
Ciprofloxacin
Cocaine
Cromolyn
Doxycycline
Enalapril
Ganciclovir
Interferons, alfa-2
Methazolamide
Minoxidil
Paroxetine
Pentamidine
Sparfloxacin
Terbinafine

Aphthous stomatitis

Aldesleukin
Asparaginase
Aspirin
Azathioprine
Azelastine
Aztreonam
Captopril
Cidofovir
Co-trimoxazole
Cyclosporine
Delavirdine
Diclofenac
Diflunisal
Doxepin
Fenoprofen
Fluoxetine
Flurbiprofen
Gold & gold compounds
Ibuprofen
Indinavir
Indomethacin
Interferons, alfa-2
Ketoprofen
Ketorolac
Losartan
Meclofenamate
Mirtazapine
Naproxen
Olanzapine
Pantoprazole
Paroxetine
Penicillamine
Piroxicam
Rofecoxib
Sertraline
Sulfamethoxazole
Sulfasalazine
Sulfisoxazole
Sulindac
Terbinafine
Tolmetin
Trientine
Zalcitabine
Zaleplon

Black tongue

Amitriptyline
Amoxapine
Amoxicillin
Ampicillin
Bacampicillin
Benztropine
Carbenicillin
Chloramphenicol
Clarithromycin
Clomipramine
Clonazepam
Cloxacillin
Co-trimoxazole
Corticosteroids
Desipramine
Dicloxacillin
Fluoxetine
Griseofulvin
Imipramine
Isocarboxazid
Lansoprazole
Maprotiline
Methicillin
Methyldopa
Mezlocillin
Minocycline
Nafcillin
Nortriptyline
Oxacillin
Oxytetracycline
Penicillins
Phenelzine
Protriptyline
Streptomycin
Sulfamethoxazole
Tetracycline
Thiothixene
Ticarcillin
Tranylcypromine

Bullous eruption

Acetazolamide
Acitretin
Aldesleukin
Alitretinoin
Aminocaproic acid
Aminosalicylate sodium
Amitriptyline
Amobarbital
Ampicillin
Arsenic
Aspirin
Atropine sulfate
Benactyzine
Bleomycin
Bumetanide
Buspirone
Busulfan
Butabarbital
Butalbital
Captopril
Carbamazepine
Carbenicillin
Cetirizine
Cevimeline
Chloral hydrate
Chloramphenicol
Chlorothiazide
Chlorpromazine
Chlorpropamide
Ciprofloxacin
Clopidogrel
Co-trimoxazole
Cocaine
Codeine
Colchicine
Corticosteroids
Cyanocobalamin
Cyclamate
Cyclosporine
Cytarabine
Dalteparin
Dapsone
Demeclocycline

Denileukin
Dexfenfluramine
Dextromethorphan
Diazepam
Diclofenac
Dicloxacillin
Dicumarol
Diethylstilbestrol
Diflunisal
Digoxin
Dirithromycin
Disulfiram
Ephedrine
Estrogens
Ethambutol
Ethchlorvynol
Ethotoin
Etodolac
Felbamate
Fenoprofen
Fluconazole
Fluorouracil
Fluoxetine
Flutamide
Fluvoxamine
Fosphenytoin
Furosemide
Ganciclovir
Glyburide
Gold & gold compounds
Griseofulvin
Hydralazine
Hydrochlorothiazide
Hydroxychloroquine
Ibuprofen
Ibutilide
Idarubicin
Imipramine
Indapamide
Indomethacin
Insulin
Interferons, alfa-2
Isoniazid
Ivermectin
Ketoprofen
Leflunomide
Lidocaine
Lisinopril
Lithium
Mechlorethamine
Meclofenamate
Meloxicam
Mephenytoin
Meprobamate
Methicillin
Methotrexate
Methoxsalen
Mezlocillin
Miconazole
Minoxidil
Mitomycin
Nabumetone
Nafcillin
Nalidixic acid
Naproxen
Neomycin
Nifedipine
Nitrofurantoin
Norfloxacin
Ofloxacin
Omeprazole
Oral contraceptives
Oxacillin
Penicillamine
Pentamidine
Pentobarbital
Pentostatin
Phenobarbital
Phenolphthalein
Phenytoin
Piperacillin
Promethazine
Propranolol
Pyridoxine
Pyrimethamine
Quinapril
Quinethazone
Quinidine
Quinine
Reserpine
Rifampin
Risperidone
Ritonavir
Rivastigmine
Rofecoxib
Saquinavir
Sertraline
Sparfloxacin
Streptomycin
Sulfadoxine
Sulfamethoxazole
Sulfasalazine
Sulfisoxazole
Tacrine
Temazepam
Tetracycline
Thalidomide
Thiopental
Ticarcillin
Tolbutamide
Tolmetin
Trimethadione
Trioxsalen
Urokinase
Vancomycin
Vasopressin
Vinblastine
Warfarin
Zalcitabine
Zidovudine
Zolpidem

Bullous pemphigoid

Aldesleukin
Amoxicillin
Ampicillin
Bumetanide
Captopril
Chloroquine
Ciprofloxacin
Dactinomycin
Enalapril
Fosinopril
Furosemide
Gold & gold compounds
Ibuprofen
Mefenamic acid
Methoxsalen
Nadolol
Omeprazole
Penicillamine
Penicillins
Potassium iodide
Psoralens
Risperidone
Sulfasalazine
Tiopronin
Tolbutamide

Candidiasis

Ampicillin
Cefaclor
Cefadroxil
Cefdinir
Cefepime
Cefixime
Cefmetazole
Cefonicid
Cefoperazone
Cefotaxime
Cefotetan
Cefoxitin
Cefpodoxime
Cefprozil
Ceftazidime
Ceftibuten
Ceftizoxime
Ceftriaxone
Celecoxib
Cephalothin
Cephapirin
Chlorotrianisene
Ciprofloxacin
Demeclocycline
Diazoxide
Fluoxetine
Gatifloxacin
Griseofulvin
Heroin
Imipenem/cilastatin
Infliximab
Interferons, alfa-2
Lansoprazole
Levofloxacin
Loracarbef
Methotrexate
Metronidazole
Minocycline
Moxifloxacin
Ofloxacin
Olanzapine
Oral contraceptives
Pamidronate
Paroxetine
Pentostatin
Piperacillin
Quetiapine
Quinupristin/dalfopristin
Riluzole
Saquinavir
Tetracycline
Tizanidine
Trovafloxacin
Venlafaxine

Cheilitis

Acitretin
Atorvastatin
Bexarotene
Busulfan
Clofazimine
Clomipramine
Cyanocobalamin
Dactinomycin
Eflornithine
Gatifloxacin
Gold & gold compounds
Grepafloxacin
Indinavir
Isotretinoin
Methoxsalen
Methyldopa
Psoralens
Ritonavir
Saquinavir
Simvastatin
Streptomycin
Sulfasalazine
Tetracycline
Trovafloxacin
Vitamin A
Zaleplon

Chills

Albuterol
Allopurinol
Amifostine
Amphotericin B
Anistreplase
Asparaginase
Azathioprine
Bexarotene
Bleomycin
Ceftriaxone
Cidofovir
Cilostazol
Dantrolene
Daunorubicin
Denileukin
Dexchlorpheniramine
Dextroamphetamine
Didanosine
Dolasetron
Droperidol
Enoxacin
Estazolam
Ethacrynic acid
Ethambutol
Fludarabine
Fosphenytoin
Ganciclovir
Gatifloxacin
Gemtuzumab
Goserelin
Heparin
Hydralazine
Infliximab
Interferons, alfa-2

Irbesartan
Irinotecan
Ketoconazole
Lamivudine
Lomefloxacin
Metolazone
Miconazole
Mifepristone
Mirtazapine
Modafinil
Moxifloxacin
Nifedipine
Nisoldipine
Nitrofurantoin
Ofloxacin
Ondansetron
Pergolide
Perindopril
Pilocarpine
Procainamide
Promethazine
Rabeprazole
Riluzole
Ritodrine
Rituximab
Rizatriptan
Sirolimus
Spectinomycin
Spironolactone
Stanozolol
Stavudine
Sufentanil
Sulfadiazine
Terconazole
Triamterene
Trihexyphenidyl
Urokinase
Vancomycin
Zaleplon

Contact dermatitis

Acetaminophen
Acyclovir
Albendazole
Albuterol
Amantadine
Aminocaproic acid
Aminophylline
Amoxicillin
Amphotericin B
Ampicillin
Amyl nitrite
Apraclonidine
Arsenic
Atorvastatin
Atropine sulfate
Azathioprine
Azelastine
Bacampicillin
Bendroflumethiazide
Betaxolol
Biperiden
Bumetanide
Captopril
Carbamazepine
Carmustine
Carteolol
Cefazolin
Cephalexin
Chloramphenicol
Chlorhexidine
Chloroquine
Chlorpheniramine
Chlorpromazine
Chlorpropamide
Cisplatin
Clindamycin
Clomipramine
Clonidine
Cloxacillin
Codeine
Corticosteroids
Cromolyn
Cyanocobalamin
Cyclophosphamide
Cyproheptadine
Daunorubicin
Dexchlorpheniramine
Diazepam
Diclofenac
Diphenhydramine
Disulfiram
Docusate
Dorzolamide
Doxepin
Doxorubicin
Eflornithine
Ephedrine
Epinephrine
Epoetin alfa
Erythromycin
Estrogens
Ethambutol
Ethanolamine
Famotidine
Fluorouracil
Fluoxetine
Fluoxymesterone
Fluphenazine
Flurbiprofen
Furazolidone
Gentamicin
Gold & gold compounds
Haloperidol
Heparin
Heroin
Hydroxychloroquine
Hydroxyzine
Ibuprofen
Ibutilide
Indinavir
Indomethacin
Insulin
Interferons, alfa-2
Ipratropium
Isoniazid
Ketoconazole
Ketoprofen
Labetalol
Lamivudine
Levobunolol
Lidocaine
Lincomycin
Mechlorethamine
Mesoridazine
Methoxsalen
Methyltestosterone
Metronidazole
Mezlocillin
Miconazole
Minoxidil
Mitomycin
Neomycin
Niacin
Nicotine
Nitrofurantoin
Nitroglycerin
Nizatidine
Norfloxacin
Nystatin
Olanzapine
Oxcarbazepine
Oxytetracycline
Pantoprazole
Paroxetine
Penicillamine
Penicillins
Pentostatin
Perphenazine
Phenoxybenzamine
Phenylephrine
Phytonadione
Pilocarpine
Piroxicam
Promethazine
Propantheline
Propranolol
Pseudoephedrine
Psoralens
Pyridoxine
Quinacrine
Quinidine
Quinine
Ranitidine
Rifampin
Ritonavir
Rivastigmine
Rofecoxib
Scopolamine
Sildenafil
Sparfloxacin
Spectinomycin
Spironolactone
Streptomycin
Succinylcholine
Terbinafine
Terbutaline
Testosterone
Thiabendazole
Thiamine
Tiagabine
Timolol
Tiopronin
Tobramycin
Tolazoline
Tolbutamide
Trifluoperazine
Venlafaxine
Vitamin A
Vitamin E
Zaleplon

Dermatitis (sic)

Acebutolol
Acetaminophen
Acitretin
Acyclovir
Aldesleukin
Alprazolam
Altretamine
Amantadine
Amikacin
Aminocaproic acid
Aminophylline
Amitriptyline
Amlodipine
Amoxapine
Amyl nitrite
Apraclonidine
Arsenic
Aspartame
Astemizole
Atenolol
Baclofen
Benazepril
Beta-carotene
Bleomycin
Capecitabine
Carbamazepine
Carmustine
Carteolol
Cefaclor
Ceftriaxone
Celecoxib
Cetirizine
Cevimeline
Chloral hydrate
Chloramphenicol
Chlordiazepoxide
Chlorhexidine
Chlorotrianisene
Chlorpheniramine
Chlorpromazine
Citalopram
Clofibrate
Clomiphene
Clomipramine
Clonazepam
Clorazepate
Clozapine
Co-trimoxazole
Colestipol
Corticosteroids
Cromolyn
Cyclobenzaprine
Cycloserine
Cyproheptadine
Dactinomycin
Dantrolene
Deferoxamine
Delavirdine
Diazepam
Diclofenac
Dicloxacillin
Dicumarol
Diltiazem

Disopyramide
Donepezil
Ephedrine
Estazolam
Estrogens
Ethambutol
Etodolac
Famciclovir
Fluorouracil
Fluphenazine
Flurazepam
Fluvoxamine
Folic acid
Foscarnet
Gemfibrozil
Gold & gold compounds
Guanethidine
Guanfacine
Hydrochlorothiazide
Hydroxyurea
Ifosfamide
Indinavir
Irbesartan
Ivermectin
Ketorolac
Leflunomide
Leuprolide
Levamisole
Lithium
Loratadine
Lorazepam
Losartan
Loxapine
Meprobamate
Mercaptopurine
Methotrexate
Misoprostol
Mitomycin
Naratriptan
Nelfinavir
Neomycin
Nifedipine
Nystatin
Ofloxacin
Orlistat
Oxazepam
Penicillins
Pentazocine
Pentostatin
Phenindamine
Prazepam
Probenecid
Procainamide
Procarbazine
Progestins
Promazine
Promethazine
Propylthiouracil
Protriptyline
Pseudoephedrine
Pyrilamine
Pyrimethamine
Quazepam
Ramipril
Risperidone
Ropinirole
Saccharin
Salsalate
Saquinavir
Scopolamine
Sertraline
Sulfamethoxazole
Sulfasalazine
Sulfinpyrazone
Sulindac
Tacrine
Telmisartan
Temazepam
Tetracycline
Thalidomide
Thioridazine
Ticlopidine
Timolol
Tolazamide
Topiramate
Toremifene
Triazolam
Trientine
Trimeprazine
Trovafloxacin
Verapamil
Vinblastine
Vitamin A
Vitamin E
Warfarin
Zalcitabine
Zolpidem

Dermatitis herpetiformis

Amitriptyline
Aspirin
Cyclophosphamide
Diclofenac
Doxorubicin
Flurbiprofen
Ibuprofen
Indomethacin
Interferons, alfa-2
Levothyroxine
Lithium
Oral contraceptives
Potassium iodide
Vincristine

Diaphoresis

Acebutolol
Acetaminophen
Acetohexamide
Acitretin
Acyclovir
Albuterol
Allopurinol
Alprazolam
Alprostadil
Amiloride
Aminophylline
Amiodarone
Amitriptyline
Amlodipine
Amoxapine
Amphotericin B
Amyl nitrite
Anistreplase
Asparaginase
Aspirin
Atenolol
Atorvastatin
Atovaquone
Azatadine
Aztreonam
Baclofen
Benazepril
Bendroflumethiazide
Betaxolol
Bethanechol
Bicalutamide
Bisacodyl
Bisoprolol
Bretylium
Bromfenac
Bumetanide
Buspirone
Butorphanol
Candesartan
Capecitabine
Carbamazepine
Carisoprodol
Carteolol
Carvedilol
Cefamandole
Cefpodoxime
Ceftazidime
Ceftriaxone
Celecoxib
Cetirizine
Cevimeline
Chlordiazepoxide
Chlorpheniramine
Cidofovir
Ciprofloxacin
Cisplatin
Citalopram
Cladribine
Clemastine
Clofibrate
Clomiphene
Clomipramine
Clonazepam
Clonidine
Clorazepate
Clozapine
Cocaine
Codeine
Corticosteroids
Cyclobenzaprine
Cyclophosphamide
Cyproheptadine
Danazol
Dantrolene
Delavirdine
Denileukin
Desipramine
Desmopressin
Dexchlorpheniramine
Dexfenfluramine
Dexmedetomidine
Dextroamphetamine
Diazepam
Diazoxide
Diclofenac
Didanosine
Diethylpropion
Diflunisal
Digoxin
Diltiazem
Dimenhydrinate
Diphenhydramine
Diphenoxylate
Dipyridamole
Dirithromycin
Disulfiram
Docusate
Dofetilide
Dolasetron
Donepezil
Doxapram
Doxazosin
Doxepin
Dronabinol (THC)
Droperidol
Edrophonium
Enalapril
Enoxacin
Entacapone
Ephedrine
Epinephrine
Eprosartan
Esmolol
Estazolam
Ethambutol
Ethchlorvynol
Etodolac
Etoposide
Felbamate
Felodipine
Fenfluramine
Fenoprofen
Fentanyl
Flecainide
Flumazenil
Fluoxetine
Fluphenazine
Flurazepam
Flurbiprofen
Flutamide
Fluvoxamine
Foscarnet
Fosinopril
Furosemide
Ganciclovir
Gatifloxacin
Gemcitabine
Glimepiride
Goserelin
Granulocyte colony-stimulating factor (GCSF)
Grepafloxacin
Guanfacine
Haloperidol
Hydralazine
Hydrochlorothiazide
Hydrocodone
Hydromorphone
Hydroxyzine
Ibuprofen
Imipenem/cilastatin

Imipramine
Indapamide
Indinavir
Indomethacin
Insulin
Interferons, alfa-2
Irinotecan
Isocarboxazid
Isoproterenol
Isosorbide dinitrate
Isosorbide mononitrate
Isotretinoin
Isradipine
Ketoprofen
Ketorolac
Labetalol
Lamotrigine
Lansoprazole
Leflunomide
Letrozole
Leuprolide
Levodopa
Levofloxacin
Levothyroxine
Liothyronine
Lisinopril
Lomefloxacin
Loratadine
Lorazepam
Losartan
Loxapine
Maprotiline
Mazindol
Medroxyprogesterone
Mefenamic acid
Meperidine
Mesalamine
Methadone
Methamphetamine
Methylphenidate
Metoprolol
Mexiletine
Mibefradil
Mirtazapine
Misoprostol
Modafinil
Moexipril
Moricizine
Morphine
Moxifloxacin
Mycophenolate
Nabumetone
Nadolol
Naloxone
Naproxen
Naratriptan
Nelfinavir
Nicotine
Nifedipine
Nimodipine
Nisoldipine
Nitroglycerin
Nizatidine
Norfloxacin
Nortriptyline
Octreotide
Ofloxacin
Olanzapine
Omeprazole
Oxaprozin
Oxazepam
Oxcarbazepine
Oxycodone
Pantoprazole
Paroxetine
Penbutolol
Penicillins
Pentagastrin
Pentazocine
Pentostatin
Pentoxifylline
Pergolide
Perindopril
Perphenazine
Phendimetrazine
Phenelzine
Phenindamine
Phenolphthalein
Phentermine
Phytonadione
Pilocarpine
Pimozide
Pindolol
Piroxicam
Potassium iodide
Pramipexole
Prazepam
Praziquantel
Prazosin
Procarbazine
Prochlorperazine
Progestins
Promethazine
Propafenone
Propantheline
Propoxyphene
Propranolol
Protriptyline
Pseudoephedrine
Pyrilamine
Quazepam
Quetiapine
Quinapril
Quinine
Quinupristin/dalfopristin
Rabeprazole
Raloxifene
Ramipril
Rifampin
Risperidone
Ritodrine
Ritonavir
Rituximab
Rivastigmine
Rizatriptan
Rofecoxib
Ropinirole
Saquinavir
Selegiline
Sertraline
Sibutramine
Sildenafil
Simvastatin
Sirolimus
Sotalol
Sparfloxacin
Spironolactone
Stavudine
Streptokinase
Sulfasalazine
Sulindac
Sumatriptan
Tacrine
Tacrolimus
Tamoxifen
Telmisartan
Temazepam
Terazosin
Terbutaline
Terfenadine
Tetracycline
Thalidomide
Thiamine
Thiothixene
Tiagabine
Ticlopidine
Timolol
Tirofiban
Tizanidine
Tocainide
Tolazamide
Tolcapone
Tolmetin
Topiramate
Toremifene
Tramadol
Tranylcypromine
Trazodone
Triamterene
Triazolam
Trifluoperazine
Trihexyphenidyl
Trimeprazine
Trimipramine
Tripelennamine
Triprolidine
Trovafloxacin
Urokinase
Ursodiol
Vasopressin
Venlafaxine
Verapamil
Yohimbine
Zalcitabine
Zaleplon
Zidovudine
Zolmitriptan
Zolpidem
Zonisamide

Dysgeusia

Acebutolol
Acetaminophen
Acetazolamide
Acyclovir
Albuterol
Aldesleukin
Alendronate
Allopurinol
Alosetron
Alprazolam
Amifostine
Amiloride
Amiodarone
Amitriptyline
Amlodipine
Amoxapine
Amoxicillin
Amprenavir
Apraclonidine
Aspirin
Astemizole
Atorvastatin
Atovaquone
Atropine sulfate
Azelastine
Aztreonam
Bacampicillin
Baclofen
Benazepril
Benzthiazide
Benztropine
Betaxolol
Bisoprolol
Bromfenac
Bromocriptine
Buspirone
Busulfan
Butorphanol
Calcitonin
Captopril
Carbamazepine
Carbenicillin
Carteolol
Cefaclor
Cefamandole
Cefmetazole
Cefpodoxime
Ceftazidime
Ceftibuten
Ceftriaxone
Celecoxib
Cerivastatin
Cetirizine
Cevimeline
Chloral hydrate
Chlorhexidine
Chlormezanone
Chlorothiazide
Cholestyramine
Cidofovir
Cinoxacin
Ciprofloxacin
Citalopram
Clarithromycin
Clidinium
Clindamycin
Clofazimine
Clofibrate
Clomipramine
Clonazepam
Clonidine
Clozapine
Co-trimoxazole
Codeine

Cromolyn
Cyclobenzaprine
Cyproheptadine
Dacarbazine
Dantrolene
Delavirdine
Desipramine
Dexfenfluramine
Dextroamphetamine
Diazoxide
Diclofenac
Dicloxacillin
Dicyclomine
Diethylpropion
Dihydroergotamine
Dihydrotachysterol
Diltiazem
Dipyridamole
Dirithromycin
Disulfiram
Docusate
Dolasetron
Donepezil
Dorzolamide
Doxazosin
Doxepin
Doxycycline
Efavirenz
Enalapril
Enoxacin
Entacapone
Esmolol
Estazolam
Ethchlorvynol
Ethionamide
Etidronate
Etoposide
Famotidine
Felbamate
Fenfluramine
Fenoprofen
Fentanyl
Flecainide
Fluconazole
Fludarabine
Fluorouracil
Fluoxetine
Flurazepam
Flurbiprofen
Fluvastatin
Fluvoxamine
Foscarnet
Fosinopril
Fosphenytoin
Ganciclovir
Gatifloxacin
Gemfibrozil
Glyburide
Glycopyrrolate
Gold & gold compounds
Granisetron
Grepafloxacin
Griseofulvin
Guanabenz
Guanfacine
Hydrochlorothiazide
Hydroflumethiazide
Hydromorphone
Hydroxychloroquine
Imipenem/cilastatin
Imipramine
Indinavir
Interferons, alfa-2
Ipratropium
Irinotecan
Isotretinoin
Ketoprofen
Ketorolac
Labetalol
Lamotrigine
Lansoprazole
Leflunomide
Leuprolide
Levodopa
Levofloxacin
Linezolid
Lisinopril
Lithium
Lomefloxacin
Loratadine
Losartan
Lovastatin
Maprotiline
Mazindol
Mechlorethamine
Meclofenamate
Meloxicam
Mesalamine
Mesna
Metformin
Methamphetamine
Methantheline
Methazolamide
Methicillin
Methimazole
Methocarbamol
Methotrexate
Methyclothiazide
Metolazone
Metoprolol
Metronidazole
Mexiletine
Midazolam
Minoxidil
Mirtazapine
Modafinil
Moexipril
Moricizine
Moxifloxacin
Nadolol
Nafcillin
Naratriptan
Nefazodone
Nicotine
Nifedipine
Nisoldipine
Norfloxacin
Nortriptyline
Ofloxacin
Olanzapine
Omeprazole
Oxacillin
Oxaprozin
Oxcarbazepine
Pamidronate
Pantoprazole
Paroxetine
Penbutolol
Penicillamine
Penicillins
Pentazocine
Pentostatin
Pentoxifylline
Pergolide
Perindopril
Phendimetrazine
Phentermine
Phytonadione
Pilocarpine
Pimozide
Pindolol
Pirbuterol
Plicamycin
Potassium iodide
Pramipexole
Pravastatin
Procainamide
Propafenone
Propantheline
Propofol
Propranolol
Propylthiouracil
Protriptyline
Pyrimethamine
Quazepam
Quinapril
Quinidine
Ramipril
Ranitidine
Ribavirin
Rifabutin
Riluzole
Rimantadine
Risperidone
Ritonavir
Rivastigmine
Saccharin
Saquinavir
Selegiline
Sertraline
Sibutramine
Simvastatin
Sotalol
Sparfloxacin
Sulfamethoxazole
Sulfasalazine
Sulfisoxazole
Sulindac
Sumatriptan
Tacrine
Tamoxifen
Temazepam
Terbinafine
Terbutaline
Thiothixene
Tiagabine
Ticarcillin
Timolol
Tocainide
Tolazamide
Tolbutamide
Tolmetin
Topiramate
Tramadol
Trazodone
Triamterene
Triazolam
Trimethoprim
Trimipramine
Trovafloxacin
Ursodiol
Vancomycin
Venlafaxine
Vinblastine
Vincristine
Vinorelbine
Zalcitabine
Zidovudine
Zolpidem
Zonisamide

Ecchymoses

Allopurinol
Alprostadil
Alteplase
Amiodarone
Amoxicillin
Anistreplase
Atorvastatin
Bacampicillin
Benactyzine
Beta-carotene
Bromfenac
Buspirone
Carbenicillin
Celecoxib
Chlorzoxazone
Cholestyramine
Cilostazol
Cloxacillin
Corticosteroids
Delavirdine
Denileukin
Desipramine
Dexfenfluramine
Dicloxacillin
Dicumarol
Diltiazem
Donepezil
Enoxaparin
Etodolac
Etoposide
Fluvoxamine
Fosphenytoin
Gatifloxacin
Gemtuzumab
Heparin
Indomethacin
Interferons, alfa-2
Irbesartan
Lamotrigine
Latanoprost
Leuprolide
Levetiracetam
Losartan

Meprobamate
Mesalamine
Methicillin
Methotrexate
Mezlocillin
Modafinil
Nafcillin
Naproxen
Nefazodone
Nisoldipine
Ofloxacin
Olanzapine
Oxacillin
Oxaprozin
Pantoprazole
Paroxetine
Penicillamine
Pentosan
Pentostatin
Perindopril
Piperacillin
Piroxicam
Plicamycin
Rabeprazole
Reteplase
Risedronate
Ritonavir
Sibutramine
Sirolimus
Sparfloxacin
Streptokinase
Sulindac
Tacrolimus
Thiotepa
Tiagabine
Ticarcillin
Ticlopidine
Tiopronin
Tizanidine
Urokinase
Vasopressin
Venlafaxine
Verapamil
Warfarin
Zaleplon
Zidovudine
Zolmitriptan
Zonisamide

Eczema (sic)

Acetohexamide
Ascorbic acid
Astemizole
Atorvastatin
Azelastine
Bisoprolol
Cevimeline
Citalopram
Clopidogrel
Dexfenfluramine
Diclofenac
Diphenhydramine
Doxazosin
Efavirenz
Eprosartan
Erythromycin
Esmolol
Estrogens
Ethionamide
Fluoxetine
Fluphenazine
Flurbiprofen
Gemfibrozil
Glipizide
Glyburide
Ketoconazole
Lamotrigine
Latanoprost
Leflunomide
Lidocaine
Lithium
Lomefloxacin
Mesalamine
Mesoridazine
Metformin
Nefazodone
Olanzapine
Omeprazole
Oral contraceptives
Oxcarbazepine
Pantoprazole
Paroxetine
Pentostatin
Perphenazine
Prochlorperazine
Riluzole
Ritonavir
Ropinirole
Saquinavir
Simvastatin
Tacrine
Telmisartan
Terbinafine
Tiagabine
Tolcapone
Topiramate
Trifluoperazine
Venlafaxine
Zaleplon
Zonisamide

Edema

Abacavir
Acebutolol
Acyclovir
Aldesleukin
Alitretinoin
Allopurinol
Alprazolam
Alprostadil
Amantadine
Aminocaproic acid
Amiodarone
Amlodipine
Amoxapine
Amoxicillin
Amyl nitrite
Apraclonidine
Asparaginase
Astemizole
Atenolol
Atorvastatin
Atracurium
Azatadine
Azithromycin
Benactyzine
Betaxolol
Bicalutamide
Bisoprolol
Bromfenac
Bumetanide
Buspirone
Butorphanol
Candesartan
Capecitabine
Carbamazepine
Carbenicillin
Carisoprodol
Carteolol
Carvedilol
Cefaclor
Cefamandole
Cefpodoxime
Ceftazidime
Cerivastatin
Cetirizine
Cevimeline
Chlorambucil
Chlordiazepoxide
Chlormezanone
Chlorotrianisene
Chlorpropamide
Chlortetracycline
Cholestyramine
Cidofovir
Cilostazol
Cinoxacin
Ciprofloxacin
Cisapride
Cladribine
Clemastine
Clomiphene
Clomipramine
Clonidine
Clopidogrel
Clozapine
Colestipol
Cromolyn
Cyclosporine
Cyproheptadine
Danazol
Deferoxamine
Delavirdine
Denileukin
Desipramine
Desmopressin
Dexchlorpheniramine
Dexfenfluramine
Diazoxide
Diclofenac
Diethylstilbestrol
Diflunisal
Dihydroergotamine
Diltiazem
Dimenhydrinate
Diphenhydramine
Dipyridamole
Dirithromycin
Disopyramide
Docetaxel
Dofetilide
Dolasetron
Dorzolamide
Doxazosin
Doxepin
Doxercalciferol
Enoxacin
Enoxaparin
Ephedrine
Epoetin alfa
Esmolol
Estazolam
Estramustine
Estrogens
Etodolac
Felbamate
Felodipine
Fentanyl
Flecainide
Fludarabine
Fluoxymesterone
Fluphenazine
Flurbiprofen
Flutamide
Fluvoxamine
Foscarnet
Fosinopril
Ganciclovir
Gatifloxacin
Gemcitabine
Gentamicin
Glimepiride
Glipizide
Goserelin
Grepafloxacin
Guanabenz
Guanfacine
Heroin
Hydralazine
Hydrocodone
Hydroxyzine
Ibuprofen
Imipramine
Indomethacin
Infliximab
Insulin
Interferons, alfa-2
Irinotecan
Isoproterenol
Isosorbide dinitrate
Isosorbide mononitrate
Isotretinoin
Isradipine
Itraconazole
Ivermectin
Kanamycin
Ketorolac
Labetalol
Lansoprazole
Leuprolide
Levamisole
Levofloxacin
Lidocaine
Lisinopril
Lithium
Lomefloxacin

Losartan
Maprotiline
Mazindol
Meclofenamate
Medroxyprogesterone
Mefenamic acid
Meloxicam
Melphalan
Mephenytoin
Mercaptopurine
Mesalamine
Mesoridazine
Methadone
Methenamine
Methimazole
Methoxsalen
Methyldopa
Methylphenidate
Methyltestosterone
Metolazone
Metoprolol
Mexiletine
Minoxidil
Mirtazapine
Mitomycin
Molindone
Morphine
Moxifloxacin
Mycophenolate
Nabumetone
Nadolol
Nafarelin
Naproxen
Naratriptan
Nicardipine
Nicotine
Nifedipine
Nimodipine
Nitroglycerin
Nizatidine
Norfloxacin
Nortriptyline
Octreotide
Ofloxacin
Olanzapine
Omeprazole
Oral contraceptives
Oxaprozin
Oxazepam
Oxcarbazepine
Pamidronate
Pantoprazole
Paroxetine
Penicillamine
Pentamidine
Pentoxifylline
Pergolide
Perindopril
Phenazopyridine
Phenelzine
Phenobarbital
Pilocarpine
Pindolol
Pioglitazone
Piperacillin
Pirbuterol
Piroxicam
Pramipexole
Praziquantel
Prazosin
Procarbazine
Progestins
Promazine
Propafenone
Propofol
Propranolol
Propylthiouracil
Protriptyline
Psoralens
Quetiapine
Quinapril
Quinestrol
Rabeprazole
Raloxifene
Ramipril
Reserpine
Riluzole
Rimantadine
Risedronate
Risperidone
Ritonavir
Rivastigmine
Rofecoxib
Ropinirole
Rosiglitazone
Scopolamine
Sertraline
Sibutramine
Sildenafil
Sirolimus
Sotalol
Sparfloxacin
Stanozolol
Streptomycin
Streptozocin
Sulfinpyrazone
Sulindac
Tacrine
Tacrolimus
Tamoxifen
Terazosin
Testosterone
Thalidomide
Tiagabine
Timolol
Tiopronin
Tirofiban
Tizanidine
Tolazoline
Tolcapone
Tolmetin
Topiramate
Toremifene
Torsemide
Trandolapril
Tranylcypromine
Trazodone
Triamterene
Trimeprazine
Tripelennamine
Triprolidine
Troglitazone
Trovafloxacin
Venlafaxine
Verapamil
Vincristine
Zalcitabine
Zaleplon
Zolmitriptan
Zolpidem
Zonisamide

Erythema

Acarbose
Acetaminophen
Acetohexamide
Acitretin
Albuterol
Aldesleukin
Alendronate
Aminoglutethimide
Amitriptyline
Amobarbital
Amphotericin B
Aprotinin
Ascorbic acid
Atracurium
Azithromycin
Betaxolol
Busulfan
Capecitabine
Carboplatin
Carmustine
Cefadroxil
Cefonicid
Chloral hydrate
Chlorotrianisene
Chlortetracycline
Cisplatin
Cladribine
Clomiphene
Clomipramine
Clonidine
Clozapine
Corticosteroids
Cromolyn
Cyproheptadine
Cytarabine
Dacarbazine
Dactinomycin
Dantrolene
Daunorubicin
Deferoxamine
Delavirdine
Desipramine
Diclofenac
Diltiazem
Dobutamine
Docetaxel
Donepezil
Doxepin
Eflornithine
Enalapril
Enoxaparin
Epirubicin
Esmolol
Etanercept
Etoposide
Felodipine
Fentanyl
Fluorouracil
Fluphenazine
Flutamide
Folic acid
Gatifloxacin
Gentamicin
Glimepiride
Glipizide
Glyburide
Granulocyte colony-stimulating factor (GCSF)
Heparin
Imipramine
Interferons, alfa-2
Irbesartan
Kanamycin
Ketamine
Lamotrigine
Leucovorin
Levobunolol
Levofloxacin
Lisinopril
Lithium
Losartan
Lovastatin
Maprotiline
Mefloquine
Mesalamine
Mesna
Mesoridazine
Metformin
Methohexital
Methotrexate
Methoxsalen
Metronidazole
Miconazole
Minoxidil
Mitomycin
Modafinil
Nabumetone
Naratriptan
Niacin
Nicotine
Nifedipine
Nitroglycerin
Norfloxacin
Nortriptyline
Omeprazole
Oral contraceptives
Oxaprozin
Pentamidine
Pentostatin
Perindopril
Perphenazine
Phenindamine
Phytonadione
Piroxicam
Prochlorperazine
Protriptyline
Psoralens
Quinestrol
Quinine
Ramipril
Ritodrine
Rofecoxib

Saquinavir
Scopolamine
Sertraline
Spironolactone
Succinylcholine
Sufentanil
Sulindac
Sumatriptan
Tacrolimus
Thalidomide
Thiopental
Ticlopidine
Tiopronin
Tolazamide
Tolbutamide
Tolterodine
Topotecan
Trifluoperazine
Vinblastine
Vinorelbine
Vitamin A

Erythema annulare centrifugum

Amitriptyline
Ampicillin
Chloroquine
Cimetidine
Gold & gold compounds
Hydrochlorothiazide
Hydroxychloroquine
Penicillins
Piroxicam
Spironolactone

Erythema multiforme

Acarbose
Acebutolol
Acetaminophen
Acetazolamide
Alendronate
Allopurinol
Amantadine
Aminosalicylate sodium
Amlodipine
Amoxapine
Amoxicillin
Amphotericin B
Ampicillin
Arsenic
Aspirin
Atenolol
Atovaquone
Atropine sulfate
Azathioprine
Aztreonam
Bacampicillin
Benactyzine
Bumetanide
Busulfan
Butabarbital
Butalbital
Carbamazepine
Carbenicillin
Carisoprodol
Cefaclor
Cefadroxil
Cefamandole
Cefazolin
Cefdinir
Cefepime
Cefixime
Cefonicid
Cefoperazone
Cefotaxime
Cefotetan
Cefpodoxime
Cefprozil
Ceftazidime
Ceftriaxone
Cefuroxime
Celecoxib
Cephalexin
Cephalothin
Cephapirin
Cephradine
Cerivastatin
Chloral hydrate
Chlorambucil
Chloramphenicol
Chlordiazepoxide
Chlormezanone
Chloroquine
Chlorothiazide
Chlorotrianisene
Chlorpromazine
Chlorpropamide
Chlorthalidone
Chlorzoxazone
Cimetidine
Cinoxacin
Ciprofloxacin
Clindamycin
Clofibrate
Clomiphene
Clonazepam
Cloxacillin
Clozapine
Co-trimoxazole
Codeine
Corticosteroids
Cyclophosphamide
Dactinomycin
Danazol
Dapsone
Deferoxamine
Delavirdine
Dexfenfluramine
Diclofenac
Dicloxacillin
Didanosine
Diethylpropion
Diethylstilbestrol
Diflunisal
Diltiazem
Dipyridamole
Doxycycline
Enalapril
Enoxacin
Erythromycin
Estrogens
Ethambutol
Ethosuximide
Etodolac
Etoposide
Famotidine
Fenoprofen
Fluconazole
Fluorouracil
Fluoxetine
Flurbiprofen
Fluvastatin
Fosphenytoin
Furazolidone
Furosemide
Gemfibrozil
Glucagon
Gold & gold compounds
Griseofulvin
Hydrochlorothiazide
Hydrocodone
Hydroxychloroquine
Hydroxyurea
Hydroxyzine
Ibuprofen
Imipenem/cilastatin
Indapamide
Indinavir
Indomethacin
Isoniazid
Isotretinoin
Itraconazole
Ketoprofen
Lamotrigine
Levamisole
Levofloxacin
Lidocaine
Lincomycin
Lithium
Loracarbef
Loratadine
Lorazepam
Lovastatin
Maprotiline
Mechlorethamine
Meclofenamate
Mefenamic acid
Mefloquine
Meloxicam
Mephenytoin
Meprobamate
Methenamine
Methicillin
Methotrexate
Methsuximide
Methyclothiazide
Methyldopa
Methylphenidate
Metoprolol
Mezlocillin
Minocycline
Minoxidil
Mitomycin
Mitotane
Nabumetone
Nadolol
Nafcillin
Nalidixic acid
Naproxen
Neomycin
Nifedipine
Nitrofurantoin
Norfloxacin
Nystatin
Ofloxacin
Omeprazole
Oral contraceptives
Oxacillin
Oxaprozin
Oxazepam
Oxcarbazepine
Oxybutynin
Pantoprazole
Paramethadione
Penicillamine
Penicillins
Pentobarbital
Phenobarbital
Phenolphthalein
Phensuximide
Phenytoin
Pindolol
Piroxicam
Pravastatin
Primidone
Probenecid
Progestins
Promethazine
Propranolol
Pyrazinamide
Pyrimethamine
Quinidine
Quinine
Ramipril
Ranitidine
Ribavirin
Rifampin
Ritodrine
Saquinavir
Scopolamine
Sertraline
Simvastatin
Spironolactone
Streptomycin
Sulfadiazine
Sulfadoxine
Sulfamethoxazole
Sulfasalazine
Sulfisoxazole
Sulindac
Tamsulosin
Terbinafine
Tetracycline
Thiabendazole
Thiopental
Thioridazine
Ticarcillin
Ticlopidine
Timolol
Tiopronin
Tobramycin
Tocainide
Tolbutamide
Tolcapone
Tolmetin
Trazodone

Trimethadione
Trimethoprim
Troleandomycin
Trovafloxacin
Vancomycin
Verapamil
Vinblastine
Vitamin A
Vitamin E
Zalcitabine
Zidovudine

Erythema nodosum

Acetaminophen
Acyclovir
Aldesleukin
Amiodarone
Arsenic
Aspirin
Azathioprine
Busulfan
Carbamazepine
Carbenicillin
Cefdinir
Chlordiazepoxide
Chlorotrianisene
Chlorpropamide
Ciprofloxacin
Clomiphene
Co-trimoxazole
Codeine
Dapsone
Diclofenac
Dicloxacillin
Diethylstilbestrol
Disopyramide
Enoxacin
Estrogens
Fluoxetine
Furosemide
Glucagon
Gold & gold compounds
Granulocyte colony-stimulating factor (GCSF)
Hydralazine
Hydroxychloroquine
Ibuprofen
Indomethacin
Isotretinoin
Levofloxacin
Meclofenamate
Medroxyprogesterone
Meprobamate
Mesalamine
Methicillin
Methimazole
Methyldopa
Mezlocillin
Minocycline
Montelukast
Naproxen
Nifedipine
Nitrofurantoin
Ofloxacin
Omeprazole
Oral contraceptives
Oxacillin
Paroxetine
Penicillamine
Penicillins
Piperacillin
Progestins
Propylthiouracil
Sparfloxacin
Streptomycin
Sulfamethoxazole
Sulfasalazine
Sulfisoxazole
Thalidomide
Ticarcillin
Ticlopidine
Trimethoprim
Verapamil
Zileuton

Erythroderma

Aldesleukin
Amitriptyline
Aspirin
Captopril
Carbamazepine
Chloroquine
Cimetidine
Ciprofloxacin
Clofazimine
Co-trimoxazole
Colchicine
Cytarabine
Dapsone
Dicloxacillin
Diflunisal
Hydroxychloroquine
Lansoprazole
Meclofenamate
Methotrexate
Minoxidil
Nitroglycerin
Nystatin
Omeprazole
Pentostatin
Phenobarbital
Phenytoin
Piroxicam
Sulfamethoxazole
Sulfasalazine
Terbinafine
Thalidomide
Timolol
Vincristine
Zalcitabine
Zidovudine

Exanthems

Abacavir
Acebutolol
Acetaminophen
Acetazolamide
Acetohexamide
Acitretin
Acyclovir
Albuterol
Aldesleukin
Alendronate
Allopurinol
Alprazolam
Altretamine
Amantadine
Amikacin
Amiloride
Aminocaproic acid
Aminoglutethimide
Aminophylline
Aminosalicylate sodium
Amiodarone
Amitriptyline
Amlodipine
Amobarbital
Amoxapine
Amoxicillin
Amphotericin B
Ampicillin
Amprenavir
Anistreplase
Aprobarbital
Aprotinin
Arsenic
Asparaginase
Aspartame
Aspirin
Astemizole
Atenolol
Atorvastatin
Atovaquone
Atropine sulfate
Azatadine
Azathioprine
Azelastine
Azithromycin
Aztreonam
Bacampicillin
Baclofen
Benactyzine
Benazepril
Bendroflumethiazide
Benztropine
Betaxolol
Bexarotene
Bicalutamide
Biperiden
Bisacodyl
Bisoprolol
Bleomycin
Bromfenac
Bromocriptine
Brompheniramine
Bumetanide
Buspirone
Busulfan
Butabarbital
Butalbital
Butorphanol
Calcitonin
Candesartan
Captopril
Carbamazepine
Carbenicillin
Carboplatin
Carisoprodol
Carmustine
Carteolol
Carvedilol
Cefaclor
Cefadroxil
Cefamandole
Cefazolin
Cefdinir
Cefepime
Cefoperazone
Cefotetan
Cefoxitin
Cefprozil
Ceftazidime
Ceftriaxone
Cefuroxime
Celecoxib
Cephalexin
Cephalothin
Cephradine
Cetirizine
Cevimeline
Chloral hydrate
Chlorambucil
Chloramphenicol
Chlordiazepoxide
Chlormezanone
Chloroquine
Chlorothiazide
Chlorpromazine
Chlorpropamide
Chlorthalidone
Chlorzoxazone
Cholestyramine
Cimetidine
Ciprofloxacin
Cisapride
Cisplatin
Cladribine
Clarithromycin
Clemastine
Clindamycin
Clofazimine
Clofibrate
Clomiphene
Clomipramine
Clonazepam
Clonidine
Clopidogrel
Clorazepate
Cloxacillin
Clozapine
Co-trimoxazole
Codeine
Colchicine
Colestipol
Corticosteroids
Cromolyn
Cyanocobalamin
Cyclamate
Cyclophosphamide
Cycloserine
Cyclosporine
Cyclothiazide
Cyproheptadine
Cytarabine
Dacarbazine
Dactinomycin
Dalteparin

Danazol
Dantrolene
Dapsone
Daunorubicin
Deferoxamine
Delavirdine
Demeclocycline
Denileukin
Desipramine
Dexfenfluramine
Diazepam
Diazoxide
Diclofenac
Dicloxacillin
Dicumarol
Dicyclomine
Didanosine
Diethylpropion
Diethylstilbestrol
Diflunisal
Digoxin
Dihydrotachysterol
Diltiazem
Dimenhydrinate
Diphenhydramine
Dipyridamole
Disopyramide
Disulfiram
Docetaxel
Docusate
Dopamine
Doxazosin
Doxepin
Doxorubicin
Doxycycline
Efavirenz
Enalapril
Enoxacin
Ephedrine
Epinephrine
Epoetin alfa
Eprosartan
Erythromycin
Estramustine
Estrogens
Ethacrynic acid
Ethambutol
Ethionamide
Ethosuximide
Etodolac
Etoposide
Famotidine
Felodipine
Fenfluramine
Fenofibrate
Fenoprofen
Fentanyl
Finasteride
Flavoxate
Flecainide
Fluconazole
Flucytosine
Fludarabine
Fluorouracil
Fluoxetine
Fluoxymesterone
Fluphenazine
Flurazepam
Flurbiprofen
Flutamide
Fluvoxamine
Folic acid
Foscarnet
Fosfomycin
Fosphenytoin
Furazolidone
Furosemide
Gabapentin
Ganciclovir
Gatifloxacin
Gemcitabine
Gemfibrozil
Gentamicin
Glimepiride
Glipizide
Glucagon
Glyburide
Gold & gold compounds
Granisetron
Granulocyte colony-stimulating factor (GCSF)
Grepafloxacin
Griseofulvin
Guanethidine
Guanfacine
Haloperidol
Halothane
Heparin
Heroin
Hydralazine
Hydrochlorothiazide
Hydrocodone
Hydromorphone
Hydroxychloroquine
Hydroxyurea
Hydroxyzine
Ibuprofen
Idarubicin
Imipenem/cilastatin
Imipramine
Indapamide
Indinavir
Indomethacin
Insulin
Interferons, alfa-2
Ipodate
Ipratropium
Isocarboxazid
Isoniazid
Isotretinoin
Isradipine
Itraconazole
Ivermectin
Kanamycin
Ketamine
Ketoconazole
Ketoprofen
Ketorolac
Labetalol
Lamivudine
Lamotrigine
Lansoprazole
Letrozole
Leuprolide
Levamisole
Levodopa
Lidocaine
Lincomycin
Lisinopril
Lithium
Lomefloxacin
Loratadine
Lorazepam
Losartan
Lovastatin
Loxapine
Maprotiline
Marihuana
Mazindol
Mebendazole
Mechlorethamine
Meclizine
Meclofenamate
Medroxyprogesterone
Mefenamic acid
Mefloquine
Meloxicam
Melphalan
Mephenytoin
Mephobarbital
Meprobamate
Mercaptopurine
Mesalamine
Mesna
Metformin
Methadone
Methantheline
Methazolamide
Methenamine
Methicillin
Methimazole
Methocarbamol
Methohexital
Methotrexate
Methoxsalen
Methsuximide
Methyclothiazide
Methyldopa
Methylphenidate
Methyltestosterone
Methysergide
Metoclopramide
Metolazone
Metoprolol
Metronidazole
Mexiletine
Mezlocillin
Miconazole
Midazolam
Minocycline
Minoxidil
Misoprostol
Mitomycin
Mitotane
Moexipril
Moricizine
Morphine
Nabumetone
Nadolol
Nafarelin
Nafcillin
Nalidixic acid
Naloxone
Naproxen
Naratriptan
Nefazodone
Neomycin
Nevirapine
Niacin
Nicardipine
Nifedipine
Nimodipine
Nisoldipine
Nitrofurantoin
Nitroglycerin
Nizatidine
Norfloxacin
Nortriptyline
Nystatin
Octreotide
Ofloxacin
Olanzapine
Olsalazine
Omeprazole
Ondansetron
Oral contraceptives
Orphenadrine
Oxacillin
Oxaprozin
Oxazepam
Oxcarbazepine
Oxytetracycline
Pamidronate
Pantoprazole
Pantothenic acid
Paramethadione
Paroxetine
Pemoline
Penbutolol
Penicillamine
Penicillins
Pentagastrin
Pentamidine
Pentazocine
Pentobarbital
Pentostatin
Pentoxifylline
Pergolide
Perindopril
Perphenazine
Phenazopyridine
Phenelzine
Phenobarbital
Phenolphthalein
Phenytoin
Phytonadione
Pimozide
Pindolol
Piperacillin
Piroxicam
Plicamycin
Polythiazide
Potassium iodide
Pravastatin

Prazepam
Prazosin
Primaquine
Primidone
Procainamide
Procarbazine
Prochlorperazine
Progestins
Promazine
Promethazine
Propafenone
Propantheline
Propofol
Propoxyphene
Propranolol
Protamine
Protriptyline
Pseudoephedrine
Pyrazinamide
Pyrimethamine
Quinacrine
Quinapril
Quinethazone
Quinidine
Quinine
Quinupristin/dalfopristin
Ramipril
Ranitidine
Reserpine
Ribavirin
Rifampin
Ritodrine
Ritonavir
Rituximab
Rivastigmine
Rofecoxib
Ropinirole
Rosiglitazone
Saccharin
Salmeterol
Salsalate
Saquinavir
Scopolamine
Secobarbital
Sertraline
Simvastatin
Sotalol
Sparfloxacin
Spectinomycin
Spironolactone
Stanozolol
Streptokinase
Streptomycin
Streptozocin
Succinylcholine
Sucralfate
Sulfadiazine
Sulfadoxine
Sulfamethoxazole
Sulfasalazine
Sulfinpyrazone
Sulfisoxazole
Sulindac
Sumatriptan
Tacrine
Tacrolimus
Tamoxifen
Temazepam
Terazosin
Terbinafine
Terbutaline
Terfenadine
Testosterone
Tetracycline
Thalidomide
Thiabendazole
Thiamine
Thioguanine
Thiopental
Thioridazine
Thiothixene
Tiagabine
Ticarcillin
Ticlopidine
Timolol
Tiopronin
Tizanidine
Tobramycin
Tocainide
Tolazamide
Tolazoline
Tolbutamide
Tolmetin
Topiramate
Torsemide
Tramadol
Tranylcypromine
Trazodone
Triamterene
Triazolam
Trichlormethiazide
Trifluoperazine
Trimeprazine
Trimethadione
Trimethoprim
Trimetrexate
Trimipramine
Triprolidine
Troleandomycin
Trovafloxacin
Urokinase
Vancomycin
Vasopressin
Venlafaxine
Verapamil
Vinblastine
Vincristine
Vitamin A
Vitamin E
Warfarin
Zalcitabine
Zaleplon
Zidovudine
Zonisamide

Exfoliative dermatitis

Acebutolol
Acetaminophen
Aldesleukin
Alitretinoin
Allopurinol
Aminoglutethimide
Aminophylline
Aminosalicylate sodium
Amiodarone
Amitriptyline
Amobarbital
Amoxicillin
Amphotericin B
Ampicillin
Aprobarbital
Arsenic
Aspirin
Atropine sulfate
Aztreonam
Bacampicillin
Benactyzine
Bendroflumethiazide
Betaxolol
Bexarotene
Bisoprolol
Bumetanide
Butabarbital
Butalbital
Capecitabine
Captopril
Carbamazepine
Carbenicillin
Carteolol
Carvedilol
Cefdinir
Cefoxitin
Chlorambucil
Chloroquine
Chlorothiazide
Chlorpromazine
Chlorpropamide
Chlorthalidone
Cimetidine
Ciprofloxacin
Cisplatin
Clofazimine
Clofibrate
Cloxacillin
Co-trimoxazole
Codeine
Cromolyn
Cytarabine
Dapsone
Demeclocycline
Desipramine
Diazepam
Diclofenac
Dicloxacillin
Diethylstilbestrol
Diflunisal
Diltiazem
Doxorubicin
Doxycycline
Enalapril
Enoxacin
Ephedrine
Epirubicin
Esmolol
Estrogens
Ethambutol
Ethosuximide
Etodolac
Fenoprofen
Fentanyl
Flecainide
Fluconazole
Fluoxetine
Fluphenazine
Flurbiprofen
Fluvoxamine
Fosinopril
Fosphenytoin
Furosemide
Ganciclovir
Gemfibrozil
Gentamicin
Gold & gold compounds
Granulocyte colony-stimulating factor (GCSF)
Grepafloxacin
Griseofulvin
Guanfacine
Haloperidol
Hydrochlorothiazide
Hydroxychloroquine
Imipramine
Indomethacin
Isoniazid
Ketoconazole
Ketoprofen
Ketorolac
Labetalol
Levamisole
Lidocaine
Lincomycin
Lithium
Meclofenamate
Mefenamic acid
Mefloquine
Mephenytoin
Mephobarbital
Meprobamate
Mesoridazine
Methantheline
Methicillin
Methimazole
Methoxsalen
Methsuximide
Methylphenidate
Metolazone
Metoprolol
Mexiletine
Mezlocillin
Mibefradil
Minocycline
Mirtazapine
Mitomycin
Nadolol
Nafcillin
Nalidixic acid
Naproxen
Nifedipine
Nisoldipine
Nitrofurantoin
Nitroglycerin
Nizatidine
Norfloxacin
Ofloxacin
Omeprazole

Oxacillin
Oxaprozin
Oxytetracycline
Paramethadione
Penicillamine
Penicillins
Pentobarbital
Pentostatin
Perphenazine
Phenobarbital
Phenolphthalein
Phenytoin
Pindolol
Piperacillin
Piroxicam
Primidone
Procarbazine
Prochlorperazine
Propranolol
Propylthiouracil
Pseudoephedrine
Pyrimethamine
Quinacrine
Quinapril
Quinidine
Quinine
Rifampin
Riluzole
Risperidone
Rivastigmine
Secobarbital
Sildenafil
Sparfloxacin
Streptomycin
Sulfadiazine
Sulfadoxine
Sulfamethoxazole
Sulfasalazine
Sulfisoxazole
Sulindac
Tetracycline
Thalidomide
Thiopental
Thioridazine
Tiagabine
Ticarcillin
Ticlopidine
Timolol
Tizanidine
Tobramycin
Tocainide
Trazodone
Trifluoperazine
Trimethadione
Trimethoprim
Vancomycin
Venlafaxine
Verapamil
Vitamin A
Warfarin
Yohimbine
Zalcitabine

Fixed eruption

Acetaminophen
Acyclovir
Albendazole
Alendronate
Allopurinol
Aminosalicylate sodium
Amitriptyline
Amoxicillin
Amphotericin B
Ampicillin
Arsenic
Aspirin
Atenolol
Atropine sulfate
Azathioprine
Azithromycin
Bacampicillin
Benactyzine
Bisacodyl
Butabarbital
Butalbital
Cabergoline
Carbamazepine
Carisoprodol
Cefazolin
Cephalexin
Chloral hydrate
Chloramphenicol
Chlordiazepoxide
Chlorhexidine
Chlormezanone
Chloroquine
Chlorothiazide
Chlorpromazine
Chlorpropamide
Cimetidine
Ciprofloxacin
Clarithromycin
Co-trimoxazole
Codeine
Colchicine
Dacarbazine
Dapsone
Demeclocycline
Dextromethorphan
Diazepam
Diflunisal
Dimenhydrinate
Diphenhydramine
Disulfiram
Docetaxel
Doxycycline
Ephedrine
Epinephrine
Erythromycin
Estrogens
Ethchlorvynol
Ethotoin
Etodolac
Fluconazole
Flurbiprofen
Foscarnet
Ganciclovir
Gold & gold compounds
Griseofulvin
Guanethidine
Heparin
Heroin
Hydralazine
Hydrochlorothiazide
Hydroxychloroquine
Hydroxyurea
Hydroxyzine
Ibuprofen
Imipramine
Indapamide
Indomethacin
Isotretinoin
Itraconazole
Ketoconazole
Levamisole
Lidocaine
Lorazepam
Meclofenamate
Mefenamic acid
Meprobamate
Mesna
Metaxalone
Methenamine
Methimazole
Methyldopa
Methylphenidate
Metronidazole
Minocycline
Naproxen
Neomycin
Niacin
Nifedipine
Nitrofurantoin
Norfloxacin
Nystatin
Ofloxacin
Omeprazole
Ondansetron
Oral contraceptives
Oxaprozin
Oxazepam
Oxytetracycline
Penicillins
Pentobarbital
Phenobarbital
Phenolphthalein
Phenytoin
Piroxicam
Procarbazine
Prochlorperazine
Promethazine
Propofol
Pseudoephedrine
Pyrazinamide
Pyridoxine
Pyrimethamine
Quinacrine
Quinidine
Quinine
Ranitidine
Rifampin
Saccharin
Saquinavir
Scopolamine
Sertraline
Sildenafil
Streptomycin
Sulfadiazine
Sulfamethoxazole
Sulfasalazine
Sulfisoxazole
Sulindac
Temazepam
Terbinafine
Terfenadine
Tetracycline
Thiabendazole
Thiopental
Ticlopidine
Tolbutamide
Trifluoperazine
Trimethadione
Trimetrexate
Tripelennamine
Triprolidine

Flushing

Acetaminophen
Albuterol
Alitretinoin
Alprostadil
Amifostine
Amiloride
Aminophylline
Amiodarone
Amitriptyline
Amlodipine
Amoxapine
Amphotericin B
Amyl nitrite
Anistreplase
Ascorbic acid
Asparaginase
Aspirin
Atracurium
Atropine sulfate
Azatadine
Azelastine
Baclofen
Benazepril
Betaxolol
Bethanechol
Biperiden
Bisoprolol
Bretylium
Bromocriptine
Buspirone
Butorphanol
Calcitonin (human & salmon)
Captopril
Carisoprodol
Carmustine
Carteolol
Cefaclor
Cefamandole
Cefoxitin
Cefpodoxime
Ceftazidime
Ceftriaxone
Cerivastatin
Cetirizine
Chloral hydrate
Chlormezanone
Chlorpropamide
Chlorzoxazone
Ciprofloxacin

Cisplatin
Clemastine
Clidinium
Clomiphene
Clomipramine
Co-trimoxazole
Codeine
Colchicine
Corticosteroids
Cromolyn
Cyclobenzaprine
Cyclophosphamide
Cyclosporine
Cyproheptadine
Dacarbazine
Danazol
Daunorubicin
Deferoxamine
Denileukin
Desipramine
Desmopressin
Diazepam
Diazoxide
Diclofenac
Dicyclomine
Diethylpropion
Diethylstilbestrol
Diflunisal
Diltiazem
Dimenhydrinate
Diphenoxylate
Dipyridamole
Disulfiram
Docetaxel
Dolasetron
Donepezil
Doxapram
Doxazosin
Doxepin
Doxorubicin
Dronabinol (THC)
Edrophonium
Efavirenz
Enalapril
Epinephrine
Esmolol
Estazolam
Estramustine
Estrogens
Etodolac
Etoposide
Famotidine
Felbamate
Felodipine
Fenfluramine
Fentanyl
Flecainide
Flumazenil
Fluoxetine
Fluoxymesterone
Flurazepam
Flurbiprofen
Fluvastatin
Folic acid
Foscarnet
Fosinopril
Furazolidone
Furosemide
Glipizide
Glyburide
Glycopyrrolate
Granulocyte colony-stimulating factor (GCSF)
Griseofulvin
Haloperidol
Hydralazine
Hydrocodone
Hydromorphone
Hydroxyzine
Ibuprofen
Imipenem/cilastatin
Imipramine
Indapamide
Indinavir
Indomethacin
Insulin
Ipratropium
Irbesartan
Irinotecan
Isoniazid
Isoproterenol
Isosorbide dinitrate
Isosorbide mononitrate
Isotretinoin
Isradipine
Ketorolac
Labetalol
Lamotrigine
Leuprolide
Levodopa
Levothyroxine
Lisinopril
Lomefloxacin
Lomustine
Loratadine
Losartan
Maprotiline
Medroxyprogesterone
Meperidine
Mesna
Mesoridazine
Methadone
Methantheline
Methocarbamol
Methyltestosterone
Methysergide
Metoclopramide
Metronidazole
Mibefradil
Miconazole
Minoxidil
Mitotane
Moexipril
Morphine
Nafarelin
Nefazodone
Niacin
Nicardipine
Nicotine
Nifedipine
Nimodipine
Nisoldipine
Nitrofurantoin
Nitroglycerin
Nortriptyline
Octreotide
Ondansetron
Orphenadrine
Oxybutynin
Penbutolol
Penicillamine
Pentagastrin
Pentazocine
Pentostatin
Pentoxifylline
Phendimetrazine
Phenindamine
Phentolamine
Phytonadione
Pilocarpine
Plicamycin
Pravastatin
Probenecid
Procainamide
Procarbazine
Progestins
Promethazine
Propafenone
Propofol
Propoxyphene
Propranolol
Protamine
Protriptyline
Pyrazinamide
Pyrilamine
Quinapril
Quinidine
Quinine
Ramipril
Reserpine
Rifampin
Risperidone
Rituximab
Rivastigmine
Rizatriptan
Rofecoxib
Ropinirole
Scopolamine
Sertraline
Sildenafil
Simvastatin
Spironolactone
Streptokinase
Succinylcholine
Sulfamethoxazole
Sulfasalazine
Sulfinpyrazone
Sulfisoxazole
Sumatriptan
Tacrine
Tacrolimus
Tamoxifen
Telmisartan
Terbutaline
Terfenadine
Testosterone
Thiabendazole
Tolazoline
Tolbutamide
Topiramate
Trandolapril
Tranylcypromine
Triamterene
Trihexyphenidyl
Trimetrexate
Tripelennamine
Triprolidine
Trovafloxacin
Urokinase
Vancomycin
Verapamil
Vinorelbine
Yohimbine
Zalcitabine
Zolmitriptan
Zolpidem

Galactorrhea

Alprazolam
Amitriptyline
Amoxapine
Buspirone
Chlordiazepoxide
Chlorpromazine
Cimetidine
Citalopram
Clomipramine
Cyclobenzaprine
Desipramine
Doxepin
Estrogens
Fluphenazine
Haloperidol
Imipramine
Isotretinoin
Loxapine
Maprotiline
Medroxyprogesterone
Mesoridazine
Methyldopa
Metoclopramide
Minocycline
Molindone
Nitrofurantoin
Nortriptyline
Octreotide
Oral contraceptives
Paroxetine
Perphenazine
Pimozide
Prochlorperazine
Progestins
Promazine
Promethazine
Protriptyline
Risperidone
Sertraline
Tamoxifen
Terfenadine
Thalidomide
Thioridazine
Thiothixene
Toremifene
Trazodone
Trifluoperazine

Trimipramine
Verapamil

Gingival hyperplasia

Amlodipine
Cevimeline
Co-trimoxazole
Cyclosporine
Diltiazem
Erythromycin
Estrogens
Ethosuximide
Ethotoin
Felodipine
Fosphenytoin
Isradipine
Ketoconazole
Lamotrigine
Lithium
Mephenytoin
Methsuximide
Mycophenolate
Nicardipine
Nifedipine
Nisoldipine
Oral contraceptives
Oxcarbazepine
Phensuximide
Phenytoin
Primidone
Sertraline
Sirolimus
Tacrolimus
Tiagabine
Topiramate
Verapamil
Zonisamide

Glossitis

Aldesleukin
Amitriptyline
Amoxapine
Amoxicillin
Ampicillin
Atorvastatin
Azelastine
Bacampicillin
Betaxolol
Bleomycin
Captopril
Carbamazepine
Carbenicillin
Cefaclor
Cefadroxil
Cefamandole
Cefpodoxime
Cefprozil
Ceftazidime
Ceftriaxone
Chloramphenicol
Chlorhexidine
Clarithromycin
Clomipramine
Cloxacillin
Co-trimoxazole
Cyclosporine
Demeclocycline
Dicloxacillin
Doxepin
Doxycycline
Enalapril
Estazolam
Etidronate
Etodolac
Felbamate
Fluoxetine
Fluvoxamine
Gabapentin
Gatifloxacin
Gold & gold compounds
Grepafloxacin
Guanadrel
Guanethidine
Imipenem/cilastatin
Imipramine
Lansoprazole
Lincomycin
Mefenamic acid
Mercaptopurine
Methicillin
Methotrexate
Metronidazole
Minocycline
Mirtazapine
Moxifloxacin
Nabumetone
Nafcillin
Nefazodone
Nisoldipine
Olanzapine
Oxacillin
Pantoprazole
Paroxetine
Penicillamine
Penicillins
Phenelzine
Pirbuterol
Protriptyline
Pyrimethamine
Quetiapine
Rabeprazole
Riluzole
Risedronate
Rivastigmine
Ropinirole
Saquinavir
Sertraline
Sildenafil
Streptomycin
Sulfadoxine
Sulfamethoxazole
Sulfasalazine
Sulfisoxazole
Sulindac
Tacrine
Tetracycline
Tiagabine
Ticarcillin
Tolmetin
Triamterene
Triazolam
Trihexyphenidyl
Trimethoprim
Trimipramine
Venlafaxine
Zalcitabine
Zaleplon
Zonisamide

Gynecomastia

Alprazolam
Amiloride
Amitriptyline
Amlodipine
Amoxapine
Amprenavir
Arsenic
Atorvastatin
Bendroflumethiazide
Bicalutamide
Busulfan
Captopril
Carmustine
Cerivastatin
Chlordiazepoxide
Chlorotrianisene
Chlorpromazine
Cimetidine
Ciprofloxacin
Citalopram
Clofibrate
Clomiphene
Clomipramine
Clonidine
Cyclobenzaprine
Cyclosporine
Delavirdine
Desipramine
Dexfenfluramine
Diazepam
Diethylpropion
Diethylstilbestrol
Digoxin
Diltiazem
Disopyramide
Doxepin
Enalapril
Estazolam
Estramustine
Estrogens
Ethionamide
Etodolac
Famotidine
Felodipine
Fenfluramine
Finasteride
Fluoxetine
Fluoxymesterone
Fluphenazine
Flutamide
Fluvastatin
Foscarnet
Fosinopril
Goserelin
Griseofulvin
Guanabenz
Haloperidol
Ibuprofen
Imipramine
Indinavir
Indomethacin
Isoniazid
Isotretinoin
Itraconazole
Ketoconazole
Ketoprofen
Lansoprazole
Latanoprost
Leuprolide
Loratadine
Lovastatin
Loxapine
Maprotiline
Medroxyprogesterone
Meprobamate
Mesoridazine
Methotrexate
Methyldopa
Methyltestosterone
Metoclopramide
Metronidazole
Minocycline
Minoxidil
Mirtazapine
Misoprostol
Molindone
Morphine
Nafarelin
Nefazodone
Nifedipine
Nisoldipine
Nizatidine
Nortriptyline
Octreotide
Omeprazole
Penicillamine
Pentostatin
Perphenazine
Phenytoin
Pimozide
Pravastatin
Procarbazine
Prochlorperazine
Progestins
Promazine
Promethazine
Protriptyline
Pyrilamine
Quinestrol
Rabeprazole
Ranitidine
Reserpine
Risperidone
Ropinirole
Saquinavir
Sertraline
Sildenafil
Simvastatin
Spironolactone
Stanozolol
Stavudine
Sulindac
Terfenadine
Testosterone
Thioridazine
Thiothixene
Tiagabine

Tolmetin
Topiramate
Trazodone
Triamterene
Trifluoperazine
Trimeprazine
Trimipramine
Venlafaxine
Verapamil
Vitamin E
Zonisamide

Hair – alopecia

Acebutolol
Acetaminophen
Acetohexamide
Acitretin
Acyclovir
Albendazole
Aldesleukin
Alitretinoin
Allopurinol
Amantadine
Amiloride
Aminophylline
Aminosalicylate sodium
Amiodarone
Amitriptyline
Amlodipine
Amoxapine
Amphotericin B
Arsenic
Asparaginase
Aspirin
Astemizole
Atenolol
Atorvastatin
Azathioprine
Bendroflumethiazide
Betaxolol
Bexarotene
Bicalutamide
Bisoprolol
Bleomycin
Bromfenac
Bromocriptine
Buspirone
Busulfan
Capecitabine
Captopril
Carbamazepine
Carboplatin
Carmustine
Carteolol
Carvedilol
Celecoxib
Cerivastatin
Cetirizine
Cevimeline
Chlorambucil
Chloramphenicol
Chlordiazepoxide
Chloroquine
Chlorothiazide
Chlorotrianisene
Chlorpropamide
Cidofovir
Cimetidine
Cisplatin
Citalopram
Clofibrate
Clomiphene
Clomipramine
Clonazepam
Clonidine
Colchicine
Cyclobenzaprine
Cyclophosphamide
Cyclosporine
Cytarabine
Dacarbazine
Dactinomycin
Danazol
Daunorubicin
Delavirdine
Desipramine
Dexfenfluramine
Diazoxide
Diclofenac
Dicumarol
Didanosine
Diethylpropion
Diethylstilbestrol
Diflunisal
Digoxin
Diltiazem
Disopyramide
Docetaxel
Donepezil
Dopamine
Doxazosin
Doxepin
Doxorubicin
Efavirenz
Eflornithine
Enalapril
Epinephrine
Epirubicin
Esmolol
Estramustine
Estrogens
Ethambutol
Ethionamide
Ethosuximide
Etidronate
Etodolac
Etoposide
Famotidine
Felbamate
Fenfluramine
Fenofibrate
Fenoprofen
Flecainide
Fluconazole
Fludarabine
Fluorouracil
Fluoxetine
Fluoxymesterone
Flurbiprofen
Fluvastatin
Fluvoxamine
Foscarnet
Gabapentin
Ganciclovir
Gemcitabine
Gemfibrozil
Gentamicin
Gold & gold compounds
Granisetron
Granulocyte colony-stimulating factor (GCSF)
Grepafloxacin
Guanethidine
Guanfacine
Haloperidol
Halothane
Heparin
Hydromorphone
Hydroxychloroquine
Hydroxyurea
Ibuprofen
Idarubicin
Ifosfamide
Imipramine
Indinavir
Indomethacin
Interferons, alfa-2
Ipratropium
Irinotecan
Isoniazid
Isotretinoin
Itraconazole
Ketoconazole
Ketoprofen
Labetalol
Lamivudine
Lamotrigine
Lansoprazole
Leflunomide
Letrozole
Leuprolide
Levamisole
Levobunolol
Levodopa
Levothyroxine
Liothyronine
Lisinopril
Lithium
Lomustine
Loratadine
Lorazepam
Losartan
Lovastatin
Loxapine
Maprotiline
Mebendazole
Mechlorethamine
Meclofenamate
Medroxyprogesterone
Mefloquine
Melphalan
Mephenytoin
Mercaptopurine
Mesalamine
Mesoridazine
Metformin
Methimazole
Methotrexate
Methsuximide
Methyldopa
Methylphenidate
Methyltestosterone
Methysergide
Metoprolol
Mexiletine
Minocycline
Minoxidil
Misoprostol
Mitomycin
Mitotane
Moexipril
Mycophenolate
Nabumetone
Nadolol
Nalidixic acid
Naproxen
Naratriptan
Nefazodone
Neomycin
Nifedipine
Nimodipine
Nisoldipine
Nitrofurantoin
Nortriptyline
Octreotide
Olanzapine
Omeprazole
Ondansetron
Oral contraceptives
Oxaprozin
Oxcarbazepine
Pantoprazole
Paramethadione
Paroxetine
Penbutolol
Penicillamine
Penicillins
Pentosan
Pentostatin
Pergolide
Phensuximide
Phentermine
Phenytoin
Pindolol
Pirbuterol
Piroxicam
Pravastatin
Prazepam
Prazosin
Probenecid
Procarbazine
Progestins
Propafenone
Propranolol
Propylthiouracil
Protriptyline
Pyrimethamine
Quazepam
Quinacrine
Quinapril
Quinidine
Rabeprazole
Ramipril
Ranitidine
Ribavirin

Riluzole
Risperidone
Rivastigmine
Rofecoxib
Ropinirole
Saquinavir
Selegiline
Sertraline
Simvastatin
Sotalol
Sparfloxacin
Spironolactone
Stanozolol
Sulfasalazine
Sulfisoxazole
Sulindac
Tacrine
Tacrolimus
Tamoxifen
Terbinafine
Terfenadine
Testosterone
Thalidomide
Thioguanine
Thioridazine
Thiotepa
Thiothixene
Tiagabine
Timolol
Tiopronin
Tizanidine
Tocainide
Tolcapone
Topiramate
Topotecan
Trazodone
Triazolam
Trimethadione
Trimipramine
Ursodiol
Vasopressin
Venlafaxine
Verapamil
Vinblastine
Vincristine
Vinorelbine
Vitamin A
Warfarin
Zalcitabine
Zaleplon
Zidovudine
Zonisamide

Hair – alopecia areata

Clomipramine
Cyclosporine
Fluvoxamine
Haloperidol
Imipramine
Interferons, alfa-2
Lithium
Oral contraceptives
Terbinafine

Hair – hirsutism

Acetazolamide
Aminoglutethimide
Chlorotrianisene
Clonazepam
Corticosteroids
Danazol
Dexfenfluramine
Diethylstilbestrol
Diltiazem
Donepezil
Estrogens
Ethosuximide
Fluoxetine
Fluoxymesterone
Gemfibrozil
Isotretinoin
Lamotrigine
Lorazepam
Medroxyprogesterone
Methsuximide
Methyltestosterone
Minoxidil
Nafarelin
Olanzapine
Oral contraceptives
Penicillamine
Pergolide
Phensuximide
Phenytoin
Prazepam
Progestins
Quazepam
Sertraline
Sirolimus
Spironolactone
Stanozolol
Tacrolimus
Tamoxifen
Testosterone
Tiagabine
Triazolam
Venlafaxine
Zonisamide

Hair – hypertrichosis

Amantadine
Amiodarone
Betaxolol
Cetirizine
Citalopram
Clomiphene
Clomipramine
Corticosteroids
Cyclosporine
Diazoxide
Epoetin alfa
Interferons, alfa-2
Latanoprost
Methoxsalen
Minoxidil
Phenytoin
Psoralens
Risperidone
Selegiline
Streptomycin
Tamoxifen
Thioridazine
Tiopronin
Trioxsalen
Verapamil
Zidovudine

Herpes simplex

Azathioprine
Azelastine
Butabarbital
Butalbital
Celecoxib
Chlorambucil
Cidofovir
Clonidine
Corticosteroids
Cyclosporine
Eflornithine
Eprosartan
Fluoxetine
Flurbiprofen
Foscarnet
Gemtuzumab
Grepafloxacin
Indinavir
Interferons, alfa-2
Methotrexate
Methoxsalen
Mirtazapine
Modafinil
Nisoldipine
Pantoprazole
Pentobarbital
Pentostatin
Perindopril
Phenobarbital
Psoralens
Ribavirin
Rivastigmine
Rofecoxib
Ropinirole
Saquinavir
Sibutramine
Sildenafil
Sparfloxacin
Tacrine
Tacrolimus
Tiagabine
Tizanidine
Tolcapone
Trioxsalen
Venlafaxine
Zolpidem

Herpes zoster

Acyclovir
Azathioprine
Celecoxib
Chlorambucil
Corticosteroids
Cyclosporine
Cytarabine
Enalapril
Fluoxetine
Flurbiprofen
Gold & gold compounds
Griseofulvin
Indinavir
Isoniazid
Mechlorethamine
Mercaptopurine
Methoxsalen
Nisoldipine
Pantoprazole
Pentostatin
Procarbazine
Psoralens
Rabeprazole
Rofecoxib
Ropinirole
Saquinavir
Tacrine
Tiagabine
Tizanidine
Tolcapone
Trioxsalen
Venlafaxine
Zolpidem

Hirsutism **see Hair – hirsutism**

Hot flashes

Bicalutamide
Cabergoline
Cefmetazole
Celecoxib
Cevimeline
Citalopram
Clomiphene
Doxazosin
Efavirenz
Epirubicin
Eprosartan
Estramustine
Fenoprofen
Flumazenil
Fluoxetine
Flurbiprofen
Flutamide
Ganirelix
Goserelin
Granisetron
Hydrocodone
Ibuprofen
Indomethacin
Interferons, alfa-2
Ketoprofen
Lamotrigine
Letrozole
Leuprolide
Levodopa
Meclofenamate
Medroxyprogesterone
Mefenamic acid
Meloxicam
Mexiletine
Modafinil
Nabumetone
Nafarelin
Naproxen
Oxcarbazepine
Oxybutynin
Piroxicam
Raloxifene
Rivastigmine
Rizatriptan
Sulindac
Sumatriptan
Tamoxifen

Tolmetin
Topiramate
Toremifene
Zolmitriptan
Zolpidem

Hyperpigmentation

Acebutolol
Ciprofloxacin
Clonidine
Corticosteroids
Cyclosporine
Doxorubicin
Enoxacin
Etodolac
Isotretinoin
Mechlorethamine
Niacin
Pentazocine
Pimozide
Quinine
Stanozolol
Vinblastine

Hypersensitivity

Abacavir
Acetaminophen
Alendronate
Allopurinol
Aminophylline
Aminosalicylate sodium
Amitriptyline
Amobarbital
Amoxicillin
Ampicillin
Anistreplase
Aprotinin
Asparaginase
Azathioprine
Azithromycin
Aztreonam
Bacampicillin
Benazepril
Bleomycin
Calcitonin (human & salmon)
Capecitabine
Carbamazepine
Carbenicillin
Carboplatin
Cefaclor
Cefadroxil
Cefamandole
Cefazolin
Cefepime
Cefixime
Cefmetazole
Cefonicid
Cefoperazone
Cefotaxime
Cefotetan
Cefpodoxime
Cefprozil
Ceftazidime
Ceftibuten
Ceftriaxone
Cefuroxime
Cephalexin
Cephapirin
Cephradine
Cerivastatin
Chloral hydrate
Chlorambucil
Chloramphenicol
Chlorhexidine
Chlorpheniramine
Chlorzoxazone
Cimetidine
Cinoxacin
Ciprofloxacin
Clarithromycin
Clemastine
Clindamycin
Cloxacillin
Co-trimoxazole
Colchicine
Corticosteroids
Cromolyn
Cyanocobalamin
Cyclamate
Cyclophosphamide
Cytarabine
Dacarbazine
Dapsone
Denileukin
Desipramine
Diazoxide
Diclofenac
Dicloxacillin
Dicumarol
Didanosine
Diflunisal
Diltiazem
Diphenhydramine
Docetaxel
Doxycycline
Edrophonium
Efavirenz
Enoxacin
Enoxaparin
Epirubicin
Epoetin alfa
Erythromycin
Ethambutol
Ethchlorvynol
Etidronate
Etoposide
Flavoxate
Fluconazole
Fluoxetine
Fluoxymesterone
Flurbiprofen
Gatifloxacin
Glyburide
Gold & gold compounds
Goserelin
Granisetron
Grepafloxacin
Heparin
Heroin
Hydralazine
Hydroxyzine
Ibuprofen
Imipenem/cilastatin
Inamrinone
Indomethacin
Infliximab
Insulin
Ipodate
Isoniazid
Kanamycin
Ketoconazole
Ketorolac
Labetalol
Lamotrigine
Lansoprazole
Leucovorin
Levobunolol
Levothyroxine
Lidocaine
Liothyronine
Lomefloxacin
Lovastatin
Mechlorethamine
Meclofenamate
Melphalan
Meprobamate
Mesalamine
Methazolamide
Methicillin
Methyldopa
Methylphenidate
Methyltestosterone
Metronidazole
Mezlocillin
Minocycline
Nafarelin
Nafcillin
Nevirapine
Nicotine
Nisoldipine
Nitrofurantoin
Nystatin
Ondansetron
Orphenadrine
Oxacillin
Oxcarbazepine
Oxytetracycline
Pamidronate
Penicillamine
Penicillins
Pentagastrin
Pentobarbital
Phenobarbital
Phenylephrine
Phytonadione
Pilocarpine
Piperacillin
Pravastatin
Primidone
Probenecid
Procarbazine
Promethazine
Propylthiouracil
Protamine
Protease inhibitors
Pyrazinamide
Pyridoxine
Pyrimethamine
Quinapril
Quinethazone
Quinidine
Quinine
Ramipril
Ranitidine
Salmeterol
Secobarbital
Simvastatin
Sparfloxacin
Spectinomycin
Succinylcholine
Sulfadiazine
Sulfadoxine
Sulfamethoxazole
Sulfasalazine
Sulfisoxazole
Sulindac
Terbinafine
Testosterone
Tetracycline
Thiabendazole
Thioridazine
Ticarcillin
Tobramycin
Tocainide
Tolbutamide
Trazodone
Trimethobenzamide
Trimetrexate
Trovafloxacin
Vancomycin
Vitamin A
Warfarin
Zidovudine
Zonisamide

Hyprtrichosis – see Hair – Hypertrichosis

Jarisch–Herxheimer reaction

Amoxicillin
Bacampicillin
Carbenicillin
Ceftriaxone
Cefuroxime
Cloxacillin
Dicloxacillin
Griseofulvin
Ketoconazole
Methicillin
Mezlocillin
Nafcillin
Oxacillin
Penicillins
Pentamidine
Piperacillin
Thiabendazole
Ticarcillin

Kaposi's sarcoma

Aldesleukin
Aminocaproic acid
Azathioprine
Busulfan
Captopril
Chlorambucil
Corticosteroids
Cyclosporine
Heroin
Interferons, alfa-2

Lichen planus
Allopurinol
Amitriptyline
Arsenic
Captopril
Doxazosin
Felbamate
Gemfibrozil
Gold & gold compounds
Hydroxyurea
Imipramine
Indomethacin
Interferons, alfa-2
Labetalol
Levobunolol
Lithium
Mesalamine
Methyldopa
Naproxen
Omeprazole
Penicillamine
Phenytoin
Prazosin
Procainamide
Psoralens
Quinidine
Quinine
Simvastatin
Spironolactone
Sulfasalazine
Sulindac
Trovafloxacin
Ursodiol

Lichenoid eruption
Acebutolol
Acetohexamide
Acyclovir
Aminosalicylate sodium
Amlodipine
Aspirin
Atenolol
Atorvastatin
Azathioprine
Captopril
Carbamazepine
Chloral hydrate
Chloroquine
Chlorothiazide
Chlorpromazine
Chlorpropamide
Co-trimoxazole
Colchicine
Cycloserine
Cyclosporine
Cyproheptadine
Dapsone
Demeclocycline
Diazoxide
Diclofenac
Diflunisal
Diltiazem
Enalapril
Epoetin alfa
Ethambutol
Fluoxetine
Fluoxymesterone
Furosemide
Glipizide
Glyburide
Gold & gold compounds
Griseofulvin
Hydrochlorothiazide
Hydroxychloroquine
Hydroxyurea
Isoniazid
Labetalol
Lansoprazole
Levamisole
Lisinopril
Mercaptopurine
Metformin
Methamphetamine
Methyldopa
Methyltestosterone
Metoprolol
Minocycline
Nadolol
Naproxen
Nifedipine
Omeprazole
Oral contraceptives
Pantoprazole
Penicillamine
Phenytoin
Pindolol
Piroxicam
Pravastatin
Prazosin
Propranolol
Propylthiouracil
Pyrimethamine
Quinacrine
Quinidine
Quinine
Ranitidine
Risperidone
Sildenafil
Simvastatin
Sotalol
Sparfloxacin
Spironolactone
Streptomycin
Sulfamethoxazole
Temazepam
Terazosin
Testosterone
Tetracycline
Timolol
Tiopronin
Tolazamide
Tolbutamide
Torsemide
Trichlormethiazide
Tripelennamine
Triprolidine
Venlafaxine
Verapamil

Linear IgA bullous dermatosis
Aldesleukin
Amiodarone
Ampicillin
Captopril
Cefamandole
Co-trimoxazole
Diclofenac
Furosemide
Glyburide
Granulocyte colony-stimulating factor (GCSF)
Interferons, alfa-2
Lithium
Penicillins
Phenytoin
Piroxicam
Rifampin
Sulfamethoxazole
Sulfisoxazole
Vancomycin

Livedo reticularis
Amantadine
Anistreplase
Arsenic
Bromocriptine
Ciprofloxacin
Dihydrotachysterol
Diphenhydramine
Estrogens
Felbamate
Heparin
Ibuprofen
Minocycline
Quinidine
Warfarin

Lupus erythematosus
Acebutolol
Acetazolamide
Albuterol
Allopurinol
Aminoglutethimide
Aminosalicylate sodium
Amiodarone
Amitriptyline
Atenolol
Betaxolol
Bisoprolol
Butabarbital
Butalbital
Captopril
Carbamazepine
Carteolol
Cerivastatin
Chlorambucil
Chlordiazepoxide
Chlorothiazide
Chlorpromazine
Chlorpropamide
Chlorthalidone
Cimetidine
Clofibrate
Clonidine
Clozapine
Co-trimoxazole
Corticosteroids
Cyclosporine
Cyproheptadine
Danazol
Dapsone
Demeclocycline
Diclofenac
Diethylstilbestrol
Diltiazem
Disopyramide
Doxazosin
Doxycycline
Enalapril
Estrogens
Ethambutol
Ethionamide
Ethosuximide
Ethotoin
Felbamate
Fluoxetine
Fluoxymesterone
Fluphenazine
Flutamide
Fluvastatin
Fosphenytoin
Furosemide
Gemfibrozil
Gold & gold compounds
Griseofulvin
Guanethidine
Hydralazine
Hydrochlorothiazide
Hydroxyurea
Ibuprofen
Imipramine
Infliximab
Interferons, alfa-2
Isoniazid
Labetalol
Lamotrigine
Leuprolide
Levodopa
Lidocaine
Lisinopril
Lithium
Lovastatin
Meclofenamate
Mephenytoin
Meprobamate
Mercaptopurine
Mesalamine
Mesoridazine
Methimazole
Methoxsalen
Methsuximide
Methyldopa
Methyltestosterone
Methysergide
Metoprolol
Mexiletine
Minocycline
Minoxidil
Nadolol
Nalidixic acid
Naproxen
Nifedipine
Nitrofurantoin
Olsalazine
Omeprazole
Oral contraceptives
Oxcarbazepine
Oxytetracycline

Paramethadione
Penicillamine
Penicillins
Pentobarbital
Perphenazine
Phenelzine
Phenindamine
Phenobarbital
Phenolphthalein
Phensuximide
Phenytoin
Pindolol
Piroxicam
Potassium iodide
Pravastatin
Prazosin
Primidone
Procainamide
Prochlorperazine
Promethazine
Propafenone
Propranolol
Propylthiouracil
Psoralens
Pyrilamine
Quinidine
Quinine
Reserpine
Rifabutin
Sertraline
Simvastatin
Spironolactone
Streptomycin
Sulfadiazine
Sulfadoxine
Sulfamethoxazole
Sulfasalazine
Sulfisoxazole
Terbinafine
Terfenadine
Testosterone
Tetracycline
Thioridazine
Ticlopidine
Timolol
Tiopronin
Tocainide
Tolazamide
Triamterene
Trichlormethiazide
Trientine
Trifluoperazine
Trimeprazine
Trimethadione
Trioxsalen
Tripelennamine
Vancomycin
Verapamil
Vitamin E
Yohimbine
Zafirlukast
Zonisamide

Mastodynia

Azelastine
Aztreonam
Betaxolol
Bexarotene
Bicalutamide
Bromfenac
Cabergoline
Celecoxib
Cetirizine
Chlorotrianisene
Chlorpromazine
Citalopram
Clomiphene
Clomipramine
Clozapine
Dexfenfluramine
Diethylstilbestrol
Dipyridamole
Doxazosin
Estramustine
Estrogens
Fenoprofen
Finasteride
Fluoxetine
Fluoxymesterone
Fluphenazine
Fluvoxamine
Ganciclovir
Gatifloxacin
Goserelin
Haloperidol
Lansoprazole
Leuprolide
Lisinopril
Loratadine
Medroxyprogesterone
Mesoridazine
Methyltestosterone
Metoclopramide
Minoxidil
Mirtazapine
Nafarelin
Nefazodone
Nitrofurantoin
Pantoprazole
Pergolide
Perphenazine
Prochlorperazine
Promazine
Promethazine
Quinestrol
Raloxifene
Riluzole
Risperidone
Rivastigmine
Sparfloxacin
Spironolactone
Temozolomide
Testosterone
Thioridazine
Thiothixene
Tiagabine
Topiramate
Trifluoperazine
Venlafaxine
Zaleplon
Zolpidem

Melanoma

Arsenic
Clomiphene
Cyclosporine
Diazepam
Gemfibrozil
Interferons, alfa-2
Levodopa
Methotrexate
Oral contraceptives
Paroxetine
Psoralens
Tacrine
Trioxsalen

Myalgia

Abacavir
Abciximab
Acebutolol
Aldesleukin
Alitretinoin
Allopurinol
Aminocaproic acid
Aminoglutethimide
Amphotericin B
Anistreplase
Apraclonidine
Aspirin
Astemizole
Atorvastatin
Azatadine
Azathioprine
Azelastine
Aztreonam
Benazepril
Betaxolol
Bexarotene
Bicalutamide
Bisoprolol
Bromfenac
Brompheniramine
Buspirone
Candesartan
Capecitabine
Captopril
Carteolol
Carvedilol
Cefonicid
Celecoxib
Cerivastatin
Cetirizine
Cevimeline
Chloroquine
Chlorpheniramine
Cidofovir
Cilostazol
Cimetidine
Cisapride
Citalopram
Cladribine
Clemastine
Clofibrate
Clomiphene
Clomipramine
Co-trimoxazole
Colesevelam
Cromolyn
Cyclosporine
Cyproheptadine
Cytarabine
Dacarbazine
Dactinomycin
Dantrolene
Delavirdine
Denileukin
Dexchlorpheniramine
Dexfenfluramine
Dicloxacillin
Didanosine
Diethylpropion
Dihydroergotamine
Dihydrotachysterol
Dimenhydrinate
Diphenhydramine
Dipyridamole
Dirithromycin
Docetaxel
Dolasetron
Doxazosin
Dronabinol (THC)
Efavirenz
Enalapril
Enoxacin
Epirubicin
Epoetin alfa
Eprosartan
Ergocalciferol
Estazolam
Famotidine
Felbamate
Felodipine
Fenfluramine
Fenofibrate
Flecainide
Fludarabine
Fluoxetine
Fluvastatin
Fluvoxamine
Foscarnet
Fosfomycin
Fosinopril
Gabapentin
Ganciclovir
Gatifloxacin
Gemcitabine
Gemfibrozil
Glipizide
Glyburide
Granulocyte colony-stimulating factor (GCSF)
Grepafloxacin
Guanethidine
Hydralazine
Hydroxyzine
Indinavir
Infliximab
Interferons, alfa-2
Isotretinoin
Itraconazole
Ivermectin
Ketoprofen
Ketorolac
Lamivudine
Lamotrigine
Lansoprazole

Leflunomide
Leuprolide
Levamisole
Levofloxacin
Levothyroxine
Liothyronine
Lisinopril
Lomefloxacin
Loratadine
Losartan
Lovastatin
Meclizine
Mefloquine
Mesalamine
Methimazole
Methotrexate
Methyldopa
Methysergide
Minocycline
Mirtazapine
Mitotane
Modafinil
Moexipril
Moxifloxacin
Mycophenolate
Nabumetone
Nafarelin
Naproxen
Nebivolol
Nefazodone
Nelfinavir
Nevirapine
Nicardipine
Nicotine
Nifedipine
Nitrofurantoin
Nizatidine
Norfloxacin
Ofloxacin
Olanzapine
Omeprazole
Orlistat
Pamidronate
Pantoprazole
Paroxetine
Pentamidine
Pentostatin
Pergolide
Perindopril
Phentermine
Pilocarpine
Pimozide
Pindolol
Pioglitazone
Pramipexole
Pravastatin
Procainamide
Procarbazine
Promethazine
Propofol
Propranolol
Propylthiouracil
Pyrazinamide
Quetiapine
Quinapril
Quinidine
Quinupristin/dalfopristin
Rabeprazole
Raloxifene
Ranitidine
Ribavirin
Rifabutin
Rifampin
Risedronate
Risperidone
Ritonavir
Rituximab
Rivastigmine
Rizatriptan
Rofecoxib
Salmeterol
Sibutramine
Sildenafil
Simvastatin
Sirolimus
Sotalol
Sparfloxacin
Stavudine
Succinylcholine
Sulfasalazine
Sulfisoxazole
Sumatriptan
Tacrine
Tacrolimus
Telmisartan
Temozolomide
Terazosin
Terfenadine
Tiagabine
Timolol
Tocainide
Tolcapone
Tolmetin
Topiramate
Torsemide
Trandolapril
Trazodone
Trimeprazine
Tripelennamine
Triprolidine
Trovafloxacin
Ursodiol
Venlafaxine
Vinblastine
Vincristine
Vinorelbine
Zafirlukast
Zalcitabine
Zaleplon
Zanamivir
Zileuton
Zolmitriptan
Zolpidem
Zonisamide

Nails – onycholysis

Acebutolol
Allopurinol
Atenolol
Bleomycin
Captopril
Clofazimine
Cloxacillin
Demeclocycline
Diflunisal
Docetaxel
Doxorubicin
Doxycycline
Estrogens
Etoposide
Fluorouracil
Gold & gold compounds
Hydroxyurea
Ibuprofen
Indomethacin
Isoniazid
Isotretinoin
Ketoprofen
Methotrexate
Metoprolol
Minocycline
Nadolol
Nitrofurantoin
Oral contraceptives
Pindolol
Piroxicam
Propranolol
Tetracycline
Timolol

Nails – pigmentation

Arsenic
Betaxolol
Bleomycin
Busulfan
Chloroquine
Chlorpromazine
Cyclophosphamide
Dacarbazine
Daunorubicin
Demeclocycline
Docetaxel
Doxorubicin
Epirubicin
Fluorouracil
Flurbiprofen
Gold & gold compounds
Hydroxychloroquine
Hydroxyurea
Ketoconazole
Methotrexate
Methoxsalen
Minocycline
Oxytetracycline
Phenytoin
Psoralens
Quinacrine
Timolol
Trioxsalen
Zidovudine

Onycholysis — see Nails – onycholysis

Oral candidiasis

Amoxicillin
Ampicillin
Atovaquone
Bacampicillin
Capecitabine
Carbenicillin
Cefaclor
Cefadroxil
Cefamandole
Cefazolin
Cefepime
Cefpodoxime
Cefprozil
Ceftazidime
Ceftibuten
Ceftizoxime
Cefuroxime
Cephalexin
Cidofovir
Ciprofloxacin
Clarithromycin
Cloxacillin
Dicloxacillin
Erythromycin
Gatifloxacin
Grepafloxacin
Griseofulvin
Leflunomide
Linezolid
Mesalamine
Methicillin
Mezlocillin
Mirtazapine
Mycophenolate
Nafcillin
Nefazodone
Olanzapine
Omeprazole
Oxacillin
Pantoprazole
Penicillins
Piperacillin
Quinupristin/dalfopristin
Riluzole
Ritonavir
Sirolimus
Sparfloxacin
Tacrolimus
Ticarcillin

Oral ulceration

Abacavir
Aldesleukin
Alendronate
Allopurinol
Alprazolam
Aminoglutethimide
Aspirin
Atorvastatin
Azathioprine
Aztreonam
Betaxolol
Bleomycin
Butabarbital
Butalbital
Capecitabine
Captopril
Cefadroxil
Chloral hydrate
Chlorambucil
Chloramphenicol
Chlorpromazine
Cidofovir
Cisplatin

Clofibrate
Clonazepam
Clorazepate
Co-trimoxazole
Codeine
Colesevelam
Cyclosporine
Cytarabine
Delavirdine
Dexfenfluramine
Diclofenac
Dicumarol
Diflunisal
Dirithromycin
Doxorubicin
Enalapril
Epirubicin
Erythromycin
Estazolam
Ethionamide
Ethosuximide
Fenoprofen
Flavoxate
Fluconazole
Fluoxetine
Foscarnet
Ganciclovir
Gatifloxacin
Gold & gold compounds
Grepafloxacin
Hydralazine
Hydroxyurea
Ibuprofen
Imipramine
Indomethacin
Irinotecan
Lamotrigine
Leflunomide
Levamisole
Lithium
Meclofenamate
Mefenamic acid
Melphalan
Meprobamate
Mesalamine
Methimazole
Methotrexate
Methsuximide
Methyldopa
Metronidazole
Minocycline
Mitomycin
Modafinil
Nabumetone
Naproxen
Nefazodone
Nelfinavir
Nisoldipine
Olanzapine
Paroxetine
Penicillamine
Penicillins
Pentobarbital
Pentosan
Phenobarbital
Phensuximide
Phenytoin
Promethazine
Propranolol
Propylthiouracil
Quazepam
Quetiapine
Quinidine
Quinine
Rabeprazole
Ritonavir
Rofecoxib
Saquinavir
Sirolimus
Sparfloxacin
Streptomycin
Sulfadoxine
Sulfamethoxazole
Sulfasalazine
Sulfisoxazole
Sulindac
Terbutaline
Tetracycline
Tiagabine
Tiopronin
Tolcapone
Tolmetin
Venlafaxine
Vincristine
Warfarin
Zalcitabine
Zaleplon
Zidovudine
Zonisamide

Paresthesias

Acetazolamide
Acetohexamide
Acitretin
Acyclovir
Alitretinoin
Allopurinol
Alprazolam
Amikacin
Amiloride
Amiodarone
Amitriptyline
Amlodipine
Amoxapine
Amphotericin B
Amprenavir
Apraclonidine
Aspirin
Astemizole
Atorvastatin
Azatadine
Aztreonam
Baclofen
Benactyzine
Benazepril
Bendroflumethiazide
Benzthiazide
Benztropine
Betaxolol
Bicalutamide
Biperiden
Bisoprolol
Bleomycin
Bromfenac
Bromocriptine
Brompheniramine
Buspirone
Butorphanol
Cabergoline
Calcitonin (human & salmon)
Candesartan
Capecitabine
Captopril
Carisoprodol
Carteolol
Carvedilol
Cefaclor
Cefamandole
Cefotaxime
Cefpodoxime
Cefprozil
Ceftazidime
Ceftibuten
Ceftizoxime
Celecoxib
Cephapirin
Cerivastatin
Cetirizine
Cevimeline
Chloramphenicol
Chlordiazepoxide
Chlorothiazide
Chlorpheniramine
Chlorpropamide
Cholestyramine
Cidofovir
Cilostazol
Cinoxacin
Ciprofloxacin
Citalopram
Clemastine
Clomipramine
Clonazepam
Clopidogrel
Clorazepate
Codeine
Cromolyn
Cyanocobalamin
Cyclamate
Cyclobenzaprine
Cycloserine
Cyclosporine
Cyclothiazide
Cyproheptadine
Dacarbazine
Danazol
Delavirdine
Demeclocycline
Denileukin
Desipramine
Dexchlorpheniramine
Dexfenfluramine
Diazepam
Diazoxide
Diclofenac
Didanosine
Diflunisal
Dihydroergotamine
Diltiazem
Dimenhydrinate
Diphenhydramine
Diphenoxylate
Dipyridamole
Dirithromycin
Disopyramide
Disulfiram
Dobutamine
Docetaxel
Dofetilide
Dolasetron
Donepezil
Doxapram
Doxazosin
Doxepin
Doxycycline
Dronabinol (THC)
Efavirenz
Eflornithine
Enalapril
Enoxacin
Epoetin alfa
Eprosartan
Esmolol
Estazolam
Ethambutol
Ethchlorvynol
Etidronate
Etodolac
Etoposide
Famciclovir
Famotidine
Felbamate
Felodipine
Fenofibrate
Fentanyl
Flecainide
Fluconazole
Flucytosine
Fludarabine
Flumazenil
Fluorouracil
Fluoxetine
Fluoxymesterone
Flurazepam
Flurbiprofen
Flutamide
Fluvastatin
Fluvoxamine
Foscarnet
Fosfomycin
Fosinopril
Fosphenytoin
Furosemide
Gabapentin
Ganciclovir
Gatifloxacin
Gemcitabine
Gemfibrozil
Gentamicin
Glipizide
Glyburide
Grepafloxacin
Griseofulvin
Guanadrel
Guanethidine

Guanfacine
Hydralazine
Hydrochlorothiazide
Hydroflumethiazide
Hydromorphone
Ibuprofen
Imipenem/cilastatin
Imipramine
Indapamide
Indinavir
Indomethacin
Infliximab
Insulin
Interferons, alfa-2
Ipratropium
Irbesartan
Isoniazid
Isradipine
Kanamycin
Ketoconazole
Ketoprofen
Ketorolac
Labetalol
Lamivudine
Lamotrigine
Lansoprazole
Leflunomide
Leuprolide
Levamisole
Levetiracetam
Levodopa
Levofloxacin
Lidocaine
Lisinopril
Lomefloxacin
Loratadine
Lorazepam
Losartan
Lovastatin
Loxapine
Mazindol
Meclizine
Meclofenamate
Medroxyprogesterone
Meloxicam
Meprobamate
Mesalamine
Mesoridazine
Methazolamide
Methimazole
Methyclothiazide
Methyldopa
Methyltestosterone
Methysergide
Metoclopramide
Metolazone
Metoprolol
Metronidazole
Mexiletine
Mibefradil
Midazolam
Minocycline
Minoxidil
Mirtazapine
Mitomycin
Modafinil
Moricizine
Moxifloxacin
Mycophenolate
Nabumetone
Nadolol
Nafarelin
Nalidixic acid
Naratriptan
Nebivolol
Nefazodone
Nelfinavir
Nevirapine
Niacin
Niacinamide
Nicardipine
Nicotine
Nifedipine
Nisoldipine
Nitrofurantoin
Nizatidine
Norfloxacin
Nortriptyline
Ofloxacin
Omeprazole
Ondansetron
Orphenadrine
Oxazepam
Oxytetracycline
Pantoprazole
Paramethadione
Paroxetine
Penbutolol
Pentagastrin
Pentazocine
Pentostatin
Pentoxifylline
Pergolide
Perindopril
Phenylephrine
Phenytoin
Pindolol
Pirbuterol
Piroxicam
Polythiazide
Potassium iodide
Pramipexole
Pravastatin
Prazepam
Prazosin
Procarbazine
Promethazine
Propafenone
Propranolol
Propylthiouracil
Protriptyline
Pyridoxine
Pyrilamine
Quazepam
Quetiapine
Quinapril
Quinethazone
Quinupristin/dalfopristin
Rabeprazole
Ramipril
Repaglinide
Rifabutin
Riluzole
Risedronate
Risperidone
Ritonavir
Rivastigmine
Rizatriptan
Rofecoxib
Ropinirole
Salmeterol
Saquinavir
Selegiline
Sertraline
Sibutramine
Sildenafil
Simvastatin
Sirolimus
Sotalol
Sparfloxacin
Spironolactone
Stavudine
Streptomycin
Sulindac
Sumatriptan
Tacrine
Tacrolimus
Telmisartan
Temazepam
Temozolomide
Terazosin
Terfenadine
Testosterone
Tetracycline
Thalidomide
Thiabendazole
Thiamine
Thioridazine
Thiothixene
Tiagabine
Timolol
Tizanidine
Tobramycin
Tocainide
Tolazamide
Tolbutamide
Tolcapone
Tolterodine
Topiramate
Topotecan
Tramadol
Trandolapril
Tranylcypromine
Trazodone
Triamterene
Triazolam
Trichlormethiazide
Trihexyphenidyl
Trimeprazine
Trimethadione
Trimipramine
Tripelennamine
Triprolidine
Trovafloxacin
Vancomycin
Venlafaxine
Verapamil
Vinblastine
Vincristine
Vinorelbine
Zalcitabine
Zaleplon
Zidovudine
Zileuton
Zolmitriptan
Zolpidem
Zonisamide

Parkinsonism

Amitriptyline
Diltiazem
Doxepin
Flucytosine
Fluphenazine
Haloperidol
Lithium
Loxapine
Maprotiline
Methyldopa
Metoclopramide
Nabumetone
Nortriptyline
Olanzapine
Pemoline
Perphenazine
Phenelzine
Prochlorperazine
Promazine
Promethazine
Protriptyline
Reserpine
Risperidone
Tacrine
Thioridazine
Thiothixene
Trifluoperazine
Trimethobenzamide
Trimipramine
Verapamil

Parosmia

Alosetron
Aminophylline
Amiodarone
Amlodipine
Apraclonidine
Atorvastatin
Buspirone
Cetirizine
Cevimeline
Clarithromycin
Doxazosin
Efavirenz
Fluoxetine
Flurbiprofen
Fluvoxamine
Gatifloxacin
Grepafloxacin
Levamisole
Mirtazapine
Ofloxacin
Propafenone
Rimantadine
Ritonavir
Sumatriptan
Terbinafine

Tiagabine
Tiopronin
Tocainide
Tolcapone
Topiramate
Venlafaxine
Zalcitabine
Zaleplon
Zolmitriptan
Zonisamide

Pemphigus

Acetaminophen
Aldesleukin
Amoxicillin
Ampicillin
Aspirin
Captopril
Cefadroxil
Cefazolin
Ceftriaxone
Cefuroxime
Cephalexin
Diclofenac
Enalapril
Glyburide
Gold & gold compounds
Heroin
Indomethacin
Interferons, alfa-2
Isotretinoin
Levamisole
Levodopa
Lisinopril
Meprobamate
Moexipril
Penicillamine
Penicillins
Phenobarbital
Phenytoin
Piroxicam
Propranolol
Quinapril
Ramipril
Rifampin
Tiopronin
Trandolapril

Periorbital edema

Aspirin
Cabergoline
Cefmetazole
Chlorambucil
Clozapine
Diltiazem
Donepezil
Ethosuximide
Famotidine
Foscarnet
Furosemide
Ibuprofen
Indomethacin
Methsuximide
Moricizine
Nifedipine
Omeprazole
Phensuximide
Phenylephrine
Pimozide
Rivastigmine
Sertraline
Streptokinase
Sulfadiazine
Sulfadoxine
Sulfasalazine
Sulfisoxazole
Trovafloxacin
Urokinase
Zolpidem

Peripheral edema

Abciximab
Acyclovir
Aldesleukin
Alendronate
Amantadine
Amlodipine
Benazepril
Bexarotene
Bicalutamide
Cabergoline
Candesartan
Carteolol
Carvedilol
Celecoxib
Cerivastatin
Cevimeline
Chlorotrianisene
Chlorpromazine
Cilostazol
Clonidine
Cyproheptadine
Delavirdine
Diclofenac
Diethylstilbestrol
Diflunisal
Dirithromycin
Dofetilide
Dolasetron
Doxazosin
Efavirenz
Enoxaparin
Eprosartan
Estrogens
Etodolac
Felodipine
Fenoprofen
Fluoxetine
Fluphenazine
Flurbiprofen
Foscarnet
Gabapentin
Gatifloxacin
Gemcitabine
Gemtuzumab
Granulocyte colony-stimulating factor (GCSF)
Grepafloxacin
Guanadrel
Guanethidine
Guanfacine
Heparin
Indapamide
Indomethacin
Isocarboxazid
Isosorbide dinitrate
Isradipine
Itraconazole
Ivermectin
Ketoprofen
Labetalol
Leflunomide
Leuprolide
Lisinopril
Loratadine
Meclofenamate
Meprobamate
Mesalamine
Mesoridazine
Methyldopa
Methysergide
Metoprolol
Mibefradil
Midazolam
Minoxidil
Mirtazapine
Moexipril
Molindone
Montelukast
Morphine
Moxifloxacin
Mycophenolate
Naproxen
Nefazodone
Nicardipine
Nifedipine
Nimodipine
Nisoldipine
Nitroglycerin
Olanzapine
Omeprazole
Pantoprazole
Paroxetine
Penbutolol
Penicillamine
Pentostatin
Pergolide
Perphenazine
Phenelzine
Phentermine
Pindolol
Piroxicam
Pramipexole
Prochlorperazine
Propranolol
Quinapril
Quinestrol
Quinupristin/dalfopristin
Rabeprazole
Raloxifene
Reserpine
Rifapentine
Riluzole
Risedronate
Ritonavir
Rituximab
Rivastigmine
Rofecoxib
Ropinirole
Selegiline
Sertraline
Sibutramine
Sildenafil
Sirolimus
Sotalol
Sparfloxacin
Tacrine
Tacrolimus
Tamoxifen
Telmisartan
Temozolomide
Terazosin
Terbinafine
Testosterone
Thioridazine
Thiothixene
Tiagabine
Tranylcypromine
Trifluoperazine
Trimeprazine
Tripelennamine
Troglitazone
Trovafloxacin
Venlafaxine
Verapamil
Zaleplon
Zonisamide

Petechiae

Abciximab
Aldesleukin
Alendronate
Allopurinol
Amitriptyline
Amlodipine
Amoxapine
Amoxicillin
Aspirin
Atorvastatin
Aztreonam
Benactyzine
Carbamazepine
Chlorzoxazone
Cladribine
Clozapine
Cytarabine
Danazol
Delavirdine
Denileukin
Desipramine
Diltiazem
Fluconazole
Fluoxetine
Gemcitabine
Gemfibrozil
Gemtuzumab
Griseofulvin
Heparin
Imipramine
Indomethacin
Lamotrigine
Maprotiline
Melphalan
Meprobamate
Mercaptopurine
Methyldopa
Minocycline
Mirtazapine

Nisoldipine
Nortriptyline
Octreotide
Ofloxacin
Pentostatin
Piroxicam
Plicamycin
Procarbazine
Protriptyline
Riluzole
Simvastatin
Sparfloxacin
Tacrine
Thioguanine
Tiagabine
Ticlopidine
Tizanidine
Trimethadione
Trimipramine
Zonisamide

Peyronie's disease

Acebutolol
Atenolol
Betaxolol
Bisoprolol
Carteolol
Labetalol
Methotrexate
Metoprolol
Nadolol
Penbutolol
Phenytoin
Pindolol
Propranolol
Ropinirole
Timolol

Photosensitivity

Acetaminophen
Acetazolamide
Acetohexamide
Aldesleukin
Alitretinoin
Allopurinol
Alprazolam
Amantadine
Amiloride
Aminosalicylate sodium
Amiodarone
Amitriptyline
Amobarbital
Amoxapine
Arsenic
Astemizole
Atenolol
Atorvastatin
Atropine sulfate
Azatadine
Azathioprine
Azithromycin
Benazepril
Bendroflumethiazide
Benzthiazide
Benztropine
Betaxolol
Bexarotene
Bisoprolol
Brompheniramine
Bumetanide
Butabarbital
Butalbital
Capecitabine
Captopril
Carbamazepine
Carisoprodol
Carteolol
Carvedilol
Cefazolin
Ceftazidime
Celecoxib
Cerivastatin
Cetirizine
Cevimeline
Chlorambucil
Chlordiazepoxide
Chlorhexidine
Chloroquine
Chlorothiazide
Chlorotrianisene
Chlorpheniramine
Chlorpromazine
Chlorpropamide
Chlortetracycline
Chlorthalidone
Cinoxacin
Ciprofloxacin
Citalopram
Clemastine
Clofazimine
Clofibrate
Clomipramine
Clorazepate
Clozapine
Co-trimoxazole
Cromolyn
Cyclamate
Cyclobenzaprine
Cyclothiazide
Cyproheptadine
Dacarbazine
Danazol
Dantrolene
Dapsone
Demeclocycline
Desipramine
Dexchlorpheniramine
Diazoxide
Diclofenac
Diflunisal
Diltiazem
Dimenhydrinate
Diphenhydramine
Disopyramide
Docetaxel
Doxepin
Doxycycline
Enalapril
Enoxacin
Epirubicin
Epoetin alfa
Estazolam
Estrogens
Ethacrynic acid
Ethambutol
Ethionamide
Etodolac
Felbamate
Fenofibrate
Flucytosine
Fluorouracil
Fluoxetine
Fluphenazine
Flurbiprofen
Flutamide
Fluvastatin
Fluvoxamine
Fosinopril
Furazolidone
Furosemide
Ganciclovir
Gatifloxacin
Gentamicin
Glimepiride
Glipizide
Glyburide
Glycopyrrolate
Gold & gold compounds
Grepafloxacin
Griseofulvin
Haloperidol
Heroin
Hydralazine
Hydrochlorothiazide
Hydroflumethiazide
Hydroxychloroquine
Hydroxyurea
Hydroxyzine
Ibuprofen
Imipramine
Indapamide
Interferons, alfa-2
Isocarboxazid
Isoniazid
Isotretinoin
Kanamycin
Ketoconazole
Ketoprofen
Ketotifen
Lamotrigine
Leuprolide
Levofloxacin
Lincomycin
Lisinopril
Lomefloxacin
Loratadine
Losartan
Loxapine
Maprotiline
Meclizine
Meclofenamate
Medroxyprogesterone
Mefenamic acid
Meloxicam
Meprobamate
Mercaptopurine
Mesalamine
Mesoridazine
Metformin
Methazolamide
Methenamine
Methotrexate
Methoxsalen
Methyclothiazide
Methyldopa
Methylphenidate
Metolazone
Minocycline
Mirtazapine
Mitomycin
Moexipril
Molindone
Moxifloxacin
Nabumetone
Nalidixic acid
Naproxen
Naratriptan
Nefazodone
Nifedipine
Nisoldipine
Nitrofurantoin
Norfloxacin
Nortriptyline
Ofloxacin
Olanzapine
Oral contraceptives
Oxaprozin
Oxcarbazepine
Oxytetracycline
Paroxetine
Pentobarbital
Pentosan
Pentostatin
Perphenazine
Phenelzine
Phenindamine
Phenobarbital
Pimozide
Piroxicam
Polythiazide
Pravastatin
Procarbazine
Prochlorperazine
Procyclidine
Promazine
Promethazine
Propranolol
Propylthiouracil
Protriptyline
Psoralens
Pyridoxine
Pyrilamine
Pyrimethamine
Quetiapine
Quinacrine
Quinapril
Quinestrol
Quinethazone
Quinidine
Quinine
Rabeprazole
Ramipril
Ranitidine
Ribavirin
Riluzole
Risperidone

Ritonavir
Rofecoxib
Ropinirole
Saccharin
Saquinavir
Scopolamine
Selegiline
Sertraline
Sildenafil
Simvastatin
Sotalol
Sparfloxacin
Spironolactone
Streptomycin
Sulfadiazine
Sulfadoxine
Sulfamethoxazole
Sulfasalazine
Sulfisoxazole
Sulindac
Sumatriptan
Tacrolimus
Terbinafine
Terfenadine
Tetracycline
Thioguanine
Thioridazine
Thiothixene
Tiagabine
Timolol
Tiopronin
Tolazamide
Tolbutamide
Topiramate
Torsemide
Tranylcypromine
Trazodone
Triamterene
Triazolam
Trichlormethiazide
Trifluoperazine
Trihexyphenidyl
Trimeprazine
Trimethadione
Trimethoprim
Trimetrexate
Trimipramine
Trioxsalen
Tripelennamine
Triprolidine
Trovafloxacin
Venlafaxine
Verapamil
Vinblastine
Vitamin A
Zalcitabine
Zaleplon
Zolmitriptan
Zolpidem

Phototoxic reaction

Acitretin
Alprazolam
Bendroflumethiazide
Captopril
Cetirizine
Chlorpromazine
Ciprofloxacin
Demeclocycline
Doxycycline
Enoxacin
Fenofibrate
Fluorouracil
Fluoxetine
Furosemide
Glipizide
Grepafloxacin
Hydrochlorothiazide
Itraconazole
Lomefloxacin
Methoxsalen
Nabumetone
Naproxen
Norfloxacin
Nortriptyline
Ofloxacin
Oxaprozin
Prochlorperazine
Promazine
Propranolol
Protriptyline
Psoralens
Sparfloxacin
Sulfisoxazole
Sulindac
Terazosin
Tetracycline
Thioridazine
Trioxsalen
Trovafloxacin
Vinblastine

Pigmentation

Amiodarone
Amitriptyline
Amphotericin B
Arsenic
Azathioprine
Betaxolol
Bisoprolol
Bleomycin
Busulfan
Captopril
Carbamazepine
Carboplatin
Carmustine
Carteolol
Cerivastatin
Chloroquine
Chlorpromazine
Cidofovir
Cisplatin
Citalopram
Clofazimine
Clomipramine
Corticosteroids
Cyclophosphamide
Dactinomycin
Dapsone
Daunorubicin
Deferoxamine
Demeclocycline
Desipramine
Diazepam
Dicumarol
Donepezil
Doxorubicin
Doxycycline
Epirubicin
Esmolol
Estrogens
Etoposide
Fluorouracil
Fluoxetine
Fluphenazine
Fluvoxamine
Foscarnet
Ganciclovir
Gold & gold compounds
Griseofulvin
Haloperidol
Heroin
Hydroxychloroquine
Ifosfamide
Imipramine
Indinavir
Insulin
Irinotecan
Ketoconazole
Ketoprofen
Labetalol
Leflunomide
Leuprolide
Lidocaine
Loxapine
Mephenytoin
Mercaptopurine
Mesoridazine
Methamphetamine
Methimazole
Methotrexate
Methoxsalen
Methyldopa
Metoprolol
Minocycline
Minoxidil
Mitomycin
Mitotane
Molindone
Nisoldipine
Ofloxacin
Olanzapine
Oral contraceptives
Oxytetracycline
Paroxetine
Pentostatin
Perphenazine
Phenazopyridine
Phenolphthalein
Phenytoin
Procarbazine
Prochlorperazine
Promazine
Promethazine
Propylthiouracil
Psoralens
Pyrimethamine
Quinacrine
Quinidine
Quinine
Rabeprazole
Rifabutin
Rifapentine
Risperidone
Ropinirole
Sparfloxacin
Spironolactone
Sulfadiazine
Sulfasalazine
Tetracycline
Thioridazine
Thiotepa
Thiothixene
Tiagabine
Timolol
Tolcapone
Topiramate
Toremifene
Trifluoperazine
Trioxsalen
Vinorelbine
Vitamin A
Zaleplon
Zidovudine

Pigmented nails – see Nails – pigmentation

Pityriasis rosea

Acetaminophen
Ampicillin
Arsenic
Aspirin
Captopril
Clonidine
Codeine
Corticosteroids
Dexfenfluramine
Gold & gold compounds
Griseofulvin
Isotretinoin
Ketotifen
Meprobamate
Metronidazole
Mitomycin
Naproxen
Omeprazole
Penicillins
Terbinafine
Tiopronin
Tripelennamine

Priapism

Alprostadil
Bromocriptine
Chlorpromazine
Citalopram
Clozapine
Cocaine
Dicumarol
Fluoxetine
Fluoxymesterone
Fluphenazine
Fluvoxamine
Guanethidine
Haloperidol
Heparin
Hydroxyzine
Labetalol

Levodopa
Loxapine
Mesoridazine
Methyltestosterone
Nefazodone
Olanzapine
Oxcarbazepine
Paroxetine
Pergolide
Perphenazine
Phenelzine
Phenoxybenzamine
Phentolamine
Prazosin
Prochlorperazine
Promazine
Promethazine
Quetiapine
Risperidone
Sertraline
Sildenafil
Stanozolol
Terazosin
Testosterone
Thioridazine
Thiothixene
Toremifene
Tranylcypromine
Trazodone
Trifluoperazine
Vancomycin
Warfarin

Pruritus

Abciximab
Acebutolol
Acetaminophen
Acetazolamide
Acetohexamide
Acitretin
Acyclovir
Albendazole
Albuterol
Aldesleukin
Alendronate
Alfentanil
Alitretinoin
Allopurinol
Alprazolam
Altretamine
Amantadine
Amikacin
Amiloride
Aminocaproic acid
Aminoglutethimide
Aminophylline
Aminosalicylate sodium
Amiodarone
Amitriptyline
Amlodipine
Amoxapine
Amoxicillin
Amphotericin B
Ampicillin
Amprenavir
Apraclonidine
Aprotinin
Arsenic
Asparaginase
Aspartame
Aspirin
Astemizole
Atenolol
Atorvastatin
Atovaquone
Atracurium
Atropine sulfate
Azithromycin
Aztreonam
Bacampicillin
Baclofen
Benactyzine
Benazepril
Bendroflumethiazide
Benztropine
Betaxolol
Bexarotene
Bicalutamide
Bisoprolol
Bleomycin
Bromfenac
Bumetanide
Buspirone
Butabarbital
Butalbital
Butorphanol
Cabergoline
Calcitonin (human & salmon)
Capecitabine
Captopril
Carbamazepine
Carbenicillin
Carboplatin
Carisoprodol
Carteolol
Carvedilol
Cefaclor
Cefadroxil
Cefamandole
Cefazolin
Cefdinir
Cefepime
Cefixime
Cefmetazole
Cefonicid
Cefoperazone
Cefotaxime
Cefotetan
Cefoxitin
Cefpodoxime
Cefprozil
Ceftazidime
Ceftibuten
Ceftizoxime
Ceftriaxone
Cefuroxime
Celecoxib
Cephalexin
Cephalothin
Cephapirin
Cephradine
Cerivastatin
Cetirizine
Cevimeline
Chloral hydrate
Chlorambucil
Chloramphenicol
Chlordiazepoxide
Chlormezanone
Chloroquine
Chlorothiazide
Chlorpromazine
Chlorpropamide
Chlortetracycline
Chlorzoxazone
Cidofovir
Cilostazol
Cimetidine
Cinoxacin
Ciprofloxacin
Cisapride
Cisplatin
Citalopram
Cladribine
Clarithromycin
Clindamycin
Clofazimine
Clofibrate
Clomiphene
Clomipramine
Clonazepam
Clonidine
Clopidogrel
Clorazepate
Cloxacillin
Clozapine
Co-trimoxazole
Codeine
Colchicine
Corticosteroids
Cromolyn
Cyanocobalamin
Cyclamate
Cyclobenzaprine
Cyclophosphamide
Cycloserine
Cyclosporine
Cytarabine
Dactinomycin
Dalteparin
Danazol
Dantrolene
Dapsone
Daunorubicin
Deferoxamine
Delavirdine
Demeclocycline
Denileukin
Desipramine
Dexfenfluramine
Diazepam
Diazoxide
Diclofenac
Dicloxacillin
Dicumarol
Dicyclomine
Didanosine
Diethylpropion
Diethylstilbestrol
Diflunisal
Digoxin
Dihydroergotamine
Dihydrotachysterol
Diltiazem
Diphenhydramine
Diphenoxylate
Dipyridamole
Dirithromycin
Disopyramide
Dobutamine
Docetaxel
Dolasetron
Donepezil
Dopamine
Doxapram
Doxazosin
Doxepin
Doxercalciferol
Doxorubicin
Efavirenz
Eflornithine
Enalapril
Enoxacin
Epirubicin
Epoetin alfa
Eprosartan
Ergocalciferol
Erythromycin
Estazolam
Estramustine
Estrogens
Etanercept
Ethambutol
Ethchlorvynol
Ethosuximide
Etidronate
Etodolac
Etoposide
Famciclovir
Famotidine
Felbamate
Felodipine
Fenfluramine
Fenofibrate
Fenoprofen
Fentanyl
Flecainide
Fluconazole
Flucytosine
Fluorouracil
Fluoxetine
Fluoxymesterone
Fluphenazine
Flurazepam
Flurbiprofen
Fluvastatin
Fluvoxamine
Folic acid
Foscarnet
Fosfomycin
Fosinopril
Fosphenytoin
Furazolidone
Furosemide
Gabapentin

Ganciclovir
Ganirelix
Gatifloxacin
Gemcitabine
Gemfibrozil
Gentamicin
Glimepiride
Glipizide
Glyburide
Gold & gold compounds
Granulocyte colony-stimulating factor (GCSF)
Grepafloxacin
Griseofulvin
Guanabenz
Guanfacine
Haloperidol
Heparin
Heroin
Hydralazine
Hydrochlorothiazide
Hydrocodone
Hydromorphone
Hydroxychloroquine
Hydroxyurea
Ibuprofen
Imipenem/cilastatin
Imipramine
Indapamide
Indinavir
Indomethacin
Infliximab
Insulin
Interferons, alfa-2
Ipodate
Ipratropium
Irbesartan
Isocarboxazid
Isoniazid
Isoproterenol
Isosorbide mononitrate
Isotretinoin
Isradipine
Itraconazole
Ivermectin
Kanamycin
Ketoconazole
Ketoprofen
Ketorolac
Ketotifen
Labetalol
Lamivudine
Lamotrigine
Lansoprazole
Latanoprost
Leflunomide
Letrozole
Leucovorin
Leuprolide
Levamisole
Levobunolol
Levofloxacin
Levothyroxine
Lidocaine
Lincomycin
Linezolid
Lisinopril
Lithium
Lomefloxacin
Loracarbef
Loratadine
Lorazepam
Losartan
Lovastatin
Loxapine
Maprotiline
Marihuana
Mebendazole
Mechlorethamine
Meclofenamate
Medroxyprogesterone
Mefenamic acid
Mefloquine
Meloxicam
Melphalan
Meperidine
Mephenytoin
Meprobamate
Mercaptopurine
Mesalamine
Mesna
Mesoridazine
Metaxalone
Metformin
Methadone
Methazolamide
Methenamine
Methicillin
Methimazole
Methocarbamol
Methotrexate
Methoxsalen
Methsuximide
Methyldopa
Methylphenidate
Methyltestosterone
Methysergide
Metolazone
Metoprolol
Metronidazole
Mexiletine
Mezlocillin
Miconazole
Midazolam
Minocycline
Minoxidil
Mirtazapine
Mitomycin
Mitotane
Modafinil
Moexipril
Molindone
Moricizine
Morphine
Moxifloxacin
Mycophenolate
Nabumetone
Nadolol
Nafarelin
Nafcillin
Nalidixic acid
Naloxone
Naproxen
Nefazodone
Nelfinavir
Neomycin
Nevirapine
Niacin
Niacinamide
Nicotine
Nifedipine
Nimodipine
Nisoldipine
Nitrofurantoin
Nizatidine
Norfloxacin
Nortriptyline
Nystatin
Octreotide
Ofloxacin
Olanzapine
Olsalazine
Omeprazole
Ondansetron
Oral contraceptives
Orphenadrine
Oxacillin
Oxaprozin
Oxazepam
Oxycodone
Oxytetracycline
Pantoprazole
Pantothenic acid
Paramethadione
Paroxetine
Penbutolol
Penicillamine
Penicillins
Pentagastrin
Pentamidine
Pentazocine
Pentobarbital
Pentosan
Pentostatin
Pentoxifylline
Pergolide
Perindopril
Perphenazine
Phenazopyridine
Phenelzine
Phenobarbital
Phenolphthalein
Phensuximide
Phenytoin
Pilocarpine
Pimozide
Pindolol
Piperacillin
Pirbuterol
Piroxicam
Pramipexole
Pravastatin
Prazepam
Praziquantel
Prazosin
Primaquine
Probenecid
Procainamide
Procarbazine
Prochlorperazine
Progestins
Propafenone
Propofol
Propoxyphene
Propranolol
Propylthiouracil
Protriptyline
Psoralens
Pyrazinamide
Pyrimethamine
Quazepam
Quinacrine
Quinapril
Quinethazone
Quinidine
Quinine
Quinupristin/dalfopristin
Rabeprazole
Ramipril
Ranitidine
Reserpine
Ribavirin
Rifampin
Rifapentine
Riluzole
Risedronate
Risperidone
Ritonavir
Rituximab
Rizatriptan
Rofecoxib
Ropinirole
Salmeterol
Salsalate
Saquinavir
Sertraline
Sibutramine
Sildenafil
Simvastatin
Sirolimus
Sotalol
Sparfloxacin
Spectinomycin
Spironolactone
Streptokinase
Streptomycin
Streptozocin
Succinylcholine
Sucralfate
Sufentanil
Sulfadiazine
Sulfadoxine
Sulfamethoxazole
Sulfasalazine
Sulfisoxazole
Sulindac
Sumatriptan
Tacrine
Tacrolimus
Tamoxifen
Tamsulosin
Telmisartan
Temazepam
Temozolomide

Terazosin
Terbinafine
Terbutaline
Terconazole
Terfenadine
Testosterone
Tetracycline
Thalidomide
Thiabendazole
Thiamine
Thioguanine
Thiopental
Thiotepa
Thiothixene
Tiagabine
Ticarcillin
Ticlopidine
Timolol
Tiopronin
Tizanidine
Tobramycin
Tocainide
Tolazamide
Tolbutamide
Tolcapone
Tolmetin
Tolterodine
Topiramate
Toremifene
Torsemide
Tramadol
Trandolapril
Tranylcypromine
Trazodone
Triamterene
Triazolam
Trifluoperazine
Trimeprazine
Trimethadione
Trimethoprim
Trimetrexate
Trimipramine
Trioxsalen
Troleandomycin
Trovafloxacin
Urokinase
Ursodiol
Vancomycin
Venlafaxine
Verapamil
Vidarabine
Vincristine
Vinorelbine
Vitamin A
Warfarin
Zalcitabine
Zaleplon
Zidovudine
Zileuton
Zolmitriptan
Zolpidem
Zonisamide

Pseudolymphoma

Alprazolam
Amitriptyline
Atenolol
Carbamazepine
Cefixime
Chlorpromazine
Cimetidine
Clarithromycin
Clonazepam
Clonidine
Co-trimoxazole
Cyclosporine
Desipramine
Diltiazem
Doxepin
Fluoxetine
Furosemide
Gemfibrozil
Gold & gold compounds
Lamotrigine
Lithium
Lorazepam
Losartan
Methotrexate
Nizatidine
Perphenazine
Phenytoin
Ranitidine
Sulfamethoxazole
Sulfasalazine
Terfenadine
Thioridazine

Psoriasis

Acebutolol
Acitretin
Aldesleukin
Amiodarone
Amoxicillin
Ampicillin
Arsenic
Aspirin
Atenolol
Betaxolol
Bisoprolol
Captopril
Carbamazepine
Carteolol
Carvedilol
Celecoxib
Chlorambucil
Chloroquine
Chlorthalidone
Cimetidine
Citalopram
Clarithromycin
Clomipramine
Clonidine
Co-trimoxazole
Cyclosporine
Dexfenfluramine
Diclofenac
Digoxin
Diltiazem
Dipyridamole
Doxycycline
Enalapril
Esmolol
Flecainide
Fluoxetine
Fluoxymesterone
Foscarnet
Ganciclovir
Gemfibrozil
Glimepiride
Glipizide
Glyburide
Gold & gold compounds
Granulocyte colony-stimulating factor (GCSF)
Hydroxychloroquine
Ibuprofen
Indomethacin
Interferons, alfa-2
Ketoprofen
Labetalol
Letrozole
Levamisole
Lithium
Meclofenamate
Mefloquine
Mesalamine
Methyltestosterone
Metoprolol
Modafinil
Nadolol
Omeprazole
Oral contraceptives
Penbutolol
Penicillamine
Pentostatin
Perindopril
Pindolol
Primaquine
Propranolol
Psoralens
Quinidine
Quinine
Rabeprazole
Ranitidine
Risperidone
Ritonavir
Rivastigmine
Ropinirole
Sotalol
Sulfamethoxazole
Sulfasalazine
Tacrine
Terbinafine
Terfenadine
Testosterone
Tetracycline
Thiabendazole
Thioguanine
Tiagabine
Timolol
Trazodone
Venlafaxine
Zaleplon

Purpura

Acetaminophen
Acetazolamide
Acitretin
Aldesleukin
Allopurinol
Alprazolam
Alteplase
Amiloride
Aminocaproic acid
Aminoglutethimide
Aminosalicylate sodium
Amiodarone
Amitriptyline
Amlodipine
Amobarbital
Amoxapine
Amoxicillin
Amphotericin B
Ampicillin
Anistreplase
Aprobarbital
Arsenic
Aspartame
Aspirin
Atenolol
Azatadine
Azathioprine
Aztreonam
Bendroflumethiazide
Benzthiazide
Beta-carotene
Betaxolol
Bisoprolol
Bromocriptine
Bumetanide
Buspirone
Busulfan
Butabarbital
Butalbital
Capecitabine
Captopril
Carbamazepine
Carbenicillin
Carteolol
Carvedilol
Cefaclor
Cefamandole
Cefdinir
Cefmetazole
Cefonicid
Cefoxitin
Ceftriaxone
Cefuroxime
Cephalexin
Cephalothin
Cephradine
Cerivastatin
Cetirizine
Chloral hydrate
Chlorambucil
Chloramphenicol
Chlordiazepoxide
Chlorothiazide
Chlorpromazine
Chlorpropamide
Chlorthalidone
Cilostazol
Cimetidine
Ciprofloxacin
Citalopram
Cladribine
Clemastine

Clindamycin
Clofibrate
Clomiphene
Clomipramine
Clonazepam
Clopidogrel
Clorazepate
Clozapine
Co-trimoxazole
Colchicine
Corticosteroids
Cyclobenzaprine
Cyclophosphamide
Cyclosporine
Cyclothiazide
Cyproheptadine
Danazol
Dapsone
Deferoxamine
Delavirdine
Demeclocycline
Denileukin
Desipramine
Dexfenfluramine
Diazepam
Diazoxide
Diclofenac
Dicloxacillin
Dicumarol
Didanosine
Diethylpropion
Diethylstilbestrol
Diflunisal
Digoxin
Diltiazem
Diphenhydramine
Dipyridamole
Disopyramide
Disulfiram
Dolasetron
Doxazosin
Doxepin
Doxorubicin
Doxycycline
Enalapril
Enoxacin
Entacapone
Ephedrine
Eprosartan
Esmolol
Estazolam
Estramustine
Estrogens
Ethacrynic acid
Ethambutol
Ethchlorvynol
Ethionamide
Ethosuximide
Ethotoin
Etodolac
Etoposide
Famotidine
Felbamate
Felodipine
Fenoprofen
Fluconazole
Flucytosine
Fluoxetine
Fluoxymesterone
Fluphenazine
Flurazepam
Flurbiprofen
Fluvastatin
Fluvoxamine
Furosemide
Gabapentin
Ganciclovir
Gentamicin
Glipizide
Glyburide
Gold & gold compounds
Griseofulvin
Guanethidine
Guanfacine
Haloperidol
Heparin
Heroin
Hydralazine
Hydrochlorothiazide
Hydroflumethiazide
Hydroxychloroquine
Hydroxyurea
Hydroxyzine
Ibuprofen
Imipramine
Indapamide
Indomethacin
Insulin
Interferons, alfa-2
Ipodate
Isoniazid
Itraconazole
Ketoconazole
Ketoprofen
Ketorolac
Labetalol
Leflunomide
Leuprolide
Levamisole
Levodopa
Levofloxacin
Lidocaine
Lincomycin
Lisinopril
Lithium
Lomefloxacin
Loratadine
Lorazepam
Losartan
Lovastatin
Loxapine
Maprotiline
Mechlorethamine
Meclofenamate
Mefenamic acid
Meloxicam
Melphalan
Mephenytoin
Mephobarbital
Meprobamate
Mercaptopurine
Metformin
Methadone
Methazolamide
Methicillin
Methimazole
Methotrexate
Methoxsalen
Methsuximide
Methyclothiazide
Methyldopa
Methylphenidate
Methyltestosterone
Metolazone
Metoprolol
Mexiletine
Miconazole
Minocycline
Mitomycin
Nalidixic acid
Naproxen
Naratriptan
Nifedipine
Nimodipine
Nitrofurantoin
Nitroglycerin
Nortriptyline
Octreotide
Ofloxacin
Omeprazole
Oral contraceptives
Oxaprozin
Oxazepam
Oxcarbazepine
Oxytetracycline
Paroxetine
Penbutolol
Penicillamine
Penicillins
Pentagastrin
Pentamidine
Pentobarbital
Pentosan
Pentostatin
Pentoxifylline
Perindopril
Perphenazine
Phenindamine
Phenobarbital
Phensuximide
Phentermine
Phenytoin
Pindolol
Piperacillin
Pirbuterol
Piroxicam
Plicamycin
Polythiazide
Potassium iodide
Pravastatin
Prazepam
Procainamide
Procarbazine
Prochlorperazine
Promazine
Promethazine
Propafenone
Propranolol
Propylthiouracil
Protriptyline
Pyrazinamide
Pyridoxine
Pyrilamine
Pyrimethamine
Quazepam
Quinethazone
Quinidine
Quinine
Rabeprazole
Ramipril
Ranitidine
Reserpine
Reteplase
Rifampin
Rifapentine
Riluzole
Risperidone
Rivastigmine
Ropinirole
Salsalate
Secobarbital
Sertraline
Simvastatin
Sirolimus
Sparfloxacin
Spironolactone
Streptokinase
Streptomycin
Streptozocin
Sulfadiazine
Sulfadoxine
Sulfamethoxazole
Sulfasalazine
Sulfinpyrazone
Sulfisoxazole
Tacrine
Tacrolimus
Tamoxifen
Temazepam
Terfenadine
Tetracycline
Thalidomide
Thiamine
Thioguanine
Thiopental
Thioridazine
Ticarcillin
Ticlopidine
Timolol
Tizanidine
Tobramycin
Tolazamide
Tolbutamide
Tolmetin
Topiramate
Topotecan
Torsemide
Trazodone
Triamterene
Triazolam
Trichlormethiazide
Trifluoperazine
Trimeprazine
Trimethadione

Trimipramine
Tripelennamine
Triprolidine
Urokinase
Vancomycin
Vasopressin
Verapamil
Vinblastine
Warfarin
Zaleplon
Zidovudine
Zolpidem
Zonisamide

Pustular eruption

Acetazolamide
Amoxicillin
Ampicillin
Azithromycin
Bacampicillin
Bexarotene
Carbamazepine
Cefaclor
Cefazolin
Cefoxitin
Cefuroxime
Cephalexin
Cephradine
Chloramphenicol
Chloroquine
Chlorpromazine
Clarithromycin
Clomipramine
Co-trimoxazole
Dactinomycin
Diltiazem
Disulfiram
Erythromycin
Felbamate
Fluoxetine
Furosemide
Heroin
Hydroxychloroquine
Imipenem/cilastatin
Isoniazid
Ivermectin
Lithium
Lomefloxacin
Minocycline
Nadolol
Naproxen
Nisoldipine
Norfloxacin
Olanzapine
Oxytetracycline
Phenytoin
Pyrimethamine
Quinidine
Ranitidine
Ritodrine
Simvastatin
Sparfloxacin
Streptomycin
Sulfadoxine
Sulfamethoxazole
Sulfasalazine
Sulfisoxazole
Tacrolimus
Terbinafine
Tetracycline
Venlafaxine
Zaleplon
Zonisamide

Pustular psoriasis

Acetazolamide
Aminoglutethimide
Amiodarone
Amoxicillin
Ampicillin
Aspirin
Atenolol
Chloroquine
Cimetidine
Corticosteroids
Cyclosporine
Diclofenac
Diltiazem
Hydroxychloroquine
Indomethacin
Lithium
Methicillin
Penicillins
Potassium iodide
Propranolol
Terbinafine

Radiation recall

Bleomycin
Buspirone
Capecitabine
Co-trimoxazole
Codeine
Dactinomycin
Doxorubicin
Epirubicin
Etoposide
Fluorouracil
Gemcitabine
Hydroxyurea
Idarubicin
Mercaptopurine
Methotrexate
Simvastatin
Sulfamethoxazole
Tamoxifen
Vinblastine

Rash (sic)

Abacavir
Acarbose
Acebutolol
Acetaminophen
Acetazolamide
Acetohexamide
Acitretin
Acyclovir
Albendazole
Aldesleukin
Alendronate
Alfentanil
Alitretinoin
Allopurinol
Alprazolam
Alprostadil
Alteplase
Altretamine
Amantadine
Amifostine
Amikacin
Amiloride
Aminocaproic acid
Aminoglutethimide
Aminophylline
Amiodarone
Amitriptyline
Amlodipine
Amobarbital
Amoxapine
Amoxicillin
Amphotericin B
Ampicillin
Amprenavir
Amyl nitrite
Anistreplase
Aprobarbital
Aprotinin
Asparaginase
Aspartame
Aspirin
Astemizole
Atenolol
Atorvastatin
Atovaquone
Atropine sulfate
Azatadine
Azathioprine
Azithromycin
Aztreonam
Bacampicillin
Baclofen
Benazepril
Bendroflumethiazide
Benzthiazide
Benztropine
Betaxolol
Bexarotene
Bicalutamide
Biperiden
Bisoprolol
Bretylium
Bromfenac
Bromocriptine
Brompheniramine
Bumetanide
Buspirone
Butabarbital
Butalbital
Butorphanol
Calcitonin (human & salmon)
Candesartan
Captopril
Carbamazepine
Carbenicillin
Carboplatin
Carisoprodol
Carteolol
Carvedilol
Cefaclor
Cefadroxil
Cefamandole
Cefazolin
Cefdinir
Cefepime
Cefixime
Cefmetazole
Cefonicid
Cefoperazone
Cefotetan
Cefoxitin
Cefpodoxime
Cefprozil
Ceftazidime
Ceftibuten
Ceftizoxime
Ceftriaxone
Cefuroxime
Celecoxib
Cephalexin
Cephalothin
Cephapirin
Cephradine
Cerivastatin
Cetirizine
Cevimeline
Chloral hydrate
Chlorambucil
Chloramphenicol
Chlordiazepoxide
Chlormezanone
Chlorothiazide
Chlorotrianisene
Chlorpromazine
Chlorpropamide
Chlortetracycline
Chlorthalidone
Chlorzoxazone
Cholestyramine
Cidofovir
Cilostazol
Cimetidine
Cinoxacin
Ciprofloxacin
Cisapride
Cisplatin
Citalopram
Cladribine
Clarithromycin
Clemastine
Clindamycin
Clofazimine
Clofibrate
Clomiphene
Clomipramine
Clonazepam
Clonidine
Clopidogrel
Clorazepate
Cloxacillin
Clozapine
Co-trimoxazole
Codeine
Colchicine
Cromolyn
Cyclobenzaprine
Cyclophosphamide
Cycloserine
Cyclosporine

Cyclothiazide
Cyproheptadine
Cytarabine
Dacarbazine
Dalteparin
Danazol
Dantrolene
Dapsone
Daunorubicin
Deferoxamine
Delavirdine
Denileukin
Desipramine
Desmopressin
Dexchlorpheniramine
Dexfenfluramine
Dextroamphetamine
Diazepam
Diazoxide
Diclofenac
Dicloxacillin
Dicumarol
Dicyclomine
Didanosine
Diethylpropion
Diethylstilbestrol
Diflunisal
Digoxin
Diltiazem
Dimenhydrinate
Diphenhydramine
Dipyridamole
Dirithromycin
Disopyramide
Disulfiram
Docetaxel
Docusate
Dofetilide
Dolasetron
Dorzolamide
Doxacurium
Doxazosin
Doxepin
Doxorubicin
Doxycycline
Edrophonium
Efavirenz
Eflornithine
Enalapril
Enoxacin
Epirubicin
Epoetin alfa
Eprosartan
Erythromycin
Esmolol
Estazolam
Estramustine
Estrogens
Etanercept
Ethacrynic acid
Ethambutol
Ethchlorvynol
Ethionamide
Ethosuximide
Ethotoin
Etidronate
Etodolac
Etoposide
Famotidine
Felbamate
Felodipine
Fenfluramine
Fenofibrate
Fenoprofen
Fentanyl
Finasteride
Flavoxate
Flecainide
Fluconazole
Flucytosine
Fludarabine
Flumazenil
Fluoxetine
Fluphenazine
Flurazepam
Flurbiprofen
Flutamide
Fluvastatin
Fluvoxamine
Folic acid
Foscarnet
Fosfomycin
Fosinopril
Fosphenytoin
Furazolidone
Furosemide
Gabapentin
Ganciclovir
Gatifloxacin
Gemcitabine
Gemfibrozil
Gemtuzumab
Gentamicin
Glimepiride
Glipizide
Glucagon
Glyburide
Glycopyrrolate
Gold & gold compounds
Goserelin
Granisetron
Granulocyte colony-stimulating factor (GCSF)
Grepafloxacin
Griseofulvin
Guanabenz
Guanfacine
Haloperidol
Heparin
Hydralazine
Hydrochlorothiazide
Hydrocodone
Hydroflumethiazide
Hydromorphone
Hydroxychloroquine
Hydroxyurea
Hydroxyzine
Ibuprofen
Idarubicin
Imipenem/cilastatin
Imipramine
Indapamide
Indinavir
Indomethacin
Infliximab
Interferons, alfa-2
Ipodate
Ipratropium
Irbesartan
Irinotecan
Isocarboxazid
Isoniazid
Isoproterenol
Isosorbide
Isosorbide mononitrate
Isotretinoin
Isradipine
Itraconazole
Ivermectin
Kanamycin
Ketamine
Ketoconazole
Ketoprofen
Ketorolac
Ketotifen
Labetalol
Lamivudine
Lamotrigine
Lansoprazole
Leflunomide
Leucovorin
Leuprolide
Levamisole
Levetiracetam
Levobunolol
Levodopa
Levofloxacin
Levothyroxine
Lidocaine
Lincomycin
Linezolid
Liothyronine
Lisinopril
Lithium
Lomefloxacin
Lomustine
Loracarbef
Loratadine
Lorazepam
Losartan
Lovastatin
Loxapine
Maprotiline
Mazindol
Mebendazole
Mechlorethamine
Meclizine
Meclofenamate
Medroxyprogesterone
Mefenamic acid
Mefloquine
Meloxicam
Melphalan
Meperidine
Mephobarbital
Meprobamate
Mercaptopurine
Mesalamine
Mesna
Mesoridazine
Metaxalone
Metformin
Methadone
Methamphetamine
Methazolamide
Methenamine
Methicillin
Methimazole
Methocarbamol
Methohexital
Methotrexate
Methoxsalen
Methsuximide
Methyclothiazide
Methyldopa
Methylphenidate
Methysergide
Metoclopramide
Metolazone
Metoprolol
Metronidazole
Mexiletine
Mezlocillin
Mibefradil
Miconazole
Midazolam
Miglitol
Minocycline
Minoxidil
Mirtazapine
Misoprostol
Mitomycin
Mitotane
Modafinil
Moexipril
Molindone
Montelukast
Moricizine
Morphine
Moxifloxacin
Mycophenolate
Nabumetone
Nadolol
Nafarelin
Nafcillin
Nalidixic acid
Naloxone
Naproxen
Naratriptan
Nefazodone
Nelfinavir
Neomycin
Nevirapine
Niacin
Niacinamide
Nicardipine
Nicotine
Nifedipine
Nimodipine
Nisoldipine
Nitrofurantoin
Nitroglycerin
Nizatidine

Norfloxacin
Nortriptyline
Nystatin
Octreotide
Ofloxacin
Olanzapine
Olsalazine
Omeprazole
Ondansetron
Orlistat
Orphenadrine
Oxacillin
Oxaprozin
Oxazepam
Oxcarbazepine
Oxybutynin
Oxycodone
Pamidronate
Pantoprazole
Paroxetine
Pemoline
Penbutolol
Penicillamine
Penicillins
Pentagastrin
Pentamidine
Pentazocine
Pentobarbital
Pentosan
Pentostatin
Pentoxifylline
Pergolide
Perindopril
Perphenazine
Phenazopyridine
Phenelzine
Phenindamine
Phenobarbital
Phensuximide
Phentermine
Phenytoin
Phytonadione
Pilocarpine
Pimozide
Pindolol
Piperacillin
Pirbuterol
Piroxicam
Polythiazide
Potassium iodide
Pramipexole
Pravastatin
Prazepam
Praziquantel
Prazosin
Primidone
Probenecid
Procainamide
Procarbazine
Prochlorperazine
Procyclidine
Progestins
Promazine
Promethazine
Propafenone
Propantheline
Propofol
Propoxyphene
Propranolol
Propylthiouracil
Protriptyline
Psoralens
Pyrazinamide
Pyrilamine
Pyrimethamine
Quazepam
Quetiapine
Quinapril
Quinestrol
Quinethazone
Quinidine
Quinine
Quinupristin/dalfopristin
Rabeprazole
Raloxifene
Ramipril
Ranitidine
Reserpine
Ribavirin
Rifabutin
Rifampin
Rifapentine
Rimantadine
Risedronate
Risperidone
Ritodrine
Ritonavir
Rituximab
Rivastigmine
Rofecoxib
Ropinirole
Salmeterol
Salsalate
Saquinavir
Scopolamine
Secobarbital
Selegiline
Sertraline
Sibutramine
Sildenafil
Simvastatin
Sirolimus
Sotalol
Sparfloxacin
Spectinomycin
Spironolactone
Stavudine
Streptokinase
Streptomycin
Succinylcholine
Sucralfate
Sufentanil
Sulfadiazine
Sulfadoxine
Sulfamethoxazole
Sulfasalazine
Sulfinpyrazone
Sulfisoxazole
Sulindac
Sumatriptan
Tacrine
Tacrolimus
Tamoxifen
Tamsulosin
Telmisartan
Temazepam
Temozolomide
Terazosin
Terbinafine
Terfenadine
Testosterone
Tetracycline
Thalidomide
Thiabendazole
Thiamine
Thioguanine
Thiopental
Thioridazine
Thiotepa
Thiothixene
Tiagabine
Ticarcillin
Ticlopidine
Timolol
Tiopronin
Tirofiban
Tizanidine
Tobramycin
Tocainide
Tolazamide
Tolazoline
Tolbutamide
Tolcapone
Tolmetin
Tolterodine
Topiramate
Torsemide
Tramadol
Trandolapril
Tranylcypromine
Trazodone
Triamterene
Triazolam
Trichlormethiazide
Trifluoperazine
Trihexyphenidyl
Trimeprazine
Trimethoprim
Trimetrexate
Trimipramine
Tripelennamine
Triprolidine
Troleandomycin
Trovafloxacin
Urokinase
Ursodiol
Vancomycin
Vasopressin
Venlafaxine
Verapamil
Vidarabine
Vinblastine
Vincristine
Vinorelbine
Warfarin
Zalcitabine
Zaleplon
Zidovudine
Zolmitriptan
Zolpidem
Zonisamide

Raynaud's phenomenon

Acebutolol
Amphotericin B
Atenolol
Azathioprine
Betaxolol
Bisoprolol
Bleomycin
Bromocriptine
Carteolol
Cisplatin
Clonidine
Cyclosporine
Dopamine
Doxorubicin
Estrogens
Ethosuximide
Gemfibrozil
Interferons, alfa-2
Labetalol
Methysergide
Metoprolol
Minocycline
Nadolol
Octreotide
Phentermine
Pindolol
Propofol
Propranolol
Sotalol
Spironolactone
Sulfasalazine
Sulindac
Sumatriptan
Thiothixene
Timolol
Vinblastine
Vincristine

Scleroderma

Aldesleukin
Azathioprine
Bleomycin
Bromocriptine
Cocaine
Dapsone
Diethylpropion
Docetaxel
Estrogens
Fosinopril
Heparin
Medroxyprogesterone
Melphalan
Mephenytoin
Methoxsalen
Methysergide
Metoprolol
Penicillamine
Pentazocine
Phenytoin
Phytonadione
Psoralens
Sotalol
Trioxsalen

Seborrhea
- Acitretin
- Atorvastatin
- Bromfenac
- Cetirizine
- Clomipramine
- Danazol
- Delavirdine
- Doxycycline
- Fluoxetine
- Fluoxymesterone
- Fluphenazine
- Flurbiprofen
- Fluvoxamine
- Foscarnet
- Gemfibrozil
- Indinavir
- Loxapine
- Mesoridazine
- Methyltestosterone
- Minoxidil
- Mirtazapine
- Nafarelin
- Olanzapine
- Oral contraceptives
- Pentostatin
- Pergolide
- Perphenazine
- Prochlorperazine
- Risperidone
- Ritonavir
- Tacrine
- Testosterone
- Thioridazine
- Tolcapone
- Topiramate
- Trifluoperazine
- Trovafloxacin

Seborrheic dermatitis
- Buspirone
- Chlorpromazine
- Cimetidine
- Ethionamide
- Fluorouracil
- Fluoxymesterone
- Gold & gold compounds
- Griseofulvin
- Haloperidol
- Interferons, alfa-2
- Lithium
- Methoxsalen
- Methyldopa
- Methyltestosterone
- Psoralens
- Saquinavir
- Stanozolol
- Testosterone
- Thiothixene
- Trioxsalen

Serum sickness
- Amobarbital
- Amoxicillin
- Ampicillin
- Anistreplase
- Aprobarbital
- Asparaginase
- Azathioprine
- Bacampicillin
- Carbamazepine
- Carbenicillin
- Cefaclor
- Cefadroxil
- Cefamandole
- Cefazolin
- Cefdinir
- Cefixime
- Cefmetazole
- Cefonicid
- Cefoperazone
- Cefotaxime
- Cefotetan
- Cefoxitin
- Cefpodoxime
- Cefprozil
- Ceftazidime
- Ceftibuten
- Ceftizoxime
- Ceftriaxone
- Cefuroxime
- Cephalexin
- Cephalothin
- Cephapirin
- Cephradine
- Ciprofloxacin
- Cloxacillin
- Co-trimoxazole
- Cromolyn
- Diclofenac
- Dicloxacillin
- Doxycycline
- Fluoxetine
- Furazolidone
- Gatifloxacin
- Griseofulvin
- Heroin
- Ibuprofen
- Indomethacin
- Ipodate
- Isoniazid
- Itraconazole
- Lincomycin
- Loracarbef
- Meclofenamate
- Mephobarbital
- Mercaptopurine
- Methicillin
- Methimazole
- Metronidazole
- Mezlocillin
- Minocycline
- Nafcillin
- Nizatidine
- Ofloxacin
- Oxacillin
- Oxaprozin
- Penicillamine
- Penicillins
- Pentoxifylline
- Phenytoin
- Piperacillin
- Piroxicam
- Potassium iodide
- Propranolol
- Rifampin
- Secobarbital
- Sparfloxacin
- Streptokinase
- Sulfadiazine
- Sulfamethoxazole
- Sulfasalazine
- Sulfisoxazole
- Sulindac
- Terbinafine
- Tetracycline
- Ticarcillin
- Ticlopidine
- Tolmetin
- Trovafloxacin
- Verapamil

Sialorrhea
- Acitretin
- Alprazolam
- Amiodarone
- Amitriptyline
- Amoxapine
- Betaxolol
- Bethanechol
- Buspirone
- Cetirizine
- Cevimeline
- Chlordiazepoxide
- Citalopram
- Clomipramine
- Clonazepam
- Clorazepate
- Clozapine
- Delavirdine
- Diazepam
- Diazoxide
- Edrophonium
- Estazolam
- Ethionamide
- Etodolac
- Fluoxetine
- Fluphenazine
- Flurazepam
- Fluvoxamine
- Gabapentin
- Gentamicin
- Guanabenz
- Guanethidine
- Guanfacine
- Haloperidol
- Ifosfamide
- Imipenem/cilastatin
- Irinotecan
- Kanamycin
- Ketamine
- Ketoprofen
- Lamotrigine
- Levodopa
- Lithium
- Loratadine
- Lorazepam
- Maprotiline
- Mefenamic acid
- Mesoridazine
- Methohexital
- Midazolam
- Mirtazapine
- Modafinil
- Molindone
- Nabumetone
- Nefazodone
- Nicotine
- Olanzapine
- Oxazepam
- Pantoprazole
- Paroxetine
- Pentoxifylline
- Perphenazine
- Pilocarpine
- Pimozide
- Potassium iodide
- Pramipexole
- Prazepam
- Prochlorperazine
- Propofol
- Quazepam
- Quetiapine
- Ramipril
- Reserpine
- Risperidone
- Rivastigmine
- Ropinirole
- Sertraline
- Succinylcholine
- Tacrine
- Temazepam
- Thiothixene
- Tiagabine
- Tobramycin
- Tolcapone
- Trazodone
- Triazolam
- Trovafloxacin
- Venlafaxine
- Zaleplon

Stevens–Johnson syndrome
- Acetaminophen
- Acetazolamide
- Acyclovir
- Albendazole
- Allopurinol
- Aminophylline
- Amiodarone
- Amobarbital
- Amoxicillin
- Ampicillin
- Amprenavir
- Aprobarbital
- Arsenic
- Aspirin
- Astemizole
- Atropine sulfate
- Azithromycin
- Bacampicillin
- Bleomycin
- Butabarbital
- Butalbital
- Captopril
- Carbamazepine
- Carbenicillin
- Carvedilol

Cefaclor
Cefadroxil
Cefamandole
Cefazolin
Cefdinir
Cefepime
Cefixime
Cefmetazole
Cefonicid
Cefoperazone
Cefotaxime
Cefotetan
Cefoxitin
Cefpodoxime
Cefprozil
Ceftazidime
Ceftibuten
Ceftizoxime
Ceftriaxone
Cefuroxime
Celecoxib
Cephalexin
Cephalothin
Cephapirin
Cephradine
Cerivastatin
Chlorambucil
Chloramphenicol
Chlormezanone
Chloroquine
Chlorothiazide
Chlorpropamide
Chlorthalidone
Cimetidine
Cinoxacin
Ciprofloxacin
Cisplatin
Clarithromycin
Clindamycin
Clofibrate
Cloxacillin
Clozapine
Co-trimoxazole
Cyclophosphamide
Cycloserine
Danazol
Dapsone
Delavirdine
Demeclocycline
Dexfenfluramine
Diclofenac
Dicloxacillin
Didanosine
Diflunisal
Diltiazem
Dipyridamole
Doxycycline
Enalapril
Enoxacin
Erythromycin
Ethambutol
Ethosuximide
Etidronate
Etodolac
Etoposide
Felbamate
Fenoprofen
Fluconazole
Fluoxetine
Flurbiprofen
Fluvastatin
Fluvoxamine
Fosphenytoin
Furosemide
Gabapentin
Ganciclovir
Gatifloxacin
Griseofulvin
Hydrochlorothiazide
Hydrocodone
Ibuprofen
Indapamide
Indinavir
Indomethacin
Isoniazid
Itraconazole
Ketoprofen
Ketorolac
Lamotrigine
Leflunomide
Levamisole
Levofloxacin
Lidocaine
Lincomycin
Lisinopril
Lomefloxacin
Loracarbef
Lorazepam
Lovastatin
Maprotiline
Mebendazole
Mechlorethamine
Meclofenamate
Mefenamic acid
Mefloquine
Meloxicam
Mephenytoin
Mephobarbital
Meprobamate
Methazolamide
Methicillin
Methotrexate
Methsuximide
Methyclothiazide
Methyldopa
Metolazone
Mexiletine
Mezlocillin
Minocycline
Minoxidil
Nabumetone
Nafcillin
Naproxen
Nevirapine
Nifedipine
Nitrofurantoin
Norfloxacin
Nystatin
Ofloxacin
Omeprazole
Oral contraceptives
Oxacillin
Oxaprozin
Oxcarbazepine
Pantoprazole
Penicillamine
Penicillins
Pentamidine
Pentobarbital
Phenobarbital
Phenolphthalein
Phensuximide
Phenytoin
Piperacillin
Piroxicam
Pravastatin
Promethazine
Propranolol
Pyrimethamine
Quinine
Ranitidine
Rifampin
Ritonavir
Saquinavir
Secobarbital
Sertraline
Simvastatin
Sparfloxacin
Streptomycin
Sulfadiazine
Sulfadoxine
Sulfamethoxazole
Sulfasalazine
Sulfisoxazole
Sulindac
Terbinafine
Tetracycline
Thiabendazole
Thiopental
Tiagabine
Ticarcillin
Ticlopidine
Tocainide
Tolmetin
Torsemide
Trimethadione
Trimethoprim
Trovafloxacin
Vancomycin
Verapamil
Vitamin A
Zidovudine
Zonisamide

Stomatitis

Acitretin
Aldesleukin
Allopurinol
Amitriptyline
Amoxapine
Amoxicillin
Amphotericin B
Ampicillin
Arsenic
Atorvastatin
Azathioprine
Azelastine
Bacampicillin
Benactyzine
Bleomycin
Bromfenac
Busulfan
Capecitabine
Carbamazepine
Carbenicillin
Carboplatin
Carmustine
Cefdinir
Celecoxib
Cetirizine
Cevimeline
Chloral hydrate
Chlorambucil
Chloramphenicol
Chlorhexidine
Chloroquine
Cidofovir
Ciprofloxacin
Citalopram
Clarithromycin
Clofibrate
Clomipramine
Cloxacillin
Co-trimoxazole
Cyclobenzaprine
Cyclophosphamide
Cyclosporine
Cytarabine
Dacarbazine
Dactinomycin
Daunorubicin
Delavirdine
Desipramine
Diclofenac
Dicloxacillin
Diflunisal
Docetaxel
Doxepin
Doxorubicin
Enalapril
Enoxacin
Epirubicin
Ethionamide
Etidronate
Etodolac
Etoposide
Fenoprofen
Fludarabine
Fluorouracil
Fluoxetine
Fluoxymesterone
Flurbiprofen
Fluvoxamine
Foscarnet
Gabapentin
Gatifloxacin
Gemcitabine
Gemtuzumab
Gentamicin
Gold & gold compounds
Granulocyte colony-stimulating factor (GCSF)
Grepafloxacin
Hydroxyurea
Ibuprofen

Idarubicin
Ifosfamide
Imipramine
Interferons, alfa-2
Ipratropium
Irinotecan
Ketoprofen
Ketorolac
Lamotrigine
Lansoprazole
Leflunomide
Levamisole
Lidocaine
Lincomycin
Lithium
Lomustine
Loratadine
Lovastatin
Maprotiline
Meclofenamate
Melphalan
Mephenytoin
Meprobamate
Mercaptopurine
Methenamine
Methicillin
Methotrexate
Methyltestosterone
Metronidazole
Mezlocillin
Mirtazapine
Mitomycin
Moxifloxacin
Nabumetone
Nafcillin
Naproxen
Nefazodone
Nicotine
Norfloxacin
Nortriptyline
Olanzapine
Olsalazine
Oxacillin
Oxaprozin
Oxcarbazepine
Pamidronate
Pantoprazole
Paroxetine
Penicillamine
Penicillins
Pentostatin
Piroxicam
Plicamycin
Pravastatin
Procarbazine
Protriptyline
Pyrilamine
Quetiapine
Quinupristin/dalfopristin
Rabeprazole
Rifampin
Riluzole
Rimantadine
Risperidone
Ropinirole
Saquinavir
Sertraline
Sildenafil
Sirolimus
Sparfloxacin
Streptokinase
Streptomycin
Sulfadiazine
Sulfadoxine
Sulfamethoxazole
Sulfasalazine
Sulfisoxazole
Sulindac
Tacrine
Terbinafine
Terfenadine
Testosterone
Thioguanine
Thiotepa
Tiagabine
Ticarcillin
Tiopronin
Tocainide
Tolmetin
Topiramate
Topotecan
Tramadol
Triazolam
Trimeprazine
Trimetrexate
Trimipramine
Tripelennamine
Trovafloxacin
Ursodiol
Venlafaxine
Vinblastine
Vincristine
Vinorelbine
Zalcitabine
Zaleplon
Zonisamide

Stomatodynia

Amoxicillin
Bacampicillin
Benztropine
Biperiden
Carbenicillin
Dicloxacillin
Erythromycin
Ethionamide
Griseofulvin
Lithium
Methicillin
Mezlocillin
Nafcillin
Oxacillin
Piperacillin
Potassium iodide
Ticarcillin
Triamterene
Vitamin A

Telangiectases

Amlodipine
Carmustine
Corticosteroids
Estrogens
Felodipine
Hydroxyurea
Interferons, alfa-2
Isocarboxazid
Isotretinoin
Lisinopril
Lithium
Methotrexate
Methysergide
Nifedipine
Oral contraceptives
Phenelzine
Progestins
Thiothixene

Tendinitis

Amlodipine
Celecoxib
Cevimeline
Ciprofloxacin
Eprosartan
Gatifloxacin
Grepafloxacin
Levofloxacin
Minoxidil
Moxifloxacin
Orlistat
Rofecoxib

Tendon rupture

Ciprofloxacin
Enoxacin
Gatifloxacin
Grepafloxacin
Leflunomide
Levofloxacin
Lomefloxacin
Mirtazapine
Moxifloxacin
Norfloxacin
Ofloxacin
Sparfloxacin
Trovafloxacin

Toxic epidermal necrolysis

Acebutolol
Acetaminophen
Acetazolamide
Aldesleukin
Allopurinol
Alprostadil
Aminosalicylate sodium
Amiodarone
Amobarbital
Amoxapine
Amoxicillin
Ampicillin
Asparaginase
Aspirin
Atenolol
Atorvastatin
Azathioprine
Aztreonam
Betaxolol
Butabarbital
Butalbital
Captopril
Carbamazepine
Carbenicillin
Cefaclor
Cefadroxil
Cefamandole
Cefazolin
Cefdinir
Cefepime
Cefmetazole
Cefonicid
Cefoperazone
Cefotaxime
Cefotetan
Cefoxitin
Cefpodoxime
Cefprozil
Ceftazidime
Ceftibuten
Ceftizoxime
Ceftriaxone
Cefuroxime
Celecoxib
Cephalexin
Cephalothin
Cephapirin
Cephradine
Cerivastatin
Chlorambucil
Chloramphenicol
Chlormezanone
Chloroquine
Chlorothiazide
Chlorpromazine
Chlorpropamide
Chlorthalidone
Cimetidine
Cinoxacin
Ciprofloxacin
Cladribine
Clindamycin
Clofibrate
Co-trimoxazole
Codeine
Colchicine
Cyclophosphamide
Cyclosporine
Cytarabine
Dactinomycin
Dapsone
Deferoxamine
Demeclocycline
Dextroamphetamine
Diclofenac
Dicloxacillin
Diflunisal
Diltiazem
Diphenhydramine
Dipyridamole
Disulfiram
Doxycycline
Enalapril
Enoxacin
Erythromycin
Ethambutol
Etidronate
Etodolac
Famotidine
Felbamate
Fenoprofen

Fluconazole
Fluoxetine
Fluphenazine
Flurbiprofen
Flutamide
Fluvastatin
Fluvoxamine
Foscarnet
Fosphenytoin
Gatifloxacin
Gentamicin
Gold & gold compounds
Grepafloxacin
Griseofulvin
Heparin
Heroin
Hydrochlorothiazide
Hydrocodone
Hydroxychloroquine
Ibuprofen
Imipenem/cilastatin
Indapamide
Indomethacin
Isoniazid
Isotretinoin
Ketoprofen
Ketorolac
Lamotrigine
Leflunomide
Levofloxacin
Lisinopril
Lovastatin
Meclofenamate
Mefenamic acid
Mefloquine
Meloxicam
Meperidine
Mephenytoin
Meprobamate
Mercaptopurine
Methazolamide
Methicillin
Methotrexate
Methyldopa
Metolazone
Metoprolol
Metronidazole
Mezlocillin
Nabumetone
Nadolol
Nafcillin
Nalidixic acid
Naproxen
Neomycin
Nevirapine
Nifedipine
Nitrofurantoin
Norfloxacin
Ofloxacin
Omeprazole
Oxacillin
Oxaprozin
Oxcarbazepine
Pantoprazole
Paroxetine
Penicillamine
Penicillins
Pentamidine
Pentazocine
Pentobarbital
Phenobarbital
Phenolphthalein
Phenytoin
Pindolol
Piperacillin
Piroxicam
Plicamycin
Pravastatin
Primidone
Procarbazine
Prochlorperazine
Promethazine
Propranolol
Pyridoxine
Pyrimethamine
Quinidine
Quinine
Ranitidine
Reserpine
Rifampin
Simvastatin
Sparfloxacin
Streptomycin
Streptozocin
Sulfadiazine
Sulfadoxine
Sulfamethoxazole
Sulfasalazine
Sulfisoxazole
Sulindac
Terbinafine
Terconazole
Tetracycline
Thalidomide
Thiabendazole
Thiopental
Thioridazine
Ticarcillin
Timolol
Tiopronin
Tolbutamide
Tolmetin
Trimethoprim
Trovafloxacin
Vancomycin
Vinorelbine
Zidovudine
Zonisamide

Urticaria

Acarbose
Acebutolol
Acetaminophen
Acetazolamide
Acetohexamide
Acitretin
Acyclovir
Albendazole
Albuterol
Aldesleukin
Alfentanil
Allopurinol
Alprazolam
Alprostadil
Alteplase
Amantadine
Amikacin
Amiloride
Aminocaproic acid
Aminoglutethimide
Aminophylline
Aminosalicylate sodium
Amiodarone
Amitriptyline
Amlodipine
Amobarbital
Amoxapine
Amoxicillin
Amphotericin B
Ampicillin
Anistreplase
Aprobarbital
Aprotinin
Arsenic
Asparaginase
Aspartame
Aspirin
Astemizole
Atenolol
Atorvastatin
Atracurium
Atropine sulfate
Azatadine
Azathioprine
Azithromycin
Aztreonam
Bacampicillin
Baclofen
Benactyzine
Benazepril
Bendroflumethiazide
Benzthiazide
Benztropine
Betaxolol
Biperiden
Bisacodyl
Bisoprolol
Bleomycin
Bromfenac
Bromocriptine
Bumetanide
Buspirone
Busulfan
Butabarbital
Butalbital
Butorphanol
Calcitonin (human & salmon)
Captopril
Carbamazepine
Carbenicillin
Carboplatin
Carisoprodol
Cefaclor
Cefadroxil
Cefamandole
Cefazolin
Cefdinir
Cefepime
Cefixime
Cefmetazole
Cefonicid
Cefoperazone
Cefotaxime
Cefotetan
Cefoxitin
Cefpodoxime
Cefprozil
Ceftazidime
Ceftibuten
Ceftizoxime
Ceftriaxone
Cefuroxime
Celecoxib
Cephalexin
Cephalothin
Cephapirin
Cephradine
Cerivastatin
Cetirizine
Chloral hydrate
Chlorambucil
Chloramphenicol
Chlordiazepoxide
Chlorhexidine
Chlormezanone
Chloroquine
Chlorothiazide
Chlorotrianisene
Chlorpromazine
Chlorpropamide
Chlorthalidone
Chlorzoxazone
Cholestyramine
Cidofovir
Cilostazol
Cimetidine
Cinoxacin
Ciprofloxacin
Cisapride
Cisplatin
Citalopram
Clarithromycin
Clemastine
Clidinium
Clindamycin
Clofazimine
Clofibrate
Clomiphene
Clomipramine
Clonazepam
Clonidine
Clopidogrel
Clorazepate
Cloxacillin
Clozapine
Co-trimoxazole
Cocaine
Codeine
Colchicine
Colestipol
Corticosteroids
Cromolyn
Cyanocobalamin
Cyclamate
Cyclobenzaprine

Cyclophosphamide
Cycloserine
Cyclosporine
Cyclothiazide
Cyproheptadine
Cytarabine
Dacarbazine
Dactinomycin
Danazol
Dantrolene
Dapsone
Daunorubicin
Deferoxamine
Delavirdine
Demeclocycline
Denileukin
Desipramine
Dexchlorpheniramine
Dexfenfluramine
Dextroamphetamine
Diazepam
Diazoxide
Diclofenac
Dicloxacillin
Dicumarol
Dicyclomine
Didanosine
Diethylpropion
Diethylstilbestrol
Diflunisal
Digoxin
Diltiazem
Dimenhydrinate
Diphenhydramine
Diphenoxylate
Dipyridamole
Dirithromycin
Disopyramide
Disulfiram
Docetaxel
Dolasetron
Donepezil
Dopamine
Doxacurium
Doxazosin
Doxepin
Doxorubicin
Doxycycline
Edrophonium
Efavirenz
Enalapril
Enoxacin
Enoxaparin
Ephedrine
Epinephrine
Epirubicin
Epoetin alfa
Erythromycin
Esmolol
Estazolam
Estramustine
Estrogens
Ethacrynic acid
Ethambutol
Ethchlorvynol
Ethionamide
Ethosuximide
Etidronate
Etodolac
Etoposide
Famotidine
Felbamate
Felodipine
Fenfluramine
Fenofibrate
Fenoprofen
Fentanyl
Finasteride
Flavoxate
Flecainide
Fluconazole
Flucytosine
Flumazenil
Fluorouracil
Fluoxetine
Fluoxymesterone
Fluphenazine
Flurazepam
Flurbiprofen
Flutamide
Fluvastatin
Fluvoxamine
Folic acid
Foscarnet
Fosinopril
Furazolidone
Furosemide
Gabapentin
Ganciclovir
Gatifloxacin
Gemfibrozil
Gentamicin
Glimepiride
Glipizide
Glucagon
Glyburide
Glycopyrrolate
Gold & gold scompounds
Goserelin
Granisetron
Granulocyte colony-stimulating factor (GCSF)
Grepafloxacin
Griseofulvin
Guanethidine
Guanfacine
Haloperidol
Halothane
Heparin
Heroin
Hydralazine
Hydrochlorothiazide
Hydrocodone
Hydroflumethiazide
Hydromorphone
Hydroxychloroquine
Hydroxyurea
Hydroxyzine
Ibuprofen
Idarubicin
Imipenem/cilastatin
Imipramine
Indapamide
Indinavir
Indomethacin
Infliximab
Insulin
Interferons, alfa-2
Ipodate
Ipratropium
Irbesartan
Isoniazid
Isoproterenol
Isotretinoin
Isradipine
Itraconazole
Ivermectin
Kanamycin
Ketoconazole
Ketoprofen
Ketorolac
Labetalol
Lamivudine
Lamotrigine
Lansoprazole
Leflunomide
Leucovorin
Leuprolide
Levamisole
Levobunolol
Levodopa
Levofloxacin
Levothyroxine
Lidocaine
Lincomycin
Liothyronine
Lisinopril
Lithium
Lomefloxacin
Loracarbef
Loratadine
Lorazepam
Losartan
Lovastatin
Loxapine
Maprotiline
Marihuana
Mazindol
Mebendazole
Mechlorethamine
Meclizine
Meclofenamate
Medroxyprogesterone
Mefenamic acid
Mefloquine
Meloxicam
Melphalan
Meperidine
Mephenytoin
Mephobarbital
Meprobamate
Mercaptopurine
Mesalamine
Mesna
Mesoridazine
Metaxalone
Metformin
Methadone
Methamphetamine
Methantheline
Methazolamide
Methenamine
Methicillin
Methimazole
Methocarbamol
Methohexital
Methotrexate
Methoxsalen
Methsuximide
Methyclothiazide
Methyldopa
Methylphenidate
Methyltestosterone
Methysergide
Metoclopramide
Metolazone
Metoprolol
Metronidazole
Mexiletine
Mezlocillin
Miconazole
Midazolam
Minocycline
Minoxidil
Mitomycin
Mitotane
Moexipril
Montelukast
Moricizine
Moxifloxacin
Nabumetone
Nadolol
Nafarelin
Nafcillin
Nalidixic acid
Naloxone
Naproxen
Naratriptan
Nefazodone
Nelfinavir
Neomycin
Niacin
Nicardipine
Nicotine
Nifedipine
Nisoldipine
Nitrofurantoin
Nitroglycerin
Nizatidine
Norfloxacin
Nortriptyline
Nystatin
Octreotide
Ofloxacin
Olanzapine
Olsalazine
Omeprazole
Ondansetron
Oral contraceptives
Orphenadrine
Oxacillin
Oxaprozin
Oxazepam

Oxybutynin
Oxycodone
Oxytetracycline
Pantoprazole
Pantothenic acid
Paroxetine
Penicillamine
Penicillins
Pentagastrin
Pentamidine
Pentazocine
Pentobarbital
Pentosan
Pentostatin
Pentoxifylline
Pergolide
Perphenazine
Phendimetrazine
Phenelzine
Phenindamine
Phenobarbital
Phenolphthalein
Phentermine
Phenytoin
Phytonadione
Pilocarpine
Pimozide
Pindolol
Piperacillin
Piroxicam
Polythiazide
Potassium iodide
Pravastatin
Prazepam
Praziquantel
Prazosin
Primaquine
Primidone
Probenecid
Procainamide
Procarbazine
Prochlorperazine
Procyclidine
Progestins
Promazine
Promethazine
Propafenone
Propantheline
Propofol
Propoxyphene
Propranolol
Propylthiouracil
Protamine
Protriptyline
Pseudoephedrine
Psoralens
Pyrazinamide
Pyrilamine
Pyrimethamine
Quazepam
Quinacrine
Quinapril
Quinestrol
Quinethazone
Quinidine
Quinine
Quinupristin/dalfopristin
Rabeprazole
Ramipril
Ranitidine
Reserpine
Ribavirin
Riboflavin
Rifabutin
Rifampin
Rifapentine
Risperidone
Ritodrine
Ritonavir
Rituximab
Rivastigmine
Rofecoxib
Ropinirole
Saccharin
Salmeterol
Salsalate
Saquinavir
Scopolamine
Secobarbital
Secretin
Sertraline
Sildenafil
Simvastatin
Sotalol
Sparfloxacin
Spectinomycin
Spironolactone
Stanozolol
Streptokinase
Streptomycin
Succinylcholine
Sucralfate
Sufentanil
Sulfadiazine
Sulfadoxine
Sulfamethoxazole
Sulfasalazine
Sulfisoxazole
Sulindac
Sumatriptan
Tacrine
Tamoxifen
Temazepam
Terbinafine
Terbutaline
Terfenadine
Testosterone
Tetracycline
Thalidomide
Thiabendazole
Thiamine
Thiopental
Thioridazine
Thiotepa
Thiothixene
Tiagabine
Ticarcillin
Ticlopidine
Timolol
Tiopronin
Tirofiban
Tizanidine
Tobramycin
Tolazamide
Tolazoline
Tolbutamide
Tolcapone
Tolmetin
Topiramate
Torsemide
Tramadol
Tranylcypromine
Trazodone
Triamterene
Triazolam
Trichlormethiazide
Trifluoperazine
Trihexyphenidyl
Trimeprazine
Trimethadione
Trimipramine
Tripelennamine
Triprolidine
Troleandomycin
Trovafloxacin
Urokinase
Ursodiol
Vancomycin
Vasopressin
Venlafaxine
Verapamil
Vinblastine
Vincristine
Vitamin E
Warfarin
Zalcitabine
Zanamivir
Zidovudine
Zolmitriptan
Zolpidem
Zonisamide

Vaginal candidiasis
Ampicillin
Aztreonam
Cefamandole
Cefdinir
Cefixime
Cefpodoxime
Ceftazidime
Celecoxib
Chlorotrianisene
Delavirdine
Diethylstilbestrol
Dirithromycin
Enoxacin
Estrogens
Lamotrigine
Leflunomide
Lomefloxacin
Metronidazole
Norfloxacin
Paroxetine
Riluzole
Ropinirole
Sibutramine
Sparfloxacin
Tizanidine
Venlafaxine

Vaginitis
Acyclovir
Amitriptyline
Amoxapine
Amoxicillin
Azithromycin
Aztreonam
Bacampicillin
Carbenicillin
Cefaclor
Cefadroxil
Cefamandole
Cefazolin
Cefdinir
Cefepime
Cefixime
Cefmetazole
Cefonicid
Cefotaxime
Cefpodoxime
Cefprozil
Ceftazidime
Ceftibuten
Ceftizoxime
Ceftriaxone
Cefuroxime
Celecoxib
Cephalexin
Cephapirin
Cephradine
Cetirizine
Cevimeline
Chlorotrianisene
Cilostazol
Ciprofloxacin
Cisapride
Clomipramine
Cloxacillin
Dicloxacillin
Dirithromycin
Donepezil
Doxycycline
Enoxacin
Fenofibrate
Fluvoxamine
Fosfomycin
Gatifloxacin
Gold & gold compounds
Grepafloxacin
Imipramine
Lamotrigine
Leuprolide
Levofloxacin
Lincomycin
Lomefloxacin
Loratadine
Medroxyprogesterone
Methicillin
Mezlocillin
Mifepristone
Mirtazapine
Moxifloxacin
Nafarelin
Nafcillin
Nefazodone
Nisoldipine

Nortriptyline
Octreotide
Ofloxacin
Olanzapine
Orlistat
Oxacillin
Oxcarbazepine
Pantoprazole
Paroxetine
Pentostatin
Perindopril
Piperacillin
Quinupristin/dalfopristin
Raloxifene
Rivastigmine
Sertraline
Sparfloxacin
Tetracycline
Tiagabine
Ticarcillin
Tolcapone
Topiramate
Trovafloxacin
Venlafaxine
Zaleplon
Zileuton
Zolpidem

Vasculitis

Acebutolol
Acetaminophen
Acyclovir
Allopurinol
Amiloride
Aminosalicylate sodium
Amiodarone
Amitriptyline
Amlodipine
Amoxapine
Amoxicillin
Ampicillin
Anistreplase
Aspartame
Aspirin
Atenolol
Azathioprine
Bendroflumethiazide
Benzthiazide
Bromocriptine
Bumetanide
Busulfan
Butabarbital
Butalbital
Captopril
Carbamazepine
Carbenicillin
Cefdinir
Cerivastatin
Cevimeline
Chloramphenicol
Chlordiazepoxide
Chloroquine
Chlorothiazide
Chlorpromazine
Chlorpropamide
Cimetidine
Ciprofloxacin
Clarithromycin
Clindamycin
Clomipramine
Clorazepate
Clozapine
Co-trimoxazole
Cocaine
Colchicine
Corticosteroids
Cromolyn
Cyclophosphamide
Cyclosporine
Cyclothiazide
Cyproheptadine
Cytarabine
Dacarbazine
Delavirdine
Desipramine
Diazepam
Diclofenac
Dicloxacillin
Didanosine
Diflunisal
Digoxin
Diltiazem
Diphenhydramine
Disulfiram
Doxepin
Doxycycline
Enalapril
Ephedrine
Erythromycin
Estrogens
Ethacrynic acid
Etodolac
Famotidine
Fluoxetine
Flurbiprofen
Fluvastatin
Fosinopril
Furosemide
Gatifloxacin
Gemcitabine
Gemfibrozil
Gentamicin
Glucagon
Glyburide
Gold & gold compounds
Granulocyte colony-stimulating factor (GCSF)
Griseofulvin
Guanethidine
Heparin
Heroin
Hydralazine
Hydrochlorothiazide
Hydroflumethiazide
Hydroxychloroquine
Hydroxyurea
Ibuprofen
Imipenem/cilastatin
Imipramine
Indapamide
Indomethacin
Insulin
Interferons, alfa-2
Isoniazid
Isotretinoin
Itraconazole
Ketoconazole
Leflunomide
Levamisole
Lisinopril
Lithium
Lomefloxacin
Lovastatin
Maprotiline
Meclofenamate
Mefenamic acid
Mefloquine
Meloxicam
Melphalan
Meprobamate
Mercaptopurine
Mesalamine
Metformin
Methazolamide
Methicillin
Methimazole
Methotrexate
Methoxsalen
Methyldopa
Methylphenidate
Metolazone
Mezlocillin
Minocycline
Mitotane
Nabumetone
Nafcillin
Naproxen
Nicotine
Nifedipine
Nizatidine
Norfloxacin
Nortriptyline
Ofloxacin
Oxacillin
Oxaprozin
Oxytetracycline
Penicillamine
Penicillins
Pentamidine
Pentobarbital
Pergolide
Phenobarbital
Phenytoin
Phytonadione
Piperacillin
Piroxicam
Polythiazide
Potassium iodide
Pravastatin
Procainamide
Propylthiouracil
Protriptyline
Psoralens
Pyridoxine
Pyrimethamine
Quinapril
Quinethazone
Quinidine
Quinine
Ramipril
Ranitidine
Rifampin
Ritodrine
Simvastatin
Sotalol
Sparfloxacin
Spironolactone
Streptokinase
Streptomycin
Sulfamethoxazole
Sulfasalazine
Sulfisoxazole
Sulindac
Tamoxifen
Terbutaline
Tetracycline
Thalidomide
Thiamine
Ticarcillin
Ticlopidine
Tocainide
Torsemide
Trazodone
Triamterene
Trichlormethiazide
Trimethadione
Trioxsalen
Trovafloxacin
Vancomycin
Verapamil
Warfarin
Zidovudine

Vesicular eruption

Acyclovir
Amoxicillin
Amphotericin B
Carbenicillin
Colchicine
Denileukin
Dicumarol
Dicloxacillin
Enoxaparin
Letrozole
Penicillamine
Penicillins
Piperacillin
Piroxicam
Propylthiouracil
Pyridoxine
Warfarin

Xerosis

Acebutolol
Acitretin
Aldesleukin
Alprazolam
Amiloride
Amlodipine
Amoxapine
Amphotericin B
Apraclonidine
Atenolol
Atorvastatin
Atropine sulfate
Benztropine
Betaxolol

Bexarotene
Bicalutamide
Bisoprolol
Bleomycin
Buspirone
Busulfan
Capecitabine
Captopril
Carteolol
Celecoxib
Cerivastatin
Cetirizine
Cevimeline
Chlorpromazine
Chlortetracycline
Cidofovir
Cilostazol
Cimetidine
Citalopram
Clindamycin
Clofazimine
Clofibrate
Clomipramine
Delavirdine
Desipramine
Dexmedetomidine
Diazoxide
Dicyclomine
Disopyramide
Docetaxel
Doxazosin
Eflornithine
Estazolam
Estramustine
Famotidine
Fluorouracil
Fluoxetine
Fluphenazine
Flurbiprofen
Fluvastatin
Fluvoxamine
Foscarnet
Gemfibrozil
Glycopyrrolate
Gold & gold compounds
Grepafloxacin
Hydroxyurea
Imipramine
Indinavir
Interferons, alfa-2
Isotretinoin
Ketoconazole
Labetalol
Lamotrigine
Leflunomide
Leuprolide
Levamisole
Levothyroxine
Liothyronine
Lithium
Loratadine
Losartan
Mechlorethamine
Medroxyprogesterone
Mesalamine
Mesoridazine
Methantheline
Methoxsalen
Metolazone
Metoprolol
Mexiletine
Minoxidil
Mirtazapine
Modafinil
Moricizine
Moxifloxacin
Nabumetone
Nadolol
Naratriptan
Nefazodone
Niacin
Nisoldipine
Nizatidine
Nortriptyline
Olanzapine
Omeprazole
Orlistat
Oxybutynin
Pantoprazole
Paroxetine
Penicillamine
Pentamidine
Pentostatin
Pergolide
Perindopril
Perphenazine
Pindolol
Prochlorperazine
Procyclidine
Promazine
Propantheline
Propranolol
Protriptyline
Quetiapine
Rabeprazole
Ranitidine
Risperidone
Ritonavir
Rofecoxib
Saquinavir
Scopolamine
Sertraline
Sparfloxacin
Spironolactone
Sulfasalazine
Tacrine
Tamoxifen
Thalidomide
Thioridazine
Tiagabine
Timolol
Tizanidine
Tolterodine
Topiramate
Trifluoperazine
Trihexyphenidyl
Trioxsalen
Ursodiol
Venlafaxine
Vitamin A
Zalcitabine
Zaleplon
Zonisamide

Xerostomia

Acebutolol
Acetazolamide
Acitretin
Albendazole
Albuterol
Alprazolam
Alprostadil
Amantadine
Amiloride
Amitriptyline
Amlodipine
Amoxapine
Amoxicillin
Amphotericin B
Apraclonidine
Astemizole
Atropine sulfate
Azatadine
Azathioprine
Azelastine
Bacampicillin
Baclofen
Benactyzine
Bendroflumethiazide
Benztropine
Betaxolol
Bexarotene
Bicalutamide
Biperiden
Bisoprolol
Bromfenac
Bromocriptine
Brompheniramine
Buclizine
Bumetanide
Buspirone
Butorphanol
Cabergoline
Captopril
Carbamazepine
Carbenicillin
Carisoprodol
Carteolol
Carvedilol
Cefixime
Ceftibuten
Celecoxib
Cerivastatin
Cetirizine
Cevimeline
Chloramphenicol
Chlordiazepoxide
Chlormezanone
Chlorpheniramine
Chlorpromazine
Chlortetracycline
Cidofovir
Cimetidine
Ciprofloxacin
Cisapride
Citalopram
Clemastine
Clidinium
Clomipramine
Clonazepam
Clonidine
Clorazepate
Clozapine
Codeine
Cromolyn
Cyclobenzaprine
Cyproheptadine
Delavirdine
Desipramine
Dexchlorpheniramine
Dexfenfluramine
Dextroamphetamine
Diazepam
Diazoxide
Diclofenac
Dicloxacillin
Dicyclomine
Didanosine
Diethylpropion
Diflunisal
Dihydroergotamine
Dihydrotachysterol
Diltiazem
Dimenhydrinate
Diphenhydramine
Diphenoxylate
Dirithromycin
Disopyramide
Donepezil
Doxazosin
Doxepin
Dronabinol (THC)
Efavirenz
Enalapril
Enoxacin
Entacapone
Ephedrine
Epinephrine
Eprosartan
Ergocalciferol
Esmolol
Estazolam
Ethacrynic acid
Ethionamide
Etodolac
Famotidine
Felbamate
Felodipine
Fenfluramine
Fenoprofen
Fentanyl
Flavoxate
Flecainide
Fluconazole
Flucytosine
Flumazenil
Fluoxetine
Fluphenazine
Flurazepam
Flurbiprofen
Fluvoxamine
Foscarnet
Fosfomycin
Fosinopril
Fosphenytoin

Furosemide
Gabapentin
Ganciclovir
Glycopyrrolate
Grepafloxacin
Griseofulvin
Guanabenz
Guanadrel
Guanethidine
Guanfacine
Haloperidol
Hydrochlorothiazide
Hydrocodone
Hydromorphone
Hydroxyzine
Ibuprofen
Imipramine
Indapamide
Indinavir
Indomethacin
Interferons, alfa-2
Ipratropium
Isocarboxazid
Isoetharine
Isoniazid
Isoproterenol
Isosorbide dinitrate
Isotretinoin
Isradipine
Itraconazole
Ketoprofen
Ketorolac
Labetalol
Lamotrigine
Lansoprazole
Leflunomide
Levodopa
Levofloxacin
Lisinopril
Lithium
Lomefloxacin
Loratadine
Lorazepam
Losartan
Lovastatin
Loxapine
Maprotiline
Mazindol
Mebendazole
Meclizine
Meclofenamate
Mefenamic acid
Meloxicam
Meperidine
Meprobamate
Mesoridazine
Methadone
Methamphetamine
Methantheline
Methazolamide
Methicillin
Methyldopa
Methylphenidate
Metoclopramide
Metolazone
Metronidazole
Mexiletine
Mezlocillin
Mirtazapine
Modafinil
Moexipril
Molindone
Moricizine
Morphine
Moxifloxacin
Nabumetone
Nadolol
Nafcillin
Naproxen
Nefazodone
Niacin
Nicardipine
Nicotine
Nifedipine
Nisoldipine
Nitrofurantoin
Nitroglycerin
Nizatidine
Norfloxacin
Nortriptyline
Octreotide
Ofloxacin
Olanzapine
Omeprazole
Ondansetron
Orphenadrine
Oxacillin
Oxazepam
Oxcarbazepine
Oxybutynin
Oxycodone
Pantoprazole
Paroxetine
Penicillins
Pentamidine
Pentazocine
Pentoxifylline
Pergolide
Perindopril
Perphenazine
Phendimetrazine
Phenelzine
Phenindamine
Phenobarbital
Phenoxybenzamine
Phentermine
Pimozide
Pirbuterol
Piroxicam
Pramipexole
Prazepam
Prazosin
Procarbazine
Prochlorperazine
Procyclidine
Promazine
Promethazine
Propafenone
Propantheline
Propofol
Propoxyphene
Propranolol
Protriptyline
Pseudoephedrine
Pyrilamine
Pyrimethamine
Quazepam
Quetiapine
Quinapril
Quinethazone
Rabeprazole
Ramipril
Reserpine
Riluzole
Rimantadine
Risperidone
Ritonavir
Rivastigmine
Rizatriptan
Rofecoxib
Ropinirole
Saquinavir
Scopolamine
Selegiline
Sertraline
Sibutramine
Sildenafil
Sotalol
Sparfloxacin
Spironolactone
Sucralfate
Sulfasalazine
Sulindac
Sumatriptan
Tacrine
Tamoxifen
Telmisartan
Temazepam
Terazosin
Terbutaline
Terfenadine
Thalidomide
Thiabendazole
Thioguanine
Thioridazine
Thiothixene
Tiagabine
Ticarcillin
Tiopronin
Tizanidine
Tocainide
Tolcapone
Tolmetin
Tolterodine
Topiramate
Torsemide
Tramadol
Trandolapril
Tranylcypromine
Trazodone
Triamterene
Triazolam
Trichlormethiazide
Trifluoperazine
Trihexyphenidyl
Trimeprazine
Trimipramine
Tripelennamine
Triprolidine
Trovafloxacin
Venlafaxine
Verapamil
Vitamin A
Zalcitabine
Zaleplon
Zolmitriptan
Zolpidem
Zonisamide

DESCRIPTION OF THE 29 MOST COMMON REACTION PATTERNS

Acanthosis nigricans

Acanthosis nigricans (AN) is a process characterized by a soft, velvety, brown or grayish-black thickening of the skin that is symmetrically distributed over the axillae, neck, inguinal areas and other body folds.

While most cases of AN are seen in obese and prepubertal children, it can occur as a marker for various endocrinopathies as well as in female patients with elevated testosterone levels, irregular menses, and hirsutism.

It is frequently a concomitant of an underlying malignant condition, principally an adenocarcinoma of the intestinal tract.

Acneform lesions

Acneform eruptions are inflammatory follicular reactions that resemble acne vulgaris and that are manifested clinically as papules or pustules. They are monomorphic reactions, have a monomorphic appearance, and are found primarily on the upper parts of the body. Unlike acne vulgaris, there are rarely comedones present. Consider a drug-induced acneform eruption if:

- The onset is sudden
- There is a worsening of existing acne lesions
- The extent is considerable from the outset
- The appearance is monomorphic
- The localization is unusual for acne as, for example, when the distal extremities are involved
- The patient's age is unusual for regular acne
- There is an exposure to a potentially responsible drug.

The most common drugs responsible for acneform eruptions are: ACTH, androgenic hormones, anticonvulsants (hydantoin derivatives, phenobarbital, trimethadione), corticosteroids, danazol, disulfiram, halogens (bromides, chlorides, iodides), lithium, oral contraceptives, tuberculostatics (ethionamide, isoniazid, rifampin), vitamins B_2, B_6, and B_{12}.

Acute generalized exanthematous pustulosis

Arising on the face or intertriginous areas, acute generalized exanthematous pustulosis (AGEP) is characterized by a rapidly evolving, widespread, scarlatiniform eruption covered with hundreds of small superficial pustules.

Often accompanied by a high fever, AGEP is most frequently associated with penicillin and macrolide antibiotics, and usually occurs within 24 hours of the drug exposure.

Alopecia

Many drugs have been reported to occasion hair loss. Commonly appearing as a diffuse alopecia, it affects women more frequently than men and is limited in most instances to the scalp. Axillary and pubic hairs are rarely affected except with anticoagulants.

The hair loss from cytostatic agents, which is dose-dependent and begins about 2 weeks after the onset of therapy, is a result of the interruption of the anagen (growing) cycle of hair. With other drugs the hair loss does not begin until 2–5 months after the medication has been begun. With cholesterol-lowering drugs, diffuse alopecia is a result of interference with normal keratinization.

The scalp is normal and the drug-induced alopecia is almost always reversible within 1–3 months after the therapy has been discontinued. The regrown hair is frequently depigmented and occasionally more curly.

The most frequent offenders are cytostatic agents and anticoagulants, but hair loss can occur with a variety of common drugs, including hormones, anticonvulsants, amantadine, amiodarone, captopril, cholesterol-lowering drugs, cimetidine, colchicine, etretinate, isotretinoin, ketoconazole, heavy metals, lithium, penicillamine, valproic acid, and propranolol.

Angioedema

Angioedema is a term applied to a variant of urticaria in which the subcutaneous tissues, rather than the dermis, are mainly involved.

Also known as Quincke's edema, giant urticaria, and angioneurotic edema, this acute, evanescent, skin-colored, circumscribed edema usually affects the most distensible tissues: the lips, eyelids, earlobes, and genitalia. It can also affect the mucous membranes of the tongue, mouth, and larynx.

Symptoms of angioedema, frequently unilateral, asymmetrical and non-pruritic, last for an hour or two but can persist for 2–5 days.

The etiological factors associated with angioedema are as varied as that of urticaria (which see).

Aphthous stomatitis

Aphthous stomatitis – also known as canker sores – is a common disease of the oral mucous membranes.

Arising as tiny, discrete or grouped, papules or vesicles, these painful lesions develop into small (2–5 mm in diameter), round, shallow ulcerations having a grayish, yellow base surrounded by a thin red border.

Located predominantly over the labial and buccal mucosae, these aphthae heal without scarring in 10–14 days. Recurrences are common.

Black hairy tongue (lingua villosa nigra)

Black hairy tongue (BHT) represents a benign hyperplasia of the filiform papillae of the anterior two-thirds of the tongue.

These papillary elongations, usually associated with black, brown, or yellow pigmentation attributed to the overgrowth of pigment-producing bacteria, may be as long as 2 cm.

Occurring only in adults, BHT has been associated with the administration of oral antibiotics, poor dental hygiene, and excessive smoking.

Bullous eruptions

Bullous and vesicular drug eruptions are diseases in which blisters and vesicles occur as a complication of the administration of drugs. Blisters are a well-known manifestation of cutaneous reactions to drugs.

In many types of drug reactions, bullae and vesicles may be found in addition to other manifestations. Bullae are usually noted in erythema multiforme, Stevens–Johnson syndrome, toxic epidermal necrolysis, fixed eruptions when very intense, urticaria, vasculitis, porphyria cutanea tarda, and phototoxic reactions (from furosemide and nalidixic acid). Tense, thick-walled bullae can be seen in bromoderma and iododerma as well as in barbiturate overdosage.

Common drugs that cause bullous eruptions and bullous pemphigoid are: nadalol, penicillamine, piroxicam, psoralens, rifampin, clonidine, furosemide, diclofenac, mefenamic acid, bleomycin, and others.

Erythema multiforme and Stevens–Johnson syndrome

Erythema multiforme is a relatively common, acute, self-limited, inflammatory reaction pattern that is often associated with a preceding herpes simplex or mycoplasma infection. Other causes are associated with connective tissue disease, physical agents, X-ray therapy, pregnancy and internal malignancies, to mention a few. In 50% of the cases, no cause can be found. In a recent prospective study of erythema multiforme, only 10% were drug related.

The eruption rapidly occurs over a period of 12 to 24 hours. In about half the cases there are prodromal symptoms of an upper respiratory infection accompanied by fever, malaise, and varying degrees of muscular and joint pains.

Clinically, bluish-red, well-demarcated, macular, papular, or urticarial lesions, as well as the classical 'iris' or 'target lesions', sometimes with central vesicles, bullae, or purpura, are distributed preferentially over the distal extremities, especially over the dorsa of the hands and extensor aspects of the forearms. Lesions tend to spread peripherally and may involve the palms and trunk as well as the mucous membranes of the mouth and genitalia. Central healing and overlapping lesions often lead to arciform, annular and gyrate patterns. Lesions appear over the course of a week or 10 days and resolve over the next 2 weeks.

The Stevens–Johnson syndrome (erythema multiforme major), a severe and occasionally fatal variety of erythema multiforme, has an abrupt onset and is accompanied by any or all of the following: fever, myalgia, malaise, headache, arthralgia, ocular involvement, with occasional bullae and erosions covering less than 10% of the body surface. Painful stomatitis is an early and conspicuous symptom. Hemorrhagic bullae may appear over the lips, mouth and genital mucous membranes. Patients are often acutely ill with high fever. The course from eruption to the healing of the lesions may extend up to 6 weeks.

The following drugs have been most often associated with erythema multiforme and Stevens–Johnson syndrome: allopurinol, anticonvulsants (phenytoin), barbiturates, carbamazepine, estrogens/progestins, gold, NSAIDs, penicillamine, sulfonamides, tetracycline, and tolbutamide.

Erythema nodosum

Erythema nodosum is a cutaneous reaction pattern characterized by erythematous, tender or painful subcutaneous nodules commonly distributed over the anterior aspect of the lower legs, and occasionally elsewhere.

More common in young women, erythema nodosum is often associated with increased estrogen levels as occurs during pregnancy and with the ingestion of oral contraceptives. It is also an occasional manifestation of streptococcal infection, sarcoidosis, secondary syphilis, tuberculosis, certain deep fungal infections, Hodgkin's disease, leukemia, ulcerative colitis, and radiation therapy and is often preceded by fever, fatigue, arthralgia, vomiting, and diarrhea.

The incidence of erythema nodosum due to drugs is low and it is impossible to distinguish clinically between erythema nodosum due to drugs and that caused by other factors.

Some of the drugs that are known to occasion erythema nodosum are: antibiotics, estrogens, amiodarone, gold, NSAIDs, oral contraceptives, sulfonamides, and opiates.

Exanthems

Exanthems, commonly resembling viral rashes, represent the most common type of cutaneous drug eruption. Described as maculopapular or morbilliform eruptions, these flat, barely raised, erythematous patches, from one to several millimeters in diameter, are usually bilateral and symmetrical. They commonly begin on the head and neck or upper torso and progress downward to the limbs. They may present or develop into confluent areas and may be accompanied by pruritus and a mild fever.

The exanthems caused by drugs can be classified as either:

- Morbilliform eruptions: fingernail-sized erythematous patches
- Scarlatiniform eruptions: punctate, pinpoint, or pinhead-sized lesions in erythematous areas that have a tendency to coalesce. Circumoral pallor and the subsequent appearance of scaling may also be noted.

Maculopapular drug eruptions usually fade with desquamation and, occasionally, postinflammatory hyperpigmentation, in about 2 weeks. They invariably recur on rechallenge.

Exanthems often have a sudden onset during the first 2 weeks of administration, except for semisynthetic penicillins that frequently develop after the first 2 weeks following the initial dose.

The drugs most commonly associated with exanthems are: amoxicillin, ampicillin, bleomycin, captopril, carbamazepine, chlorpromazine, cotrimoxazole, gold, nalidixic acid, naproxen, phenytoin, penicillamine, and piroxicam.

Exfoliative dermatitis

Exfoliative dermatitis is a rare but serious reaction pattern that is characterized by erythema, pruritus and scaling over the entire body (erythroderma).

Drug-induced exfoliative dermatitis usually begins a few weeks or longer following the administration of a culpable drug. Beginning as erythematous, edematous patches, often on the face, it spreads to involve the entire integument. The skin becomes swollen and scarlet and may ooze a straw-colored fluid; this is followed in a few days by desquamation.

High fever, severe malaise and chills, along with enlargement of lymph nodes, often coexist with the cutaneous changes.

One of the most dangerous of all reaction patterns, exfoliative dermatitis can be accompanied by any or all of the following: hypothermia, fluid and electrolyte loss, cardiac failure, and gastrointestinal hemorrhage. Death may supervene if the drug is continued after the onset of the eruption. Secondary infection often complicates the course of the disease. Once the active dermatitis has receded, hyperpigmentation as well as loss of hair and nails may ensue. The following drugs, among others, can bring about exfoliative dermatitis: barbiturates, captopril, carbamazepine, cimetidine, furosemide, gold, isoniazid, lithium, nitrofurantoin, NSAIDs, penicillamine, phenytoin, pyrazolons, quinidine, streptomycin, sulfonamides, and thiazides.

Fixed eruptions

A fixed eruption is an unusual hypersensitivity reaction characterized by one or more well-demarcated erythematous plaques that recur at the same cutaneous (or mucosal) site or sites each time exposure to the offending agent occurs. The sizes of the lesions vary from a few millimeters to as much as 20 centimeters in diameter. Almost any drug that is ingested, injected, inhaled, or inserted into the body can trigger this skin reaction.

The eruption typically begins as a sharply marginated, solitary edematous papule or plaque – occasionally surmounted by a large bulla – which usually develops 30 minutes to 8 hours following the administration of a drug. If the offending agent is not promptly eliminated, the inflammation intensifies, producing a dusky red, violaceous or brown patch that may crust, desquamate, or blister within 7 to 10 days. The lesions are rarely pruritic. Favored sites are the hands, feet, face, and genitalia – especially the glans penis.

The reason for the specific localization of the skin lesions in a fixed drug eruption is unknown. The offending drug cannot be detected at the skin site. Certain drugs cause a fixed eruption at specific sites, for example, tetracycline and ampicillin often elicit a fixed eruption on the penis, whereas aspirin usually causes skin lesions on the face, limbs and trunk.

Common causes of fixed eruptions are: ampicillin, aspirin, barbiturates, dapsone, metronidazole, NSAIDs, oral contraceptives, phenolphthalein, phenytoin, quinine, sulfonamides, and tetracyclines.

Gingival hyperplasia

Gingival hyperplasia, a common, undesirable, non-allergic drug reaction begins as a diffuse swelling of the interdental papillae.

Particularly prevalent with phenytoin therapy, gingival hyperplasia begins about 3 months after the onset of therapy, and occurs in 30 to 70% of patients receiving it. The severity of the reaction is dose-dependent and children and young adults are more frequently affected. The most severe cases are noted in young women.

In many cases, gingival hyperplasia is accompanied by painful and bleeding gums. There is often superimposed secondary bacterial gingivitis. This can be so extensive that the teeth of the maxilla and mandible are completely overgrown.

While it is characteristically a side-effect of hydantoin derivatives, it may occur during the administration of phenobarbital, nifedipine, diltiazem and other medications.

Lichenoid (lichen planus-like) eruptions

Lichenoid eruptions are so called because of their resemblance to lichen planus, a papulosquamous disorder that characteristically presents as multiple, discrete, violaceous, flat-topped papules, often polygonal in shape and which are extremely pruritic.

Not infrequently, lichenoid lesions appear weeks or months following exposure to the responsible drug. As a rule, the symptoms begin to recede a few weeks following the discontinuation of the drug.

Common drug causes of lichenoid eruptions are: antimalarials, beta-blockers, chlorpropamide, furosemide, gold, methyldopa, phenothiazines, quinidine, thiazides, and tolazamide.

Lupus erythematosus

A reaction, clinically and pathologically resembling idiopathic systemic lupus erythematosus (SLE), has been reported in association with a large variety of drugs. There is some evidence that drug-induced SLE, invariably accompanied by a positive ANA reaction with 90% having antihistone antibodies, may have a genetically determined basis. These symptoms of SLE, a relatively benign form of lupus, recede within days or weeks following the discontinuation of the responsible drug. Skin lesions occur in about 20% of cases. Drugs cause fewer than 8% of all cases of systemic LE.

The following drugs have been commonly associated with inducing, aggravating or unmasking SLE: beta-blockers, carbamazepine, chlorpromazine, estrogens, griseofulvin, hydralazine, isoniazid (INH), lithium, methyldopa, minoxidil, oral contraceptives, penicillamine, phenytoin (diphenylhydantoin), procainamide, propylthiouracil, quinidine, and testosterone.

Onycholysis

Onycholysis, the painless separation of the nail plate from the nail bed, is one of the most common nail disorders.

The unattached portion, which is white and opaque, usually begins at the free margin and proceeds proximally, causing part or most of the nail plate to become separated. The attached, healthy portion of the nail, by contrast, is pink and translucent.

Pemphigus vulgaris

Pemphigus vulgaris (PV) is a rare, serious, acute or chronic, blistering disease involving the skin and mucous membranes.

Characterized by thin-walled, easily-ruptured, flaccid bullae that are seen to arise on normal or erythematous skin and over mucous membranes, the lesions of PV appear initially in the mouth (in about 60% of the cases) and then spread, after weeks or months, to involve the axillae and groin, the scalp, face and neck. The lesions may become generalized.

Because of their fragile roofs, the bullae rupture leaving painful erosions and crusts may develop principally over the scalp.

Photosensitivity

A photosensitive reaction is a chemically induced change in the skin that makes an individual unusually sensitive to electromagnetic radiation (light). On absorbing light of a specific wavelength, an oral, injected or topical drug may be chemically altered to produce a reaction ranging from macules and papules, vesicles and bullae, edema, urticaria, or an acute eczematous reaction.

Any eruption that is prominent on the face, the dorsa of the hands, the 'V' of the neck, and the presternal area should suggest an adverse reaction to light. The distribution is the key to the diagnosis.

Initially the eruption, which consists of erythema, edema, blisters, weeping and desquamation, involves the forehead, rims of the ears, the nose, the malar eminences and cheeks, the sides and back of the neck, the extensor surfaces of the forearms and the dorsa of the hands. These reactions commonly spare the shaded areas: those under the chin, under the nose, behind the ears and inside the fold of the upper eyelids. There is usually a sharp cut-off at the site of jewelry and at clothing margins. All light-exposed areas need not be affected equally.

There are two main types of photosensitive reactions: the phototoxic and the photoallergic reaction.

Phototoxic reactions, the most common type of drug-induced photosensitivity, resemble an exaggerated sunburn and occur within 5 to 20 hours after the skin has been exposed to a photosensitizing substance and light of the proper wavelength and intensity. It is not a form of allergy – prior sensitization is not required – and, theoretically, could occur in anyone given enough drug and light. Phototoxic reactions are dose-dependent both for drug and sunlight. Patients with phototoxicity reactions are commonly sensitive to ultraviolet A (UVA radiation), the so-called 'tanning rays' at 320–400 nm. Phototoxic reactions may cause onycholysis, as the nail bed is particularly susceptible because of its lack of melanin protection.

Patients with a true photoallergy (the interaction of drug, light and the immune system), a less common form of drug-induced photosensitivity, are often sensitive to UVB radiation, the so-called 'burning rays' at 290–320 nm. Photoallergic reactions, unlike phototoxic responses, represent an immunologic change and require a latent period of from 24 to 48 hours during which sensitization occurs. They are not dose-related.

If the photosensitizer acts internally, it is a photodrug reaction; if it acts externally, it is photocontact dermatitis.

Drugs that are likely to cause phototoxic reactions are: amiodarone, nalidixic acid, various NSAIDs, phenothiazines (especially chlorpromazine), and tetracyclines (particularly demeclocycline).

Photoallergic reactions may occur as a result of exposure to systemically-administered drugs such as griseofulvin, NSAIDs, phenothiazines, quinidine, sulfonamides, sulfonylureas, and thiazide diuretics as well as to external agents such as para-aminobenzoic acid (found in sunscreens), bithionol (used in soaps and cosmetics), paraphenylenediamine, and others.

Pigmentation

Drug-induced pigmentation on the skin, hair, nails, and mucous membranes is a result of either melanin synthesis, increased lipofuscin synthesis, or post-inflammatory pigmentation.

Color changes, which can be localized or widespread, can also be a result of a deposition of bile pigments (jaundice), exogenous metal compounds, and direct deposition of elements such as carotene or quinacrine.

Post-inflammatory pigmentation can follow a variety of drug-induced inflammatory cutaneous reactions; fixed eruptions are known to leave a residual pigmentation that can persist for months.

The following is a partial list of those drugs that can cause various pigmentary changes: anticonvulsants, antimalarials, cytostatics, hormones, metals, tetracyclines, phenothiazine tranquilizers, psoralens, amiodarone, etc.

Pityriasis rosea-like eruptions

Pityriasis rosea, commonly mistaken for ringworm, is a unique disorder that usually begins as a single, large, round or oval pinkish patch known as the 'mother' or 'herald' patch. The most common sites for this solitary lesion are the chest, the back, or the abdomen. This is followed in about 2 weeks by a blossoming of small, flat, round or oval, scaly patches of similar color, each with a central collarette scale, usually distributed in a Christmas tree pattern over the trunk and, to a lesser degree, the extremities. This eruption seldom itches and usually limits itself to areas from the neck to the knees.

While the etiology of idiopathic pityriasis rosea is unknown, we do know that various medications have been reported to give rise to this friendly disorder. These are: barbiturates, beta-blockers, bismuth, captopril, clonidine, gold, griseofulvin, isotretinoin, labetalol, meprobamate, metronidazole, penicillin, and tripelennamine.

In drug-induced pityriasis rosea, the 'herald patch' is usually absent, and the eruption will often not follow the classic pattern.

Pruritus

Generalized itching, without any visible signs, is one of the least common adverse reactions to drugs. More frequently than not, drug-induced itching – moderate or severe – is fairly generalized.

For most drugs it is not known in what way they elicit pruritus; some drugs can cause itching directly or indirectly through cholestasis. Pruritus may develop by different pathogenetic mechanisms: allergic, pseudoallergic (histamine release), neurogenic, by vasodilatation, cholestatic effect, and others.

A partial list of those drugs that can cause pruritus are as follows: aspirin, NSAIDs, penicillins, sulfonamides, chloroquine, ACE-inhibitors, amiodarone, nicotinic acid derivatives, lithium, bleomycin, tamoxifen, interferons, gold, penicillamine, methoxsalen, isotretinoin, etc.

Psoriasis

Many drugs, as a result of their pharmacological action, have been implicated in the precipitation or exacerbation of psoriasis or psoriasiform eruptions.

Psoriasis is a common, chronic, papulosquamous disorder of unknown etiology with characteristic histopathological features and many biochemical, physiological, and immunological abnormalities.

Drugs that can precipitate psoriasis are, among others, beta-blockers and lithium. Drugs that are reported to aggravate psoriasis are antimalarials, beta-blockers, lithium, NSAIDs, quinidine, and photosensitizing drugs. The effect and extent of these drug-induced psoriatic eruptions are dose dependent.

Purpura

Purpura, a result of hemorrhage into the skin, can be divided into thrombocytopenic purpura and non-thrombocytopenic purpura (vascular purpura). Both thrombocytopenic and vascular purpura may be due to drugs, and most of the drugs producing purpura may do so by giving rise to vascular damage and thrombocytopenia. In both types of purpura, allergic or toxic (nonallergic) mechanisms may be involved.

Some drugs combine with platelets to form an antigen, stimulating formation of antibody to the platelet–drug combination. Thus, the drug appears to act as a hapten; subsequent antigen–antibody reaction causes platelet destruction leading to thrombocytopenia.

The purpuric lesions are usually more marked over the lower portions of the body, notably the legs and dorsal aspects of the feet in ambulatory patients.

Other drug-induced cutaneous reactions – erythema multiforme, erythema nodosum, fixed eruption, necrotizing vasculitis, and others – can have a prominent purpuric component.

A whole host of drugs can give rise to purpura, the most common being: NSAIDs, thiazide diuretics, phenothiazines, cytostatics, gold, penicillamine, hydantoins, thiouracils, and sulfonamides.

Raynaud's phenomenon

Raynaud's phenomenon is the paroxysmal, cold-induced constriction of small arteries and arterioles of the fingers and, less often, the toes.

Occurring more frequently in women, Raynaud's phenomenon is characterized by blanching, pallor, and cyanosis. In severe cases, secondary changes may occur: thinning and ridging of the nails, telangiectases of the nail folds, and, in the later stages, sclerosis and atrophy of the digits.

Toxic epidermal necrolysis (TEN)

Also known as Lyell's syndrome, toxic epidermal necrolysis is a rare, serious, acute exfoliative, bullous eruption of the skin and mucous membranes that usually develops as a reaction to diverse drugs. TEN can also be a result of a bacterial or viral infection and can develop after radiation therapy or vaccinations.

In the drug-induced form of TEN, a morbilliform eruption accompanied by large red, tender areas of the skin will develop shortly after the drug has been administered. This progresses rapidly to blistering, and a widespread exfoliation of the epidermis develops dramatically over a very short period accompanied by high fever. The hairy parts of the body are usually spared. The mucous membranes and eyes are often involved.

The clinical picture resembles an extensive second-degree burn; the patient is acutely ill. Fatigue, vomiting, diarrhea and angina are prodromal symptoms. In a few hours the condition becomes grave.

TEN is a medical emergency and unless the offending agent is discontinued immediately, the outcome may be fatal in the course of a few days.

Drugs that are the most common cause of TEN are: allopurinol, ampicillin, amoxicillin, carbamazepine, NSAIDs, phenobarbital, pentamidine, phenytoin (diphenylhydantoin), pyrazolons, and sulfonamides.

Urticaria

Urticaria induced by drugs is, after exanthems, the second most common type of drug reaction. Urticaria, or hives, is a vascular reaction of the skin characterized by pruritic, erythematous wheals. These welts – or wheals – caused by localized edema, can vary in size from one millimeter in diameter to large palm-sized swellings, favor the covered areas (trunk, buttocks, chest), and are, more often than not, generalized. Urticaria usually develops within 36 hours following the administration of the responsible drug. Individual lesions rarely persist for more than 24 hours.

Urticaria may be the only symptom of drug sensitivity, or it may be a concomitant or followed by the manifestations of serum sickness. Urticaria may be accompanied by angioedema of the lips or eyelids. It may, on rare occasions, progress to anaphylactoid reactions or to anaphylaxis.

The following are the most common causes of drug-induced urticaria: antibiotics, notably penicillin (more commonly following parenteral administration than by ingestion), barbiturates, captopril, levamisole, NSAIDs, quinine, rifampin, sulfonamides, thiopental, and vancomycin.

Vasculitis

Drug-induced cutaneous necrotizing vasculitis, a clinicopathologic process characterized by inflammation and necrosis of blood vessels, often presents with a variety of small, palpable purpuric lesions most frequently distributed over the lower extremities: urticaria-like lesions, small ulcerations, and occasional hemorrhagic vesicles and pustules. The basic process involves an immunologically mediated response to antigens that result in vessel-wall damage.

Beginning as small macules and papules, they ultimately eventuate into purpuric lesions and, in the more severe cases, into hemorrhagic blisters and frank ulcerations. A polymorphonuclear infiltrate and fibrinoid changes in the small dermal vessels characterize the vasculitic reaction.

Drugs that are commonly associated with vasculitis are: ACE-inhibitors, amiodarone, ampicillin, cimetidine, coumadin, furosemide, hydantoins, hydralazine, NSAIDs, pyrazolons, quinidine, sulfonamides, thiazides, and thiouracils.

Xerostomia

Xerostomia is a dryness of the oral cavity that makes speaking, chewing and swallowing difficult.

Resulting from a partial or complete absence of saliva production, xerostomia can be caused by a variety of medications.

Index of Generic and Trade Names

Generic drug names are in **bold**

Hylorel **guanadrel**
Hylutin **progestins**
Hyperstat **diazoxide**
Hytakerol **dihydrotachysterol**
Hytrin **terazosin**
Hyzaar **losartan**

I-Pilopine **pilocarpine**
ibuprofen Advil, Genpril, Haltran, Medipren, Midol 220, Motrin, Nuprin, Pamprin, Profen, Rufen, Trendar, Uni-Proc
ibutilide Corvert
Idamycin **idarubicin**
idarubicin Idamycin
Ifex **ifosfamide**
ifosfamide Ifex
Iletin Lente **insulin**
Ilosone **erythromycin**
Ilotycin **erythromycin**
Imdur **isosorbide mononitrate**
imipenem/cilastatin Primaxin
imipramine Tofranil
Imitrex **sumatriptan**
Imodium **loperamide**
Imuran **azathioprine**
inamrinone Inocor
indapamide Lozol
Inderal **propranolol**
Inderide **propranolol**
indinavir Crixivan
Indocin **indomethacin**
indomethacin Indocin
Infasurf **calfactant**
Infergen **interferons, alfa-2**
infliximab Remicade
Infumorph **morphine**
Inocor **inamrinone**
insulin Humulin, Iletin Lente, Novolin R, NPH, Protamine, Velosulin
Intal **cromolyn**
Integrilin **eptifibatide**
interferons, alfa-2 Alferon N, Infergen, Intron A, Rebetron, Roferon-A
Intron A **interferons, alfa-2**
Intropin **dopamine**
Invirase **saquinavir**
Ionamin **phentermine**
Iopidine **apraclonidine**
ipodate Bilivist, Oragrafin
ipratropium Atrovent, Combivent
irbesartan Avalide, Avapro
irinotecan Camptosar
Ismelin **guanethidine**
Ismo **isosorbide mononitrate**
Ismotic **isosorbide**
isocarboxazid Marplan
isoetharine Arm-a-Med, Beta-2, Bronkomed, Bronkometer, Bronkosol, Dey-Lute
isoniazid Rifamate, Rifater
isoproterenol Aerolone, Arm-a-Med, Isuprel, Medihaler-ISO, Norisodrine
Isoptin **verapamil**
Isopto Carpine **pilocarpine**
Isopto Frin **phenylephrine**
Isopto Hyoscine Ophthalmic **scopolamine**
Isordil **isosorbide dinitrate**
isosorbide Ismotic
isosorbide dinitrate Dilatrate-SR, Isordil, Sorbitrate
isosorbide mononitrate Imdur, Ismo, Monoket
isotretinoin Accutane
isoxsuprine Vasodilan, Voxsuprine
isradipine DynaCirc
Isuprel **isoproterenol**
itraconazole Sporanox
ivermectin Stromectol

Jenamicin **gentamicin**
Jenest **oral contraceptives**

Kabikinase **streptokinase**
Kadian **morphine**
Kaletra **lopinavir**
kanamycin Kantrex
Kantrex **kanamycin**
Keflex **cephalexin**
Keflin **cephalothin**
Keftab **cephalexin**
Kefurox **cefuroxime**
Kefzol **cefazolin, cephalothin**
Kemadrin **procyclidine**
Kenalog **corticosteroids**
Keppra **levetiracetam**
Kerlone **betaxolol**
Ketalar **ketamine**
ketamine Ketalar
ketoconazole Nizoral
ketoprofen Orudis, Oruvail
ketorolac Acular, Toradol
ketotifen Zaditor
Kevadon **thalidomide**
Kie **potassium iodide**
Klavikordal **nitroglycerin**
Klonopin **clonazepam**
Konakion **phytonadione**
Kytril **granisetron**

L-Phrine **phenylephrine**
labetalol Normodyne, Normozide, Trandate
Lamictal **lamotrigine**
Lamisil **terbinafine**
lamivudine Combivir, Epivir
lamotrigine Lamictal
Lamprene **clofazimine**
Lanoxicaps **digoxin**
Lanoxin **digoxin**
lansoprazole Prevacid
Lariam **mefloquine**
Larotid **penicillins**
Lasix **furosemide**
latanoprost Xalatan
Ledercillin **penicillins**
leflunomide Arava
Legatrin **quinine**
Lescol **fluvastatin**
letrozole Femara
Leucovorin **leucovorin**
leucovorin Leucovorin
Leukeran **chlorambucil**
leuprolide Lupron
Leustatin **cladribine**
levamisole Ergamisol
levaquin **levofloxacin**
Levatol **penbutolol**
levetiracetam Keppra
Levlen **oral contraceptives**
Levo-T **levothyroxine**
levobunolol AKBeta, Betagan
levodopa Atamet, Sinemet
levofloxacin **levaquin**
Levothyroid **levothyroxine**
levothyroxine Eltroxin, Levo-T, Levothyroid, Levoxyl, Synthroid
Levoxyl **levothyroxine**

trimethobenzamide Arrestin, Benzacot, Bio-Gan, Navogan, Stemetic, T-Gene, Tebamide, Tegamide, Ticon, Tigan, Triban, Tribenzagen, Trimazide
trimethoprim Bactrim
trimetrexate Neutrexin
trimipramine Surmontil
Trimox **penicillins**
Trinalin **azatadine, pseudoephedrine**
Triofed **triprolidine**
Triostat **liothyronine**
trioxsalen Trisoralen
tripelennamine PBZ
Triphasil **oral contraceptives**
Triposed **triprolidine**
triprolidine Actagen, Actidil, Actifed, Allerphed, Cenafed, Genac, Myidil, Trifed, Triofed, Triposed
Triptone **dimenhydrinate**
Trisonex **arsenic**
Trisoralen **psoralens, trioxsalen**
Trobicin **spectinomycin**
Trocal **dextromethorphan**
troglitazone Rezulin
troleandomycin TAO
trovafloxacin Trovan
Trovan **trovafloxacin**
Truphylline **aminophylline**
Trusopt **dorzolamide**
Tubasal **aminosalicylate sodium**
Tussar-2 **codeine**
Tussgen **hydrocodone**
Tussi-Organidin **codeine**
Tussionex **hydrocodone**
Tussogest **hydrocodone**
Tylenol **acetaminophen**
Tylox **oxycodone**

Ultram **tramadol**
Unasyn **penicillins**
Uni-Proc **ibuprofen**
Unipen **penicillins**
Uniretic **moexipril**
Univasc **moexipril**
Urecholine **bethanechol**
Urex **methenamine**
Urised **methenamine**
Urispas **flavoxate**
urokinase Abbokinase
Uroqid **methenamine**
Urso **ursodiol**
ursodiol Actigall, Urso

V-Cillin **penicillins**
Valadol **acetaminophen**
Valdrene **diphenhydramine**
Valium **diazepam**
Vancocin **vancomycin**
vancomycin Vancocin
Vaniqua **eflornithine**
Vanquish **aspirin**
Vantin **cefpodoxime**
Vascor **bepridil**
Vasodilan **isoxsuprine**
vasopressin Pitressin
Vasotec **enalapril**
Velban **vinblastine**
Velosef **cephradine**
Velosulin **insulin**
venlafaxine Effexor
Ventolin **albuterol**
VePesid **etoposide**
verapamil Calan, Covera-HS, Isoptin, Tarka, Verelan
Verelan **verapamil**
Vermox **mebendazole**
Versed **midazolam**
Vertab **dimenhydrinate**
Viagra **sildenafil**
Vibazine **buclizine**
Vibra-Tabs **doxycycline**
Vibramycin **doxycycline**
Vicks Formula 44 **dextromethorphan**
Vicks Sinest, etc. **phenylephrine**
Vicks Vatronol **ephedrine**
Vicodin **acetaminophen, hydrocodone**
Vicoprofen **hydrocodone**
vidarabine Vira-A Ophthalmic
Videx **didanosine**
vinblastine Velban
Vincasar **vincristine**
vincristine Oncovin, Vincasar
vinorelbine Navelbine
Vioxx **rofecoxib**
Vira-A Ophthalmic **vidarabine**
Viracept **nelfinavir**
Viramune **nevirapine**
Virazole **ribavirin**
Virilon **methyltestosterone**
Visken **pindolol**
Vistaril **hydroxyzine**
Vistide **cidofovir**
Vita Plus E **vitamin E**
Vita-C **ascorbic acid**
vitamin A Aquasol A, Del-Vi-A, Palmitate A
Vitamin B_{12} **cyanocobalamin**
Vitamin D **ergocalciferol**
vitamin E Aquasol E, E-Vitamin Succinate, Eprolin, Pheryl-E, Vita Plus E, Vitec
Vitamin K_1 **phytonadione**
Vitec **vitamin E**
Vivactil **protriptyline**
Volmax **albuterol**
Voltaren **diclofenac**
Voxsuprine **isoxsuprine**

warfarin Coumadin
Wehamine **dimenhydrinate**
Welchol **colesevelam**
Wellbutrin **bupropion**
Winstrol **stanozolol**
Wintrocin **erythromycin**
Wyamicin S **erythromycin**
Wycillin **penicillins**
Wymox **penicillins**
Wytensin **guanabenz**

Xalatan **latanoprost**
Xanax **alprazolam**
Xeloda **capecitabine**
Xenical **orlistat**
Xylocaine **lidocaine**

Yocon **yohimbine**
yohimbine Actibine, Aphrodyne, Yocon, Yohimex, Yomax
Yohimex **yohimbine**
Yomax **yohimbine**
Yutopar **ritodrine**

Zaditor **ketotifen**
zafirlukast Accolate
Zagam **sparfloxacin**
zalcitabine Hivid

Drug Eruptions Illustrated

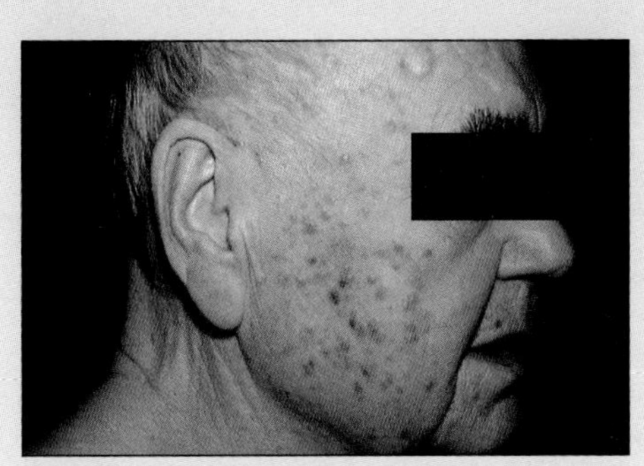

Acne (ciprofloxacin)

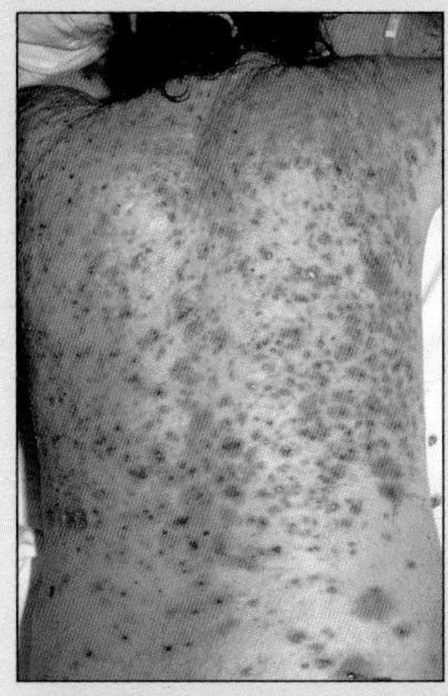

Acne fulminans

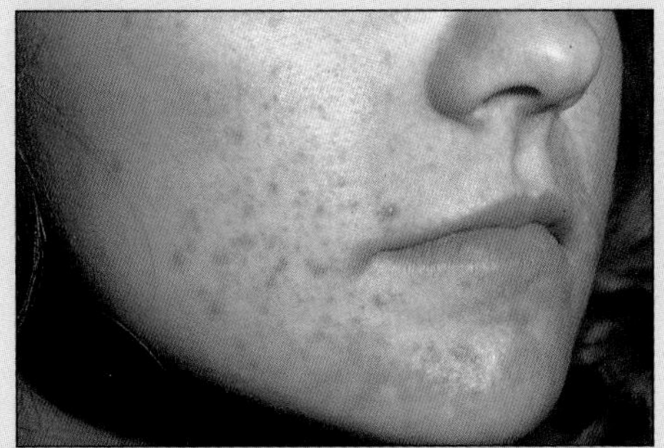

Acne (systemic corticosteroids)

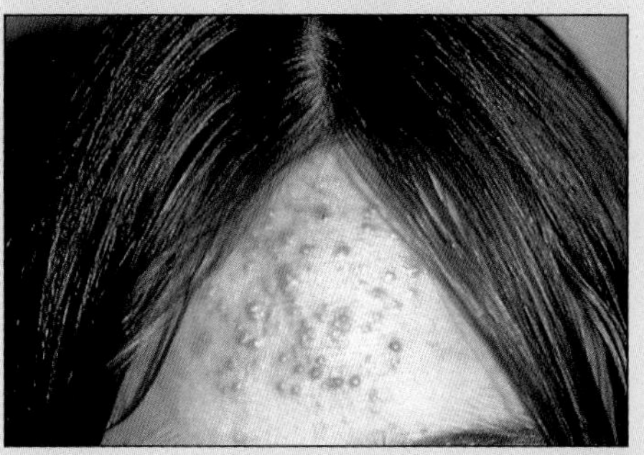

Acne (iodine)

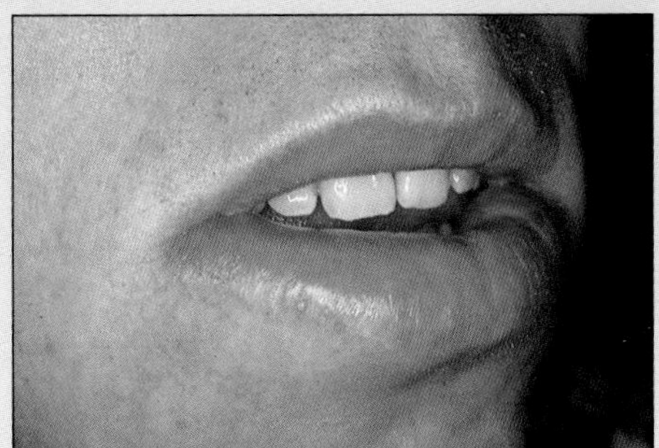

Angioedema

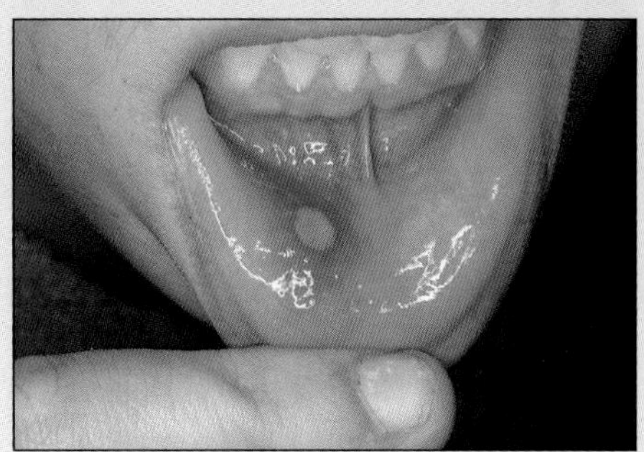

Aphthous stomatitis

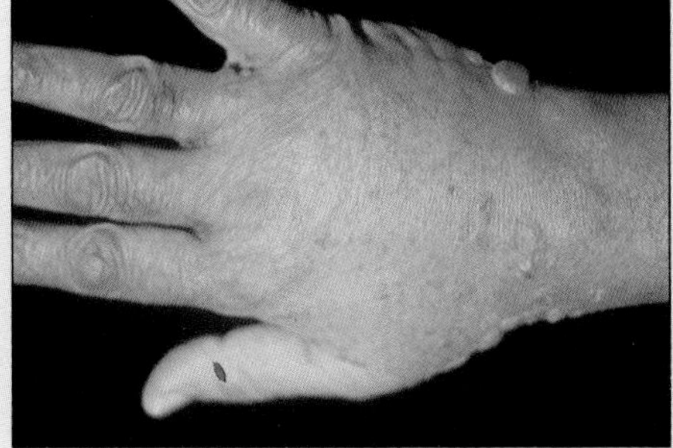

Bullous pemphigoid

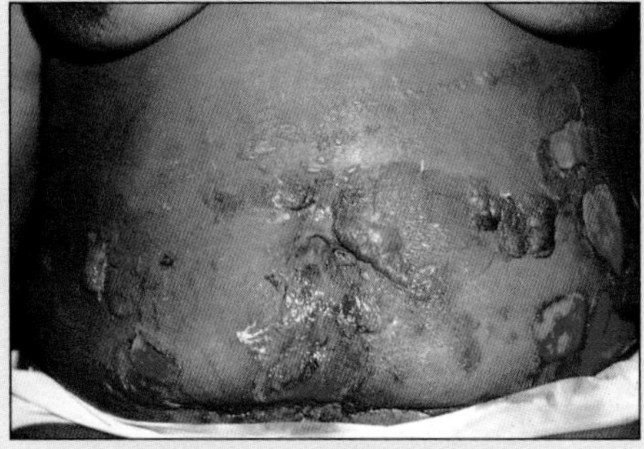

Bullous pemphigoid

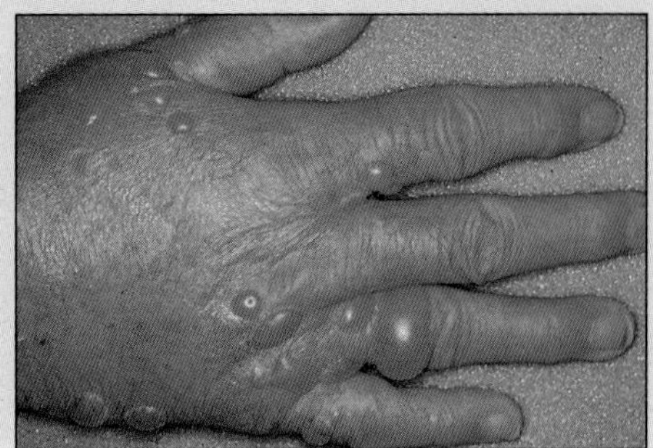

Bullous pemphigoid

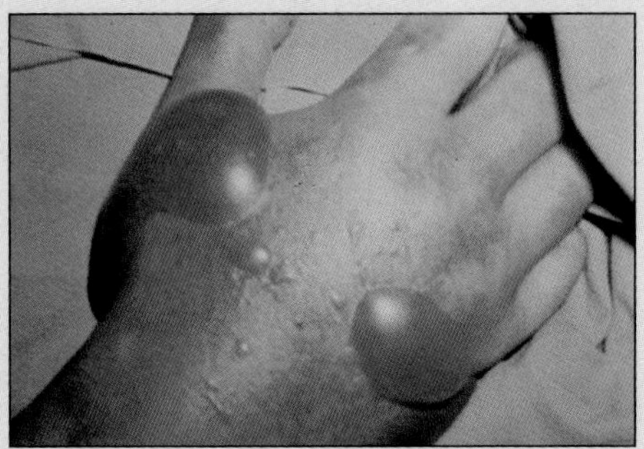

Bullous drug eruption

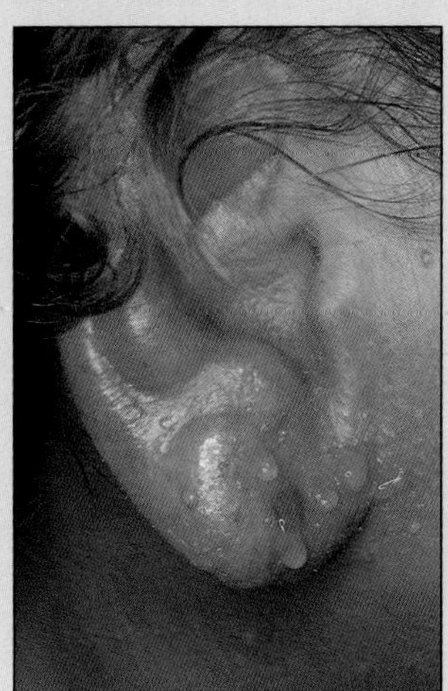

Contact (neomycin)

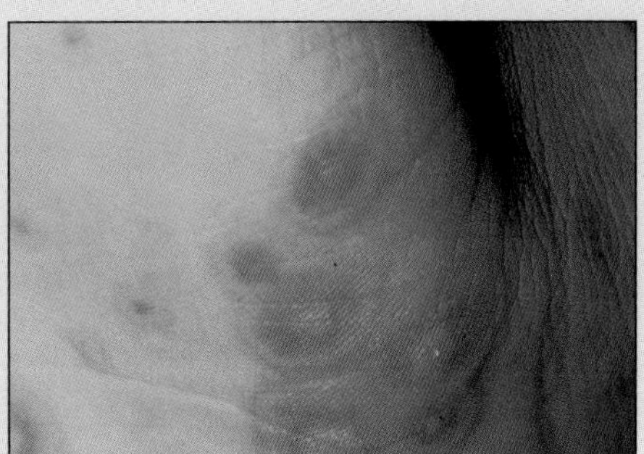

Erythema multiforme

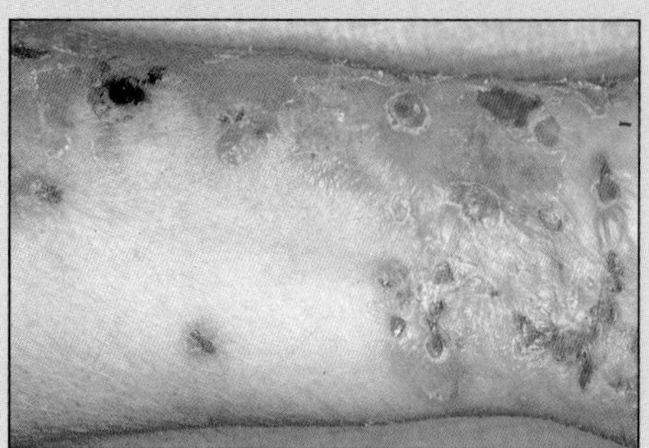

Bullous pemphigoid

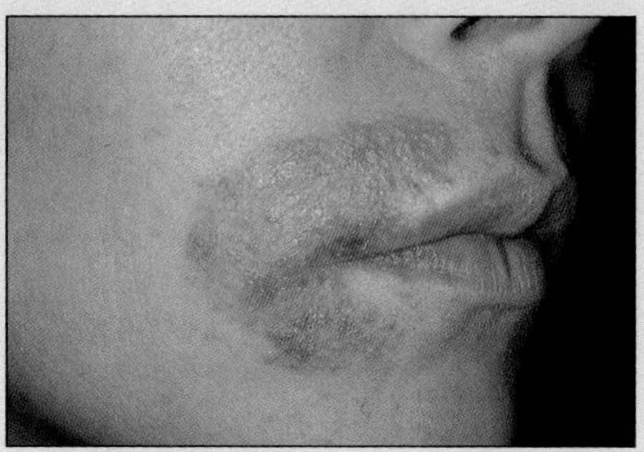

Contact (mycolog cream)

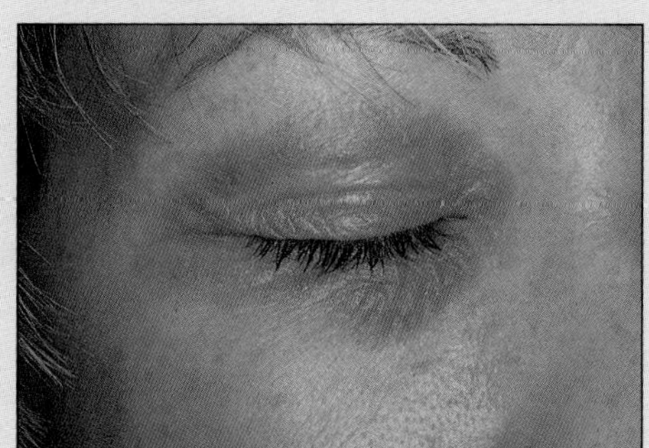

Contact (vitamin E cream)

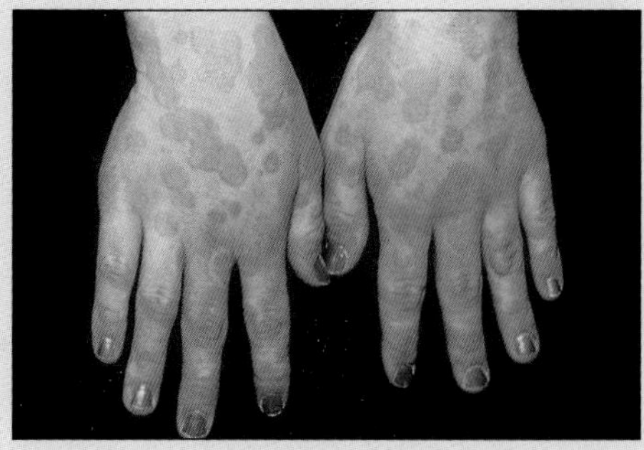

Erythema multiforme

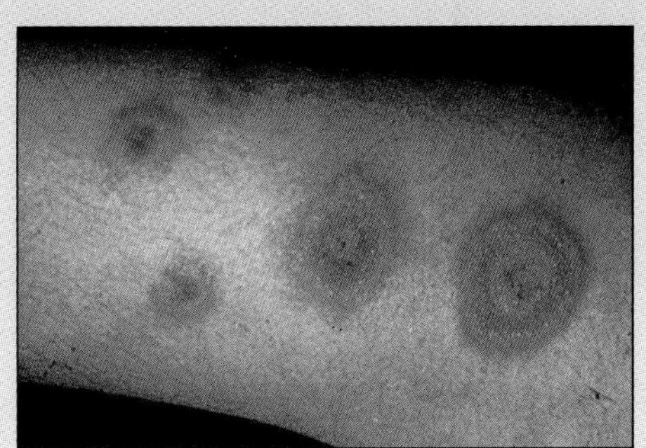

Erythema multiforme

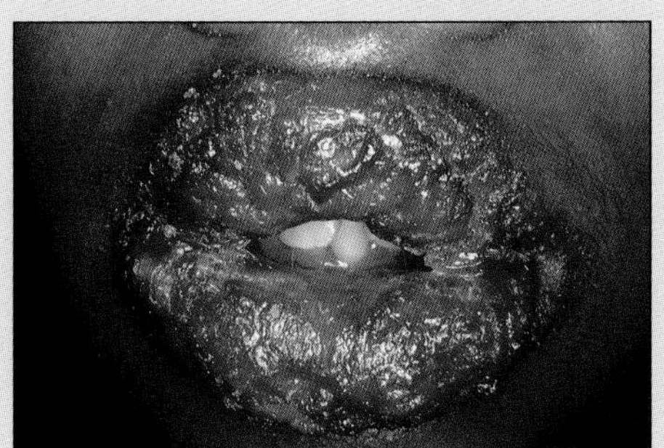

Erythema multiforme

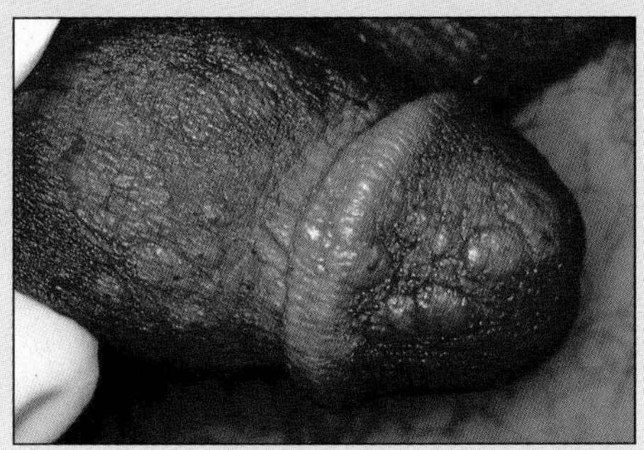

Erythema multiforme

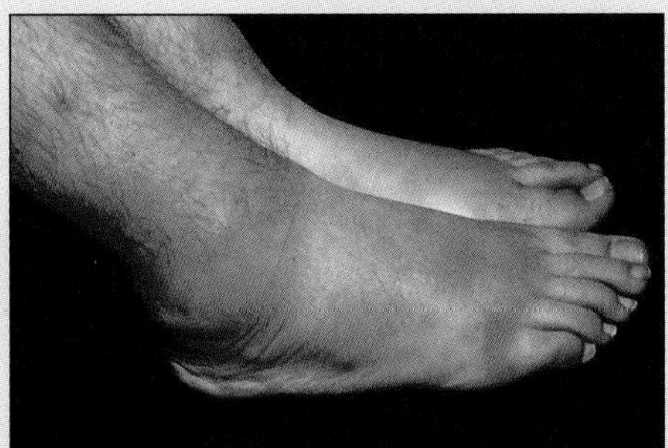

Erythema nodosum

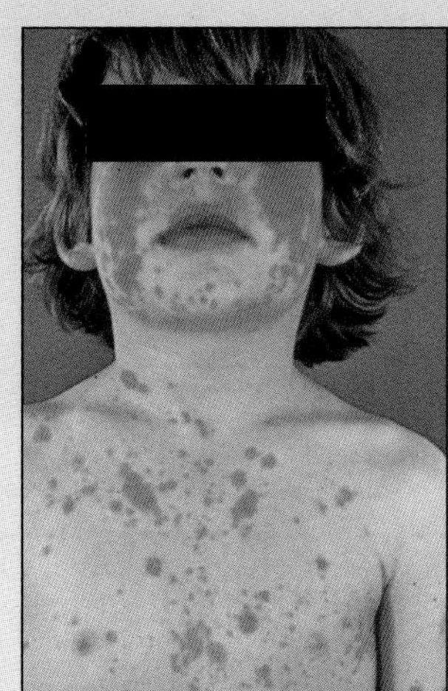

Erythema multiforme

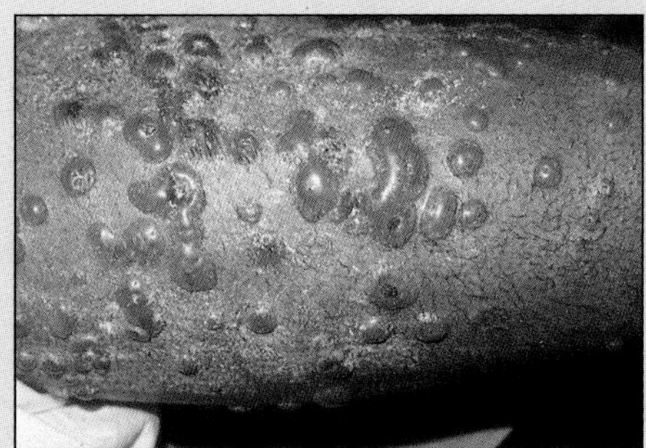

Erythema multiforme

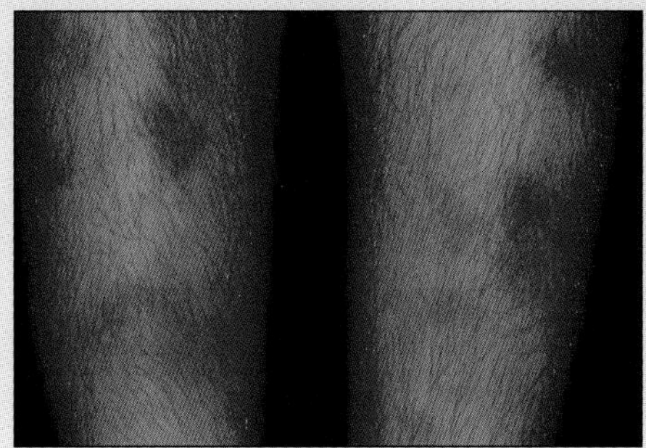

Erythema nodosum

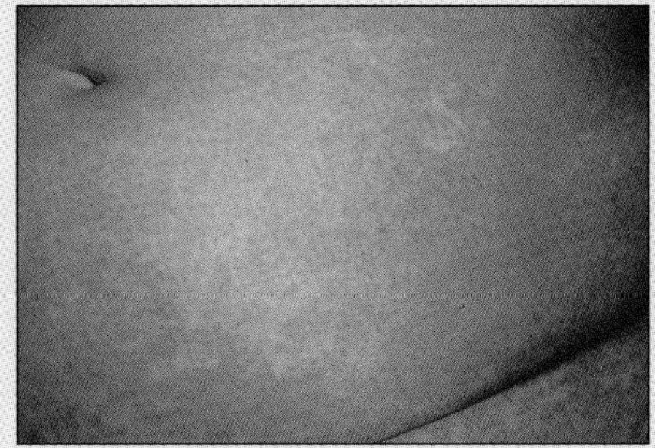

Erythroderma

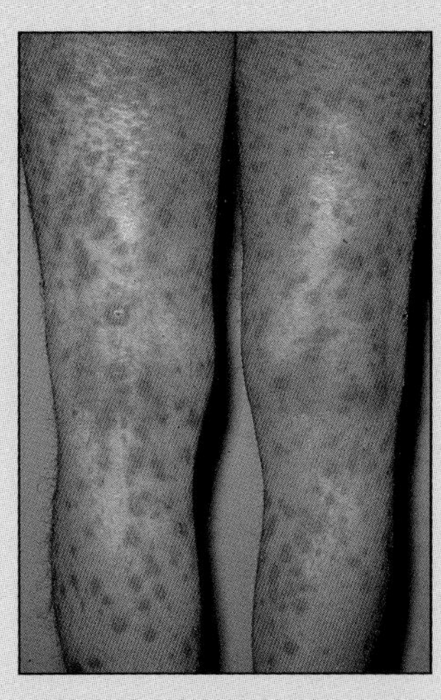
Exanthem (phenobarbital)

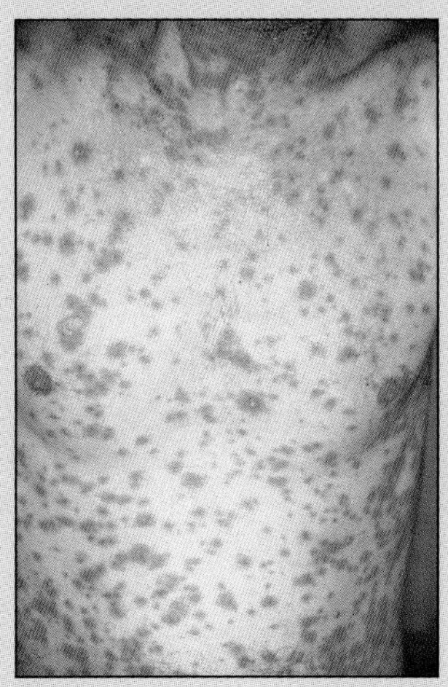
Exanthem (griseofulvin)

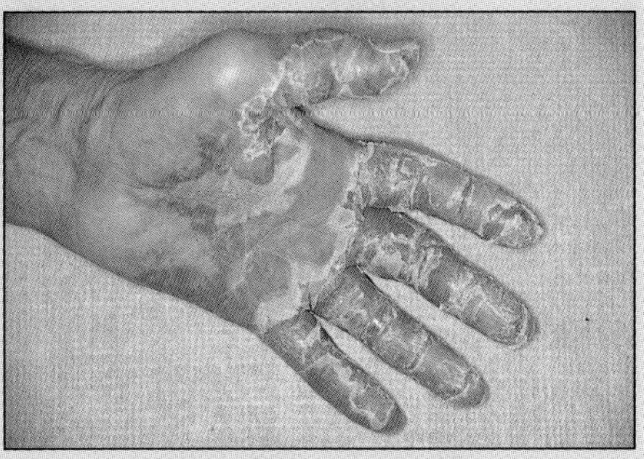
Exfoliative dermatitis

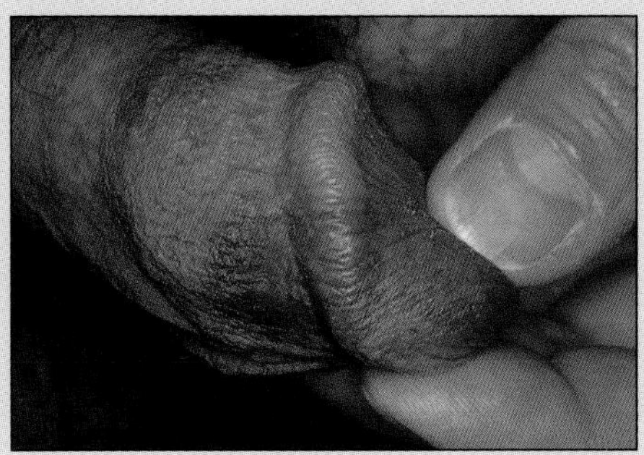
Fixed eruption

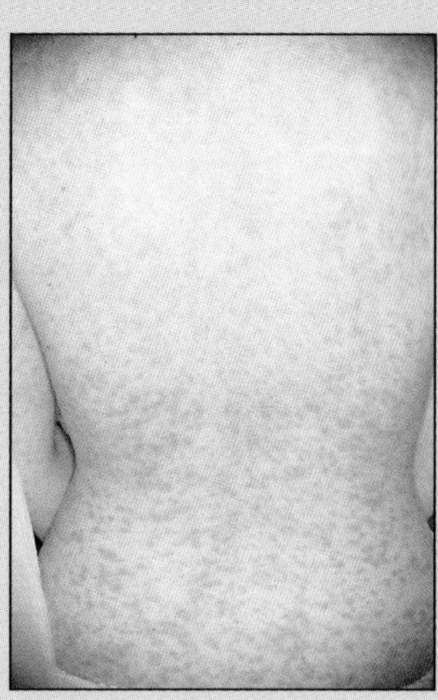
Exanthem (ampicillin)

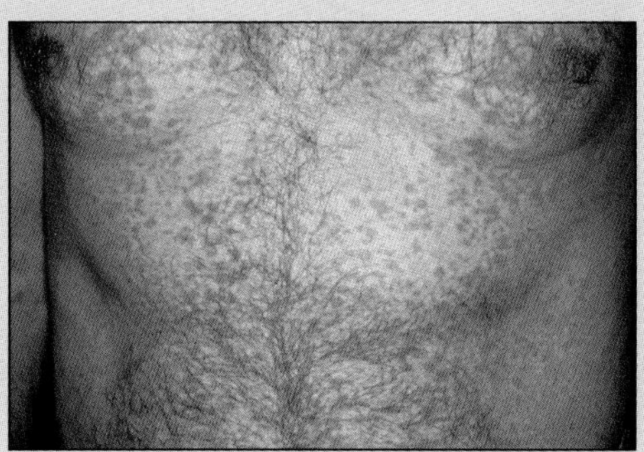
Exanthem (cotrimoxazole)

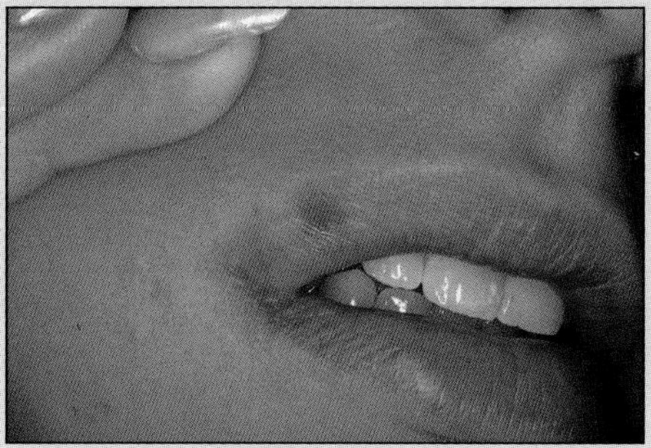
Fixed eruption

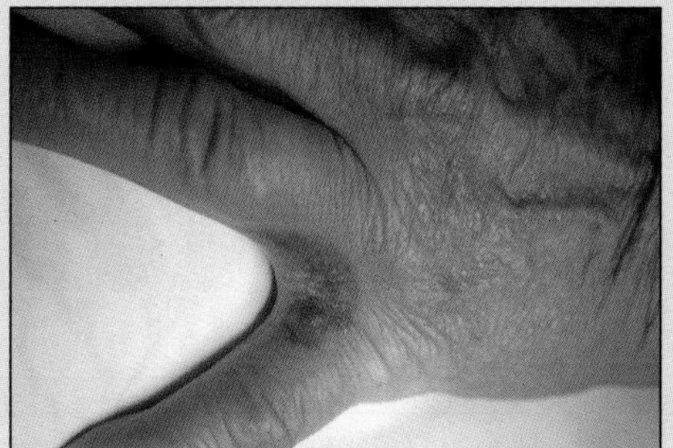
Fixed eruption

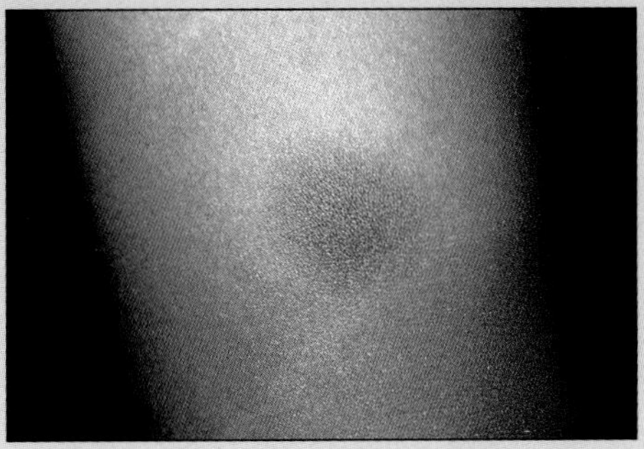
Fixed eruption (cyclophosphamide)

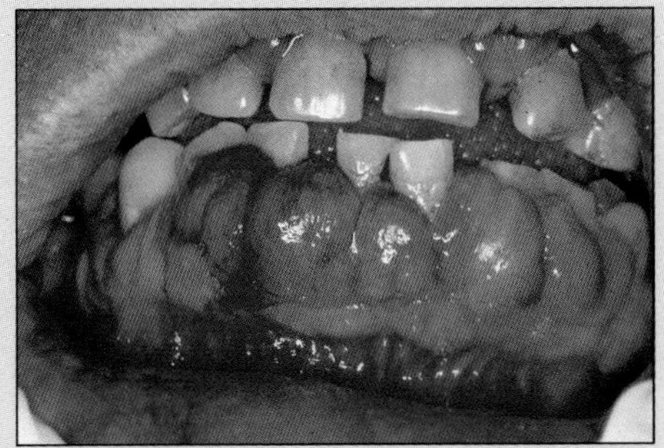
Gingival hyperplasia (verapamil)

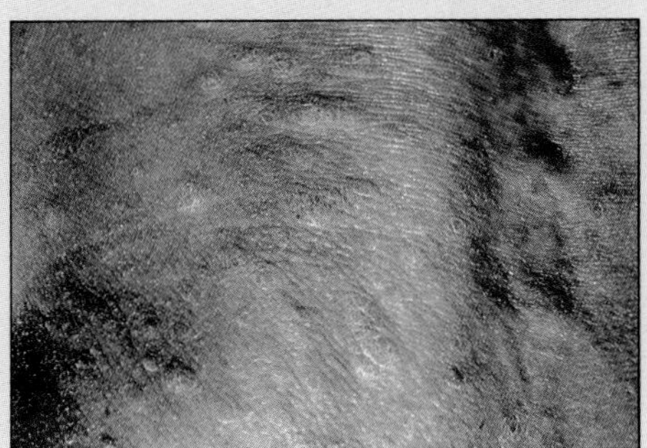
Lichenoid eruption

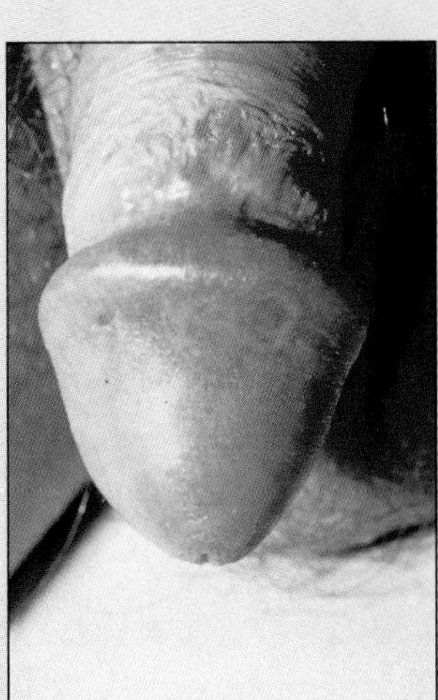
Lichen planus

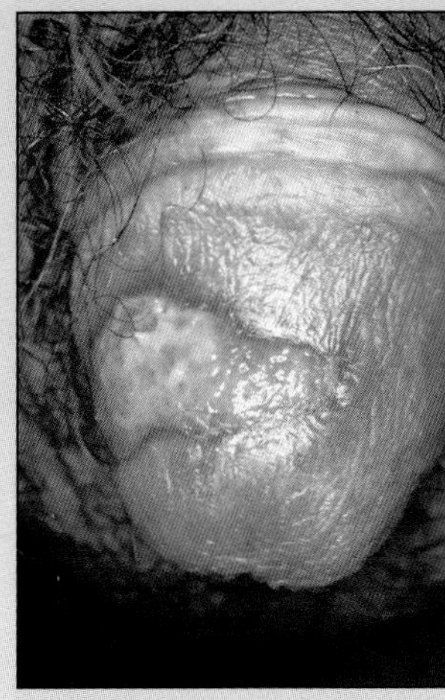
Fixed eruption

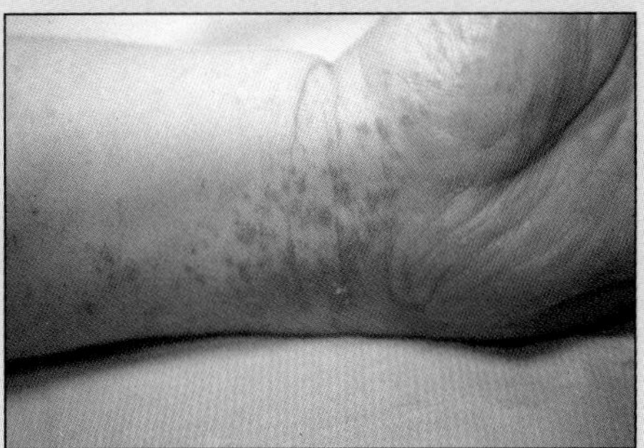
Lichenoid eruption

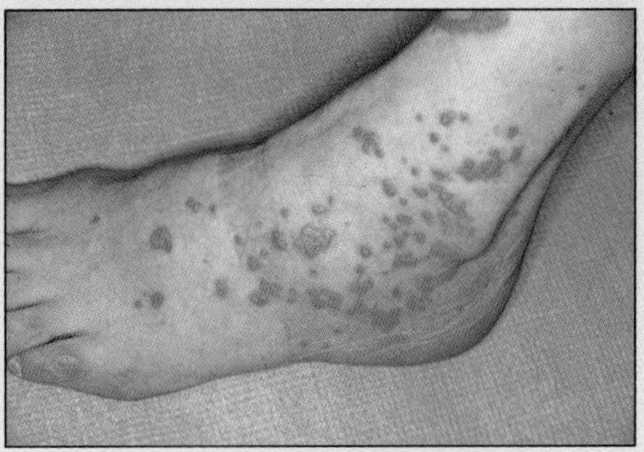
Lichen planus

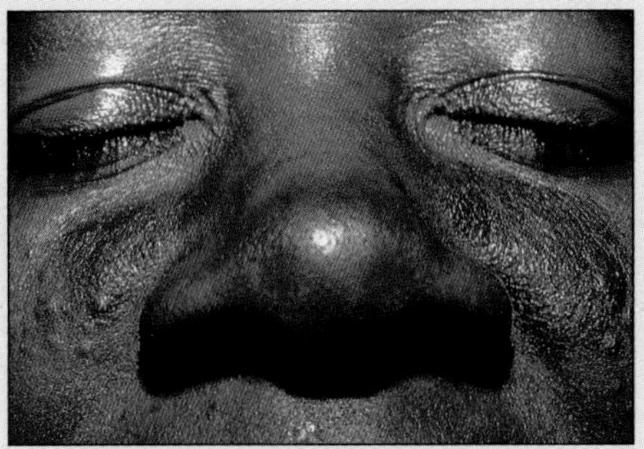
Lupus erythematosus

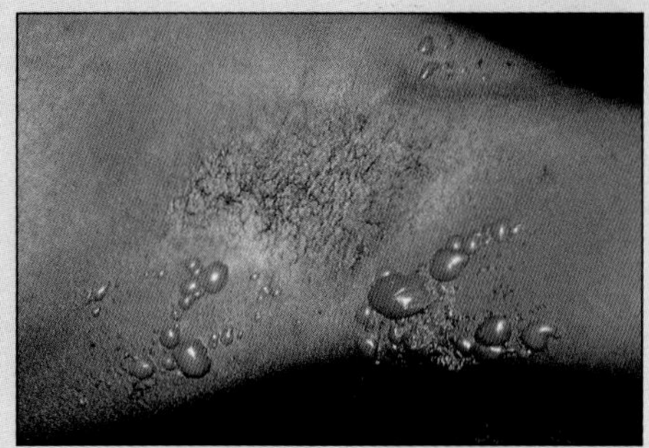
Bullous lupus erythematosus

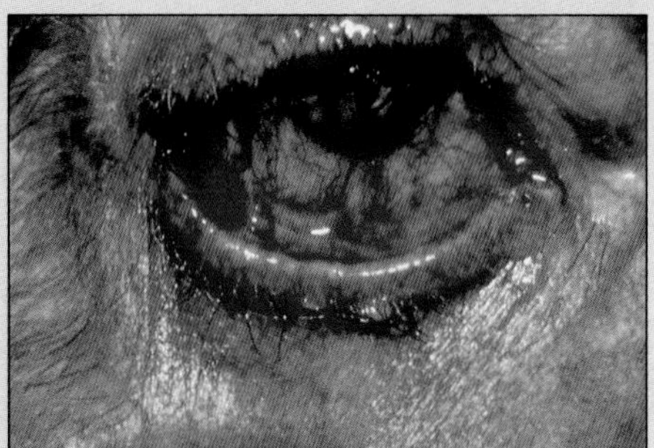
Cicatricial pemphigoid

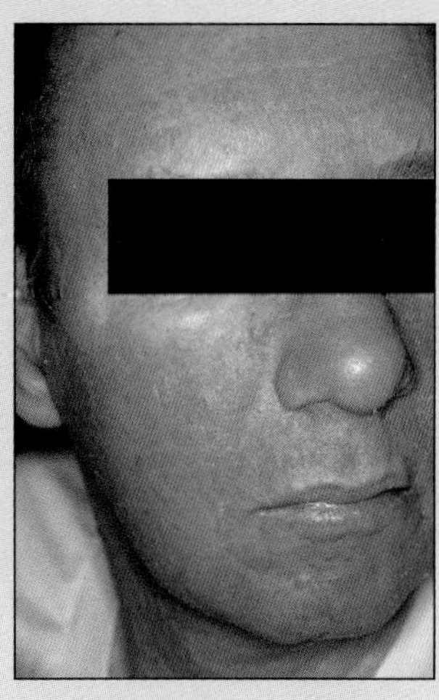
Photosensitivity

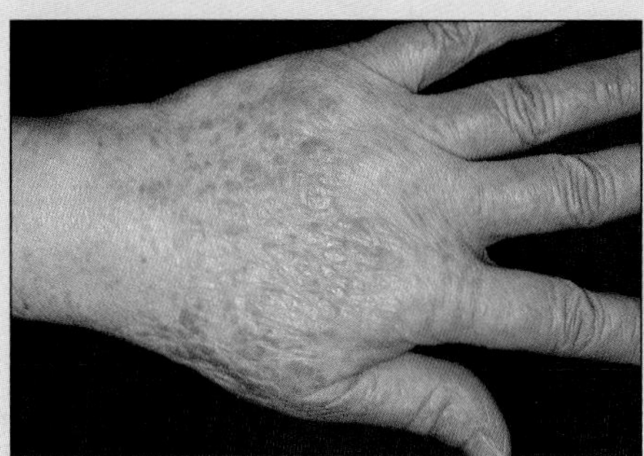
Photosensitivity (lichenoid)

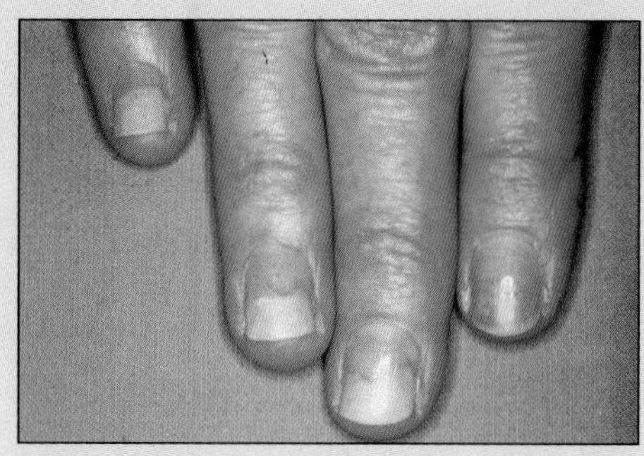
Photo-onycholysis (tetracycline)

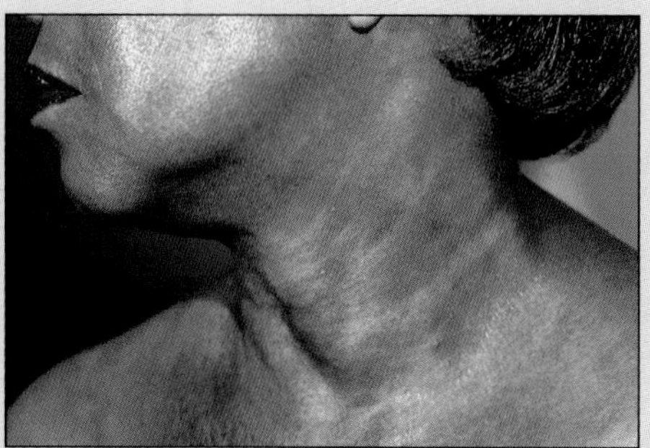
Photocontact dermatitis

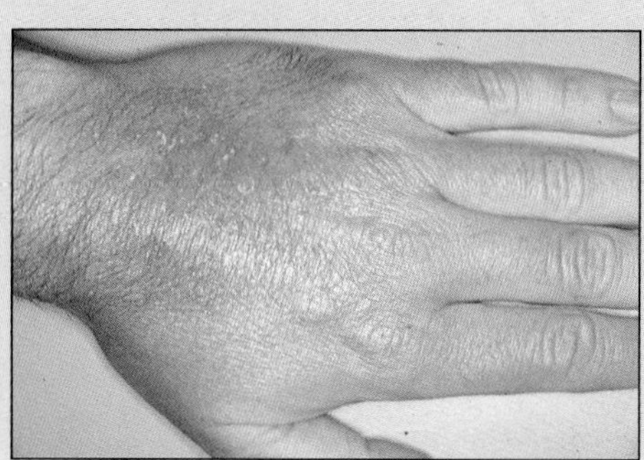
Photosensitivity

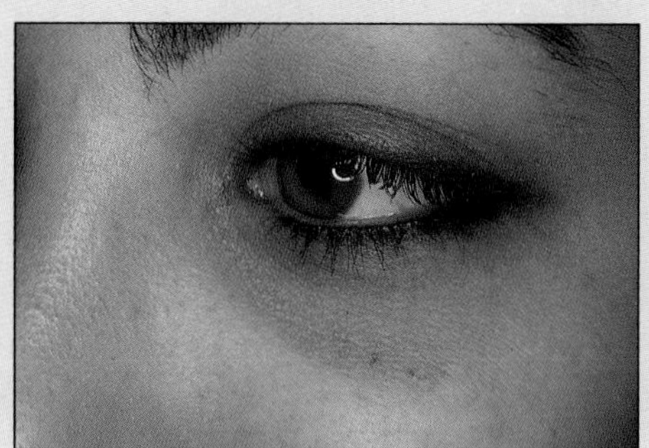
Pigmentation

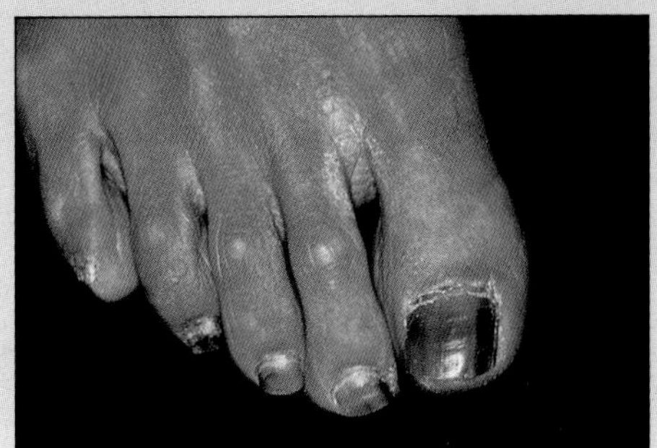
Pigmentation (zidovudine)

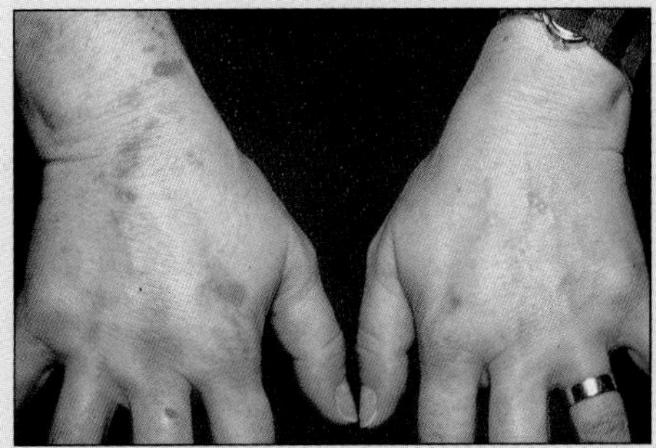
Porphyria (estrogens)

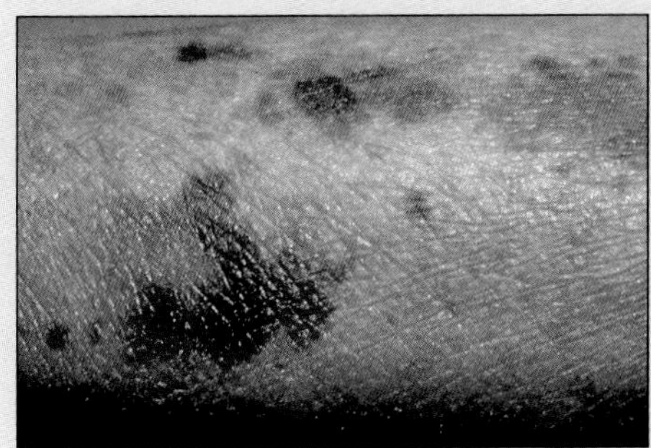
Purpura (aspirin)

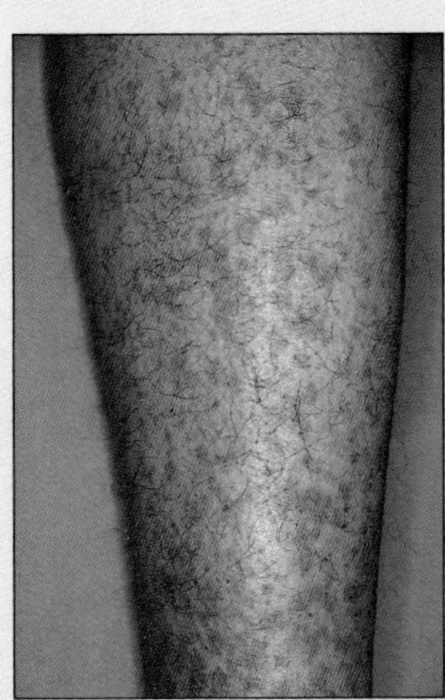
Purpura (naproxen)

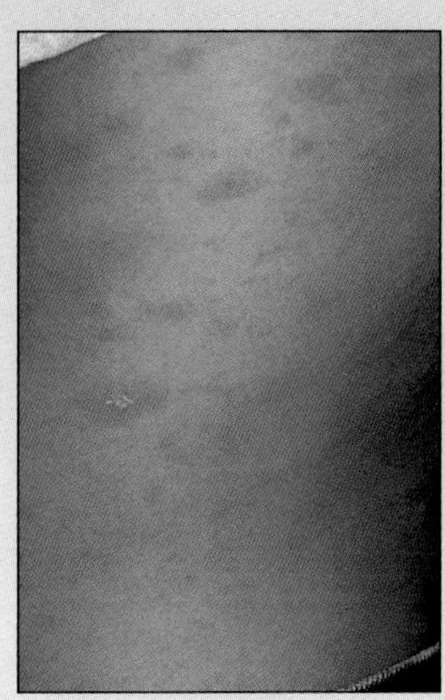
Pityriasis rosea

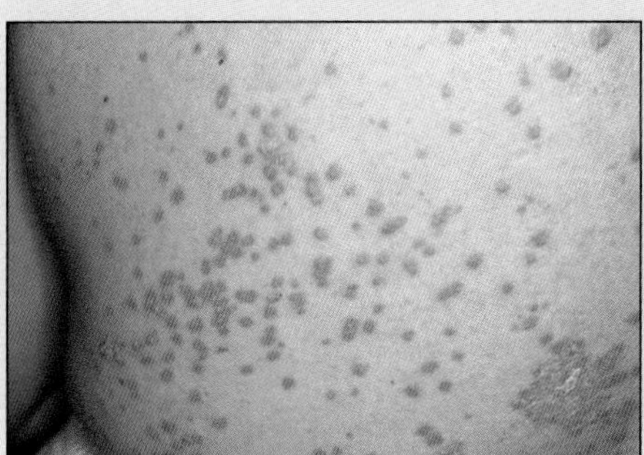
Psoriasis

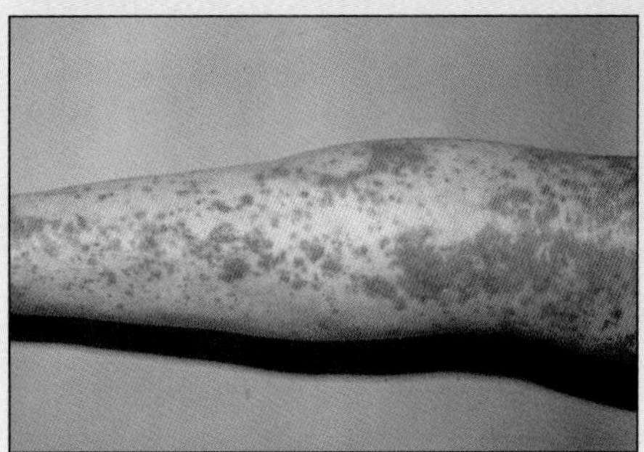
Purpura

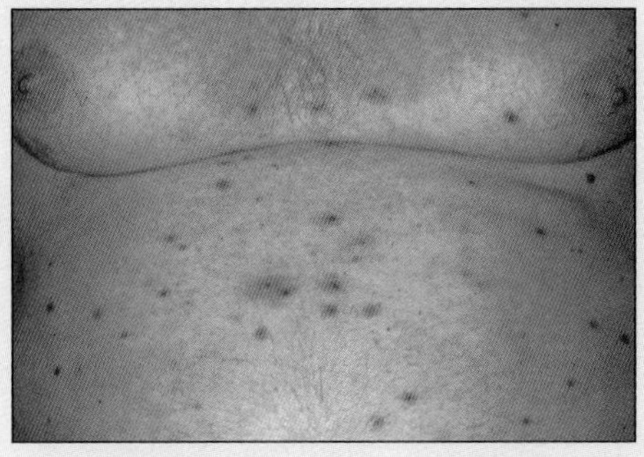
Pustular eruption (lithium)

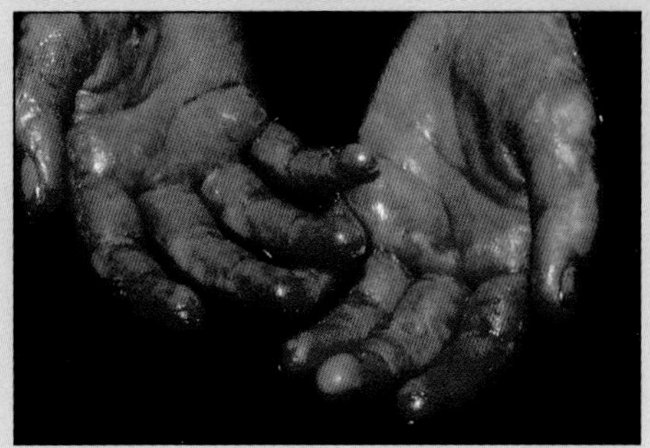
Stevens–Johnson syndrome (dilantin)

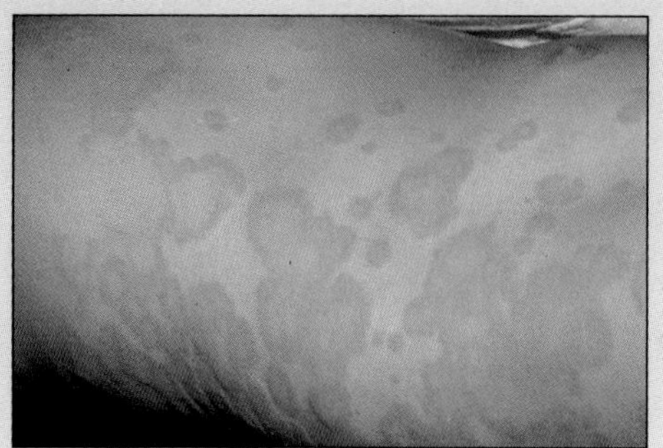
Urticaria

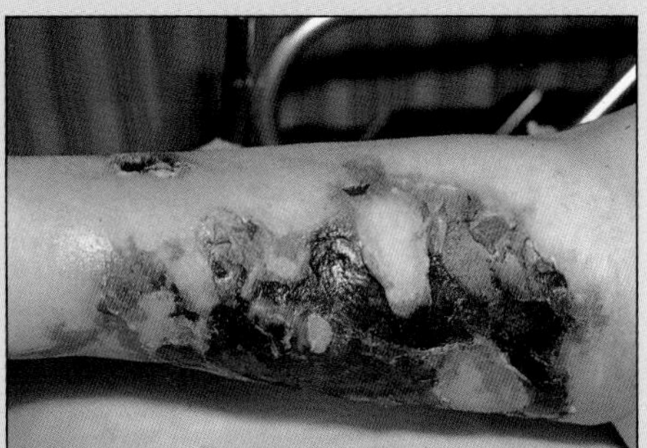
Necrosis

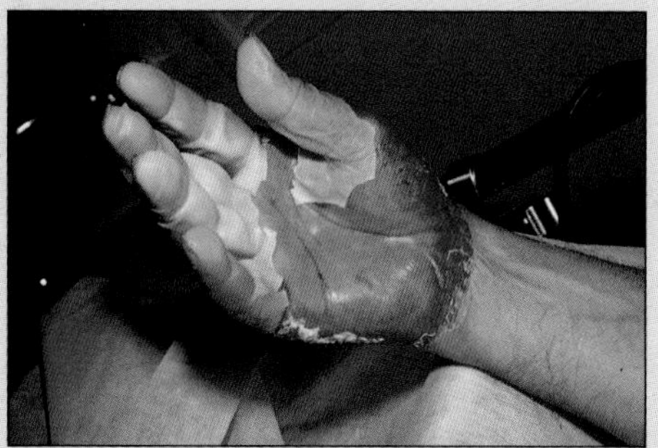
Toxic epidermal necrolysis

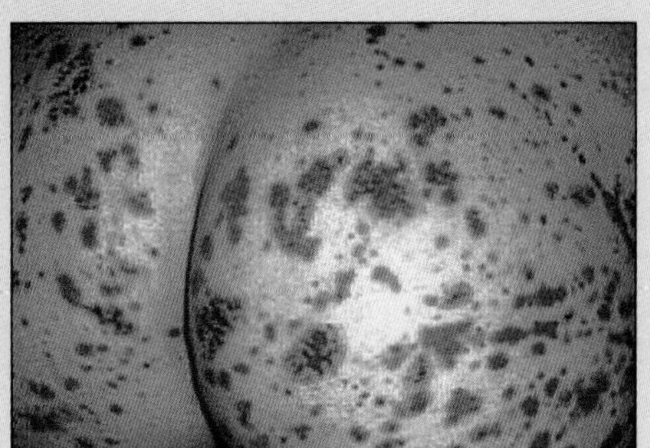
Vasculitis

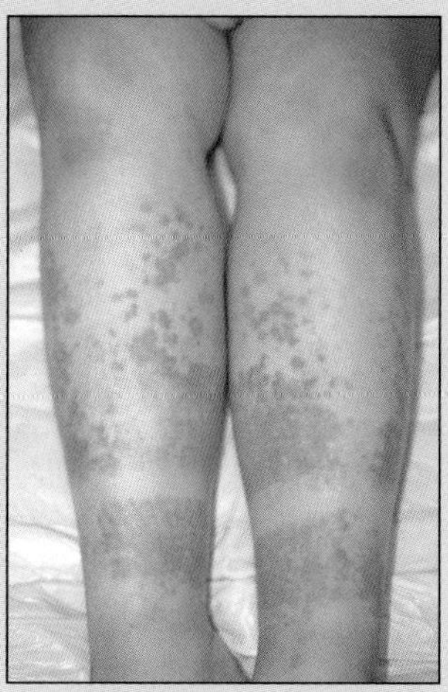
Vasculitis

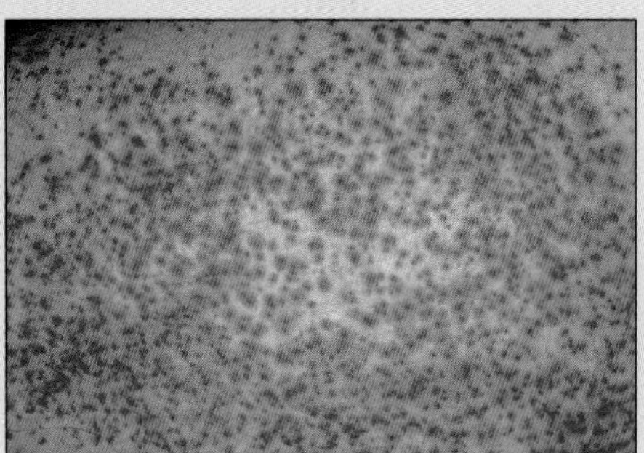
Leukocytoclastic vasculitis

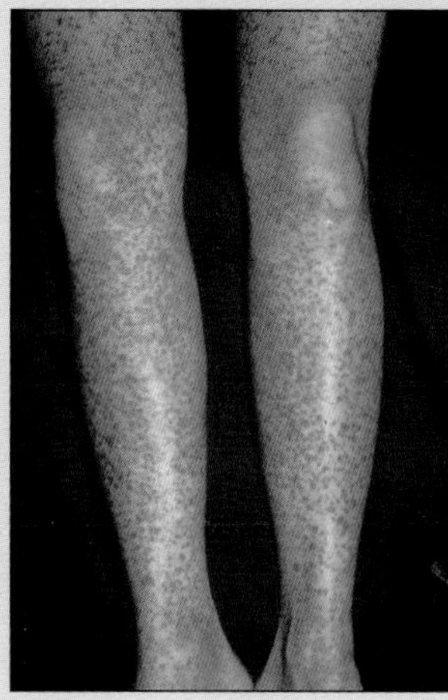
Vasculitis